Rheumatoid Arthritis

Rheumatoid Arthritis

Marc C. Hochberg, MD, MPH
Professor of Medicine
Head, Division of Rheumatology and Clinical Immunology
University of Maryland School of Medicine
Baltimore, Maryland

Alan J. Silman, MD, FRCP
Medical Director, Arthritis Research Campaign
Chesterfield, United Kingdom
Professor, Rheumatic Diseases Epidemiology
University of Manchester
Manchester, United Kingdom

Josef S. Smolen, MD
Professor of Medicine
Medical University of Vienna, Austria
Chairman, Department of Internal Medicine
Chairman, Division of Rheumatology
Medical University of Vienna
Vienna, Austria

Michael E. Weinblatt, MD
John R. and Eileen K. Riedman Professor of Medicine
Harvard Medical School
Co-Director of Clinical Rheumatology
Brigham and Women's Hospital
Boston, Massachusetts

Michael H. Weisman, MD
Director, Division of Rheumatology
Cedars-Sinai Medical Center
Professor of Medicine
University of California, Los Angeles School of Medicine
Los Angeles, California

MOSBY

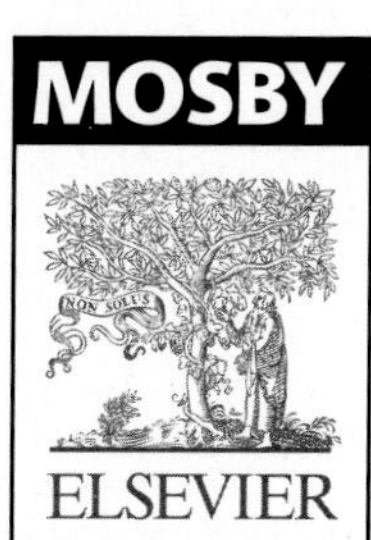

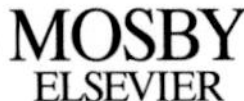

1600 John F. Kennedy Blvd.
Ste 1800
Philadelphia, PA 19103-2899

RHEUMATOID ARTHRITIS ISBN: 978-0-323-05475-1

Notice

Knowledge and best practice in this field are constantly changing. As new research and experience broaden our knowledge, changes in practice, treatment and drug therapy may become necessary or appropriate. Readers are advised to check the most current information provided (i) on procedures featured or (ii) by the manufacturer of each product to be administered, to verify the recommended dose or formula, the method and duration of administration, and contraindications. It is the responsibility of the practitioner, relying on their own experience and knowledge of the patient, to make diagnoses, to determine dosages and the best treatment for each individual patient, and to take all appropriate safety precautions. To the fullest extent of the law, neither the Publisher nor the Editors assume any liability for any injury and/or damage to persons or property arising out of or related to any use of the material contained in this book.

The Publisher

Library of Congress Cataloging-in-Publication Data
Rheumatoid arthritis / [edited by] Marc C. Hochberg ... [et al.]. — 1st ed.
p. ; cm.
Includes bibliographical references.
ISBN 978-0-323-05475-1
1. Rheumatoid arthritis. I. Hochberg, Marc C.
[DNLM: 1. Arthritis, Rheumatoid—diagnosis. 2. Arthritis, Rheumatoid—therapy. WE 346 R47357 2009]

RC933.R423 2009
616.7'227—dc22

2008010947

Acquisitions Editor: Pamela Hetherington
Developmental Editor: John Ingram
Design Direction: Lou Forgione

Printed in China

Last digit is the print number: 9 8 7 6 5 4 3 2 1

We would like to dedicate this book to our parents (living or of blessed memory), and our wives, children, and grandchildren.

Susan Hochberg, Francine and Jeffrey Guiffrida, and Jennifer Hochberg
Ruth Silman, Joanna, Timothy, and David Silman
Alice Smolen, and Eva, Nina, and Daniel Smolen
Barbara Weinblatt, Hillary and Jason Chapman, and Courtney Weinblatt
Betsy Weisman, Greg, Nicole, Mia and Joey Weisman, Lisa, Andrew, David and Thomas Cope, and Annie and Bill Macomber

Foreword

According to the philosopher Søren Kierkegaard, "life can only be understood backward; but it must be lived forwards."[1] Much the same is true about individual diseases. The origins of rheumatoid arthritis are hazy and in dispute, but the disease that A. J. Landre-Beauvais called "goutte asthenique primitive" (primary asthenic gout) in his 1800 doctoral dissertation, based on studies of the exclusively female population of the Paris asylum and hospital for incurable conditions, is considered the first description.[2] His intention was to emancipate this entity from generalized gout, a generic term used for centuries to designate specific diseases of the joints and rheumatism (acute rheumatic fever). Features that Landre-Beauvais recognized as distinctive included the predominance in women, a chronic course, multiple joints involved simultaneously, and finally the absence of tophi, recognized as a fairly common accompaniment of ordinary gout. He emphasized that in primary asthenic gout the changes observed resulted from the swelling, softening, and coalescence of bones and suppuration within joints.

J. M. Charcot's dissertation in 1853,[3] based on a statistical analysis of 41 women from the same Paris hospital (La Salpetriere), and his illustrations of the hand deformities in these patients, leaves little doubt that rheumatoid arthritis was the entity being described. Subsequently, he alluded frequently to this form of chronic arthritis and was the first to draw attention to Sydenham's earlier descriptions (1753) of typical hyperextension deformities of finger joints.[4]

In 18th century England, gout had become such a popular disorder that descriptions of alternative forms of joint disease were either overlooked or dismissed until the posthumous publication of William Heberden's *Commentaries* (1802), which contained observations on forms of arthritis other than gout.[5] Later, Alfred Baring Garrod, the influential clinician and scientist who used his famous thread test for the demonstration of uric acid crystals in human blood, compared gouty patients with those suffering from other arthropathies; included among these were acute (rheumatic fever) and chronic rheumatic gout. In an accompanying book he wrote, "If we agree to name a disease simply by its external characters then I admit that the term rheumatic gout is not appropriate." Then he proposed the term *rheumatoid arthritis*, "by which name I wish to imply an inflammatory affectation of the joints, not unlike rheumatism in some of its characters, but differing materially in its pathology."[6]

As the years passed rheumatoid arthritis escaped from the grasp of gout and osteoarthritis, but luminaries such as Alfred Garrod, the son of the great man, still worried that "perhaps several maladies have been confused together under the term rheumatoid arthritis. For this name, which was introduced by my father, I have a pious respect, but I am fully alive to its shortcomings." And he asked "whether the condition so called is rather a syndrome which, like malignant endocarditis, might originate in infections by several kinds of bacteria."[7]

In the early part of the 20th century, attempts to distinguish rheumatoid arthritis from other forms of chronic inflammatory polyarthritis, for example, psoriatic arthritis, postinfectious arthritis, childhood forms of arthritis, and rheumatoid spondylitis (spondyloarthropathy), were pursued. The latter proved particularly troublesome. Previously the names of Strumpell, von Bechterew, and Marie were associated with what each believed to be independent types of spinal arthritis. Their view that rheumatoid spondylitis constituted a separate disease *sui generis* was supported by a number of distinctive clinical and radiological features: namely, a preponderance of males, earlier age of onset, increased frequency of uveitis, and the absence of subcutaneous nodules. Arguing against this position were clinical similarities between patients with spondylitis and rheumatoid arthritis—that is, the frequent peripheral joint involvement, including the small finger articulations and the indistinguishable pathological appearance of the synovium in joints and diarthrodial articulations of the spine. American authorities such as Walter Bauer argued that in the absence of specific etiologic or genetic differences spondylitis was best considered "rheumatoid arthritis of the spine."[8] This position was subsequently rendered moot by laboratory studies that failed to show typical rheumatoid arthritis autoantibodies (rheumatoid factors [see following discussion]) in the blood of patients with spondylitis and the frequent genetic association of the HLA-B27 locus with the disease.[9]

The observation that the serum of patients with rheumatoid arthritis contained material(s) that could potentiate the clumping of sheep red cells coated with subagglutinating doses of rabbit antibodies or similarly coated bacteria introduced the science of immunology to the study of rheumatoid arthritis.[10,11] It was quickly recognized that the principals reactive with both rabbit and human gamma globulin antibodies resided in the high-molecular-weight fractions of serum gamma globulins (IgM) and that these soluble IgG-IgM antibody complexes were a regular, but not exclusive, feature of some patients with rheumatoid arthritis: hence, the term *rheumatoid factors* (RFs). When these subsequently were shown to be synthesized in response to antigenic determinants on the Fc fraction of "self" immunoglobulins whose confirmation had been altered after reacting with an antigen (thus, autoantibodies), rheumatoid arthritis was incorporated into the universe of autoimmune diseases. The serum of about 70% of patients with rheumatoid arthritis contains RF. The antibody is undoubtedly important in disease pathogenesis because patients who are sero-positive, especially those with high titers, have a more aggressive disease with greater joint destruction, nodules, vasculitis, and extra-articular features.[12] Conversely, because some normal individuals (10% to 20%) and patients with a variety of chronic viral infections and certain other autoimmune and hematologic diseases have detectable RF in the absence of arthritis, its pathogenicity has been challenged. What about an etiologic role? Theoretical stimuli for RF synthesis include (1) immunization with antigen-antibody complexes during anamnestic immune responses, (2) polyclonal B-cell activation, and (3) chronic viral infections. All have been extensively analyzed, but they failed to provide insights until genetic studies suggested a possible explanation.

Rheumatoid arthritis was known to appear in families, suggesting a role for genetic factors. The observation that the admixture of lymphocytes from different individuals with rheumatoid arthritis elicited less of a proliferative response than when these same patient's lymphocytes were cultured together with lymphocytes from normal individuals suggested they shared a similarity in certain histocompatability genes. Stastny subsequently pointed in the direction of the HLA system with the observation of an association of the B-cell alloantigen DR4 with rheumatoid arthritis.[13] Rapid advances in the molecular understanding of the allelic polymorphisms in the HLA-D region over the next two decades showed that rheumatoid arthritis was associated with a short sequence of amino acids (Q/RKRAA) at a site in the α helix that influences T-cell receptor–HLA interactions and the binding of peptide antigens.[14] This disease-associated HLA-DRB1 polymorphism predicted onset, severity, and patterns of disease in a number of populations and was thereafter known as the "shared epitope" (SE).

In the 1960s and 1970s occasional reports of highly specific antibodies for rheumatoid arthritis appeared. Initially they were referred to as antifillagrin antibodies, but after several decades of research they were recognized as members of a diverse group of autoantibodies that targeted different deiminated (citrullinated) proteins.[15] Such anticitrullinated protein antibodies (ACPAs) are found in 60% to 70% of rheumatoid arthritis patients, often before the appearance of clinical disease.[16] Besides their diagnostic and prognostic import, ACPAs are at the center of contemporary thinking about the pathogenesis of rheumatoid arthritis because of the finding that SE alleles are associated only with patients who are ACPA positive and not patients with rheumatoid arthritis who are ACPA negative.[17]

Gene–environment interactions are important as etiologic factors in a number of diseases. Smoking is a powerful environmental risk factor for the development of rheumatoid arthritis,[18,19] but only in association with a number of recognized host factors. For instance, HLA-DR SE genes are risk factors in smokers, but this effect is limited to patients who are RF positive.[20] The occurrence and quantity of anticitrulline antibodies is associated in a dose-dependent fashion with a history of previous smoking. Bronchoalveolar lavage cells from smokers immunostain for citrullinated proteins. Based on these findings, Klareskog has proposed that the etiology of some cases of rheumatoid arthritis can be explained by a hypothesis that incorporates several factors: namely, a known environmental trigger (smoking), which in a host with an appropriate genetic constitution (SE), will initiate an immune response (ACPAs) with the potential to contribute to disease.[21]

Thus, future studies of rheumatoid arthritis are likely to be based on subsets of patients with well-characterized biomarkers (such as ACPAs and RFs) and genetic factors. These will provide insights into causation and predict disease outcomes and treatment responses. The current excellent text already hints at these developments, but undoubtedly they will become even more prominent in future editions.

Nathan J. Zvaifler, MD
Professor of Medicine
University of California, San Diego
School of Medicine
San Diego, California

REFERENCES

1. The Journals of Søren Kierkegaard. *Wikiquote.* 10 July 2008, from: http://en.wikiquote.org/wiki/Soren_Kierkegaard
2. Landre-Beauvais AJ. The first description of rheumatoid arthritis. Unabridged text of the doctoral dissertation presented in 1800. *Joint Bone Spine* 2001;68:130–143.
3. Fraser KJ. Anglo-French contributions to the recognition of rheumatoid arthritis. *Ann Rheum Dis* 1982;41: 335–343.
4. Short C. The antiquity of rheumatoid arthritis. *Arthritis Rheum* 1974;17:193–205.
5. Heberden W. Commentaries on the history and cure of diseases. London: Payne, 1802.
6. Garrod AB. A treatise on gout and rheumatic gout. In *Rheumatoid Arthritis,* 3rd ed. London: Longmans, Green, 1875.
7. Garrod AE. Discussion on the 'aetiology and treatment of osteoarthritis and rheumatoid arthritis'. *Proc R Soc Med* 1923;17:1–4.
8. Short C, Bauer W, Reynolds WE. Rheumatoid arthritis. A definition of the disease and a clinical description based on a numerical study of 293 patients and controls. Commonwealth Fund. The Harvard University Press, 1957, pages 24–26.
9. Brewerton DA, Hart FD, Nicholls A, et al. Ankylosing spondylitis and HL-A 27. *Lancet* 1973;1:904–907

10. Waaler E. On the occurrence of a factor in human serum activating the specific agglutination of sheep red corpuscles. *Acta Pathol Microbiol Scand* 1940;17:172–176.
11. Rose HM, Ragan C, Pearce E, Lipman MO. Diffferential agglutination of normal and sensitized sheep erythrocytes by sera of patients with rheumatoid arthritis. *Proc Soc Exp Biol Med* 1949;68:1–10.
12. Carson DA, Chen PP, Kipps TJ. New roles for rheumatoid factor. *J Clin Invest* 1991;87:379–383.
13. Stastny P. Association of the B-cell alloantigen DR4 with rheumatoid arthritis. *New Engl J Med* 1978;298:869–875.
14. Gregersen PK, Silver J, Winchester RJ. The shared epitope hypothesis. An approach to understanding the molecular genetics of susceptibility to rheumatoid arthritis. *Arthritis Rheum* 1987;30:1205–1213.
15. Schellekens GA, de Jong BA, van den Hoogen FH, et al. Citrulline is an essential constituent of antigenic determinants recognized by rheumatoid arthritis–specific auto antibodies. *J Clin Invest* 1998;101: 273–281.
16. Rantapaa-Dahlqvist S, de Jong BEW, Berglin E, et al. Antibodies against cyclic citrulllinated peptide and IgA rheumatoid factor predicts the development of rheumatoid arthritis. *Arthritis Rheum* 2003;48:2741–2749.
17. van der Helm-van Mil AH, Verpoort KN, Breedvelt FC, et al. The HLA-DRB1 shared epitope alleles are primarily a risk factor for anti-CCP antibodies and are not an independent risk factor to develop RA. *Arthritis Rheum* 2006;54: 1117–1121.
18. Heliovaara M, Aho K, Aromaa A, et al. Smoking and risk of rheumatoid arthritis. *J Rheumatol* 1993;20:1830–1835.
19. Silman AJ, Newman J, MacGregor, AJ. Cigarette smoking increases the risks of rheumatoid arthritis: results from a nationwide study of disease–discordant twins. *Arthritis Rheum* 1996;39:732–735.
20. Stoit P, Bengtsson C, Nordmark B, et al. Quantification of the influence of cigarette smoking on rheumatoid arthritis. *Ann Rheum Dis* 2003;62:835–841.
21. Klareskog L, Stoit P, Lundberg I, et al. A new model for an etiology of rheumatoid arthritis: smoking may trigger HLA-DR (shared epitope)-restricted immune reactions to autoantigens modified by citrullination. *Arthritis Rheum* 2006;54:38–46.

Contributors

Daniel Aletaha, MD, MSC
Associate Professor of Medicine
Division of Rheumatology
Medical University of Vienna
Vienna, Austria

Lars Alfredsson, MD
Professor of Epidemiology
Institute of Environmental Medicine
Karolinska Institutet
Head, Epidemiology Unit
Stockholm Center for Public Health
Karolinska University
Stockholm, Sweden

Marina Backhaus, MD, PhD
Head of Department of Rheumatology and Clinical Immunology
Charité University Medicine
Berlin, Germany

Joan M. Bathon, MD
Professor of Medicine
Johns Hopkins University School of Medicine
Baltimore, Maryland

Johannes W. J. Bijlsma, MD, PhD
Professor and Head
Department of Rheumatology and Clinical Immunology
University Medical Center Utrecht
Utrecht, the Netherlands

Maarten Boers, MSc, MD, PhD
Professor of Clinical Epidemiology
Department of Clinical Epidemiology and Biostatistics
VU University Medical Center
Amsterdam, the Netherlands

Ferdinand C. Breedveld, MD
Department of Rheumatology
Leiden University Medical Center
Leiden, the Netherlands

Gerd R. Burmester, MD
Professor of Medicine
Department of Rheumatology and Clinical Immunology
Charité University Medicine
Berlin, Germany

Nicholas D. Bushar
Graduate Student
University of Maryland
Baltimore, Maryland

Frank Buttgereit, MD
Professor and Deputy Director
Department of Rheumatology and Clinical Immunology
Charité University Medicine
Berlin, Germany

Philip G. Conaghan, MBBS, PhD, FRACP, FRCP
Professor of Musculoskeletal Medicine
Academic Unit of Musculoskeletal Disease
Chapel Allerton Hospital
Leeds, United Kingdom

Shouvik Dass, MA, MRCP
Research Fellow
Academic Unit of Musculoskeletal Disease
University of Leeds
Specialist Registrar in Rheumatology
Leeds Teaching Hospitals NHS Trust
Leeds, United Kingdom

Kevin D. Deane, MD
Assistant Professor of Medicine
University of Colorado Denver School of Medicine
Denver, Colorado

Thomas Dörner, MD
Professor
Charité University Medicine
Berlin, Germany

Paul Emery, MA, MD, FRCP
Professor of Rheumatology
Faculty of Medicine and Health
Leeds Institute of Molecular Medicine
Academic Unit of Musculoskeletal Disease
Leeds, United Kingdom

John M. Esdaile, MD, MPH, FRCPC
Professor of Medicine
University of British Columbia
Scientific Director
Arthritis Research Centre of Canada
Vancouver, Canada

Donna L. Farber, MD
Department of Surgery
University of Maryland School of Medicine
Baltimore, Maryland

Jane E. Freeston, MB, BChir, MA, MRCP
Special Registrar and Research Fellow in Rheumatology
Academic Unit of Musculoskeletal Disease
University of Leeds
Chapel Allerton Hospital
Leeds, United Kingdom

Steffen Gay, MD
Professor of Rheumatology
University Hospital
University of Zurich
Zurich, Switzerland

Daniëlle M. Gerlag, MD
Assistant Professor of Medicine
Academic Medical Center/University of Amsterdam
Amsterdam, the Netherlands

Mary B. Goldring, PhD
Senior Scientist
The Hospital for Special Surgery
Joan and Sanford Weill College of Medicine at Cornell University
New York, New York

Mavis Goycochea, MD
Research Scientiest
Unidad de Epidemiología Clínica
Hospital Regional No. 1 Instituto Mexicana del Seguro Social
Distrito Federal, Mexico

Désirée van der Heijde, MD, PhD
Professor of Rheumatology
Leiden University Medical Center
Leiden, the Netherlands

Marc C. Hochberg, MD, MPH
Professor of Medicine
Head, Division of Rheumatology and Clinical Immunology
University of Maryland School of Medicine
Baltimore, Maryland

V. Michael Holers, MD
Professor of Medicine and Immunology
University of Colorado Denver School of Medicine
Aurora, Colorado

Axel J. Hueber, MD
Clinical Research Fellow
Centre for Rheumatic Diseases
Division of Immunology, Infection and Inflammation
Glasgow Biomedical Research Centre
University of Gasgow
Glasgow, United Kingdom

Tom W. J. Huizinga, MD
Chairman, Department of Rheumatology
Leiden University Medical Center
Leiden, the Netherlands

Alyssa K. Johnsen, MD PhD
Instructor
Division of Rheumatology, Allergy, and Immunology
Brigham and Women's Hospital
Harvard Medical School
Boston, Massachusetts

Arthur Kavanaugh, MD
Professor of Medicine
Division of Rheumatology, Allergy, and Immunology
University of California, San Diego
La Jolla, California

Edward Keystone, MD, FRCP(C)
Professor of Medicine, University of Toronto
Consultant Rheumatologist, Mount Sinai Hospital
Director, The Rebecca MacDonald Centre for Arthritis and Autoimmune Diseases
Chairman, The Canadian Rheumatology Research Consortium
Toronto, Canada

Hans P. Kiener, MD
Professor of Rheumatology
Department of Medicine III
Medical University of Vienna
Vienna, Austria

Raimund W. Kinne, MD
Head, Research/Experimental Rheumatology Unit
Department of Orthopedics
University Hospital Jena
Friedrich Schiller University
Jena, Germany

Lars Klareskog, MD, PhD
Professor of Rheumatology
Senior Consultant, Rheumatology Unit
Karolinska University Hospital, Solna
Stockhold, Sweden

Gisela Kobelt, MBA, PhD
Visiting Professor
Department of Orthopedics
University of Lund
Lund, Sweden
President, European Health Economics SAD
Mulhouse, France

Alisa E. Koch, MD
Frederick G.L. Huetwell and William D. Robinson, MD Professor of Rheumatology
Division of Rheumatology
University of Michigan
Ann Arbor, Michigan

Joel Kremer, MD
Professor of Medicine
Albany Medical College
The Center for Rheumatology
Albany, New York

Tore K. Kvien, MD
Department of Rheumatology
Diakonhjemmet Hospital
Oslo, Norway

Diane Lacaille, MD, MHSc, FRCPC
Assistant Professor of Medicine
University of British Columbia
Research Scientist
Arthritis Research Centre of Canada
Vancouver, Canada

Robert Landewe, MD
Professor of Rheumatology
Maastricht University Medical Center
Maastricht, the Netherlands
Consultant in Rheumatology
Atrium Medical Center
Heerlen, the Netherlands

David M. Lee, MD, PhD
Assistant Professor of Medicine
Division of Rheumatology, Immunology and Allergy
Harvard Medical School
Brigham & Women's Hospital
Boston, Massachusetts

Peter E. Lipsky, MD
National Institutes of Health
National Institute of Arthritis and Musculoskeletal and Skin Diseases
Autoimmunity Branch
Bethesda, Maryland

Klaus P. Machold, MD
Associate Professor of Medicine
Deputy Head, Division of Rheumatology
Medical University of Vienna
Vienna, Austria

C. Ronald MacKenzie, MD
Associate Professor of Medicine
Cornell Weill Medical College
Associate Attending Physician
Hospital for Special Surgery
New York Presbyterian Hospital
New York, New York

Eric L. Matteson, MD
Professor of Medicine
Mayo Clinic College of Medicine
Consultant in Rheumatology
Rochester, Minnesota

Iain B. McInnes, FRCP, PhD, FRSE
Professor of Experimental Medicine
University of Glasgow
Professor of Rheumatology
Glasgow Royal Infirmary
Glasgow, United Kingdom

Christopher G. Meyer, MD
Rheumatology Fellow
Duke University
Durham, North Carolina

Toru Mima, MD, PhD
Associate Professor
Laboratory of Immune Regulation
Graduate School of Frontier Biosciences
Osaka University
Osaka, Japan

Hoda Mirjafari, MD
Clinical Research Fellow
ARC Epidemiology Unit
University of Manchester
Manchester, United Kingdom

Larry W. Moreland, MD
Margaret J. Miller Endowed Professor for Arthritis Research
Chief, Division of Rheumatology and Clinical Immunology
University of Pittsburgh School of Medicine
Pittsburgh, Pennsylvania

Kamal D. Moudgil, MD, PhD
Associate Professor
Division of Rheumatology, Department of Medicine
Department of Microbiology and Immunology
University of Maryland School of Medicine
Baltimore, Maryland

Peter A. Nigrovic, MD
Instructor in Medicine
Harvard Medical School
Staff Rheumatologist
Brigham and Women's Hospital
Children's Hospital Boston
Boston, Massachusetts

Norihiro Nishimoto, MD, PhD
Professor
Laboratory of Immune Regulation
Graduate School of Frontier Biosciences
Osaka University
Osaka, Japan

Sarah Okada, MD
Clinical Team Leader
FDA/CDER/OND/ODE II/DAARP
Division of Anesthesia, Analgesia, and Rheumatology Products
Silver Spring, Maryland

Francesca I. Okoye, MD
Department of Surgery
University of Maryland School of Medicine
Baltimore, Maryland

Jacqueline E. Oliver, MSc, PhD
Research Associate
University of Manchester
Manchester, United Kingdom

Caroline Ospelt, MD
Professor of Rheumatology
University Hospital
University of Zurich
Zurich, Switzerland

Stephen A. Paget, MD
Joseph P. Routh Professor of Medicine
Weill Cornell Medical College
Chairman, Division of Rheumatology
Hospital for Special Surgery, New York Presbyterian Hospital
New York, New York

Saparna Pai, MD
Arthritis Foundation of Queensland Research Laboratory
Diamantina Institute for Cancer
Immunology and Metabolic Medicine
University of Queensland
Princess Alexandra Hospital
Brisbane, Australia

Thomas Pap, MD
Director, Institute of Experimental Musculoskeletal Medicine
University Hospital Münster
Münster, Germany

Dimitrios A. Pappas, MD
Post Doctoral Fellow in Rheumatology
Johns Hopkins University School of Medicine
Baltimore, Maryland

Sarah Kaprove Penn, MD
Clinical Fellow
University of Pittsburgh Medical Center
Pittsburgh, Pennsylvania

Robert M. Plenge, MD, PhD
Assistant Professor of Medicine
Harvard-Partners Center for Genetics & Genomics
Harvard Medical School
Director, Genetics & Genomics
Division of Rheumatology, Immunology and Allergy
Brigham and Women's Hospital
Boston, Massachusetts

Jana Posalski, MD
Rheumatology Fellow
Cedars-Sinai Medical Center
Los Angeles, California

Rajesh Rajaiah, PhD
Post Doctoral Researcher
Department of Microbiology and Immunology
University of Maryland School of Medicine
Baltimore, Maryland

Kurt Redlich, MD
Associate Professor of Medicine
Division of Rheumatology
Medical University of Vienna
Vienna, Austria

Johan Rönnelid, MD, PhD
Associate Professor and Consultant in Clinical Immunology
Unit of Clinical Immunology
Uppsala University Hospital
Uppsala University
Uppsala, Sweden

Clemens Scheinecker, MD
Associate Professor
Division of Rheumatology
Internal Medicine III
Medical University of Vienna
Vienna, Austria

Georg Schett, MD
Professor and Chairman
Department of Internal Medicine III
Institute for Clinical Immunology
Erlangen, Germany

David L. Scott, MD
Professor of Clinical Rheumatology
Department of Rheumatology
Kings College London School of Medicine
Honorary Consultant Rheumatologist
Kings College Hospital
London, United Kingdom

Jeffrey N. Siegel, MD
Clinical Team Leader
FDA/CDER/OND/ODE II/DAARP
Division of Anesthesia, Analgesia, and Rheumatology Products
Silver Spring, Maryland

Alan J. Silman, MD, FRCP
Medical Director, Arthritis Research Campaign
Chesterfield, United Kingdom
Professor, Rheumatic Diseases Epidemiology
University of Manchester
Manchester, United Kingdom

Lee S. Simon, MD
Associate Clinical Professor of Medicine
Harvard Medical School
Beth Israel Deaconess Medical Center
Boston, Massachusetts

Jasvinder A. Singh, MBBS, MPH
Assistant Professor of Medicine
University of Minnesota Medical School
Staff Physician, Minneapolis VA Medical Center
Minneapolis, Minnesota
Visiting Scientist
Department of Health Sciences and Orthopedic Surgery
Mayo Clinic School of Medicine
Rochester, Minnesota

Josef S. Smolen, MD
Professor of Medicine
Medical University of Vienna, Austria
Chairman, Department of Internal Medicine
Chairman, Division of Rheumatology
Medical University of Vienna
Vienna, Austria

Daniel H. Solomon, MD, MPH
Associate Professor of Medicine
Harvard Medical School
Chief, Section of Clinical Sciences
Brigham and Women's Hospital
Boston, Massachusetts

E. William St. Clair, MD
Professor of Medicine and Immunology
Duke University Medical Center
Durham, North Carolina

Günter Steiner, PhD
Division of Rheumatology
Department of Medicine III
Medical University of Vienna
Vienna, Austria
Charité University Medicine
Universitätsmedizin Berlin, Free University and Humboldt-University of Berlin
Berlin, Germany

Vibeke Strand, MD
Clinical Professor of Immunology/Rheumatology
Stanford University School of Medicine
Biopharmaceutical Consultant
Stanford, California

Bruno Stuhlmüller, PhD
Universitätsmedizin Berlin, Free University and Humboldt-University of Berlin
Department of Rheumatology and Clinical Immunology
Charité University Medicine
Berlin, Germany

Deborah Symmons, MD, FFPH, FRCP
Professor of Rheumatology and Musculoskeletal Epidemiology
School of Translational Medicine
Honorary Consultant Rheumatologist
University of Manchester
Manchester, United Kingdom

Zoltán Szekanecz, MD, PhD
Professor of Medicine, Rheumatology, and Immunology
University of Debrecen Medical Center
Institute of Medicine
Rheumatology Division
Debrecen, Hungary

Paul Peter Tak, MD, PhD
Professor of Medicine
Director, Division of Clinical Immunology and Rheumatology
Academic Medical Center/University of Amsterdam
Amsterdam, the Netherlands

Peter C. Taylor, MA, PhD, FRCP
Professor of Experimental Rheumatology and Honorary Consultant Physician
Head of Clinical Trials, Kennedy Institute of Rheumatology
Imperial College London
London, United Kingdom

Ranjeny Thomas, FRACP, MD
Professor of Rheumatology
Diamantina Institute
University of Queensland
Consultant Rheumatology
Princess Alexandra Hospital
Brisbane, Australia

Carl Turesson, MD, PhD
Associate Professor of Rheumatology
Malmö University Hospital
Malmö, Sweden
Research Collaborator
Mayo Clinic College of Medicine
Rochester, Minnesota

Edward M. Vital, MD
Professor of Rheumatology
Faculty of Medicine and Health
Leeds Institute of Molecular Medicine
Academic Unit of Musculoskeletal Disease
Leeds, United Kingdom

Michael M. Ward, MD, MPH
National Institute of Arthritis and Musculoskeletal and Skin Diseases
National Institutes of Health
Bethesda, Maryland

Deborah Weber, RN, CCRC
Mount Sinai Hospital
Toronto, Canada

Michael E. Weinblatt, MD
John R. and Eileen K. Riedman Professor of Medicine
Harvard Medical School
Co-Director of Clinical Rheumatology
Brigham and Women's Hospital
Boston, Massachusetts

Michael H. Weisman, MD
Director, Division of Rheumatology
Cedars-Sinai Medical Center
Professor of Medicine
University of California, Los Angeles School of Medicine
Los Angeles, California

Sterling G. West, MD
Professor of Medicine
University of Colorado Denver
Health Sciences Center
Aurora, Colorado

Kevin L. Winthrop, MD, MPH
Assistant Professor of Infectious Diseases, Public Health, and Preventive Medicine
Oregon Health and Science University
Portland, Oregon

Angela Zink, MD
Professor of Rheumatology
Charité University Medicine
Head, Epidemiology Unit
German Rheumatism Research Center
Berlin, Germany

Nathan J. Zvaifler, MD
Professor of Medicine
University of California, San Diego School of Medicine
San Diego, California

Acknowledgments

We would like to acknowledge the tremendous work of the contributors to ***Rheumatoid Arthritis***, without whom this book would not have been possible. In addition, we would like to acknowledge our mentors: Drs. Eva Alberman, Harry Currey (deceased), Lawrence E. Schulman, Carl Steffen (deceased), Alfred D. Steinberg, Mary Betty Stevens (deceased), and Nathan Zvaifler.

We would also like to acknowledge the excellent team at Elsevier: Kim Murphy, Pamela Hetherington, and John Ingram, as well as our secretaries and administrative assistants (Margarita Cook, Johanna Leibl, and Robin Nichols) for all of their hard work and diligence. Last, but certainly not least, we want to acknowledge our patients who continue to provide stimulating challenges to us in our clinical practices.

Contents

Section IV
Outcome Measurement of Rheumatoid Arthritis

Section V
Treatment of Rheumatoid Arthritis

Section VI
Clinical Trials

Epidemiology of Rheumatoid Arthritis

SECTION I

Classification Criteria

Deborah Symmons and Hoda Mirjafari

CHAPTER 1

Methodology for Development of Classification Criteria

Classification criteria are needed in population studies to establish the epidemiology of disease, and as part of the entry criteria for clinical trials. In practice they are also used in the legal system and by government bodies to evaluate whether individuals have the specific disease, and as an aid to teaching medical students. The methodology of development of classification criteria has gradually been refined over the last 50 years or so.

Felson and Anderson[1] defined a number of steps in the development of criteria (Table 1-1). Generally speaking, the physician's opinion has been taken as the gold standard against which criteria sets have been evaluated. A comprehensive list of potential diagnostic tests must then be developed—often using a systematic literature search followed by the Delphi technique—as this enables a large number of investigators to be involved and for a consensus to be reached by adopting an iterative approach. It may also be important to seek input from patients with the disease. Each test must be precisely defined and then evaluated in a series of cases and controls.[2] Each of the potential criteria should be reliable, precise, and easy to measure.

The cases used should be representative of the whole spectrum of disease and be drawn from primary, secondary, and tertiary care. Perhaps the most important step in testing the individual potential diagnostic tests and later the evaluation of the complete criteria set is the selection of the control group. This should comprise individuals with conditions that need to be distinguished from rheumatoid arthritis (RA). The most appropriate control group may depend on the setting in which the criteria are to be used. Thus, in a population survey, the important task is to be able to distinguish individuals with RA from those with no arthritis or with osteoarthritis (OA). However, in an early arthritis clinic, the important step may be to distinguish individuals with RA from those with other inflammatory disorders such as reactive arthritis and connective tissue diseases. It may thus be desirable to have more than one set of controls. The sensitivity and specificity of each of the potential diagnostic tests is then evaluated. All but one of any tests that are closely correlated should be removed. Statisticians should be involved in selecting the best combination and weighting of items that discriminate between cases and controls. Alternatively the classification and regression tree (CART) computer program based on the work of Brieman et al.[3] can be used. This software searches for the value of an individual diagnostic test that identifies a subgroup comprised almost entirely of cases or controls. In this context the same criterion can be used more than once at different stages of the "classification tree." It is also possible to explore the possibility of substitution if the value for a particular variable is missing in some individuals.

The validity (Table 1-2) of the proposed criteria is then tested in a new set of cases and controls. In order to avoid circularity the proposed criteria set should be evaluated by a different set of physicians and using different cases and controls from those in which they were originally developed.

In composite criteria the weakest item, that is, that which is least standardized, is the limiting factor. Thus, if a single criterion lacks reliability, precision, or feasibility, then the whole criteria set is undermined.[4]

In order to be able to use classification criteria for diagnostic purposes it is essential to have very high specificity and good sensitivity.

Table 1-1. Steps in Development of Classification Criteria	
1.	Specify the conceptual construct of the disease, that is, determine the gold standard
2.	Create a list of potential diagnostic tests, such as rheumatoid factor, anti—cyclic-citrullinated peptide (anti-CCP), joint counts, nodules
3.	Identify a large group of people with the disease and controls without disease
4.	Test to see which test or combination of tests best discriminates between those with and without disease
5.	Evaluate the validity of the proposed criteria set in an independent set of cases and controls

Adapted from Felson DT, Anderson JJ. Methodological and statistical approaches to criteria development in rheumatic diseases. *Baillieres Clin Rheumatol* 1995;9(2):253–266.

Table 1-2. Types of Validity Relevant to Classification Criteria	
Construct validity	Assessed against the predefined gold standard (often the physician's opinion). Assessed by measuring sensitivity and specificity.
Face validity	Assesses credibility.
Content validity	Also called comprehensiveness. Are all the domains of disease sampled?
Criterion validity	Do the criteria predict or correlate with other endpoints of disease, such as radiologic erosions?

The 1958 American Rheumatism Association Criteria

In 1956 a subcommittee of the American Rheumatism Association (ARA) developed a set of criteria for RA.[5–7] Although called "diagnostic criteria," it was acknowledged that these criteria were not a diagnostic tool but a set of classification criteria, intended to facilitate comparisons between groups of patients with RA and as an aid to epidemiologic surveys. Three levels of certainty were described: definite and probable RA (intended to study the course, characteristics, and treatment of RA) and possible RA (intended to study early atypical cases). The criteria were based on the experience of five members of the subcommittee who assembled a set of 332 cases and controls from 19 cities across the United States and Canada. Each participating physician was asked to contribute data from their five most recent cases of classical RA, their five most recent cases of probable RA, and five rheumatology cases without RA. Disease characteristics were then chosen that showed high specificity (for definite/probable RA) or high sensitivity (for possible RA). There was no validation of the individual items or of the final criteria set.

After subsequent discussion the committee decided that these criteria were not sufficiently rigorous. The subsequent revision, known as the 1958 ARA diagnostic criteria for RA, were adopted and used widely for many years (Table 1-3). This revision added a fourth category of classical RA, which required 7 of the 11 criteria to be positive. Agammaglobulinemia was added to the list of exclusions. Concern had been expressed about the nonstandardization of rheumatoid factor (RF) estimation, and so the

Table 1-3. 1958 American Rheumatism Association Criteria for Rheumatoid Arthritis
Criteria
1. Morning stiffness.
2. Pain on motion or tenderness of at least one joint (observed by a physician).
3. Swelling (soft tissue thickening or fluid) in at least one joint (observed by a physician).
4. Swelling of at least one other joint (observed by a physician); any interval between the involvement of the two joints should not exceed 3 months.
5. Symmetrical joint swelling (observed by a physician) with simultaneous involvement of the same joint on both sides of the body. (Bilateral involvement of proximal interphalangeal, metacarpophalangeal, or metatarsophalangeal joints is acceptable without absolute symmetry.) Terminal interphalangeal joint involvement will not satisfy this criterion.
6. Subcutaneous nodules (observed by a physician) over bony prominences, on extensor surfaces or in juxta-articular regions.
7. X-ray changes typical of rheumatoid arthritis (which must include at least bony decalcification localized to or greatest around involved joints).
8. Positive agglutination test—demonstration of rheumatoid factor by any test that, in two laboratories, has been positive in not more than 5% of normal controls.
9. Poor mucin clot from synovial fluid.
10. Characteristic histologic changes in synovial membrane with three or more of the following:
• Marked villous hypertrophy
• Proliferation of superficial synovial cells often with pallisading
• Marked infiltration of chronic inflammatory cells (lymphocytes of plasma cells predominating) with tendency to form lymphoid follicles
• Deposition of compact fibrin either on the surface or interstitially
• Foci of cell necrosis
11. Characteristic histologic changes in nodules showing granulomatous foci with central zones of cell necrosis, surrounded by proliferating fixed cells and peripheral fibrosis and chronic inflammatory cell infiltration, predominantly perivascular.
Classical Rheumatoid Arthritis
At least seven criteria must be present. For criteria 1 to 5, the joint signs or symptoms must have been continuous for at least 6 weeks. None of the features listed under exclusions should be present.
Definite Rheumatoid Arthritis
At last five criteria must be present. For criteria 1 to 5, the joint signs or symptoms must have been continuous for at least 6 weeks. None of the features listed under exclusions should be present.
Probable Rheumatoid Arthritis
At least three criteria must be present. In at least one of criteria 1 to 5, the joint signs or symptoms must have been continuous for at least 6 weeks. None of the features listed under exclusions should be present.

Table 1-3. 1958 American Rheumatism Association Criteria for Rheumatoid Arthritis—cont'd
Possible Rheumatoid Arthritis
This diagnosis requires at least two of the following. The total duration of symptoms must be at least 3 weeks.
1. Morning stiffness.
2. Tenderness or pain on motion of at least one joint (observed by a physician).
3. History of observation of joint swelling.
4. Subcutaneous nodules (observed by a physician).
5. Raised ESR or CRP.
6. Iritis.
Exclusions
1. The typical rash of systemic lupus erythematosus with butterfly distribution, follicle plugging, and areas of atrophy.
2. High concentrations of LE cells.
3. Histologic evidence of polyarteritis nodosa.
4. Weakness of neck, trunk, and pharangeal muscles or persistent muscle swelling of dermatomyositis.
5. Definite scleroderma, not confined to the fingers.
6. Clinical picture characteristic of rheumatic fever.
7. Clinical picture characteristic of gouty arthritis.
8. Tophi.
9. Clinical picture characteristic of acute infectious arthritis of bacterial or viral origin.
10. Tubercle bacilli in joints or histologic evidence of joint tuberculosis.
11. Clinical picture characteristic of Reiter's syndrome.
12. Clinical picture characteristic of the shoulder–hand syndrome.
13. Clinical picture characteristic of hypertrophic pulmonary osteoarthropathy.
14. Clinical picture characteristic of neuroarthrophy with condensation and destruction of bones of involved joints and with associated neurologic findings.
15. Homogentisic acid in the urine.
16. Histologic evidence of sarcoidosis or a positive Kveim test.
17. Multiple myeloma.
18. Characteristic skin lesions of erythema nodosum.
19. Leukemia or lymphoma.
20. Agammaglobulinemia.
From Ropes MW, Bennett GA, Cobb S, et al. 1958 Revision of diagnostic criteria for rheumatoid arthritis. *Bull Rheum Dis* 1958;9(4):175–176.

committee specified the use of a method that was positive in fewer than 5% of healthy controls in at least two independent laboratories. The symptoms and signs had to be present for at least 6 weeks for classical, definite, and probable RA, and for at least 3 weeks for possible RA.

The use of exclusion rules for the 1958 criteria meant that it was not possible for individuals to be classified as having more than one rheumatic disease (e.g., RA and gout). Nevertheless, reflecting the understanding of the conditions at the time, ankylosing spondylitis (then often called rheumatoid spondylitis), psoriatic arthritis, arthritis associated with inflammatory bowel disease, and childhood arthritis were all included in this classification scheme.

Rome Criteria

The 1958 ARA criteria were reviewed at a symposium on Population Studies in Relation to Chronic Rheumatism sponsored by the Council for International Organizations of Medical Sciences (CIOMS) held in Rome in 1961.[8] The meeting made three major recommendations to address what were perceived as weaknesses of the 1958 criteria. The first was to remove the last three criteria that were considered invasive and impractical, particularly for epidemiologic studies. Ankylosing spondylitis was added to the list of exclusions. The resulting criteria set was known as the Rome (active) criteria set.

Within the context of epidemiologic studies, it is also important to be able to identify cases with evidence of past, but currently inactive, disease. A second set of criteria known as the Rome (inactive) criteria was, therefore, developed for this purpose (Table 1-4). It included two categories: definite and probable.

New York Criteria

The Third International Symposium on Population Studies of the Rheumatic Diseases was held in New York in 1966.[9,10] It was noted that the frequency of many of the items in the Rome criteria had never been established in the normal population. Lawrence and Wood[11] had examined data from surveys conducted by the Arthritis and Rheumatism Council Epidemiology Research Unit between 1954 and 1961. They concluded that the 1958 criteria were not sufficiently sensitive or specific and, in particular, that patients with OA were often misclassified as having RA. The meeting expanded on the format of the Rome inactive criteria (Table 1-4), and included the 13 most important clinical variables that contributed to a clinical diagnosis of RA. Items of low prevalence, such as nodules, were excluded. These stricter criteria for the classification of RA, known as the New York Criteria[9] were later published (Table 1-5). The New York criteria set is the only set developed specifically for use in epidemiologic studies. It recognizes inactive disease at the current examination. However, this criteria set has a number of major weaknesses. First, no rules are given as to how many of the four criteria need to be satisfied to classify an individual as

Table 1-4. Rome (Inactive) Criteria
1. Past history of polyarthritis.
2. Symmetrical deformity of peripheral joints consisting of ankylosis or irreducible subluxation, especially of the lateral MTP or MCP joints; there must be some involvement of one hand or foot. Involvement limited to large joints, such as the elbows or knees does not satisfy this criterion.
3. Radiologic changes of RA of grade 2 or more.
4. Positive serologic test for RA.
Note: Definite RA requires three of four criteria, and probable RA requires two of four criteria. Adapted from Kellgren JH. Diagnostic criteria for population studies. *Bull Rheum Dis* 1962;13:291–292.

Table 1-5. New York Criteria for Diagnosis of Rheumatoid Arthritis

1. A history, past or present, of an episode of joint pain involving three or more limb joints, without stipulation as to duration. The joints on either side are counted separately, but joints that occur in groups (e.g., PIPs, MCPs) are counted as only one joint even if more than one of them is involved on the same side.
2. Involvement by swelling, limitation, subluxation, or ankylosis of at least three limb joints (excluding DIPs, fifth PIPs, first carpo-metacarpal joints, hip, and first MTPs) with symmetry of at least one joint pair. There must be involvement of one hand, wrist, or foot as involvement of large joints such as elbows or knees does not satisfy this criterion. Subluxation of the lateral MTPs must be irreducible.
3. X-ray features of grade 2 or more erosive arthritis in the hands, wrists, or feet.
4. Positive serologic reaction for rheumatoid factor, determined by a method that is controlled by periodic testing of reference sera and by change of sera with other laboratories.

From Bennett PD, Burch TA. New York symposium on population studies in the rheumatic diseases: A new diagnostic criteria. *Bull Rheum Dis* 1967;17:453–458.

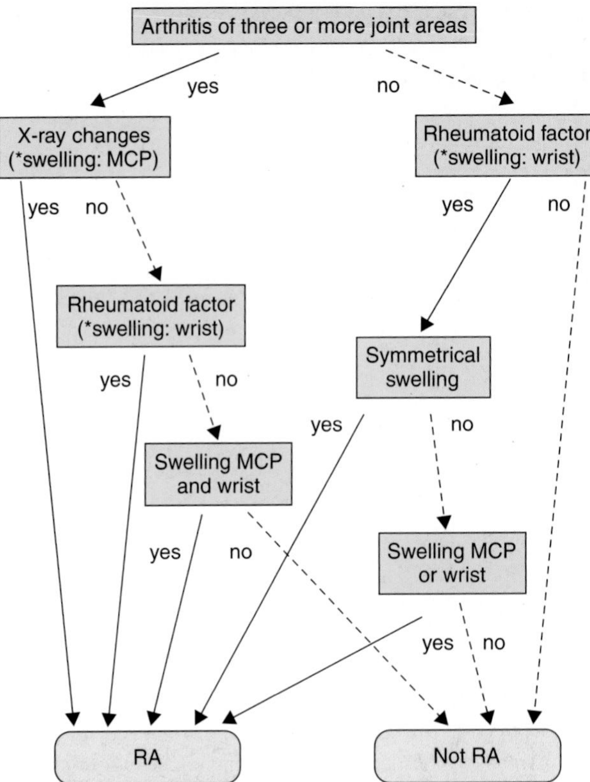

Figure 1-1. 1987 ARA decision tree for RA classification. (Adapted from Arnett FC, Edworthy SM, Bloch DA, et al. The American Rheumatism Association 1987 revised criteria for the classification of rheumatoid arthritis. *Arthritis Rheum* 1988;31:315–324.) *Variables in parentheses can be used when data on the first listed variable are not available.

having RA. The individual criteria are felt to be too descriptive and cumbersome for practical use. Two of the four criteria are based on the results of investigations, and so the set is vulnerable to missing data with no rules as to how this situation should be handled.

The 1987 American College of Rheumatology Criteria

The 1958 criteria set and their offspring the Rome criteria were widely used in clinical and epidemiologic studies for almost 30 years. However, during that time, the construct of RA evolved as did the methodology for criteria development. In particular, rheumatologists were unhappy because the spondyloarthritides, calcium pyrophosphate deposition disease, polymyalgia rheumatica, and Lyme arthritis were all included within seronegative RA; several of the 1958 criteria were invasive and so seldom used; and the distinctions among the different categories of RA (classical, definite, probable, and possible) did not reflect clinical judgment.

In addition, many of the individual criteria of the 1958 set had no definitions, and so it was impossible to be sure that they were being used in a standardized fashion.

The development process for the 1987 American College of Rheumatology (ACR) criteria had many similarities with that for 1958. A total of 41 rheumatologists from university and private practice were asked to provide details of patients aged 16 years and older whom they considered to have RA and of the next consecutive patient who did not have RA or a localized rheumatic condition.[12] The data items from the 1958 and New York criteria, as well as potential criteria proposed by the subcommittee, were collected from 262 RA cases and 262 controls. The average disease duration of the RA cases was 7 years. The majority of control subjects had established diagnoses such as osteoarthritis, fibromyalgia, or systemic lupus erythematosus. The sensitivity and specificity of the individual items and various combinations were tested. In addition the technique of recursive partitioning[3] was used to develop a classification tree (Figure 1-1).

The committee appropriately chose to use the term "classification" rather than "diagnostic" criteria. The 1987 criteria exist in two formats: the "list" and the "tree." The "list" (Table 1-6) comprises seven items—at least four of which should be positive. The "list" format recognizes only one category of RA (effectively combining definite and classical RA and excluding probable and possible RA). There are no exclusions.

The classification tree consists of eight subsets of patients, five of which are classified as RA. It allows substitution for missing data, which makes it particularly useful for epidemiologic studies.

Use of 1987 Criteria in Population Studies

Like the 1958 criteria, the 1987 criteria predominantly identify patients with active RA—requiring, for example, evidence of active joint inflammation rather than past joint damage. Patients in remission or using effective therapy may not currently experience morning stiffness, although it may have been a prominent feature in the past.

Table 1-6. Revised 1987 American Rheumatism Association Criteria

1.	Morning stiffness	Morning stiffness in and around the joints, lasting at least 1 hour before maximal improvement.
2.	Arthritis in three or more joint areas[a]	Soft tissue swelling or fluid (not bony overgrowth) observed by a physician, present simultaneously for at least 6 weeks.
3.	Arthritis of hand joints	Swelling of wrist MCP or PIP for at least 6 weeks
4.	Symmetrical arthritis	Simultaneous involvement of the same joint areas (defined in 2) on both sides of the body (bilateral involvement of PIPs, MCPs, or MTPs is acceptable without absolute symmetry for at least 6 weeks.
5.	Rheumatoid nodules	Subcutaneous nodules over bony prominences, or extensor surfaces, or in juxta-articular regions, observed by a physician.
6.	Rheumatoid factor	Detected by a method positive in less than 5% normal controls.
7.	Radiographic changes	Typical of RA on posteroanterior hand and wrist radiographs which must include erosions or unequivocal bony decalcification localized to or most marked adjacent to the involved joints (osteoarthritis changes alone do not qualify).

Notes: At least four criteria must be fulfilled for classification as RA. Patients with two clinical diagnoses are not excluded.
[a]Proposed areas: right or left PIP, MCP, wrist, elbow, knee, ankle, MTP.
Adapted from Arnett FC, Edworthy SM, Bloch DA, et al. The American Rheumatism Association 1987 revised criteria for the classification of rheumatoid arthritis. *Arthritis Rheum* 1988;31:315–324.

Table 1-7. Proposed Modified Format for Application of Revised 1987 American Rheumatism Association Criteria to Population and Family Studies

1.	Morning stiffness	Morning stiffness in and around the joints, lasting at least 1 hour before maximal improvement at any time in the disease course.
2.	Arthritis in at least three joint areas[a]	Soft tissue swelling or fluid observed by a physician, with swelling at current examination or deformity and a documented history of swelling.
3.	Arthritis of hands	Swelling of wrist, MCP, or PIP with swelling at current examination or deformity and a documented history of swelling.
4.	Symmetric arthritis	Simultaneous involvement of the same joint areas (defined in 2) on both sides of the body (bilateral involvement of PIPs, MCPs, or MTPs is acceptable without absolute symmetry) with swelling at current examination or deformity and a documented history of swelling.
5.	Rheumatoid nodules	Over bony prominences or extensor surfaces, or in juxta-articular regions, observed by a physician and present at current examination or documented in the past.
6.	Rheumatoid factor	Detected by a method positive in less than 5% normal controls at current examination or documented to have been positive in the past by any assay method.
7.	Radiographic changes	Typical of RA on posteroanterior hand and wrist radiographs which must include erosions or unequivocal bony decalcification localized to or most marked adjacent to the involved joints (osteoarthritis changes alone do not qualify).

Note: At least four criteria must be fulfilled for classification as RA.
[a]As defined in Table 1-6.
Adapted from MacGregor AJ, Bamber S, Silman AJ. A comparison of the performance of different methods of disease classification for rheumatoid arthritis. Results of an analysis from a nationwide twin study. *J Rheumatol* 1994;21(8):1420–1426 and Arnett FC, Edworthy SM, Bloch DA, et al. The American Rheumatism Association 1987 revised criteria for the classification of rheumatoid arthritis. *Arthritis Rheum* 1988;31:315–324.

MacGregor et al.,[13] in the context of a nationwide twin study, studied 283 individuals using the physician diagnosis of RA as the gold standard. They examined the performance of the Rome active criteria, the New York criteria, and the 1987 criteria. They proposed an adaptation of the 1987 criteria (Table 1-7) that would enable inactive cases of RA to be identified. Using sensitivity and specificity analyses as well as kappa statistics, they concluded that their adaptation of the 1987 criteria had similar properties to the New York (two out of four) criteria.

Past and Current Criticisms of 1987 Criteria

It is generally accepted that the 1987 criteria are more specific but less sensitive than the 1958 criteria. There was an overlap between the physicians who developed the criteria and those who provided cases in which the criteria were assessed. This introduces a circularity that is not ideal. The joint examination is confined to 14 joint areas (7 on each side) and does not include the shoulders or the ankles. Only 18% of the RA cases had disease duration of less than 1 year.

The radiologic criterion only includes hand x-rays. A number of groups have explored the consequences of excluding feet x-rays.[14,15] In a prospective study conducted by Bernelot Moens et al.,[16] there were 17 patients who were classified as having RA by their rheumatologist but not by the 1987 ACR criteria (i.e., false negatives); 12 of these had erosions in their metatarsophalangeal (MTP) joints but not in their hands.

Validation of Existing Criteria Sets

The 1956 ARA criteria have never been subjected to external validation. The 1958 criteria were not validated at the time but have subsequently been assessed in a number of studies. For example, in the 1960s, O'Sullivan and Cathcart[17,18] surveyed 4552 people in Sudbury, Massachusetts; 0.87% met the 1958 ARA criteria and 0.37% the New York criteria at baseline. Only 36% of participants who originally satisfied the 1958 ARA criteria for probable or definite RA still met the criteria 3 to 5 years later, whereas 65% who satisfied the New York criteria still appeared to have the disease 3 to 5 years later.

Mitchell and Fries[19] studied 840 RA patients aged over 16 years. They defined seven disease subsets on the basis of the 1958 ARA criteria. They reported a close association between the number of criteria satisfied and the severity of disease.

The publication of the 1987 ACR criteria[12] led to a flurry of validation studies. Bernelot Moens et al.[16] examined the properties of the 1958 and 1987 criteria sets in two cohorts of patients assembled by the Jan van Breemen Institute in Amsterdam. The first cohort comprised 1338 patients seen since 1984 with a clinical diagnosis of RA who had data available on RF. They examined data collected at baseline and all data collected during the course of the disease. The second cohort comprised 93 RA cases and 1357 non-RA cases seen between September 1987 and September 1988; 43 patients were in both cohorts. The 1987 criteria have also been externally validated by Kobayashi et al.,[20] Kaarela et al.,[21] and Levin et al.[22] While Bernelot Moens et al.[16] concluded that it was appropriate not to have a list of excluded conditions, Levin et al.[22] noted a high proportion of false positives among patients with SLE, psoriatic arthritis, and gout. In addition, in a study of 270 patients with early arthritis from Brittany, Saraux et al.[23] found that some patients who satisfied the ACR criteria at baseline and after 2 years did not have RA, and concluded that it would be helpful to have some exclusion criteria.

Relatively little work has been done to validate the "tree" version of the criteria despite its apparent advantages. Lunt et al.[24] followed 848 subjects with recent-onset inflammatory polyarthritis (IP) for 5 years. They applied the "tree" criteria at baseline (using permitted surrogates for missing data) and the "list" criteria cumulatively. Although RA prevalence was higher at baseline with the "tree" version (63% vs 47%), it was similar at 5 years using either approach (69% vs 72%). Sixty-four percent satisfied both formats of the criteria at 5 years. Although there was poor agreement between the surrogate measure and the real data (e.g., metacarpophalangeal joint [MCP] swelling and radiologic erosions in the hand), the use of the surrogate data produced good to very good agreement in categorizing subjects as having RA.

There has been no attempt to validate the 1987 criteria in non-Caucasian populations in which the prevalence of RA may be lower.

Problem Posed by Early Inflammatory Polyarthritis

One consistent criticism of the 1987 criteria has been poor performance, and in particular, low sensitivity in patients with early inflammatory arthritis. This lack of sensitivity in early disease was acknowledged in the original paper. It has been shown that applying the "list" format to patients with new-onset IP is not useful in predicting the future development of persistent, disabling, or erosive disease.[23,25] The "tree" format performs rather better but is seldom used.[24] However, the process of developing new criteria for what might be called "early RA" poses a number of important intellectual challenges. Rheumatologists are not proficient at identifying early RA on the basis of signs and symptoms alone. Thus, it is difficult to identify a construct that could be used as a gold standard. Paradoxically, there has been a trend for rheumatologists to use the 1987 ACR criteria as diagnostic criteria to tell them which patients with IP have evolved into RA.[26] Additional problems in the classification of early IP are a possible secular trend with RA becoming milder (and thus less easy to diagnose) and the trend toward ever earlier and more effective treatment that prevents the development of the pathognomonic features of RA—in particular radiologic erosions.

All previous classification criteria have required the symptoms and signs of disease to be present for at least 6 weeks before the criteria were applied. Thus, by definition, it is impossible to have early RA of less than 6 weeks duration. Because many of the existing criteria such as radiologic erosions and nodules are not present in early disease, it may take time for the patient to satisfy the criteria. These observations raise the philosophical question as to whether patients who eventually satisfy the 1987 ACR criteria have had RA since the first day of symptoms or whether all early arthritis is in fact undifferentiated and that patients evolve into RA.[27] In other words, there may be different genetic and environmental risk factors for susceptibility to inflammatory arthritis from those that determine persistence and evolution into RA. There may be yet another set of determinants of severity, given persistence.

Therefore, in the context of individuals with early arthritis, the predictive properties of potential criteria may be important. The SIGN guidelines group conducted a comprehensive review of prognostic marker studies in patients with early arthritis (Table 1-8). They identified higher joint counts, high erythrocyte sedimentation rate (ESR) and/or C-reactive protein (CRP), early radiologic erosions, poor physical function at presentation, low socioeconomic status, and lower educational level as important predictors of a worse outcome. These would therefore all be contenders to be included in a list of potential diagnostic tests for early RA.

In early disease, one is looking for clinical features or biomarkers that identify individuals likely to develop persistent arthritis or radiologic erosions. In recent years there have been a number of studies of cohorts of patients with early arthritis that have attempted to identify predictors of either persistence/remission or of particular outcomes such as radiological erosions or physical function; unfortunately the results are very diffuse (Tables 1-9 and 1-10). In addition, some studies have attempted to predict those patients who would eventually satisfy the ACR criteria for RA (Table 1-11). Indeed, Visser et al.[28] developed an algorithm in patients with early arthritis that predicted firstly persistence and then, given persistence, the development of erosions. As yet it remains impossible to identify a biomarker signature that identifies those patients destined to develop RA. See Chapters 4 and 6 for further discussion of these issues.

Recent Developments in Understanding of Inflammatory Polyarthritis with Implications for Classification

Should Anti-CCP Antibody Status Replace Rheumatoid Factor Status?

The presence of rheumatoid factor (RF) is a strong predictor of persistence and the development of erosions. However, RF is relatively nonspecific, as it is positive in many chronic inflammatory

Table 1-8. Studies of Remission and Persistence Prognostic Markers in Early Inflammatory Arthritis ($n \geq 100$)

Name of Study	Inclusion Criteria	Patients (*n*)	Length of Follow-up	Outcome of Interest	Predictors Identified
NOAR The Norfolk Arthritis Register Est. 1989[32]	Age ≥16 years Synovitis ≥2 joints Duration ≥4 weeks	579	3 years	Remission	Male gender <6 joints tender at baseline
Leiden Early Arthritis Clinic Est. 1993[33]	Symptoms <2 years Arthritis ≥1 joint Arthritis diagnosis by rheumatologist	296 RA = 158 UA = 138	2 years	Remission	RAP model much better predictor than SE model Absence of HLA-DQ and DR DERAA-DRB1
The Austrian Early Arthritis Action Est. 1995[34]	Symptoms <3 months Nontraumatic synovitis >1 joint ESR >20 mm CRP >0.5 mg/dl	200	>6 month/ <9 years	Persistence	RF –ve / low titer
SONORA Study of New Onset Rheumatoid Arthritis[35]	3–12 month symptoms Rheumatologist diagnosis	343	5 years	Disease severity (ACR %)	Smoking affected remission in females only
Schumacher et al., 2004[36]	Symptoms <1 year Inflammatory arthritis ≥1 joint	121	>1 year (Median = 5 years)	Persistent erosive disease	Polyarticular disease Hand involvement Fulfilling ACR criteria
Stockman et al., 2006[37]	Symptoms ≤5 years ≥2 swollen and tender joints ≥2 weeks Consecutive patients presenting to the community with IA	159	3 years	Remission Persistence	Age ≥60 years RF –ve 2 SE alleles (only if RF-positive) ≥4 ACR criteria feet/knee involvement at baseline

ACR, American College of Rheumatology; *RF,* rheumatoid factor; *SE,* shared epitope; *UA,* undifferentiated arthritis.

conditions including systemic lupus erythematosus (SLE), primary Sjögren's syndrome, and chronic osteomyelitis, and in up to 5% of the normal population.

Citrullination (or deimination) is the post-translational conversion of the amino acid arginine to citrulline. Arginine is positively charged and citrulline is neutral. This change in charge results in unfolding of the protein concerned. Myelin basic protein, filagrin, and some histones normally include citrulline residues. Other proteins, including fibrin and vimentin may become citrullinated as a consequence of inflammation, cell injury, or cell death. Citrullinated proteins have been found in inflamed synovium and the lungs of smokers. However, the presence of citrullinated proteins does not automatically lead to the development of autoantibodies directed against them. Anti-CCP antibody formation is much more likely in individuals who are shared epitope positive.

There is considerable but not absolute overlap between RF and anti-CCP antibodies in patients with arthritis. In a recent systematic review, Avouac et al.[29] reported that, overall, anti-CCP antibodies have a sensitivity of 70% to 80% and a specificity of 95% to 98% for RA. Thus, they are considerably more specific for RA than RF. Anti-CCP antibodies are more strongly associated with erosions than RF, but less strongly associated with extra-articular features.[30]

Some have argued that anti-CCP positive arthritis is a distinct disease entity. If this is so, then it becomes particularly important to establish the nature of the disease experienced by patients with IP who are anti-CCP negative (i.e., the majority at presentation). One-quarter of patients with early RA who are anti-CCP antibody negative will satisfy the 1987 ACR criteria for RA within 3 years of presentation.[31]

It is probably too early to decide the exact role of anti-CCP testing in the classification of RA. It would certainly be against the principle of classification criteria development just to substitute anti-CCP tests for RF tests in the list of criteria. More work is needed on the relative information concerning prognosis and phenotype conveyed by RF and anti-CCP. That information can then be fed into the re-evaluation of a new set of classification criteria for RA.

New Imaging Modalities for Detection of Cartilage and Bone Damage

Joint damage in RA has historically been assessed using plain radiographs of the hands and feet, as reflected in the 1958 and 1987 criteria. However, newer imaging techniques such as ultrasound and magnetic resonance imaging (MRI) may be able to detect signs indicative of damage long before changes are apparent on plain x-ray. Again work is still in

Table 1-9. Studies of Predictors of Physical Function and Disability Persistence in Early Inflammatory Arthritis ($n \geq 100$)

Name of Study	Inclusion Criteria	Patients (*n*)	Length of Follow-up	Outcome of Interest	Predictors Identified
ERAS The Early Rheumatoid Arthritis Cohort Est. 1986[38–40]	Symptoms <2 years No DMARDs	*n* = 732 732 985	5 years 5 years	Disability (Steinbrocker, HAQ) Work disability Disability	Predictors at baseline: Female gender Age >60 at baseline HAQ >1 at presentation Manual disability HAQ in first year[49] Predictors at 1 year: HAQ Socioeconomic status Hb Radiographic score DAS
NOAR The Norfolk Arthritis Register Est. 1989[41,42]	Age ≥16 years Synovitis ≥2 joints Duration ≥4 weeks	381 528	1 year 2 years 5 years	Disability (HAQ) Disability (HAQ) Disability (HAQ)	High baseline HAQ Large joint involvement Female sex Longer disease duration Female >65 years in age No. of damaged joints RF +ve Nodules at baseline Age at symptom onset at 1 year HAQ score at 1 year Nodules at 1 year Joint tenderness at 1 year
NIH National Institute of Health cohort Est. 1994[43]	Peripheral synovitis ≥6/52 <12/12 Minimum of one joint	n = 238	1 year	Function (HAQ)	Number of active joints Not meeting criteria for RA Independent of RF

Table 1-10. Studies Investigating Predictors of Erosive Disease in Early Inflammatory Arthritis ($n \geq 100$)

Name of Study	Inclusion Criteria	Patients (*n*)	Length of Follow-up	Outcome of Interest	Predictors Identified
Swedish study Est. 1985[44]	Symptoms <2 years	183	5–15 years	Erosions	Persistent disease
NOAR The Norfolk Arthritis Register Est. 1989[45]	Age ≥16 years Synovitis ≥2 joints Duration ≥4 weeks	532	2 years	Erosions (Larsen)	Baseline CRP SE
CPR The Western Consortium of Practicing Rheumatologists Est. 1993[46]	Duration <1 year RF +ve ≥6 swollen joints ≥9 tender joints No DMARDs	276	6 years	Radiographic progression (Sharp score)	Radiographs taken in first 6 months not correlated X-rays at 7–18 months weakly correlated Correlation increases with time and maximum at 6 years
Leiden Early Arthritis Clinic Est. 1993[28,33,47–49]	Symptoms <2 years Arthritis ≥1 joint Arthritis diagnosis by rheumatologist As above As above	285 467 296 RA = 158 UA = 138	2 years 4 years 2 years	Erosions (Sharp) Erosions (Sharp) Erosions (Sharp)	IL-16(60) Knee arthritis at presentation (predictive of small joint erosion later)[57] IL-10 genotype[37,58] Anti-CCP2 > anti-CCP1 RAP model much better predictor than SE model HLA-DQ and DR Absence of DERAA-DRB1

Table 1-10. Studies Investigating Predictors of Erosive Disease in Early Inflammatory Arthritis ($n \geq 100$)—cont'd

Name of Study	Inclusion Criteria	Patients (*n*)	Length of Follow-up	Outcome of Interest	Predictors Identified
van der Heijde et al., 1992[50]	Symptoms <1 year	147	2 years	Erosions (Sharp)	Baseline: CRP/ESR/DAS DR4/DR2 RF 6 months: DAS
Gough et al., 1994[51]	Early inflammatory arthritis DMARD naive	170	1 year	Erosions (method not specified)	HVR3 DRB1 RF All except one patients with DW4/DW14 developed erosions
The Austrian Early Arthritis Action Est. 1995[52]	Symptoms <3 months Nontraumatic synovitis ≥1 joint ESR >20 mm CRP >0.5 mg/dl Morning stiffness ≥60 minutes	200	>6 month/ <9 years	Erosions (Larsen)	Anti-RA33 Ab
Listing et al., 2000[53]	Symptoms <2 years Rx with DMARDs 3 years	139	4 years	Erosions (Rantigen radiographic score)	DRB1*04/01 RF at baseline High CRP at baseline
Goldbach-Mansky et al., 2005[54]	Symptoms <1 year ≥1 joint ≥6 weeks duration Mix of RA/UA/ spondyloarthropathy	257	1 year	Erosions (method not specified)	Raised granzyme B level if RF +ve only
Jansen et al., 2002[55]	Age ≥18 Peripheral arthritis ≥2 joints Symptoms <3 years No DMARDs Diagnosis of RA made by experienced rheumatologist at second clinic visit and patients classified as RA or UA. UA patients were followed up to look for radiographic progression	280 RA = 203 UPA = 77	1 year	Erosions (Sharp)	Baseline variables: Disease severity (DAS) Increased age Hand involvement

CCP, cyclic-citrullinated peptide; *DMARDs,* disease-modifying antirheumatic drugs; *UA,* undifferentiated arthritis.

progress to define the exact signs that would support the classification into RA.

Conclusion

The 1958 ARA classification criteria were used for approximately 30 years before being revised. The 1987 ACR criteria are now 20 years old. Is there any indication that they are becoming obsolete? There seems little doubt that new criteria are needed to enable those patients with early IP likely to evolve into RA to be identified. This will likely comprise some sort of "biomarker signature." It is hoped that some combination of genetic and serologic status, perhaps with understanding of the cytokine profile, may help to identify such patients with a good degree of certainty. In terms of established RA the case for review seems less pressing. Certainly the role of anti-CCP antibody status needs to be addressed—but this is probably of greater significance in early disease. Similarly, the place of new imaging techniques needs to be established. Classification criteria should ideally include investigations that are readily available, particularly if the criteria are to be used in the population setting.

Table 1-11. Studies of Predictors of Diagnosis of Rheumatoid Arthritis Markers in Early Inflammatory Arthritis ($n \geq 100$)

Name of Study	Inclusion Criteria	Patients (n)	Length of Follow-up	Outcome of Interest	Predictors Identified
NIH National Institute of Health cohort Est. 1994[43]	Peripheral synovitis ≥6/52 <12/12 min one joint	238	1 year	Physician diagnosis	RF Anti-Sa and Antifilaggrin Ab and Anti-CCP = specificity >90% but sensitivity <50% therefore no additional diagnostic benefit
Leiden Early Arthritis Clinic Est. 1993[28,31,49,56]	Symptoms <2 years Arthritis ≥1 joint diagnosis by rheumatologist As above As above As above	524 RA = 30% UA = 26% Crystal = 11% OA = 6% Sarcoid = 5% Spondyloarthropathy = 4% Reactive arthritis = 3% Other = 15% 936 RA = 22% at baseline UA = 37% at baseline 155 All RA as per ACR criteria at 1 year—others excluded 467	1–2 years (only follow-up for year 2 if persistent disease at year 1 r/v) 1 year 1 year 4 years	Physician diagnosis Fulfilment of the ACR criteria at 1 year Fulfillment of ACR criteria at 1 year Physician diagnosis	Symptom duration at first visit Symptom >6/52 at presentation predicts persistent arthritis Morning stiffness Arthritis ≥3 joint groups Small joint start Symmetrical start I IgM RF Anti-CCP Ab SE homozygous DQ RA homozygous DQ RA heterozygous DQ3 and DQ5 predict RA DQ3 and DQ5 with DERAA motif protects against RA[67] Anti-CCP1 Anti-CCP2 Anti-CCP2 > anti-CCP1
The Austrian Early Arthritis Action Est. 1995[34]	Symptoms <3 months Nontraumatic synovitis >1 joint ESR >20 mm CRP >0.5 mg/dl	200	>6 month/ <9 years	Physician diagnosis	RF especially high titer Anti-CCP Ab Anti-RA33 Ab

Saraux et al., 2001[23,57,58]	Symptoms <1 year Swelling ≥1 joint Age ≥16 years Diagnosis by 5 rheu-matologists at final visit As above As above	270 As above As above	2 years As above As above	Physician diagnosis As above As above	ACR criteria equivalent to clinician diagnosis >1 year only Morning stiffness sens = 68% spec = 65% arthritis ≥3 areas sens = 80% spec = 43% arthritis of hands sens = 81% spec = 46% symmetrical arthritis sens = 77% spec = 37% rh nodules sens = 3% spec = 100% RF sens = 59% spec = 93% radiographic change sens = 22% spec = 98%(69) IgM RF (ELISA) IgG AKA latex test above 3 in combination = strongest predictors Anti-CCP (53 UI) Ab APF AKA
Devauchelle et al., 2001[59] Devauchelle et al., 2004[60]	Age ≥16 years Swelling ≥1 joint Symptoms <1 year	270 149	2 years 30 months (mean)	Physician diagnosis Physician diagnosis	No additional help from hand x-rays at baseline Erosions in hands Erosions on feet Erosions on hands/feet sens = 32% spec = 95%
Nielen et al.[61]	Age ≥18 Arthritis ≥2 joints Symptoms ≥2 years No DMARDs previously	379 RA = 258 UA = 121	1 year	Physician diagnosis at 1 year	Anti-citrullinated human fibrinogen Ab (ACF) Anti-CCP IgM RF
Jansen et al., 2002[62]	Arthritis ≥2 joints Symptoms <3 years	379 RA = 258 UPA = 121	Variable <3 years	Physician diagnosis at 1 year	IgM RF >30 IgA RF >10 Anti-CCP >50 IgM RF >40 IgM RF >30 + IgA RF >10 Sens = 46.5% spec = 96.7% IgM RF >40 + anti-CCP >50 Sens = 33.3% spec = 97.5%

References

1. Felson DT, Anderson JJ. Methodological and statistical approaches to criteria development in rheumatic diseases. *Baillieres Clin Rheumatol* 1995;9(2):253–266.
2. Dougados M, Gossec L. Classification criteria for rheumatic diseases: Why and how? *Arthritis Rheum* 2007;57(7):1112–1115.
3. Brieman L, Friedman JH, Olsken RA. *Classification and Regression Trees*. Belmont CA: Wadsworth, 1984.
4. Johnson SR, Goek ON, Singh-Grewal D, et al. Classification criteria in rheumatic diseases: A review of methodologic properties. *Arthritis Rheum* 2007;57(7):1119–1133.
5. Bennett GA, Cobb S, Jacox R, et al. Proposed diagnostic criteria for rheumatoid arthritis. *Bull Rheum Dis* 1956;7(4):121–124.
6. Ropes MW, Bennett GA, Cobb S, et al. Proposed diagnostic criteria for rheumatoid arthritis. *Ann Rheum Dis* 1957;16(1):118–125.
7. Ropes MW. Conservative therapy in rheumatoid arthritis. *J Chronic Dis* 1957;5(6):697–705.
8. Kellgren JH. Diagnostic criteria for population studies. *Bull Rheum Dis* 1962;13:291–292.
9. Bennett PD, Burch TA. New York symposium on population studies in the rheumatic diseases. A new diagnostic criteria. *Bull Rheum Dis* 1967;17:453–458.
10. Bennett PH, Burch TA. The epidemiological diagnosis of ankylosing spondylitis. In: Bennett PH, Wood PHN, eds. *Population Studies of the Rheumatic Diseases*. Amsterdam: Excerpta Medica, 1968: 305–313.
11. Lawrence JS, Allander E. Report from the sub-committee on diagnostic criteria for rheumatoid arthritis. In: Bennett PH, Wood PHN, National Institute of Arthritis and Metabolic Diseases, Arthritis Foundation Conference, eds. *Population Studies of the Rheumatic Diseases: Proceedings of the Third International Symposium, New York, June 5–10, 1966*. Sponsored by the National Institute of Arthritis and Metabolic Diseases and the Arthritis Foundation. Amsterdam: Excerpta Medica Foundation, 1968:175–178.
12. Arnett FC, Edworthy SM, Bloch DA, et al. The American Rheumatism Association 1987 revised criteria for the classification of rheumatoid arthritis. *Arthritis Rheum* 1988;31:315–324.
13. MacGregor AJ, Bamber S, Silman AJ. A comparison of the performance of different methods of disease classification for rheumatoid arthritis. Results of an analysis from a nationwide twin study. *J Rheumatol* 1994;21(8):1420–1426.
14. Paimela L. The radiographic criterion in the 1987 revised criteria for rheumatoid arthritis. Reassessment in a prospective study of early disease. *Arthritis Rheum* 1992;35(3):255–258.
15. Symmons DP, Barrett EM, Bankhead CR, et al. The incidence of rheumatoid arthritis in the United Kingdom: Results from the Norfolk Arthritis Register. *Br J Rheumatol* 1994;33(8):735–739.
16. Bernelot Moens HJ, van de Laar MA, van der Korst JK. Comparison of the sensitivity and specificity of the 1958 and 1987 criteria for rheumatoid arthritis. *J Rheumatol* 1992;19(2):198–203.
17. Cathcart ES, O'Sullivan JB. Rheumatoid arthritis in a New England town. A prevalence study in Sudbury, Massachusetts. *N Engl J Med* 1970;282(8):421–424.
18. O'Sullivan JB, Cathcart ES. The prevalence of rheumatoid arthritis. Follow-up evaluation of the effect of criteria on rates in Sudbury, Massachusetts. *Ann Intern Med* 1972;76(4):573–577.
19. Mitchell DM, Fries JF. An analysis of the American Rheumatism Association criteria for rheumatoid arthritis. *Arthritis Rheum* 1982;25(5):481–487.
20. Kobayashi S, Sugawara M, Takahashi H, et al. [Evaluation of the 1987 revised ARA criteria for rheumatoid arthritis in Japan]. *Ryumachi* 1989;29(2):97–104.
21. Kaarela K, Kauppi MJ, Lehtinen KE. The value of the ACR 1987 criteria in very early rheumatoid arthritis. *Scand J Rheumatol* 1995;24(5):279–281.
22. Levin RW, Park J, Ostrov B, et al. Clinical assessment of the 1987 American College of Rheumatology criteria for rheumatoid arthritis. *Scand J Rheumatol* 1996;25(5):277–281.
23. Saraux A, Berthelot JM, Chales G, et al. Ability of the American College of Rheumatology 1987 criteria to predict rheumatoid arthritis in patients with early arthritis and classification of these patients two years later. *Arthritis Rheum* 2001;44(11):2485–2491.
24. Lunt M, Symmons DP, Silman AJ. An evaluation of the decision tree format of the American College of Rheumatology 1987 classification criteria for rheumatoid arthritis: Performance over five years in a primary care-based prospective study. *Arthritis Rheum* 2005; 52(8):2277–2283.
25. Harrison BJ, Symmons DP, Barrett EM, et al. The performance of the 1987 ARA classification criteria for rheumatoid arthritis in a population based cohort of patients with early inflammatory polyarthritis. American Rheumatism Association. *J Rheumatol* 1998; 25(12):2324–2330.
26. Symmons DP, Hazes JM, Silman AJ. Cases of early inflammatory polyarthritis should not be classified as having rheumatoid arthritis. *J Rheumatol* 2003;30(5):902–904.
27. Dixon WG, Symmons DP. Does early rheumatoid arthritis exist? *Clin RheumatolBest Pract Res Clin Rheumatol* 2005;19(1):37–53.
28. Visser H, le Cessie S, Vos K, et al. How to diagnose rheumatoid arthritis early: A prediction model for persistent (erosive) arthritis. *Arthritis Rheum* 2002;46(2):357–365.
29. Avouac J, Gossec L, Dougados M. Diagnostic and predictive value of anti-cyclic citrullinated protein antibodies in rheumatoid arthritis: A systematic literature review. *Ann Rheum Dis* 2006;65(7):845–851.
30. De Rycke L, Peene I, Hoffman IE, et al. Rheumatoid factor and anticitrullinated protein antibodies in rheumatoid arthritis: Diagnostic value, associations with radiological progression rate, and extra-articular manifestations. *Ann Rheum Dis* 2004;63(12): 1587–1593.
31. van Gaalen FA, Linn-Rasker SP, van Venrooij WJ, et al. Autoantibodies to cyclic citrullinated peptides predict progression to rheumatoid arthritis in patients with undifferentiated arthritis: A prospective cohort study. *Arthritis Rheum* 2004;50(3):709–715.
32. Harrison B, Symmons D. Early inflammatory polyarthritis: Results from the Norfolk Arthritis Register with a review of the literature. II. Outcome at three years. *Rheumatology (Oxford)* 2000;39(9):939–949.
33. Vos K, Visser H, Schreuder GM, et al. Human leukocyte antigen-DQ and DR polymorphisms predict rheumatoid arthritis outcome better than DR alone. *Hum Immunol* 2001;62(11):1217–1225.
34. Nell VP, Machold KP, Stamm TA, et al. Autoantibody profiling as early diagnostic and prognostic tool for rheumatoid arthritis. *Ann Rheum Dis* 2005;64(12):1731–1736.
35. Massarotti E, Gregersen P, Bombardier C, et al. Clinical markers of disease progression in the SONORA cohort: Effects of rheumatoid factor and smoking history. *Ann Rheum Dis* 2003;62:194.
36. Schumacher HR, Jr., Habre W, Meador R, et al. Predictive factors in early arthritis: Long-term follow-up. *Semin Arthritis Rheum* 2004; 33(4):264–272.
37. Stockman A, Tait BD, Wolfe R, et al. Clinical, laboratory and genetic markers associated with erosions and remission in patients with early inflammatory arthritis: A prospective cohort study. *Rheumatol Int* 2006;26(6):500–509.
38. Young A, Dixey J, Cox N, et al. How does functional disability in early rheumatoid arthritis (RA) affect patients and their lives? Results of 5 years of follow-up in 732 patients from the Early RA Study (ERAS). *Rheumatology (Oxford)* 2000;39(6):603–611.
39. Young A, Dixey J, Kulinskaya E, et al. Which patients stop working because of rheumatoid arthritis? Results of five years' follow-up in 732 patients from the Early RA Study (ERAS). *Ann Rheum Dis* 2002;61(4):335–340.

40. Bansback N, Young A, Brennan A, et al. A prognostic model for functional outcome in early rheumatoid arthritis. *J Rheumatol* 2006;33(8):1503–1510.
41. Harrison BJ, Symmons DP, Brennan P, et al. Inflammatory polyarthritis in the community is not a benign disease: Predicting functional disability one year after presentation. *J Rheumatol* 1996;23(8): 1326–1331.
42. Wiles NJ, Dunn G, Barrett EM, et al. One year follow-up variables predict disability 5 years after presentation with inflammatory polyarthritis with greater accuracy than at baseline. *J Rheumatol* 2000;27(10):2360–2366.
43. Gerber LH, Furst G, Yarboro C, et al. Number of active joints, not diagnosis, is the primary determinant of function and performance in early synovitis. *Clin Exp Rheumatol* 2003;21(5 Suppl 31):S65–S70.
44. Eberhardt K, Fex E. Clinical course and remission rate in patients with early rheumatoid arthritis: Relationship to outcome after 5 years. *Br J Rheumatol* 1998;37(12):1324–1329.
45. Harrison B, Thomson W, Symmons D, et al. The influence of HLA-DRB1 alleles and rheumatoid factor on disease outcome in an inception cohort of patients with early inflammatory arthritis. *Arthritis Rheum* 1999;42(10):2174–2183.
46. Paulus HE, Oh M, Sharp JT, et al. Correlation of single time-point damage scores with observed progression of radiographic damage during the first 6 years of rheumatoid arthritis. *J Rheumatol* 2003; 30(4):705–713.
47. Linn-Rasker SP, van der Helm-van Mil AH, Breedveld FC, et al. Arthritis of the large joints—in particular, the knee—at first presentation is predictive for a high level of radiological destruction of the small joints in rheumatoid arthritis. *Ann Rheum Dis* 2007;66(5): 646–650.
48. Lard LR, van Gaalen FA, Schonkeren JJ, et al. Association of the -2849 interleukin-10 promoter polymorphism with autoantibody production and joint destruction in rheumatoid arthritis. *Arthritis Rheum* 2003;48(7):1841–1848.
49. van Gaalen FA, Visser H, Huizinga TW. A comparison of the diagnostic accuracy and prognostic value of the first and second anti-cyclic citrullinated peptides (CCP1 and CCP2) autoantibody tests for rheumatoid arthritis. *Ann Rheum Dis* 2005;64(10):1510–1512.
50. van der Heijde DM, van Riel PL, van Leeuwen MA, et al. Prognostic factors for radiographic damage and physical disability in early rheumatoid arthritis. A prospective follow-up study of 147 patients. *Br J Rheumatol* 1992;31(8):519–525.
51. Gough A, Faint J, Salmon M, et al. Genetic typing of patients with inflammatory arthritis at presentation can be used to predict outcome. *Arthritis Rheum* 1994;37(8):1166–1170.
52. Machold KP, Stamm TA, Nell VP, et al. Very recent onset rheumatoid arthritis: Clinical and serological patient characteristics associated with radiographic progression over the first years of disease. *Rheumatology (Oxford)* 2007;46(2):342–349.
53. Listing J, Rau R, Muller B, et al. HLA-DRB1 genes, rheumatoid factor, and elevated C-reactive protein: Independent risk factors of radiographic progression in early rheumatoid arthritis. Berlin Collaborating Rheumatological Study Group. *J Rheumatol* 2000;27(9):2100–2109.
54. Goldbach-Mansky R, Suson S, Wesley R, et al. Raised granzyme B levels are associated with erosions in patients with early rheumatoid factor positive rheumatoid arthritis. *Ann Rheum Dis* 2005;64(5): 715–721.
55. Jansen LM, van SD, van der Horst-Bruinsma IE, et al. One-year outcome of undifferentiated polyarthritis. *Ann Rheum Dis* 2002; 61(8):700–703.
56. van der Horst-Bruinsma IE, Visser H, Hazes JM, et al. HLA-DQ–associated predisposition to and dominant HLA-DR–associated protection against rheumatoid arthritis. *Hum Immunol* 1999;60(2): 152–158.
57. Saraux A, Berthelot JM, Chales G, et al. Value of laboratory tests in early prediction of rheumatoid arthritis. *Arthritis Rheum* 2002;47(2): 155–165.
58. Saraux A, Berthelot JM, Devauchelle V, et al. Value of antibodies to citrulline-containing peptides for diagnosing early rheumatoid arthritis. *J Rheumatol* 2003;30(12):2535–2539.
59. Devauchelle Pensec V, Saraux A, Berthelot JM, et al. Ability of hand radiographs to predict a further diagnosis of rheumatoid arthritis in patients with early arthritis. *J Rheumatol* 2001;28(12):2603–2607.
60. Devauchelle Pensec V, Saraux A, Berthelot JM, et al. Ability of foot radiographs to predict rheumatoid arthritis in patients with early arthritis. *J Rheumatol* 2004;31(1):66–70.
61. Nielen MM, van der Horst AR, van Schaardenburg D, et al. Antibodies to citrullinated human fibrinogen (ACF) have diagnostic and prognostic value in early arthritis. *Ann Rheum Dis* 2005;64(8): 1199–1204.
62. Jansen AL, van der Horst-Bruinsma I, van Schaardenburg D, et al. Rheumatoid factor and antibodies to cyclic citrullinated peptide differentiate rheumatoid arthritis from undifferentiated polyarthritis in patients with early arthritis. *J Rheumatol* 2002;29(10):2074–2076.

Descriptive Epidemiology of Rheumatoid Arthritis

CHAPTER 2

Alan J. Silman and Marc C. Hochberg

This chapter will discuss the methodologic aspects behind the measurement of the incidence and prevalence of rheumatoid arthritis (RA) in various populations. Variations in the incidence of RA in European and U.S. populations will be discussed and the effect of age on incidence will be shown. The prevalence of RA in European and U.S. populations and variations with age will also be covered. Studies also show how the incidence of RA has changed over time, and this will be examined by looking at studies by calendar year and birth cohort studies. Variations in the geographic occurrence of RA will also be covered discussing how estimates of RA vary both between and within countries.

Methodologic Aspects

The occurrence of RA has been widely studied in different populations. The incidence of RA is the number of new cases arising in the population at risk over a given time period. Prevalence represents all the existing cases of RA at a given point in time (point prevalence) or period of time (period prevalence). Methods used to ascertain the incidence and prevalence of RA in some recent studies are summarized in Tables 2-1 and 2-2, respectively. Older studies faced methodologic issues resulting in large differences in both the incidence and prevalence of RA in different populations. Prolonged observation results in more reliable estimates of the true epidemiology of RA and more recent studies have been more consistent in their estimates of RA. However, it can still be difficult to directly compare data from different studies as investigators do not always distinguish between the prevalence of active disease (or receiving therapy) and the prevalence of ever been diagnosed. Furthermore, although the criteria for diagnosing RA are well established, they were not designed for epidemiologic studies.[1]

Incidence in European and U.S. Populations

The incidence of RA varies by populations (Table 2-3). Low incidence rates (8.8/100,000) have been reported in a recent study from France.[2] The rates in Scandinavian countries are higher at 24 to 36 per 100,000.[3–7] The highest recently reported incidence rates (42–45/100,000) were observed in the United States.[8,9] The most recent data on the incidence of RA in the United States come from the Rochester Epidemiology Project, a record linkage system that allows access to medical records of all residents of Rochester, Minnesota, who obtained care from local health care providers, including the Mayo Clinic and affiliated hospitals.[9] An inception cohort of all cases of RA first diagnosed between January 1, 1955 and December 31, 1994, and followed up until January 1, 2000, was identified; the incidence date was defined as the first date of fulfillment of the American College of Rheumatology (ACR) criteria. There were a total of 609 incident cases, including 445 women and 164 men. The overall age- and sex-adjusted average annual incidence of RA was 44.6 per 100,000 per year (95% confidence interval [CI]: 41.0–48.2); the average annual incidence rates were 57.8 (95% CI: 52.4–63.2) and 30.4 (95% CI: 25.6–35.1) per 100,000 per year for women and men, respectively.

Wiles and colleagues[10] recently summarized the difficulties in ascertaining the true incidence of RA in populations. They studied how the delay between symptom onset to notification to a population-based arthritis register affected the estimates of incidence. Allowing 12 months from symptom onset to notification to the register gave incidence estimates of 30.8/100,000 for women and 12.7/100,000 for men. If 5 years elapsed between symptom onset and notification, these estimates rose by 45% for women and 36% for men. Additionally, if the criteria were applied cumulatively, the estimates rose by 75% for women and 93% for men. They concluded that accurate estimates of incidence can only be gained by long-term observation.

Influence of Age

In most populations, the incidence of RA increases with age until the eighth decade where it starts to decline again. RA is more common in women and is uncommon in young men (<35 years). The difference between genders is not consistent and changes with increasing age. Figure 2-1 shows the age distribution of the annual incidence of RA in the Rochester Epidemiology Project patient cohort.[9] The overall age-specific average annual incidence rates increased with age until 85 years; sex-specific rates peaked at a younger age group in women, 55 to 64 years, than in men, aged 75 to 84 years (Figure 2-1). The ratio of age- and sex-specific average annual incidence rates varied significantly according to age group, with a fourfold higher rate in women in the 35- to 44-year age group compared with an almost identical rate in the 75- to 84-year age group. The average annual age- and sex-adjusted incidence rate fell progressively over four decades of study, from 61.2 (95% CI: 51.2–71.3) per 100,000 per year in 1955 to 1964, to 32.7 (95% CI: 27.3–38.0) per 100,000 per year in 1985 to 1994; this decline in RA incidence was more marked in women than in men (Figure 2-2).

Table 2-1. Methods Used to Measure Prevalence

Sample	Questionnaire	RA Diagnosis Confirmed by:
Cross-sectional survey	Structured interview	Physical examination and laboratory investigation
Stratified sample		Clinical investigation
County patient register	Postal survey	
Two housing blocks	Structured interview	Clinical investigation
GP registers	Postal survey	Rheumatologist practice
House-to-house survey	Questionnaires	
GP (contact by phone/letter)	Structured interview by rheumatologist	Examined by rheumatologist and GP
Electoral register	Self-questionnaire	
National telephone directory/next-birthday method	Validated questionnaire	Patient's rheumatologist or clinical examination
Primary care setting	Postal questionnaire	Clinical examination
Arthritis registries, computerized database, local health care providers		
Censuses of 20 municipalities (random sample)	Structured interview by rheumatologist	

Table 2-2. Methods Used to Ascertain Incidence

Drug reimbursement entitlement
Referrals to rheumatology department/private rheumatologists
Hospital records for joint aspirates
Prospective population-based register
Review of medical records
Inception cohort
Norwegian RA register
Prospective case–control study
Regional media announcements

Prevalence in European and U.S. Populations

Studies that have reported the prevalence of RA in the last two decades are summarized in Table 2-4. Low prevalence (<0.2%) has been observed in Yugoslavia.[11] Some European countries such as Italy[12] and France[13] have reported low prevalence ratios around 0.3%. UK estimates are higher at around 0.8%[14] and similar to ratios in Finland.[15] Higher prevalence has been observed in the United States (1.1%).[16] Data from Rochester, Minnesota suggest an overall prevalence of RA on January 1, 1985, of 1.07 per 100

Table 2-3. Incidence of Rheumatoid Arthritis in Epidemiologic Studies from 1990 Onward

Year (Study years)	Country	Reference	Type of Study	Age	Incidence/100,000
1999 (1985–1996)	Japan	24	Longitudinal population-based study	All	8 (0–17) Women: 0; Men: 16
1994 (1986–1989)	France	2	Identified from in- and out-patients at various practitioners	20–70	8.8 Women: 12.7; Men: 4.7
1997 (1985–1995)	Greece	36	Patient record review	≥16	15–36
2002 (1999–2000)	Sweden	4	Hospital referrals	>16	24 Women: 29; Men: 18
1998	Norway	5	Postal survey	20–79	25.7 Women: 36.7; Men: 13.8
1987–1996	Norway	3	Hospital records	≥20	28.7 Women: 36; Men: 21.4
2001 (1995)	Finland	6	Central hospital districts	>16	31.7 (95% CI: 29.2 to 34.4) Women: 40 (36–44.2); Men: 23.2 (20.2–26.7)
2003 (2000)	Finland	7		≥16	36
1994 (1990/1991)	UK	37	Prospective population survey	15+	Women: 36; Men: 14
1993 (1987/1990)	United States	8	Review of medical records	≥18	42 (23–60) Women: 60 (46–75) , Men: 22 (13–32)
2002	United States	9	Inception cohort of Rochester residents	≥18	44.6 (41–48.2) Women: 57.8 (52.4–63.2), Men: 30.4 (25.6–35.1)

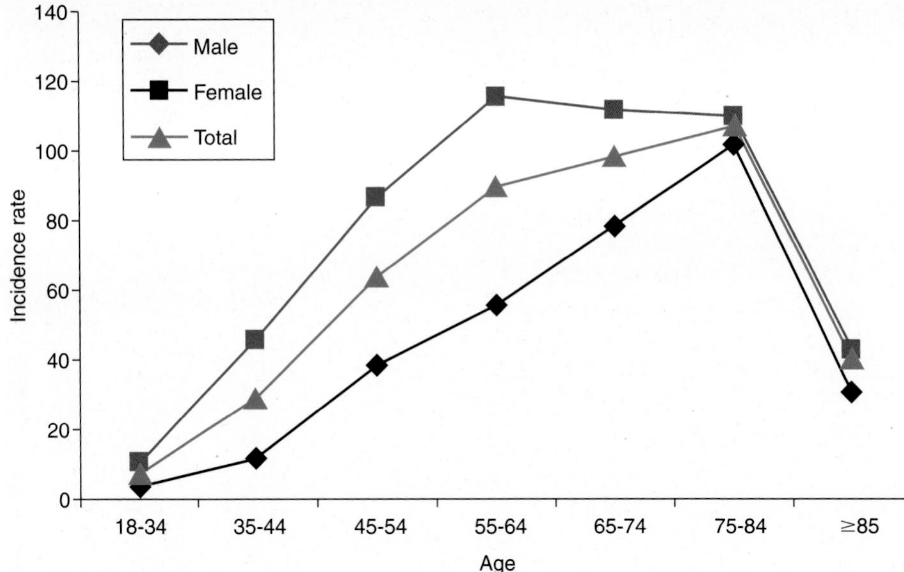

Figure 2-1. Age distribution of the annual incidence of RA in Rochester, Minnesota by gender. (Data from Doran MF, Pond GR, Crowson CS, O'Fallon WM, Gabriel SE. Trends in incidence and mortality in rheumatoid arthritis in Rochester, Minnesota, over a forty-year period. *Arthritis Rheum* 2002;46(3):625–631.)

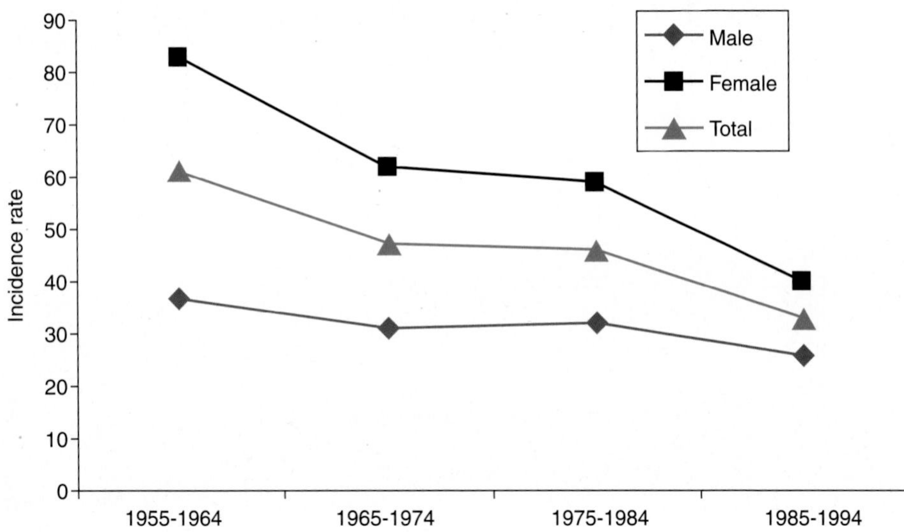

Figure 2-2. Decrease in RA incidence in Rochester, Minnesota by gender and time period. (Data from Doran MF, Pond GR, Crowson CS, O'Fallon WM, Gabriel SE. Trends in incidence and mortality in rheumatoid arthritis in Rochester, Minnesota, over a forty-year period. *Arthritis Rheum* 2002;46(3):625–631.)

persons aged 35 and older (95% CI: 0.94–1.20); prevalence among women was approximately double that in men at 1.37 compared to 0.74 per 100.[16] A more recent update of this population-based data set reported a decline in overall prevalence to 0.85 per 100 persons aged 35 and older as of January 1, 1995 (95% CI: 0.75–0.95). The most recent estimates from the United States using data from Rochester, Minnesota, and Census population estimates from 2005 show that 0.6% of American adults (1.293 million) have RA.[17] A higher prevalence of RA has also been noted in Mexican Americans compared to both whites and blacks.[18] The prevalence of RA is between two- to five-fold higher in women compared to men (Table 2-5).

Influence of Age

The prevalence of a nonlethal disease such as RA will increase with age as new cases in younger people who survive will then add to the "prevalence pool." In a recent study from the UK, sex-specific estimates for RA were calculated by conducting a two-stage population-based survey.[14] Researchers found that RA prevalence increased in females from 0.12% in the 16-44 year age band to 2.99% in the 75-plus age band (Figure 2-3). Increases were also shown in males from 0.58% in the 45- to 64-year age group to 2.18% in the 75-plus group. These figures represent the minimum estimates of prevalence assuming that none of the nonresponders had RA. Assuming that those who declined to be examined had the same rate of RA as those who agreed to be examined produced higher estimates. In females, the prevalence increased from 0.21% in the 16- to 44-year-olds to 5.36% in the 75-plus age group. In males, prevalence was 0.94% for the 45- to 64-year-olds and increased to 3.08% in the 75-plus age band.

The prevalence of RA in older Americans was recently estimated using data from the Third National Health and Nutrition Examination Survey (NHANES III).[18] The overall prevalence of RA among people aged 60 and older was quite similar in the three different case identification strategies: 2.03 per 100 (95% CI: 1.30–2.76), 2.15 per 100 (95% CI: 1.43–2.87) and 2.34 per 100 (95% CI: 1.66–3.02), respectively. The prevalence of RA was generally greater in women, ranging from 2.35 to 2.71 per 100,

Table 2-4. Prevalence of Rheumatoid Arthritis in Epidemiologic Studies (1990 to Date)

Year (Study years)	Country	Reference	Type of Study	Age (years)	Prevalence (%) (95% confidence interval)
1998 (1990/1991)	Yugoslavia	11	Cross-sectional survey	≥20	0.18 (0.17–0.20)
1998	Saudi Arabia	28		≥16	0.22
2003 (1997/1998)	China	29	Random selection, COPCORD Questionnaire	>15	0.28 (0.15–0.41)
2005 (2001)	France	13	Telephone survey	≥18	0.31 (0.18–0.48)
1998 (1991–1992)	Italy	12	Postal questionnaire	≥16	0.33 (0.13–0.53)
1993	Urbanized Chinese	38	Structured interview	≥16	0.35
1991	Sultanate of Oman	39	House-to-house survey	≥16	0.36 0.84[a]
2005	Hungary	40	Survey	14–65	0.37 (0.26–0.51)
2005 (2000/2001)	Turkey	41	Cross-sectional study (randomized cluster)	≥16	0.38 (0.16–0.59)
2001 (1987–1996)	Norway	3	1987 ARA criteria	>20	0.39 in 1989 0.47 in 1994
1997	Norway	42	Postal population survey/County patient register	20–79	0.44 (0.41–0.46)
2005 (2002/2003)	Italy, Sardinia	43	Rheumatologist—structured interview	≥18	0.46
2004	Turkey	44	Interview	≥20	0.49 (0.27–0.83)
2002	Spain	45	Census and screening interview	≥20	0.5 (0.25–0.85)
1999	Ireland	46	Random electoral register		0.5
1999	Sweden	47	Questionnaire	20–74	0.51 (0.31–0.79)
2008 (2005)	United States	48		≥18	0.6
1999	France	49	Questionnaire	≥18	0.62 (0.33–0.91)
2006	Greece	50	Standardized questionnaire	≥19	0.68 (0.51–0.85)
1993	India	51	House-to-house survey	>16	0.75
1993	Finland	15	National Sickness Insurance Register	>16	0.8
2002	UK	14	NOAR	≥16	0.81
1999 (1985)	United States	16	Inception cohort	≥35	1.1 (0.9–1.2).
1996	Japan	24		All ages	1.7 (0.3–3.1)
2002 (1998/1999)	Argentina	30	Outpatient and hospitalization medical records	≥16	1.97 (1.8–2)

[a]Adjusted for population structure.

Table 2-5. Prevalence of Rheumatoid Arthritis by Gender in Studies Published Since 1990

Year	Country	Reference	Age (years)		Prevalence (%) (95% confidence interval)
2005	Hungary	40	14–65	Men Women	0.23 (0.15–0.35) 0.48 (0.35–0.64)
2005 (2002/2003)	Italy, Sardinia	43	≥18	Men Women	0.19 0.73
2002	Spain	45	≥20	Men Women	0.2 0.8 (0.4–1.1)
2002 (1998/1999)	Argentina	30	≥16	Men Women	0.6 (0.49–0.73) 3.2 (2.9–3.5)
2002	UK	14	≥16	Men Women	0.44 1.16
1999	France	49	≥18	Men Women	0.32 (0.01–0.63) 0.86 (0.39–1.33)
1996	Japan	24	All ages	Men Women	(0–2.6) 2.4 (0.1–4.7)

Table 2-5. Prevalence of Rheumatoid Arthritis by Gender in Studies Published Since 1990—cont'd

Year	Country	Reference	Age (years)		Prevalence (%) (95% confidence interval)
1998 (1991–1992)	Italy	12	≥16	Men	0.13 (0–0.31)
				Women	0.51 (0.18–0.84)
1998 (1990/1991)	Yugoslavia	11	≥20	Men	0.09 (0.07–0.10)
				Women	0.29 (0.26–0.31)
2001 (1987–1996)	Norway	3	>20	Men	0.24 (in 1989)–0.30 (in 1993)
				Women	0.54 (in 1989)–0.63 (in 1993)
1997	Norway	42	20–79	Men	1.9
				Women	6.7
2003 (1997/1998)	China	29	>15	Men	1.4
				Women	4.1
1999 (1985)	United States	16	≥35	Men	0.74 (0.56–0.91)
				Women	1.4 (1.2–1.6)
1993	Finland	15	>16	Men	0.61
				Women	1.0
2005 (2001)	France	13	≥18	Men	0.09 (0.02–0.2)
				Women	0.51 (0.27–0.82)
2004	Turkey	44	≥20	Men	0.15 (0.02–0.60)
				Women	0.77 (0.40–1.35)

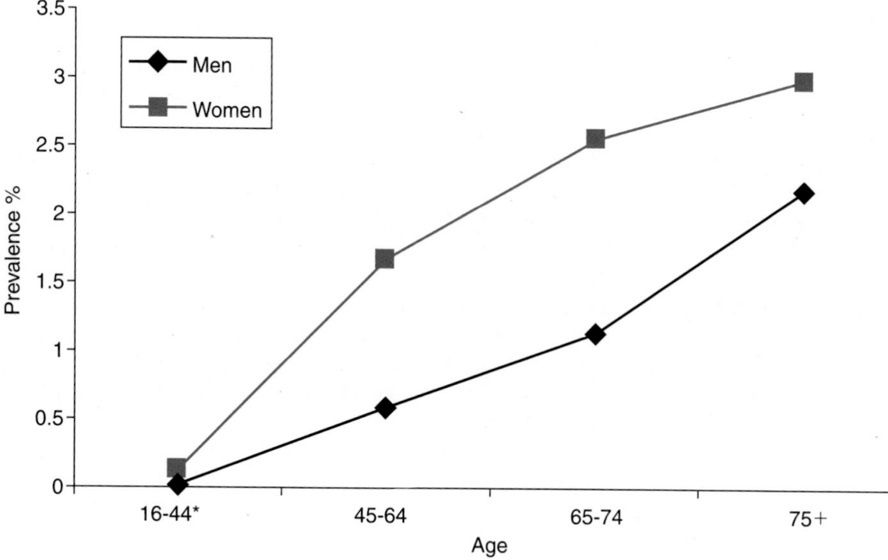

Figure 2-3. Prevalence by age band in the United Kingdom. *Males aged 16 to 44 years were not included in the study. This is an estimate calculated by assuming the female:male ratio of RA is the same as that observed in the Norfolk Arthritis Register. (From Symmons D, Turner G, Webb R, Asten P, Barrett E, Lunt M, et al. The prevalence of rheumatoid arthritis in the United Kingdom: New estimates for a new century. *Rheumatology* 2002; 41(7):793–800.)

than in men, ranging from 1.59 to 1.85 per 100, and in people aged 70 and older, ranging from 2.46 to 2.80 per 100, than in persons aged 60 to 69 years, ranging from 1.59 to 1.89 per 100.

Time Influence

Trends of Incidence by Calendar Year

It has been suggested that the incidence of RA is on the decline.[19–21] Doran and colleagues[9] studied a population cohort in Rochester, Minnesota over 40 years. They found that the incidence of RA fell from 61.2/100,000 in 1955 to 1964, to 32.7/100,000 in 1985 to 1994 (Figure 2-2). A decrease in the U.S. incidence has also been reported by Dugowson and colleagues,[22] who found that incidence rates were 44.7% lower than previous estimates. A Finnish study also observed a significant decline in the number of rheumatoid factor (RF)–negative RA cases of approximately 40%.[23] Jacobsson and colleagues[19] studied trends in RA incidence in the Pima Indians, living in the state of Arizona, over a 25-year period. They found that the incidence declined by 55% in men and by 57% in women. They concluded that this may implicate an environmental factor in the pathogenesis of RA.

In Japan, a decline in RA incidence has also been reported.[24] The total incidence decreased significantly from 0.39 per 1000 person-years in 1965 to 1975 to 0.08 per 1000 person-years in 1985 to 1996. The decrease was a consequence of the decline observed in women with no significant decrease in men over the same time period. However, Riise and colleagues[3] have found no evidence to support a decline in incidence in their Norwegian study between the time periods 1987–1991 and 1992–1996.

Table 2-6. Regional Differences in Rheumatoid Arthritis Incidence in Finnish Study, 1995[6]

	Incidence/100,000 (95% confidence interval)		
Region	**All**	**Men**	**Women**
Vaasa	16.3 (9.8–24.3)	9.4 (3.4–20.3)	23.2 (13.5–38.2)
Tampere	26.6 (21.5–31.5)	25.1 (17.9–33.6)	30.6 (23.3–39.9)
Lahti	27.9 (20.6–37.3)	12.5 (6.0–23.1)	41.7 (29.7–58.2)
Savonlinna	28.6 (16.0–45.5)	15.4 (3.9–36.8)	39.8 (21.1–71.4)
Seinäjoki	28.9 (21.3–38.9)	20.0 (10.9–32.2)	38.7 (26.0–54.3)
Mikkeli	29.9 (19.9–44.0)	28.2 (14.4–48.6)	31.7 (18.2–53.6)
Kotka	31.1 (23.1–41.5)	24.3 (14.3–38.2)	35.9 (23.6–51.3)
Hämeenlinna	34.3 (24.8–45.4)	21.3 (12.1–37.1)	46.0 (31.7–65.4)
Kuopio	36.3 (28.7–45.7)	25.1 (16.2–36.9)	44.2 (32.6–59.0)
Jyväskylä	43.1 (34.4–52.9)	30.0 (20.3–42.9)	54.5 (41.9–70.3)
Joensuu	44.8 (34.6–57.3)	32.5 (20.8–49.3)	56.1 (40.5–76.7)

From Kaipiainen-Seppanen O, Aho K, Nikkarinen M. Regional differences in the incidence of rheumatoid arthritis in Finland in 1995. *Ann Rheum Dis* 2001;60(2):128–132.

Trends of Incidence by Year of Birth

Enzer and colleagues[25] found a strong birth-cohort effect in the Pima Indians, in which those born at the end of the nineteenth century were more likely to be seropositive for RF, again implicating environmental factors in the development of RA. Data from Rochester, Minnesota has shown decreasing incidence rates in successive cohorts. Unusually high incidence rates were found in people born in the 1880s and 1890s in their eighth decades of life and in women born in the 1890s in their seventh decade of life.[9] In a recent study from Japan, an increased age at the time of disease onset has been reported. Two groups were compared: the first from 1960 to 1965 and the second from 1985 to 1990. The mean age at time of disease onset increased significantly from 37.5 years in the first group to 46.9 in the second group.[26] A recent Finnish study also reported that there has been a shift in the mean age at diagnosis from 50.2 years in 1975 to 57.8 years in 1990.[27]

Geographic Influence

The epidemiology of RA is known to differ geographically. Low prevalence (<0.3%) has been observed in Saudi Arabia[28] and China,[29] while higher prevalence has been observed in Japan (1.7%)[24] and Argentina (2.0%).[30] The highest prevalence estimates for RA have been observed in Native-American populations, including the Inupiat, Chippewa, and Pima Indians.[31,32] The prevalence in African populations is often low. A study of Afro-Caribbeans living in inner-city Manchester found they had a lower prevalence (0.29%) than whites in the same area (0.8%).[33]

Regional Differences within Countries

Roux and colleagues in a recent study in France[34] found higher prevalence in the south (0.59%–0.66%) compared to the north of the country (0.14%–0.24%). The average national prevalence rate was 0.31% (95% CI: 0.18–0.48). In Pakistani communities, the prevalence of RA was found to be lower in poor (0.09 95% CI: 0.02–0.36) compared to the affluent areas (0.20 95% CI: 0.06–0.51).[35] Boyer and colleagues[31] studied the prevalence rates in indigenous, circumpolar populations. They found higher ratios in both the Alaskan Inupiat (1.78%) and the Siberian Eskimos (1.42%), and lower ratios in the Alaskan Yupiks (0.62%) and Russian Chukchis (0.73%).

Regional differences in the incidence of RA in Norway were reported by studying patients who were entitled to drug reimbursement for RA in central hospital districts (Table 2-6).[6] Incidence varied from a low of 16.3 per 100,000 in the Vaasa region to a high of 44.8 per 100,000 in the Joensuu region. Variation was noted in both sexes among regions with incidence varying from 9.4 to 32.5 per 100,000 in men and from 23.2 to 56.1 per 100,000 in women.

Conclusion

There is a considerable amount of epidemiologic data on the occurrence of RA worldwide. There are important differences in incidence between populations and intriguing evidence of a recent decline. These observations provide possible clues to the contribution of both genetic and environmental influences on disease etiology.

References

1. Macgregor AJ, Silman AJ. A reappraisal of the measurement of disease occurrence in rheumatoid arthritis. *J Rheumatol* 1992;19(8): 1164–1166.
2. Guillemin F, Briancon S, Klein JM, et al. Low incidence of rheumatoid arthritis in France. Scan *J Rheumatol* 1994;23(5): 264–268.
3. Riise T, Jacobsen BK, Gran JT. Incidence and prevalence of rheumatoid arthritis in the county of Troms, northern Norway. *J Rheumatol* 2000;27(6):1386–1389.
4. Soderlin MK, Borjesson O, Kautiainen H, et al. Annual incidence of inflammatory joint diseases in a population based study in southern Sweden. *Ann Rheum Dis* 2002;61(10):911–915.

5. Uhlig T, Kvien TK, Glennas A, et al. The incidence and severity of rheumatoid arthritis. Results from a county register in Oslo, Norway. *J Rheumatol* 1998;25(6):1078–1084.
6. Kaipiainen-Seppanen O, Aho K, Nikkarinen M. Regional differences in the incidence of rheumatoid arthritis in Finland in 1995. *Ann Rheum Dis* 2001;60(2):128–132.
7. Savolainen E, Kaipiainen-Seppanen O, Kroger L, Luosujarvi R. Total incidence and distribution of inflammatory joint diseases in a defined population: Results from the kuopio 2000 arthritis survey. *J Rheumatol* 2003;30(11):2460–2468.
8. Chan KW, Felson DT, Yood RA, Walker AM. Incidence of rheumatoid arthritis in central Massachusetts. *Arthritis Rheum* 1993;36(12): 1691–1696.
9. Doran MF, Pond GR, Crowson CS, et al. Trends in incidence and mortality in rheumatoid arthritis in Rochester, Minnesota, over a forty-year period. *Arthritis Rheum* 2002;46(3):625–631.
10. Wiles N, Symmons DPM, Harrison B, et al. Estimating the incidence of rheumatoid arthritis—trying to hit a moving target? *Arthritis Rheum* 1999;42(7):1339–1346.
11. Stojanovic R, Vlajinac H, Palic-Obradovic D, et al. Prevalence of rheumatoid arthritis in Belgrade, Yugoslavia. *Br J Rheumatol* 1998; 37(7):729–732.
12. Cimmino MA, Parisi M, Moggiana G, et al. Prevalence of rheumatoid arthritis in Italy: The Chiavari study. *Ann Rheum Dis* 1998; 57(5):315–318.
13. Guillemin F, Saraux A, Guggenbuhl P, et al. Prevalence of rheumatoid arthritis in France: 2001. *Ann Rheum Dis* 2005;64(10): 1427–1430.
14. Symmons D, Turner G, Webb R, et al. The prevalence of rheumatoid arthritis in the United Kingdom: New estimates for a new century. *Rheumatology* 2002;41(7):793–800.
15. Hakala M, Pollanen R, Nieminen P. The ARA 1987 revised criteria select patients with clinical rheumatoid arthritis from a population-based cohort of subjects with chronic rheumatic diseases registered for drug reimbursement. *J Rheumatol* 1993;20(10): 1674–1678.
16. Gabriel SE, Crowson CS, O'Fallon WM. The epidemiology of rheumatoid arthritis in Rochester, Minnesota, 1955–1985. *Arthritis Rheum* 1999;42(3):415–420.
17. Helmick CG, Felson DT, Lawrence RC, et al. Estimates of the prevalence of arthritis and other rheumatic conditions in the United States: Part I. *Arthritis Rheum* 2008;58(1):15–25.
18. Rasch EK, Hirsch R, Paulose-Ram R, Hochberg MC. Prevalence of rheumatoid arthritis in persons 60 years of age and older in the United States—effect of different methods of case classification. *Arthritis Rheum* 2003;48(4):917–926.
19. Jacobsson LT, Hanson RL, Knowler WC, et al. Decreasing incidence and prevalence of rheumatoid arthritis in Pima Indians over a twenty-five-year period. *Arthritis Rheum* 1994;37(8): 1158–1165.
20. Silman AJ. The changing face of rheumatoid arthritis: Why the decline in incidence? *Arthritis Rheum* 2002;46(3):579–581.
21. Uhlig T, Kvien TK. Is rheumatoid arthritis disappearing? *Ann Rheum Dis* 2005;64(1):7–10.
22. Dugowson CE, Koepsell TD, Voigt LF, et al. Rheumatoid arthritis in women—incidence rates in group health cooperative, Seattle, Washington, 1987–1989. *Arthritis Rheum* 1991;34(12):1502–1507.
23. KaipiainenSeppanen O, Aho K, Isomaki H, Laakso M. Incidence of rheumatoid arthritis in Finland during 1980–1990. *Ann Rheum Dis* 1996;55(9):608–611.
24. Shichikawa K, Inoue K, Hirota S, et al. Changes in the incidence and prevalence of rheumatoid arthritis in Kamitonda, Wakayama, Japan, 1965–1996. *Ann Rheum Dis* 1999;58(12):751–756.
25. Enzer I, Dunn G, Jacobsson L, et al. An epidemiologic study of trends in prevalence of rheumatoid factor seropositivity in Pima Indians: Evidence of a decline due to both secular and birth-cohort influences. *Arthritis Rheum* 2002;46(7):1729–1734.
26. Imanaka T, Shichikawa K, Inoue K, et al. Increase in age at onset of rheumatoid arthritis in Japan over a 30-year period. *Ann Rheum Dis* 1997;56(5):313–316.
27. KaipiainenSeppanen O, Aho K, Isomaki H, Laakso M. Shift in the incidence of rheumatoid arthritis toward elderly patients in Finland during 1975–1990. *Clin Exp Rheumatol* 1996;14(5): 537–542.
28. Al-Dalaan A, Al Ballaa S, Bahabri S, et al. The prevalence of rheumatoid arthritis in the Qassim region of Saudi Arabia. *Ann Saudi Med* 1998;18(5):396–397.
29. Dai SM, Han XH, Zhao DB, et al. Prevalence of rheumatic symptoms, rheumatoid arthritis, ankylosing spondylitis, and gout in Shanghai, China: A COPCORD study. *J Rheumatol* 2003;30(10): 2245–2251.
30. Spindler A, Bellomio V, Berman A, et al. Prevalence of rheumatoid arthritis in Tucuman, Argentina. *J Rheumatol* 2002;29(6): 1166–1170.
31. Boyer GS, Benevolenskaya LI, Templin DW, et al. Prevalence of rheumatoid arthritis in circumpolar native populations. *J Rheumatol* 1998;25(1):23–29.
32. Peschken CA, Esdaile JM. Rheumatic diseases in North America's indigenous peoples. *Semin Arthritis Rheum* 1999;28(6):368–391.
33. Macgregor AJ, Riste LK, Hazes JMW, Silman AJ. Low prevalence of Rheumatoid Arthritis in black-Caribbean compared with whites in inner-city Manchester. *Ann Rheum Dis* 1994;53(5): 293–297.
34. Roux CH, Saraux A, Le Bihan E, et al. Rheumatoid arthritis and spondyloarthropathies: Geographical variations in prevalence in France. *J Rheumatol* 2007;34(1):117–122.
35. Hameed K, Gibson T, Kadir M, et al. The prevalence of rheumatoid arthritis in affluent and poor urban communities of Pakistan. *Br J Rheumatol* 1995;34(3):252–256.
36. Drosos AA, Alamanos I, Voulgari PV, et al. Epidemiology of adult rheumatoid arthritis in northwest Greece 1987–1995. *J Rheumatol* 1997;24(11):2129–2133.
37. Symmons DP, Barrett EM, Bankhead CR, et al. The incidence of rheumatoid arthritis in the United Kingdom: Results from the Norfolk Arthritis Register. *Br J Rheumatol* 1994;33(8): 735–739.
38. Lau E, Symmons D, Bankhead C, et al. Low prevalence of rheumatoid arthritis in the urbanized Chinese of Hong Kong. *J Rheumatol* 1993;20(7):1133–1137.
39. Pountain G. The prevalence of rheumatoid arthritis in the Sultanate of Oman. *Br J Rheumatol* 1991;30(1):24–28.
40. Kiss CG, Lovei C, Suto G, et al. Prevalence of rheumatoid arthritis in the South-Transdanubian region of Hungary based on a representative survey of 10,000 inhabitants. *J Rheumatol* 2005;32(9): 1688–1690.
41. Kacar C, Gilgil E, Tuncer T, et al. Prevalence of rheumatoid arthritis in Antalya, Turkey. *Clin Rheumatol* 2005;24(3):212–214.
42. Kvien TK, Glennas A, Knudsrod OG, et al. The prevalence and severity of rheumatoid arthritis in Oslo—Results from a county register and a population survey. *Scand J Rheumatol* 1997;26(6): 412–428.
43. Marotto D, Nieddu ME, Cossu A, Carcassi A. [Prevalence of rheumatoid arthritis in North Sardinia: The Tempio Pausania's study.]. *Reumatismo* 2005;57(4):273–276.
44. Akar S, Birlik M, Gurler O, et al. The prevalence of rheumatoid arthritis in an urban population of Izmir-Turkey. *Clin Exp Rheumatol* 2004;22(4):416–420.
45. Carmona L, Villaverde V, Hernandez-Garcia C, et al. The prevalence of rheumatoid arthritis in the general population of Spain. *Rheumatology* 2002;41(1):88–95.
46. Power D, Codd M, Ivers L, et al. Prevalence of rheumatoid arthritis in Dublin, Ireland: A population based survey. *Ir J Med Sci* 1999; 168(3):197–200.

47. Simonsson M, Bergman S, Jacobsson LT, et al. The prevalence of rheumatoid arthritis in Sweden. Scan *J Rheumatol* 1999;28(6):340–343.
48. Helmick CG, Felson DT, Lawrence RC, et al. Estimates of the prevalence of arthritis and other rheumatic conditions in the United States: Part I. *Arthritis Rheum* 2008;58(1):15–25.
49. Saraux A, Guedes C, Allain J, et al. Prevalence of rheumatoid arthritis and spondyloarthropathy in Brittany, France. *J Rheumatol* 1999;26(12):2622–2627.
50. Andrianakos A, Trontzas P, Christoyannis F, et al. Prevalence and management of rheumatoid arthritis in the general population of Greece—the ESORDIG study. *Rheumatology* 2006;45(12):1549–1554.
51. Malaviya AN, Kapoor SK, Singh RR, et al. Prevalence of rheumatoid arthritis in the adult Indian population. *Rheumatol Int* 1993;13(4):131–134.

The Genetic Basis of Rheumatoid Arthritis

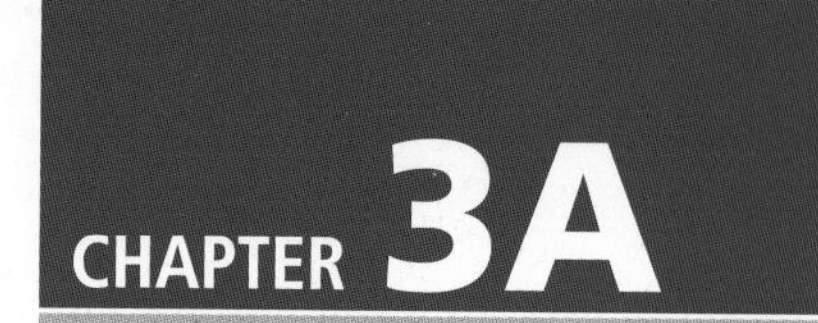

Robert M. Plenge

The genetic contribution to RA susceptibility in humans has been demonstrated through twin studies,[1] family studies,[2] and genome-wide linkage scans.[3–9] Heritability refers to the amount of phenotypic variation due to additive genetic factors, rather than common environmental factors, stochastic variation, gene–environment interactions, and gene–gene interactions. One such study demonstrated that approximately 60% of disease variability is inherited.[1] Another measure of genetic contribution to disease activity is to compare prevalence of disease in family members versus the general population. Whereas the population risk of RA is ~1%, the monozygotic (MZ) twin of a patient with RA has a risk of ~15%.[10–12] Moreover, the relative risk to the sibling of a proband with RA is ~5 for RA,[13–15] although the number varies depending on the population studied.[3]

MHC-Region and *HLA-DRB1* Susceptibility Alleles

The major histocompatibility complex (MHC) region spans ~3.6 megabases (Mb) on the short arm of human chromosome 6, and contains hundreds of genes, including many involved in immune function. It has been estimated that the MHC region of the human genome accounts for approximately one-third of the overall genetic component of RA risk.[14,16] Genome-wide linkage scans using both microsatellite[3–7] and single nucleotide polymorphism (SNP) markers[8] have identified consistently this region as important in RA pathogenesis. These genome-wide scans have demonstrated that the MHC region has the largest genetic contribution in RA.[3,5]

Much, but probably not all, of the risk attributable to the MHC region is associated with alleles within the *HLA-DRB1* gene. An association between RA and the class II HLA proteins was first noted in the 1970's, when the mixed lymphocyte culture (MLC) type Dw4 (related to the serological subtype DR4) was observed to be more common among patients with RA compared to controls.[17,18] Subsequently, investigation of the molecular diversity of Class II proteins (subunits of HLA-DR, -DQ, and -DP) localized the serological Dw4 subtype to the *HLA-DRB1* gene.[19] When the susceptible DR subtypes were considered as a group, Gregersen et al.[20] noted a shared amino acid (a.a.) sequence at positions 70–74 of the HLA-DRB1 protein. These residues are important in peptide binding, and thus it was hypothesized that RA-associated alleles bind specific peptides, which in turn facilitates the development of autoreactive T cells. These alleles are now known collectively as "shared epitope" alleles due to the related sequence composition in the third hypervariable region: the susceptibility alleles result in missense a.a. changes, where the shared susceptibility a.a. motif is ^{70}Q/R-K/R-R-A-A.[74]

Since the initial observation, a large number of population studies have confirmed the association between RA and allelic variants at *HLA-DRB1*. At the level of DNA, the most common (>5% population frequency) *HLA-DRB1* shared epitope–susceptibility alleles include *0101, *0401, and *0404 in individuals of European ancestry, and *0405 and *0901 in individuals of Asian ancestry; less common shared epitope alleles include *0102, *0104, *0408, *0413, *0416, *1001, and *1402. Of note, the *0901 allele observed among Asian populations does not strictly conform to the SE a.a. sequence motif (^{70}R-R-R-A-E^{74}), and the classic SE alleles may not contribute to risk in African-American and Hispanic-American RA populations.[21,22] Thus, additional exploration of the molecular basis of *HLA-DRB1* susceptibility alleles is needed in the future.

While *HLA-DRB1* susceptibility alleles are often considered as a group, the strength of the genetic association to RA susceptibility differs across the *DRB1* alleles. There are at least two classes of *HLA-DRB1* risk alleles (high and moderate). In general, DRB1*0401 and *0405 alleles exhibit a high level of risk, with a relative risk (RR) of approximately 3. The DRB1*0101, *0404, *0901, and *1001 alleles exhibit a more moderate relative risk in the range of 1.5.

It is becoming increasingly clear that *HLA-DRB1* shared epitope alleles only influence the development of seropositive RA, and more specifically anti-CCP+ RA.[23,24] Collectively, the shared epitope alleles have an odds ratio (OR) of over 5 if CCP+ RA patients are compared to matched healthy controls. These alleles are quite common in the general population (collectively, allele frequency of ~40% in individuals of European ancestry).

Numerous studies have shown that *HLA-DRB1* susceptibility alleles influence disease severity in long-standing disease, particularly the development of bony erosions (e.g., Moxley and Cohen,[25] Chen et al.,[26] and Gorman et al.[27]). More recently, however, it has been suggested that this association is primarily due to the presence of CCP autoantibodies.[23] It remains to be determined whether *HLA-DRB1* alleles contribute additional risk of developing erosive disease independent of CCP autoantibodies.[28] This more recent observation may be an important explanation for why some studies have demonstrated that SE alleles predict erosive changes, but only in RF− patients.[29,30] One hypothesis to explain this observation is that RF− patients in these older studies are actually CCP+ (and it is known that SE alleles have a stronger association with CCP+ than RF+ RA[24]). In the future, it will be important to assess the relationship between *HLA-DRB1* alleles and clinical outcome, controlling for the effect of CCP as well as other important clinical variables.

Despite decades of research, it is not fully known how the *HLA-DRB1* alleles cause risk of RA, and direct functional proof has been difficult. Hypotheses include that the SE alleles influence (1) thresholds for T-cell activation (based on avidity between the T-cell receptor, MHC, and peptide, especially in the context of post-translational modification events important in RA pathogenesis; (2) thymic selection of high-affinity, self-reactive T cells (based on the T-cell synovial repertoire); and (3) molecular mimicry of microbial antigens. It is worthwhile noting that the third hypervariable region of the protein (location of SE allelic variants) contains a peptide-binding groove that serves to present peptides to CD4+ T cells, and that citrullination of certain peptides triggers a strong immune response to citrullinated peptides in *HLA-DRB1* *0401 transgenic mice.[31]

Other MHC-Region Genes

Several studies suggest that additional genes within the MHC likely contribute to disease susceptibility, once the effect of *HLA-DRB1* has been taken into consideration.[32–36] For example, an extended haplotype that includes *HLA-DRB1* DR3 alleles may be associated with RA.[32] The associated haplotype spans ~500 kilobases (kb), and contains Class III MHC genes, including the TNF-alpha region implicated in other studies.[35] One study suggests that this association is restricted to CCP− patients.[24]

No single study has yet comprehensively tested DNA variants within the MHC in a patient population large enough to detect subtle effects beyond *HLA-DRB1* alleles. Only recently have genetic linkage disequilibrium maps become available to thoroughly test the hypothesis that non–*HLA-DRB1* alleles influence the risk of developing RA. Application of high-density SNP genotyping in large patient collections should provide additional insight into the role of the MHC region in susceptibility and severity of RA.

Non-MHC Genes

The identity of genes contributing to RA that lie outside the MHC region has been more elusive. A sizeable portion of genetic variation is attributable to such non-HLA genes—up to two-thirds in some studies. In 2004, a variant within the gene *PTPN22* was identified as contributing to risk of RA.[37] More recently, advances in human genetics have led to the discovery of several new RA susceptibility loci (e.g., *STAT4*, *TRAF1-C5*, and *6q23*), with mounting evidence that many more will be discovered in the near future.

It is important to consider the statistical evidence in support of a genetic association. Many genetic association studies conducted in small patient collections (e.g., <1000 samples) are false-positive results. Accordingly, replication in independent patients is crucial. If the observed odds ratio is modest (e.g., <1.50), then thousands of patients are required to detect a *p*-value that is sufficient to overcome the multiple hypothesis testing burden of the ~1 million uncorrelated common genetic variants across the genome. If a genetic variant is reproducibly associated across multiple sample collections, then it is considered a "confirmed" association. If a variant is associated in some but not all studies, then it is considered a "suggestive" association.

It is also important to emphasize that most genetic associations are to regions of the genome (also referred to as loci) that may contain no genes, or may contain many genes. While it is convenient to refer to these loci by stating the name of the gene (e.g., *STAT4*), there is often little evidence linking a specific associated genetic variant to altered gene function. For some confirmed genetic associations, a locus contains several promising biologic candidate genes (e.g., *TRAF1* and *C5*). Other confirmed loci (e.g., *6q23*, which refers to chromosomal location) may be in the vicinity of a plausible candidate gene (e.g., *TNFAIP3*), although the associated variant lies outside the protein coding sequence of the gene itself.

Figure 3A-1 contains a list of confirmed and suggestive loci associated with risk of RA, together with their possible function in RA pathogenesis. The figure provides an oversimplified view of the role these loci play in RA pathogenesis. Nonetheless, it provides a useful framework for listing the confirmed and suggestive genetic associations.

The most convincing non-HLA locus associated with RA is *PTPN22*.[37] This genetic association has been replicated across multiple independent studies. The susceptibility allele is a missense variant that changes an arginine to tryptophan amino acid (R620W), resulting in alteration of T-cell activation.[37,38] The magnitude of the genetic effect, as measured by the odds ratio, is substantially less than for *HLA-DRB1*0401* but similar to other SE alleles (*PTPN22* OR ~1.75). Interestingly, this allele is absent for East Asians, and thus not associated with susceptibility in Japanese populations.[39] As with *HLA-DRB1* alleles, *PTPN22* only associates with seropositive RA. There is some evidence that *PTPN22* influences age of onset,[40] and may have a more significant effect in males compared to females,[40,41] but no evidence that it influences disease activity or radiographic erosions.[42,43]

A confirmed association of a genetic variant at the *STAT4* locus was identified from a study of candidate genes under a linkage peak on chromosome 2.[44] The risk allele is common in individuals of Asian, African, and European ancestry, where the frequency ranges from ~20% to 30% in the general population, and provides a 1.25-fold increase risk in RA per copy of the susceptibility allele. The variant most strongly associated with risk lies within a large third intron, and there is no obvious protein coding polymorphism. *STAT4* is an important transcription factor in the differentiation of naïve T cells into Th-1 helper cells. More recent evidence suggests that *STAT4* may be involved in the differentiation of a Th-17 cells.

One of the first RA genome-wide association studies (see below) led to the identification of the *TRAF1-C5* locus.[45] An independent study based on a candidate gene approach identified the same locus.[46] A single genetic variant is associated with risk, with an OR of ~1.25. The risk variant is common in the general population (~35%–50% in all ethnic groups studied). The associated locus contains two strong biologic candidate genes: *TRAF1* and *C5*. The *TRAF1* gene encodes an intracellular protein that mediates signal transduction through tumor

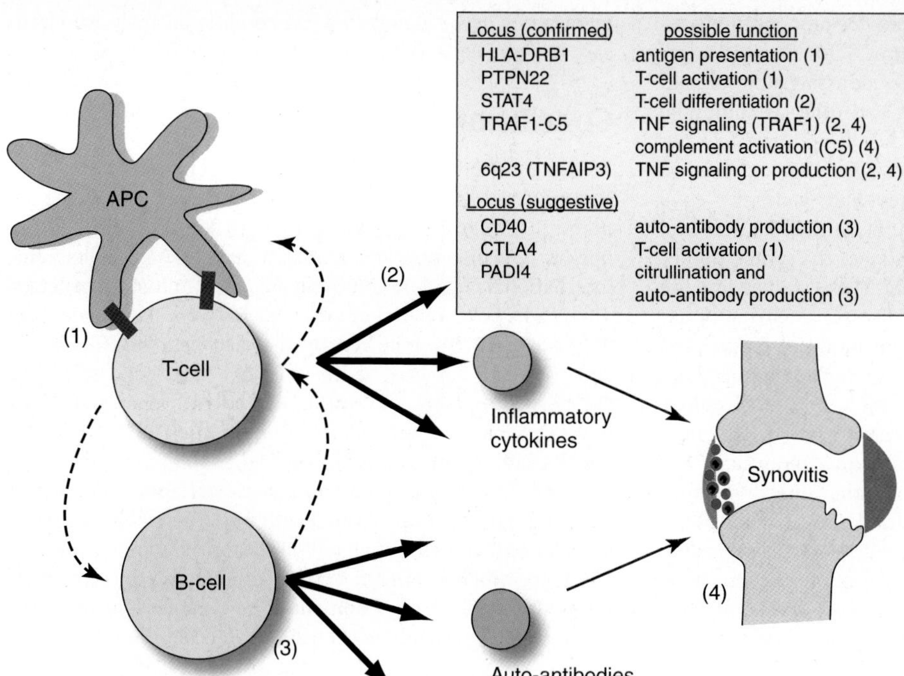

Figure 3A-1. Gene loci associated with RA susceptibility and possible role in RA pathogenesis.

necrosis factor receptors 1 and 2, and through CD40. *TRAF1* knockout mice exhibit exaggerated T-cell proliferation and activation in response to TNF or when stimulated through the T-cell receptor (TCR) complex, suggesting that TRAF1 acts as a negative regulator of these signaling pathways. TRAF1 binds several intracellular proteins, including the NF-κB inhibitory protein *TNFAIP3*. C5 is a component of the complement pathway, which has been implicated in RA pathogenesis for over 30 years. Complement activation leading to significant depletion of complement components has been demonstrated in synovial fluid of RA patients. C5 cleavage generates the potently proinflammatory anaphylatoxin C5a as well as C5b, which initiates generation of the membrane attack complex. C5-deficient mice are resistant to inflammatory arthritis in models with a dominant humoral component (e.g., collagen-induced arthritis and K/BxN serum transfer model).

Two independent genome-wide association studies identified a locus on chromosome 6q23 associated with RA risk.[47,48] Interestingly, there are at least two distinct alleles that confer risk at this locus,[47] both with ORs of ~1.25. The associated variants do not fall within any known gene. However, a good candidate gene, *TNFAIP3*, is located ~185 kb away from the associated region. *Tumor necrosis factor, alpha-induced protein 3* (*TNFAIP3*), also known as *A20*, is a potent inhibitor of NF-kappaB signaling and is required for termination of TNF-induced signals. Mice lacking *Tnfaip3* demonstrate chronic inflammation, consistent with loss of function of this gene playing a role in autoimmunity. Whether the associated variants influence *TNFAIP3* or another gene at this locus will require additional investigation.

In addition to these loci, several other loci have suggestive evidence of genetic association. One locus, which contains the *CD40* gene, was identified as part of a genome-wide association study.[45] This result has not yet been widely replicated. CD40, which is a member of the TNF-receptor superfamily, is a costimulatory protein found on antigen presenting cells (APC), most notably B cells. This receptor is essential in mediating a variety of B-cell responses, including B-cell proliferation and differentiation, T-cell–dependent immunoglobulin isotype switching, germinal center formation, and stimulation of the humoral memory response.

The association between variants with *CTLA4* and susceptibility to autoimmunity is most convincing in type 1 diabetes and autoimmune thyroiditis. CTLA4 is a negative regulator of T-cell activation. In these diseases, an allele in the 3' untranslated region (UTR) of the gene causes a modest increase in disease risk (OR ~1.2–1.5). Several studies have extended these findings to RA,[40,49] where the magnitude of the genetic effect is again modest (~1.15).

PADI4 encodes for an enzyme that post-translationally modifies arginine to citrulline, and may therefore be important in generating anti-CCP autoantibodies. An initial report in Japanese patients implicated a common variant (population allele frequency ~35%) in disease risk[50]; subsequent reports have been less convincing statistically, but nonetheless support an association with RA susceptibility.[51]

Genome-Wide Association Studies

Candidate gene studies in RA, as with many other complex diseases, highlight the current challenge of genetic association studies.[52] First, most candidate gene studies test a small fraction of genetic variation in the human genome. It is estimated that over 10 million common variants (population allele frequency >1%) exist in the human genome; most candidate gene studies test a vanishingly small fraction of these variants. Second, the expected genetic effect for most disease alleles is quite modest (OR <1.3). Therefore, thousands of patients are required to detect the genetic effect—and most studies have been conducted on far fewer, limiting power to detect a true positive association.

Advances in human genetics now provide an opportunity to test hundreds of thousands of common SNPs across the genome. These studies, termed "genome-wide association studies," have recently been conducted in RA and other autoimmune diseases with encouraging success.[45,47,48] If appropriately designed and interpreted,[53] it is expected that these studies will continue to expand the list of RA susceptibility genes.

While creating an exciting opportunity in human genetics, there are several important limitations to contemporary genome-wide association studies. First, these studies test the role of common variants in human disease; as currently designed, very few rare variants (with population frequency <1%) or copy number variants (CNVs) are including on these genotyping platforms (also referred to as arrays or chips). Second, not all common genetic variants are represented on the genotyping arrays. It is estimated that more than 90% of known common SNPs are captured either directly or indirectly (through correlated patterns of linkage disequilibrium). And third, once a common SNP has been associated reproducibly with disease risk, it is necessary to refine the statistical signal. This requires cataloguing all common genetic variants across the locus (through re-sequencing of cases and controls), followed by dense genotyping and conditional analysis in large case–control collections.

Conclusion

A bottleneck in the ability to translate genetics to improved patient care has been the ability to identify regions of the genome that reproducibly associate with RA risk. This bottleneck is now being broken, thanks to large patient collections, international collaborations, and advances in human genetics. The *HLA-DRB1* "shared epitope" alleles were first recognized in the late 1970's, followed by the discovery of *PTPN22* in 2004. In 2007, at least three new loci have been identified (*STAT4, TRAF1-C5*, and *6q23*), with several other loci showing promise but not yet definitive confirmation (*CD40, CTLA4*, and *PADI4*). Going forward, the field should continue to expect the discovery of common genetic variants with modest effect sizes (OR <1.30). Armed with a list of confirmed genetic associations, the challenge will be to determine if confirmed RA susceptibility variants also (1) predict response to treatment, (2) guide the development of new small molecule treatments, and (3) provide novel insights into RA etiology.

References

1. MacGregor AJ, Snieder H, Rigby AS, et al. Characterizing the quantitative genetic contribution to rheumatoid arthritis using data from twins. *Arthritis Rheum* 2000;43:30–37.
2. Bali D, Gourley S, Kostyu DD, et al. Genetic analysis of multiplex rheumatoid arthritis families. *Genes Immun* 1999;1:28–36.
3. Jawaheer D, Seldin MF, Amos CI, et al. A genomewide screen in multiplex rheumatoid arthritis families suggests genetic overlap with other autoimmune diseases. *Am J Hum Genet* 2001;68:927–936.
4. Jawaheer D, Seldin MF, Amos CI, et al. Screening the genome for rheumatoid arthritis susceptibility genes: A replication study and combined analysis of 512 multicase families. *Arthritis Rheum* 2003;48:906–916.
5. Cornelis F, Faure S, Martinez M, et al. New susceptibility locus for rheumatoid arthritis suggested by a genome-wide linkage study. *Proc Natl Acad Sci U S A* 1998;95:10746–10750.
6. MacKay K, Eyre S, Myerscough A, et al. Whole-genome linkage analysis of rheumatoid arthritis susceptibility loci in 252 affected sibling pairs in the United Kingdom. *Arthritis Rheum* 2002;46:632–639.
7. Shiozawa S, Hayashi S, Tsukamoto Y, et al. Identification of the gene loci that predispose to rheumatoid arthritis. *Int Immunol* 1998;10:1891–1895.
8. Amos CI, Chen WV, Lee A, et al. High-density SNP analysis of 642 Caucasian families with rheumatoid arthritis identifies two new linkage regions on 11p12 and 2q33. *Genes Immun* 2006;7:277–286.
9. Etzel CJ, Chen WV, Shepard N, et al. Genome-wide meta-analysis for rheumatoid arthritis. *Hum Genet* 2006;119:634–641.
10. Silman AJ, MacGregor AJ, Thomson W, et al. Twin concordance rates for rheumatoid arthritis: Results from a nationwide study. *Br J Rheumatol* 1993;32:903–907.
11. Aho K, Koskenvuo M, Tuominen J, Kaprio J. Occurrence of rheumatoid arthritis in a nationwide series of twins. *J Rheumatol* 1986;13:899–902.
12. Jarvinen P, Aho K. Twin studies in rheumatic diseases. *Semin Arthritis Rheum* 1994;24:19–28.
13. Wolfe F, Kleinheksel SM, Khan MA. Prevalence of familial occurrence in patients with rheumatoid arthritis. *Br J Rheumatol* 1988;27(Suppl 2):150–152.
14. Deighton CM, Walker DJ, Griffiths ID, Roberts DF. The contribution of HLA to rheumatoid arthritis. *Clin Genet* 1989;36:178–182.
15. Hasstedt SJ, Clegg DO, Ingles L, Ward RH. HLA-linked rheumatoid arthritis. *Am J Hum Genet* 1994;55:738–746.
16. Rigby AS, Silman AJ, Voelm L, et al. Investigating the HLA component in rheumatoid arthritis: An additive (dominant) mode of inheritance is rejected, a recessive mode is preferred. *Genet Epidemiol* 1991;8:153–175.
17. Stastny P. Association of the B-cell alloantigen DRw4 with rheumatoid arthritis. *N Engl J Med* 1978;298:869–871.
18. Stastny P, Fink CW. HLA-Dw4 in adult and juvenile rheumatoid arthritis. *Transplant Proc* 1977;9:1863–1866.
19. Gregersen PK, Moriuchi T, Karr RW, et al. Polymorphism of HLA-DR beta chains in DR4, -7, and -9 haplotypes: Implications for the mechanisms of allelic variation. *Proc Natl Acad Sci U S A* 1986;83:9149–9153.
20. Gregersen PK, Silver J, Winchester RJ. The shared epitope hypothesis. An approach to understanding the molecular genetics of susceptibility to rheumatoid arthritis. *Arthritis Rheum* 1987;30:1205–1213.
21. McDaniel DO, Alarcon GS, Pratt PW, Reveille JD. Most African-American patients with rheumatoid arthritis do not have the rheumatoid antigenic determinant (epitope). *Ann Intern Med* 1995;123:181–187.
22. Teller K, Budhai L, Zhang M, et al. HLA-DRB1 and DQB typing of Hispanic American patients with rheumatoid arthritis: The "shared epitope" hypothesis may not apply. *J Rheumatol* 1996;23:1363–1368.
23. Huizinga TW, Amos CI, van der Helm-van Mil AH, et al. Refining the complex rheumatoid arthritis phenotype based on specificity of the HLA-DRB1 shared epitope for antibodies to citrullinated proteins. *Arthritis Rheum* 2005;52:3433–3438.
24. Irigoyen P, Lee AT, Wener MH, et al. Regulation of anti-cyclic citrullinated peptide antibodies in rheumatoid arthritis: Contrasting effects of HLA-DR3 and the shared epitope alleles. *Arthritis Rheum* 2005;52:3813–3818.
25. Moxley G, Cohen HJ. Genetic studies, clinical heterogeneity, and disease outcome studies in rheumatoid arthritis. *Rheum Dis Clin North Am* 2002;28:39–58.

26. Chen JJ, Mu H, Jiang Y, et al. Clinical usefulness of genetic information for predicting radiographic damage in rheumatoid arthritis. *J Rheumatol* 2002;29:2068–2073.
27. Gorman JD, Lum RF, Chen JJ, et al. Impact of shared epitope genotype and ethnicity on erosive disease: A meta-analysis of 3,240 rheumatoid arthritis patients. *Arthritis Rheum* 2004;50:400–412.
28. van der Helm-van Mil AH, Verpoort KN, Breedveld FC, et al. The HLA-DRB1 shared epitope alleles are primarily a risk factor for anti-cyclic citrullinated peptide antibodies and are not an independent risk factor for development of rheumatoid arthritis. *Arthritis Rheum* 2006;54:1117–1121.
29. Mattey DL, Hassell AB, Dawes PT, et al. Independent association of rheumatoid factor and the HLA-DRB1 shared epitope with radiographic outcome in rheumatoid arthritis. *Arthritis Rheum* 2001;44: 1529–1533.
30. El-Gabalawy HS, Goldbach-Mansky R, Smith D 2nd, et al. Association of HLA alleles and clinical features in patients with synovitis of recent onset. *Arthritis Rheum* 1999;42:1696–1705.
31. Hill JA, Southwood S, Sette A, et al. Cutting edge: The conversion of arginine to citrulline allows for a high-affinity peptide interaction with the rheumatoid arthritis-associated HLA-DRB1*0401 MHC class II molecule. *J Immunol* 2003;171:538–541.
32. Jawaheer D, Li W, Graham RR, et al. Dissecting the genetic complexity of the association between human leukocyte antigens and rheumatoid arthritis. *Am J Hum Genet* 2002;71:585–594.
33. Zanelli E, Jones G, Pascual M, et al. The telomeric part of the HLA region predisposes to rheumatoid arthritis independently of the class II loci. *Hum Immunol* 2001;62:75–84.
34. Singal DP, Li J, Lei K. Genetics of rheumatoid arthritis (RA): Two separate regions in the major histocompatibility complex contribute to susceptibility to RA. *Immunol Lett* 1999;69:301–306.
35. Mulcahy B, et al. Genetic variability in the tumor necrosis factor-lymphotoxin region influences susceptibility to rheumatoid arthritis. *Am J Hum Genet* 1996;59:676–683.
36. Kochi Y, Waldron-Lynch F, McDermott MF, et al. Analysis of single-nucleotide polymorphisms in Japanese rheumatoid arthritis patients shows additional susceptibility markers besides the classic shared epitope susceptibility sequences. *Arthritis Rheum* 2004;50: 63–71.
37. Begovich AB, Carlton VE, Honigberg LA, et al. A missense single-nucleotide polymorphism in a gene encoding a protein tyrosine phosphatase (PTPN22) is associated with rheumatoid arthritis. *Am J Hum Genet* 2004;75:330–337.
38. Vang T, Congia M, Macis MD, et al. Autoimmune-associated lymphoid tyrosine phosphatase is a gain-of-function variant. *Nat Genet* 2005;37:1317–1319.
39. Ikari K, Momohara S, Inoue E, et al. Haplotype analysis revealed no association between the PTPN22 gene and RA in a Japanese population. *Rheumatology (Oxford)* 2006;45:1345–1348.
40. Plenge RM, Padyukov L, Remmers EF, et al. Replication of putative candidate-gene associations with rheumatoid arthritis in >4,000 samples from North America and Sweden: Association of susceptibility with PTPN22, CTLA4, and PADI4. *Am J Hum Genet* 2005; 77:1044–1060.
41. Pierer M, Kaltenhäuser S, Arnold S, et al. Association of PTPN22 1858 single-nucleotide polymorphism with rheumatoid arthritis in a German cohort: Higher frequency of the risk allele in male compared to female patients. *Arthritis Res Ther* 2006;8:R75.
42. Wesoly J, van der Helm-van Mil AH, Toes RE, et al. Association of the PTPN22 C1858T single-nucleotide polymorphism with rheumatoid arthritis phenotypes in an inception cohort. *Arthritis Rheum* 2005;52:2948–2950.
43. Harrison P, Pointon JJ, Farrar C, et al. Effects of PTPN22 C1858T polymorphism on susceptibility and clinical characteristics of British Caucasian rheumatoid arthritis patients. *Rheumatology (Oxford)* 2006;45:1009–1011.
44. Remmers EF, Plenge RM, Lee AT, et al. STAT4 and the risk of rheumatoid arthritis and systemic lupus erythematosus. *N Engl J Med* 2007;357:977–986.
45. Plenge RM, et al. TRAF1-C5 as a risk locus for rheumatoid arthritis—a genomewide study. *N Engl J Med* 2007;357:1199–1209.
46. Kurreeman FA, et al. A candidate gene approach identifies the TRAF1/C5 region as a risk factor for rheumatoid arthritis. *PLoS Med* 2007;4:e278.
47. Plenge RM, Seielstad M, Padyukov L, et al. Two independent alleles at 6q23 associated with risk of rheumatoid arthritis. *Nat Genet*; 39:1477–1482.
48. Thomson W, Barton A, Ke X, et al. Rheumatoid arthritis association at 6q23. *Nat Genet*;39:1431–1433.
49. Lei C, Dongqing Z, Yeqing S, et al. Association of the CTLA-4 gene with rheumatoid arthritis in Chinese Han population. Eur J *Hum Genet* 2005;13:823–828.
50. Suzuki A, Yamada R, Chang X, et al. Functional haplotypes of PADI4, encoding citrullinating enzyme peptidylarginine deiminase 4, are associated with rheumatoid arthritis. *Nat Genet* 2003;34: 395–402.
51. Iwamoto T, Ikari K, Nakamura T, et al. Association between PADI4 and rheumatoid arthritis: A meta-analysis. *Rheumatology (Oxford)* 2006;45:804–807.
52. Plenge R, Rioux JD. Identifying susceptibility genes for immunological disorders: Patterns, power, and proof. *Immunol Rev* 2006; 210:40–51.
53. Hirschhorn JN, Daly MJ. Genome-wide association studies for common diseases and complex traits. *Nat Rev Genet* 2005;6:95–108.

Environmental Risk Factors for Rheumatoid Arthritis

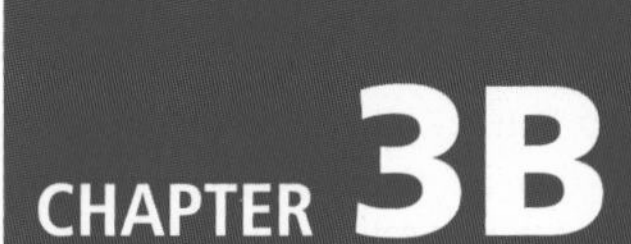

Lars Klareskog, Johan Rönnelid, and Lars Alfredsson

Risk factors for rheumatoid arthritis (RA) comprise a combination of genetic, environmental, and stochastic factors, as is the case for all multifactorial complex genetic diseases. Whereas the relative contributions from genetic versus other factors can be roughly estimated for the entity we call RA, it is more difficult to separate the contributions from stochastic and environmental factors. Thus, twin studies have estimated the genetic risk for RA to be about 50% with the rest being environmental and stochastic.[1–3]

One major weakness with this reasoning has, however, been obvious in recent years, following the recognition that RA can be divided in at least two distinct subsets defined in large part by the presence/absence of anti-citrullinated protein/peptide antibodies (ACPA).[4–7] Thus, known genetic as well as environmental risk factors differ dramatically between these two subsets of RA. The main genetic risk factors defined so far, that is, HLA-DR alleles,[6–9] PTPN22 risk alleles,[10–14] and TRAF1/C5-related genes[15–17] are all confined to the ACPA-positive subset of disease, whereas other genetic risk factors, notably IRF-5, appear to be mainly associated with ACPA-negative disease.[18] Also, the main known environmental risk factor, smoking, is a risk factor mainly or only for the ACPA-positive form of RA,[6,19,20] which largely overlaps with the rheumatoid factor (RF)–positive form previously shown to be associated with smoking.[21–23] It can be anticipated that heredity as well as influence of environmental factors other than smoking may also differ between these two major subsets, and possibly also within these subsets.

This information emphasizes that we are only at the beginning of an era where it will be possible to disentangle the complex interactions between environmental and genetic risk factors and to understand pathology-associated immune reactions that may be triggered in the context of various combinations of genes and environmental factors. We have to carefully separate different subsets of RA in studies and descriptions of how environmental factors interact with genes in providing the basis for the onset of—and disease course for—different forms of RA.

Having provided this general comment on the complexity as well as promise for studies on environmental factors and RA, the rest of this chapter will be devoted to description of what has hitherto been learned concerning the role of environment in this disease. Notably, however, almost all such studies have been conducted without dividing RA into subsets, and most studies on environment have not taken the genetics into account.

We must also acknowledge that the effect of a certain factor on disease onset may be different from the same factor's effect on disease progression and on comorbidities. So far, very few studies have been performed addressing effects from environmental agents on disease progression and comorbidities. Such studies are needed, as they might provide the patient as well as the treating physician with critical information about what the patient might be able to do in order to reduce disease severity and comorbidities.

Environmental Risk Factors: What Is the Evidence and How Good Is the Evidence?

Studies of the impact of environmental factors on the risk of developing RA, as well as many other multifactorial diseases, are associated with several methodologic as well as practical problems, and the literature on environment and RA is therefore relatively scarce with a frequent lack of reproduction of findings. Thus, this review focuses mainly on risk factors that have either been well reproduced in several studies or have been performed using large population-based case–control or cohort studies.

The most methodologically attractive studies concerning environment should, however, come from studies of disease-discordant monozygotic twins, who are also discordant for the environmental exposure we want to investigate. So far, only one such study has been published, but this investigation gave a very convincing result[24]: In a study of the UK twin registry, 13 monozygotic and RA discordant twin pairs were identified who were also discordant for smoking. In these 13 twin pairs, the smoker was the one with RA in 12 of the 13 cases. This result thus clearly demonstrates what major impact an environmental agent—in this case, smoking—may have in defined genetic contexts.

The other two major acceptable methods, population-based case–control studies and cohort studies have delivered most of our current knowledge on environmental factors in RA, and often both types of studies have arrived at the same results. Case–control studies are in most cases the best powered and can provide quantification of effects of environmental exposures. In addition, case–control studies allow the division of RA into subsets and make studies of gene–environment interactions possible. The drawback is the risk of bias in recruitment of cases as well as recall bias in responses from patients and controls. Thus, the best case–control studies are carried out in newly diagnosed cases (to reduce recall bias) and where both cases and controls are recruited from the same defined study population (to reduce recruitment bias). The cohort studies are usually less subject to both these biases, but have most often a low power. Optimally, results from the two approaches should be combined. For the environmental risk factors described in the following, the evidence is in most cases based on combined results from both case-control and cohort studies.

"Environmental influence" is also an ambiguous notion that encompasses physical exposures from distinct environmental agents and associations with certain lifestyles and preceding life events, as well as associations with various socioeconomic conditions. In addition, factors such as medication, including hormones, may be considered under this heading. These latter factors will, however, not be discussed in this chapter.

Environmental Risk Factors

Silica Dust Exposure

Silica dust is the exposure with the longest-term known risk for RA. This risk has been demonstrated mainly in studies of miners, where RA has been more common in those exposed to silica than in those not exposed[25–27]; the results from these studies are also in agreement with previous reports on an association between silicosis and RA.[28] Mechanisms responsible for the relationship between stone dust exposure and occurrence of RA have thus far not been studied systematically, but preliminary data indicate that silica exposure is mainly a risk factor for ACPA-positive RA.[29] No studies have been published concerning the effects of silica exposure on the disease course.

Smoking

Smoking is by now the most well-established environmental risk factor for RA, but the relationship was not evident until in 1987 when the increased risk of RA in smokers was observed by serendipity in a study with an unrelated objective.[30] Since then a large number of epidemiologic studies have confirmed the increased risk for RA in smokers.[21–23,31,36]

It was not until relatively recently, however, that the influence of smoking was related to subsets of RA as well as to a genetic context. These investigations revealed a number of interesting features of smoking which indicated that smoking might have a quite specific role in triggering a particular variant of RA rather than unspecifically delivering a signal that activates any type of inflammation.

First, it was shown that smoking is a risk factor only for either RF- or ACPA-positive RA; there was no or very little risk for RF- or ACPA-negative RA.[6,19–21,23,36,37] Second, smoking exerts its effects over a long time period before RA onset, and cessation of smoking reverts the increased risk only after 10 to 20 years.[35,36] This indicates that smoking exerts its biologic effects predisposing for ACPA/RF positive RA several years before onset of disease. Third, smoking interacts profoundly with the major susceptibility genes for ACPA-positive RA, that is, HLA DRB1 alleles that contain the shared epitope (SE)–associated motif.[6,19,20,38] The results from these studies demonstrate that the risk of developing ACPA-positive RA is between 10 and 40 times higher in individuals who are smokers and carry HLA-DRB1 SE allele(s) as compared with those who do not carry the DRB1 SE and have not smoked. These interactions have now been described in Swedish and Danish as well as Dutch studies and confirmed in U.S. studies, although with notably lower risk figures.[39] Smoking may also be a risk factor for RA in individuals lacking HLA-DRB1 SE alleles, although the risk there is considerably less.[38] Additional data have indicated that smoking may be particularly important as a risk factor for extra-articular RA.[40–42]

Whether passive smoking is a risk factor is an interesting but yet largely unanswered question. Only one preliminary report has addressed this issue, indicating that there may be an increase in RA incidence after passive exposure to smoking.[43] One interesting recent study, however, suggested that smoking by the mother during pregnancy may influence the future risk for RA in the offspring.[44]

A few studies have been concerned with the effects of smoking on the disease course, and here the data are less consistent than in the case of disease induction. Thus, some reports suggest a more severe course in smokers,[45,46] whereas one recent report did not find any such effect.[47] Most of these studies are, however, cross-sectional, which means that it is difficult to determine to what extent smoking exerts a continuous adverse effect on the course of a disease. Also, with one exception, these studies have not considered the effects of smoking on disease course in the context of new information on interactions with genetic determinants and in the context of the RA subsets. The exception is a recent study by Anne Barton and colleagues, where the risk for development of cardiovascular disease in RA patients was shown to be dependent on smoking, and presence of HLA-DRB1 SE genes as well as ACPA.[48]

Mineral Oils and Other Adjuvants

Mineral oils belong to a broad category of compounds with adjuvant actions, that is, agents with the ability to directly activate the innate immune system via pattern recognition molecules, and indirectly to activation of the adaptive immune system via enhanced antigen presentation. One interesting feature of these adjuvants is their ability to induce arthritis in certain strains of rodents.[49–52] Such arthritis induction has been observed both after single injections of adjuvants into the skin (e.g., in the back of the tail and at a distance from involved joints), or even via topical applications of the mineral oils to the skin.[53] This rodent arthritis is very dependent on the genetic background of the animals, and disease development appears to be dependent on activation of macrophages and then T cells in the regional lymph nodes, rather than from inflammation and immune activation in the skin.[52]

These observations of an arthritis-inducing function of agents with adjuvant actions, which are very common in the human environment, have created an interest in studies of the effects of adjuvants also for human RA. A few case series indicating that adjuvants may have this role also in humans have been published,[54,55] but so far only a few systematic studies have appeared focusing on this question in humans. In one such study using case–control methodology, exposure to several different mineral oils, in particular hydraulic oils, was seen to be associated with an increased risk of RA.[56] The affected individuals were mainly men with high levels of occupational exposure. Whether other adjuvants may exert similar actions in humans is still unknown. Possibly, associations between certain occupations (and farming in particular) and an increased risk for RA[57–59] may be due to increased exposure to agents with adjuvant actions.

Infections

Much interest has been paid to the possibility that infections might trigger development of RA, but little solid evidence exists that distinct infectious organisms may cause or contribute to the syndrome we call RA. The potentials for infectious agents to be involved in the pathogenesis, as well as the problems in detecting such contributions have been reviewed elsewhere.[60,61] One possibility is that infections may contribute to RA via their adjuvant actions, similar to adjuvant arthritis in rodents,[49,52] and the demonstration of arthritis after administration of mycobacteria as adjuvants in tumor treatment or as vaccinations provide some indirect support for this notion.[54,55] Still, the possibility definitely exists that parts of the RA syndrome may become associated with a distinct microbial trigger, as in the case for Lyme arthritis, where tick-borne *Borrelia* was demonstrated to be the trigger for a disease with many similarities to RA, but now defined as a separate entity.[62,63]

Blood Transfusions

Blood transfusion as a risk factor for RA has been described in a single important report, which indicated a fivefold risk increase.[22] This report obviously needs to be confirmed; debate has included speculation on infectious origins as well as adjuvant actions and the formation of genetic chimerism.

Dietary Factors

Much interest has been devoted to the issue of food as a risk factor of RA as well as for dietary agents influencing the course of RA. This area was recently reviewed by Pattisson et al.[64] Thus far, studies addressing this issue have, however, not been widely reproduced and many uncertainties remain. There are suggestions that red meat may cause an increased risk for RA,[65] and that intake of fruit[66] and oily fish may protect against RA,[67,68] but all these reports need confirmation. Circumstantial evidence of potential importance is that both very high and very low body mass index appear to be associated with an increased risk for RA.[22,69] These observations thus may have to be taken into account when considering effects of different diets. Several vegetarian and vegan diets have been suggested to influence the course of RA,[70–73] but so far the influence of these diets on eventual onset of RA has not been investigated.

Coffee

Conflicting reports exist concerning coffee consumption as a possible risk factor for development of RA. A few reports have suggested that coffee is a risk factor,[74,75] whereas others have not been able to verify this association.[76] Also, different forms of coffee (including decaffeinated coffee) have been associated with an increased risk for RA,[75] but these data are somewhat contradictory. In some but not all of the studies on coffee consumption and RA, cigarette smoking has been carefully considered as a confounder. In summary, the issue of coffee consumption and risk for RA remains unclear, and no suggestions for the mechanisms involved have been suggested or investigated.

Socioeconomic Factors

Socioeconomic factors have long been suspected to be associated with risk for development of RA, as is the case for many different chronic diseases. The data for RA are, however, somewhat conflicting. In one major study from the UK, no influence of socioeconomic factors on RA was seen,[77] and similar results were obtained from Norway.[23] In contrast, a recent report from a Swedish case–control study found a moderate influence for education level on RA risk, even after careful adjustment for smoking habits and various occupational exposures.[78] Which components of socioeconomic background may be responsible for the increased RA risk are unknown.

General Considerations on Gene–Environment Interactions and Environmental Risk Factors

As discussed earlier, interactions between genes and environment and stochastic factor contributions together comprise the basis for understanding the etiology of a complex genetic disease like RA. Nevertheless, knowledge of which interactions exist in RA is very scarce, and the methodologies for determining such interactions are less well established. Thus, a short discussion of both methodologies and their application on hitherto described examples of interactions is warranted.

Interactions between two or more factors that may influence the risk to develop a defined disease state can be quantified using a few different methods. The classical method in epidemiology was originally described by Rothman,[79,80] where the observed combined risk conferred by two different factors is compared with the sum of the independent effects of the two factors. If the risk of disease among those with the former is higher than the sum of independent effects, then interaction exists (according to this definition of interaction as departure from additivity of effects). This deviation can be quantified and the proportion of the combined risk that is attributable to the interaction per se, is called "attributable proportion due to interaction."[81,82] This way of calculating the interactions between two risk factors, which has been used for many years in epidemiology, is relatively new in the field of gene–environment interactions as well as in the field of gene–gene interactions. Interaction according to this notion implies the existence of at least one pathway toward disease that requires the involvement of both risk factors.

Another common method for quantifying interactions is based on the product term of the two risk factors in a logistic regression model (multiplicative interaction).[79] In relation to the notion of interaction given above, interaction may be detected by means of departure from a multiplicativity model as well, although this detection will have a lower sensitivity and higher specificity in relation to the corresponding detection by means of departure from additivity.

Gene-environment interactions have been recorded regarding risk of RA. A few examples exist where both the additive and multiplicative methods for determining gene-environment interactions have been utilized. The main examples are those that focused on interactions between smoking and HLA-DRB1 risk alleles. Here, several studies have demonstrated an interaction using the Rothman departure from additively criterion as well as the departure from multiplicativity criterion.[14,39] Another example is the interaction between smoking and glutathione-S-transferase M1 locus regarding risk of RA.[83] Taken together, the existing data demonstrate how different methods for calculation of interactions may yield different results, and that we are in need for further methodologic development in this area.

Using Genetic Epidemiology to Generate Hypotheses on Molecular Pathogenesis

We postulate that events triggered by specific environmental triggers in the context of specific genes determine the evolution of disease—and induce pathogenic immune and inflammatory reactions. Accordingly, we should use the existing as well as forthcoming data on gene–environment interactions as a basis for most studies on pathogenesis of RA. First, such studies must obviously take into account that there is a profound difference between the known risk factors for ACPA-positive and ACPA-negative RA. Second they should attempt to encompass the known environmental and genetic risk factors in a model that can be tested in molecular systems. Obviously, knowledge of genetic epidemiology is still quite scarce in this context, but we will illustrate the concept with what has emerged from the studies on environmental factors and gene–environment interactions described above (for a more detailed discussion, see Klareskog, et al.[84]). MHC class II–dependent T-cell activation should thus be of critical importance for the ACPA-positive, but not necessarily for the ACPA-negative subset of RA. Whether the critical effects of MHC class II–T-cell interactions occur at the level of activation in lymphoid systems, in the target organ, or at the level of T-cell education in the thymus, however, cannot be deduced from genetic epidemiology. The second feature, the interaction between the PTPN22 risk allele and DRB1 alleles, indicates that a functional variant of the tyrosine phosphatase N22 (coded by the PTPN22 gene), present in a pathway involved in T-cell signaling,[10] is part of the same molecular pathways involving antigen presentation and T-cell activation (or T-cell tolerization).

Smoking may obviously interact with this proposed T-cell–dependent immune activation at several stages—as an adjuvant as well as a generator of antigens that are recognized by MHC class II–dependent T cells (for a general discussion of different possibilities, see Harel-Meir, et al.[85]). The latter possibility is particularly attractive in the context of RA, provided that the interaction between DRB1 alleles, PTPN22 alleles, and smoking takes place exclusively in the subset of RA characterized by the presence of antibodies to citrullinated protein antigens. The hypothesis that can now be subject to further experimental testing is that smoking may activate peptidyl arginine deminases to produce citrullinated proteins in the lung, and that SE-containing DRB1 molecules, in particular 0401 and 0404,[86,87] can function as restriction elements for such immune activation. As citrulline-modified proteins are present also in synovial tissue during a series of unspecific inflammatory events in the joint,[88,89] one can postulate a series of events from smoke in the lung to the immune events that are dependent on the susceptibility genes, to the effector phase that follows several years after the first encounter with the environmental exposure. Interestingly, this scenario is compatible with the observations of RA-specific autoantibodies, including ACPA several years before disease onset.[90–92] They are also compatible with the previous demonstration that smoking is able to trigger production of rheumatoid factors.[31,93] As immunity to citrullinated proteins in some experimental systems has been demonstrated to contribute to arthritis,[94,95] it appears that the genetic epidemiology, at least in the present scenario, produces a basis for molecular experiments aimed at disentangling the molecular pathology for a subset of RA. We would assume that several additional potential pathways will be identified when both genes and environmental stimuli are considered in concert.

Conclusions

Understanding which environmental agents may contribute to triggering immune events that determine disease onset, the continuation and chronicity of the disease, and the comorbidities associated with RA, is of fundamental importance for any effort aiming to preventing the disease and its consequences. Thus far, we have only made small advances in this respect, which may owe to the fact that only relatively minor resources have been devoted to systematic studies in this area of rheumatology. Our shortcomings may also be due to the fact that we have only recently investigated the environmental influences in the contexts of genetic determinants and subdivision of RA into relevant subsets. Nevertheless, the findings already made for smoking can most probably be used more efficiently than today in both health care and in the society in general. It has been estimated (from both Swedish and Danish studies) that 20% to 25% of all RA cases would never have occurred if the smoking habit had not existed (Pedersen,[96] and L. Alfredsson, unpublished observation). This information should be distributed more efficiently among clinicians and researchers as well as patients; everyone should be encouraged to do what they can to diminish the risk for RA, that is, stop or never begin smoking. This measure might be particularly efficient in individuals with a genetic predisposition for RA.

Lastly, we also want to reiterate the need to consider environment, genes, and the interactions between them in all forthcoming studies on genetics and molecular immunology of the various subsets of the syndrome we call RA.

References

1. Aho K, Koskenvuo M, Tuominen J, et al. Occurrence of rheumatoid arthritis in a nationwide series of twins. *J Rheumatol* 1986;13(5):899–902.
2. Silman AJ, MacGregor AJ, Thomson W, et al. Twin concordance rates for rheumatoid arthritis: Results from a nationwide study. *Br J Rheumatol* 1993;32(10):903–907.
3. MacGregor AJ, Snieder H, Rigby AS, et al. Characterizing the quantitative genetic contribution to rheumatoid arthritis using data from twins. *Arthritis Rheum* 2000;43(1):30–37.
4. Schellekens GA, de Jong BA, van den Hoogen FH, et al. Citrulline is an essential constituent of antigenic determinants recognized by rheumatoid arthritis-specific autoantibodies. *J Clin Invest* 1998;101(1):273–281.
5. Schellekens GA, Visser H, de Jong BA, et al. The diagnostic properties of rheumatoid arthritis antibodies recognizing a cyclic citrullinated peptide. *Arthritis Rheum* 2000;43(1):155–163.
6. Klareskog L, Stolt P, Lundberg K, et al. A new model for an etiology of rheumatoid arthritis: smoking may trigger HLA-DR (shared

epitope)-restricted immune reactions to autoantigens modified by citrullination. *Arthritis Rheum* 2006;54(1):38–46.

7. van der Helm-van Mil AH, Verpoort KN, Breedveld FC, et al. The HLA-DRB1 shared epitope alleles are primarily a risk factor for anti-cyclic citrullinated peptide antibodies and are not an independent risk factor for development of rheumatoid arthritis. *Arthritis Rheum* 2006;54(4):1117–1121.
8. Stastny P. Association of the B-cell alloantigen DRw4 with rheumatoid arthritis. *N Engl J Med* 1978;298(16):869–871.
9. Gregersen PK, Silver J, Winchester RJ. The shared epitope hypothesis. An approach to understanding the molecular genetics of susceptibility to rheumatoid arthritis. *Arthritis Rheum* 1987;30(11):1205–1213.
10. Begovich AB, Carlton VE, Honigberg LA, et al. A missense single-nucleotide polymorphism in a gene encoding a protein tyrosine phosphatase (PTPN22) is associated with rheumatoid arthritis. *Am J Hum Genet* 2004;75(2):330–337.
11. Plenge RM, Padyukov L, Remmers EF, et al. Replication of putative candidate-gene associations with rheumatoid arthritis in >4,000 samples from North America and Sweden: Association of susceptibility with PTPN22, CTLA4, and PADI4. *Am J Hum Genet* 2005; 77(6):1044–1060.
12. Kokkonen H, Johansson M, Innala L, et al. The PTPN22 1858C/T polymorphism is associated with anti-cyclic citrullinated peptide antibody–positive early rheumatoid arthritis in northern Sweden. *Arthritis Res Ther* 2007;9(3):R56.
13. Kokkonen H, Johansson M, Innala L, et al. Correction: The PTPN22 1858C/T polymorphism is associated with anti-cyclic citrullinated peptide antibody-positive early rheumatoid arthritis in northern Sweden. *Arthritis Res Ther* 2007;9(5):403.
14. Källberg H, Padyukov L, Plenge RM, et al. Gene–gene and gene–environment interactions involving HLA-DRB1, PTPN22, and smoking in two subsets of rheumatoid arthritis. *Am J Hum Genet* 2007;80(5):867–875.
15. Kurreeman FA, Padyukov L, Marques RB, et al. A candidate gene approach identifies the TRAF1/C5 region as a risk factor for rheumatoid arthritis. *PLoS Med* 2007;4(9):e278.
16. Plenge RM, Seielstad M, Padyukov L, et al. TRAF1-C5 as a risk locus for rheumatoid arthritis—a genomewide study. *N Engl J Med* 2007;357(12):1199–1209.
17. Potter C, Eyre S, Cope A, et al. Investigation of association between the TRAF family genes and RA susceptibility. *Ann Rheum Dis* 2007; 66(10):1322–1326.
18. Sigurdsson S, Padyukov L, Kurreeman FA, et al. Association of a haplotype in the promoter region of the interferon regulatory factor 5 gene with rheumatoid arthritis. *Arthritis Rheum* 2007;56(7): 2202–2210.
19. Linn-Rasker SP, van der Helm-van Mil AH, van Gaalen FA, et al. Smoking is a risk factor for anti-CCP antibodies only in rheumatoid arthritis patients who carry HLA-DRB1 shared epitope alleles. *Ann Rheum Dis* 2006;65(3):366–371.
20. Pedersen M, Jacobsen S, Garred P, et al. Strong combined gene–environment effects in anti-cyclic citrullinated peptide-positive rheumatoid arthritis: A nationwide case–control study in Denmark. *Arthritis Rheum* 2007;56(5):1446–1453.
21. Heliovaara M, Aho K, Aromaa A, et al. Smoking and risk of rheumatoid arthritis. *J Rheumatol* 1993;20(11):1830–1835.
22. Symmons DP, Bankhead CR, Harrison BJ, et al. Blood transfusion, smoking, and obesity as risk factors for the development of rheumatoid arthritis: Results from a primary care–based incident case–control study in Norfolk, England. *Arthritis Rheum* 1997;40(11): 1955–1961.
23. Uhlig T, Hagen KB, Kvien TK. Current tobacco smoking, formal education, and the risk of rheumatoid arthritis. *J Rheumatol* 1999;26(1):47–54.
24. Silman AJ, Newman J, MacGregor AJ. Cigarette smoking increases the risk of rheumatoid arthritis. Results from a nationwide study of disease-discordant twins. *Arthritis Rheum* 1996;39(5):732–735.
25. Klockars M, Koskela RS, Jarvinen E, et al. Silica exposure and rheumatoid arthritis: A follow up study of granite workers 1940–1981. *Br Med J (Clin Res Ed)* 1987;294(6578):997–1000.
26. Turner S, Cherry N. Rheumatoid arthritis in workers exposed to silica in the pottery industry. *Occup Environ Med* 2000;57(7):443–447.
27. Steenland K, Sanderson W, Calvert GM. Kidney disease and arthritis in a cohort study of workers exposed to silica. *Epidemiology* 2001;12(4):405–412.
28. Sluis-Cremer GK, Hessel PA, Hnizdo E, et al. Relationship between silicosis and rheumatoid arthritis. *Thorax* 1986;41(8):596–601.
29. Stolt P, Padyukov L, Lundberg I, et al. Silica exposure is associated with increased risk of a restricted sub-group of RA: Results from the Swedish EIRA study. *Ann Rheum Dis* 2005;64:582–586.
30. Vessey MP, Villard-Mackintosh L, Yeates D. Oral contraceptives, cigarette smoking and other factors in relation to arthritis. *Contraception* 1987;35(5):457–464.
31. Tuomi T, Heliovaara M, Palosuo T, et al. Smoking, lung function, and rheumatoid factors. *Ann Rheum Dis* 1990;49(10):753–756.
32. Hernandez Avila M, Liang MH, Willett WC, et al. Reproductive factors, smoking, and the risk for rheumatoid arthritis. *Epidemiology* 1990;1(4):285–291.
33. Karlson EW, Lee IM, Cook NR, et al. A retrospective cohort study of cigarette smoking and risk of rheumatoid arthritis in female health professionals. *Arthritis Rheum* 1999;42(5):910–917.
34. Hutchinson D, Shepstone L, Moots R, et al. Heavy cigarette smoking is strongly associated with rheumatoid arthritis (RA), particularly in patients without a family history of RA. *Ann Rheum Dis* 2001;60(3):223–227.
35. Criswell LA, Merlino LA, Cerhan JR, et al. Cigarette smoking and the risk of rheumatoid arthritis among postmenopausal women: Results from the Iowa Women's Health Study. *Am J Med* 2002; 112(6):465–471.
36. Stolt P, Bengtsson C, Nordmark B, et al. Quantification of the influence of cigarette smoking on rheumatoid arthritis: Results from a population based case–control study, using incident cases. *Ann Rheum Dis* 2003;62(9):835–841.
37. Padyukov L, Silva C, Stolt P, et al. A gene-environment interaction between smoking and shared epitope genes in HLA-DR provides a high risk of seropositive rheumatoid arthritis. *Arthritis Rheum* 2004;50(10):3085–3092.
38. Verpoort KN, Papendrecht-van der Voort EA, van der Helm-van Mil AH, et al. Association of smoking with the constitution of the anti-cyclic citrullinated peptide response in the absence of HLA-DRB1 shared epitope alleles. *Arthritis Rheum* 2007;56(9):2913–2918.
39. Lee HS, Irigoyen P, Kern M, et al. Interaction between smoking, the shared epitope, and anti-cyclic citrullinated peptide: A mixed picture in three large North American rheumatoid arthritis cohorts. *Arthritis Rheum* 2007;56(6):1745–1753.
40. Turesson C, Jacobsson LT. Epidemiology of extra-articular manifestations in rheumatoid arthritis. *Scand J Rheumatol* 2004;33(2):65–72.
41. Nyhäll-Wåhlin BM, Jacobsson LT, Petersson IF, et al. Smoking is a strong risk factor for rheumatoid nodules in early rheumatoid arthritis. *Ann Rheum Dis* 2006;65(5):601–606.
42. Turesson C, Schaid DJ, Weyand CM, et al. Association of HLA-C3 and smoking with vasculitis in patients with rheumatoid arthritis. *Arthritis Rheum* 2006;54(9):2776–2783.
43. Karlson EW, Costenbader KH, Mandl LA. Secondhand smoke exposure and the risk of rheumatoid arthritis: Data from the nurses' health study study. *Arthritis Rheum* 2004;50:S267 (Abstract).
44. Jaakkola JJ, Gissler M. Maternal smoking in pregnancy as a determinant of rheumatoid arthritis and other inflammatory polyarthropathies during the first 7 years of life. *Int J Epidemiol* 2005;34(3): 664–671.
45. Papadopoulos NG, Alamanos Y, Voulgari PV, et al. Does cigarette smoking influence disease expression, activity and severity in early rheumatoid arthritis patients? *Clin Exp Rheumatol* 2005; 23(6):861–866.

46. Manfredsdottir VF, Vikingsdottir T, Jonsson T, et al. The effects of tobacco smoking and rheumatoid factor seropositivity on disease activity and joint damage in early rheumatoid arthritis. *Rheumatology (Oxford)* 2006;45(6):734–740.
47. Finckh A, Dehler S, Costenbader KH, et al. Cigarette smoking and radiographic progression in rheumatoid arthritis. *Ann Rheum Dis* 2007;66(8):1066–1071.
48. Farragher TM, Goodson NJ, Naseem H, et al. Association of the HLA-DRB1 gene with premature death, particularly from cardiovascular disease, in patients with rheumatoid arthritis and inflammatory polyarthritis. *Arthritis Rheum* 2008;58(2):359–369.
49. Pearson CM. Development of arthritis, periarthritis and periostitis in rats given adjuvants. *Proc Soc Exp Biol Med* 1956;91(1): 95–101.
50. Kleinau S, Erlandsson H, Holmdahl R, et al. Adjuvant oils induce arthritis in the DA rat. I. Characterization of the disease and evidence for an immunological involvement. *J Autoimmun* 1991;4(6): 871–880.
51. Cannon GW, Woods ML, Clayton F, et al. Induction of arthritis in DA rats by incomplete Freund's adjuvant. *J Rheumatol* 1993;20(1):7–11.
52. Holmdahl R, Lorentzen JC, Lu S, et al. Arthritis induced in rats with nonimmunogenic adjuvants as models for rheumatoid arthritis. *Immunol Rev* 2001;184:184–202.
53. Kleinau S, Erlandsson H, Klareskog L. Percutaneous exposure of adjuvant oil causes arthritis in DA rats. *Clin Exp Immunol* 1994;96(2):281–284.
54. Torisu M, Miyahara T, Shinohara N, et al. A new side effect of BCG immunotherapy—BCG-induced arthritis in man. *Cancer Immunol Immunother* 1978;5:77–83.
55. Hughes RA, Allard SA, Maini RN. Arthritis associated with adjuvant mycobacterial treatment for carcinoma of the bladder. *Ann Rheum Dis* 1989;48(5):432–434.
56. Sverdrup B, Källberg H, Bengtsson C, et al. Association between occupational exposure to mineral oil and rheumatoid arthritis: Results from the Swedish EIRA case–control study. *Arthritis Res Ther* 2005;7(6):R1296–1303.
57. Lundberg I, Alfredsson L, Plato N, et al. Occupation, occupational exposure to chemicals and rheumatological disease. A register based cohort study. *Scand J Rheumatol* 1994;23(6):305–310.
58. Olsson AR, Skogh T, Wingren G. Occupational determinants for rheumatoid arthritis. *Scand J Work Environ Health* 2000;26(3): 243–249.
59. Olsson AR, Skogh T, Axelson O, et al. Occupations and exposures in the work environment as determinants for rheumatoid arthritis. *Occup Environ Med* 2004;61(3):233–238.
60. Carty SM, Snowden N, Silman AJ. Should infection still be considered as the most likely triggering factor for rheumatoid arthritis? *J Rheumatol* 2003;30(3):425–429.
61. Molina V, Shoenfeld Y. Infection, vaccines and other environmental triggers of autoimmunity. *Autoimmunity* 2005;38(3):235–245.
62. Steere AC, Grodzicki RL, Kornblatt AN, et al. The spirochetal etiology of Lyme disease. *N Engl J Med* 1983;308(13):733–740.
63. Feder HM Jr, Johnson BJ, O'Connell S, et al. A critical appraisal of "chronic Lyme disease." *N Engl J Med* 2007;357(14):1422–1430.
64. Pattison DJ, Harrison RA, Symmons DP. The role of diet in susceptibility to rheumatoid arthritis: A systematic review. *J Rheumatol* 2004;31(7):1310–1319.
65. Pattison DJ, Symmons DP, Lunt M, et al. Dietary risk factors for the development of inflammatory polyarthritis: Evidence for a role of high level of red meat consumption. *Arthritis Rheum* 2004; 50(12):3804–3812.
66. Pattison DJ, Silman AJ, Goodson NJ, et al. Vitamin C and the risk of developing inflammatory polyarthritis: prospective nested case–control study. *Ann Rheum Dis* 2004;63(7):843–847.
67. Shapiro JA, Koepsell TD, Voigt LF, et al. Diet and rheumatoid arthritis in women: A possible protective effect of fish consumption. *Epidemiology* 1996;7(3):256–263.
68. Pedersen M, Stripp C, Klarlund M, et al. Diet and risk of rheumatoid arthritis in a prospective cohort. *J Rheumatol* 2005;32(7): 1249–1252.
69. Pedersen M, Jacobsen S, Klarlund M, et al. Environmental risk factors differ between rheumatoid arthritis with and without autoantibodies against cyclic citrullinated peptides. *Arthritis Res Ther* 2006;8(4):R133.
70. Kjeldsen-Kragh J, Haugen M, Forre O. Diet therapy in rheumatoid arthritis. *Lancet* 1992;339(8787):250.
71. Hafström I, Ringertz B, Spångberg A, et al. A vegan diet free of gluten improves the signs and symptoms of rheumatoid arthritis: The effects on arthritis correlate with a reduction in antibodies to food antigens. *Rheumatology (Oxford)* 2001;40(10):1175–1179.
72. McKellar G, Morrison E, McEntegart A, et al. A pilot study of a Mediterranean-type diet intervention in female patients with rheumatoid arthritis living in areas of social deprivation in Glasgow. *Ann Rheum Dis* 2007;66(9):1239–1243.
73. Muller H, de Toledo FW, Resch KL. Fasting followed by vegetarian diet in patients with rheumatoid arthritis: A systematic review. *Scand J Rheumatol* 2001;30(1):1–10.
74. Heliovaara M, Aho K, Knekt P, et al. Coffee consumption, rheumatoid factor, and the risk of rheumatoid arthritis. *Ann Rheum Dis* 2000;59(8):631–635.
75. Mikuls TR, Cerhan JR, Criswell LA, et al. Coffee, tea, and caffeine consumption and risk of rheumatoid arthritis: Results from the Iowa Women's Health Study. *Arthritis Rheum* 2002;46(1):83–91.
76. Karlson EW, Mandl LA, Aweh GN, et al. Coffee consumption and risk of rheumatoid arthritis. *Arthritis Rheum* 2003;48(11):3055–3060.
77. Bankhead C, Silman A, Barrett B, et al. Incidence of rheumatoid arthritis is not related to indicators of socioeconomic deprivation. *J Rheumatol* 1996;23(12):2039–2042.
78. Bengtsson C, Nordmark B, Klareskog L, et al. Socioeconomic status and the risk of developing rheumatoid arthritis: Results from the Swedish EIRA study. *Ann Rheum Dis* 2005;64(11):1588–1594.
79. Ahlbom A, Alfredsson L. Interaction: A word with two meanings creates confusion. *Eur J Epidemiol* 2005;20(7):563–564.
80. Rothman KJ. *Epidemiology: An Introduction.* Oxford: Oxford University Press, 2002.
81. Hosmer DW, Lemeshow S. Confidence interval estimation of interaction. *Epidemiology* 1992;3(5):452–456.
82. Andersson T, Alfredsson L, Källberg H, et al. Calculating measures of biological interaction. *Eur J Epidemiol* 2005;20(7):575–579.
83. Mattey DL, Hutchinson D, Dawes PT, et al. Smoking and disease severity in rheumatoid arthritis: Association with polymorphism at the glutathione S-transferase M1 locus. *Arthritis Rheum* 2002; 46(3):640–646.
84. Klareskog L, Rönnelid J, Lundberg K, et al. Immunity to citrullinated proteins in rheumatoid arthritis. *Annu Rev Immunol* 2008.
85. Harel-Meir M, Sherer Y, Shoenfeld Y. Tobacco smoking and autoimmune rheumatic diseases. *Nat Clin Pract Rheumatol* 2007; 3(12):707–715.
86. Hill JA, Southwood S, Sette A, et al. The conversion of arginine to citrulline allows for a high-affinity peptide interaction with the rheumatoid arthritis–associated HLA-DRB1*0401 MHC class II molecule. *J Immunol* 2003;171(2):538–541.
87. Auger I, Sebbag M, Vincent C, et al. Influence of HLA-DR genes on the production of rheumatoid arthritis-specific autoantibodies to citrullinated fibrinogen. *Arthritis Rheum* 2005;52(11):3424–3432.
88. Chapuy-Regaud S, Sebbag M, Baeten D, et al. Fibrin deimination in synovial tissue is not specific for rheumatoid arthritis but commonly occurs during synovitides. *J Immunol* 2005;174(8):5057–5064.
89. Cantaert T, De Rycke L, Bongartz T, et al. Citrullinated proteins in rheumatoid arthritis: Crucial but not sufficient! *Arthritis Rheum* 2006;54(11):3381–3389.
90. Aho K, Palosuo T, Heliovaara M, et al. Antifilaggrin antibodies within "normal" range predict rheumatoid arthritis in a linear fashion. *J Rheumatol* 2000;27(12):2743–2746.

91. Rantapää-Dahlqvist S, de Jong BA, Berglin E, et al. Antibodies against cyclic citrullinated peptide and IgA rheumatoid factor predict the development of rheumatoid arthritis. *Arthritis Rheum* 2003;48(10):2741–2749.
92. Nielen MM, van Schaardenburg D, Reesink HW, et al. Specific autoantibodies precede the symptoms of rheumatoid arthritis: A study of serial measurements in blood donors. *Arthritis Rheum* 2004;50(2):380–386.
93. Masdottir B, Jonsson T, Manfredsdottir V, et al. Smoking, rheumatoid factor isotypes and severity of rheumatoid arthritis. *Rheumatology (Oxford)* 2000;39(11):1202–1205.
94. Lundberg K, Nijenhuis S, Vossenaar ER, et al. Citrullinated proteins have increased immunogenicity and arthritogenicity and their presence in arthritic joints correlates with disease severity. *Arthritis Res Ther* 2005;7(3):R458–R467.
95. Kuhn KA, Kulik L, Tomooka B, et al. Antibodies against citrullinated proteins enhance tissue injury in experimental autoimmune arthritis. *J Clin Invest* 2006;116(4):961–973.
96. Pedersen M. *Risk Factors for Rheumatoid Arthritis. A Case–Control Study*. Copenhagen: Copenhagen University, 2006.

Risk Factors for Rheumatoid Arthritis: Other Nongenetic Host Factors

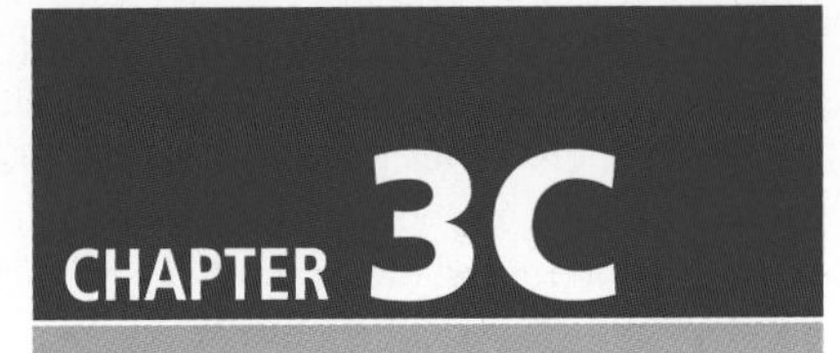

Marc C. Hochberg, Jacqueline E. Oliver, and Alan J. Silman

There are a number of nongenetic host factors that have been widely studied and linked to the development of rheumatoid arthritis (RA). This chapter will discuss how both lifestyle (smoking, diet, occupation, etc.) and constitutional factors that are not directly genetic (hormones, pregnancy, obesity) are thought to be linked to the development of RA.

Lifestyle Factors

Social Class

There have been several studies that have examined the effect of socioeconomic status on the risk of RA.[1–4] In a large population-based case–control study in Sweden (the EIRA study), the risk of RA was studied vis-à-vis levels of formal education; people without a university degree had an increased risk of RA (relative risk [RR] = 1.4, 95% confidence interval [CI]: 1.2–1.8) compared to those with a degree.[4] A Danish case–control study also found a significant inverse relationship between level of education and risk of RA; subjects with the longest time in formal education had a reduced risk compared to those with the lowest education level (OR = 0.43, 95% CI: 0.24–0.76).[1] However, Uhlig and colleagues[2] failed to find an association between level of education and risk of RA. The Norfolk Arthritis Register (a large prospective population-based register) reported that none of five indicators of socioeconomic status were associated with increased incidence of RA.[3]

Smoking

Smoking has been linked to an increased risk of RA.[5] In a large study of female health professionals, the duration of smoking was linked to an increased risk of RA; women who had smoked for more than 20 years were found to have a 39% increased risk and this was increased to 49% for seropositive RA.[6] In a large-cohort study of adult Finns, smoking increased the risk of seropositive RA in male ex-smokers (RR = 2.6, 95% CI: 1.3–5.3) and male current smokers (RR = 3.8, 95% CI: 2–6.9) compared to men who had never smoked.[7] The increased risk of seropositive but not seronegative RA was also reported in a Swedish study.[8] Data from a twin study reported a strong association between ever smoking and RA in both monozygotic twins (OR = 12, 95% CI: 1.8–513) and dizygotic twins (OR = 2.5, 95% CI: 0.92–7.9).[9] Costenbader and colleagues[10] analyzed data from the Nurses Health Study. A total of 680 RA cases, diagnosed from 1976 and 2002, were confirmed using a questionnaire and medical record review. After age adjustment, the RR of RA was significantly elevated among both current (RR = 1.43, 95% CI: 1.16–1.75) and past smokers (RR = 1.47, 95% CI: 1.23–1.76) compared with never smokers. There was a significant linear dose–response relationship between increased risk of RA with increasing pack-years of smoking ($p < 0.01$). The effect of smoking was much stronger among RF-positive cases than among RF-negative cases, and the risk remained elevated in past smokers until 20 years or more after cessation. No difference for risk for developing RA during premenopausal years versus postmenopausal women was seen among even smokers. The authors concluded that one-quarter of the 680 new cases of RA diagnosed after the age of 35 in this large cohort could have been prevented if none of these women had ever smoked. The association between cigarette smoking and development of RA was also examined in the Iowa Women's Health Study.[5] This study included 31,336 women in Iowa, age 55 to 69 years of which 158 cases of RA were identified and validated between 1987 and 1997. This study concluded that smoking led to an approximately twofold increased risk of RA among postmenopausal women (RR = 2.0, 95% CI: 1.3–2.9) and that this risk persists for about 10 years for former smokers (RR = 1.8, 95% CI: 1.1–3.1). These investigators estimated that about 18% of cases of RA in postmenopausal women can be attributed to smoking.

A recent study has found that the risk of RA may be determined by exposures occurring when in the womb. Jaakkola and Gissler[11] found that high exposure to tobacco smoke increases the risk of both RA (OR = 4.64, 95% CI: 1.94–11.07) and inflammatory polyarthritis (OR = 6.76, 95% CI: 2.00–22.9).[11] However this effect was only observed in girls.

Several reports have reported on the gene–environment interaction between smoking and RA.[12–16] A large Swedish population-based case–control study studied different gene/smoking combinations.[12] They reported that the risk of RF seropositive RA was greatest in current smokers with SE genes (RR = 7.5, 95% CI: 4.2–13.1). For those with double copies of SE genes, the risk increased further (RR = 15.7, 95% CI: 7.2–34.2). This interaction between smoking and SE genes was significant. This interaction has been expanded further to examine the connection with the presence of anti-CCP antibodies. Patients who both smoked and had the SE gene had an increased risk of anti-CCP antibodies (OR = 5.27).[13] Klareskog and colleagues[14] have also reported on this hypothesis; they found that smoking and carrying two copies of the SE genes increased the risk by 21-fold of anti-citrulline–positive RA.[14]

Diet

There is an increasing amount of scientific literature concerning the effect of dietary factors on the risk of RA.[17] The benefits of consuming a high proportion of oily fish and vegetables, the so-called Mediterranean diet, may offer a protective role against the development of RA. In a prospective, population-based case–control study, the association of antioxidants was studied.[18] Authors found that lower intakes of fruit and vegetables increased the risk of inflammatory polyarthritis. This risk was over three-fold for low vitamin C intake (OR = 3.3, 95% CI: 1.4–7.9). Consumption of a high intake of red meat has been associated with an increased risk of inflammatory polyarthritis.[19] Increased risks were found for those that had the highest levels of red meat consumption (OR = 1.9, 95% CI: 0.9–4.0), meat and meat products (OR = 2.3, 95% CI: 1.1–4.9), and total protein (OR = 2.9, 95% CI: 1.1–7.5). Not all studies agree; Pedersen and colleagues,[19a] for instance, found that intake of a range of dietary factors including fruit, vitamins, or meat had no association with the risk of RA. They did, however, link the intake of oily fish with a reduced risk of RA. Linos and colleagues[20] found that the risk of RA was inversely associated with consumption of cooked vegetables (OR = 0.39) and olive oil (OR = 0.39).[20]

There is also evidence that high consumption of the antioxidants (β-cryptoxanthin and zeaxanthin) found in some fruits and vegetables may reduce the risk. Strong evidence in support of this came from a prospective case–control study using dietary data from a 7-day diet diary.[21] Two further studies support this finding. Aho and Heliovaara[22] noted that selenium, alpha-tocopherol, beta-carotene, and an overall antioxidant index were inversely associated with the later development of RA. The relationship of vitamins C and E, carotenoids, and antioxidant trace elements from foods and supplements with the incidence of RA in older women was also evaluated using data from the Iowa Women's Health Study.[23] After adjustment for other risk factors for RA, including cigarette smoking, intake of beta-cryptoxanthin was associated with a reduced incidence of RA (RR = 0.56, 95% CI: 0.39–0.90), while no associations were found with other carotenoids (total carotenoids, alpha- or beta-carotene, lycopene, or lutein/zeaxanthin).

Caffeine intake has also been studied with no consensus on its role in the development of RA. In data from the Iowa Women's Health Study, women drinking four or more cups of decaffeinated coffee per day were found to have an increased risk of RA (RR = 2.58, 95% CI: 1.63–4.06).[24] They also found a protective role for tea consumption where women drinking more than three cups per day had a decreased risk of RA (RR = 0.4, 95% CI: 0.16–0.97). Daily caffeine intake was not associated with RA. However, data from a large prospective study found no association with the consumption of decaffeinated or caffeinated coffee or tea and risk of RA.[25]

Infection

Virus

The most widely studied and strongest associations have been found with the Epstein Barr virus (EBV).[26–28] Both higher levels of anti-EBV antibodies and higher EBV loads in peripheral blood lymphocytes have been found in RA patients[29] and the virus is frequently found in the synovial tissue of RA patients,[30–32] although not all studies confirm this.[33] Deiminated EBV sequences are recognized by anti-CCP antibodies suggesting that EBV infection may have a role in inducing these antibodies found in the sera of RA patients.[34] Parvovirus B19 has also been found to be significantly higher in RA patients.[35] However, results from a twin study suggested that there was no overall increased susceptibility to RA from exposure to the parvovirus B19. Interestingly there was an association in two subgroups; affected twin was RF negative (OR = 2.0, 95% CI: 0.9–12.4) and in opposite-sex twins where affected twin was female (OR = 3.0, 95% CI: 0.9–11.6).[36] There are also case reports of RA developing after infection with Hepatitis C[37] and HIV.[38] These two cases were both positive for HLA subtypes, which may suggest that they were already genetically susceptible to the disease.

Other Organisms

In a recent case–control study, the presence of antibodies against *Mycoplasma pneumoniae* were associated with the risk of RA (OR = 2.34, $p < 0.001$).[39] *Proteus* has also been linked to an increased risk of RA.[40] There are also case reports of RA or juvenile RA developing after infection with *Bartonella*[41] and *Chlamydia*.[42] *Borrelia burgdorferi* has previously been implicated as a risk factor for RA. However, this was not supported by results from a recent case–control study where no evidence for increased seropositivity was found in subjects with RA.[42a]

Occupation

A number of occupations have been linked to an increased risk of RA including farming, mining, and exposure to chemicals.[43,44] One of the greatest occupational risks is silica exposure.[45,46] The Swedish EIRA study reported that men who were exposed to silica had an increased risk of RA: in 18- to 70-year-olds (OR = 2.2, 95% CI: 1.2–3.9), 50- to 70-year-olds (OR = 2.7, 95% CI: 1.2–5.8). Men with high exposure to silica (rock drilling and stone crushing) were three times more likely to develop RA (OR = 3.0, 95% CI: 1.2–7.6) compared to silica-exposed men in general.[47]

A population-based case–control study in Sweden found that exposure to mineral oil in men increased the risk of RA (RR = 1.3, 95% CI: 1–1.7).[48] Manual employees and assistant/intermediate nonmanual employees have been reported to be 20% more likely to develop RA than nonmanual employees.[4] The increased risk of RA when working in the agricultural industry was studied by De Roos and colleagues[49] recently in a nested case–control study in females. They found no strong evidence of increased risk through applying or working with pesticides, but found that there was an increased risk with welding (OR = 2.1, 95% CI: 0.8–5.4).

Medical Interventions

Lymphoid Surgery

In the past, there have been a number of reports which suggested that surgery to remove tonsils or the appendix may be associated with an increased risk of RA. However, in a questionnaire survey of over 1500 patients with RA, no significant association could be found.[50]

Contraceptive Pill

A number of studies have examined the use of the oral contraceptive pill (OCP) in the development of RA. About two-thirds of the studies have found that the OCP has a protective role,[51,52] while the other third have found no association.[53,54] One study suggested that it was only current OCP use that had a protective role.[55] However, meta-analyses have suggested that its role is not conclusive.[56,57] While, the bulk of the evidence points to a protective role for oral contraceptives in the development of RA, additional research is needed to resolve this controversy.

Blood Transfusions

Data from the Norfolk Arthritis Register showed that there was an increased risk of developing of RA after a blood transfusion (OR = 4.83, 95% CI: 1.29–18.07).[58] However, the opposite effect has been reported by Cerhan and colleagues.[59] In a prospective cohort study of women aged 55 to 69 years, they found that a previous blood transfusion was inversely related to the risk of RA (RR = 0.72, 95% CI: 0.48–1.08). The association was greater in women who developed RF-positive RA (RR = 0.59, 95% CI: 0.35–1.0).

Constitutional Factors

Hormonal

The significantly higher incidence of RA in women and onset during childbearing years suggests that there may be a hormonal basis for the disease, and this has been the subject of many studies.

Fertility and Adverse Outcomes

Nulliparity may be a risk factor for the development of RA, although conflicting results have been reported. There is some evidence that women who develop RA have decreased fecundity prior to disease onset.[60] One study reported nulliparous women had an increased risk of RA (OR = 1.8),[52] and the risk of RA in women who have ever been pregnant is halved,[61] indicating a protective effect of pregnancy. However, other studies have found that although there was an increased trend in nulliparity in RA patients, it was not statistically significant.[62]

Adverse pregnancy outcomes prior to disease onset have been proposed to have a role in RA development. van Dunne and colleagues[63] found that patients who had one or more miscarriages had a significant increase in joint damage. Termination of pregnancy has been associated with an increased risk of developing RA (OR = 3.74, 95% CI: 1.4–9.9).[64] However, Nelson and colleagues[65] reported that neither of these events significantly increased the risk of RA. A large cohort study of over 31,000 women aged 55 to 69 years followed up for 11 years found that the only reproductive factor that had a strong association with RA was polycystic ovary syndrome (RR = 2.58, 95% CI: 1.06–6.3).[66] The Nurses Health Study examined a number of hormonal factors and their relationship with RA.[67] Very irregular menstrual cycles (RR = 1.4, 95% CI: 1.0–2.0) were associated with an increased risk of RA. Early age at menarche (RR = 1.6, 95% CI: 1.1–24) was associated with an increased risk of seropositive RA. The other factors examined—parity, number of children, age at first birth, and OCP use—did not increase the risk of RA. Data from the Iowa Women's' Health Study also examined the relationship of reproductive risk factors to development of RA in elderly women.[66] After age adjustment, few reproductive factors were significantly associated with RA in this age group. There was an inverse association with later age at menopause and RA, women who underwent menopause after age 51 had an RR of 0.64 (95% CI: 0.41–1.00) compared with women who underwent menopause before age 45 suggesting that a delay in menopause might have a potentially protective effect against RA development. In this cohort, women who self-reported physician-diagnosed polycystic ovary syndrome (PCOS) had the most consistently elevated risk for RA (RR = 2.58, 95% CI: 1.06–6.30). A possible biologic explanation might be the elevated levels of androgens found in PCOS. A nonsignificant elevated risk was also associated with a self-reported, physician-diagnosed history of endometriosis (RR = 1.72, 95% CI: 0.93–3.18); endometriosis also is characterized by elevated androgen levels and has been associated with autoimmunity.

There was no evidence of a significant effect for age at menarche, history of hysterectomy or oophorectomy, use of oral contraceptives, history of pregnancy and breast-feeding, history of infertility, ever being pregnant, number of miscarriages, parity, and total number of pregnancies or number of children breast-fed. The investigators concluded that female reproductive factors are not likely to be major determinants of RA risk, at least in the age group of older women; however, this does not exclude the possibility that hormonal factors might have a stronger influence in younger women.

Breast-Feeding

Another hormonal effect that has been widely studied is the role of breast-feeding in the development of RA. Again not all studies have produced consistent results. A large population-based cohort study found that increased lactation time had a protective role.[68] This effect was also noted in a large cohort study of over 100,000 nurses and was dose dependent.[67] A recent study has linked cortisol levels with duration of breast-feeding.[69] Women who breast-fed for more than 12 months had significantly higher cortisol levels, and this association was greater in women with three or more births, which may have a relevance for autoimmune disease such as RA. Breast-feeding after a first pregnancy significantly increases the risk of RA (OR = 5.4, 95% CI: 2.5–11.4).[70] This risk decreases after a second pregnancy (OR = 2.0) and there is no increased risk after a third pregnancy. For women who were RF positive with erosive disease the risk was greatest. Jorgensen and colleagues[51] found that duration of breast-feeding was linked with the development of more severe disease, and having more than three breast-fed children increased the risk more than threefold of a poor disease outcome. Parity was also associated with disease outcome, and having more than three children increased the risk nearly fivefold of severe disease.

Body Shape/Obesity

The risk of RA may also be associated with obesity. Data from the Norfolk Arthritis Register showed that having a body mass index of 30 or more increased the risk of developing RA (OR = 3.74, 95% CI: 1.14–12.27).[58] This increased risk of RA in obese women was also reported by Voigt and colleagues.[71] In a prospective cohort study of older women, neither body mass index nor body fat distribution were linked with RA.[59]

Other Comorbidities

Atopy

The prevalence of atopy in RA patients has been widely studied, and there is some evidence that it protects against the future development of RA. This is thought to be due to the mutual antagonism of T-helper cell (Th) diseases. Th1 cells exist in RA patients, whereas Th2 cells predominate in atopic disorders.

A cross-sectional study found the atopic disorders of hay fever, atopic dermatitis, and asthma were reduced in RA patients.[72] In a recent case–control study of 300 RA patients, the cumulative incidence (RA 7.5%, controls 18.8%; $p < 0.01$) and the point prevalence (RA 3.5%, controls 16.2%; $p < 0.0001$) of atopy was found to be significantly lower in RA patients compared to controls.[73] A similar finding was reported in a recent study where there was a lower occurrence of hay fever (2.3% vs 24.2%, $p < 0.0001$) and house mite dust sensitivity (3.1% vs 12.2% $p < 0.003$) in patients compared to controls. They also reported that the severity of RA was less in patients with atopy.[74] The prevalence of hay fever in RA patients was also reduced (RR = 0.48) in a study of outpatients[75]; this study also reported lower disease activity in RA patients with hay fever.

However, other studies do not confirm these results. A Canadian population study reported that a history of allergy was positively associated with RA in women (OR = 1.57, 95% CI: 1.43–1.73) and in men (OR = 1.55, 95% CI: 1.36–1.77).[76] There was no difference in the prevalence of RA in Turkish patients compared to the general population.[77] An inverse relationship between the presence of rhinitis and RA has also been reported but this study found no negative association between RA and asthma or eczema.[78]

Schizophrenia

Schizophrenia and RA are also reported to have a negative association,[79] and the majority of studies confirm this negative finding.[80] Some studies have reported that no association exists.[81] A meta-analysis of the data estimated that the rate of RA in patients with schizophrenia was only 29% of the rate in patients with other psychiatric problems.[82] A large population-based case–control study was carried out using the Danish Psychiatric Care Register (20,495 cases and 204,912 age- and gender-matched controls). Patients with schizophrenia were found to have a reduced risk of RA (OR = 0.44, 95% CI: 0.24–0.81).[83] However, the authors reported that other musculoskeletal disorders were also significantly reduced, and RA incidence in bipolar patients was similar to the controls. They suggest that the negative association may be due to ascertainment bias and selection due to the reporting and treatment of medical illness.

Conclusion

Although a number of hormonal and environmental factors have been implicated in the development of RA, conflicting results are still being reported for many of these risk factors. Such results highlight the need for more robustly designed studies.

References

1. Pedersen M, Jacobsen S, Klarlund M, Frisch M. Socioeconomic status and risk of rheumatoid arthritis: A Danish case–control study. *J Rheumatol* 2006;33(6):1069–1074.
2. Uhlig T, Hagen KB, Kvien TK. Current tobacco smoking, formal education, and the risk of rheumatoid arthritis. *J Rheumatol* 1999; 26(1):47–54.
3. Bankhead C, Silman A, Barrett B, et al. Incidence of rheumatoid arthritis is not related to indicators of socioeconomic deprivation. *J Rheumatol* 1996;23(12):2039–2042.
4. Bengtsson C, Nordmark B, Klareskog L, et al. Socioeconomic status and the risk of developing rheumatoid arthritis: Results from the Swedish EIRA study. *Ann Rheum Dis* 2005;64(11):1588–1594.
5. Criswell LA, Merlino LA, Cerhan JR, et al. Cigarette smoking and the risk of rheumatoid arthritis among postmenopausal women: Results from the Iowa Women's Health Study. *Am J Med* 2002; 112(6):465–471.
6. Karlson EW, Lee IM, Cook NR, et al. A retrospective cohort study of cigarette smoking and risk of rheumatoid arthritis in female health professionals. *Arthritis Rheum* 1999;42(5):910–917.
7. Heliovaara M, Aho K, Aromaa A, et al. Smoking and risk of rheumatoid arthritis. *J Rheumatol* 1993;20(11):1830–1835.
8. Stolt P, Bengtsson C, Nordmark B, et al. Quantification of the influence of cigarette smoking on rheumatoid arthritis: Results from a population based case-control study, using incident cases. *Ann Rheum Dis* 2003;62(9):835–841.
9. Silman AJ, Newman J, MacGregor AJ. Cigarette smoking increases the risk of rheumatoid arthritis. Results from a nationwide study of disease-discordant twins. *Arthritis Rheum* 1996;39(5):732–735.
10. Costenbader KH, Feskanich D, Mandl LA, Karlson EW. Smoking intensity, duration, and cessation, and the risk of rheumatoid arthritis in women. *Am J Med* 2006;119(6):503–509.
11. Jaakkola JJ, Gissler M. Maternal smoking in pregnancy as a determinant of rheumatoid arthritis and other inflammatory polyarthropathies during the first 7 years of life. *Int J Epidemiol* 2005; 34(3):664–671.
12. Padyukov L, Silva C, Stolt P, et al. A gene–environment interaction between smoking and shared epitope genes in HLA-DR provides a high risk of seropositive rheumatoid arthritis. *Arthritis Rheum* 2004;50(10):3085–3092.
13. Linn-Rasker SP, van der Helm-van Mil AH, van Gaalen FA, et al. Smoking is a risk factor for anti-CCP antibodies only in rheumatoid arthritis patients who carry HLA-DRB1 shared epitope alleles. *Ann Rheum Dis* 2006;65(3):366–371.
14. Klareskog L, Stolt P, Lundberg K, et al. A new model for an etiology of rheumatoid arthritis: smoking may trigger HLA-DR (shared epitope)–restricted immune reactions to autoantigens modified by citrullination. *Arthritis Rheum* 2006;54(1):38–46.
15. Criswell LA, Saag KG, Mikuls TR, et al. Smoking interacts with genetic risk factors in the development of rheumatoid arthritis among older Caucasian women. *Ann Rheum Dis* 2006;65(9):1163–1167.
16. Kallberg H, Padyukov L, Plenge RM, et al. Gene–gene and gene–environment interactions involving HLA-DRB1, PTPN22, and smoking in two subsets of rheumatoid arthritis. *Am J Hum Genet* 2007;80(5):867–875.
17. Pattison DJ, Harrison RA, Symmons DP. The role of diet in susceptibility to rheumatoid arthritis: A systematic review. *J Rheumatol* 2004;31(7):1310–1319.
18. Pattison DJ, Silman AJ, Goodson NJ, et al. Vitamin C and the risk of developing inflammatory polyarthritis: prospective nested case–control study. *Ann Rheum Dis* 2004;63(7):843–847.
19. Pattison DJ, Symmons DP, Lunt M, et al. Dietary risk factors for the development of inflammatory polyarthritis: Evidence for a role of high level of red meat consumption. *Arthritis Rheum* 2004; 50(12):3804–3812.

19a. Pedersen M, Stripp C, Klarlund M, et al. Diet and risk of rheumatoid arthritis in a prospective cohort. *J Rheumatol* 2005;32(7): 1249–1252.

20. Linos A, Kaklamani VG, Kaklamani E, Koumantaki Y, et al. Dietary factors in relation to rheumatoid arthritis: A role for olive oil and cooked vegetables? *Am J Clin Nutr* 1999;70(6):1077–1082.

21. Pattison DJ, Symmons DP, Lunt M, et al. Dietary beta-cryptoxanthin and inflammatory polyarthritis: Results from a population-based prospective study. *Am J Clin Nutr* 2005;82(2):451–455.
22. Aho K, Heliovaara M. Risk factors for rheumatoid arthritis. *Ann Med* 2004;36(4):242–251.
23. Cerhan JR, Saag KG, Merlino LA, et al. Antioxidant micronutrients and risk of rheumatoid arthritis in a cohort of older women. *Am J Epidemiol* 2003;157(4):345–354.
24. Mikuls TR, Cerhan JR, Criswell LA, et al. Coffee, tea, and caffeine consumption and risk of rheumatoid arthritis: Results from the Iowa Women's Health Study. *Arthritis Rheum* 2002;46(1):83–91.
25. Karlson EW, Mandl LA, Aweh GN, Grodstein F. Coffee consumption and risk of rheumatoid arthritis. *Arthritis Rheum* 2003;48(11): 3055–3060.
26. Costenbader KH, Karlson EW. Epstein-Barr virus and rheumatoid arthritis: Is there a link? *Arthritis Res Ther* 2006;8(1):204.
27. Balandraud N, Roudier J, Roudier C. Epstein-Barr virus and rheumatoid arthritis. *Autoimmun Rev* 2004;3(5):362–367.
28. Toussirot E, Roudier J. Pathophysiological links between rheumatoid arthritis and the Epstein-Barr virus: An update. *Joint Bone Spine* 2007;74:418–426.
29. Balandraud N, Meynard JB, Auger I, et al. Epstein-Barr virus load in the peripheral blood of patients with rheumatoid arthritis: Accurate quantification using real-time polymerase chain reaction. *Arthritis Rheum* 2003;48(5):1223–1228.
30. Takeda T, Mizugaki Y, Matsubara L, et al. Lytic Epstein-Barr virus infection in the synovial tissue of patients with rheumatoid arthritis. *Arthritis Rheum* 2000;43(6):1218–1225.
31. Blaschke S, Schwarz G, Moneke D, et al. Epstein-Barr virus infection in peripheral blood mononuclear cells, synovial fluid cells, and synovial membranes of patients with rheumatoid arthritis. *J Rheumatol* 2000;27(4):866–873.
32. Takei M, Mitamura K, Fujiwara S, et al. Detection of Epstein-Barr virus-encoded small RNA 1 and latent membrane protein 1 in synovial lining cells from rheumatoid arthritis patients. *Int Immunol* 1997;9(5):739–743.
33. Niedobitek G, Lisner R, Swoboda B, et al. Lack of evidence for an involvement of Epstein-Barr virus infection of synovial membranes in the pathogenesis of rheumatoid arthritis. *Arthritis Rheum* 2000;43(1):151–154.
34. Pratesi F, Tommasi C, Anzilotti C, et al. Deiminated Epstein-Barr virus nuclear antigen 1 is a target of anti-citrullinated protein antibodies in rheumatoid arthritis. *Arthritis Rheum* 2006;54(3): 733–741.
35. Chen YS, Chou PH, Li SN, et al. Parvovirus B19 infection in patients with rheumatoid arthritis in Taiwan. *J Rheumatol* 2006; 33(5):887–891.
36. Hajeer AH, MacGregor AJ, Rigby AS, et al. Influence of previous exposure to human parvovirus B19 infection in explaining susceptibility to rheumatoid arthritis: An analysis of disease discordant twin pairs. *Ann Rheum Dis* 1994;53(2):137–139.
37. Hirohata S, Inoue T, Ito K. Development of rheumatoid arthritis after chronic hepatitis caused by hepatitis C virus infection. *Intern Med* 1992;31(4):493–495.
38. Wegrzyn J, Livrozet JM, Touraine JL, Miossec P. Rheumatoid arthritis after 9 years of human immunodeficiency virus infection: possible contribution of tritherapy. *J Rheumatol* 2002;29(10): 2232–2234.
39. Ramirez AS, Rosas A, Hernandez-Beriain JA, et al. Relationship between rheumatoid arthritis and *Mycoplasma pneumoniae*: A case–control study. *Rheumatology (Oxford)* 2005;44(7):912–914.
40. Ebringer A, Khalafpour S, Wilson C. Rheumatoid arthritis and proteus—a possible etiological association. *Rheumatol Int* 1989; 9(3–5):223–228.
41. Tsukahara M, Tsuneoka H, Tateishi H, et al. Bartonella infection associated with systemic juvenile rheumatoid arthritis. *Clin Infect Dis* 2001;32(1):E22–E23.
42. Jolly M, Curran JJ. Chlamydial infection preceding the development of rheumatoid arthritis: A brief report. *Clin Rheumatol* 2004; 23(5):435–453.
42a. Chary-Valckenaere I, Guillemin F, Pourel J, et al. Seroreactivity to Borrelia burgdorferi antigens in early rheumatoid arthritis: A case–control study. *Br J Rheumatol* 1997;36(9):945–949.
43. Lundberg I, Alfredsson L, Plato N, et al. Occupation, occupational exposure to chemicals and rheumatological disease — a register-based cohort study. *Scand J Rheumatol* 1994;23(6):305–310.
44. Olsson AR, Skogh T, Axelson O, Wingren G. Occupations and exposures in the work environment as determinants for rheumatoid arthritis. *Occup Environ Med* 2004;61(3):233–238.
45. Calvert GM, Rice FL, Boiano JM, et al. Occupational silica exposure and risk of various diseases: An analysis using death certificates from 27 states of the United States. *Occup Environ Med* 2003; 60(2):122–129.
46. Parks CG, Conrad K, Cooper GS. Occupational exposure to crystalline silica and autoimmune disease. *Environ Health Perspect* 1999; 107:793–802.
47. Stolt P, Kallberg H, Lundberg I, et al. Silica exposure is associated with increased risk of developing rheumatoid arthritis: Results from the Swedish EIRA study. *Ann Rheum Dis* 2005;64(4): 582–586.
48. Sverdrup B, Kallberg H, Bengtsson C, et al. Association between occupational exposure to mineral oil and rheumatoid arthritis: Results from the Swedish EIRA case–control study. *Arthritis Res Ther* 2005;7(6):R1296–R1303.
49. De Roos AJ, Cooper GS, Alavanja MC, Sandler DP. Rheumatoid arthritis among women in the agricultural health study: Risk associated with farming activities and exposures. *Ann Epidemiol* 2005;15(10):762–770.
50. Moens HB, Corstjens A, Boon C. Rheumatoid arthritis is not associated with prior tonsillectomy or appendectomy. *Clin Rheumatol* 1994;13(3):483–486.
51. Jorgensen C, Picot MC, Bologna C, Sany J. Oral contraception, parity, breast feeding, and severity of rheumatoid arthritis. *Ann Rheum Dis* 1996;55(2):94–98.
52. Spector TD, Roman E, Silman AJ. The pill, parity, and rheumatoid arthritis. *Arthritis Rheum* 1990;33(6):782–789.
53. Moskowitz MA, Jick SS, Burnside S, et al. The relationship of oral contraceptive use to rheumatoid arthritis. *Epidemiology* 1990; 1(2):153–156.
54. Drossaers-Bakker KW, Zwinderman AH, van Zeben D, et al. Pregnancy and oral contraceptive use do not significantly influence outcome in long-term rheumatoid arthritis. *Ann Rheum Dis* 2002;61(5):405–408.
55. Brennan P, Bankhead C, Silman A, Symmons D. Oral contraceptives and rheumatoid arthritis: Results from a primary care-based incident case–control study. *Semin Arthritis Rheum* 1997;26(6): 817–823.
56. Pladevall Vila M, Delclos GL, Varas C, et al. Controversy of oral contraceptives and risk of rheumatoid arthritis: Meta-analysis of conflicting studies and review of conflicting meta-analyses with special emphasis on analysis of heterogeneity. *Am J Epidemiol* 1996;144(1):1–14.
57. Spector TD, Hochberg MC. The protective effect of the oral-contraceptive pill on rheumatoid-arthritis—an overview of the analytic epidemiologic studies using metaanalysis. *J Clin Epidemiol* 1990;43(11):1221–1230.
58. Symmons DPM, Bankhead CR, Harrison BJ, et al. Blood transfusion, smoking, and obesity as risk factors for the development of rheumatoid arthritis—Results from a primary care-based incident case-control study in Norfolk, England. *Arthritis Rheum* 1997; 40(11):1955–1961.
59. Cerhan JR, Saag KG, Criswell LA, et al. Blood transfusion, alcohol use, and anthropometric risk factors for rheumatoid arthritis in older women. *J Rheumatol* 2002;29(2):246–254.

60. Nelson JL, Koepsell TD, Dugowson CE, et al. Fecundity before disease onset in women with rheumatoid arthritis. *Arthritis Rheum* 1993;36(1):7–14.
61. Hazes JM, Dijkmans BA, Vandenbroucke JP, de Vries RR, Cats A. Pregnancy and the risk of developing rheumatoid arthritis. *Arthritis Rheum* 1990;33(12):1770–1775.
62. Pope JE, Bellamy N, Stevens A. The lack of associations between rheumatoid arthritis and both nulliparity and infertility. *Semin Arthritis Rheum* 1999;28(5):342–350.
63. van Dunne FM, Lard LR, Rook D, et al. Miscarriage but not fecundity is associated with progression of joint destruction in rheumatoid arthritis. *Ann Rheum Dis* 2004;63(8):956–960.
64. Carette S, Surtees PG, Wainwright NW, et al. The role of life events and childhood experiences in the development of rheumatoid arthritis. *J Rheumatol* 2000;27(9):2123–2130.
65. Nelson JL, Voigt LF, Koepsell TD, et al. Pregnancy outcome in women with rheumatoid arthritis before disease onset. *J Rheumatol* 1992;19(1):18–21.
66. Merlino LA, Cerhan JR, Criswell LA, et al. Estrogen and other female reproductive risk factors are not strongly associated with the development of rheumatoid arthritis in elderly women. *Semin Arthritis Rheum* 2003;33(2):72–82.
67. Karlson EW, Mandl LA, Hankinson SE, Grodstein F. Do breast-feeding and other reproductive factors influence future risk of rheumatoid arthritis? Results from the Nurses' Health Study. *Arthritis Rheum* 2004;50(11):3458–3467.
68. Brun JG, Nilssen S, Kvale G. Breast-feeding, other reproductive factors and rheumatoid-arthritis—a prospective study. *Br J Rheumatol* 1995;34(6):542–546.
69. Lankarani-Fard A, Kritz-Silverstein D, Barrett-Connor E, Goodman-Gruen D. Cumulative duration of breast-feeding influences cortisol levels in postmenopausal women. *J Womens Health Gend Based Med* 2001;10(7):681–687.
70. Brennan P, Silman A. Breast-feeding and the onset of rheumatoid arthritis. *Arthritis Rheum* 1994;37(6):808–813.
71. Voigt LF, Koepsell TD, Nelson JL, et al. Smoking, obesity, alcohol-consumption, and the risk of rheumatoid-arthritis. *Epidemiology* 1994;5(5):525–532.
72. Rudwaleit M, Andermann B, Alten R, et al. Atopic disorders in ankylosing spondylitis and rheumatoid arthritis. *Ann Rheum Dis* 2002;61(11):968–974.
73. Hilliquin P, Allanore Y, Coste J, et al. Reduced incidence and prevalence of atopy in rheumatoid arthritis. Results of a case–control study. *Rheumatology (Oxford)* 2000;39(9):1020–1026.
74. Hartung AD, Bohnert A, Hackstein H, et al. Th2-mediated atopic disease protection in Th1-mediated rheumatoid arthritis. *Clin Exp Rheumatol* 2003;21(4):481–484.
75. Verhoef CM, van Roon JAG, Vianen ME, et al. Mutual antagonism of rheumatoid arthritis and hay fever: A role for type 1 type 2 T cell balance. *Ann Rheum Dis* 1998;57(5):275–280.
76. Karsh J, Chen Y, Lin M, Dales R. The association between allergy and rheumatoid arthritis in the Canadian population. *Eur J Epidemiol* 2005;20(9):783–787.
77. Kaptanoglu E, Akkurt I, Sabin O, et al. Prevalence of atopy in rheumatoid arthritis in Sivas, Turkey. A prospective clinical study. *Rheumatol Int* 2004;24(5):267–271.
78. Olsson AR, Wingren G, Skogh T, et al. Allergic manifestations in patients with rheumatoid arthritis. *APMIS* 2003;111(10):940–944.
79. Torrey EF, Yolken RH. The schizophrenia–rheumatoid arthritis connection: Infectious, immune, or both? *Brain Behav Immun* 2001;15(4):401–410.
80. Eaton WW, Hayward C, Ram R. Schizophrenia and rheumatoid arthritis: A review. *Schizophr Res* 1992;6(3):181–192.
81. Lauerma H, Lehtinen V, Joukamaa M, et al. Schizophrenia among patients treated for rheumatoid arthritis and appendicitis. *Schizophr Res* 1998;29(3):255–261.
82. Oken RJ, Schulzer M. At issue: Schizophrenia and rheumatoid arthritis—the negative association revisited. *Schizophr Bull* 1999;25(4):625–638.
83. Mors O, Mortensen PB, Ewald H. A population-based register study of the association between schizophrenia and rheumatoid arthritis. *Schizophr Res* 1999;40(1):67–74.

Clinical Features of Rheumatoid Arthritis

SECTION II

The Onset of Rheumatoid Arthritis

CHAPTER 4

Tom W.J. Huizinga and Ferdinand C. Breedveld

Rheumatoid arthritis (RA) is a chronic potentially destructive arthritis that is defined by the presence of four out of the seven criteria that were developed by the American College of Rheumatology (ACR) in 1987. As mentioned in detail in Chapter 1, the criteria were formulated by experts based on characteristics of patients with long-standing RA (mean disease duration of 8 years).[1] Intuitively, one understands that the patients who fulfill these criteria may have different pathogenetic entities that independently lead to fulfillment of this syndrome. Indeed, data suggest that the risk factors for autoantibody-positive disease and autoantibody-negative disease may differ. Thus, the issue of when RA starts needs to be considered in the light of the different entities present in the syndrome of RA. Current evidence indicates that the identified genetic risk factors do not predispose to all RA, but only to a specific subset of the disease based on autoantibodies, and in particular ACPA (antibodies against citrinullated protein antigens), which are the most specific antibodies for RA.[2]

The current knowledge on genetic variants involved in the severity of RA is reviewed elsewhere (see Chapter 3A), but in summary, three genetic and one environmental risk factors have been identified for ACPA-positive disease and one genetic risk factor for ACPA-negative disease with an indication that the IRF5 gene is also a risk factor for ACPA-negative disease and CTLA4 and stat-4 variants are genetic risk factors for ACPA-positive disease as well[3–9] (Figure 4-1).

Pre-Disease Processes

The knowledge on pre-disease processes originates from case–control studies in which pre-disease blood samples are available. A number of abnormalities have been observed in these pre-disease samples that can be distinguished in the onset of autoantibodies, the onset of an inflammatory response, and the onset of lipid abnormalities.

Autoantibodies

In studies from Finland from the 1970s,[10,11] it was already identified that autoantibodies are present before disease onset. During more recent Dutch[12] and Swedish case–control studies,[13] these findings were replicated. For instance, the Swedish study consisted of early RA patients (mean ± SD symptom duration 7 ± 3 months; four ACR criteria fulfilled). The prevalence of autoantibodies was 34% for ACPA, 17% for IgG-RF, 20% for IgM-RF, and 34% for IgA-RF in the samples when these patients donated blood before disease (all highly significant compared with controls). The sensitivities for detecting these autoantibodies at more than 1.5 years and 1.5 years and less before the appearance of any RA symptoms were 25% and 52% for ACPA, 15% and 30% for IgM-RF, 12% and 27% for IgG-RF, and 29% and 39% for IgA-RF. Intriguingly, not only the number of antibodies increased in the pretreatment phase to disease, but also the titer of the antibodies, with a strong increase in titers the last year before arthritis develops. In the Dutch study,[12] it was found that the autoantibodies are present in a median of 4.5 years (range 0.1–13.8) before symptom onset.

Regarding risk factors for the presence of ACPA in patients before they developed RA, it was demonstrated that the main genetic risk factors like the HLA class II alleles, which form the shared epitope (SE) (for explanation, see Chapter 3A), and PTPN22 are in fact risk factors for the ACPA response instead of for RA.[13] Data to support that is that the influence of the SE allelesand ACPA on the progression from recent-onset undifferentiated arthritis (UA) to RA was determined in 570 patients

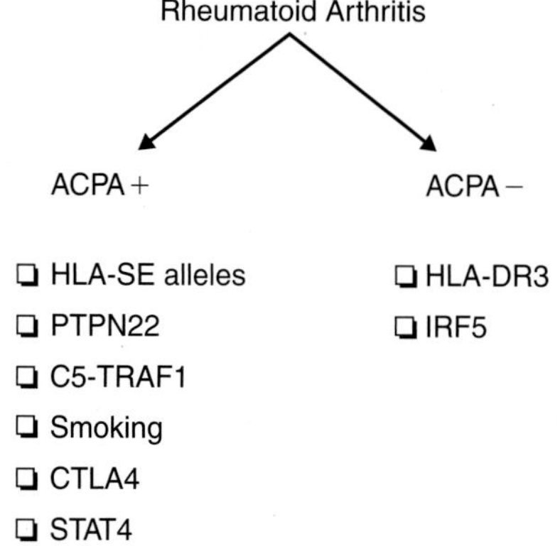

Figure 4-1. Differences in risk factors for susceptibility to ACPA-positive and ACPA-negative RA. (For explanation of the individual genes, see Chapter 3A.)

with recent-onset undifferentiated arthritis at the 2-week visit of a population-based inception cohort, the Leiden Early Arthritis Cohort[14] (Figure 4-2). A total of 177 patients with UA developed RA during the 1-year follow-up, whereas the disease in 393 patients remained unclassified or was given other diagnoses. The SE alleles correlated with the presence of ACPA. Both in SE-positive and in SE-negative patients with UA, the presence of ACPA was significantly associated with the development of RA. More intriguingly, however, no apparent contribution of the SE alleles to the progression to RA was found when analyses were stratified according to the presence of anti-CCP antibodies. Thus, the SE alleles do not independently contribute to the progression to RA from UA, but rather contribute to the development of ACPA. Very similar data have been reported for the PTPN22 gene variants, but the current studies have been underpowered to prove that PTPN22 is a risk factor for the occurrence of the ACPA response rather than for the occurrence of ACPA-positive RA.[15] For smoking as well as for the C5-TRAF polymorphism, these data are not available yet, although a recent Finish study in pre-disease samples from RA patients suggested that smoking by itself was not a risk factor for the occurrence of ACPA.[16]

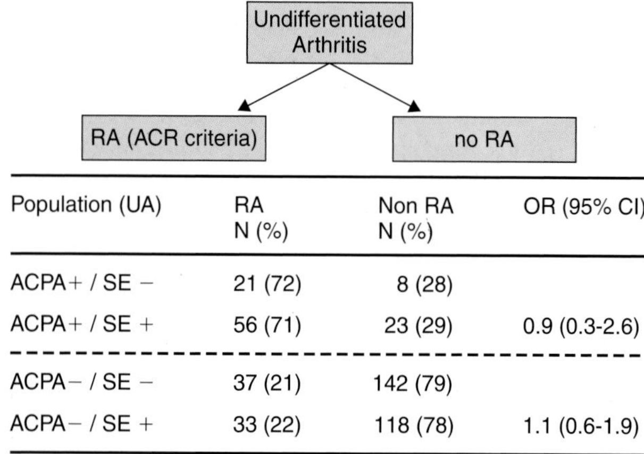

Population (UA)	RA N (%)	Non RA N (%)	OR (95% CI)
ACPA+ / SE −	21 (72)	8 (28)	
ACPA+ / SE +	56 (71)	23 (29)	0.9 (0.3-2.6)
ACPA− / SE −	37 (21)	142 (79)	
ACPA− / SE +	33 (22)	118 (78)	1.1 (0.6-1.9)

Figure 4-2. Shared epitope alleles are risk factors for ACPA, not for development of RA.

Inflammatory Markers

In the pre-disease samples of patients, more signs of preclinical disease activity have been demonstrated such as increased presence of inflammatory parameters as measured by serial measurements of C-reactive protein (CRP).[17] In the Dutch case–control study that compared pre-disease samples of RA patients with samples taken from healthy donors from the same time period, the median CRP concentration was increased in the patient group before the onset of symptoms compared with the control group. The CRP concentration increased significantly over time in patients with preclinical RA. It is somewhat controversial whether this increase is observed both in patients with and without ACPA. In the Dutch study, it was observed that although the levels in patients with ACPA were higher than in those without, in both subsets the concentration of the acute-phase response increased in pre-disease patients. In a follow-up study[18] of the same group, it was found that in the ACPA-positive subgroup a close connection in time was observed between the occurrence of serologic abnormalities and the occurrence of autoantibodies such as ACPA. However, in the Swedish study,[19] no differences in CRP levels were found in pre-disease patient samples, but for another marker of the acute-phase response, MCP1, a clear difference was found but only in the ACPA-positive patients. Monocyte chemotactic protein-1 [MCP-1] is a chemokine expressed in the synovium in patients with RA and is associated with leukocyte migration.

Whether increased levels of C-reactive protein (CRP) are associated with increased risk of subsequent RA has been evaluated.[20] In about 28,000 women of the Women's Health Study in the United States, 398 had a new diagnosis of RA. Of these, 90 cases fulfilled the ACR criteria. In age-adjusted analysis, the relative risks for developing confirmed, incident RA associated with increasing tertiles of CRP (first, second, and third) were 1.00 (reference value), 0.94 (0.54–1.61), and 1.29 (0.78–2.12). Further adjustment for randomized treatment, age, body mass index, and smoking demonstrated corresponding identical relative risks. When CRP levels were analyzed to determine whether they predicted incident RA within 4 years, between 5 to 8 years, and 9 or more years after CRP measurement, no significant associations for any time period were observed. In conclusion, the case–control studies that use healthy blood donors indicate that some dysregulation of the inflammatory response is present before disease, but the clinical relevance of such an increased acute-phase response in pre-disease patients is absent.

Atherosclerotic Events

Recent-onset RA is associated with dyslipidemia.[21] In the Dutch pre-disease samples, whether atherogenic risk factors are present before arthritis occurs has been investigated.[22] The samples of patients who later developed RA showed, on average, 4% higher total cholesterol, 9% lower HDL cholesterol, 17% higher triglyceride, and 6% higher apo B levels than matched controls ($p \leq 0.05$). Thus, the patients who later developed rheumatoid arthritis had a considerably more atherogenic lipid profile than matched blood donors at least 10 years before onset of symptoms. The authors attempted to find differences for the ACPA-positive and ACPA-negative subsets, but were not able to find differences in these relatively small groups of patients, suggesting that the atherogenetic risk profile is similar in ACPA-positive and ACPA-negative RA.

Definitions of Early Arthritis and Undifferentiated Arthritis

As it is conceivable that in the near future, clinical trials will be designed to assess treatment efficacy in patients with early undifferentiated arthritis (UA), the definition of UA, the natural course of UA, clinical characteristics that predict the progression from UA to RA, and pathophysiological differences between UA and RA are of utmost relevance.

The published trials evaluating treatment strategies in RA all include patients classified according to the 1987 ACR criteria for RA. In clinical practice, patients presenting with an early arthritis frequently have an undifferentiated disease that in time may progress to a polyarthritis fulfilling the ACR criteria for RA or may have a more benign disease course. The ACR criteria have been criticized, as they have low discriminative ability in patients presenting with a recent onset arthritis[23–27] (see also Chapter 1). This is not surprising, considering the method by which the criteria were formulated and the components of the ACR criteria. One of the criteria is the presence of erosions on the radiographs of hands and wrists. In the early phases of RA, only 13% of the patients have erosive disease.[28] Additionally, erosions often initially present in the small joints of the feet and appear in the small joints of the hands at a later point in the disease course.[29] Also, rheumatoid nodules are very rare in the early phases of RA and rheumatoid factor is present in only 50% of the patients with early RA.[30] This indicates that at present a set of criteria is needed that applies to early undifferentiated arthritis and that differentiate the UA patients that will progress to RA from those that will have a more benign disease course. Before the characteristics that predict the disease outcome in UA patients can be identified, a general acceptance on the definition for early UA is needed. In the literature, several terms that refer to arthritis of recent onset are used, but they refer to distinct categories of patients and should therefore be separated. The most frequently used terms are "early arthritis," "early RA," and UA. Early arthritis is the description of a state in which there is a mono-, oligo-, or poly-arthritis that has a recent onset. In the case of early arthritis, the disease can be undifferentiated or differentiated (Figure 4-3).

For example, about 20% of the patients that present with an early arthritis directly fulfill the ACR criteria, and thus can be classified as RA. Since the ACR criteria also state that the patients fulfill the criteria for at least 6 weeks, a disease duration of less than 6 weeks is by definition impossible in case of early RA. Patients with an early arthritis may also fulfill classification criteria for other diagnoses. Finally, those early arthritis patients that cannot be classified according to ACR criteria and in whom the arthritis is not septic or reactive in origin have per exclusion an undifferentiated arthritis. Discerning UA from early arthritis and early RA is relevant when comparing studies that describe models that predict the disease outcome or studies that assess therapeutic efficacy as the generalizability of these studies depends on the patient group that is included.

As stated above, the syndrome RA can now be identified in ACPA-positive and ACPA-negative disease. This applies to UA as well with a different disease course in these two syndromes with a much higher chance to develop RA in the ACPA-positive UA patients.[31]

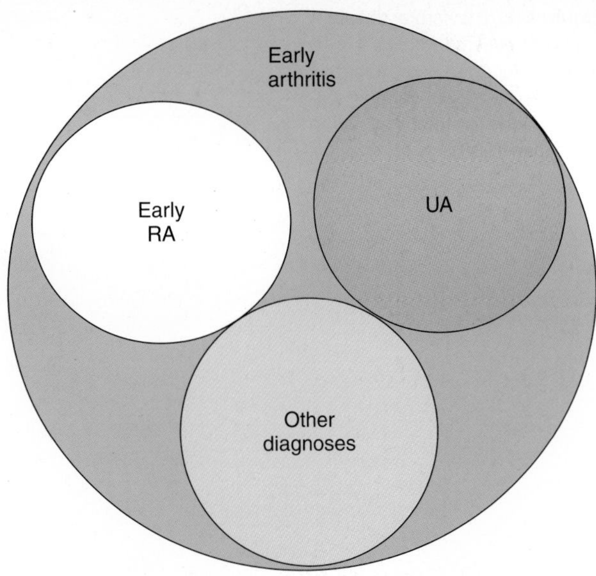

Figure 4-3. The term "early arthritis" may refer to early UA, early RA, and other classified diagnoses.

Natural Disease Course of Undifferentiated Arthritis

The natural disease course of UA is variably reported in several inception cohorts. This is due not only to the use of different definitions for UA, but also to differences in inclusion criteria for several early arthritis cohorts. For example, inclusion in the Norfolk Arthritis Registry (NOAR) (UK) required the presence of at least two swollen joints,[29] whereas inclusion in the Leeds early arthritis clinic (UK)[30] or the arthritis cohort from Wichita (United States), the presence of synovitis was not required.[32] On the other hand, some early arthritis clinics did not include patients with UA but only patients who fulfilled the criteria for RA.[33,34] Inclusion criteria from early arthritis cohorts differ not only in the presence/absence of arthritis, but also in the maximum allowed symptom duration. Patients could be included in the NOAR when the arthritis was present for at least 4 weeks, whereas symptom duration of more than 12 weeks was an exclusion criterion for the early arthritis cohort from Birmingham. Different inclusion and exclusion criteria instigate the enrollment of different groups of patients, and clarify that different results are observed when the natural disease course is studied.

Early arthritis cohorts that included all patients with at least one swollen joint reported that at initial presentation, about 20% of the patients fulfilled the criteria for RA and 35% to 54% of the patients presented with UA.[35,36] In the case of UA, the disease course was diverse: 40% to 55% remitted spontaneously,[37,38] 35% to 50%[37] developed RA, and the remaining patients developed other diagnoses or remained undifferentiated (Figure 4-4).

These data also illustrate that when evaluating studies on UA patients, the duration of symptoms are of importance for the outcome of the patient group. In other words UA from recent onset (several weeks) has a different natural course than an arthritis that after 1 year of follow-up is still unclassified (persistent undifferentiated arthritis). In the Leiden Early Arthritis Clinic, only a minority of patients who had persistent

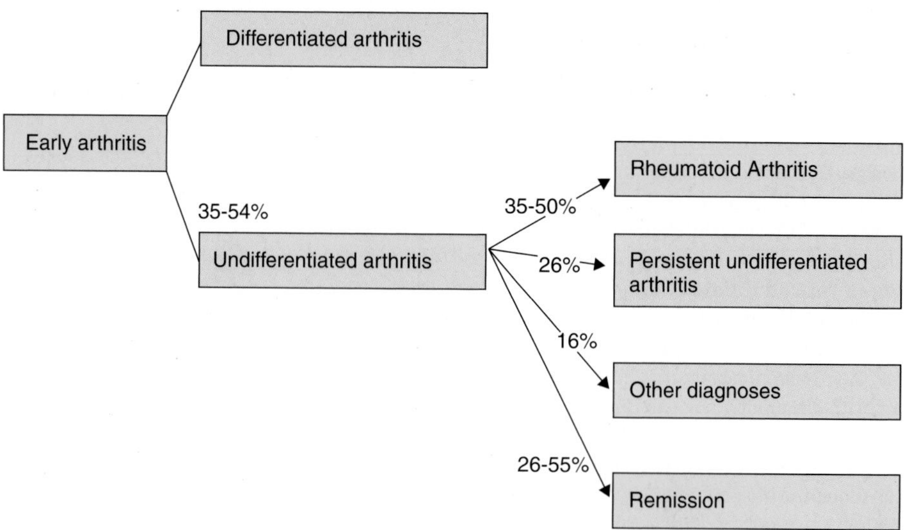

Figure 4-4. The natural disease course of patients with early arthritis and UA. Reported percentages differ among early arthritis cohorts, which explains why the total may add to more than 100%.

UA after 1 year of follow-up developed RA later in the disease course.

Intriguingly, the reported rates of spontaneous remission patients with UA are importantly different from those in RA. Whereas remission was achieved in 40% to 55% of the patients with recent-onset undifferentiated arthritis, the remission rate in RA is less than 10% to 15%.[39–41] Apparently, the chance to achieve a natural remission becomes smaller when the disease process is more mature. This supports the notion that chronicity might be more easily reversed in the UA phase.

Predicting Progression from Undifferentiated Arthritis to Rheumatoid Arthritis

As UA has a variable disease course and disease-modifying antirheumatic drug (DMARD) therapy is potentially toxic, only the UA patients that have a high probability of developing RA are preferentially treated with DMARDs, whereas the patients who will achieve a spontaneous remission will preferentially not receive these drugs. This underlines the need for a model able to predict the disease outcome in individual patients with UA. Initial attempts to define such prognostic criteria have been made by Visser et al.[42] based on the Leiden Early Arthritis Cohort. This model predicts disease persistency and development of erosions. For the development of this model, all early arthritis patients were included and not only patients with UA. As the model of Visser et al. was not developed using specifically patients with UA, this model is not optimal for guiding individualized treatment decisions in UA. Recently, a model that predicts the disease outcome in individual patients with UA was developed, also based on the Leiden Early Arthritis Cohort.[43] From a total cohort of 1700 early arthritis patients, 570 patients presented with UA. After 1 year of follow-up, 31% of the UA patients had progressed to RA. The remaining two-thirds had developed other diagnoses (16%), achieved spontaneous remission (26%), or remained unclassified (26%). Clinical characteristics between the UA patients that had and had not developed RA were compared; using logistic regression analysis, the variables that were independent predictors for the development of RA were selected. This resulted in the construction of a prediction rule[43] (Tables 4-1 and 4-2).

The discriminative ability of this prediction rule was assessed by the area under the receiver operator curve, which was 0.89 for the derivation cohort and 0.97 for the replication cohort.

Table 4-1. Form Used to Calculate Prediction Score in Points for Individual Patients with Undifferentiated Arthritis

1.	Age in years	Multiply by 0.02	
2.	Gender	If female	1 point
3.	Distribution of involved joints	If small joints in hands/feet	0.5 point
		If symmetric	0.5 point
		If upper extremities	1 point
		If upper and lower extremities	1.5 points
4.	Length of VAS morning stiffness (range 0–100 mm)	If 26–90 mm	1 point
		If >90 mm	2 points
5.	Number of tender joints	If 4–10	0.5 point
		If ≥11	1 point
6.	Number of swollen joints	If 4–10	0.5 point
		If ≥11	1 point
7.	C-reactive protein level (mg/L)	If 5–50	0.5 point
		If ≥51	1.5 points
8.	Positive rheumatoid factor	If yes	1 point
9.	Positive anti-CCP antibodies	If yes	2 points
	Total score		

Table 4-2. Observed Chances to Progress to Rheumatoid Arthritis for Various Prediction Scores

Prediction Score	Non-RA n	(%)	RA n	(%)
0	1	(100)	0	(0)
1	8	(100)	0	(0)
2	42	(100)	0	(0)
3	58	(100)	0	(0)
4	78	(93)	6	(7)
5	73	(85)	13	(15)
6	63	(74)	22	(26)
7	37	(49)	38	(51)
8	16	(33)	33	(67)
9	6	(14)	36	(86)
10	5	(23)	17	(77)
11	0	(0)	8	(100)
12	0	(0)	1	(100)
13	0	(0)	1	(100)
14	0		0	
Total	387		175	

The total prediction score ranged between 0 and 14. All patients with a score of less than 4 did not progress and all patients with a score of more than 10 did progress to RA. With the cut-off levels less than 6 and more than 8, the negative and positive predictive values were 91% and 84%, respectively. As this prediction rule consists of nine variables that are regularly assessed at the outpatient clinic (age, gender, distribution of involved joints, morning stiffness severity, number of tender and swollen joints, C-reactive proteins, rheumatoid factor, and anti-CCP antibodies), this prediction rule can be easily applied in daily practice. Moreover, as the prediction rule estimates the chance for an individual patient to progress to RA as a percentage, application of this rule might facilitate the involvement of patients themselves in treatment decision making. This model was recently replicated in both Germany and the UK.[44] As can be seen from the prediction models the chance of progression of RA is higher in ACPA positive disease than in ACPA negative disease, strongly pointing to differences in disease course in these different disease subsets.[3,9,31]

Presentation Patterns of ACPA+ Versus ACPA– Disease

The various risk factors for ACPA-positive disease (smoking, shared epitope, PTPN22, and C5-TRAF) and ACPA-negative disease, as well as the difference in progression rates between ACPA-positive and ACPA-negative UA, raise the question of whether anti-CCP–positive and –negative RA are different disease entities with distinct clinical characteristics. In a detailed study in which 228 incident RA patients with and 226 without ACPA were extensively compared with regard to clinical characteristics, no differences were observed.[45] After 4 years of follow-up, patients with ACPA had more swollen joints and more severe radiologic destruction. In conclusion, the phenotype of RA patients with or without ACPA is similar with respect to clinical presentation but differs with respect to disease course.[45] In contrast to the absence of clinical characteristics, differences have been observed in the comparison of synovial tissue infiltrate of patients with ACPA-positive versus ACPA-negative RA.[46] Although it is obviously not easy to compare histology when arthritis develops, an attempt was made by comparing biopsies from early and late disease. Synovial tissue from 34 ACPA-positive patients had a higher number of infiltrating lymphocytes (61.6 vs 31.4 per HPF [400x], $p = 0.01$), less extensive fibrosis (1.2 vs 1.9, $p = 0.04$) and a thinner synovial lining layer (2.1 vs 3.3, $p < 0.01$) than the tissues from 23 ACPA-negative patients. Synovial tissues from the ACPA-positive patients expressed more CD3, CD8, CD45RO, and CXCL-12. Joint damage, assessed using the Kellgren and Lawrence (K&L) grade on standard anteroposterior radiographs, was greater in ACPA-positive than ACPA-negative patients. The difference in lymphocyte count was already present 3.8 years before the index biopsy (76.7 vs 26.7 in the ACPA positive vs the ACPA-negative patients; $p = 0.008$), and independent of disease duration and K&L score. These data indicate that the risk factors, the chance of progression from UA to RA, and histology are different for ACPA-positive and ACPA-negative disease.

Biologic Differences from Pre-Disease States to Undifferentiated Arthritis and Rheumatoid Arthritis

A number of studies have looked at serum markers to study the specific processes during the disease course. These studies point that the evolution of pre-disease to undifferentiated arthritis to RA reflects an ongoing immune response during which the disease process acquires different characteristics.

In one study from the United States,[47] it was shown that the rheumatoid factor isotypes IgM, IgA, and IgG appeared a median of 3.8, 3.2, and 0.9 years prior to diagnosis, respectively, and that the ACPA appeared a median of 3.3 years prior to diagnosis. The median times of appearance of ACPA and all cytokines/chemokines tested were within 2 years of diagnosis. The median time of symptom onset prior to diagnosis was 0.5 years. These data indicate that first tolerance to autoantigens is broken during the preclinical period of RA development (as measured by early RF-IgM and ACPA positivity) followed by sequential abnormalities in class-switched RF, cytokines/chemokines, and CRP as onset of symptomatic disease approached.

The evolution of the autoantibody response has been analyzed in detail during development of RA in the Leiden cohort from the Netherlands in patients with UA, recent-onset RA, and RA after long disease duration.[48] Figure 4-5 shows that a lower number of isotypes were observed in UA compared to RA. Intriguingly, when the patients with UA were divided in those who developed RA within 3 months compared to those who developed RA after 1 year, it was clearly shown that the number of isotypes used reflects the development of RA fulfilling the ACR criteria.

These data indicate development into full usage of the ACPA isotype repertoire early in the disease process. The sustained presence of IgM ACPA indicates an ongoing recruitment of

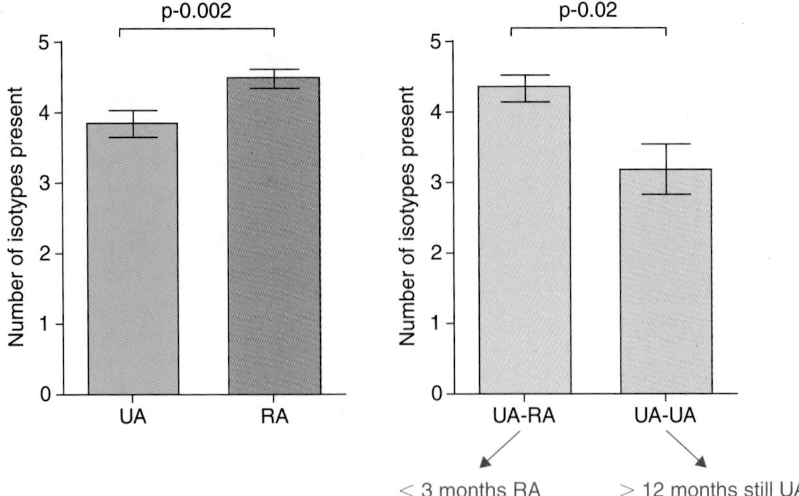

Figure 4-5. The ACPA reaction in UA patients that progress to RA display a broader isotype usage.

new B cells into the ACPA response, reflecting a continuous (re)activation of the RA-specific ACPA response during the disease course. Similar data have been presented with regard to the development of the specificity of the ACPA response, both in the Leiden cohort as in the pre-disease samples of the American army, it was observed that the immune response as measured by the reactivity of ACPA to a number of citrinullated peptides became broader during the development of the pre-disease stage to UA to RA.[49,50]

In conclusion, the biological mechanisms underlying UA and RA differ both in quantity (e.g., level of proinflammatory cytokines) and quality (e.g., isotype usage and specificity of the autoantibody response). Apparently, UA patients that have more of these quantitative or qualitative traits have a concomitant higher risk to progress to RA.

Outcomes of Treatment in Undifferentiated Arthritis

Almost all clinical trials of therapeutic strategies have included patients with (early or long-standing) RA. At present there is one study that assessed the efficacy of methotrexate (MTX) in patients with UA.[51,52] In this double-blind clinical trial, patients were randomized for treatment with either methotrexate or placebo. Patients were followed for 30 months and both progression toward RA and level of joint destruction were measured. A significantly lower number of MTX-treated UA patients had progressed to RA compared to the placebo-treated patients. In addition, the UA patients that were treated with methotrexate had a significantly lower lever of radiologic joint destruction, indicating a less severe disease course. Interestingly, after the cessation of methotrexate at 18 months, the difference in the number of patients who developed RA remained statistically significant but the difference became smaller. This suggests that in some patients methotrexate had hampered the progression of the disease, but had not been able to totally stop the underlying pathophysiologic mechanisms. These data have to be replicated in other studies, and hopefully future targeted therapies will be able to fully halt the development of persistent arthritis. Nevertheless, the data of this study are promising as they indicate that treatment in an early phase of RA, before the disease is established, is effective. Treatment trials in the pre-disease stages have been proposed, but no data have been presented yet.

Conclusion

The question of when RA develops can partly be answered for the ACPA-positive subset. The autoantibody response develops on average about 4 years[12] before RA. Subsequently, the autoantibody response develops by wider isotype usage and broader reactivity and the occurrence of inflammatory markers and dyslipidemia. Next, UA develops, and by a further ongoing immune response the patients will develop RA over time. Treatment trials in UA indicate that interference in this stage is possible. Prediction rules to prevent overtreatment in UA patients have been developed and validated in several European countries, and can be used in clinical practice to prevent overtreatment in these patients in which a substantial portion of patients achieve a spontaneous remission as well.

References

1. Harrison BJ, Symmons DP, Barrett EM, Silman AJ. The performance of the 1987 ARA classification criteria for rheumatoid arthritis in a population based cohort of patients with early inflammatory polyarthritis. American Rheumatism Association. *J Rheumatol* 1998;25(12):2324–2330.
2. Nishimura K, Sugiyama D, Kogata Y, et al. Meta-analysis: Diagnostic accuracy of anti-cyclic citrullinated peptide antibody and rheumatoid factor for rheumatoid arthritis. *Ann Intern Med* 2007;146(11):797–808.
3. Huizinga TW, Amos CI, van der Helm-van Mil AH, et al. Refining the complex rheumatoid arthritis phenotype based on specificity of the HLA-DRB1 shared epitope for antibodies to citrullinated proteins. *Arthritis Rheum* 2005;52(11):3433–3438.
4. Van der Helm-van Mil AH, Verpoort KN, Breedveld FC, et al. The HLA-DRB1 shared epitope alleles are primarily a risk factor for anti-CCP antibodies and are not an independent risk factor to develop RA. *Arthritis Rheum* 2006;54(4):1117–1121.

5. Begovich AB, Carlton VE, Honigberg LA, et al. A missense single-nucleotide polymorphism in a gene encoding a protein tyrosine phosphatase (PTPN22) is associated with rheumatoid arthritis. *Am J Hum Genet* 2004;75(2):330–337.
6. Van Oene M, Wintle RF, Liu X, et al. Association of the lymphoid tyrosine phosphatase R620W variant with rheumatoid arthritis, but not Crohn's disease, in Canadian populations. *Arthritis Rheum* 2005;52(7):1993–1998.
7. Gomez LM, Anaya JM, Gonzalez CI, et al. PTPN22 C1858T polymorphism in Colombian patients with autoimmune diseases. *Genes Immun* 2005;6(7):628–631.
8. Wesoly J, van der Helm-van Mil AH, Toes RE, et al. Association of the PTPN22 C1858T single-nucleotide polymorphism with rheumatoid arthritis phenotypes in an inception cohort. *Arthritis Rheum* 2005;52(9):2948–2950.
9. Kallberg H, Padyukov L, Plenge RM, et al. Gene-gene and gene-environment interactions involving HLA-DR, PTPN22 and smoking in two subsets of rheumatoid arthritis. *Am J Hum Genet* 2007;80(5):867–875.
10. Aho K, Heliovaara M, Maatela J, et al. Rheumatoid factors antedating clinical rheumatoid arthritis. *J Rheumatol* 1991;18: 1282–1284.
11. Aho K, von Essen R, Kurki P, et al. Antikeratin antibody and antiperinuclear factor as markers for subclinical rheumatoid disease process. *J Rheumatol* 1993;20:1278–1281.
12. Nielen MM, van Schaardenburg D, Reesink HW, et al. Specific autoantibodies precede the symptoms of rheumatoid arthritis: A study of serial measurements in blood donors. *Arthritis Rheum* 2004;50:380–386.
13. Rantapaa-Dahlqvist S, de Jong BA, Berglin E, et al. Antibodies against cyclic citrullinated peptide and IgA rheumatoid factor predict the development of rheumatoid arthritis. *Arthritis Rheum* 2003;48(10):2741–2749.
14. Van der Helm-van Mil AH, Verpoort KN, Breedveld FC, et al. The HLA-DRB1 shared epitope alleles are primarily a risk factor for anti-cyclic citrullinated peptide antibodies and are not an independent risk factor for development of rheumatoid arthritis. *Arthritis Rheum* 2006;54(4):1117–1121.
15. Feitsma AL, Toes RE, Begovich AB, et al. *Rheumatology (Oxford)* Risk of progression from undifferentiated arthritis to rheumatoid arthritis: The effect of the PTPN22 1858T-allele in anti-citrullinated peptide antibody positive patients. *Rheumatology (Oxford)* 2007; 46(7):1092–1095.
16. Koivula MK, Heliövaara M, Ramberg J, et al. Autoantibodies binding to citrullinated telopeptide of type II collagen and to cyclic citrullinated peptides predict synergistically the development of seropositive rheumatoid arthritis. *Ann Rheum Dis* 2007;66: 1450–1455.
17. Nielen MM, van Schaardenburg D, Reesink HW, et al. Increased levels of C-reactive protein in serum from blood donors before the onset of rheumatoid arthritis. *Arthritis Rheum* 2004;50: 2423–2427.
18. Nielen MM, van Schaardenburg D, Reesink HW, et al. Simultaneous development of acute phase response and autoantibodies in preclinical rheumatoid arthritis. *Ann Rheum Dis* 2006;65(4): 535–537.
19. Rantapaa-Dahlqvist S, Boman K, Tarkowski A, et al. Up regulation of monocyte chemoattractant protein-1 expression in anti-citrulline antibody and immunoglobulin M rheumatoid factor positive subjects precedes onset of inflammatory response and development of overt rheumatoid arthritis. *Ann Rheum Dis* 2007; 66(1):121–123.
20. Shadick NA, Cook NR, Karlson EW, et al. C-reactive protein in the prediction of rheumatoid arthritis in women. *Arch Intern Med* 2006;166(22):2490–2494.
21. Georgiadis AN, Papavasiliou EC, Lourida ES, et al. Atherogenic lipid profile is a feature characteristic of patients with early rheumatoid arthritis: effect of early treatment—a prospective, controlled study. *Arthritis Res Ther* 2006;8(3):R82.
22. van Halm VP, Nielen MM, Nurmohamed MT, et al. Lipids and inflammation: serial measurements of the lipid profile of blood donors who later developed rheumatoid arthritis. *Ann Rheum Dis* 2007;66(2):184–188.
23. Pincus T, Callahan LF. What is the natural history of rheumatoid arthritis? *Rheum Dis Clin North Am* 1993;19(1):123–151.
24. Harrison B, Symmons D. Early inflammatory polyarthritis: Results from the Norfolk Arthritis Register with a review of the literature. II. Outcome at three years. *Rheumatology (Oxford)* 2000;39(9): 939–949.
25. Symmons DP, Hazes JM, Silman AJ. Cases of early inflammatory polyarthritis should not be classified as having rheumatoid arthritis. *J Rheumatol* 2003;30(5):902–904.
26. Green M, Marzo-Ortega H, McGonagle D, et al. Persistence of mild, early inflammatory arthritis: The importance of disease duration, rheumatoid factor, and the shared epitope. *Arthritis Rheum* 1999;42:2184–2188.
27. Machold KP, Stamm TA, Eberl GJ, et al. Very recent onset arthritis—clinical, laboratory, and radiological findings during the first year of disease. *J Rheumatol* 2002;29(11):2278–2287.
28. Van der Heijde DM, van Leeuwen MA, van Riel PL. Radiographic progression on radiographs of hands and feet during the first 3 years of rheumatoid arthritis measured according to Sharp's method (van der Heijde modification). *J Rheumatol* 1995;22(9): 1792–1796.
29. Symmons DP, Silman AJ. The Norfolk Arthritis Register (NOAR). *Clin Exp Rheumatol* 2003;21(5 Suppl 31):S94–S99.
30. Quinn MA, Green MJ, Marzo-Ortega H, et al. Prognostic factors in a large cohort of patients with early undifferentiated inflammatory arthritis after application of a structured management protocol. *Arthritis Rheum* 2003;48(11):3039–3045.
31. Van Gaalen FA, Linn-Rasker SP, van Venrooij WJ, et al. Autoantibodies to cyclic citrullinated peptides predict progression to rheumatoid arthritis in patients with undifferentiated arthritis: A prospective cohort study. *Arthritis Rheum* 2004;50(3):709–715.
32. Wolfe F, Ross K, Hawley DJ, et al. The prognosis of rheumatoid arthritis and undifferentiated polyarthritis syndrome in the clinic: A study of 1141 patients. *J Rheumatol* 1993;20(12):2005–2009.
33. Sokka T. Early rheumatoid arthritis in Finland. *Clin Exp Rheumatol* 2003;21(5 Suppl 31):S133–S137.
34. Kvien TK, Uhlig T. The Oslo experience with arthritis registries. *Clin Exp Rheumatol* 2003;21(5 Suppl 31):S118–S122.
35. Van Aken J, van Bilsen JH, Allaart CF, et al. The Leiden Early Arthritis Clinic. *Clin Exp Rheumatol* 2003;21(5 Suppl 31):S100–S105.
36. Hulsemann JL, Zeidler H. Undifferentiated arthritis in an early synovitis out-patient clinic. *Clin Exp Rheumatol* 1995;13(1):37–43.
37. Van Aken J, Van Dongen H, le Cessie S, et al. Long-term outcome of rheumatoid arthritis that presented with undifferentiated arthritis compared to rheumatoid arthritis at presentation—an observational cohort study. *Ann Rheum Dis* 2006;65(1):20–25.
38. Tunn EJ, Bacon PA. Differentiating persistent from self-limiting symmetrical synovitis in an early arthritis clinic. *Br J Rheumatol* 1993;32(2):97–103.
39. Harrison BJ, Symmons DP, Brennan P, et al. Natural remission in inflammatory polyarthritis: Issues of definition and prediction. *Br J Rheumatol* 1996;35(11):1096–1100.
40. Linn-Rasker SP, Allaart CF, Kloppenburg M, et al. Sustained remission in a cohort of patients with RA: Association with absence of IgM-rheumatoid factor and absence of anti-CCP antibodies. *Int J Adv Rheumatol* 2004:2(4):4–6.
41. Van der Helm-van Mil AH, Dieude P, Schonkeren JJ, et al. No association between tumour necrosis factor receptor type 2 gene polymorphism and rheumatoid arthritis severity: A comparison of the extremes of phenotypes. *Rheumatology (Oxford)* 2004;43(10): 1232–1234.

42. Visser H, le Cessie S, Vos K, et al. How to diagnose rheumatoid arthritis early: A prediction model for persistent (erosive) arthritis. *Arthritis Rheum* 2002;46(2):357–365.
43. Van der Helm-van Mil AH, le Cessie S, van Dongen H, et al. A rule to predict disease outcome in patients with recent-onset undifferentiated arthritis to guide individual treatment decisions. *Arthritis Rheum* 2007;56(2):433–440.
44. Van der Helm-van Mil AHM, Detert J, le Cessie S, et al. Moving towards individualized treatment decision making: Validation of a prediction rule for disease outcome in patients with recent-onset undifferentiated arthritis. Arthritis Rheum, 2008, in press.
45. Van der Helm-van Mil AH, Verpoort KN, Breedveld FC, et al. Antibodies to citrullinated proteins and differences in clinical progression of rheumatoid arthritis. *Arthritis Res Ther* 2005;7(5): R949–R958.
46. Van Oosterhout M, Bajema I, Levarht EW, et al. Differences in synovial tissue infiltrates between anti-cyclic citrullinated peptide-positive rheumatoid arthritis and anti-cyclic citrullinated peptide-negative rheumatoid arthritis. *Arthritis Rheum* 2008;58(1): 53–60.
47. Deane KD, Hueber W, Lazar AM, et al. Autoantibodies precede cytokine/chemokine and C-reactive protein elevations in the preclinical period of rheumatoid arthritis (RA) development. *Arthritis Rheum* 2007;56(9, suppl):s319 [abstract 748].
48. Verpoort KN, Jol-van der Zijde CM, Papendrecht-van der Voort EAM, et al. Isotype distribution of anti-citrullinated peptide antibodies (ACPA) in undifferentiated arthritis and rheumatoid arthritis reflects an ongoing immune response. *Arthritis Rheum* 2006; 54(12):3799–3808.
49. Verpoort KN, Cheung K, Ioan-Facsinay A, et al. Fine-specificity of the ACPA response is influenced by shared epitope alleles. *Arthritis Res Ther* 2007;9(Suppl 3):P16.
50. Hueber WJ, Tomooka BH, Deane K, et al. Autoantibody profiling in pre-disease RA samples. *Arthritis Rheum* 2007;56(9, suppl):s517 [abstract 1289].
51. Van Gaalen F, Ioan-Facsinay A, Huizinga TW, et al. The devil in the details: The emerging role of anticitrulline autoimmunity in rheumatoid arthritis. *J Immunol* 2005;175(9):5575–5580.
52. Van Dongen H, van Aken J, Lard LR, et al. Efficacy of methotrexate treatment in patients with probable rheumatoid arthritis: A double-blind, randomized, placebo-controlled trial. *Arthritis Rheum* 2007; 56(5):1424–1432.

Articular and Periarticular Manifestations of Established Rheumatoid Arthritis

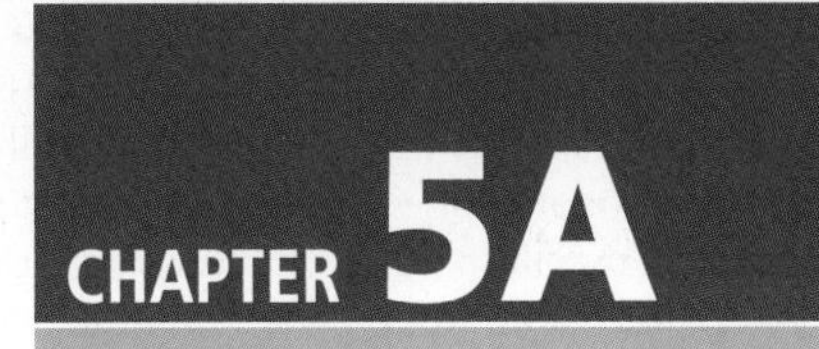

Jana Posalski and Michael H. Weisman

It is critical to have an appreciation for when true rheumatoid arthritis (RA) begins and separates itself from other forms of arthritis that are self-limiting or represent another diagnosis. Several recent studies indicate the value of early diagnosis and prompt appropriate intervention in patients with rheumatoid arthritis (RA) in order to avoid the development of irreversible joint damage and creation of functional disability.[1,2]

Recognizing the features of early RA can be challenging. Lessons from early arthritis clinics reveal that self-limited disease can present with mono-, oligo-, or polyarticular inflammatory arthritis and can closely mimic the onset of RA. In the Leiden Early Arthritis Clinic, at 2 weeks, only 10% of patients met criteria for established RA, and one third were considered undifferentiated arthritis (UA). Only about a third of these UA patients ended up evolving into RA, and the rest remitted spontaneously, continued to be UA, or developed into other chronic rheumatic diseases.[3]

ACR classification criteria identify those patients with established disease; these criteria cannot be used to identify early presenters.[4] Several studies have attempted to characterize the clinical features of early RA patients that could predict the development of persistent established disease.[5–9] Visser and colleagues[5] devised a clinical prediction model, developed from the Leiden Early Arthritis Cohort, for the purpose of distinguishing between self-limited and persistent disease (see Chapter 4 for detailed discussion). By using scores based on symptom duration at first visit, morning stiffness, arthritis in three or more joints, compression pain in bilateral MTPs, presence of IgM-RF (rheumatoid factor), anti-CCP antibodies, and erosions on hand and foot radiographs, they were able to determine the probability of self-limited versus persistent nonerosive or persistent erosive disease. The symptom duration criterion was the strongest predictor of persistent disease; patterns of joint involvement were not predictive.[5] Schumacher et al. also evaluated predictive factors in early arthritis and observed that patients with polyarticular disease and those with hand involvement were most likely to be persistent.[6]

In the Leiden clinic, these investigators observed that the number of swollen joints, male gender, and negative tests for rheumatoid factor and CCP antibody were more predictive of self-limited disease, while the presence of HLA class II alleles, especially the shared epitope, were more associated with persistent disease. In a small study intended to establish risk of RA outcome at 1 year for patients who had mild forms of arthritis at presentation, Green et al.[8] noted that duration of signs and symptoms at more than 3 months was the strongest predictor of RA, with little effect noted for either number of active joints at presentation or their distribution. Similarly, Quinn et al.[9] evaluated 100 consecutive patients with early undifferentiated arthritis of the hands, and found that the best predictor of patients who would require future disease-modifying antirheumatic drug (DMARD) therapy was persistent synovitis at 12 weeks.

It is safe to argue from the present state of our knowledge (although not necessarily comforting to know) that only duration of signs and symptoms for a minimum 3 months, without necessarily specifying any particular joint distribution, remains the most important clinical criteria that identify patients who are most likely to result in having established RA. Therefore it is in this group of patients where the risk of aggressive treatment is most justified.

What are the Clinical Features of Established Rheumatoid Arthritis?

The course of established RA can range from mild disease to rapidly progressive multisystem inflammation. About 70% of patients who have RA display a slow, insidious disease onset; 20% have an intermediate onset; and 10% have a sudden acute onset.[9] Patients predominantly complain of pain, stiffness, and swelling of their peripheral joints as the cardinal features of the disease. Physical examination of the joints reveals tenderness to palpation, synovial thickening, joint effusion, and sometimes erythema and warmth. With longer duration of disease, there may be decreased range of motion with the much later possibility of joint ankylosis and subluxation.[10] Initial involvement occurs in the upper extremities in over half of patients, with multiple joints affected in one-third and hand only involvement in about one-quarter of the cases. Joint symptoms are initially symmetric in 70% of patients or become symmetric by 1 year after onset in 85%.[9] The joints most commonly affected are the proximal interphalangeal (PIP) and metacarpophalangeal (MCP) joints of the hands and wrists, followed by the metatarsophalangeal (MTP) joints of the feet, ankles, and shoulders.[11] It has been observed that the distal interphalangeal (DIP) joints of the fingers are not affected initially in most patients.

There appear to be patterns of joint complaints mixed in with laboratory abnormalities that may have some prognostic significance; for example, patients with early patterns of large proximal joints coupled with MCP I and II involvement appear to have a worse prognosis. Older patients who have shoulder, elbow, wrist, and knee complaints and are seropositive tend to have more serious outcomes, and the association of MCP I and II involvement alone with seropositivity appears to result in more severe as well as erosive disease. Those with MCP II, III, IV, and V involvement tend to be younger and have a more benign disease process. Those with MTPs II, III, IV, and V and ankle and midtarsal joints have been shown to have greater risk for erosive disease.[11]

Once the disease is established, laboratory tests and imaging provide data to monitor patients' status, and some of these measures appear to have prognostic significance as well. Lindqvist et al. observed that the erythrocyte sedimentation rate (ESR) and IgA-RF were the strongest predictors of joint damage in both hands and feet after 5 years of disease, and that anti-CCP antibodies were the only significant predictor of damage after 10 years of disease.[12] Anti-CCP antibodies are particularly important in seronegative patients, as they confer an increased likelihood of radiographic erosive disease and disability.[13] Future studies may prove that anti-MCV (modified citrullinated vimentin) antibodies are more sensitive than anti-CCP as a susceptibility as well as a severity marker for RA.[14]

Radiographic evidence of joint destruction from synovitis is seen in more than 70% of patients within their first 2 years of disease.[10] Radiographic damage appears to take place most rapidly over the first few years, but patients continue to show progressive joint damage for over 20 years.[15] The hallmarks of RA on radiography are symmetric alignment abnormalities, periarticular osteoporosis, joint space narrowing with marginal erosions, periarticular soft tissue swelling, and possibly rheumatoid nodules and synovial cysts in some patients (Figure 5A-1). Other modalities such as ultrasound, computed tomography (CT), and magnetic resonance imaging (MRI) can also be helpful diagnostically when physical findings are equivocal or plain radiography is normal. Ultrasound can help to evaluate soft tissue pathology, aid in aspiration of synovial fluid or injection of medications into the joint, or to assess for erosions. CT resolution has improved greatly for musculoskeletal imaging of certain areas where three-dimensional imaging is important, and MRI can evaluate bone and all the articular structures without exposing the patient to ionizing radiation.[16] Recent studies of MRI versus CT have found similarities in detection of bony erosions in RA.[17] MRI can reveal synovial hypertrophy, bone edema, and early erosive changes as early as 4 months after disease onset[10] (Figures 5A-2 and 5A-3). Recent studies have shown that both bone erosions and bone marrow edema on MRI are due to inflammatory infiltrates,[18] and bone marrow edema on MRI is associated with erosive progression and poor functional outcome.[19]

There are several RA subsets that have subtle differences distinguishing them from classic seropositive RA. Seronegative RA is diagnosed in as many as 15% to 20% of RA patients. These patients ultimately meet all of the usual criteria for RA; however, they are RF-negative.[20] Histologically, there appear to be no significant differences in objective measures of synovial inflammation.[21] Palindromic rheumatism is a disease characterized by acute, recurrent "palindromic" attacks of oligoarticular arthritis with prominent peri- and para-articular tissue inflammation, sometimes associated with nodules; however, no bone or cartilage destruction takes place, and a favorable long-term prognosis is the typical course. Nearly 50% of cases, however, eventually turn into typical RA with RF positivity.[22]

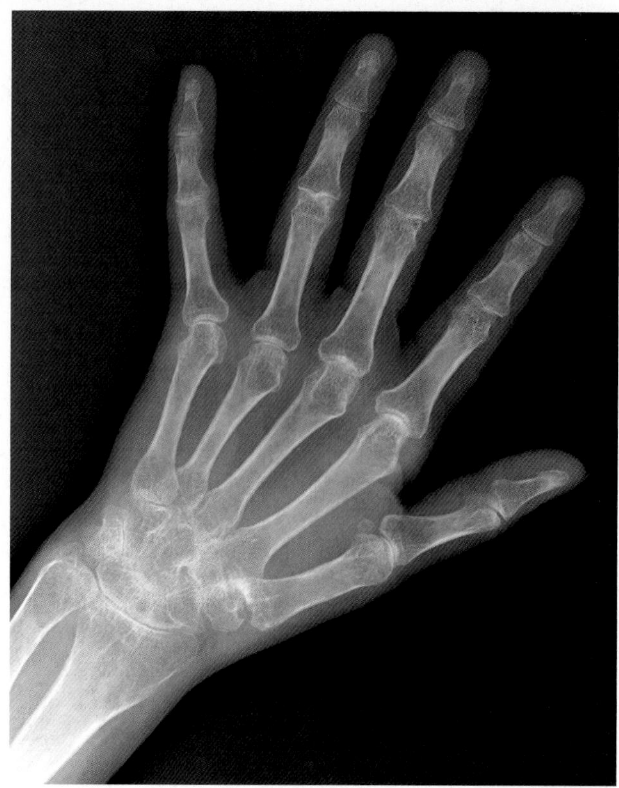

Figure 5A-1. Typical abnormalities of RA are illustrated in this radiograph of the left hand. Soft tissue swelling is present around the metacarpophalangeal joints and wrist with diffuse narrowing of MCP, PIP, and radiocarpal joint spaces. Erosions are seen at the first CMC joint and distal ulna. Periarticular osteopenia surrounds all of the articulations.

The issue of RA in the elderly has been the subject of debate as to whether it is a distinct disease from classic, younger-onset RA. In the population of people aged 60 years and older, the prevalence of RA is about 2%,[23] and these patients usually have a more acute onset with disabling morning stiffness and pain in the upper extremities, especially in the shoulder joints. They possess very high elevations of ESR, and the female predominance is not as strong as in younger-onset RA. The RF test may have more limited diagnostic utility in these cases since false-positive tests for RF increase with age; however, CCP may be more specific[23] and diagnostically useful. Although polymyalgia rheumatica may share the DR4 haplotype and could present with peripheral arthritis, it is characterized by a very acute onset of pain, stiffness and myalgias in the hip and shoulder girdle, negative RF and anti-CCP tests, and markedly elevated ESR, and usually responds rapidly to low-dose prednisone. This constellation of signs and symptoms typically occur in patients older than 50 years.[24] Remitting seronegative symmetric synovitis with pitting edema (RS3PE) is an acute onset of symmetric polysynovitis involving peripheral joints and flexor digitorum tendons associated with pitting

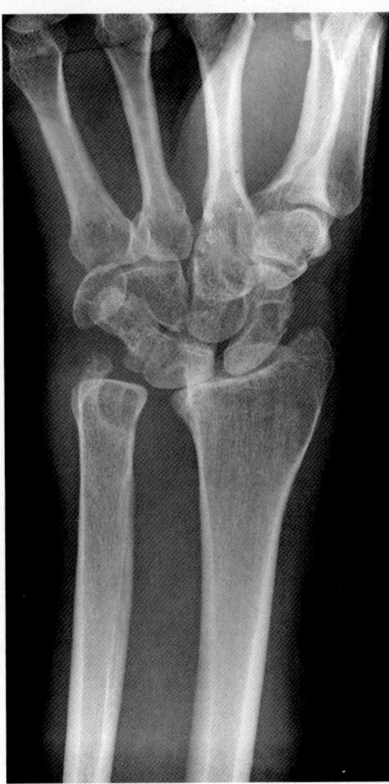

Figure 5A-2. Radiograph of the left wrist reveals soft-tissue swelling with narrowing about the radial carpal joint associated with early reactive sclerosis involving the radial articular surface. There is widening of the distal radial–ulnar joint and cysts are present within the carpal navicular and distal ulna.

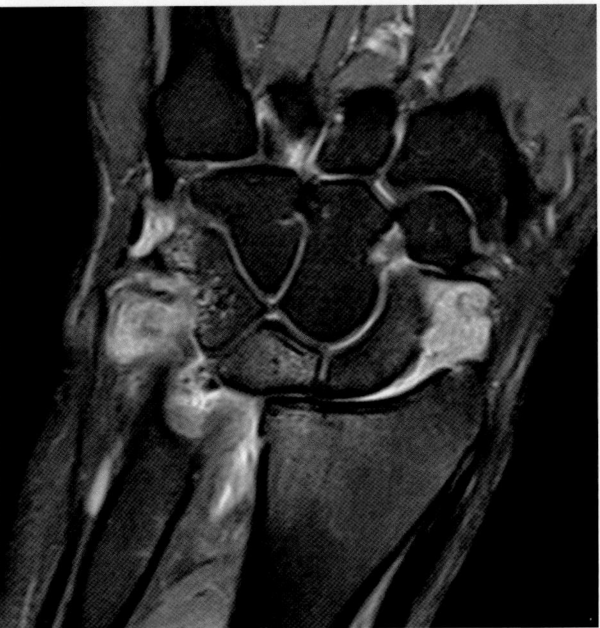

Figure 5A-3. An MRI of the left wrist of the same patient in Figure 5A-2 reveals multiple bony erosions in the ulna, lunate, triquetrum, and distal radius. Complete loss of articular cartilage is noted within the radiocarpal articulation with slight ulnar shift of the carpus. Exuberant synovial proliferation with inflamed synovium is seen to enter the large erosion within the distal ulna, illustrating the extensive synovitis that is missed on conventional radiography.

edema of the dorsum of the hands and feet (Figure 5A-4). The onset is so acute that patients often recall the exact time they were first affected. These patients are seronegative, and there are no erosive changes on radiography. Patients usually completely remit with only mild flexion deformities and without functional impairment.[25]

Adult-onset Still's disease can mimic RA when patients present with arthritis, but the typical patient comes to medical attention with major systemic signs and symptoms of high spiking fevers returning to normal in each 24-hour period, evanescent salmon-pink colored rash (Figure 5A-5) associated with the fevers, impressive leukocytosis and thrombocytosis, and with the minor criteria of sore throat, lymphadenopathy, splenomegaly, liver dysfunction, and seronegativity.[26] Additionally, very elevated levels of ferritin and glycosylated ferritin can aid with diagnosis.[27] It is the authors' repeated observation that the diagnosis is usually made in a hospitalized patient after an exasperating search for a diagnosis by both oncologists and infectious disease specialists is unsuccessful.

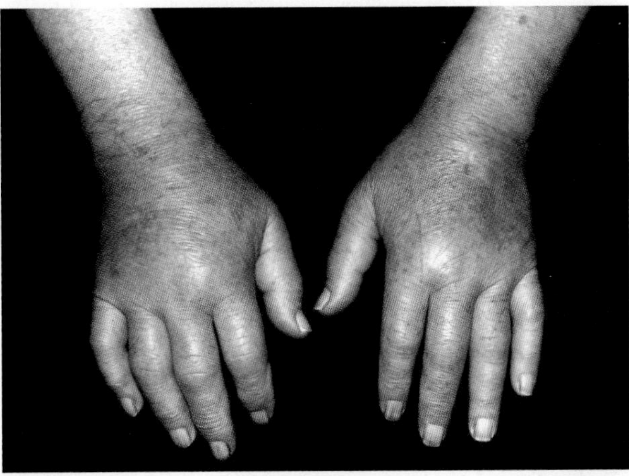

Figure 5A-4. Diffuse swelling of the hand with polyarthritis of the MCPs, PIPs, and wrists seen in remitting seronegative symmetric synovitis with pitting edema, or RS3PE syndrome.

Upper Extremity

Hand

RA affecting the hands almost always presents with pain and swelling of the MCP and PIP joints. The findings are usually symmetric and patients will complain of pain and stiffness markedly worse in the morning that requires a few hours of movement or a hot shower to loosen them up. Stiffness occurs most probably because inflammation-related swelling and edema of the synovium and periarticular structures limits the motion of the joints. It is most pronounced after long periods of inactivity because the fluid appears to slowly build from the underlying synovial inflammation. This phenomenon is termed "gelling" and can dominate the

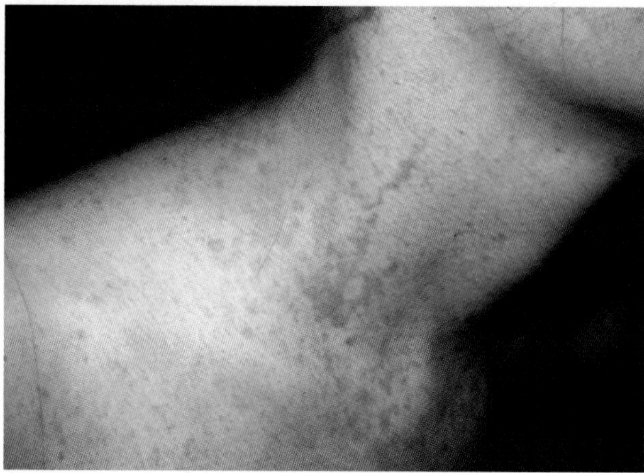

Figure 5A-5. Evanescent salmon-pink rash seen in a patient with adult-onset Still's disease.

clinical picture in some patients. It is postulated that with movement, the fluid is resorbed or moved to other compartments by dynamic pressures.[28] Physical examination of the joints is an important guide to efficacy of patient management; examination of the bilateral hands will account for 20 of the 28 joints in the modified disease activity score. This calculation requires an assessment of the total number of swollen joints and the total number of tender joints separately.[29]

Clinical exam may reveal warm, erythematous joints with effusions, soft tissue swelling around the MCP and PIP joints, and even decreased grip strength (Figure 5A-6). Radiographs of early RA typically show joint space narrowing of MCP and PIP joints and soft tissue swelling related to joint effusion, synovitis, and periarticular edema. The presence of periarticular osteopenia may be noted. If erosions are detected at the onset of presentation of the patient, they are noted as irregularities of the white cortical bone usually seen first at the second MCP[16]; however, there is typically a lag time from disease onset to evidence of radiographic erosions. As the disease progresses, the dominant hand frequently shows significantly more joint destruction.[30] DIP joint involvement with erosion is infrequently observed in seropositive RA patients, and is usually a manifestation of coexisting erosive osteoarthritis.[31] Evaluation of finger joints by ultrasound may not perform as accurately as the clinical exam for detecting overall abnormalities, but it has been shown by some investigators to improve upon radiography for detecting erosions.[32] Ultrasound may be more operator dependent compared to other imaging modalities. MRI is most sensitive in detecting bone changes in the early stages of the disease.[33]

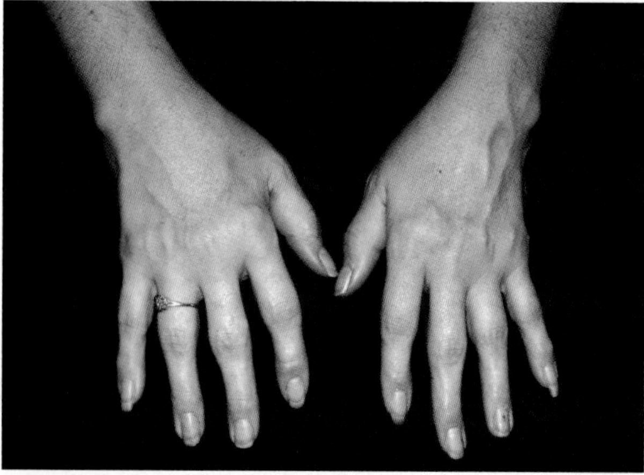

Figure 5A-6. Swelling indicating synovitis of the MCPs, PIPs, and wrists in a patient with early stages of RA.

With ongoing inflammation, evidence of clinical hypertrophy of the synovial lining and inflammation of periarticular structures will occur. One can detect synovial thickening on physical exam by feeling a bogginess of the joint on palpation (Figure 5A-7). Tenosynovitis presents with tenderness, warmth, and swelling along the flexor or extensor digital tendons and this process affects up to 55% of rheumatoid patients; the third flexor tendon is most frequently involved, followed by the second and then the fourth.[34] Patients can also suffer tendon ruptures from tendons rubbing against bony prominences from eroded bone; this often presents as a painless, sudden loss of extension or flexion. The most frequent site for extensor tendon rupture is at the distal end of the ulna with loss of movement of the third, fourth, and/or fifth fingers.[28] It is the authors' impression that tendon rupture is not as common an event in the modern era of aggressive disease management; most rheumatologists hardly see this complication any more. Tenosynovitis is

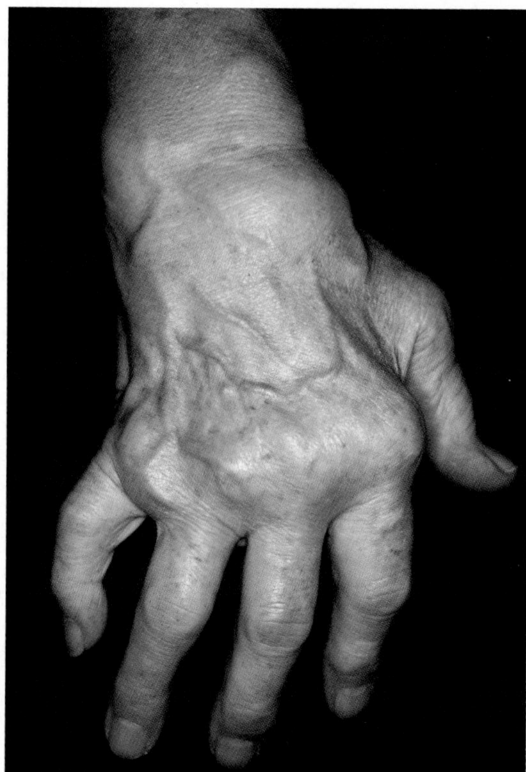

Figure 5A-7. Marked synovial thickening and hypertrophy associated with ongoing inflammation in an RA patient. Joints will feel boggy and very tender and warm on physical examination. Early deformities (radial deviation of the wrist, ulnar deviation of the digits) of the hands are emerging.

inflammation of the synovial fluid-filled sacs that surround tendon sheaths, and this process can connect to the joint space with enlargement from fluid coming from the joint causing formation of a synovial cyst. These cysts can distend, rupture, become infected, and cause local compressive symptoms.[35] Synovial cysts are sometimes confused with rheumatoid nodules; these rheumatoid nodules can also occur on tendons and cause triggering whereby the nodule gets trapped as the tendon moves through its sheath.[28]

Late manifestations of RA of the hands are anatomic disruptions of the integrity of the joint surfaces causing the visible joint deformities that subsequently lead to loss of function and disability (Figure 5A-8). Abnormal alignment results from the changing biomechanical forces affecting tendons and ligaments along eroded bone. This results in subluxations at the MCP joints, the boutonniere and swan neck deformities, and the Z deformity of the thumb.[16] The Boutonniere deformity is a nonreducible flexion at the PIP joint with hyperextension at the DIP joint. This process occurs when the central extensor tendon is stretched, the PIP is pulled through the tendon, and the lateral bands are displaced. With time the tendon shortens and the DIP becomes hyperflexed.[28] The swan-neck deformity is the opposite of the boutonniere. It is hyperextension at the PIP joint and flexion of the DIP joint; this process takes place either when the extensor tendon is affected and a shortening of the central extensor tendon occurs or when the PIP joint capsule herniates from weakening due to synovitis.[28]

Wrist

Early involvement of the wrist is common in RA patients, with pain, swelling, and limited range of motion as prominent signs and symptoms. Similar to the hands, the wrist findings are usually symmetric, and patients complain of pain and stiffness that is worse in the morning. Swelling is most prominent dorsally as well as over the ulnar styloid, and a typical feature is often visible swelling and rope-like thickening of the extensor carpi ulnaris tendon sheath. Loss of wrist extension is most prominent at the early stages.[36]

Ongoing inflammation can lead to erosions, tenosynovitis, and nerve compression. Early erosions occur in the pisiform, triqetrum, and ulnar styloid areas. Trentham and Masi[37] devised a measurement, later validated by Alarcon and Koopman,[38] in order to assess the progression of carpal involvement in RA called the carpo:metacarpal ratio: the ratio of the length of the carpus to the length of the third metacarpal bone. A decreased ratio correlates well with the overall radiographic stages of RA, and likely results from the cartilage loss and bone compaction at the radial to lunate, lunate to capitate, and capitate to third metacarpal articulations.[38] As inflammation continues, cartilage and bone destruction cause diffuse carpal narrowing, and the normal 2-mm wide articulations between the individual carpal bones are lost.[16] Progressive tenosynovitis can also lead to erosions, usually over the ulnar styloid from the inflammation of the extensor carpi ulnaris tendon and sheath.[16] Tenosynovitis can also be present in the common sheath of the abductor pollicis longus and extensor pollicis brevis tendons, called de Quervain's tenosynovitis. In this situation, patients feel pain on the radial aspect of the wrist and the pain can radiate proximally.[28] Both carpal tunnel syndrome and ulnar nerve entrapment can result from synovitis around the flexor tendons. With median nerve entrapment in the carpal tunnel, the palmar aspect of the first, second, third, and radial side of the fourth digits have decreased sensation with numbness and tingling especially in the night-time hours. Continued entrapment leads to motor loss and thenar muscle atrophy.[28] Ulnar nerve involvement causes numbness and tingling over the fifth and ulnar side of the fourth digits.[28]

Chronic inflammation at the wrist leads to deformities, loss of function, and bony attrition, affecting adjacent tendons that may result in tendon rupture (Figure 5A-9). A zigzag deformity is formed by the combination of the ulnar deviation of the phalanges at the metacarpal–phalangeal joints coupled with rotation of the navicular bone and radial deviation of the carpal bones at the distal radius and ulna articulations. With continued radial drift of the carpal bones and volar subluxation of the carpus, the ulnar styloid becomes more prominent.[36] The greater the degree of radial deviation at the wrist, the worse the ulnar

Figure 5A-8. Deformities in late RA are illustrated by enlarged MCP joints with subluxation and ulnar deviation of the phalanges associated with Z-deformities of thumbs and swan-neck deformities most obvious on the right second through fourth digits.

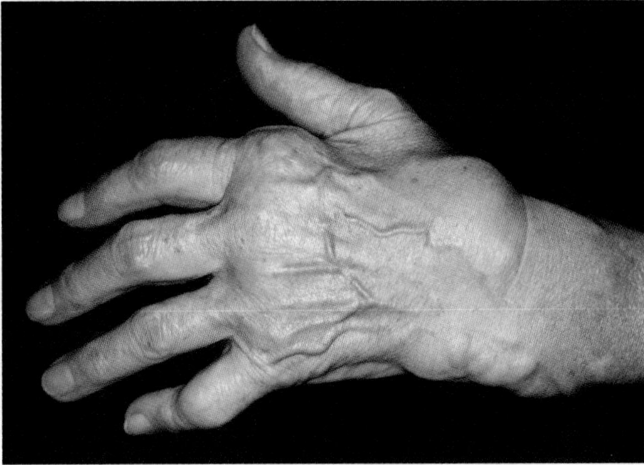

Figure 5A-9. Marked swelling of the wrist as well as the extensor carpi ulnaris tendon sheath illustrates the proliferative nature of the RA process.

deviation is for the phalanges.[39] Radial deviation at the wrist can be readily seen on a PA radiograph when more than half of the lunate articular surface is no longer articulating with the radius.[16] Paradoxically, some RA patients have ulnar deviation at the wrist and radial deviation of the fingers. In these patients, a greater degree of their ulnar wrist deviation is also associated with worse radial drift at the phalanges.[39] RA patients also display an increased rate of collapse of the carpal height with an associated decrease in the ratio of carpal height to radial width.[39] Tendon ruptures appear to occur from a combination of factors including progressive inflammation, tendon thickening, and decreased movement of tendon through its peritendonous sheath. These ruptures can lead to subluxation and may be associated with additional adjacent tendon ruptures. Unfortunately, neither clinical exam nor symptom severity can predict which patients will get tendon ruptures.[40] Investigators using MRI to evaluate the distribution and extent of tendon abnormalities in patients with active RA observed that the tendon sheaths on the volar aspect of the wrist have less peritendonous effusion, while the dorsal and ulnar compartments display more moderate to high degrees of effusions and/or pannus, tendonitis, and partial and complete tears.[40]

Elbow

One of the earliest clinical findings in RA is loss of full extension at the elbow. Patients are often unaware of this as they quite easily compensate for overall arm function and movement with their wrists and shoulders. Soft tissue changes are seen early on radiographs with joint effusions displacing the anterior and posterior fat pads.[16] In a cohort of patients with seropositive, erosive RA, 61% had erosive involvement of their elbows, and 40% had bilateral elbow involvement.[41] The incidence of mild (Larson grade 2) erosions were 33% and 18% for severe (Larson grade 3–5) erosions.[41] One of the initial positional changes that takes place as the disease progresses is an anterior, anterolateral, or ventral subluxation of the radial head in relation to the capitellum of the humerus.[42] This is followed gradually by progressive proximal migration and subluxation of the ulna. Also, whereas the normal joint has a humero-ulnar angle of approximately 10 degrees, or a slight valgus angle, as RA begins to affect the elbow, the angle enlarges to become even more valgus.[42] Patients may develop mild flexion contractures and nodule formation on the extensor surface of the elbow, and these subcutaneous rheumatoid nodules can cause cortical bone erosions in the underlying ulna and radius and appear like scalloped defects.[43]

With continued inflammation, the valgus angulation can become three times greater than normal with severe flexion contractures leading to functional disability.[42] Simultaneously, the olecranon process moves proximally in relation to the humerus and can lead to an almost 1-cm difference between a normal and severely affected joint. At Larson grade 5, the valgus angulation collapses into a more neutral position from bony destruction and disruption of the ligaments, and the proximal migration of the olecranon can cause medial compression forces that increase the risk for stress fracture of the medial ridge. These changes can ultimately lead to complete dislocation of the joint.[42] Erosions are most observed on the capitellum, the lateral epicondyle, and the olecranon.[41] Late radiographic changes of joint destruction of the elbow are narrowing of the humeroradial and humeroulnar joint spaces, and marked bone destruction of both the humerus and the olecranon bones at their articulating surfaces.[44,45]

Shoulder

Involvement of articular and periarticular tissues of the shoulder is extremely common, and is one of the most disabling features in patients, especially because of its effect on sleep. Patients may present with shoulder pain and stiffness, decreased range of motion, difficulty sleeping, and less commonly, swollen, warm joints. The shoulder joint, rotator cuff muscles, and shoulder bursa can be affected with the initial symptoms, usually a result of a combination of synovitis, tendonitis, and/or bursitis. Synovitis may present with an anterior effusion resembling a mass. Subdeltoid, subacromial, and scapulothoracic bursitis can occur. The subacromial bursa lies below the acromion and above the rotator cuff musculature. With subacromial bursitis, patients have pain with abduction of the shoulder as the acromion impinges on the bursa, and there may be a localized swelling under the deltoid muscle.[46] Bicipital tendonitis commonly occurs and invokes the feared complication of tendon rupture with the "pop-eye" sign, the contraction of the belly of the biceps muscle.[47]

With chronic, untreated subacromial bursitis due to RA, inflammation can progress to destruction of the rotator cuff muscles, superior subluxation of the humeral head, and extension of the pannus into the glenohumeral joint.[46] Erosions of the glenohumeral joints are seen in 55% of seropositive, erosive RA patients after 15 years of disease. Mild erosions (Larson grade 2) are seen in 27% and severe erosions (Larson grade 3–5) in 21%. Erosions occur first at the superolateral articular margin of the humerus where the rotator cuff muscles attach. The next most common site of erosion is the anatomic neck of the humerus.[48] With continued chronic inflammation, weakening of the rotator cuff muscles will cause superior subluxation of the humeral head. In addition, commonly seen and correlating well with glenohumeral joint destruction is acromioclavicular joint damage.[49] Erosions here can lead to resorption of the distal clavicle.[16] Although less commonly observed, glenoid erosions can take place, and they are more central versus posterior as seen in conditions that cause osteoarthritis of the shoulder.[50] After more marked erosive destruction occurs in the shoulder, a late finding on radiography is glenohumeral-joint space narrowing.[51] When there is progressive upward migration of the humerus with subacromial space narrowing, concern for rotator cuff damage or disruption is imminent. Physical exam may reveal limited abduction and external rotation of the affected arm. Evaluation with ultrasound or MRI is warranted to evaluate the rotator cuff musculature foı atrophy or tear.[52] MRI arthrography can be helpful to assess the rotator cuff or labral tears. Rarely, when the pressure from a shoulder joint effusion is coupled with activity of the arm, it may exceed the ability of the joint capsule to maintain its integrity (especially at the inferior surface), and an acute shoulder joint rupture can lead to a pseudothrombotic syndrome resembling venous obstruction.[53]

Lower Extremity

Foot and Ankle

Initial involvement of the feet and ankles in RA is quite common; 13% of patients develop symptoms in their feet as the first sign of disease onset.[9] At some time during the course of disease, it has been demonstrated that 90% of patients will have foot and ankle manifestations.[54] Patients may complain of pain on weight-bearing movement and walking, and often the swelling will cause their shoes to be tight and an increased shoe size becomes evident. The forefoot is the most common painful area.[55] On examination, swelling in the synovium and soft tissues of the metatarsal–phalangeal joints may cause patients toes to splay laterally so that you could see light shining between their toes (the "daylight sign") (Figure 5A-10). A slight squeeze across the MTP joints may prove very tender.

It is important to examine the feet and ankles for alignment, swelling, pain, and deformities while the patient is both on the exam table as well as standing to avoid compensation for abnormalities in the more proximal knee and hip joints. Also it is important to observe the gait as pain and malalignment may change based on how a patient loads her weight. Patients may complain of paresthesias if synovitis compresses the tarsal tunnel where the posterior tibial nerve runs. They may not be able to do a heel-rise if there is edema or swelling of the posterior tibialis tendon.[55] Pain at the arch of the foot, with plantar flexion and dorsiflexion of the ankle, indicates involvement of the talonavicular joint.[56] The earliest changes on radiograph are similar to the hands, with periarticular osteopenia and soft tissue swelling.[54] The forefoot usually displays the earliest changes with the lateral fifth metatarsal head first to show an erosion as well as the medial side of the first interphalangeal joint.[16] Diffuse joint space narrowing of the ankle and tarsal articulations may also be observed.[16] Lateral radiographs allow evaluation of the alignment of the forefoot to the hindfoot by drawing a line in the longitudinal axis of the first metatarsal to the longitudinal axis of the talus, as well as evaluation of the subtalar, talonavicular, and calcaneocuboid joints. Anteroposterior weight-bearing radiographs evaluate abnormalities of the forefoot, talonavicular, and calcaneocuboid joints, as well as the ability to assess for talar tilt indicating ankle involvement.[55]

With continued synovitis and weight bearing, ligaments, tendons, and bones of the feet and ankles are all affected, and can lead to deformity, pain, and disability in an untreated or partially treated patient. Of those afflicted with foot and ankle disease, 90% have forefoot disease, 66% have subtalar involvement, and 9% have ankle disease[54] (Figure 5A-11). Tenosynovitis is most common in the peronaei and the tibialis posterior tendons.[57] Initially, inflammation in the forefoot leads to weakening of the capsular and ligamentous structures in the MTPs causing decreased stabilization. The intermetatarsophalangeal joint ligaments stretch and the fibrofatty cushion weakens and is displaced anteriorly.[58] With the continued dorsiflexion during walking, the second to fifth MTP joints begin to sublux and eventually the extensor tendons shorten and the proximal phalanges can dislocate entirely.[54] The dislocated proximal phalanges rest on the dorsal aspect of their metatarsals and the metatarsal heads then herniate through the plantar capsule and become the site of weight bearing on the bottom of the foot. Callus formation over the metatarsal heads ensues.[54] The most pressure in the forefoot is under the second and third metatarsal heads; lesions under these heads are noted in 40% of patients.[58] As the metatarsal joints dislocate, their digital flexor tendons are displaced into the intermetatarsal spaces and cause pulling of the MTPs into extension. This leads to hammer mallet or claw-toe deformities.[54] "Cock-up" toe is a hyperextension at the metatarsophalangeal joint with subluxation of the phalange above the metatarasal head so that the toe is elevated and the toe pad does not usually touch the floor. "Hammer toe" is flexion of the distal and/or proximal interphalangeal joints with the distal phalange pointing downward.[57]

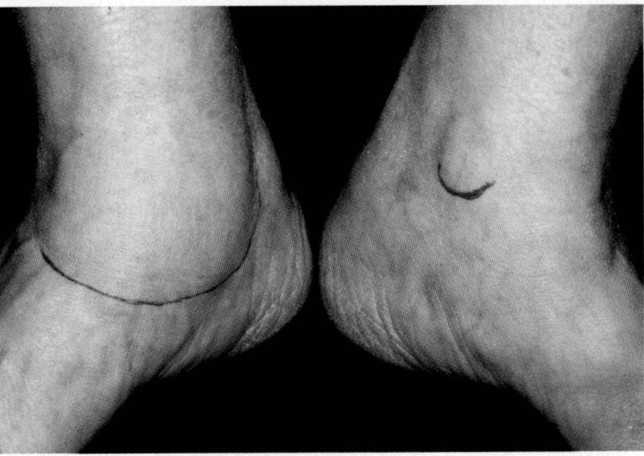

Figure 5A-11. Obvious subtalar joint swelling is present on the medial side of the hindfoot of this RA patient.

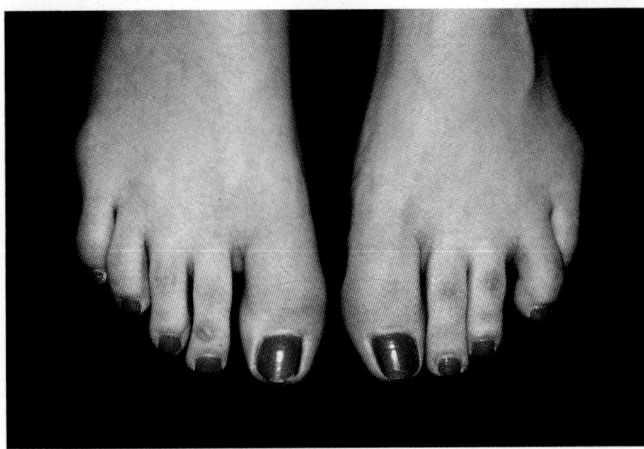

Figure 5A-10. Swelling of the synovium and soft tissues of the MTP joints causes toes to splay laterally and not touch each other; this is called the "daylight sign."

Progressive hallux valgus of the first MTP joint is an early manifestation in the rheumatoid foot, and is usually associated with the development of a bunion at the medial aspect of the metatarsal head.[57] Synovial cysts of the plantar aspect of the foot are rare, but can lead to pain and difficulty in weight bearing.[59] The ankle has little surrounding muscle and is therefore forced to sustain the body weight on the articular surfaces of the tibia, fibula, talus, and navicular bones, for which the talonavicular bone bears the brunt of much of this weight. With continued inflammation, the talonavicular bone collapses and causes the valgus flat foot deformity.[56] Radiographic evaluation of positional abnormalities will occur later in disease. With dislocation of the MTPs, the AP radiograph shows the proximal phalanges end-on, or the "gun-barrel sign."[54] The MTPs are both clinically and radiographically most frequently involved in established disease; however, the ankles appear to have more clinical abnormalities than radiologic joint damage.[58] MRI studies have shown that decline in walking ability in RA patients increased with the severity of destruction of the talonavicular joint.[56]

Deformities of the Forefoot

Hallux valgus is caused by the pathologic changes in the ligamentous supporting structures resulting from inflammation and is one of the most frequently encountered rheumatoid foot deformities. It is defined when the first metatarsal and the base of the first phalange are at an angle greater than 20 degrees; the angle is greater in females and with longer duration of disease. The first toe tends to lie under the second and third toes as the disease progresses. Bunions usually form medially on the metatarsal head, and in extreme cases this deformity can form a prominence, or an exotosis, covered by a pannus that can erode the adjacent bone.[57] Hallux rigidus, or arthritis in the first metatarsophalangeal joint leading to stiffness and inability to dorsiflex, is seen in 13% of females and 7% of males with RA.[57]

With decreased stability from the ligamentous structures of the MTPs, the proximal phalanges sublux and eventually dislocate such that they lie dorsally on the metatarsal heads. The plantar fat pad is attached to the proximal phalanges; upon their subluxation the fat pad is pulled distally and the MTPs have little soft-tissue cushioning. Calluses form along the plantar aspect of the metatarsal heads.[55] These metatarsal heads take one-half of the weight endured by the foot.[57] On x-ray, the metatarsal heads show progressive erosions, remineralization, and then blunt spur formation where the heads appear almost "chewed" away from advanced erosive disease.[57] With chronic inflammation, the outermost ligaments holding the forefoot together give way leading to "metatarsal spread," and the forefoot deviates laterally, called "fibular deviation."[57]

Deformities of the Midfoot

The midfoot is not commonly involved in RA, but if it is, the talonavicular and naviculocuneiform joints are usually affected. The arch of the foot is supported mostly by muscle and ligaments, and with continued inflammation and weakness and stretching with weight bearing, this process leads to deformity. As disease duration occurs, the likelihood of developing *pes planovalgus*, rigid flat foot, increases.[57] Pes planovalgus is caused by involvement of the talonavicular joint resulting in pronation and eversion of the foot. If the tibialis posterior tendon, the joint capsule, and the deltoid, calcaneonavicular, and talonavicular collateral ligaments are weakened, there can be collapse of the longitudinal arch of the foot and the talus moves forward and medially.[55]

Deformities of the Hindfoot

Heel pain is uncommon in RA, ranging from 2.5% to 16% of patients in various studies.[57] Patients will complain of ill-defined heel pain with difficulty walking on uneven ground.[55] The two areas most affected are the sub-Achilles and subplantar areas where the Achilles tendon and plantar aponeurosis insert on the calcaneus. The insertion of the Achilles tendon can itself become inflamed and thickened, or the sub-Achilles bursa can be inflamed with abnormalities seen in the normal triangular area between the Achilles and the calcaneous.[57] In addition, rheumatoid nodule formation over these areas can cause pain; spontaneous rupture of the Achilles tendon has been reported.[60] Calcaneal stress fractures can rarely occur.[61] Erosions of the calcaneus have been seen, but are not specific for RA, as they can be seen with the spondyloarthropathies as well.[57]

Knees

Lessons from the Leiden Early Arthritis Clinic have revealed that arthritis of the knees at first presentation is predictive of a more destructive course of RA.[62] Early symptoms of RA in the knee are due to synovial proliferation and effusion, and knee joint effusions limit flexion of the knee associated with patients' complaints of restriction of movement. Synovial hypertrophy can be palpated, and effusions can be observed by patellar tap or the bulge sign (Figure 5A-12). Radiographs reveal joint effusion with enlargement of the suprapatellar bursa on lateral films.[16]

Persistent inflammation of the knee, especially in the inadequately managed patient, causes progressive cartilage damage, ligamentous laxity, and quadriceps muscle atrophy, eventually leading to weakness, contractures, and difficulty walking. Radiographs will typically show narrowing of medial and lateral knee compartments as well as bare area erosions, and valgus or varus deformities may occur.[16] Increased intra-articular pressure in the joint from increasing synovial fluid can cause damage to the adjacent articular structures and can push posteriorly leading to an outpouching of the synovial capsule. These popliteal or Baker's cysts have been shown to be connected to the joint by a one-way valvular mechanism whereby the fluid from the knee joint moves posteriorly when the pressure increases and cannot return.[63] These cysts will rupture and produce symptoms that mimic acute thrombophlebitis with a painful and swollen thigh or calf (Figure 5A-13). The rupture may also show crescentic bruising beneath the malleoli, the hemorrhagic crescent sign.[64] Popliteal cysts, historically evaluated by double-contrast arthrography, are now imaged with ultrasound or MRI.[16]

It is important from both a diagnostic as well as therapeutic standpoint to be aggressive in managing inflammation in the rheumatoid knee because of its potential for producing functional disability. Both ultrasound and MRI can be used to

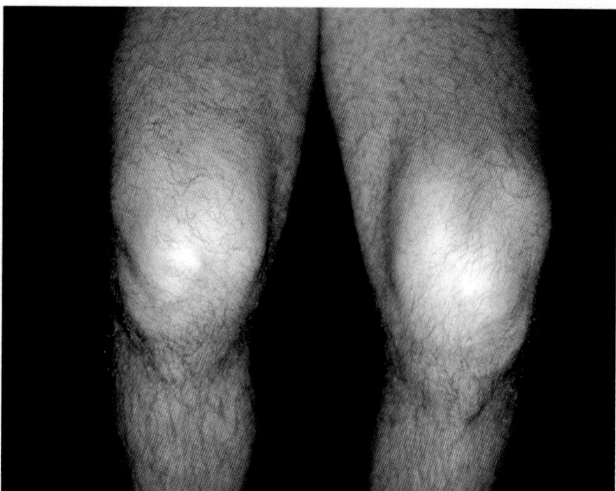

Figure 5A-12. Bilateral knee joint effusions are present in this patient. The effusions are greater on the patient's left side, illustrating the extent of expansion of the suprapatellar pouch.

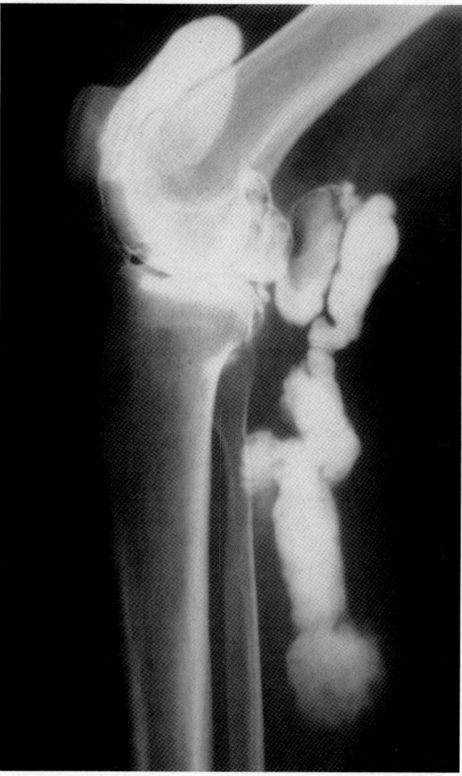

Figure 5A-13. Conventional contrast arthrography demonstrates a Baker's cyst in the popliteal space associated with rupture and fluid extending distally into the calf musculature.

evaluate the knee joint and its periarticular structures. One recent study revealed that (18)F-FDG PET scanning of the knee correlates well with MRI, ultrasound, and laboratory tests such as CRP, and MMP-3 levels in assessing the metabolic activity of knee synovitis.[65]

Hips

The incidence of hip involvement in RA varies from 10% in patients with less than 10 years of disease up to 40% in patients with longer disease durations. Those with hip disease also appear have more destructive peripheral joint disease.[66] On physical exam, patients may have stiffness and limited range of motion with internal rotation correlating best with radiographic findings. Patients may complain of groin pain or medial knee pain that is referred from the hip; however, less than 50% of patients with hip joint disease suffer any symptoms.[66] Hip involvement should be distinguished from other causes of pain in the proximal limb girdle; patients may also have pain on palpation of the lateral aspect of the hip related to inflammation of the trochanteric or iliopsoas bursas.

Destruction of the hip joint is more pronounced in those with longer disease duration, and in females; body mass index is not a risk factor.[66] Radiographs reveal diffuse joint space narrowing with erosions of the femoral head and neck. With continued inflammation and erosive disease, the femoral head and acetabulum can erode into and protrude medially through the pelvis, termed *petrusio acetabuli*.[16] Petrusio acetabuli is more frequent in females, and is associated with longer disease duration; in one retrospective study of 100 RA patients, it was observed in 23%.[67] Osteonecrosis, or avascular necrosis, of the hip has also been observed in RA patients, particularly related to a history of corticosteroid use. MR imaging is more sensitive than CT or nuclear scintigraphy for detecting early AVN; early findings include a sclerotic non–signal-producing line between the necrotic and viable bone lined by a hyperintense rim of granulation tissue, called "the double-line sign." If present, fluid within a subchondral fracture associated with AVN can be observed on T2-weighted images, and a centrally located low-signal region that is remodeled compact trabecular bone may be visualized. Abnormalities in the signal of the femoral head marrow can be noted on both T1- and T2-weighted imaging representing changes in vascularity or conversion to fatty marrow.[68] Radiographs will show femoral head collapse in the later stages of this process.[69]

Spine and Axial Joints

C-Spine

Many patients have cervical spine abnormalities, but in the modern era few develop complications related to these findings. The reported prevalence of cervical involvement varies from 17% to 88% depending on the study, but more recent observational cohorts of early arthritis patients reveal its prevalence to be much less, and it is suggested that earlier aggressive treatment has contributed to this improvement.[70] Moreover, serious complications or surgical requirement for cervical spine abnormalities are rare.[71] Risk factors for cervical spine abnormalities include multiple and severe peripheral joint involvement (especially of the hands), rheumatoid nodules, high-titer RF seropositivity, high-dose steroid treatment, longer disease duration, radiographic erosions in hands and feet, extra-articular features, and vasculitis.[72,73]

Synovitis of the cervical spine can lead to laxity of ligaments, loss of articular cartilage, and erosions into bones; the most frequently involved cervical segments are the occipito-atlantal and atlanto-axial (C1–C2) articulations. Causes of cervical instability in RA are largely due to atlantoaxial subluxation, basilar invagination, and subaxial subluxation.[72] Pannus formation can cause spinal canal stenosis; pannus surrounding the odontoid may result in cord compression.[72] The earliest symptoms of C-spine instability are pain in the neck, occiput, retro-orbital, or temporal areas. If the greater occipital nerves are compressed, occipital headaches may occur. C-spine instability can lead to radiculopathy syndromes in which nerve root compression causes pain, dysethesia, and decreased reflexes in the dermatome of the affected root. More severe cervical instability will lead in some patients to cord compression exhibited as myelopathy with weakness, a heaviness sensation in the lower extremities, gait disturbances, hand clumsiness, bowel/bladder abnormalities, increased deep tendon reflexes, dorsiflexion of the first toe with stimulation of the plantar aspect of the foot (Babinski sign), and/or electrical sensation in the neck on flexion (Lhermitte's sign).[72] Vertebrobasilar insufficiency can progress to tinnitus, vertigo, diplopia, or loss of proprioception. When the atlanto–dens interval is greater than 9 mm, there is anterior subluxation combined with basilar invagination, or the space available for the cord is 14 mm or less, there is a high likelihood of cord compression.[72]

Atlantoaxial Subluxation

Anterior subluxation is most common, observed in about 4% of patients. It occurs as a result of either odontoid erosion or laxity of the transverse, alar, and apical ligaments of C1 allowing posterior slippage of the odontoid process.[15,72] The complication can develop within 2 years of disease onset, but usually affects patients with a disease duration of 10 years or greater, active disease for more than 5 years, and early erosions in peripheral joints.[15,72] Posterior subluxation is less common and can be caused by erosions or fractures in the odontoid or an arch defect in the anterior aspect of the atlas.[72] Lateral subluxation is caused by bony erosion into the articular capsules of the lateral joints.[73]

Basilar Invagination

When bone and cartilage are eroded from the occipitoatlantal and atlantoaxial joints, the skull can descend on the cervical spine and the odontoid can enter the foramen magnum causing basilar invagination.[72] This can lead to brain stem or cord compression, vertebral artery insufficiency, and can result in sudden death. The prevalence of basilar invagination in RA patients is 5% to 32% in various studies, and it usually follows evidence for atlantoaxial subluxation. Basilar invagination can make the atlanto–dens interval look improved on radiography; therefore, clinicians must be vigilant when noting any of these changes.

Subaxial Subluxation

Late in the RA disease process, destruction of the facet joints, interspinous ligaments, and discovertebral junctions below the atlantoaxial segment leads to subaxial subluxations.[72] The changes seen in these apophyseal joints are joint space narrowing, erosion, sclerosis, and sometimes fusion. At the discovertebral joints, disc space narrowing, erosions, and sclerosis may occur.[73] These changes usually take place at several levels causing a "step ladder" deformity.[72] Cord compression is likely when anterior subluxation is 3.5 mm or more or the space available for the cord is 14 mm or less.[72]

Early radiographic changes of C-spine disease include odontoid erosions, subaxial subluxations, apophyseal joint erosion and sclerosis, disc-space-space narrowing, and osteophytosis at C4 to C7.[74] CT and MRI can increase detection with CT scans best for assessing erosions and spinal cord compression. Static and dynamic MRI will more clearly show pannus formation and changes that take place in the odontoid, foramen magnum, spinal cord, and dura.[72]

Nevertheless, many patients are asymptomatic in spite of imaging abnormalities; this creates a clinical dilemma. Should we screen every patient for C-spine involvement when only a few will suffer from complications? Should we screen all patients prior to surgical procedures requiring positional manipulations or anesthesia? Older literature recommends obtaining C-spine films on any RA patient who will undergo surgery, but the more recent literature suggests that if patients have a shorter disease duration (less than 5 years) or have little clinical activity and no neck complaints, C-spine films do not necessarily need to be obtained.[70–72] Without the known risk factors and the presence of good control of disease, presurgical x-rays may not be necessary.

Thoracic, Lumbar, and Sacral Spine

Abnormalities of the thoracolumbar and sacral joints are infrequent in RA patients. Ligament laxity, apophyseal and facet joint synovitis, and vertebral body osteoporosis predispose the RA patient to vertebral damage.[75] Deformities seen include erosions in apophyseal joints and at the discovertebral junction. Discovertebral changes may be secondary to abnormal motion at the discovertebral junction due to apophyseal joint instability or from synovial tissue extension from the apophyseal joints into the discs.[75] Alternatively, vertebral disease may be related to occult trauma at the discovertebral junction which predisposes patients to disc herniation and formation of Schmorl's nodes or granulomatous nodules in the marrow of vertebral bodies.[75]

Lumbar involvement in seropositive RA is associated with erosive disease of the hands and feet, and with cervical spine arthritis.[76] The prevalence in the lumbar spine is low, however, with 5% in males and 3% in females.[76] Subluxation, disc space narrowing without osteophytosis, apophyseal erosions, endplate erosions, facet erosions, and vertebral destruction can be observed.[76,77] Neurologic symptoms such as leg pain or numbness and/or intermittent claudication occur in 12% to 18% of patients.[77] Lesions in the upper, middle, and lower thoracic levels are infrequent, but have been reported to lead to cord compression.[77] Thoracic abnormalities are usually found in patients with severe erosive arthritis and may be related to increased the motion at thoracic levels that are compensating for a spontaneously fused cervical spine along with collapse of the vertebrae from ongoing synovitis.[77] Sacroiliac joints are rarely involved in RA and when abnormalities exist they consist of narrowing of the joint space with or without erosions, and no sclerosis. These changes are seen only after severe and long disease duration.[78] The occurrence of osteoporosis involving vertebral bodies is discussed in Chapter 5C.

Sternoclavicular and Manubriosternal Joints

Pain and swelling from sternoclavicular and manubriosternal articulations occur in about 70% of erosive RA patients, but only 10% have clinical evidence of inflammation on joint examination.[79] Sternoclavicular involvement is noted in about one-third of RA patients, usually accompanying arthritis in other joints. Symptoms are usually asymmetric but can be bilateral, and include swelling, crepitus, tenderness, hypertrophy, pain, or limitation of motion.[80] Manubriosternal joint involvement is common in RA, and is often associated with severe cervicodorsal spinal erosion and deformity; erosion, reactive sclerosis, and ankylosis of the manubriosternal joint can occur.[79] The involvement of the manubriosternal joint, although commonly seen, is often a minor clinical problem and only rare cases of subluxation or dislocation have been reported.[79]

Temporomandibular Joint

The frequency of clinical temporomandibular joint (TMJ) involvement in RA has ranged from 4.7% to 84% in various studies,[81] but the proportion of patients who need treatment for TMJ symptoms appear to be far fewer. TMJ arthritis manifests clinically with pain, swelling, crepitus, and stiffness upon mouth opening with limitation of motion.[81] Its occurrence is more likely with severe and prolonged disease duration.[81] Goupille et al.[81] found no tomographic abnormalities of the TMJ that were specific for RA versus other non-RA patients with TMJ symptoms, except that the incidence of erosions and cysts of the mandibular condyle were significantly higher in RA patients and these correlated with the severity of the disease. Radiography and CT scans of the TMJ assess bony changes reasonably well; however, the disc and surrounding soft tissues are not well visualized.

Radiographic changes are joint-space narrowing, marginal erosions, osteolysis, and destruction of the condyle. With advanced disease there is a flattening and sclerosis of the condylar head.[82] MRI can evaluate all the articular components, and with gadolinium, may visualize the inflammatory pannus and joint effusions as well.[82] MRI is the only imaging modality that can visualize severe disc destruction.[83] Ultrasound is comparable to MRI at detecting effusions.[82]

Cricoarytenoid Joint

The cricoarytenoid joint of the larynx is difficult to examine clinically, and symptoms usually go unnoticed by patients or physicians.[84] In various studies, 26% to 86% of RA patients have cricoarytenoid involvement, but it rarely has resulted in complications.[85,86] It is more common in females and with prolonged duration and severity of disease.[86,87] Pannus may erode into the arytenoid cartilage, cricoid cartilage, subchondral bone, joint capsule, and/or the surrounding ligaments. Joint space narrowing and ankylosis can occur. Subsequently, ankylosis of the cricoarytenoid joint can cause the vocal cords to be fixed in the midline and lead to upper airway obstruction.

Only 26% of patients ever experience laryngeal symptoms.[86] The most common manifestation is the sensation of a foreign body or pharyngeal fullness in the throat worse with swallowing or speaking; patients may develop a hoarse voice.[86] There may be a cough or dyspnea if there is associated laryngeal edema and/or odynophagia. If the glossopharyngeal and vagus nerves are affected, pain may radiate to the ear. Stridor can occur and may worsen while sleeping.[85] Although quite rare, the destruction of the cricoarytenoid joint can lead to airway obstruction and possibly death.[85] If a patient develops a superimposed upper respiratory infection, this underlying abnormality can also be fatal.[88]

Imaging can confirm a suspected diagnosis of cricoarytenoid involvement, though clinical symptoms do not always correlate with the imaging findings. Sore throats and difficulty during inspiration are the only symptoms that are associated with abnormalities seen on laryngoscopy, and no symptoms are associated with abnormalities on CT scan.[84] Laryngoscopic exam is usually used to confirm the diagnosis. In acute inflammation, laryngoscopy will reveal swelling and erythema of the vocal cords, or vocal cord bowing on inspiration. With chronic inflammation, vocal cords can look normal but can possess focal vocal cord lesions, asymmetric arytenoids, decreased mobility or bowing of the vocal cords, and there has been a reported case of a submucosal mass in the larynx that was confused with squamous cell cancer.[86] Neck radiography or CT can also be used to confirm the diagnosis; these modalities are often complementary to laryngoscopy. CT imaging will reveal cricoarytenoid erosions, luxation, prominence, and abnormal positioning of the vocal cords.[86] Pulmonary function tests may show an extrathoracic upper airway obstruction pattern.[85]

Ossicles of the Ear

Hearing loss has been reported in RA patients with some studies describing both transient and permanent conductive deafness, while others have reported sensorineural deafness.[89] It is unclear exactly how the interossicular joints are affected or how they contribute to hearing loss, however, it has been observed that assessment by the Grason-Stadler 1720B otoadmittance meter will show increased laxity of the conducting system in affected patients.[89] Additionally, audiologic and electroacoustic immitance measurements suggest that the etiology may be increased stiffness in the middle ear or associated increased stiffness associated with ligamentous instability.[90]

Conclusions

Many of the late stage articular and periarticular manifestations of RA described herein are not seen contemporaneously as frequently as in the past most likely due to our improved ability to diagnose and treat patients. Certainly cigarette smoking reduction may have played an additional role in changing the severity and progression of disease. With our new therapeutic armamentarium, we are able to put patients into a clinical remission much more readily. However, observations have shown patients who are in an apparent clinical remission can have progressive joint damage and evidence of subclinical synovitis. In a randomized, controlled, double-blinded clinical trial in patients with <1 year of disease at baseline, Cohen et al. noted that 16.7% of those in sustained clinical remission by DAS <1.6 criteria had radiographic progression of disease, and 20% developed erosions in a previously unaffected joint between years 3 and 5 of disease.[91] Additional observations have revealed that patients who were in apparent remission by DAS28 and/or ACR remission criteria actually continue to have progressive and persistent synovitis and bony damage on imaging studies. Brown et al. demonstrated in a cohort of patients in clinical remission that 96% had synovitis and 46% had bone marrow edema on MRI. Further, 73% had synovial hypertrophy and 43% had increased Doppler signal indicating synovitis by ultrasound.[92]

Therefore, other more sensitive modalities employed to identify sub-clinical disease activity (imaging, biomarkers, etc.) may need to be incorporated into our assessment. Although our traditional physical examination and descriptors based on those findings have disclosed a marked improvement in disease outcome over the past 10 years, we need to advance our definition of disease remission to even more effectively control disease progression.

References

1. Goekoop-Ruiterman YP, de Vries-Bouwstra JK, Allaart CF, et al. Clinical and radiographic outcomes of four different treatment strategies in patients with early rheumatoid arthritis (the BeSt study): A randomized, controlled trial. *Arthritis Rheum* 2005; 52(11):3381–3390.
2. Verstappen SM, Jacobs JW, van der Veen MJ, et al. Intensive treatment with methotrexate in early rheumatoid arthritis: Aiming for remission. Computer Assisted Management in Early Rheumatoid Arthritis (CAMERA, an open-label strategy trial). *Ann Rheum Dis* 2007;66(11):1443–1449.

3. van der Helm-van Mil AH, Breedveld FC, Huizinga TW. Aspects of early arthritis. Definition of disease states in early arthritis: Remission versus minimal disease activity. *Arthritis Res Ther* 2006;8(4):216.
4. Arnett FC, Edworthy SM, Bloch DA, et al. The American Rheumatism Association 1987 revised criteria for the classification of rheumatoid arthritis. *Arthritis Rheum* 1988;31(3):315–324.
5. Visser H, le Cessie S, Vos K, et al. How to diagnose rheumatoid arthritis early: A prediction model for persistent (erosive) arthritis. *Arthritis Rheum* 2002;46(2):357–365.
6. Schumacher HR Jr, Habre W, Meador R, Hsia EC. Predictive factors in early arthritis: Long-term follow-up. *Semin Arthritis Rheum* 2004;33(4):264–272.
7. Green M, Marzo-Ortega H, McGonagle D, et al. Persistence of mild, early inflammatory arthritis: The importance of disease duration, rheumatoid factor, and the shared epitope. *Arthritis Rheum* 1999;42(10):2184–2188.
8. Quinn MA, Green MJ, Marzo-Ortega H, et al. Prognostic factors in a large cohort of patients with early undifferentiated inflammatory arthritis after application of a structured management protocol. *Arthritis Rheum* 2003;48(11):3039–3045.
9. Fleming A, Crown JM, Corbett, M. Early rheumatoid disease. I. Onset. *Ann Rheum Dis* 19761976;35(4):357–360.
10. Lee DM, Weinblatt ME. Rheumatoid arthritis. *Lancet* 2001;358(9285): 903–911.
11. Fleming A, Benn RT, Corbett M, Wood PH. Early rheumatoid disease. II. Patterns of joint involvement. *Ann Rheum Dis* 1976; 35(4):361–364.
12. Lindqvist E, Eberhardt K, Bendtzen K, et al. Prognostic laboratory markers of joint damage in rheumatoid arthritis. *Ann Rheum Dis* 2005;64(2):196–201.
13. Quinn MA, Gough AK, Green MJ, et al. Anti-CCP antibodies measured at disease onset help identify seronegative rheumatoid arthritis and predict radiological and functional outcome. *Rheumatology (Oxford)* 2006;45(4):478–480.
14. Mathsson L, Mullazehi M, Wick MC, et al. Antibodies against citrullinated vimentin in rheumatoid arthritis: Higher sensitivity and extended prognostic value concerning future radiographic progression as compared with antibodies against cyclic citrullinated peptides. *Arthritis Rheum* 2008;58(1):36–45.
15. Sokka T. Early rheumatoid arthritis in Finland. *Clin Exp Rheumatol* 2003;21(5 Suppl 31):S133–S137.
16. Learch T. Imaging of rheumatoid arthritis. In: Hochberg M, ed., *Rheumatology*, 4th ed., vol. 1. Spain: Mosby Elsevier, 2008.
17. Dohn UM, Ejbjerg BJ, Hasselquist M, et al. Rheumatoid arthritis bone erosion volumes on CT and MRI: Reliability and correlations with erosion scores on CT, MRI and radiography. *Ann Rheum Dis* 2007;66(10):1388–1392.
18. Jimenez-Boj E, Nöbauer-Huhmann I, Hanslik-Schnabel B, et al. Bone erosions and bone marrow edema as defined by magnetic resonance imaging reflect true bone marrow inflammation in rheumatoid arthritis. *Arthritis Rheum* 2007;56(4):1118–1124.
19. McQueen FM, Ostendorf B. What is MRI bone oedema in rheumatoid arthritis and why does it matter? *Arthritis Res Ther* 2006; 8(6):222.
20. Handa R. Approach to seronegative arthritis. *J Indian Acad Clin Med* 2003;4(3):190–192.
21. Fujinami M, Sato K, Kashiwazaki S, Aotsuka S. Comparable histological appearance of synovitis in seropositive and seronegative rheumatoid arthritis. *Clin Exp Rheumatol* 1997;15(1):11–17.
22. Guerne PA, Weisman MH. Palindromic rheumatism: Part of or apart from the spectrum of rheumatoid arthritis. *Am J Med* 1992; 93(4):451–460.
23. Tutuncu Z, Kavanaugh A. Rheumatic disease in the elderly: Rheumatoid arthritis. *Rheum Dis Clin North Am* 2007;33:57–70.
24. Mandell BF. Polymyalgia rheumatica: Clinical presentation is key to diagnosis and treatment. *Cleve Clin J Med* 2004;71(6): 489–495.
25. McCarty DJ, O'Duffy JD, Pearson L, Hunter JB. Remitting seronegative symmetrical synovitis with pitting edema. RS3PE syndrome. *JAMA* 1985;254(19):2763–2767.
26. Yamaguchi M, Ohta A, Tsunematsu T, et al. Preliminary criteria for classification of adult Still's disease. *J Rheumatol* 1992;19(3): 424–430.
27. Fautrel B, Le Moël G, Saint-Marcoux B, et al. Diagnostic value of ferritin and glycosylated ferritin in adult onset Still's disease. *J Rheumatol* 2001;28(2):322–329.
28. Soeroso J. Review article: Hand deformities in rheumatoid arthritis. *Folia Med Indones* 2006;42(4):262–269.
29. Prevoo ML, van 't Hof MA, Kuper HH, et al. Modified disease activity scores that include twenty-eight-joint counts. Development and validation in a prospective longitudinal study of patients with rheumatoid arthritis. *Arthritis Rheum* 1995;38(1):44–48.
30. Owsianik WD, Kundi A, Whitehead JN, et al. Radiological articular involvement in the dominant hand in rheumatoid arthritis. *Ann Rheum Dis* 1980;39(5):508–510.
31. Jacob J, Sartoris D, Kursunoglu S, et al. Distal interphalangeal joint involvement in rheumatoid arthritis. *Arthritis Rheum* 1986;29(1): 10–15.
32. Weidekamm C, Köller M, Weber M, Kainberger F. Diagnostic value of high-resolution B-mode and doppler sonography for imaging of hand and finger joints in rheumatoid arthritis. *Arthritis Rheum* 2003;48(2):325–333.
33. McGonagle D, Conaghan PG, O'Connor P, et al. The relationship between synovitis and bone changes in early untreated rheumatoid arthritis: A controlled magnetic resonance imaging study. *Arthritis Rheum* 1999;42(8):1706–1711.
34. Gray RG, Gottlieb NL. Hand flexor tenosynovitis in rheumatoid arthritis. Prevalence, distribution, and associated rheumatic features. *Arthritis Rheum* 1977;20(4):1003–1008.
35. Martin LF, Bensen WG. An unusual synovial cyst in rheumatoid arthritis. *J Rheumatol* 1987;14(1):139–141.
36. Hastings DE, Evans JA. Rheumatoid wrist deformities and their relation to ulnar drift. *J Bone Joint Surg Am* 1975;57(7):930–934.
37. Trentham DE, Masi AT. Carpo:metacarpal ratio. A new quantitative measure of radiologic progression of wrist involvement in rheumatioid arthritis. *Arthritis Rheum* 1976;19(5):939–944.
38. Alarcon GS, Koopman WJ. The carpometarcarpal ratio: A useful method for assessing disease progression in rheumatoid arthritis. *J Rheumatol* 1985;12(5):846–848.
39. Read GO, Solomon L, Biddulph S. Relationship between finger and wrist deformities in rheumatoid arthritis. *Ann Rheum Dis* 1983; 42(6):619–625.
40. Valeri G, Ferrara C, Ercolani P, et al. Tendon involvement in rheumatoid arthritis of the wrist: MRI findings. *Skeletal Radiol* 2001; 30(3):138–143.
41. Lehtinen JT, Kaarela K, Ikävalko M, et al. Incidence of elbow involvement in rheumatoid arthritis. A 15 year endpoint study. *J Rheumatol* 2001;28(1):70–74.
42. Lehtinen JT, Kaarela K, Kauppi MJ, et al. Valgus deformity and proximal subluxation of the rheumatoid elbow: A radiographic 15 year follow up study of 148 elbows. *Ann Rheum Dis* 2001;60(8):765–769.
43. Dorfman HD, Norman A, Smith RJ. Bone erosion in relation to subcutaneous rheumatoid nodules. *Arthritis Rheum* 1970;13(1):69–73.
44. Lehtinen JT, Kaarela K, Kauppi MJ, et al. Bone destruction patterns of the rheumatoid elbow: A radiographic assessment of 148 elbows at 15 years. *J Shoulder Elbow Surg* 2002;11(3):253–258.
45. Lehtinen JT, Kaarela K, Belt EA, et al. Radiographic joint space in rheumatoid elbow joints. A 15-year prospective follow-up study in 74 patients. *Rheumatology (Oxford)* 2001;40(10):1141–1145.
46. Huston KA, Nelson AM, Hunder GG. Shoulder swelling in rheumatoid arthritis secondary to subacromial bursitis. *Arthritis Rheum* 1978;21(1):145–147.
47. Roddy E, Lim V, Fairbairn KJ, Pande I. Ruptured "Baker's-type cyst" of the arm—a case study. *Rheumatology (Oxford)* 2003;42(5):704–705.

48. Lehtinen JT, Kaarela K, Belt EA, et al. Incidence of glenohumeral joint involvement in seropositive rheumatoid arthritis. A 15-year endpoint study. *J Rheumatol* 2000;27(2):347–350.
49. Lehtinen JT, Kaarela K, Belt EA, et al. Relation of glenohumeral and acromioclavicular joint destruction in rheumatoid shoulder. A 15-year follow-up study. *Ann Rheum Dis* 2000;59(2):158–160.
50. Sperling J. Shoulder arthritis in patients with rheumatoid arthritis. *US Musculoskel Rev* 2006;2:79–80.
51. Lehtinen JT, Lehto MU, Kaarela K, et al. Radiographic joint space in rheumatoid glenohumeral joints. A 15-year prospective follow-up study in 74 patients. *Rheumatology (Oxford)* 2000;39(3):288–292.
52. Lehtinen JT, Belt EA, Lybäck CO, et al. Subacromial space in the rheumatoid shoulder: A radiographic 15-year follow-up study of 148 shoulders. *J Shoulder Elbow Surg* 2000;9(3):183–187.
53. Dejager J, Fleming A. Shoulder joint rupture and pseudothrombosis in rheumatoid arthritis. *Ann Rheum Dis* 1984;43:503–504.
54. Burra G, Katchis SD. Rheumatoid arthritis of the forefoot. *Rheum Dis Clin North Am* 1998;24(1):173–180.
55. Trieb K. Management of the foot in rheumatoid arthritis. *J Bone Joint Surg Br* 2005;87(9):1171–1177.
56. Miyamoto N, Senda M, Hamada M, et al. Talonavicular joint abnormalities and walking ability of patients with rheumatoid arthritis. *Acta Med Okayama* 2004;58(2):85–90.
57. Calabro JJ. A critical evaluation of the diagnostic features of the feet in rheumatoid arthritis. *Arthritis Rheum* 1962;5:19–29.
58. Vidigal E, Jacoby RK, Dixon AS, et al. The foot in chronic rheumatoid arthritis. *Ann Rheum Dis* 1975;34(4):292–297.
59. Bienenstock H. Rheumatoid plantar synovial cysts. *Ann Rheum Dis* 1975;34(1):98–99.
60. Rask MR. Achilles tendon rupture owing to rheumatoid disease. Case report with a nine-year follow-up. *JAMA* 1978;239(5):435–436.
61. Semba CP, Mitchell MJ, Sartoris DJ, Resnick D. Multiple stress fractures in the hindfoot in rheumatoid arthritis. *J Rheumatol* 1989;16(5):671–676.
62. Linn-Rasker SP, van der Helm-van Mil AH, Breedveld FC, Huizinga TW. Arthritis of the large joints—in particular, the knee—at first presentation is predictive for a high level of radiological destruction of the small joints in rheumatoid arthritis. *Ann Rheum Dis* 2007;66(5):646–650.
63. Jayson MI, Dixon AS. Valvular mechanisms in juxta-articular cysts. *Ann Rheum Dis* 1970;29(4):415–420.
64. Kraag G, Thevathasan EM, Gordon DA, Walker IH. The hemorrhagic crescent sign of acute synovial rupture. *Ann Intern Med* 1976;85(4):477–478.
65. Beckers C, Jeukens X, Ribbens C, et al. (18)F-FDG PET imaging of rheumatoid knee synovitis correlates with dynamic magnetic resonance and sonographic assessments as well as with the serum level of metalloproteinase-3. *Eur J Nucl Med Mol Imaging* 2006;33(3):275–280.
66. Lehtimaki MY, Kautiainen H, Hämäläinen MM, et al. Hip involvement in seropositive rheumatoid arthritis. Survivorship analysis with a 15-year follow-up. *Scand J Rheumatol* 1998;27(6):406–409.
67. Gusis S, Cocco JA, Rose CD, et al. Protrusio acetabuli in adult rheumatoid arthritis. *Clin Rheumatol* 2005;10(2):158–161.
68. Glickstein MF, Burk DL Jr, Schiebler ML, et al. Avascular necrosis versus other diseases of the hip: Sensitivity of MR imaging. *Radiology* 1988;169(1):213–215.
69. Watanabe Y, Kawai K, Hirohata K. Histopathology of femoral head osteonecrosis in rheumatoid arthritis: The relationship between steroid therapy and lipid degeneration in the osteocyte. *Rheumatol Int* 1989;9(1):25–31.
70. van Eijk IC, Nielen MM, van Soesbergen RM, et al. Cervical spine involvement is rare in early arthritis. *Ann Rheum Dis* 2006;65(7):973–974.
71. Matteson EL. Cervical spine disease in rheumatoid arthritis: How common a finding? How uncommon a problem? *Arthritis Rheum* 2003;48(7):1775–1778.
72. Rawlins BA, Girardi FP, Boachie-Adjei O. Rheumatoid arthritis of the cervical spine. *Rheum Dis Clin North Am* 1998;24(1):55–65.
73. Chellapandian D, et al. The cervical spine involvement in rheumatoid arthritis and its correlation with disease severity. *J Indian Rheumatol Assoc* 2004;12:2–5.
74. Wolfe BK, O'Keeffe D, Mitchell DM, Tchang SP. Rheumatoid arthritis of the cervical spine: Early and progressive radiographic features. *Radiology* 1987;165(1):145–148.
75. Resnick D. Thoracolumbar spine abnormalities in rheumatoid arthritis. *Ann Rheum Dis* 1978;37(4):389–391.
76. Lawrence JS, Sharp J, Ball J, Bier F. Rheumatoid arthritis of the lumbar spine. *Ann Rheum Dis* 1964;23:205–217.
77. Nakamura C, Kawaguchi Y, Ishihara H, et al. Upper thoracic myelopathy caused by vertebral collapse and subluxation in rheumatoid arthritis: Report of two cases. *J Orthop Sci* 2004;9(6):629–634.
78. Dixon AS, Lience E. Sacro-iliac joint in adult rheumatoid arthritis and psoriatic arthropathy. *Ann Rheum Dis* 1961;20:247–257.
79. Khong TK, Rooney PJ. Manubriosternal joint subluxation in rheumatoid arthritis. *J Rheumatol* 1982;9(5):712–715.
80. Yood RA, Goldenberg DL. Sternoclavicular joint arthritis. *Arthritis Rheum* 1980;23(2):232–239.
81. Goupille P, Fouquet B, Goga D, et al. The temporomandibular joint in rheumatoid arthritis: Correlations between clinical and tomographic features. *J Dent* 1993;21(3):141–146.
82. Melchiorre D, Calderazzi A, Maddali Bongi S, et al. A comparison of ultrasonography and magnetic resonance imaging in the evaluation of temporomandibular joint involvement in rheumatoid arthritis and psoriatic arthritis. *Rheumatology (Oxford)* 2003;42(5):673–676.
83. Larheim TA, Smith HJ, Aspestrand F. Temporomandibular joint abnormalities associated with rheumatic disease: Comparison between MR imaging and arthrotomography. *Radiology* 1992;183(1):221–226.
84. Lawry GV, Finerman ML, Hanafee WN, et al. Laryngeal involvement in rheumatoid arthritis. A clinical, laryngoscopic, and computerized tomographic study. *Arthritis Rheum* 1984;27(8):873–882.
85. Kolman J, Morris I. Cricoarytenoid arthritis: A cause of acute upper airway obstruction in rheumatoid arthritis. *Can J Anaesth* 2002;49(7):729–732.
86. Chen JJ, Branstetter BFT, Myers EN. Cricoarytenoid rheumatoid arthritis: An important consideration in aggressive lesions of the larynx. *Am J Neuroradiol* 2005;26(4):970–972.
87. Kamanli A, Gok U, Sahin S, et al. Bilateral cricoarytenoid joint involvement in rheumatoid arthritis: A case report. *Rheumatology (Oxford)* 2001;40(5):593–594.
88. Geterud A, Ejnell H, Månsson I, et al. Severe airway obstruction caused by laryngeal rheumatoid arthritis. *J Rheumatol* 1986;13(5):948–951.
89. Rosenberg JN, Moffat DA, Ramsden RT, et al. Middle ear function in rheumatoid arthritis. *Ann Rheum Dis* 1978;37(6):522–524.
90. Reiter D, Konkle DF, Myers AR, et al. Middle ear immittance in rheumatoid arthritis. *Arch Otolaryngol* 1980;106(2):114–117.
91. Cohen G, Gossec L, Dougados M, et al., Radiological damage in patients with rheumatoid arthritis on sustained remission. *Ann Rheum Dis* 2007;66(3):358–363.
92. Brown AK, Quinn MA, Karim Z, et al., Presence of significant synovitis in rheumatoid arthritis patients with disease-modifying antirheumatic drug-induced clinical remission: Evidence from an imaging study may explain structural progression. *Arthritis Rheum* 2006;54(12)3761–3773.

Clinical Features of Rheumatoid Arthritis: Extra-Articular Manifestations

Carl Turesson and Eric L. Matteson

Rheumatoid arthritis (RA) is a systemic, inflammatory disease. Effects of systemic inflammation contribute substantially to the risk of disease-related premature mortality. In particular, patients with extra-articular RA (ExRA) manifestations are at an increased risk of developing cardiovascular disease (CVD) or severe infections.[1,2]

Severe ExRA manifestations (including vasculitis, vasculitis-related neuropathy, Felty's syndrome, glomerulonephritis, pericarditis, pleuritis, and scleritis) develop in approximately 15% of Caucasian patients with RA during long-term follow-up, and incidence estimates from community-based RA cohorts and early RA inception cohorts have been close to 1 case per 100 person-years.[3,4] Signs of systemic inflammation in patients with RA include constitutional symptoms, such as fatigue, low-grade fever, and weight loss, and elevated levels of inflammatory biomarkers including erythrocyte sedimentation rate and C-reactive protein. Uncontrolled systemic inflammation in RA is associated with several long-term complications. For instance, rheumatoid cachexia, with a loss of lean body mass, is often a feature of long-standing, severe disease. A low body mass index has been associated with an increased mortality risk in patients with RA.[5] High disease activity and persistent elevation of inflammatory biomarker levels are associated with tissue amyloidosis and organ damage.[6]

Rheumatoid Nodules

The most frequent ExRA manifestation is the development of subcutaneous rheumatoid nodules (Figure 5B-1), which occur in 7% of patients with RA at disease onset and approximately 30% of all patients with RA at some point during the disease course.[7]

Subcutaneous nodules occur mainly in patients with RA who are seropositive for rheumatoid factor (RF).[8] Presence of the nodules may reflect the level of disease activity, but can occur in cases of relatively quiescent joint disease. Patients with rheumatoid nodules in early RA are at an increased risk of developing more severe ExRA manifestations.[8]

Rheumatoid nodules develop most commonly on pressure areas, including the elbows, finger joints, ischial and sacral prominences, the occipital scalp, and the Achilles tendon, but they can also occur in internal organ tissue, such as the myocardium, the meninges, and lung tissue.[9] The etiology of rheumatoid nodules is uncertain, but they appear to be T-helper 1 granulomata.[10] They may develop as a result of small-vessel vasculitis with fibrinoid necrosis, which forms the center of the nodule, and surrounding fibroblastic proliferation; histologically, there is focal central fibrinoid necrosis with surrounding fibroblasts.[11] In some patients, cutaneous microinfarcts overlying rheumatoid nodules may be seen (Figure 5B-2).

Hematologic Disease

Active RA is associated with anemia of chronic disease and lymphadenopathy, and also with an increased risk of non-Hodgkin lymphoma compared with the general population.[12,13] The most frequent subtype in patients with RA is large-cell, B-cell lymphoma.[13] Chronic neutropenia with splenomegaly in the absence of lymphoma occurs in patients with Felty's syndrome. However, chronic RA-related neutropenia that is otherwise clinically and immunologically similar to that seen in classic Felty's syndrome may occur in patients with RA in the absence of significant enlargement of the spleen.[14] Felty's syndrome typically occurs in patients with long-standing, seropositive, nodular, deforming RA, although patients have occasionally been reported to present with features of Felty's syndrome at disease onset.[15] The condition affects approximately 1% of patients with RA.[16]

Vasculitis

Systemic vasculitis in patients with RA may present with involvement of small- and medium-sized vessels of the skin and a progressive sensorimotor neuropathy. This may lead to mononeuritis multiplex and severe vasculitis of the lower extremities (Figure 5B-3). Without proper treatment, this infrequent phenotype can be associated with a poor prognosis. Cutaneous manifestations include nail-fold infarcts, leg ulcers, purpura, and digital gangrene. Isolated nailfold infarcts or leg ulcers may occur without associated systemic involvement. In some patients, the vasculitis may extend to involve mesenteric, coronary, and cerebral arteries. Systemic vasculitis is also associated

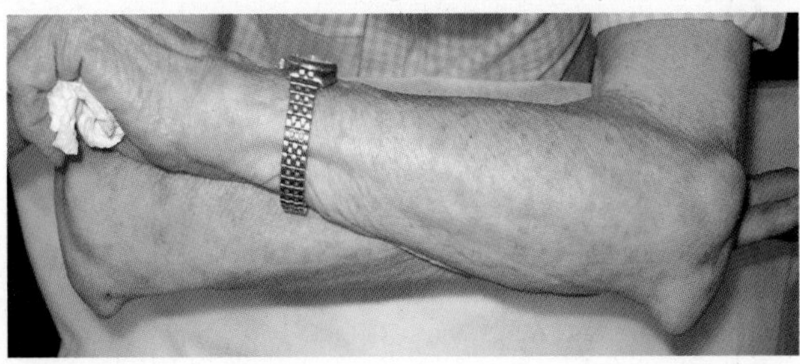

Figure 5B-1. Subcutaneous rheumatoid nodules with typical distribution.

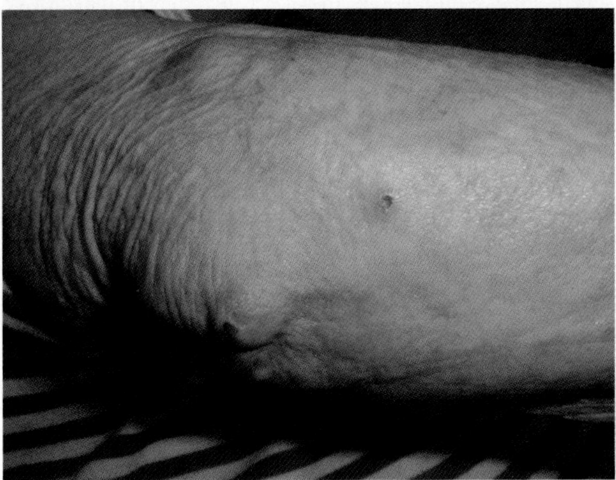

Figure 5B-2. Subcutaneous rheumatoid nodule with microinfarcts in a patient with complicated extra-articular RA.

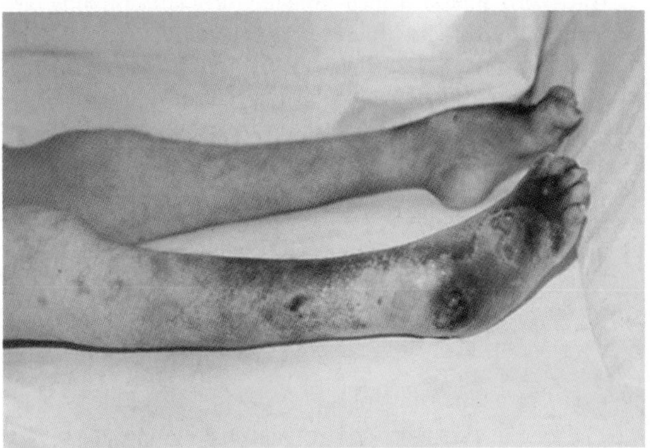

Figure 5B-3. Systemic rheumatoid vasculitis. Bilateral foot droop due to mononeuritis multiplex and bilateral lower-extremity vasculitis is seen.

with severe eye involvement and CVD.[17] Patients with rheumatoid vasculitis usually have high serum titers of RF, cryoglobulins, and circulating immune complexes, and low levels of complement.[18] In addition, they usually have an increased erythrocyte sedimentation rate, anemia, thrombocytosis, and a diminished serum albumin concentration.

Lower leg ulcers are an especially vexing clinical manifestation of severe, generally long-standing RA. The prognosis of patients with RA-associated leg ulcers is highly variable. It is likely that other factors, in addition to the vasculitis, influence the final outcome. The pathogenesis of leg ulcers is thought to be due to an underlying vasculitis that initiates the lesions, but ulcer expansion and its chronicity may be influenced by other features, including concomitant venous insufficiency, arterial insufficiency, dependent edema, trauma, superimposed infection, and long-term use of glucocorticoids.[19]

Patients with vasculitis and other severe ExRA manifestations have an increased risk of peripheral atherosclerotic vascular disease,[20] other cardiovascular events,[1] and cardiovascular death.[21] These associations are independent of smoking. Strategies to prevent vascular disease in patients with RA should include optimal antirheumatic treatment to control disease activity, and interventions aimed at traditional cardiovascular risk factors.

Rheumatoid Arthritis–Associated Lung Disease

Pulmonary involvement in RA is frequent, although not always clinically recognized.[22] Lung manifestations in RA include rheumatoid pleuritis, RA-associated interstitial pneumonitis, cryptogenic organizing pneumonia, obliterative bronchiolitis, and intrapulmonary rheumatoid nodules. Pleuritis in patients with RA may lead to progressing respiratory distress due to rapidly accumulating pleural fluid, or have an insidious course, which is detected only at routine chest radiography or at autopsy. Rheumatoid pleural effusions are usually exudates with mixed cell counts and low glucose levels.[23] The low glucose level in rheumatoid pleural effusions is a result of increased glucose consumption by inflammatory cells and impaired transport across the inflamed pleura. The presence of multinucleated giant cells in pleural fluid is highly specific for rheumatoid pleuritis, but such cells are seen in less than 50% of cases.[24] Rheumatoid pleuritis is associated with exudative pericarditis, and also with interstitial lung disease.

The prevalence of diffuse interstitial pulmonary fibrosis in RA varies, depending on the epidemiologic and diagnostic methods used to detect and evaluate the condition. In a community-based study, 6% of patients developed symptomatic interstitial lung disease within 10 years of RA onset.[25] The most common radiographic finding is bilateral basilar interstitial abnormalities, which are often asymmetric. Initially, these may appear as patchy alveolar infiltrates; with progressive disease a more reticulonodular pattern is seen.[26] High-resolution computed tomography and open lung biopsy are considered the gold-standard methods for diagnosing interstitial lung disease.[27] The clinical presentation and course of pulmonary fibrosis in RA has been reported to be similar to that of idiopathic pulmonary fibrosis, but response to immunosuppression may actually be better if pulmonary fibrosis occurs in the context of RA or other collagen diseases.[28] Histologic findings and results of bronchoalveolar lavage can be variable, ranging from lymphocytic alveolitis to neutrophilic inflammation. Histologic features from tissue obtained at lung biopsy include an inflammatory infiltrate with lymphocytes, plasma cells, and histiocytes with varying degrees of fibrosis, and may be classified as usual interstitial pneumonitis (IP) or nonspecific IP.[27] Specific stainings have

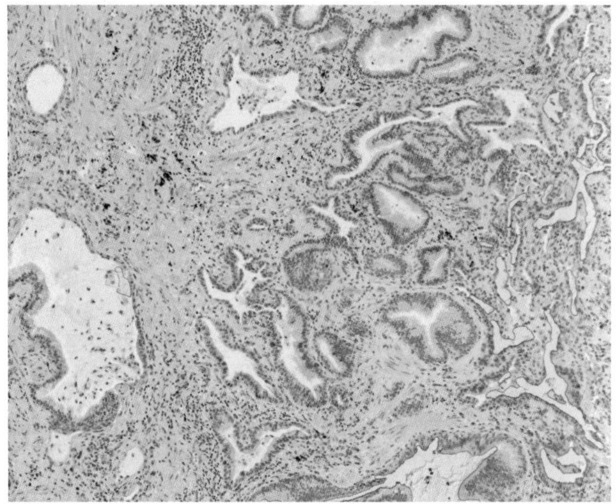

Figure 5B-4. Interstitial pneumonitis with CD4+ T cells (red stain) in a patient with RA (original magnification × 100).

suggested a role for $CD4^+$ T cells in patients with RA-associated IP, but not in patients with idiopathic IP[29] (Figure 5B-4). RA-specific dysregulation of T cells may be important in the pathogenesis of RA-associated lung disease, with potential implications for targeted therapies.[29] In addition, $CD20^+$ B cells in diffuse infiltrates and structures resembling lymphoid follicles is a prominent feature of RA associated IP. Quantification of the $CD20^+$ infiltrates has revealed them to be significantly more abundant in patients with RA-associated IP than those with idiopathic IP.[30]

RA-associated IP must be distinguished from methotrexate-induced lung toxicity, which usually has a subacute onset with rapidly progressive respiratory symptoms, less radiographic evidence of fibrosis, and a histologic pattern dominated by eosinophilia and type II pneumocyte hyperplasia.[31] Possible toxic drug reactions have also been reported in patients treated with leflunomide and tumor necrosis factor (TNF) inhibitors.[27] The possibility of a superimposed respiratory tract infection must be considered in the setting of rapid progression of pulmonary symptoms in patients with suspected RA-associated or treatment-related lung disease.

Other Manifestations

Pericarditis, which is the most frequent cardiac manifestation of RA,[32] presents as acute chest pain and dyspnea with exudative fluid, or as long-standing right-sided heart failure due to chronic constrictive pericarditis. The 30-year incidence of symptomatic and clinically detected pericarditis has been estimated to be 11%,[3] although subclinical involvement may be considerably more common and is frequently detected at autopsy.[33]

RA-associated glomerulonephritis is often of the mesangioproliferative type, and is less likely to progress to renal failure than the nephritis of systemic lupus erythematosus.[34] Scleritis and peripheral ulcerative keratitis are associated with severe, long-standing joint disease, which may or may not be active, and with ExRA manifestations involving other organs. Patients with RA may also develop milder eye manifestations such as episcleritis, often in the setting of active disease, or keratoconjunctivitis sicca in the setting of secondary Sjögren's syndrome.

Predictors and Pathogenesis

Severe ExRA manifestations share immunologic and inflammatory disease mechanisms (Table 5B-1), although local factors may also influence organ involvement. Predictors of severe ExRA include clinical, serologic, and genetic markers (Figure 5B-5). In addition to being a risk factor for the development of RA,[35] smoking is associated with early rheumatoid nodules and development of severe ExRA.[25,36] In a community-based cohort of patients with RA, the association between smoking and future development of ExRA was found to be independent of RF positivity,[25] indicating that smoking may be involved in the pathogenesis of systemic features of RA through several different mechanisms.

HLA-DRB1 alleles, which influence RA susceptibility, are also predictors of disease severity, including extra-articular organ involvement. In particular, in populations of mainly northern European descent, patients with a double dose of HLA-DRB1*04 shared epitope alleles have an increased risk of developing severe ExRA.[37,38] The gene dose phenomenon may be explained by an effect on the selection and activation of T cells through an interaction between major histocompatibility complex (MHC) class II molecules and T-cell receptors.[38] In

Table 5B-1. Pathogenetic Mechanisms in Extra-Articular Rheumatoid Arthritis

Disease Mechanism	Proposed Pathway	Organ Involvement	References
Systemic production of proinflammatory cytokines	Increased leukocyte migration Increased serum amyloid A expression with tissue deposition	Severe extra-articular manifestations overall Amyloidosis	45,49
Circulating immune complexes	Immune complex tissue deposition Complement activation	Vasculitis Felty's syndrome	41,43,44
Systemic endothelial activation	Increased tissue cell infiltration Disturbed hemostasis Local hypoxia	Severe extra-articular RA	45,46
Local T- and B-cell infiltration	Chronic inflammation with associated fibrosis	RA-associated interstitial pneumonitis	29,30
Circulating $CD28^{null}$ T cells with features of immunosenescence	Cytotoxicity Proinflammatory cytokine production	Vasculitis Severe extra-articular RA overall	50–52

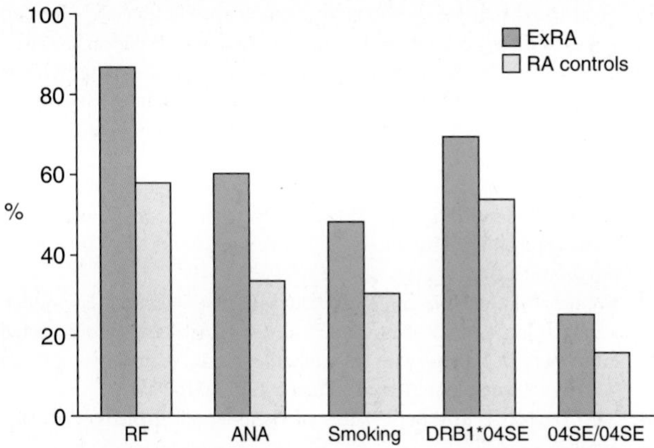

Figure 5B-5. Predictors of severe extra-articular manifestations in a large multicenter case cohort of patients with RA from Sweden and the United States. (Data from Turesson C, Schaid DJ, Weyand CM, et al. Association of smoking and HLA-C3 with vasculitis in patients with rheumatoid arthritis. *Arthritis Rheum* 2006;54:2776–2783; and Turesson C, Schaid DJ, Weyand CM, et al. The impact of HLA-DRB1 genes on extra-articular disease manifestations in rheumatoid arthritis. *Arthritis Res Ther* 2005;7:R1386–R1393.) *RF,* Rheumatoid factor; *ANA,* antinuclear antibodies; *DRB1*04 SE,* shared epitope of HLA-DRB1*04; *04 SE/04 SE,* double dose of HLA-DRB1*04 SE.

addition, MHC class I molecules have been implicated in RA-associated vasculitis. The HLA-C*03 allele has been associated with vasculitis, but not with other ExRA manifestations.[36,39] Genetic HLA-C variation could be a marker for other linked genes, or could determine MHC class I–associated immune responses.

Severe ExRA manifestations occur mainly in RF-seropositive patients,[40] and very high levels of RF and antibodies to cyclic citrullinated peptides (anti-CCP) have been found in patients with RA-associated vasculitis and Felty's syndrome,[41] and also in RA-associated IP.[42] Circulating immune complexes have been implicated in vasculitis[43] and other severe ExRA manifestations.[44] Studies of muscle tissue from patients with severe ExRA (vasculitis, pericarditis, pleuritis, or Felty's syndrome) have shown increased endothelial expression of HLA-DQ and interleukin-1α in the absence of local inflammatory infiltrates,[45] suggesting that this is a sign of generalized endothelial activation.[46] Microvascular abnormalities may play a role in a number of ExRA organ manifestations and in vascular comorbidity through effects on cell migration, tissue oxygenation, and hemostasis. The concept of extra-articular RA as a systemic vascular disorder is supported by findings of perivascular cell infiltrates in rheumatoid nodules[11] and pericarditis specimen.[47]

Loss of lean body mass in patients with RA correlates with biomarkers of inflammation,[48] and elevated serum levels of TNF have been observed in patients with systemic amyloidosis[49] and other severe ExRA organ involvement.[45] Chronic systemic inflammation in severe RA is associated with the emergence of clonally expanded, circulating T cells with features of immunosenescence, including downregulation of the costimulatory molecule CD28 and upregulation of markers of natural killer cells, including killer immunoglobulin-like receptors (KIR) and CD56.[50–52] Such cells may contribute to extra-articular organ involvement in RA.

Management of Extra-Articular Manifestations

Recommendations for treatment of systemic features of RA are based mainly on experience from treatment of RA in general, anecdotal case reports, and expert opinion and experience.[53] Proper management of patients with ExRA manifestations includes adequate long-term treatment with disease-modifying antirheumatic drugs (DMARDs), with the addition of glucocorticoids for severe organ complications. Controlled studies show improved outcomes in patients with systemic vasculitis and severe eye manifestations treated with cyclophosphamide and high-dose glucocorticoids.[17,54,55] In patients with Felty's syndrome, white blood cell counts may improve with conventional DMARD therapy, such as methotrexate.[56] Consistent with the suggested role for T cells in RA-associated IP discussed earlier, a beneficial response to cyclosporine has been described in several case reports.[53]

Although the effect of TNF inhibitors and other biologic response modifiers on ExRA manifestations has not been systematically evaluated, a number of reports of excellent responses have been published, including manifestations such as vasculitis and scleritis.[53,57] On the other hand, an induction of vasculitis and a worsening of interstitial lung disease have also been reported after treatment with TNF inhibitors.[58–60] Observational studies have yielded conflicting results. Presently, there is a need for more data on effects of TNF blockers on pulmonary disease.

Additional studies of specific treatments for ExRA are needed, particularly in patients with RA-associated IP. Cautious assessment of treatment with other biologic response modifiers directed at specific cells, such as anti–T cell and anti–B cell treatment for RA-associated lung disease, may be of value based for example on experience with anti–B-cell therapy for IP in other forms of connective tissue disorders.[61–63] Treatments directed at interfering with the fibrotic process and mast cell function being developed for other forms of IP may also be of value.

References

1. Turesson C, McClelland RL, Christianson TJ, et al. Severe extra-articular disease manifestations are associated with an increased risk of first ever cardiovascular events in patients with rheumatoid arthritis. *Ann Rheum Dis* 2007;66:70–75.
2. Doran MF, Crowson CS, Pond GR, et al. Predictors of infection in rheumatoid arthritis. *Arthritis Rheum* 2002;46:2294–2300.
3. Turesson C, O'Fallon WM, Crowson CS, et al. Occurrence of extra-articular disease manifestations is associated with excess mortality in a community based study of rheumatoid arthritis. *J Rheumatol* 2002;29:62–67.
4. Turesson C, Eberhardt K, Jacobsson LTH, Lindqvist E. Incidence and predictors of severe extra-articular disease manifestations in an

early rheumatoid arthritis inception cohort. *Ann Rheum Dis* 2007; 66:1543–1545.

5. Kremers HM, Nicola PJ, Crowson CS, et al. Prognostic importance of low body mass index in relation to cardiovascular mortality in rheumatoid arthritis. *Arthritis Rheum* 2004;50:3450–3457.
6. Schneider F. AA amyoloidosis in inflammatory rheumatic diseases. A report of clinical experiences. *Z Rheumatol* 1992;51:177–182.
7. Nyhäll-Wåhlin B, Jacobsson LT, Petersson IF, et al. Smoking is a strong risk factor for rheumatoid nodules in early rheumatoid arthritis. *Ann Rheum Dis* 2006;65:601–606.
8. Turesson C, Jacobsson L, Bergström U, et al. Predictors of extra-articular manifestations in rheumatoid arthritis. *Scand J Rheumatol* 2000;29:358–364.
9. Raven RW, Weber FP, Price LW. The necrobiotic nodules of rheumatoid arthritis. *Ann Rheum Dis* 1948;7:63–75.
10. Hessian PA, Highton J, Kean A, et al. Cytokine profile of the rheumatoid nodule suggests that it is a Th1 granuloma. *Arthritis Rheum* 2003;48:334–338.
11. Sokoloff L, McCluskey RT, Bunim JJ. Vascularity of the early subcutaneous nodule in rheumatoid arthritis. *Arch Pathol* 1953;55: 475–495.
12. Kassan SS, Chused TL, Moutsopoulos HM, et al. Increased risk of lymphoma in sicca syndrome. *Ann Intern Med* 1978;89: 888–892.
13. Baecklund E, Iliadou A, Askling J, et al. Association of chronic inflammation, not its treatment, with increased lymphoma risk in rheumatoid arthritis. *Arthritis Rheum* 2006;54:692–701.
14. Campion G, Maddison PJ, Goulding N, et al. The Felty syndrome: A case-matched study of clinical manifestations and outcome, serologic features, and immunogenetic associations. *Medicine (Baltimore)* 1990;69:69–80.
15. Turesson C. Arthritis with fever of unknown origin. *Int J Adv Rheumatol* 2006;4:72–75.
16. Saway PA, Prasthofer EF, Barton JC. Prevalence of granular lymphocyte proliferations in patients with rheumatoid arthritis and neutropenia. *Am J Med* 1989;86: 303–307.
17. Foster AC, Forstot SL, Wilson LA. Mortality rate in rheumatoid arthritis patients developing necrotizing scleritis or peripheral ulcerative keratitis: Effects of systemic immunosuppression. *Ophthalmology* 1984;91:1253–1263.
18. Scott DG, Bacon PA, Allen C, et al. IgG rheumatoid factor, complement and immune complexes in rheumatoid synovitis and vasculitis: Comparative and serial studies during cytotoxic therapy. *Clin Exp Immunol* 1981;43:54–63.
19. Pun YL, Barraclough DR, Muirden KD. Leg ulcers in rheumatoid arthritis. *Med J Aust* 1990;153:585–587.
20. Liang KP, Liang KV, Matteson EL, et al. Incidence of noncardiac vascular disease in rheumatoid arthritis and relationship to extra-articular disease manifestations. *Arthritis Rheum* 2006;54:642–648.
21. Maradit-Kremers HM, Nicola PJ, Crowson CS, et al. Cardiovascular death in rheumatoid arthritis: A population-based study. *Arthritis Rheum* 2005;52:722–732.
22. Saag KG, Kolluri S, Koehnke RK, et al. Rheumatoid arthritis lung disease. Determinants of radiographic and physiologic abnormalities. *Arthritis Rheum* 1996;39:1711–1719.
23. Walker WC, Wright V. Pulmonary lesions in rheumatoid arthritis. *Medicine* 1968;47:501–520.
24. Boddington MM, Spriggs AI, Morton JA, Mowat AG. Cytodiagnosis of rheumatoid pleural effusions. *J Clin Pathol* 1971;24: 95–106.
25. Turesson C, O'Fallon WM, Crowson CS, et al. Extra-articular disease manifestations in rheumatoid arthritis: Incidence trends and risk factors over 46 years. *Ann Rheum Dis* 2003;62:722–727.
26. Tanoue LT. Pulmonary manifestations of rheumatoid arthritis. *Clin Chest Med* 1998;19:667–685.
27. Kim DS. Interstitial lung disease in rheumatoid arthritis: Recent advances. *Curr Opin Pulm Med* 2006;12:346–353.
28. Scott DG, Bacon PA. Response to methotrexate in fibrosing alveolitis associated with connective tissue disease. *Thorax* 1980;35:725–731.
29. Turesson C, Matteson EL, Vuk-Pavlovic Z, et al. Increased CD4+ T cell infiltrates in rheumatoid arthritis-associated interstitial pneumonitis compared with idiopathic interstitial pneumonitis. *Arthritis Rheum* 2005;52:73–79.
30. Atkins SR, Turesson C, Myers JL, et al. Morphological and quantitative assessment of CD20+ B-cell infiltrates in rheumatoid arthritis associated nonspecific interstitial pneumonia and usual interstitial pneumonia. *Arthritis Rheum* 2006;54:635–641.
31. Kremer JM, Alarcón GS, Weinblatt ME, et al. Clinical, laboratory, radiographic, and histopathologic features of methotrexate-associated lung injury in patients with rheumatoid arthritis: A multicenter study with literature review. *Arthritis Rheum* 1997;40:1829–1837.
32. Kirk J, Cosh J. The pericarditis of rheumatoid arthritis. *Q J Med* 1969;38:397–423.
33. Bonfiglio T, Atwater EC. Heart disease in patients with seropositive rheumatoid arthritis: A controlled autopsy study and review. *Arch Intern Med* 1969;124:714–719.
34. Ramirez G, Lambert R, Bloomer HA. Renal pathology in patients with rheumatoid arthritis. *Nephron* 1981;28:124–126.
35. Silman AJ, Newman J, MacGregor AJ. Cigarette smoking increases the risk of rheumatoid arthritis. Results from a nationwide study of disease-discordant twins. *Arthritis Rheum* 1996;39:732–735.
36. Turesson C, Schaid DJ, Weyand CM, et al. Association of smoking and HLA-C3 with vasculitis in patients with rheumatoid arthritis. *Arthritis Rheum* 2006;54:2776–2783.
37. Turesson C, Schaid DJ, Weyand CM, et al. The impact of HLA-DRB1 genes on extra-articular disease manifestations in rheumatoid arthritis. *Arthritis Res Ther* 2005;7:R1386–R1393.
38. Turesson C, Weyand CM, Matteson EL. Genetics of rheumatoid arthritis—is there a pattern predicting extra-articular manifestations? *Arthritis Care Res* 2004;51:853–863.
39. Yen JH, Moore BE, Nakajima T, et al. Major histocompatibility complex class I–recognizing receptors are disease risk genes in rheumatoid arthritis. *J Exp Med* 2001;193:1159–1167.
40. Voskuyl AE, Zwinderman AH, Westedt ML, et al. Factors associated with the development of rheumatoid vasculitis: Results of a case control study. *Ann Rheum Dis* 1996;55:190–192.
41. Turesson C, Jacobsson LT, Sturfelt G, et al. Rheumatoid factor and antibodies to cyclic citrullinated peptides are associated with severe extra-articular manifestations in rheumatoid arthritis. *Ann Rheum Dis* 2007;66:59–64.
42. Bongartz T, Cantaert T, Atkins SR, et al. Citrullination in extra-articular manifestations in rheumatoid arthritis. *Rheumatology (Oxford)* 2007;46:70–75.
43. Scott DG, Bacon PA, Allen C, et al. IgG rheumatoid factor, complement and immune complexes in rheumatoid synovitis and vasculitis: Comparative and serial studies during cytotoxic therapy. *Clin Exp Immunol* 1981;43:54–63.
44. Melsom RD, Hornsfall AC, Schrieber L, et al. Anti-C1q affinitiy associated circulating immune complexes correlate with extra-articular rheumatoid disease. *Rheumatol Int* 1986;6:227–231.
45. Turesson C, Englund P, Jacobsson L, et al. Increased endothelial expression of HLA-DQ and Interleukin-1-α in extra-articular rheumatoid arthritis—results from immunohistochemical studies of skeletal muscle. *Rheumatology* 2001;40:1346–1354.
46. Turesson C. Endothelial expression of MHC class II molecules in autoimmune disease. *Curr Pharm Des* 2004;10:129–143.
47. Butnam S, Espinoza LR, Del Carpio J, Osterland CK. Rheumatoid pericarditis. Rapid deterioration with evidence of local vasculitis. *JAMA* 1977;238:2394–2396.
48. Roubenoff R, Roubenoff RA, Cannon JG, et al. Rheumatoid cachexia: Cytokine-driven hypermetabolism accompanying reduced body cell mass in chronic inflammation. *J Clin Invest* 1994;93:2379–2386.
49. Maury CP, Liljestrom M, Laiho K, et al. Tumor necrosis factor alpha, its soluble receptor 1, and –308 gene promoter polymorphism

in patients with rheumatoid arthritis witho or without amyloidosis—implications for the pathogenesis of nephropathy and anemia of chronic disease in reactive amyloidosis. *Arthritis Rheum* 2003;48:3069–3076.

50. Schmidt D, Goronzy JJ, Weyand CM, et al. CD4+ CD7– CD28– T cells are expanded in rheumatoid arthritis and characterized by autoreactivity. *J Clin Invest* 1996;97:2027–2037.
51. Michel JJ, Turesson C, Lemster B, et al. CD56-expressing T cells that have senescent features are expanded in rheumatoid arthritis. *Arthritis Rheum* 2007;56:43–45.
52. Martens PB, Goronzy JJ, Schaid D, et al. Expansion of unusual CD4+ T cells in severe rheumatoid arthritis. *Arthritis Rheum* 1997;40:1106–1114.
53. Turesson C, Matteson EL. Management of extra-articular disease manifestations in rheumatoid arthritis. *Curr Opin Rheumatol* 2004;16:206–211.
54. Scott DG, Bacon PA. Intravenous cyclophosphamide plus methylprednisolone in treatment of systemic rheumatoid vasculitis. *Am J Med* 1984;76:377–384.
55. Clewes AR, Dawson JK, Kaye S, et al. Peripheral ulcerative keratitis in rheumatoid arthritis: Successful use of cyclophosphamide and comparison of clinical and serological characteristics. *Ann Rheum Dis* 2005;64:961–962.
56. Fiechtner JJ, Miller RD, Starkebaum G. Reversal of neutropenia with methotrexate in patients with Felty's syndrome: Correlation of response with neutrophil-reactive IgG. *Arthritis Rheum* 1989;32:194–201.
57. Botsios C, Sfriso P, Ostuni PA, et al. Efficacy of the IL-1 receptor antagonist, anakinra, for the treatment of diffuse anterior scleritis in rheumatoid arthritis. Report of two cases. *Rheumatology* 2007;46:1042–1043.
58. Jarrett SJ, Cunnane G, Conaghan PG, et al. Anti-tumor necrosis factor-alpha induced vasculitis: Case series. *J Rheumatol* 2003;30:2287–2291.
59. Chatterjee S. Severe interstitial pneumonitis associated with infliximab therapy. *Scand J Rheumatol* 2004;33:276–277.
60. Lindsay K, Melsom R, Jacob BK, et al. Acute progression of interstitial lung disease: A complication of etanercept particularly in the presence of rheumatoid lung and methotrexate treatment. *Rheumatology (Oxford)* 2006;45:1048–1049.
61. Brulhart L, Waldburger J-M, Gabay C. Rituximab in the treatment of antisynthetase syndrome. *Ann Rheum Dis* 2006;65:974–975.
62. Levine TD. Rituximab in the treatment of dermatomyositis: An open label pilot study. *Arthritis Rheum* 2005;52:601–607.
63. Wagner SA, Mehta AC, Laber DA. Rituximab-induced interstitial lung disease. *Am J Hematol* 2007;82:916–919.

Comorbidity in Rheumatoid Arthritis

John M. Esdaile, Mavis Goycochea, and Diane Lacaille

Comorbidity is most commonly defined as "a concomitant but unrelated pathologic or disease process."[1] For example, a person with breast cancer who has chronic bronchitis due to smoking would be considered to have chronic bronchitis as a comorbid condition. In contrast to the concept that the comorbid disease is unrelated to the primary disease, comorbidity has also been used to include conditions that are actually caused by the underlying condition. As noted by Wikipedia, "this is a newer, nonstandard definition and is less well accepted."[2] The second definition of comorbidity is widely used in rheumatology. Indeed, the comorbid conditions such as infection, osteoporosis or cardiovascular disease could be considered as complications in patients with rheumatoid arthritis (RA), as they result in significant burdens in addition to the articular complications from the primary disease. All of the above are complications of RA—complications of a severe condition, the primary manifestation of which is articular, but in which the systemic features of the disease create a raft of complications, each of which carries both substantial disability and mortality risk.

Infection in Rheumatic Arthritis

Increase in Risk

Infection is a cause of significant morbidity[3] and mortality in patients with RA.[4] Despite a large literature, there are only a limited number of controlled studies. Doran et al.[3] conducted a population-based study and demonstrated that after controlling for age, sex, smoking, leucopenia, corticosteroid use, and diabetes mellitus, the incidence of confirmed infections in RA was increased 1.7-fold (95% confidence interval [CI]: 1.42–2.03), and that infections requiring hospitalization were increased 1.83-fold (95% CI: 1.52–2.21). They noted that the increase was greatest for infections of the skin, soft tissues, and respiratory tract, and particularly for the joints and bone. Septic arthritis was increased almost 15-fold and osteomyelitis was increased 10-fold compared to the general population. Overall, one in five people with RA in the Rochester, Minnesota community had an objective infection every year.

Two earlier controlled studies from clinics in the Netherlands found no increase in infections in RA.[5,6] In both studies, the controls were patients with osteoarthritis or fibromyalgia. The authors assessed infections by recall rather than objective confirmation, which may explain the difference in the results from those of Doran.

Is Therapy the Cause? Nonbiologic Disease-Modifying Antirheumatic Drugs

The reason for the increased morbidity and mortality due to infection is uncertain. Inflammation or some other aspect of the immune dysregulation of RA could increase the risk. Alternatively, RA treatment could predispose to infection, especially the use of immunosuppressive drugs.

Lacaille et al.[7] evaluated an administrative dataset of 27,710 persons with RA in British Columbia, Canada to assess the role of nonbiologic disease-modifying antirheumatic drugs (DMARDs) in causing the increase in the rate of infections. Results were adjusted for age, sex, RA duration, socioeconomic status, and corticosteroid use, comorbidity, and prior infections as time-dependent covariates. When nonbiologic DMARDs were used without corticosteroids, there was no increase in infections compared to those with RA not receiving DMARDs; in fact, there was a 10% decrease in the incidence of mild infections and a trend to a decrease in serious infections. There was no overall difference in effect between nonimmunosuppressive DMARDs and those with immunosuppressive potential. However, when the effect of individual DMARDs with immunosuppressive potential was examined, infection rates were higher with azathioprine, cyclosporine, cyclophosphamide, and leflunomide, but not with methotrexate.

In Lacaille's study,[7] corticosteroids increased the rate of both mild and serious infections. When used alone, corticosteroids almost doubled the risk of hospitalization for infection, a finding noted in a half-dozen earlier studies.[8]

Biologic Agents

While corticosteroids have been available for more than 50 years, and drugs such as methotrexate for more than a quarter century, allowing time for the accumulation of data on infection, the same is not true for biologic agents. Solid data are generally lacking. All anti-TNF agents have resulted in increased rates of tuberculosis (Tbc), other granulomatous infections, and other bacterial intracellular infections. The pattern of Tbc differs with anti-TNF therapy—there is more extrapulmonary Tbc than one would expect.[9] Pretreatment screening for Tbc appears to reduce the rate of infection.

A recent report highlights the problem. The British Society for Rheumatology Biologics Register was assessed, and the conclusion reached was that "anti-TNF therapy was not associated with increased risk of overall serious infection compared with DMARD treatment," although the authors noted that serious skin and soft-tissue infections were increased.[10]

A follow-up report noted the impact of how the relationship of the biologic of interest to the infection was modeled in the analysis.[11] The reanalysis concluded that all anti-TNF treatments increase the risk of serious infection more than fourfold in the first 90 days of use and that there is an increased risk for the 90 days following drug discontinuation. For the present, it is best to assume that all biologic agents carry an increased risk of serious infection.

Osteoporosis and Fracture in Rheumatoid Arthritis

Increase in Risk

The bone mineral density (BMD) of 394 female patients identified in the Oslo County RA Register was contrasted to European/U.S. healthy subjects.[12] BMD was reduced at the femoral neck and total hip, but not for the spine at L2–L4. The possibility that the BMD at L2–L4 was increased by osteoarthritis or fractures was noted by the authors. The rate of osteoporosis, defined as a T score of 2.5 standard deviations or less below the mean of young female controls, was doubled in the RA population.

Fracture is the outcome of concern with osteoporosis. The increased risk of hip fracture in RA has been known for more than a decade. A recent study of the British General Practice Research Database evaluated 30,262 patients with RA and three times as many controls matched for age, sex, and calendar time. The study identified an increase in risk of fractures for hip, pelvis, vertebrae, humerus, and tibia/fibula.[13] Radius/ulna fractures were not increased but if treated in the emergency or other outpatient setting they would not have been detected. The relative risk of hip fracture was 2.0 (95% CI: 1.8–2.3) and of spinal fractures was 2.4 (95% CI: 2.0–2.8).

A study of vertebral deformities in women with RA in the Oslo County RA Register was contrasted with population-based controls matched for age, gender, and residential area.[14] The risk of deformities was increased, particularly for multiple deformities (relative risk for two or more deformities was 2.6; 95% CI: 1.2–6.0).

Risk Factors

In the Oslo County RA Registry studies, BMD was predicted by older age, low body mass index (BMI), current corticosteroid use, higher modified Health Assessment Questionnaire scores, and rheumatoid factor positivity.[12] RA predicted vertebral deformities independent of bone mineral density and corticosteroid use, suggesting that disease factors are causal.[14]

In the British General Practice report, the authors presented a scoring system for calculating the risk of hip and spinal fractures.[13] For instance, they noted that a 65-year-old woman with long-standing RA and a low BMI, a previous history of fracture and use of corticosteroids had an almost 6% chance of fracture in the following 5 years. Long-standing disease and low BMI, both of which relate to disease activity, as well as corticosteroid use, were the predictors identified for hip fracture on multivariate analysis.

Can the Risk Be Reduced?

Rheumatoid arthritis is recognized as an independent risk factor for reduced BMD and fracture. Based on recommendations for bone mass measurement from the International Society for Clinical Densitometry, all postmenopausal women and men aged 50 and above with RA should have BMD measurement. In addition, premenopausal women and younger men receiving glucocorticoid therapy at doses of 5 mg per day or above should also have BMD measured.[15]

Disease activity of RA has been linked to reduced BMD and fracture, but the evidence that controlling disease activity may limit these complications is scant and relies primarily on studies of bone markers.[16] There are sufficient other reasons to treat RA disease activity aggressively and future research can illuminate whether this reduces osteoporosis and its consequences.

Calcium supplementation and vitamin D use for osteoporosis and fracture prevention are likely reasonable, especially in those with low calcium and vitamin D intakes. Vitamin D levels in RA may be reduced as a consequence of the disease.[17] Furthermore, higher serum levels of vitamin D have been hypothesized to have immunologic benefits.[18]

While there is debate as to whether there is a safe dose of corticosteroids, the consensus is that a safe dose has not been identified.[16] Studies with large sample sizes, such as those cited above, have demonstrated a definite link between corticosteroid use and fractures in RA, although other studies have found no or limited effect, perhaps due to their smaller sample size. In that other DMARDs have not been linked to osteoporosis, minimization of corticosteroid dose to the smallest necessary seems prudent.

In patients with RA receiving therapy with corticosteroids or those with osteoporosis not taking corticosteroids, calcium, vitamin D, and a nitrogen-containing bisphosphonate are the standard.[19,20] In those at very high risk of fracture, teriparatide confers an efficacy advantage over bisphosphonates, but the agent is expensive and there was an increase in mild side effects.[19,20]

Cardiovascular Disease in Rheumatoid Arthritis

Increase in Risk

Cardiovascular disease has been a well-recognized complication of RA for decades. In 2002, van Doornum et al.[21] suggested that the evidence of increased morbidity and mortality from cardiovascular disease in RA justified it being labeled as an extra-articular feature. In reviewing the literature, they noted the increased prevalence of myocardial infarction (MI), congestive heart failure, and stroke in RA compared to osteoarthritis, as well as increases in clinically silent ischemic heart disease and in subclinical vascular disease as detected by carotid artery ultrasound.

Recent epidemiologic studies have confirmed the increased risk of cardiovascular disease in RA. A study from Malmö, Sweden reported a standardized incidence ratio of 1.76 (95% CI: 1.23–2.44) for MI in RA versus the general population with similar increases in men and women.[22] There was a trend to an increase in stroke in both sexes. Solomon et al.[23] used the Nurses' Health Study data (>100,000 participants overall) to compare the incidence of cardiovascular disease in those with and without RA. The relative risk of MI was 2.0 (95% CI: 1.23–3.29) with essentially all of the increase in risk occurring after 10 years of RA (relative risk of 3.10, 95% CI: 1.64–5.87). Data from the Mayo Clinic found the relative risk of hospitalization for MI was 2.13 (95% CI: 1.13–4.03). But in contrast to the Nurses' Health Study where the risk was a late complication, in the study from the Mayo Clinic[24] the increase in risk preceded the diagnosis of RA (as defined by meeting the American College of Rheumatology criteria for RA) by 2 years, suggesting that cardiovascular disease is an integral part of RA. A recent meta-analysis found a slightly lower relative risk of MI in RA of 1.42 (95% CI: 1.22–1.64).[25]

van Doornum and colleagues[21] noted an average increase in mortality of 70% based on the mean standardized mortality ratio from a pooled analysis. Cardiovascular deaths followed by cerebrovascular deaths predominated as the causes of the excess in overall mortality in most studies. The absence of a major increase in pericarditis, coronary artery vasculitis and rheumatoid valvular heart disease led the authors to argue that the increase was due to premature atherosclerosis. They noted that the erythrocyte sedimentation rate (ESR), extra-articular features of RA, and use of corticosteroids predicted death, suggesting the role of the disease activity and its management as key players in the outcome.

Does Atherosclerosis Differ in Rheumatoid Arthritis?

While studies are limited, histologic evaluation of coronary artery involvement at autopsy by the Mayo Clinic group showed evidence of increased inflammatory change, more unstable plaque, and less multivessel atherosclerotic disease in 41 RA patients compared to 82 age- and sex-matched controls.[26] Thus, it is possible that rheumatoid ischemic heart disease differs from conventional ischemic heart disease. Additional studies are needed to illuminate both rheumatoid and nonrheumatoid cardiovascular disease.

Risk Factors

The levels of the conventional Framingham risk factors (age, gender, hypertension, diabetes, hypercholesterolemia, smoking) and BMI have been assessed in RA, and they remain as risk factors in RA as in non-RA. However, they do not explain the significantly increased rates of RA cardiovascular disease,[24,27,28] and are similar in those with and without RA.[29] Regular aspirin use and family history of early MI were not associated with the increase in risk of cardiovascular events in the Nurses' Health Study.[28] However, inflammatory markers such as CRP, fibrinogen and the like, were associated with cardiovascular events.[28] An ESR ≥60 mm/hour on three or more occasions, occurrence of RA vasculitis or RA lung disease predicted cardiovascular deaths.[30]

Beyond the fact that the extent of RA inflammation appears associated with the increase in risk of cardiovascular disease, the details of the mechanism by which it occurs are not certain. Inflammation has been linked to reduced levels of serum antioxidants—in particular carotenoids—thought to be important in atherogenesis.[29] RA patients may consume or absorb lower amounts of antioxidants and vitamins that may protect against atherosclerosis.[29] Inflammatory mediators may also cause endothelial dysfunction that results in ischemia.[31]

Can the Risk Be Reduced?

That RA is a risk factor for cardiovascular disease akin to smoking, diabetes, hypertension, and hyperlipidemia is established. The role of inflammation, at least as a marker of the RA disease process, appears associated with the increase in risk. The inevitable question is, will controlling the inflammation make a difference? Choi et al.,[32] reporting on 18 years of follow-up in 1240 RA patients, showed that methotrexate treatment reduced overall mortality by 60% (95% CI: 20–80%) and cardiovascular mortality by 70% (95% CI: 30–80%). Noncardiovascular mortality was generally unaffected. Suissa et al.[33] used an insurance claims database to demonstrate the significant benefit of methotrexate and other nonbiologic disease modifying antirheumatic drugs in reducing acute MI. Biologic agents did not reduce this outcome in this database, and corticosteroid use appeared to increase acute MI. Using the British Society for Rheumatology Biologics Register, Dixon et al.[34] showed that anti-TNF users and DMARD users had similar rates of MI, but there was a significant reduction in MI in those who responded to an anti-TNF within 6 months compared to those who did not (relative risk of MI in responders = 0.36, 95% CI: 0.19–0.69).

With cardiovascular and cerebrovascular disease the leading cause of increased death in RA, prevention is vital. Guidelines have been proposed to assist in managing these risks in individual patients.[35] In brief, the guidelines recommend a thorough assessment of traditional risk factors for cardiovascular disease in all patients, appropriate management of abnormal risk factors and aggressive control of the RA inflammatory process. Interestingly, statins may beneficially influence both RA disease activity and vascular risk.[36–38]

Conclusions

Infections, osteoporosis, and cardiovascular disease are complications of RA; they are not unrelated comorbidities.[38] RA causes these three complications. Disease activity predicts these outcomes. There is some evidence that better control of RA disease activity will reduce cardiovascular complications. While distinguishing between an adverse event of corticosteroids and the RA disease activity for which the corticosteroids are given is not completely resolved, keeping the dose of corticosteroids to a minimum seems desirable as traditional DMARDs have not been linked to these complications and corticosteroids have. Traditional DMARDs may reduce the frequency of infection and cardiovascular disease.

Additional research is needed to evaluate the link between reducing RA disease activity and reducing these complications. The impact of new biologic agents on these outcomes also needs further study. Nonetheless, the recognition that infection, osteoporosis, and cardiovascular disease are integral to the RA disease process and not unrelated comorbidities will allow prevention studies to move forward that focus on these outcomes in RA.

Acknowledgments

John Esdaile is a Kirkland Foundation Scholar, Mavis Goycochea is a CONACYT and IMSS Scholar, and Diane Lacaille is the Nancy and Peter Paul Saunders Scholar and holds an Investigator Award from the Arthritis Society of Canada. The work is funded by operating grants from the Canadian Institutes of Health Research and the Canadian Arthritis Network.

References

1. Comorbidity. *The American Heritage Medical Dictionary*. Boston: Houghton Mifflin, 2007.
2. *Comorbidity in Medicine.* Wikipedia, November 2007.
3. Doran MF, Crowson CS, Pond GR, et al. Frequency of infection in patients with rheumatoid arthritis compared with controls: A population-based study. *Arthritis Rheum* 2002;46:2287–2293.
4. Wolfe F, Mitchell DM, Sibley JT, et al. The mortality of rheumatoid arthritis. *Arthritis Rheum* 1994;37:481–494.
5. Vandenbroucke JP, Kaaks R, Valkenburg HA, et al. Frequency of infections among rheumatoid arthritis patients, before and after disease onset. *Arthritis Rheum* 1987;30:810–813.
6. van Albada-Kuipers GA, Linthorst J, Peeters EAJ, et al. Frequency of infection among patients with rheumatoid arthritis versus patients with osteoarthritis or soft tissue rheumatism. *Arthritis Rheum* 1988;31:667–671.
7. Lacaille D, Guh D, Abrahamowicz M, et al. Use of non-biologic DMARDs is not associated with an increased risk of infection in rheumatoid arthritis. *Arthritis Rheum* 2008;(in press).
8. Wolfe F, Caplan L, Michaud K. Treatment for rheumatoid arthritis and the risk of hospitalization for pneumonia. Associations with prednisone, disease-modifying antirheumatic drugs, and anti-tumor necrosis factor therapy. *Arthritis Rheum* 2006;54:628–634.
9. Keane J, Gershon S, Wise RP, et al. Tuberculosis associated with infliximab, a tumor necrosis factor alpha-neutralizing agent. *N Engl J Med* 2001;345:1098–1104.
10. Dixon WG, Watson K, Lunt M, et al. Rates of serious infection, including site-specific and bacterial intracellular infection, in rheumatoid arthritis patients receiving anti-tumor necrosis factor therapy. Results from the British Society for Rheumatology biologics register. *Arthritis Rheum* 2006;54:2368–2376.
11. Dixon WG, Symmons DPM, Lunt M, et al. Serious infection following anti-tumor necrosis factor alpha therapy in patients with rheumatoid arthritis. *Arthritis Rheum* 2007;56:2896–2904.
12. Haugeberg G, Uhlig T, Falch JA, et al. Bone mineral density and frequency of osteoporosis in female patients with rheumatoid arthritis: Results from 394 patients in the Oslo County Rheumatoid Arthritis Register. *Arthritis Rheum* 2000;43:522–530.
13. van Staa TP, Geusens P, Bijlsma JWJ, et al. Clinical assessment of the long-term risk of fracture in patients with rheumatoid arthritis. *Arthritis Rheum* 2006;54:3104–3112.
14. Ørstavik RE, Haugeberg G, Mowinckel P, et al. Vertebral deformities in rheumatoid arthritis: A comparison with population-based controls. *Arch Intern Med* 2004;164:420–425.
15. Hochberg MC: Recommendations for measurement of bone mineral density and identifying persons to be treated for osteoporosis. *Rheum Dis Clin North Am* 2006;32:681–689.
16. Haugeberg G, Ørstavik RE, Kvien TK. Effects of rheumatoid arthritis on bone. *Curr Opin Rheumatol* 2003;15:469–475.
17. Aguado P, del Campo MT, Garcés MV, et al. Low vitamin D levels in outpatient postmenopausal women from a rheumatology clinic in Madrid, Spain: Their relationship with bone mineral density. *Osteoporosis Int* 2000;11:739–744.
18. Arnson Y, Amital H, Shoenfeld Y. Vitamin D and autoimmunity: New aetiological and therapeutic considerations. *Ann Rheum Dis* 2007;66:1137–1142.
19. Saag KG, Shane E, Boonen S, et al. Teriparatide or alendronate in glucocorticoid-induced osteoporosis. *N Engl J Med* 2007;357: 2028–2039.
20. Sambrook PN. Anabolic therapy in glucocorticoid-induced osteoporosis. (Editorial.) *N Engl J Med* 2007;357:2084–2086.
21. van Doornum S, McColl G, Wicks IP. Accelerated atherosclerosis. An extraarticular feature of rheumatoid arthritis? *Arthritis Rheum* 2002;46:862–873.
22. Turesson C, Jarenros A, Jacobsson L, et al. Increased incidence of cardiovascular disease in patients with rheumatoid arthritis: Results from a community based study. *Ann Rheum Dis* 2004;63:952–955.
23. Solomon DH, Karlson EW, Rimm EB, et al. Cardiovascular morbidity and mortality in women diagnosed with rheumatoid arthritis. *Circulation* 2003;107:1303–1307.
24. Maradit-Kremers H, Crowson CS, Nicola PJ, et al. Increased unrecognized coronary heart disease and sudden deaths in rheumatoid arthritis. A population-based cohort study. *Arthritis Rheum* 2005;52:402–411.
25. Avina-Zubieta JA, Choi HK, Etminan M, et al. Risk of cardiovascular morbidity in rheumatoid arthritis: A meta-analysis of observational studies (abstract). *Arthritis Rheum* 2006;54:S107–S108.
26. Aubry M-C, Maradit-Kremers H, Reinalda MS, et al. Differences in atherosclerotic coronary heart disease between subjects with and without rheumatoid arthritis. *J Rheumatol* 2007;34:937–942.
27. del Rincon I, Williams K, Stern MP, et al. High incidence of cardiovascular events in a rheumatoid arthritis cohort not explained by traditional cardiac risk factors. *Arthritis Rheum* 2001;44: 2737–2745.
28. Solomon DH, Curham GC, Rimm E, et al. Cardiovascular risk factors in women with and without rheumatoid arthritis. *Arthritis Rheum* 2004;50:3444–3449.
29. de Pablo P, Dietrich T, Karlson EW. Antioxidants and other novel cardiovascular risk factors in subjects with rheumatoid arthritis in a large population sample. *Arthritis Rheum* 2007;57:953–962.
30. Maradit-Kremers H, Nicola PJ, Crowson CS, et al. Cardiovascular death in rheumatoid arthritis. A population-based study. *Arthritis Rheum* 2005;52:722–732.
31. van Leuven SI, Franssen R, Kastelein JJ, et al. Systemic inflammation as a risk factor for atherothrombosis. *Rheumatology* 2007; (advance access published August 16, 2007). http://rheumatology.oxfordjournals.org/cgi/content/abstract/kem202v1.
32. Choi HK, Hernan MA, Seeger JD, et al. Methotrexate and mortality in patients with rheumatoid arthritis: A prospective study. *Lancet* 2002;359:1173–1177.
33. Suissa S, Bernatsky S, Hudson M. Antirheumatic drug use and the risk of acute myocardial infarction. *Arthritis Rheum* 2006;5531–5536.
34. Dixon WG, Watson KD, Lunt M, Hyrich KL. Reduction in the incidence of myocardial infarction in patients with rheumatoid arthritis who respond to anti-tumor necrosis factor therapy. Results from the British Society for Rheumatology Biologics Register. *Arthritis Rheum* 2007;56:2905–2912.
35. Pham T, Gossec L, Constantin A, et al. Cardiovascular risk and rheumatoid arthritis clinical practice guidelines based on published evidence and expert opinion. *Joint Bone Spine* 2006;73:379–387.
36. McInnes IB, McCarey DW, Sattar N. Do statins offer therapeutic potential in inflammatory arthritis? *Ann Rheum Dis* 2004;63: 1535–1537.
37. Okamoto H, Koizumi K, Kamitsuji S, et al. Beneficial action of statins in patients with RA in a large observational cohort. *J Rheumatol* 2007;34:1–5.
38. McCarey DW, McInnes IB, Madhok R, et al. Trial of atorvastatin in rheumatoid arthritis (TARA): Double-blind, randomised placebo-controlled trial. *Lancet* 2004;363:2015–2021.
39. Hochberg MC, Johnston SS, John AK. The incidence and prevalence of extra-articular and systemic manifestations in a cohort of newly-diagnosed patients with rheumatoid arthritis between 1999 and 2006. *Curr Med Res Opin* 2008;24(2):469–480.

Early (Rheumatoid) Arthritis

Klaus P. Machold and Josef S. Smolen

CHAPTER 6

Rheumatoid arthritis (RA) is characterized by joint destruction, functional impairment, disability, and premature mortality.[1–3] Prevention of progression of the destructive processes is possible both in early and later stages of the disease,[4–8] mainly by use of steroids, "conventional" disease-modifying antirheumatic drugs (DMARDs), biologic agents, or combinations thereof.[9–18] Because bone erosions or cartilage destruction rarely, if ever, heal,[19–23] and thus damage accumulates over time, it is obvious that these agents will have better effects on outcome the earlier they are started. Also, in terms of the underlying pathogenetic (inflammatory) processes, earlier intervention may be more effective if it is interfering with the inflammatory cascade before its mechanisms are "fully established" and have not reached an "autonomous" stage that is thought to prevail in later phases of RA.[24] Therefore, it seems obvious and advisable to start treatment as early as possible, and ideally even before damage (defined as the visualized destruction of cartilage and/or bone) has occurred. The only, albeit still unresolved, obstacle to early therapy remains early diagnosis. Even if diagnosis at these early stages using published criteria does not seem possible,[25,26] early prognostication should identify patients who may benefit most from therapeutic intervention and separate them from individuals who might sustain more harm than benefit from possibly toxic treatment.

What is *Early* Arthritis?

At first glance, considering the often decades-long duration of chronic inflammatory rheumatic diseases, several weeks or even months difference in the definition of a threshold between "early" and "later" appear to be of little importance. Observations from several early arthritis patient cohorts have demonstrated a remarkably short period of time during which an arthritis (and in particular rheumatoid arthritis) may be regarded as "early."[27–39] This time-frame has also been named "window of opportunity" assuming that if an intervention such as treatment with a disease modifying drug were initiated during this time, the effect of such treatment would be much greater than at a later time during the "disease career." Support for the concept of a distinct character of the early months of RA as compared to later stages came from observations of different cytokine patterns in the synovium of early arthritis patients.[40] This suggests that the pathogenetic events may change in the course of the disease. These observations are corroborated by the finding that remission was more commonly induced in patients with disease of 4 or fewer months duration compared with longer disease duration,[41] and by observations of delayed radiologic progression if DMARD treatment was instituted at a median of 3 months versus a median of 12 months after symptom onset.[42]

In other studies, however, the comparison of early RA (defined as a symptom duration of <1 year) and established RA (>5 years), by immunohistologic analysis of the synovium, including an assessment of composition of the cellular infiltrate as well as TNF-α, IL-1β, and IL-6 expression, did not reveal any differences between early and long-standing disease.[43] Expression of IFN-γ, IL-10, and IL-12 mRNA in synovial fluid mononuclear cells were also similar between such early patients and those with established (>1 year) RA.[44]

Additional factors may promote synovial inflammation and lead to perpetuation of the disease in some patients with late-stage RA. In particular, development of mutations in the p53 tumor suppressor gene and other regulatory genes have been hypothesized to play a key role in the conversion of chronic synovitis into an autonomous disease, independent of the initial immune-mediated inflammatory process.[45,46] Furthermore, the cumulative destruction of bone and articular cartilage may result in the release of fragments that enhance inflammation, similar to the process in patients with inflammatory osteoarthritis.[47–49] It remains to be determined, however, when and how this transition might occur. In clinical practice, a substantial majority of rheumatologists now adhere to a definition of "early RA" which limits its duration to 3 months.[50]

With regard to the pace of destruction occurring in RA, it has been shown that the majority of patients who developed erosive disease did so within the first year after symptom onset,[51] with approximately 75% of RA patients having joint erosions at 2 years.[52] These findings underscore the necessity to consider effective treatment well before the first year of symptoms has elapsed. On the other hand, a sizable minority of patients initially presenting with overt synovitis and arthritis of the hands had a relatively benign course with self-limiting disease or at least little, if any, damage.[33,51]

The pattern of progression in those patients who develop destructive/erosive disease has been found to be quite variable.[53] It has been suggested by Sharp et al.[54] that the pace of progression of radiologic damage slows after longer duration. However, this decline was only modest and did not appear before the third decade of the disease history, when a substantial proportion of the joints (approximately 20%) of these patients already had accrued "maximum erosion scores." Prevention of this catastrophic outcome by early effective intervention thus appears mandatory.

Diagnosis of Early Arthritis

At the time of first presentation to a physician, patients with arthritis may show a remarkable variability in clinical signs and symptoms as well as in the presence or absence of laboratory or imaging abnormalities.[55,56] Criteria that would allow differentiation of groups of patients with regard to diagnosis of their arthritis at this stage currently do not exist. Moreover, current classification criteria for "established" RA have been developed with the clinical researcher in mind, and are intended not primarily for diagnosis but rather should be used to separate groups of patients with established disease from those with other diseases and to standardize the characteristics of these patients for clinical studies.[57] Diagnostic criteria account for the results of the clinical evaluation of many more features of the disease, relate to the individual patient, and are useful primarily for the physician. In addition, given the inherent variability not only of RA, but also most other arthritides which may present clinically in a similar fashion to RA, prognostication is an important aim for the clinician and the patient in order to select the appropriate therapy.[58] The reader should see Chapter 1 for a further discussion of classification criteria for RA.

The current classification criteria for RA[59] were developed by detailed analysis of patients with established disease and were intended to "classify," rather than diagnose, patients with RA mainly for the purpose of clinical studies. These criteria are therefore neither useful for clinical studies of, nor as a surrogate of, diagnostic criteria for early RA.[60] Given the inherent uncertainty in diagnosing a disease with a variety of clinical manifestations (see below), the 1958 American Rheumatism Association criteria allow for categorization of a patient as suffering from "probable" and "possible" RA.[61] Thus, this set of criteria encompasses a broader scope of disease stages than the 1987 classification criteria.[62] Although the terms "probable" and "possible RA" would also encompass patients with earlier (i.e., not established) disease, criteria for classification or diagnosis of "early RA" have not yet been developed.[60] The need for such criteria is underlined by observations that only about half of the patients who are diagnosed with RA at 1 year from presentation fulfilled current classification criteria for RA already at the time of their first visit to the rheumatologist (within three months from onset), while approximately 20% of the non-RA patients did so[26] (Figure 6-1).

Signs and Symptoms Typical for Early Rheumatoid Arthritis

As already mentioned, currently no universally accepted definition of early RA exists. Nevertheless, if one defines established RA as a polyarticular systemic disease with symmetric involvement of joints of the upper and lower extremities, presence of autoantibodies, and with a high tendency to erode joints, at least some of the clinical characteristics will be regularly found already early on (Table 6-1).

Polyarthritis

Many patients who subsequently will be diagnosed with RA have low numbers of swollen and/or tender joints ("joint counts") at disease onset or at first presentation to the physician. In one study of a cohort of very early arthritis patients, more than 25% of the subjects who developed erosions within 1 year had five or fewer swollen joints at presentation, employing a 28 joint count.[51] In another recent study, early arthritis patients who developed RA had a median of four swollen joints and more than 25% had only up to four tender joints using a 44 joint count.[64] Recognizing the implications of these observations, recommendations of a task force of the European League against Rheumatism (EULAR) suggested considering early RA even with only one persistently swollen joint.[65]

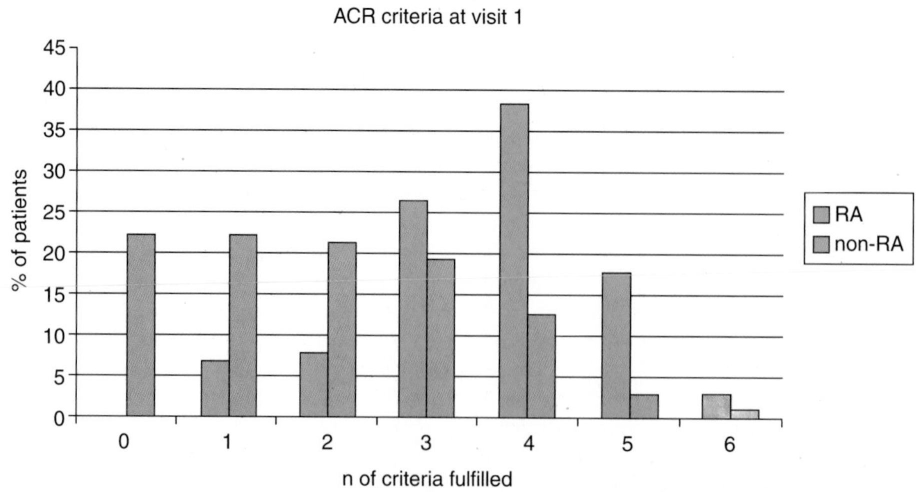

Figure 6-1. American College of Rheumatology (ACR) criteria at first visit. The percentage of RA patients fulfilling ACR criteria for RA (52%) was significantly higher at first visit compared to the non-RA patients ($p < 0.0001$). Nevertheless, a considerable percentage of patients with RA did not fulfill ACR criteria initially, while several non-RA patients had at least four criteria. (Adapted from Machold KP, Stamm TA, Eberl GJ, et al. Very recent onset arthritis—clinical, laboratory, and radiological findings during the first year of disease. *J Rheumatol* 2002;29(11): 2278–2287.)

Table 6-1. Characteristics of Established RA

Characteristic of RA	Comment (Differential Diagnosis, Clinical Use)
Inflammation (joint swelling with characteristic soft tissue involvement) Acute phase response (CRP, elevated ESR)	Osteoarthritis has usually bony swelling and rarely has signs of systemic inflammation.
Polyarthritis (involvement of >5 joints)	Seronegative spondylarthropathies are usually oligoarticular (some cases of RA may be oligoarticular at onset).
Symmetry (same joint regions of both upper and lower extremities)	Seronegative spondylarthropathies are usually asymmetric, involve mostly the lower extremity and mostly large joints (with the exception of psoriatic arthritis).
Chronicity (duration of >6 weeks)	Remission of arthritis after nonspecific treatment during the first 12 weeks confers a favorable prognosis.
Autoantibodies (RF, ACPA, anti-RA33)	Most other diseases are "seronegative" (connective tissue diseases are associated with other types of autoantibodies).
Erosions (bony destruction seen on conventional x-ray)	Most other forms of arthritis (except psoriatic arthritis) are usually nonerosive.
Absence of recent infections or comorbid conditions associated with arthritides	UT or GI infections (reactive arthritis); psoriasis (psoriatic arthritis); IBD; ankylosing spondylitis; predominant extraarticular symptoms (connective tissue diseases).
Painful MCP or MTP compression	Inflammation of MCP or MTP joints is characteristic of RA (and is rarer in other arthritides).
Morning stiffness (lasting more than a few minutes)	Morning stiffness associated with osteoarthritis rarely exceeds 30 minutes.
Genetics	RA has a characteristic genetic background. Costs and limited accuracy of analyses currently preclude routine genetic testing for use as diagnostic or prognostic tool.

Symmetric Involvement of Upper and Lower Extremity

Rheumatoid arthritis characteristically involves the small joints of hands and feet.[66] In addition, large joints of the upper and lower extremities as well as the cervical spine joints may be involved. The probability for the diagnosis of RA was three times higher if clinical involvement of both the upper and the lower extremity was present than with involvement of either.[64] Arthritis confined to the lower limbs, with or without spinal pain or spinal inflammation, is more indicative of a seronegative spondyloarthropathy.[67] Symmetric arthritis (involving the same joint areas on both sides of the body), despite being a component of both the 1958 and the 1987 American College of Rheumatology (ACR) criteria, is a variable with only mild predictive value for developing RA.[64] Frequently, symmetry is absent in early stages of the disease.[51,55,56]

Chronicity

Probably the most characteristic feature of RA is its chronic course. Any form of transient or self-limiting arthritis, therefore, is, by definition, not RA. The current RA classification criteria define a duration of symptoms of least 6 weeks,[59] and the 1958 criteria required a symptom duration of at least 3 weeks for "possible" and at least 6 weeks for "probable" or "definite" RA.[61] More recent systematic observations, however, suggest 3 months duration of arthritis as the most discriminative time point to differentiate between persistent and self-remitting disease.[68] In line with these data, with symptom duration of less than 6 weeks at presentation a patient is three times more likely not to progress to RA than to develop RA, while the presence of symptoms for more than 6 weeks (and likewise even longer duration) will increase the risk to develop RA.[64,69]

Autoantibodies

For over five decades, rheumatoid factor (RF), an antibody specific for immunoglobulin G, has been known to be one of the characteristics of RA, and has been used to diagnose, classify, and characterize patients with this disease. Between 46% and 75% of early RA patients test positive for RF.[10,26,39,70,71] Unfortunately, RF is not pathognomonic for RA, and frequently occurs in other disorders, such as connective tissue diseases or chronic infections,[72,73] as well as in healthy individuals,[74,75] mostly in low titers. High-titer RF (RF >50 IU/ml), in contrast, has been shown to be highly discriminative between RA and non-RA in patients with early arthritis.[76] More recently, antibodies to citrullinated proteins (ACPA) have been described to occur relatively specifically in RA[77]; ACPA are found in the sera of ~50% of patients with early arthritis diagnosed subsequently as RA and may be present in patients even before symptom onset.[78,79] Since the groups of patients with high-titer RF and ACPA are widely overlapping, it has been suggested to test first for RF and then if RF is negative or "low titer" (<50 IU/ml), test for ACPA to support the RA diagnosis.[76,80] Probably even more importantly, RF and/or ACPA also give some prognostic information: Presence of these antibodies is highly predictive of erosive disease and associated with more rapid progression of joint destruction.[51,81–83] Moreover, RF is associated with persistence of arthritis.[84,85]

Erosions

The presence of erosions, which occur in a majority of RA patients, is very characteristic, albeit not to be expected in the very early stages of the disease. Occurrence of erosions early after onset of symptoms is indicative of RA[26,69]; however, at a mean of 8 weeks from symptom onset, these x-ray changes are found in only up to 10% of patients.[51] Therefore, this cannot be considered a characteristic of early RA. More importantly, the very aim of early diagnosis and treatment is the prevention of erosions and other signs of (possibly irreversible) joint destruction. Thus, the diagnosis needs to be made before the appearance of evidence for joint destruction.

Other Features

Metacarpophalangeal/Metatarsophalangeal Compression Test

Inflamed joints are usually painful. Pain may be present even if joint swelling is subtle. The involvement of metacarpophalangeal (MCP) and metatarsophalangeal (MTP) joints may often be recognized by compression pain at the MCP and/or MTP level. In fact, a positive compression test provides a major contribution to diagnostic algorithms in early arthritis, and is present in more than 60% of the patients who will be diagnosed as RA.[64,69]

Morning Stiffness

Stiffness of long (more than several minutes) duration is a typical symptom of inflammatory joint disease. The 1987 classification criteria for established RA require duration of at least 1 hour. Typically, in other disorders, such as osteoarthritis, stiffness is in general much shorter and only in the order of a few minutes. Therefore, morning stiffness of more than 45 minutes may be seen as characteristic for RA.[64,86]

Acute Phase Response

Laboratory testing usually reveals higher acute-phase parameters, such as C-reactive protein (CRP) or erythrocyte sedimentation rate (ESR), in early arthritis patients destined to suffer from RA than in those who do not develop RA.[64] However, the variability among patients is considerable and makes the distinction difficult for individual patients due to the broad overlap. Moreover, initially normal tests for inflammation do not rule out later evolution of erosive disease. On the other hand, joint damage in early RA increases with increasing acute-phase reactant levels (and also increasing clinical disease activity).[51,87,88]

Imaging Abnormalities

Conventional x-ray imaging, despite being currently the only standard technique for visualizing the typical changes associated with RA, is notoriously insensitive to small and/or early changes.[89] Magnetic resonance imaging (MRI) and sonography may allow detection of erosions earlier than traditional radiographic techniques.[90–92] However, these modalities have not yet been sufficiently validated and their diagnostic value is not undisputed.[93] Nevertheless, both MRI and ultrasonography are more sensitive than clinical examination to identify synovitis and joint effusions. In an experimental animal model, the earliest phases of destructive arthritis have been shown to be characterized by juxta-articular tendonitis, which can be well visualized by MRI and sonography.[94]

Genetics

The genetic background of RA is quite characteristic,[95] at least in Caucasian populations, and differs from that of most other arthritides, in particular the seronegative spondyloarthropathies. However, costs of accurate analyses as well as the complexities of the influences of the genetic background of a given individual[96,97] currently preclude the use of genetic testing as a diagnostic or prognostic tool.

Prognostication

The major purpose of diagnosing a disease in a given patient is to guide treatment decisions on the basis of prognostic criteria. This prognosis, in turn, will determine the necessity and intensity of treatment as well as the necessary frequency of reassessment and follow-up. From the patient's view, the prognosis of his or her disease will also determine the risk that has to be taken when receiving potentially toxic drugs or unpleasant or time-consuming treatments such as wearing splints, undergoing physical therapy, or performing regular exercise.

Currently, no universally and/or easy-to-use algorithm or criteria set exists that allows predicting with sufficient confidence which patients will or will not develop persistent and/or destructive arthritis. Although several algorithms have been developed in order to predict RA or erosive disease among early arthritis patients,[69,98–100] none of these have been sufficiently validated. Furthermore, the sensitivity and specificity of currently available algorithms is insufficient to identify patients who will develop erosive RA, and thus would allow for sufficient confidence to make decisions on intensive therapies.[101] This deficiency is partly due to the abovementioned differences in inclusion criteria for early arthritis clinics: The algorithms may be at least partly dependent on the population in which they were developed. Therefore, at the present time, one may have to rely on recommendations and expert opinions,[65,86] rather than on algorithms or criteria derived from clinical studies. These recommendations, however, usually relate to speedy referral to a rheumatologist for further diagnostic workup rather than to a clinical diagnosis.

Recently, two sets of European recommendations concerning early arthritis have been developed. One of these calls for rapid referral to a rheumatologist in the event of clinical suspicion of RA. This suspicion should be supported by the presence of three characteristics: three or more swollen joints, positive compression test on MCPs or MTPs, and morning stiffness of more than 30 minutes.[86] In the other set, referral of patients with one or more swollen joints within 6 weeks of symptom onset (to prevent a longer delay of referral of patients with potential RA) is recommended. Careful history taking and clinical and laboratory examinations to exclude other diseases are also suggested. It is emphasized that the probability of persistence increases with the number of swollen and tender joints, the presence of acute-phase reactants, and autoantibody (RF, ACPA) levels; radiographs should be taken to reveal erosive disease.[65] These recommendations also suggest starting DMARD therapy in patients likely to develop persistent and/or erosive disease as early as possible.[65] In addition, it is important to recognize that the diagnosis of erosions by radiography also depends on experience of the reader. Thus, only a physician (radiologist, rheumatologist) experienced in assessing RA x-rays should perform the reading.

In an early arthritis cohort suffering from undifferentiated arthritis (i.e., arthritis that could not be classified according to ACR criteria and lasting less than 1 year), the group in Leiden, The Netherlands, has developed a scoring system that was externally validated using a control group with identical characteristics (undifferentiated arthritis of up to 1-year duration). The prediction score includes easily determinable clinical and laboratory characteristics (age, gender, distribution and symmetry of arthritis, morning stiffness, tender and swollen joint counts, CRP, RF, and ACPA), and yielded positive and negative predictive values in the validation group in the vicinity of 90%.[64] It remains to be tested whether this prediction system is useful in other settings; if so, it may guide treatment decisions, and thus fulfill the requirement of both avoiding overtreatment and initiate (even very aggressive) treatment in patients who are highly likely to develop RA.

Treatment of Early Arthritis

Nonsteroidal Anti-Inflammatory Drugs

As already mentioned, up to 60% of all patients presenting with early arthritis may have a self-limiting course.[33,69] These patients only require temporary therapy that relieves their symptoms, and may shorten the duration of the arthritis. Nonsteroidal anti-inflammatory drugs (NSAIDs) are often prescribed in these patients; however, NSAIDs do not alter the course of the arthritis and its outcome, and their long-term use may be associated with considerable side effects.

Glucocorticoids

In common clinical practice, depot corticosteroids are often used, either as local intra-articular or as systemic intramuscular injections. Alternatively, short courses of oral steroids may be prescribed in these very early arthritis patients. Unlike maintenance therapy with oral corticosteroids, the short-term intermittent use of corticosteroids is considered safe, although there is limited scientific evidence to underscore this.[102] In one of the few studies explicitly addressing the issue of treatment of very early (*not* rheumatoid) arthritis, Green et al.[68] administered a single dose of depot steroids (120 mg of methylprednisolone), either intra-articularly or intramuscularly. The results of this open study suggested that this approach was safe and resulted in a significant number of disease remissions. Clinical practice varies widely among "rheumatology schools," and there is no consensus on whether to apply corticosteroids, parenteral or oral, in these patients.

Disease-Modifying Antirheumatic Drugs

Persistent early arthritis—that is, arthritis that is continuously clinically apparent for more than 6 weeks to 3 months—represents a situation in which glucocorticoid therapy, either as a single measure or in combination with DMARDs (and NSAIDS, if necessary) is deemed appropriate. Steroids have, in this circumstance, been advocated as both safe and efficacious singly or in combination with DMARD therapy.[103–105] The superiority of early initiation of DMARDs compared to delayed treatment or treatment with NSAIDs alone has been demonstrated conclusively in this setting.[29,31,32,42,106,107] Likewise, at least in patients who at these stages were classified as having RA, a combination of corticosteroids with DMARDs appears to offer additional benefits in terms of clinical response as well as radiologic outcomes,[103,104,108] although these findings have not been universally reproducible.[109]

Considering its favorable risk–benefit ratio, methotrexate is (as in established RA) regarded to be the drug of first choice.[110–113] In "mild" cases or in case of contraindications such as the desire to become pregnant or significant comorbidities such as liver or kidney disease, other DMARDs should be considered.[112] Depending on the individual patient's circumstances, treatment with hydroxychloroquine or sulfasalazine should be started, although these compounds may be less efficacious. In general, when employing early DMARD treatment, combinations with corticosteroids appear to be beneficial.[37,114] More recently, "aggressive" treatment strategies have been proposed that used combinations of DMARDs and/or the addition of tumor necrosis factor antagonists to "conventional" DMARDs in early "criteria-positive" RA.[6,7,10,11,71,113,115–117] The results of these randomized trials indicate superior outcomes of combination therapies and/or the addition of biologic drugs compared to less aggressive "conventional" approaches. In this context, it has to be mentioned that not all combinations of (conventional) DMARDs may be superior to using the same DMARDs singly.[39,118,119] In addition, it is important to bear in mind that none of these trials has included patients who did not, at the time of inclusion, fulfill ACR RA criteria. Thus, it remains unclear whether the possibly higher risk associated with more aggressive strategies is warranted at least in the subset of patients with less destructive diseases.

A recent analysis has revealed that the fate of any DMARD treatment, MTX or biologic, can be predicted within 3 to 6 months from the start of therapy. Thus, starting patients with early RA with more traditional therapeutic approach and then switching rapidly to another compound may be the most practicable strategy.

Conclusion

Patients with early (rheumatoid) arthritis represent a substantial challenge to the clinician caring for them. The problem is not only to discriminate relatively benign disease from cases in which urgent initiation of highly active treatment is needed, but also to decide on the intensity of treatment in order to avoid subjecting patients to excessive risk associated with at least some of the therapies. Currently, no universally accepted algorithm exists to support with confidence such diagnostic and/or therapeutic decisions. Nevertheless, available evidence suggests certain prognostic indicators indicative of unfavorable prognosis: Patients presenting with polyarthritis (three or more swollen joints), positive MCP/MTP compression test, RF of at least 50 IU/ml (or ACPA), and elevated CRP appear to be at a very high risk to develop persistent (and erosive) disease. In addition, presence of erosions on initial x-rays would confirm the destructive nature of the arthritis. Persistence of arthritis (>12 weeks) and/or oligoarthritis accompanied by serologic evidence of inflammation or RF of at least 50 IU/ml (or ACPA) are likewise regarded as indicators of a high risk for developing chronic and destructive joint disease. In all instances, other diseases associated with arthritis should have been excluded (see above). The (presumed) diagnosis of RA should be followed by the institution of DMARD therapy to prevent further persistence, joint damage, and disability.

References

1. Smolen JS, Aletaha D. Patients with rheumatoid arthritis in clinical care. *Ann Rheum Dis* 2004;63(3):221–225.
2. Wolfe F, Michaud K, Gefeller O, Choi HK. Predicting mortality in patients with rheumatoid arthritis. *Arthritis Rheum* 2003;48(6): 1530–1542.
3. Pincus T, Callahan LF, Sale WG, et al. Severe functional declines, work disability, and increased mortality in seventy-five rheumatoid arthritis patients studied over nine years. *Arthritis Rheum* 1984;27: 864–872.
4. Lipsky PE, van der Heijde DM, St Clair EW, et al. Infliximab and methotrexate in the treatment of rheumatoid arthritis. Anti-Tumor Necrosis Factor Trial in Rheumatoid Arthritis with Concomitant Therapy Study Group. *N Engl J Med* 2000;343(22): 1594–1602.
5. Keystone EC, Kavanaugh AF, Sharp JT, et al. Radiographic, clinical, and functional outcomes of treatment with adalimumab (a human anti-tumor necrosis factor monoclonal antibody) in patients with active rheumatoid arthritis receiving concomitant methotrexate therapy: A randomized, placebo-controlled, 52-week trial. *Arthritis Rheum* 2004;50(5):1400–1411.
6. St Clair EW, van der Heijde DM, Smolen JS, et al. Combination of infliximab and methotrexate therapy for early rheumatoid arthritis: A randomized, controlled trial. *Arthritis Rheum* 2004;50(11): 3432–3443.
7. Breedveld FC, Weisman MH, Kavanaugh AF, et al. The PREMIER study: A multicenter, randomized, double-blind clinical trial of combination therapy with adalimumab plus methotrexate versus methotrexate alone or adalimumab alone in patients with early, aggressive rheumatoid arthritis who had not had previous methotrexate treatment. *Arthritis Rheum* 2006;54(1):26–37.
8. Aletaha D, Funovits J, Keystone EC, Smolen JS. Disease activity early in the course of treatment predicts long-term response to therapy after one year in rheumatoid arthritis patients. *Arthritis Rheum* 2007;56:3226–3235.
9. Bukhari MA, Wiles NJ, Lunt M, et al. Influence of disease-modifying therapy on radiographic outcome in inflammatory polyarthritis at five years: Results from a large observational inception study. *Arthritis Rheum* 2003;48(1):46–53.
10. Boers M, Verhoeven AC, Markusse HM, et al. Randomised comparison of combined step-down prednisolone, methotrexate and sulphasalazine with sulphasalazine alone in early rheumatoid arthritis. *Lancet* 1997;350(9074):309–318.
11. Goekoop-Ruiterman YPM, Vries-Bouwstra JK, Allaart CF, et al. Clinical and radiographic outcomes of four different treatment strategies in patients with early rheumatoid arthritis (the BeSt study): A randomized, controlled trial. *Arthritis Rheum* 2005;52(11): 3381–3390.
12. Mullan RH, Bresnihan B. Disease-modifying anti-rheumatic drug therapy and structural damage in early rheumatoid arthritis. *Clin Exp Rheumatol* 2003;(21 Suppl 31):S158–S164.
13. Pincus T, Ferraccioli G, Sokka T, et al. Evidence from clinical trials and long-term observational studies that disease-modifying anti-rheumatic drugs slow radiographic progression in rheumatoid arthritis: Updating a 1983 review. *Rheumatology (Oxford)* 2002;41(12): 1346–1356.
14. Scott DL, Strand V. The effects of disease-modifying anti-rheumatic drugs on the Health Assessment Questionnaire score. Lessons from the leflunomide clinical trials database. *Rheumatology (Oxford)* 2002;41(8):899–909.
15. Aletaha D, Smolen JS. The rheumatoid arthritis patient in the clinic: Comparing more than 1,300 consecutive DMARD courses. *Rheumatology (Oxford)* 2002;41(12):1367–1374.
16. Aletaha D, Smolen JS. Effectiveness profiles and dose dependent retention of traditional disease modifying antirheumatic drugs for rheumatoid arthritis. An observational study. *J Rheumatol* 2002; 29(8):1631–1638.
17. Choi HK, Hernan MA, Seeger JD, et al. Methotrexate and mortality in patients with rheumatoid arthritis: A prospective study. *Lancet* 2002;359(9313):1173–1177.
18. Smolen JS, Aletaha D, Koeller M, et al. New therapies for treatment of rheumatoid arthritis. *Lancet* 2007;370(9602):1861–1874.
19. Sokka T, Hannonen P. Healing of erosions in rheumatoid arthritis. *Ann Rheum Dis* 2000;59(8):647–649.
20. Rau R, Wassenberg S, Herborn G, et al. Identification of radiologic healing phenomena in patients with rheumatoid arthritis. *J Rheumatol* 2001;28(12):2608–2615.
21. Sharp JT, van der Heijde D, Boers M, Boonen A, et al. Repair of erosions in rheumatoid arthritis does occur. Results from 2 studies by the OMERACT subcommittee on healing of erosions. *J Rheumatol* 2003;30(5):1102–1107.
22. van der Heijde D, Landewe R. Imaging: do erosions heal? *Ann Rheum Dis* 2003;62:10–12.
23. Ideguchi H, Ohno S, Hattori H, et al. Bone erosions in rheumatoid arthritis can be repaired through reduction in disease activity with conventional disease-modifying antirheumatic drugs. *Arthritis Res Ther* 2006;8(3):R76.
24. Firestein GS, Zvaifler NJ. How important are T cells in chronic rheumatoid synovitis? II. T cell–independent mechanisms from beginning to end. *Arthritis Rheum* 2002;46(2):298–308.
25. Harrison BJ, Symmons DPM, Barrett EM, Silman AJ. The performance of the 1987 ARA classification criteria for rheumatoid arthritis in a population based cohort of patients with early inflammatory polyarthritis. *J Rheumatol* 1998;28:2324–2330.
26. Machold KP, Stamm TA, Eberl GJ, et al. Very recent onset arthritis—clinical, laboratory, and radiological findings during the first year of disease. *J Rheumatol* 2002;29(11):2278–2287.
27. van der Horst-Bruinsma IE, Speyer I, Visser H, et al. Diagnosis and course of early-onset arthritis: Results of a special early arthritis clinic compared to routine patient care. *Br J Rheumatol* 1998;37: 1084–1088.
28. Symmons DPM, Barrett EM, Bankhead CR, et al. The Incidence of Rheumatoid Arthritis in the United Kingdom: Results from the Norfolk Arthritis Register. *Br J Rheumatol* 1994;33(8):735–739.
29. Van der Heide A, Jacobs JW, Bijlsma JW, et al. The effectiveness of early treatment with "second-line" antirheumatic drugs. A randomized, controlled trial. *Ann Intern Med* 1996;124(8): 699–707.
30. Mottonen T, Paimela L, Ahonen J, et al. Outcome in patients with early rheumatoid arthritis treated according to the "sawtooth" strategy. *Arthritis Rheum* 1996;39:996–1005.
31. Stenger AA, van Leeuwen MA, Houtman PM, et al. Early effective suppression of inflammation in rheumatoid arthritis reduces radiographic progression. *Br J Rheumatol* 1998;37(11):1157–1163.
32. Choy EHS, Scott DL, Kingsley GH, et al. Treating rheumatoid arthritis early with disease modifying drugs reduces joint damage: A randomised double blind trial of sulphasalazine vs diclofenac sodium. *Clin Exp Rheumatol* 2002;20(3):351–358.
33. Quinn MA, Green MJ, Marzo-Ortega H, et al. Prognostic factors in a large cohort of patients with early undifferentiated inflammatory arthritis after application of a structured management protocol. *Arthritis Rheum* 2003;48(11):3039–3045.
34. Machold KP, Nell VPK, Stamm TA, et al. The Austrian Early Arthritis Registry. *Clin Exp Rheumatol* 2003;21(5):S113–S117.
35. Lindqvist E, Jonsson K, Saxne T, Eberhardt K. Course of radiographic damage over 10 years in a cohort with early rheumatoid arthritis. *Ann Rheum Dis* 2003;62(7):611–616.
36. Cush JJ. Early arthritis clinic: A USA perspective. *Clin Exp Rheumatol* 2003;21(5):S75–S78.

37. Svensson B, Ahlmen M, Forslind K. Treatment of early RA in clinical practice: A comparative study of two different DMARD/corticosteroid options. *Clin Exp Rheumatol* 2003;21(3):327–332.
38. Chan KW, Felson DT, Yood A, Walker AM. The lag time between onset of symptoms and diagnosis of rheumatoid arthritis. *Arthritis Rheum* 1994;38:448–449.
39. Dougados M, Combe B, Cantagrel A, et al. Combination therapy in early rheumatoid arthritis: A randomised, controlled, double-blind, 52-week clinical trial of sulphasalazine and methotrexate compared with the single components. *Ann Rheum Dis* 1999;58(4):220–225.
40. Raza K, Falciani F, Curnow SJ, et al. Early rheumatoid arthritis is characterized by a distinct and transient synovial fluid cytokine profile of T cell and stromal cell origin. *Arthritis Res Ther* 2005;7(4):R784–R795.
41. Mottonen T, Hannonen P, Korpela M, et al. Delay to institution of therapy and induction of remission using single-drug or combination-disease-modifying antirheumatic drug therapy in early rheumatoid arthritis. *Arthritis Rheum* 2002;46(4):894–898.
42. Nell VPK, Machold KP, Eberl G, et al. Benefit of very early referral and very early therapy with disease-modifying anti-rheumatic drugs in patients with early rheumatoid arthritis. *Rheumatology* 2004; 43(7):906–914.
43. Tak PP, Smeets TJM, Daha MR, et al. Analysis of the synovial cell infiltrate in early rheumatoid synovial tissue in relation to local disease activity. *Arthritis Rheum* 1997;40:217–225.
44. Bucht A, Larsson P, Weisbrot L, et al. Expression of interferon-gamma (IFN-gamma), IL-10, IL-12 and transforming growth factor-beta (TGF-beta) mRNA in synovial fluid cells from patients in the early and late phases of rheumatoid arthritis (RA). *Clin Exp Immunol* 1996;103(3):357–367.
45. Firestein GS, Echeverri F, Yeo M, et al. Somatic mutations in the p53 tumor suppressor gene in rheumatoid arthritis synovium. *Proc Natl Acad Sci U S A* 1997;94(20):10895–10900.
46. Tak PP, Zvaifler NJ, Green DR, Firestein GS. Rheumatoid arthritis and p53: How oxidative stress might alter the course of inflammatory diseases. *Immunol Today* 2000;21(2):78–82.
47. Tak PP. Is early rheumatoid arthritis the same disease process as late rheumatoid arthritis? *Best Pract Res Clin Rheumatol* 2001; 15(1):17–26.
48. Tak PP, Smeets TJM, Boyle DL, et al. p53 overexpression in synovial tissue from patients with early and longstanding rheumatoid arthritis compared with patients with reactive arthritis and osteoarthritis. *Arthritis Rheum* 1999;42(5):948–953.
49. Baeten D, Demetter P, Cuvelier C, et al. Comparative study of the synovial histology in rheumatoid arthritis, spondyloarthropathy, and osteoarthritis: Influence of disease duration and activity. *Ann Rheum Dis* 2000;59(12):945–953.
50. Aletaha D, Eberl G, Nell VPK, et al. Attitudes to early rheumatoid arthritis: Changing patterns. Results of a survey. *Ann Rheum Dis* 2004;63(10):1269–1275.
51. Machold KP, Stamm TA, Nell VPK, et al. Very recent onset rheumatoid arthritis: Clinical and serological patient characteristics associated with radiographic progression over the first years of disease. *Rheumatology* 2007;46(2):342–349.
52. van der Heijde DM. Joint erosions and patients with early rheumatoid arthritis. *Br J Rheumatol* 1995;(34 Suppl 2):74–78.
53. Plant MJ, Jones PW, Saklatvala J, et al. Patterns of radiological progression in early rheumatoid arthritis: Results of an 8-year prospective study. *J Rheumatol* 1998;25:417–426.
54. Sharp JT, Wolfe F, Mitchell DM, Bloch DA. The progression of erosion and joint space narrowing scores in rheumatoid arthritis during the first twenty-five years of disease. *Arthritis Rheum* 1991;34(6): 660–668.
55. Masi AT. Articular patterns in the early course of rheumatoid arthritis. *Am J Med* 1983;75(6A):16–26.
56. Rantapaa-Dahlqvist S. Diagnostic and prognostic significance of autoantibodies in early rheumatoid arthritis. *Scand J Rheumatol* 2005;34:83–96.
57. Singh JA, Solomon DH, Dougados M, et al. Development of classification and response criteria for rheumatic diseases. *Arthritis Rheum* 2006;55(3):348–352.
58. Smolen JS, Sokka T, Pincus T, Breedveld FC. A proposed treatment algorithm for rheumatoid arthritis: Aggressive therapy, methotrexate, and quantitative measures. *Clin Exp Rheumatol* 2003;21(5): S209–S210.
59. Arnett FC, Edworthy SM, Bloch DA, et al. The American Rheumatism Association 1987 revised criteria for the classification of rheumatoid arthritis. *Arthritis Rheum* 1988;31:315–324.
60. Aletaha D, Breedveld FC, Smolen JS. The need for new classification criteria for rheumatoid arthritis. *Arthritis Rheum* 2005;52(11): 3333–3336.
61. Ropes MW, Bennett GA, Cobb S, et al. 1958 revision of diagnostic criteria for rheumatoid arthritis. *Bull Rheum Dis* 1958;9:175–176.
62. Moens HJB, van de Laar MAFJ, van der Korst JK. Comparison of the sensitivity and specificity of the 1958 and 1987 criteria for rheumatoid arthritis. *J Rheumatol* 1992;19:198–203.
63. Mitchell DM, Fries JF. An analysis of the American Rheumatism Association criteria for rheumatoid arthritis. *Arthritis Rheum* 1982; 25(5):481–487.
64. van der Helm-van Mil, le Cessie S, Van Dongen H, et al. A prediction rule for disease outcome in patients with recent-onset undifferentiated arthritis—How to guide individual treatment decisions. *Arthritis Rheum* 2007;56(2):433–440.
65. Combe B, Landewe R, Lukas C, et al. EULAR recommendations for the management of early arthritis: Report of a task force of the European Standing Committee for International Clinical Studies Including Therapeutics (ESCISIT). *Ann Rheum Dis* 2007;66(1): 34–45.
66. Smolen JS, Breedveld FC, Eberl G, et al. Validity and reliability of the twenty-eight-joint count for the assessment of rheumatoid arthritis activity. *Arthritis Rheum* 1995;38(1):38–43.
67. Dougados M, van der Linden S, Juhlin R, et al. The European Spondylarthropathy Study Group preliminary criteria for the classification of spondylarthropathy. *Arthritis Rheum* 1991;34: 1218–1227.
68. Green M, Marzo-Ortega H, McGonagle D, et al. Persistence of mild, early inflammatory arthritis: The importance of disease duration, rheumatoid factor, and the shared epitope. *Arthritis Rheum* 1999;42(10):2184–2188.
69. Visser H, le Cessie S, Vos K, et al. How to diagnose rheumatoid arthritis early: A prediction model for persistent (erosive) arthritis. *Arthritis Rheum* 2002;46(2):357–365.
70. van der Heijde DMFM, van Riel PLCM, van Leeuwen MA, et al. Older versus younger onset rheumatoid arthritis: Results at onset and after 2 years of a prospective followup study of early rheumatoid arthritis. *J Rheumatol* 1991;18:1285–1289.
71. Mottonen T, Hannonen P, Leirisalo-Repo M, et al. Comparison of combination therapy with single-drug therapy in early rheumatoid arthritis: A randomised trial. FIN-RACo trial group. *Lancet* 1999; 353(9164):1568–1573.
72. Waaler E. On the occurrence of a factor in human serum activating the specific agglutination of sheep blood corpuscles. *Acta Pathol Microbiol Immunol Scand* 1939;17:172–182.
73. Steiner G, Smolen JS. Autoantibodies in rheumatoid arthritis. In: Firestein GS, Panayi GS, Wollheim FA, eds. Rheumatoid Arthritis, 2nd Edition. Oxford: Oxford University Press, 2006:193–198.
74. Mikkelsen WM, Dodge HJ, Duff IF, Kato H. Estimates of the prevalence of rheumatic diseases in the population of Tecumseh, Michigan 1959–1960. *J Chronic Dis* 1967;20(6):351–369.
75. Lichtenstein MJ, Pincus T. Rheumatoid arthritis identified in population-based cross-sectional studies: Low prevalence of rheumatoid factor. *J Rheumatol* 1991;18(7):989–993.
76. Nell VPK, Machold KP, Stamm TA, et al. Autoantibody profiling as early diagnostic and prognostic tool for rheumatoid arthritis. *Ann Rheum Dis* 2005;64(12):1731–1736.

77. Schellekens GA, Visser H, de Jong BA, et al. The diagnostic properties of rheumatoid arthritis antibodies recognizing a cyclic citrullinated peptide. *Arthritis Rheum* 2000;43(1):155–163.
78. Rantapaa-Dahlqvist S, de Jong BAW, Berglin E, et al. Antibodies against cyclic citrullinated peptide and IgA rheumatoid factor predict the development of rheumatoid arthritis. *Arthritis Rheum* 2003;48(10):2741–2749.
79. Nielen MMJ, Van Schaardenburg D, Reesink HW, et al. Specific autoantibodies precede the symptoms of rheumatoid arthritis: A study of serial measurements in blood donors. *Arthritis Rheum* 2004; 50(2):380–386.
80. Symmons DP. Classification criteria for rheumatoid arthritis—time to abandon rheumatoid factor? *Rheumatology (Oxford)* 2007;46(5): 725–726.
81. Bukhari M, Lunt M, Harrison BJ, et al. Rheumatoid factor is the major predictor of increasing severity of radiographic erosions in rheumatoid arthritis: Results from the Norfolk Arthritis Register Study, a large inception cohort. *Arthritis Rheum* 2002;46(4):906–912.
82. van Gaalen FA, van Aken J, Huizinga TW, et al. Association between HLA class II genes and autoantibodies to cyclic citrullinated peptides (CCPs) influences the severity of rheumatoid arthritis. *Arthritis Rheum* 2004;50:2113–2121.
83. Vries-Bouwstra J, le Cessie S, Allaart C, et al. Using predicted disease outcome to provide differentiated treatment of early rheumatoid arthritis. *J Rheumatol* 2006;33(9):1747–1753.
84. Harrison BJ, Symmons DP, Brennan P, et al. Natural remission in inflammatory polyarthritis: Issues of definition and prediction. *Br J Rheumatol* 1996;35:1096–1100.
85. Tunn EJ, Bacon PA. Differentiating persistent from self-limiting symmetrical synovitis in an early arthritis clinic. *Br J Rheumatol* 1993;32:97–103.
86. Emery P, Breedveld FC, Dougados M, et al. Early referral recommendation for newly diagnosed rheumatoid arthritis: Evidence-based development of a clinical guide. *Ann Rheum Dis* 2002;61(4): 290–297.
87. van Leeuwen MA, van Rijswijk MH, Sluiter WJ, et al. Individual relationship between progression of radiological damage and the acute phase response in early rheumatoid arthritis. Towards development of a decision support system. *J Rheumatol* 1997;24(1):20–27.
88. Smolen JS, van der Heijde DMFM, St.Clair EW, et al. Predictors of joint damage in patients with early rheumatoid arthritis treated with high-dose methotrexate without or with concomitant infliximab. Results from the ASPIRE trial. *Arthritis Rheum* 2006;54:702–710.
89. Backhaus M, Kamradt T, Sndrock D, et al. Arthritis of the finger joints. A comprehensive approach comparing conventional radiography, scintigraphy, ultrasound, and contrast-enhanced magnetic resonance imaging. *Arthritis Rheum* 1999;42:1232–1245.
90. Ostergaard M, Ejbjerg B, Szkudlarek M. Imaging in early rheumatoid arthritis: Roles of magnetic resonance imaging, ultrasonography, conventional radiography and computed tomography. *Best Pract Res Clin Rheumatol* 2005;19(1):91–116.
91. Keen HI, Brown AK, Wakefield RJ, Conaghan PG. MRI and musculoskeletal ultrasonography as diagnostic tools in early arthritis. *Rheum Dis Clin North Am* 2005;31(4):699–714.
92. Taylor PC. The value of sensitive imaging modalities in rheumatoid arthritis. *Arthritis Res Ther* 2003;5(5):210–213.
93. Boutry N, Hachulla E, Flipo RM, et al. MR imaging findings in hands in early rheumatoid arthritis: Comparison with those in systemic lupus erythematosus and primary Sjögren syndrome. *Radiology* 2005;236:593–600.
94. Hayer S, Redlich K, Korb A, et al. Tenosynovitis and osteoclast formation as the initial preclinical changes in a murine model of inflammatory arthritis. *Arthritis Rheum* 2007;56:79–88.
95. Gregersen PK, Silver J, Winchester RJ. The shared epitope hypothesis: An approach to understanding the molecular genetics of susceptibility to rheumatoid arthritis. *Arthritis Rheum* 1987;30(11): 1205–1213.
96. Bayley JP, Baggen JM, der Pouw-Kraan T, et al. Association between polymorphisms in the human chemokine receptor genes CCR2 and CX(3)CR1 and rheumatoid arthritis. *Tissue Antigens* 2003;62(2):170–174.
97. Huizinga TWJ, Amos CI, van der Helm-van Mil, et al. Refining the complex rheumatoid arthritis phenotype based on specificity of the HLA-DRB1 shared epitope for antibodies to citrullinated proteins. *Arthritis Rheum* 2005;52(11):3433–3438.
98. Brennan P, Harrison B, Barrett E, et al. A simple algorithm to predict the development of radiological erosions in patients with early rheumatoid arthritis: Prospective cohort study. *BMJ* 1996;313: 471–476.
99. Drossaers-Bakker KW, Zwinderman AH, Vlieland TP, et al. Long-term outcome in rheumatoid arthritis: A simple algorithm of baseline parameters can predict radiographic damage, disability, and disease course at 12-year follow-up. *Arthritis Rheum* 2002; 47(4):383–390.
100. Combe B, Dougados M, Goupille P, et al. Prognostic factors for radiographic damage in early rheumatoid arthritis: A multiparameter prospective study. *Arthritis Rheum* 2001;44(8):1736–1743.
101. Symmons DPM, Hazes JMW, Silman AJ. Cases of early inflammatory polyarthritis should not be classified as having rheumatoid arthritis. *J Rheumatol* 2003;30(5):902–904.
102. Boers M. The case for corticosteroids in the treatment of early rheumatoid arthritis. *Rheumatology* 1999;38(2):95–97.
103. Kirwan JR, Arthritis and Rheumatism Council Low-Dose Glucocorticoid Study Group. The effects of glucocorticoids on joint destruction in rheumatoid arthritis. *N Engl J Med* 1995;333: 142–146.
104. Van Everdingen AA, Jacobs JWG, Van Reesema DRS, Bijlsma JWJ. Low-dose prednisone therapy for patients with early active rheumatoid arthritis: Clinical efficacy, disease-modifying properties, and side effects. A randomized, double-blind, placebo-controlled clinical trial. *Ann Intern Med* 2002;136(1):1–12.
105. Wassenberg S, Rau R, Steinfeld P, Zeidler H. Very low-dose prednisolone in early rheumatoid arthritis retards radiographic progression over two years. A multicenter, double-blind, placebo-controlled trial. *Arthritis Rheum* 2005;52(11):3371–3380.
106. Egsmose C, Lund B, Borg C, et al. Patients with rheumatoid arthritis benefit from early 2nd line therapy: 5-year follow-up of a prospective double blind placebo controlled study. *J Rheumatol* 1995;22:2208–2213.
107. Lard LR, Visser H, Speyer I, vet al. Early versus delayed treatment in patients with recent-onset rheumatoid arthritis: comparison of two cohorts who received different treatment strategies. *Am J Med* 2001;111(6):446–451.
108. Svensson B, Boonen A, Albertsson K, et al. Low-dose prednisolone in addition to the initial disease-modifying antirheumatic drug in patients with early active rheumatoid arthritis reduces joint destruction and increases the remission rate: A two-year randomized trial. *Arthritis Rheum* 2005;52(11):3360–3370.
109. Capell HA, Madhok R, Hunter JA, et al. Lack of radiological and clinical benefit over two years of low dose prednisolone for rheumatoid arthritis: Results of a randomised controlled trial. *Ann Rheum Dis* 2004;63(7):797–803.
110. van Jaarsveld CH, Jacobs JW, van der Veen MJ, et al. Aggressive treatment in early rheumatoid arthritis: A randomised controlled trial. On behalf of the Rheumatic Research Foundation Utrecht, The Netherlands. *Ann Rheum Dis* 2000;59(6):468–477.
111. Jobanputra P, Wilson J, Douglas K, Burls A. A survey of British rheumatologists' DMARD preferences for rheumatoid arthritis. *Rheumatology* 2004;43(2):206–210.
112. Le Loet X, Berthelot JM, Cantagrel A, et al. Clinical practice decision tree for the choice of the first disease modifying antirheumatic drug for very early rheumatoid arthritis: A 2004 proposal of the French Society of Rheumatology. *Ann Rheum Dis* 2006;65(1): 45–50.

113. Verstappen SMM, Jacobs JWG, van der Veen MJ, et al. Intensive treatment with methotrexate in early rheumatoid arthritis: Aiming for remission. Computer Assisted Management in Early Rheumatoid Arthritis (CAMERA, an open-label strategy trial). *Ann Rheum Dis* 2007;66(11):1443–1449.
114. Smolen JS, Aletaha D, Keystone E. Superior efficacy of combination therapy for rheumatoid arthritis. Fact or fiction? *Arthritis Rheum* 2005;52:2975–2983.
115. Grigor C, Capell H, Stirling A, et al. Effect of a treatment strategy of tight control for rheumatoid arthritis (the TICORA study): A single-blind randomised controlled trial. *Lancet* 2004;364(9430): 263–269.
116. Bathon JM, Martin RW, Fleischmann RM, et al. A comparison of etanercept and methotrexate in patients with early rheumatoid arthritis. *N Engl J Med* 2000;343(22):1586–1593.
117. O'Dell JR, Elliott JR, Mallek JA, et al. Treatment of early seropositive rheumatoid arthritis—doxycycline plus methotrexate versus methotrexate alone. *Arthritis Rheum* 2006;54(2):621–627.
118. Haagsma CJ, van Riel PL, de Jong AJ, van de Putte LB. Combination of sulphasalazine and methotrexate versus the single components in early rheumatoid arthritis: A randomized, controlled, double-blind, 52-week clinical trial. *Br J Rheumatol* 1997;36(10): 1082–1088.
119. van den Borne BEEM, Landewe RBM, The HSG, et al. Combination therapy in recent onset rheumatoid arthritis: A randomized double-blind trial of the addition of low-dose cyclosporine to patients treated with low-dose chloroquine. *J Rheumatol* 1998;25(8): 1493–1498.

The Social and Economic Impact of Rheumatoid Arthritis

CHAPTER 7

Gisela Kobelt

The progressive nature of rheumatoid arthritis (RA) and its onset in early or mid-life means that many patients live with the disease for 30 or more years. The social and economic impact of the disease is considerable, as it is associated with chronic pain and fatigue, and leads rapidly to restrictions in functional capacity.[1–9] Based on inception cohorts, it has been estimated in the past that as many as a third of patients will be unable to work within 10 years of disease onset,[10,11] making production losses a very significant part of the economic burden of the disease.[6,8,9,12–14] The mortality and morbidity associated with RA translate into a health burden for society[15] and loss of quality of life (QoL) for patients.[9,16–18]

In this chapter, we will first discuss the social costs (health burden) for society and for patients, and then provide an overview of the economic cost of RA. For a more detailed overview of these issues, see Jönsson et al.[19] Our discussion is based on published data, and it must be emphasized that the field of RA is currently undergoing changes that are not without consequences on burden and costs. The diagnosis and management of the disease have improved, and the adoption of early treatment with disease-modifying arthritic drugs (DMARDs) in the early 1990s is likely to have changed today's outcomes and consequences of the disease compared to the 1980s when many of the epidemiologic studies were initiated. The introduction of biological treatments a decade ago has accelerated this change.[10,11] This medical progress, but also the transition in the workplace to less physically demanding jobs, may make it possible for patients with RA to remain in the workforce for a longer time. The costs of RA may thus look different from what appears in the current literature in only a few years.

Health Burden of Rheumatoid Arthritis

In this discussion, we define the burden of RA as the loss of health due to morbidity and mortality, using measurements that can be applied to any disease to allow comparison. For illustrative purposes, we will also use these measurements to estimate the intangible cost of the disease.

Disability-Adjusted Life Years

The World Health Organization has developed a measure suitable to estimate the health burden of different diseases across the world, the disability-adjusted life year (DALY).[15] The DALY combines disability (morbidity) and mortality, weighting thus a healthy life year with the impact of the disease. There has been intense discussion regarding the validity of this measure, notably relating to how the disability weights were derived, and a comprehensive review of the concept and the measurement is available.[20]

The loss of DALYs due to RA was estimated at 0.84% of all DALYs lost in Europe and at 0.69% in the United States.[20] Deaths due to RA were estimated at 0.09% and 0.12% of all deaths, respectively, indicating that the burden of RA due to morbidity is larger than that due to mortality. In Europe, the burden is higher in countries with a low income per capita (e.g., Central and Eastern Europe), in line with evidence that the disease is correlated with socioeconomic conditions.[21] Southern European countries have a somewhat lower burden, reflecting epidemiologic evidence that prevalence and disease severity may be lower.[16,22]

Quality-Adjusted Life Years

Within the field of health economics, another measure has been devised to measure the disease burden that allows comparing the impact of a disease on patients and the changes obtained with treatment. The quality-adjusted life year (QALY) combines life expectancy (years) with its quality into an index that can be used across all diseases.[23] QoL is measured as "utility," a valuation of given health states on a scale anchored between 0 (death) and 1 (full health), using decision analytic methods or specific preference-based questionnaires. The utility "weight" is then applied to time: Living 2 years with a utility of 0.5 represents 1 QALY—which is identical to living 1 year in full health.

A number of studies have measured utility in different populations of RA patients. In cross-sectional data, results will heavily depend on the sample, as QoL worsens with progressing disease.[8,9,24] However, all population-based studies, or studies with large samples covering the full disease spectrum, have found comparatively low utility scores. For instance, in a Swedish study in 541 patients with a mean Health Assessment Questionnaire (HAQ) score of 1.1, the mean utility was 0.58.[9] In a more recent study in France, mean utility was estimated at 0.5 in a sample of 1348 patients with a mean HAQ score of 1.4.[18]

As these scores are not disease-specific, they can be related to results for other diseases. A recently published "league table" showed RA to be one of the diseases with the worst utility[25,26] (Table 7-1).

As mentioned above, mean utility scores depend very much on the sample used in the study. Utilities are most influenced by the main symptoms of the disease (pain, fatigue, limitations in function), and as these worsen with progressing disease, utilities decline. Regression analysis using Swedish data showed that by far the strongest predictor of utilities is function (HAQ), but that disease activity (Disease Activity Score [DAS]) appears to

Table 7-1. Utility in Rheumatoid Arthritis Compared to Other Diseases

Disease	Mean Utility	Standard Deviation	Patients	Setting
Rheumatoid arthritis	0.500	0.307	1487	OP
Multiple sclerosis	0.555	0.320	13186	OP
Angina pectoris	0.576	0.306	284	IP
Acute myocardial infarction	0.610	0.336	251	IP
Chronic ischemic heart disease	0.636	0.293	789	IP
Gastro-esophageal reflux disease	0.671	0.301	216	IP
Cataract	0.672	0.286	748	IP
Diabetes (type 2)	0.764	0.287	159	OP
Menopausal disorders	0.703	0.317	103	OP
Malignant neoplasms of skin	0.726	0.267	273	IP

IP, Inpatient; *OP*, outpatient.
Adapted from Currie CJ, McEwan P, Peters JR, et al. The routine collation of health outcomes data from hospital treated subjects in the Health Outcomes Data Repository (HODaR): Descriptive analysis from the first 20,000 subjects. *Value Health* 2005;8(5):581–590; and Orme M, Kerrigan J, Tyas D, et al. The effect of disease, functional status and relapses on the utility of people with multiple sclerosis in the UK. *Value Health* 2007;10(1):54–60.

have an additional effect, while all other variables (age, gender, disease duration) were not significant when HAQ and DAS are included in the model.[9] This finding may partly be related to the instrument that was used to measure utilities, the EQ-5D.[27] The EQ-5D measures five domains of QoL (mobility, self-care, usual activities, pain/discomfort, anxiety/depression), and it is possible that the measure misses part of the impact of fatigue. Another utility measure, the SF6, derived from a generic QoL instrument (SF36), includes vitality as a sixth domain, as this was found to be important in the development of the measure.[28] However, due to issues with anchoring of the scales, the instrument has been shown not to adequately measure severe health states in diseases such as RA.[28]

Using the EQ-5D, utilities were found to be almost identical across different countries, as shown in Figure 7-1 with the examples from Sweden and France.[9,18] The impact of disease activity is illustrated in Figure 7-2 with utilities shown for patients at the same HAQ level, but with high and low disease activity.[9]

Intangible Costs

The methodology for studies on the cost of illness of a disease lists three types of costs that should be included: direct, indirect, and intangible costs. The latter are defined as the cost due to suffering from the disease and/or its treatment. Currently, there is discussion on how best to assign a monetary value to this suffering, and few studies have actually included these costs.

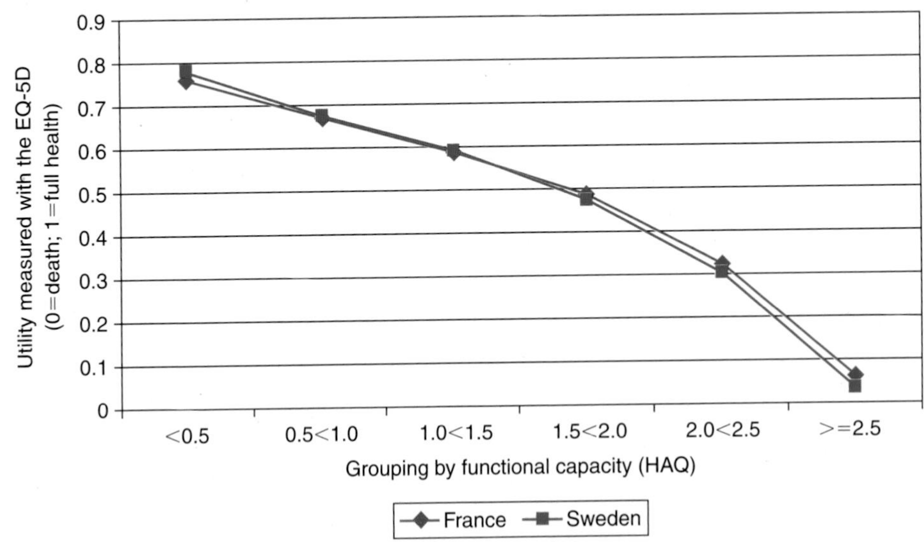

Figure 7-1. Utilities in the two most recent large cross-sectional studies in Europe measured using the EQ-5D were identical (Sweden 2002, $n = 616$; France 2005, $n = 1348$), supporting the claim that the measure is truly disease oriented and does not change by country or setting when related to a general measure of disease severity. (Adapted from Kobelt G, Lindgren P, Lindroth Y, et al. Modelling the effect of function and disease activity on costs and quality of life in rheumatoid arthritis. *Rheumatology (Oxford)* 2005;44(9):1169–1175; and Kobelt G, Woronoff A, Richard B, et al. The effect of rheumatoid arthritis on costs and quality of life of patients in France. An observational study in 1500 patients. *Joint, Bone and Spine* 2008;75(7).)

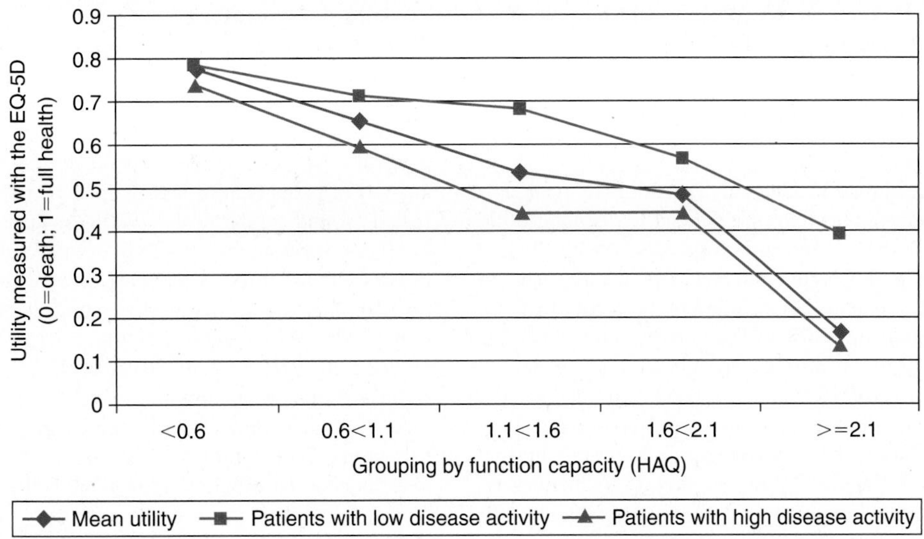

Figure 7-2. Patients were first grouped into five groups according to functional capacity (HAQ) and then separated by disease activity. Disease activity was expressed using the patient global VAS (scale 1–10) as a proxy, with a cut-off point of 4.0. The authors of the study found that this cut-off corresponded to a DAS28 of 3.2. Note that the number of patients over HAQ 2 with low disease activity was extremely small. (Adapted from Kobelt G, Lindgren P, Lindroth Y, et al. Modelling the effect of function and disease activity on costs and quality of life in rheumatoid arthritis. *Rheumatology (Oxford)* 2005;44(9):1169–1175.)

However, if we accept that the suffering is appropriately expressed in utility measurements, it is possible to compare the scores from patients to the values obtained in the general population, thus estimating the loss of utility due to the disease. This difference, over the course of 1 year, will provide the loss of QALYs experience by patients with a disease. In countries where health technology assessment (HTA) and economic evaluation are actively used in decision making, such as when deciding on the reimbursement of a new treatment, the QALY is generally used as the outcome measure due to its comparability across diseases. Although no official threshold for the willingness to pay for a QALY gained exists, it is generally implied from the way decisions have been made that treatments with an incremental cost of €50,000 per QALY gained (compared to standard treatment) are acceptable. Applying this threshold to the QALYs lost due to a disease provides one type of monetary estimate of intangible costs.

Using the most recent large cost-of-illness study in Europe,[18] we have estimated the QALY loss, compared to an age- and gender-matched population, at 0.3 QALYs, and thus an intangible cost of €15.000 per patient and year (Figure 7-3). It is interesting to note that the loss of utility is similar at all ages,

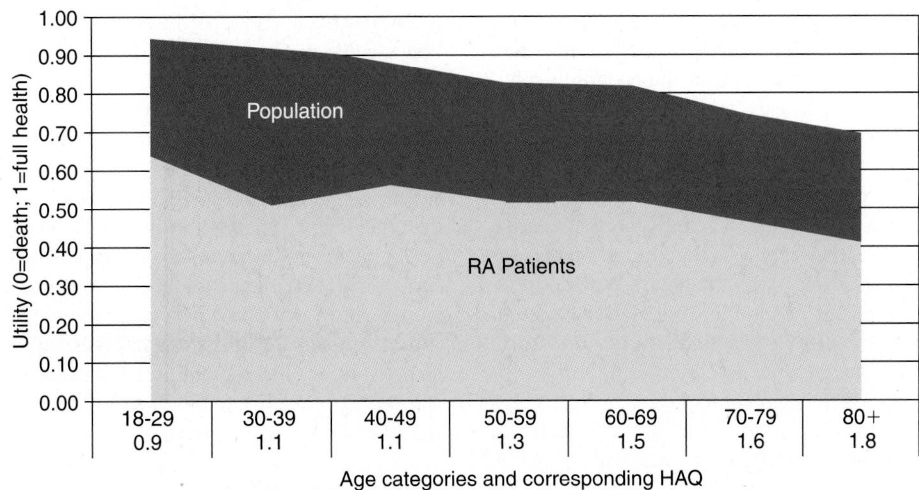

Figure 7-3. Patients were grouped by age, and the mean utility score of each group compared to scores for an age- and gender-matched sample of the general population. The loss of quality of life is evident at all ages, but it is interesting to note that the older groups with considerably worse HAQ scores have about the same loss as younger patients, demonstrating clearly the effect of coping with the disease over time. The difference translates into a loss of 0.3 QALYs per year in this sample of 1348 patients in France. (Adapted from Kobelt G, Woronoff A, Richard B, et al. The effect of rheumatoid arthritis on costs and quality of life of patients in France. An observational study in 1500 patients. *Joint, Bone and Spine* 2008;75(7).)

despite worse HAQ scores for older patients, which would demonstrate the effect of coping with the disease.

Economic Cost of Rheumatoid Arthritis

Cost Definitions

Costs of a disease should include only costs directly related to the disease. However, it is often very difficult to distinguish between costs of the disease and costs for a patient with the disease. RA highlights this issue quite well. For instance, should costs for cardiac problems be included or not? Although we know that increased mortality in RA is partly due to cardiac deaths,[29] it is difficult to distinguish whether a given patient would have no cardiac comorbidity without RA, or whether RA exacerbates existing disease. In order to answer this question, comparative studies with a control group from the normal population would be required. However, as costs are highly variable between patients because a small number of patients with severe disease use a large part of the resources, cost studies require large samples. This, in turn, makes it difficult to identify and include a control group.

Costs are defined as the quantity of resources (e.g., consultations, admissions, etc.) multiplied by price. Both can be very different from one country to another for a number of reasons, and using costs from one country to conclude on costs in another is highly problematic. Resource utilization is influenced by payment mechanisms. For instance, fee-for-service in insurance-based health care systems with private practitioners will lead to large number of visits, while national health services with only hospital specialists will lead to few visits. In the former case, tariffs will be set to influence consumption and they will thus not necessarily reflect the actual cost, while in the latter case the price will be based on actual use based on a case mix. Tradition has its own influence on consumption. For instance, inpatient admission is more frequent and length of stay longer in countries in Southern Europe compared to Northern Europe or North America. However, a stronger influence comes again from the payment systems, where payment per admission will shorten length of stay dramatically compared to a per diem payment. Across the world, however, the largest difference in costs stems from the economic environment. Spending on health care is directly related to the gross domestic product (GDP). A report by the World Bank in 1997 showed that not only do richer nations spend more on health care, they also finance a larger part of it from public sources (with the exception of the United States). In 2004, health care expenditures per capita in the United States was $6000 PPP (purchasing power parity), compared to $600 PPP in Turkey (Organization for Economic Cooperation and Development data). Clearly, neither expenditures nor unit costs can be the same, with the possible exception of pharmaceutical products that compete in a global market.

In general, we distinguish between direct costs, medical and nonmedical, and indirect costs. Medical costs are defined as health care costs, while nonmedical costs include devices or investments and services such as home care, transportation, and assistance from family members. Indirect costs represent production losses for society due to sick leave, early retirement, or premature death. Cost-of-illness studies should take the perspective of society, that is, they should include all costs regardless of who pays.

Costs in the Literature

There is an abundance of small cost studies pertaining to RA in various countries that focus on different types of patients and different objectives. It would be beyond the scope of this chapter to review all of them. A review in 2000 estimated the direct medical costs at around US$6000 per patient and year.[6] An analysis of patients aged less than 65 years in the German RA registry found similar costs (4700 euros per patient and year), but these represented only a third of total costs.[14] A recent study in France found direct health care costs of almost €12, 000 in a population-based sample, representing slightly more than half of total costs.[18] One of the major reasons for the higher costs in France compared to Germany is that the French study included a considerable proportion of patients treated with TNF inhibitors. Another review in 2005 found that mean total costs per patient in different studies could range from as little as US$1500 to as much as US$16,600 and concluded that indeed, there was no way to compare these studies.[7]

However, a number of general findings emerge from these studies. Costs increase with increasing disease severity, and in particular with functional disability. Several studies found a relation between disease activity and costs,[9,30–34] although the amplitude of the variation is small.[9,31,35] One study estimated that direct costs increase from around €600 per year for patients with low disease activity to €1200 for patients with high disease activity.[35] In contrast, total costs increase from around €5000 for patients with minimal functional disability (HAQ <0.5) to €20,000 for patients with severe disease (HAQ >2).[9,18,36] All types of costs increase as HAQ worsens, although productivity losses tend to decrease in advanced disease, as fewer patients are of working age as illustrated in a Swedish and a French study in Figure 7-4.[9,18] These two studies also illustrate differences in several countries: Patients with disabilities in Sweden receive considerable support from the health care system (direct cost) and thus require only very limited help from family members; in contrast, patients in France have to rely heavily on their families.

Nevertheless, decreased work capacity is one of the strongest drivers of costs. Early in the disease, active inflammation leads to absence from work.[9] As the disease progresses, reduced function requires patients to leave the work force. Early retirement rates vary by study sample, but also by country and the year of the study, covering a range between 25% and 40% for samples with an average disease duration of up to 10 years, and between 33% and 50% beyond 10 years.[9–11,13,14,18,36–38] Depending on the age of the sample (proportion of patients of working age) and the type of costs included in the study, productivity losses represent between 30% and 50% of total costs. As all other type of costs, early retirement is significantly correlated with HAQ. In a French study, workforce participation at HAQ levels below 1.0 appeared normal, while at HAQ 2.0 or higher, only 10% to 15% of patients of working age were actually working, compared with an expected 55% to 60% in the general population between age 50 and 60 years (Figure 7-5).[18]

Overall Cost Estimates

Recently, an economic model was used to estimate the overall cost of RA in various countries.[19] The methodology was based on an earlier study of the cost of brain disorders in Europe.[39] The authors used cost data from published studies (OECD Health Data,[40] Eurostat,[41] World Bank[42]) adjusted to the same year (2006 purchasing power parity) to render data comparable and

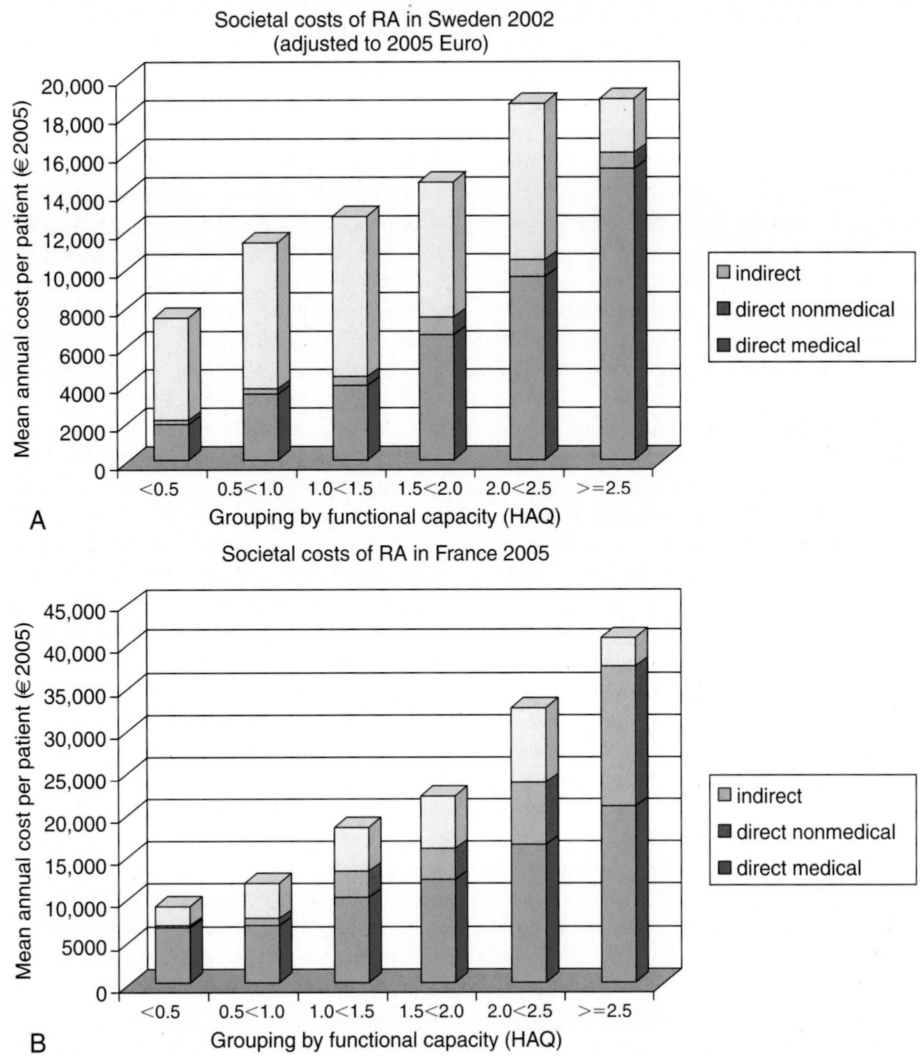

Figure 7-4. Costs are most strongly correlated with functional capacity (HAQ), with all costs increasing with worsening disease in Sweden (A) and France (B). Indirect costs, however, are also related to age: Patients with more advanced disease are most often also older, and the number of patients at working age in the most severe HAQ groups is small, thus reducing indirect costs. (Adapted from Kobelt G, Lindgren P, Lindroth Y, et al. Modelling the effect of function and disease activity on costs and quality of life in rheumatoid arthritis. *Rheumatology (Oxford)* 2005;44(9):1169–1175; and Kobelt G, Woronoff A, Richard B, et al. The effect of rheumatoid arthritis on costs and quality of life of patients in France. An observational study in 1500 patients. *Joint, Bone and Spine* 2008;75(7).)

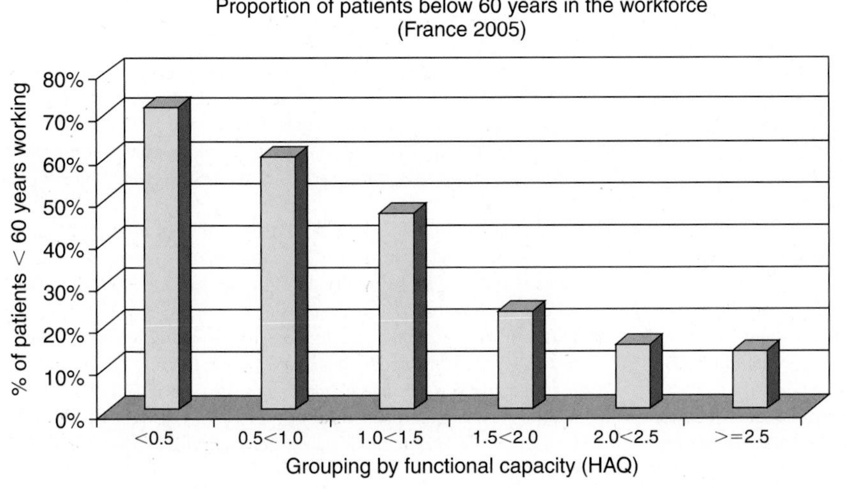

Figure 7-5. The official retirement age in France is 60 years, and workforce participation of the population in 2005 was estimated at 64% for women and 75% for men (www.insee.fr). Respective numbers for the population over 50 are 55% for women and 64% for men. Thus, early in the disease and with a low HAQ, work capacity is not impaired. However, at HAQ levels above 2 only around 15% of patients are still working. (Adapted from Kobelt G, Woronoff A, Richard B, et al. The effect of rheumatoid arthritis on costs and quality of life of patients in France. An observational study in 1500 patients. *Joint, Bone and Spine* 2008;75(7).)

extrapolated to countries where no studies were available. Cost studies were identified in PubMed, the Health Economic Evaluation Database (HEED), EuroNHEED, and various research institutions. Studies with a special focus, such as estimating the cost of a specific intervention or including a subset of patients, were excluded from the study. The most complete and most recent studies were included in the calculations. All studies selected included direct medical costs, and a large number also included productivity losses; however, nonmedical costs and informal care had to be based on a more limited number of studies. Next, although most studies included were recent and referred to years since 2000, the use of biological drugs was steadily growing and drug costs were thus heavily influenced by the study year.

Results are expressed as the average annual cost per patient, including direct health care costs, nonmedical costs, informal care, and productivity losses. Total costs per country were to be based on national prevalence estimates. However, prevalence data for RA are scarce and the study therefore assumed an average prevalence in the population of 0.66% was used for Northern countries, and 0.45% for Southern countries.

In Europe, the average annual cost per patient was estimated at €13,500, with however, a large difference between Western Europe (€17,200) and Central and Eastern Europe (€4900). In the United States, the cost per patient was €21,000, much of the difference compared to Western Europe being due to a higher penetration of TNF inhibitors. Health care costs represented 35% (of which around 40% was accounted for by drugs), nonmedical costs 14%, productivity losses 32%, and informal care 19%.

The total annual cost of RA was estimated at €45 billion in Europe for a patient population of slightly less than 3 million. Western Europe represented €42 billion for a total of 2.3 million patients. Costs in the United States were estimated at €42 billion, for slightly less than 2 million patients.

Conclusion

This chapter summarized some of the literature regarding the social and economic burden of RA. Without question, the disease is one of the most severe in terms of the impact on patients' QoL. Utilities measured in population samples are comparable only to those found for multiple sclerosis. The difference in utility scores of RA patients compared to a normal age- and gender-matched population is around 0.3 (on a scale between 0 and 1), and this difference is present at all levels of the disease. Expressed in monetary terms, the loss of QALYs leads to an intangible cost of €15,000 per year and patient. This is again very similar to what has been estimated for multiple sclerosis.

Costs outside the health care system represent the majority of costs in RA; health care costs including drugs represent only around one-third of total costs to society. The loss of functional capacity leads rapidly to the loss of work capacity, and productivity cost are estimated at one-third or more of total costs. A small number of studies has included informal care (defined as help from family and friends for performing activities of daily living), and found that these represent a substantial portion of total cost. Although family support represents "nonpaid help," studies have assigned a cost (opportunity cost of time) to this activity, as without the family, a professional from the health care sector would be required.

A recent study has estimated the total cost of RA in a number of countries (Europe, Turkey, Russian Federation, North America, and Australia) at close to €100 billion for 2006, of which €45 billion was in Europe. Health care costs (~35%) would represent an estimated 1.4% of all health care expenditures in the countries included in the study.

As management of the RA improves, and new technology such as the biologic drugs truly modifies the disease, costs will change. Health care costs are unlikely to decrease, but it is hoped that in the future, patients will be able to remain in the workforce longer and require less outside help.

References

1. Meenan R, Yelin E, Nevitt M, Epstain W. The impact of chronic disease: A socioeconomic profile of rheumatoid arthritis. *Arthritis Rheum* 1981;24:544–549.
2. Allaire S, Prashker M, Meenan R. The cost of rheumatoid arthritis. (Review.) *Pharmacoeconomics* 1995;6(6):515–522.
3. Pincus T. The underestimated long-term medical and economic consequences of rheumatoid arthritis. *Drugs* 1995;50(1):1–14.
4. Young A, Wilkinson P, Talamo J, et al. Socioeconomic factors in the presentation and outcome of early RA. Lessons for the health service? *Ann Rheum Dis* 2000;59(10):794–799.
5. Jonsson D, Husberg L. Socioeconomic costs of rheumatic diseases: Implications for technology assessment. *J Technol Assess Health Care* 2000;16:1193–1200.
6. Cooper N. Economic burden of rheumatoid arthritis: A systematic review. *Rheumatology* 2000;39(1):28–33.
7. Rosery H, Bergemann R, Maxion-Bergemann S. International variation in resource utilisation and treatment costs for rheumatoid arthritis. A systematic literature review. *Pharmacoeconomics* 2005; 23(3):243–257.
8. Kobelt G, Eberhardt K, Jönsson L, Jönsson B. Economic consequences of the progression of rheumatoid arthritis in Sweden. *Arthritis Rheum* 1999;42(2):347–356.
9. Kobelt G, Lindgren P, Lindroth Y, et al. Modelling the effect of function and disease activity on costs and quality of life in rheumatoid arthritis. *Rheumatology (Oxford)* 2005;44(9):1169–1175.
10. Young A, Dixey J, Kulinskaya E, et al. Which patients with early RA stop working. Results from a 5-year inception cohort of 547 patients. *Ann Rheum Dis* 2002;61:335–340.
11. Fex E, Larsson B-M, Nived K, Eberhardt K. Impact of rheumatoid arthritis on work status and social and leisure time activities in patients followed 8 years from onset. *J Rheumatol* 1997;25:44–50.
12. Wong J, Ramey D, Singh G. Long-term morbidity, mortality and economis of rheumatoid arthritis. *Arthritis Rheum* 2001;44(12): 2746–2749.
13. Merkesdal S, Ruof J, Schoffski O, et al. Indirect medical costs in early rheumatoid arthritis: Composition of and changes in indirect costs within the first three years of disease. *Arthritis Rheum* 2001; 44(3):528–534.
14. Huscher D, Merkesdal S, Thiele K, et al. Cost of illness in rheumatoid arthritis, ankylosing spondylitis, psoriatic arthritis and systemic lupus erythematosus in Germany. *Ann Rheum Dis* 2006;65(9):1175–1183.
15. World Health Organization. Death and DALY estimated for 2002 by cause for WHO member states. Geneva: World Health Organization, 2002.

16. Antoni C, Maini R, Grunke M. Cooperative on quality of life in rheumatic diseases: Results of a survey among 6000 patients across 11 European countries. *Arthritis Rheum* 2002;46(Suppl): S76 (abstract)
17. Hurst N, Kind P, Ruta D, et al. Measuring health-related quality of life in rheumatoid arthritis: Validity, responsiveness and reliability of EuroQol (EQ-5D). Br *J Rheumatol* 1997;36:551–559.
18. Kobelt G, Woronoff A, Richard B, et al. The effect of rheumatoid arthritis on costs and quality of life of patients in France. An observational study in 1500 patients. *Joint, Bone and Spine* 2008;75(7).
19. Jönsson B, Kobelt G, Smolen J. The burden of rheumatoid arthritis and patient access to treatment. *Eur J Health Econ* 2008;Suppl2:S33–S106.
20. Fox-Rushby J. *Disability-Adjusted Life Years (DALYs) for Decision Making? An Overview of the Literature*. London: Office of Health Economics, 2002.
21. Young A, Wilkinson P, Talamo J, et al. Socioeconomic deprivation and rheumatoid disease. What lessons for the health service? *Ann Rheum Dis* 2000;59(10):794–799.
22. Drosos AA, Lanchbury JS, Panayi GS, Moutsopoulos HM. Rheumatoid arthritis in Greek and British patients. A comparative clinical, radiologic, and serologic study. *Arthritis Rheum* 1992;35(7): 745–748.
23. Torrance G. Measurement of health state utilities for economic appraisal. A review. *J Health Econ* 1986;5:1–30.
24. Kobelt G, Jönsson L, Lindgren P, et al. Modeling the progression of rheumatoid arthritis. A Two-country model to estimate costs and consequences of rheumatoid arthritis. *Arthritis Rheum* 2002;46(9): 2310–2319.
25. Currie CJ, McEwan P, Peters JR, et al. The routine collation of health outcomes data from hospital treated subjects in the Health Outcomes Data Repository (HODaR): Descriptive analysis from the first 20,000 subjects. *Value Health* 2005;8(5):581–590.
26. Orme M, Kerrigan J, Tyas D, et al. The effect of disease, functional status and relapses on the utility of people with multiple sclerosis in the UK. *Value Health* 2007;10(1):54–60.
27. EuroQol Group. EuroQol—a new facility for the measurement of health-related quality of life. *Health Policy* 1990;16:199–208.
28. Brazier J, Roberts J, Deverill M. The estimation of a preference-based measure of health from the SF-36. *J Health Econ* 2002; 21(2):271–292.
29. Jacobsson LT, Turesson C, Gulfe A, et al. Treatment with tumor necrosis factor blockers is associated with a lower incidence of first cardiovascular events in patients with rheumatoid arthritis. *J Rheumatol* 2005;32(7):1213–1218.
30. Kobelt G, Jonsson L, Lindgren P, et al. Modeling the progression of rheumatoid arthritis: A two-country model to estimate costs and consequences of rheumatoid arthritis. *Arthritis Rheum* 2002;46(9): 2310–2319.
31. Michaud K, Messer J, Choi HK, Wolfe F. Direct medical costs and their predictors in patients with rheumatoid arthritis: A three-year study of 7,527 patients. *Arthritis Rheum* 2003;48(10):2750–2762.
32. Pugner KM, Scott DI, Holmes JW, Hieke K. The costs of rheumatoid arthritis: An international long-term view. *Semin Arthritis Rheum* 2000;29(5):305–320.
33. Kobelt G, Eberhardt K, Jonsson L, Jonsson B. Economic consequences of the progression of rheumatoid arthritis in Sweden. *Arthritis Rheum* 1999;42(2):347–356.
34. Hulsemann JL, Ruof J, Zeidler H, Mittendorf T. Costs in rheumatology: Results and lessons learned from the "Hannover Costing Study." *Rheumatol Int* 2006;26(8):704–711.
35. Hulsemann JL, Ruof J, Zeidler H, Mittendorf T. Costs in rheumatology: Results and lessons learned from the "Hannover Costing Study." *Rheumatol Int* 2005;26(8):704–711.
36. Lajas C, Abasolo L, Bellajdel B, et al. Costs and predictors of costs in rheumatoid arthritis: A prevalence-based study. *Arthritis Rheum* 2003;49(1):64–70.
37. Doeglas D, Suurmeijer T, Krol B, et al. Work disability in early rheumatoid arthritis. *Ann Rheum Dis* 1995;54(6):455–460.
38. Chorus AM, Miedema HS, Wevers CJ, van Der Linden S. Labour force participation among patients with rheumatoid arthritis. *Ann Rheum Dis* 2000;59(7):549–554.
39. Andlin-Sobocki P, Jonsson B, Wittchen HU, Olesen J. Cost of disorders of the brain in Europe. *Eur J Neurol* 2005;12(Suppl 1): 1–27.
40. Organisation for Economic Co-operation and Development. OECD Health Data 2007. Statistics and Indicators for 30 Countries. http://www.oecd.org/document/30/0,3343,en_2649_37407_12968734_1_1_1_137407,00.html.
41. European Commission. Eurostat 2007. http://epp.eurostat.ec.europa.eu.
42. World Bank. Statistics, 2007. http://www.worldbank.org.

Pathogenesis of Rheumatoid Arthritis

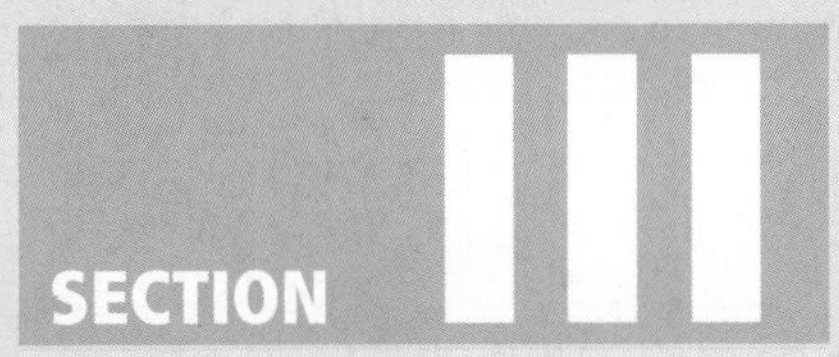

The Role of T Cells in Rheumatoid Arthritis

CHAPTER 8A

Clemens Scheinecker

T cells have long been implicated in mediating many aspects of joint inflammation. In general, $CD4^+$ T cells are recognized to drive the inflammatory response as activated proinflammatory Th1 effector cells. In addition, however, recent studies concerning the role certain T-cell subsets, such as regulatory T cells (Treg) or the newly discovered Th17 T-cell lineage, suggest an even broader involvement of T cells in the pathogenesis of RA. These insights into the immunopathogenesis of RA (RA) at the same time have generated new opportunities for the development of innovative therapeutic approaches in the treatment of RA.

T-Cell Development, Thymic Selection, and Tolerance

T cells derive from hematopoietic precursor cells in the bone marrow, and undergo differentiation in the thymus, where potentially autoagressive T cells are removed from the repertoire by "negative selection." Maturation of T cells requires "positive selection," which involves binding of the T-cell receptor to major histocompatibility complex (MHC) molecules. Positive selection ensures the successful differentiation of those immature thymocytes that are eventually able to recognize self-MHC molecules complexed with foreign antigens (peptides). Those cells that survive thymic selection leave the thymus and form the peripheral T-cell repertoire. However, clonal deletion in the thymus is not foolproof, nor should it be since a repertoire completely devoid of reactivity to self might well be devoid or reactivity to anything. Therefore, following thymic selection, additional mechanisms are required in order to maintain tolerance toward self-structures in the periphery. Failure of immunologic self-tolerance leads to the development of autoimmune diseases, as is seen in RA, which distinguishes this disease fundamentally from other inflammatory and degenerative joint diseases such as reactive arthritis or osteoarthritis.[1]

T cells that leave the thymus are then seeded to the peripheral lymphoid tissue and to the recirculating pool of lymphocytes where they need to be activated in order to exert their functional role as effector T cells.

T-Cell Activation

Central to the antigen activation of a T cell is the T-cell receptor (TCR). The TCR exists in two heterodimeric forms either consisting of alpha and beta ($\alpha\beta$ TCR) or gamma and delta ($\gamma\delta$ TCR) proteins.[2–3] The antigens recognized by the $\gamma\delta$ TCR are still being defined, whereas it has been concluded that the $\alpha\beta$ TCR binds to protein fragments presented by class I or class II MHC–encoded molecules. It appears that the $\alpha\beta$ TCR binds to both the peptide as well as polymorphic residues of MHC molecules.[4] Antigen recognition by T cells is therefore called MHC restricted. Whereas MHC class I molecules are expressed virtually on all nucleated cells, MHC class II molecule expression is restricted to so-called professional antigen-presenting cells (APC) such as B cells, dendritic cells (DCs), and monocytes/macrophages, and to activated T cells in humans (Figure 8A-1). Thus, B-cell depletion such as with antibodies against CD20 may, in part, act via elimination of antigen-presenting B cells.

The CD3 complex, which consists of four invariant transmembrane polypeptides ($\gamma,\delta,\epsilon,\epsilon$) mediates signaling and is also necessary for the surface expression of the TCR. The TCR/CD3 complex is associated with a largely intracytoplasmatic homodimer of ζ-chains that are critical for intracellular T-cell signaling.[5] The antigen recognition of cell-bound antigens by the $\alpha\beta$ TCR is facilitated by CD4 and CD8 coreceptors. They stabilize the MHC/peptide/TCR complex during T-cell activation, and thus increase the sensitivity of a T cell for activation. TCR interactions with MHC class I molecules direct $CD4^+CD8^+$ thymocytes into the $CD8^+$ lineage, whereas interactions with MHC class II molecules results in maturation into $CD4^+$ cells.[6] $CD4^+$ T cells primarily function as regulators of other immune cells either through cytokine secretion or by direct cell–cell contact and are called T *helper* (Th) cells. $CD8^+$ *(cytotoxic)* T cells are

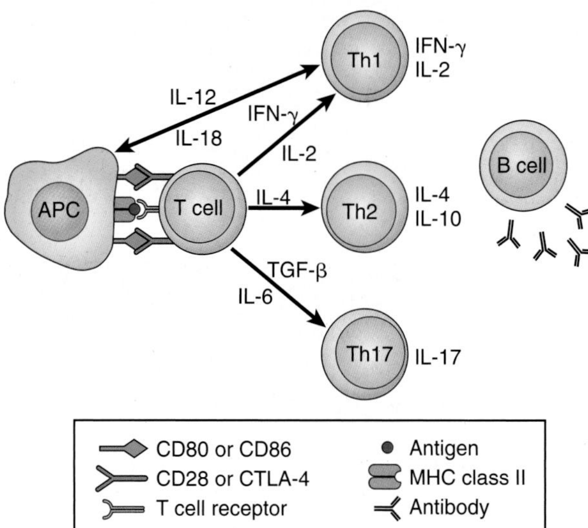

Figure 8A-1. T-cell activation in RA. Antigen-presenting cells (APC) present (auto)antigen(s) to naive T cells in the context of MHC class II molecules. T cells differentiate to Th1, Th2, or Th17 T cells, and provide help for B cells for the production of (auto)antibodies.

effector cells that kill infected target cells. In recent years, CD4$^+$ T cells have been identified that are able to inhibit immune reactions and even suppress established immunity. These cells have been called regulatory or suppressor T cells.

A key role for T cells in RA can be suspected for a number of reasons. One of the strongest arguments for T cells stems from the fact that susceptibility to RA is significantly greater in individuals with the MHC class II DR4 haplotype, owing to the QKRAA or QRRAA motifs in the hypervariable region, which were named "shared epitope." These MHC molecules may participate in disease pathogenesis by selectively binding arthritogenic peptides for presentation to autoreactive CD4$^+$ T cells. The nature of the arthritogenic Ag is not known, but recent work has identified post-translationally modified proteins containing citrulline (deiminated arginine) as specific targets of the IgG Ab response in RA patients.[7] Analysis of peptide affinity for a number of HLA alleles showed that only MHC class II molecules with the shared epitope had an increased affinity for the citrulline-containing peptide. This could result in a higher density of peptide–MHC complexes on APCs, which may exceed the biochemical margin of safety necessary for T-cell activation.[8]

Synovial T Cells

The synovium of joints affected by RA contains large numbers of activated T cells.[9] Synovial T cells express CD69, an early activation marker that correlates with disease activity, and produce CD40 ligand, a member of the tumor necrosis factor receptor (TNFR) superfamily responsible for the promotion of B-cell proliferation, immunoglobulin (Ig) production, activation of myelomonocytic cells, and DC differentiation.[10] Synovial CD4$^+$ T cells from patients express CD45RO, which characterizes them as memory T cells, while the number of naive T cells in the synovia is comparably low.[11] When transplanted into immunocompromised SCID mice, synovial T cells can transfer the disease.[12] In addition, treatment with anti-CD2 antibody depleted synovial-tissue–resident T cells, and resulted in a marked decline in the production of various proinflammatory cytokines.[13]

T cells involved in RA pathogenesis are probably polyclonal.[14] Depletion of T cells by thoracic duct drainage[15] or their modulation by immunosuppressive drugs, such as cyclosporine, has resulted in improvement, implying an important role for T cells in the inflammatory process[16] that is further supported by the observation that activated T cells may regulate osteoclast activation and thus joint destruction.[17]

Circulating antibodies to autoantigens other than IgG, including type II collagen, proteoglycans, cartilage link proteins, nuclear antigens, heat shock proteins, and heavy chain–binding proteins, can be detected in RA patients,[18] and, in some cases, T-cell reactivity was demonstrated by *in vitro* proliferation assays. However, despite extensive research, the initiating autoantigen(s) in the disease process have not yet been identified. Nevertheless, the ongoing search for antigens that might induce or perpetuate the disease has led to the identification of several novel autoantigens. Many of the reactivities to such autoantigens do not show striking specificity for RA, whether at the B-cell or the T-cell level. Remarkable exceptions are antibodies to IgG (i.e., rheumatoid factor [RF]) and citrullinated target structures on the B-cell level[19] and reactivity to the heterogeneous ribonucleoprotein A2 (RA33) on the T-cell level.[20] On the other hand, these reactivities may arise as a consequence of pathologic alterations in the joint, but they may also be related to infections. In the latter case, aside from the classical T-cell receptor (TCR) recognition of peptides presented in the context of MHC molecules, CD-1–restricted T cells, which recognize (self-)glycolipids in the context of the nonpolymorphic antigen-presenting molecule CD1, may also be involved.[21] In addition, changes in the characteristics of autoantigens due to their post-translational modification and/or aberrant processing, may further obscure the repertoire of the initially causative autoimmune response. Finally, initial autoreactive T cells may be swamped by the recruitment and expansion of nonspecific T cells.

Helper T-Cell Subsets: Th0, Th1, and Th2

CD4$^+$ helper T cells have been divided into distinct subsets based on the types of cytokines that they produce (Figure 8A-1). Th1 cells are characterized by the production of interferon (IFN)-γ and interleukin (IL)-2 but not IL-4, whereas Th2 cells produce IL-4 and IL-10. Some cytokines, such as IL-3, GM-CSF, and TNF-α, are produced by both subsets. Naive CD4$^+$ T cells are neither the Th1 nor Th2 type. When first stimulated with antigen and antigen-presenting cells (APC), CD4$^+$ T cells secrete low amounts of IL-2, IL-4, and IFN-γ. This state of differentiation is called Th0. Th0 cells polarize toward Th1 or Th2 cells within 48 hours following stimulation, although the Th1 or Th2 cytokine pattern becomes evident only upon further restimulation.[22] Several factors influence the differentiation of Th0 cells along the Th1 or Th2 pathway, including the cytokine milieu in which T-cell activation takes place, concentration of antigen, costimulatory molecules, type of APC, route of antigen entry, and presence of certain hormones.[23] Crucial for the differentiation of Th1 cells is the production of IL-12 by activated macrophages or DCs. In addition, IL-18 synergizes with IL-12 in the induction of IFN-γ–producing Th1 cells. Although IL-18 cannot induce the differentiation of Th1 cells on its own, it can potentiate and stabilize the development of Th1 cells induced by IL-12.[24] Th2 differentiation is mainly induced by IL-4 and several cell types have been reported as a source for IL-4, including mast cells, basophils, NK T cells, eosinophils, and Th2 cells themselves in an autocrine fashion. IL-6 and IL-7 have been shown to trigger the secretion of IL-4 by naive T cells, thus paralleling the effect of IL-12 on the Th1 pathway.[25]

Th1 cells trigger delayed-type hypersensitivity (DTH) reactions and direct immunoglobulin switch toward IgG2a. Th2 cells, on the other hand, trigger type I hypersensitivity reactions, and direct immunoglobulin class switching toward IgG1 and IgE.[23] Th1 cells develop preferentially during bacterial infections with intracellular pathogens. Th1 secreted cytokines activate monocytes/macrophages to produce proinflammatory cytokines, reactive oxygen intermediates, and nitric oxide. They stimulate their phagocytic function and enhance their antigen-presenting capacity by an increase in MHC class II molecule expression.

Th2 cells produce the anti-inflammatory cytokines IL-4 and IL-5, and develop during infections with gastrointestinal nematodes and helminths. Th2 T cells are thereby involved in allergic immune responses.

There is a consensus among investigators that Th1 cells cause chronic inflammatory autoimmune diseases such as multiple sclerosis, diabetes, and RA, whereas Th2 cells are protective in this aspect. In the collagen-induced arthritis model (CIA), anticollagen type II antibodies are mostly of the Th1-dependent IgG2a subclass, and disease development is markedly reduced in IL-12 knockout (KO) animals.[26,27] T-cell clones from human rheumatoid synovial tissue are predominantly IFN-γ–producing Th1 cells, and IFN-γ, in contrast to IL-4, can be detected in the majority of synovial biopsies.[28,29] On the other hand, CIA develops more rapidly and with higher severity in IFN-γ receptor KO mice as compared to their normal littermates, suggesting a protective role for IFN-γ at least during later stages of the disease.[30,31] In addition, the assessment of peripheral blood cytokine levels in RA patients has generated variable results, such as elevated IFN-γ or IL-4 levels in individual patients.[32] One explanation might be that the immune response converts from a Th1 to a Th2 cytokine pattern at different time points in the course of the disease, as observed in the CIA model of RA.[33] Differences in synovial cytokine patterns between early and established arthritis have also been observed in human RA.[34]

Signal1/Signal2

Activation of T cells requires at least two distinct signals. The first is the antigen-specific interaction between the TCR and nominal antigen presented in the context of the MHC on the surface of an APC (Figure 8A-1). The second signal can be provided by a variety of membrane-bound molecules that can positively affect a T cell and enhance activation, division, survival, and cytokine secretion. These costimulatory molecules largely fall into three main groups, namely, immunoglobulin superfamily members, TNF receptor (TNFR) superfamily members, and cytokine receptors. CD28, the inducible costimulatory molecule (ICOS), and CD2 typify costimulatory molecules of the immunoglobulin superfamily, and recent reviews have detailed their importance in many immune responses driven by T cells (e.g., Appleman and Boussiotis[35]). Cytokine receptors that can control T-cell growth or survival in some situations are also numerous, and include IL-2 receptor (IL-2R), IL-7R, IL-15R, IL-1R, and IL-6R. Lastly, signals through a number of TNFR family members have also been shown to augment T-cell responses in various settings, and these include CD40, OX40 (CD134), 4-1BB (CD137), CD27, CD30, and herpes virus entry mediator (HVEM).[36,37]

One of the most prominent T-cell costimulatory receptors is CD28. CD28 is expressed on most T cells, but, in humans, approximately 50% of CD8 T cells do not express CD28. CD28 has two well-characterized ligands, B7-1 (CD80) and B7-2 (CD86), that are expressed on potent APCs, including B cells, activated macrophages, and DCs. Interruption of the CD28–B7 interaction can block costimulatory function and prevent T-cell activation *in vitro* and *in vivo*, highlighting the importance of this interaction. Moreover, mice deficient in CD28 or B7-1 and B7-2 have markedly impaired immune responses.[38,39] CD80 and CD86 are also expressed on activated T cells and are present on T cells obtained from RA joints, suggesting a self-sustained mechanism for T-cell activation. Moreover, costimulatory molecules may be present at elevated levels in rheumatoid tissue, inducing T-cell activation even in the absence of antigen.[40]

Disruption of this dual-signal process results in T cells entering a dormant or anergic state.[41] Anergic cells do not proliferate or, if they do, they are immunologically unresponsive to subsequent antigen exposure. Conversely, costimulation triggers IL-2 production and enables proliferation and subsequent effector activity on the part of the T cells.

Cytotoxic T-lymphocyte–associated antigen 4 (CTLA-4, CD152), which is upregulated on T cells following their activation, also interacts with CD80 and CD86, providing an important control for T-cell function.[42] Its production is stimulated by CD28 activation and the subsequent release of IL-2, and it appears hours to days after the T cell has become activated. CTLA-4 does not appear to be expressed by resting T cells, but is upregulated during cell-cycle progression.[43] Due to a variety of intracellular events, only a minor proportion of total CTLA-4 is expressed at the cell surface under steady-state conditions. CTLA-4 is assumed to play a downregulatory role in T-cell activity, in that it reduces the proliferation of T cells and the production of cytokines. In addition to these effects on T-cell activity, about one-third of the amino-acid sequence of CTLA-4 is identical to that of CD28, and it binds to CD80 and CD86 on APCs at the same sites to which CD28 binds, but with much higher affinity (by a factor of about 2500 for CD80 and 570 for CD86).[42] Therefore, it also blocks CD28 binding to CD80 and CD86. The biological role for these differences in affinity is to limit T-cell responses and downregulate them. The need for this is clearly demonstrated in CTLA-4 KO mice.[44,45] These mice experience fatal T-cell hyper-responsiveness, apparently directed toward multiple self-antigens, despite normal thymic selection. These data are compatible with the hypothesis that CTLA-4 either restricts the activation of self-reactive T cells or effectively attenuates responses postactivation. A construct of CTLA-4 with an IgG-Fc, abatacept (CTLA-4Ig), presumably inhibiting T-cell costimulation, is effective in and approved for the treatment of RA.[46] However, this compound may also interfere with osteoclast activation.[47]

Interestingly, CTLA-4 is constitutively expressed on $CD25^+$ Treg.[48] There are controversial reports, however, concerning the role of CTLA-4 for Treg function; although some investigators have shown a role for CTLA-4 in Treg function,[49,50] others have not.[51,52] Taken together, three distinct functions of CTLA-4 might be relevant under different circumstances.[53] First, CTLA-4 sets the threshold for T-cell activation, and thus probably contributes to maintenance of peripheral tolerance. Second, CTLA-4 has additional functions in already activated T cells: (1) to restrain

T-cell proliferation, and (2) to initiate the survival of T cells. Finally, CTLA-4 might be involved in the control of T-cell survival and apoptosis during chronic inflammation, which could contribute to the success of the treatment of RA patients with CTLA-4Ig.[54]

Regulatory T Cells

A significant development in the field of tolerance has been the re-emergence of the concept that T-cell reactivity might be controlled indirectly by a distinct subset of T cells with a regulatory function. A small proportion of peripheral $CD4^+$ T cells that express the CD25 molecules constitute a population of potent suppressors of T-cell responses both *in vitro* and *in vivo*. These regulatory T cells (Treg) are crucial components of a complex machinery responsible for sustaining peripheral tolerance toward self-structures.[55] Depletion of $CD4^+/CD25^+$ T cells in mice results in the onset of systemic autoimmune disease, and the cotransfer of these cells with $CD4^+/CD25^-$ cells into animals prevents the development of experimentally induced autoimmune diseases such as colitis, gastritis, insulin-dependent autoimmune diabetes, and thyroiditis in susceptible strains.[49,56–58]

In the collagen-induced arthritis (CIA) model of RA in mice, depletion of $CD25^+$ Treg was found to result in an exacerbation of arthritis and an increase in collagen-II–specific antibody titers.[59] On the other hand, the adoptive transfer of $CD25^+$ Treg into animals with CIA markedly slowed disease progression.[60] Increased proportions of functionally active $CD4^+/CD25^+$ Treg have been observed in inflamed joints of patients with RA.[61] A different study demonstrated that peripheral blood $CD25^+$ Treg from RA patients, although capable of suppressing the proliferation of responder T cells, displayed a diminished capacity to suppress proinflammatory cytokine production, which was restored by anti-TNF-α treatment.[62] A direct and indirect effect of TNF-α on Treg function has further been demonstrated *in vitro* and *in vivo*. Whereas high-dose TNF-α stimulation inhibited Treg function and Foxp-3 expression via upregulation of TNFRII, anti–TNF-α therapy restored functional defects of Treg in RA patients.[63] Together, these data suggest that Treg play a role in the pathogenesis of RA and might provide a rationale for targeting T cells by modulating Treg activity in the treatment of RA.

Th17 T Cells

A subset of IL-17–producing $CD4^+$ T helper cells has been described that constitutes a new T-cell polarization state, and has been termed the Th17 lineage (Figure 8A-1). Th17 T cells are distinct from those of the Th1 lineage, and represent the third arm of the CD4 T-cell effector repertoire: Th1, Th2, and Th17.[64] IL-17 induces the release of proinflammatory mediators in a wide range of cell types. It stimulates the production of IL-6 and prostaglandin E2 locally, and synergized with other inflammatory cytokines such as IL-1α, TNF-β, IFN-γ, and CD40 ligand (reviewed in Afzali, et al.[65]). An aberrant Th17 response has been implicated in the pathogenesis of RA since IL-17 KO animals fail to develop collagen-induced arthritis,[66] and blocking IL-17 with monoclonal antibodies has been shown to ameliorate the disease in animal models of RA.[67,68] In addition, the intra-articular injection of IL-17 in mouse joints induces similar changes to RA,[69] and local overexpression of IL-17 exacerbates arthritis significantly.[70] In human RA, however, data regarding the role of Th17 T cells to date are less clear, as for example, IL17 can be detected in the synovial tissue and synovial fluid but only at low levels.[71,72] IL-17 inhibitors are in development, and combination treatment with other biologic agents should be of interest in RA as well as in other autoimmune diseases.

In summary, current concepts confirm the essential role of T cells in the induction, maintenance, and relapse of RA. Although anti-inflammatory cytokine therapies are effective in RA treatment, additional T-cell targeted approaches might be critical in particular in the treatment of patients that fail current therapies. The control of pathogenic autoreactive T cells and the restoration of functional defects in T cells with regulatory function therefore comprise a challenging future therapeutic strategy.

References

1. Medzhitov R, Janeway CA Jr. Innate immunity: The virtues of a nonclonal system of recognition. *Cell* 1997;91(3):295–298.
2. Allison JP, Lanier LL. Structure, function, and serology of the T-cell antigen receptor complex. *Annu Rev Immunol* 1987;5: 503–540.
3. Brenner MB, Strominger JL, Krangel MS. The gamma delta T cell receptor. *Adv Immunol* 1988;43:133–192.
4. Bjorkman PJ, Saper MA, Samraoui B, et al. Structure of the human class I histocompatibility antigen, HLA-A2. *Nature* 1987;329(6139): 506–512.
5. Chan AC, Iwashima M, Turck CW, Weiss A. ZAP-70: A 70-kd protein-tyrosine kinase that associates with the TCR zeta chain. *Cell* 1992;71(4):649–662.
6. Kisielow P, Bluthmann H, Staerz UD, et al. Tolerance in T-cell-receptor transgenic mice involves deletion of nonmature CD4+8+ thymocytes. *Nature* 1988;333(6175):742–746.
7. Zendman AJ, Vossenaar ER, van Venrooij WJ. Autoantibodies to citrullinated (poly)peptides: A key diagnostic and prognostic marker for rheumatoid arthritis. *Autoimmunity* 2004;37(4): 295–299.
8. Hill JA, Southwood S, Sette A, et al. Cutting edge: The conversion of arginine to citrulline allows for a high-affinity peptide interaction with the rheumatoid arthritis-associated HLA-DRB1*0401 MHC class II molecule. *J Immunol* 2003;171(2): 538–541.
9. Weyand CM, Goronzy JJ. T-cell responses in rheumatoid arthritis: Systemic abnormalities-local disease. *Curr Opin Rheumatol* 1999; 11(3):210–217.
10. MacDonald KP, Nishioka Y, Lipsky PE, Thomas R. Functional CD40 ligand is expressed by T cells in rheumatoid arthritis. *J Clin Invest* 1997;100(9):2404–2414.
11. Weyand CM. New insights into the pathogenesis of rheumatoid arthritis. *Rheumatology (Oxford)* 2000;39(Suppl 1):3–8.
12. Mima T, Saeki Y, Ohshima S, et al. Transfer of rheumatoid arthritis into severe combined immunodeficient mice. The pathogenetic implications of T cell populations oligoclonally expanding in the rheumatoid joints. *J Clin Invest* 1995;96(4):1746–1758.
13. Klimiuk PA, Yang H, Goronzy JJ, Weyand CM. Production of cytokines and metalloproteinases in rheumatoid synovitis is T cell dependent. *Clin Immunol* 1999;90(1):65–78.

14. Friou GJ. Setting the scene: A historical and personal view of immunologic diseases, autoimmunity and ANA. *Clin Exp Rheumatol* 1994;12(Suppl 11):S23–S25.
15. Vaughan JH, Fox RI, Abresch RJ, et al. Thoracic duct drainage in rheumatoid arthritis. *Clin Exp Immunol* 1984;58(3):645–653.
16. Sany J. Immunological treatment of rheumatoid arthritis. *Clin Exp Rheumatol* 1990;8(Suppl 5):81–88.
17. Kong YY, Feige U, Sarosi I, et al. Activated T cells regulate bone loss and joint destruction in adjuvant arthritis through osteoprotegerin ligand. *Nature* 1999;402(6759):304–309.
18. Smolen JS, Steiner G. Are autoantibodies active players or epiphenomena? *Curr Opin Rheumatol* 1998;10(3):201–206.
19. Goldbach-Mansky R, Lee J, McCoy A, et al. Rheumatoid arthritis associated autoantibodies in patients with synovitis of recent onset. *Arthritis Res* 2000;2(3):236–243.
20. Fritsch R, Eselbock D, Skriner K, et al. Characterization of autoreactive T cells to the autoantigens heterogeneous nuclear ribonucleoprotein A2 (RA33) and filaggrin in patients with rheumatoid arthritis. *J Immunol* 2002;169(2):1068–1076.
21. De Libero G, Moran AP, Gober HJ, et al. Bacterial infections promote T cell recognition of self-glycolipids. *Immunity* 2005;22(6):763–772.
22. Nakamura T, Kamogawa Y, Bottomly K, Flavell RA. Polarization of IL-4– and IFN-gamma–producing CD4+ T cells following activation of naive CD4+ T cells. *J Immunol* 1997;158(3):1085–1094.
23. Abbas AK, Murphy KM, Sher A. Functional diversity of helper T lymphocytes. *Nature* 1996;383(6603):787–793.
24. Robinson D, Shibuya K, Mui A, et al. IGIF does not drive Th1 development but synergizes with IL-12 for interferon-gamma production and activates IRAK and NFκB. *Immunity* 1997;7(4):571–581.
25. Lafaille JJ. The role of helper T cell subsets in autoimmune diseases. *Cytokine Growth Factor Rev* 1998;9(2):139–151.
26. McIntyre KW, Shuster DJ, Gillooly KM, et al. Reduced incidence and severity of collagen-induced arthritis in interleukin-12–deficient mice. *Eur J Immunol* 1996;26(12):2933–2938.
27. Watson WC, Townes AS. Genetic susceptibility to murine collagen II autoimmune arthritis. Proposed relationship to the IgG2 autoantibody subclass response, complement C5, major histocompatibility complex (MHC) and non-MHC loci. *J Exp Med* 1985;162(6):1878–1891.
28. Miltenburg AM, van Laar JM, de Kuiper R, et al. T cells cloned from human rheumatoid synovial membrane functionally represent the Th1 subset. *Scand J Immunol* 1992;35(5):603–610.
29. Canete JD, Martinez SE, Farres J, et al. Differential Th1/Th2 cytokine patterns in chronic arthritis: Interferon gamma is highly expressed in synovium of rheumatoid arthritis compared with seronegative spondyloarthropathies. *Ann Rheum Dis* 2000;59(4):263–268.
30. Manoury-Schwartz B, Chiocchia G, Bessis N, et al. High susceptibility to collagen-induced arthritis in mice lacking IFN-gamma receptors. *J Immunol* 1997;158(11):5501–5506.
31. Vermeire K, Heremans H, Vandeputte M, et al. Accelerated collagen-induced arthritis in IFN-gamma receptor-deficient mice. *J Immunol* 1997;158(11):5507–5513.
32. Schulze-Koops H, Lipsky PE, Kavanaugh AF, Davis LS. Elevated Th1- or Th0-like cytokine mRNA in peripheral circulation of patients with rheumatoid arthritis. Modulation by treatment with anti-ICAM-1 correlates with clinical benefit. *J Immunol* 1995;155(10):5029–5037.
33. Doncarli A, Stasiuk LM, Fournier C, Abehsira-Amar O. Conversion in vivo from an early dominant Th0/Th1 response to a Th2 phenotype during the development of collagen-induced arthritis. *Eur J Immunol* 1997;27(6):1451–1458.
34. Raza K, Falciani F, Curnow SJ, et al. Early rheumatoid arthritis is characterized by a distinct and transient synovial fluid cytokine profile of T cell and stromal cell origin. *Arthritis Res Ther* 2005;7(4):R784–R795.
35. Appleman LJ, Boussiotis VA. T cell anergy and costimulation. *Immunol Rev* 2003;192:161–180.
36. Liu Y, Janeway CA Jr. Cells that present both specific ligand and costimulatory activity are the most efficient inducers of clonal expansion of normal CD4 T cells. *Proc Natl Acad Sci U S A* 1992;89(9):3845–3849.
37. Croft M. Costimulation of T cells by OX40, 4-1BB, and CD27. *Cytokine Growth Factor Rev* 2003;14(3–4):265–273.
38. Shahinian A, Pfeffer K, Lee KP, et al. Differential T cell costimulatory requirements in CD28-deficient mice. *Science* 1993;261(5121):609–612.
39. Borriello F, Sethna MP, Boyd SD, et al. B7-1 and B7-2 have overlapping, critical roles in immunoglobulin class switching and germinal center formation. *Immunity* 1997;6(3):303–313.
40. Verwilghen J, Lovis R, De Boer M, et al. Expression of functional B7 and CTLA4 on rheumatoid synovial T cells. *J Immunol* 1994;153(3):1378–1385.
41. Schwartz RH. T cell anergy. *Annu Rev Immunol* 2003;21:305–334.
42. Karandikar NJ, Vanderlugt CL, Walunas TL, et al. CTLA-4: A negative regulator of autoimmune disease. *J Exp Med* 1996;184(2):783–788.
43. Alegre ML, Noel PJ, Eisfelder BJ, et al. Regulation of surface and intracellular expression of CTLA4 on mouse T cells. *J Immunol* 1996;157(11):4762–4770.
44. Tivol EA, Borriello F, Schweitzer AN, et al. Loss of CTLA-4 leads to massive lymphoproliferation and fatal multiorgan tissue destruction, revealing a critical negative regulatory role of CTLA-4. *Immunity* 1995;3(5):541–547.
45. Waterhouse P, Penninger JM, Timms E, et al. Lymphoproliferative disorders with early lethality in mice deficient in Ctla-4. *Science* 1995;270(5238):985–988.
46. Genovese MC, Becker JC, Schiff M, et al. Abatacept for rheumatoid arthritis refractory to tumor necrosis factor alpha inhibition. *N Engl J Med* 2005;353(11):1114–1123.
47. Axmann R, Herman S, Zaiss M, et al. CTLA-4 directly inhibits osteoclast formation. *Ann Rheum Dis* 2008 (published online January 12).
48. Sakaguchi S. Regulatory T cells: Key controllers of immunologic self-tolerance. *Cell* 2000;101(5):455–458.
49. Read S, Malmstrom V, Powrie F. Cytotoxic T lymphocyte-associated antigen 4 plays an essential role in the function of CD25(+)CD4(+) regulatory cells that control intestinal inflammation. *J Exp Med* 2000;192(2):295–302.
50. Takahashi T, Tagami T, Yamazaki S, et al. Immunologic self-tolerance maintained by CD25(+)CD4(+) regulatory T cells constitutively expressing cytotoxic T lymphocyte-associated antigen 4. *J Exp Med* 2000;192(2):303–310.
51. Levings MK, Sangregorio R, Roncarolo MG. Human cd25(+)cd4(+) T regulatory cells suppress naive and memory T cell proliferation and can be expanded in vitro without loss of function. *J Exp Med* 2001;193(11):1295–1302.
52. Shevach EM. CD4+ CD25+ suppressor T cells: more questions than answers. *Nat Rev Immunol* 2002;2(6):389–400.
53. Brunner-Weinzierl MC, Hoff H, Burmester GR. Multiple functions for CD28 and cytotoxic T lymphocyte antigen-4 during different phases of T cell responses: Implications for arthritis and autoimmune diseases. *Arthritis Res Ther* 2004;6(2):45–54.
54. Kremer JM, Westhovens R, Leon M, et al. Treatment of rheumatoid arthritis by selective inhibition of T-cell activation with fusion protein CTLA4Ig. *N Engl J Med* 2003;349(20):1907–1915.
55. Sakaguchi S. Naturally arising CD4+ regulatory T cells for immunologic self-tolerance and negative control of immune responses. *Annu Rev Immunol* 2004;22:531–562.
56. Powrie F, Mauze S, Coffman RL. CD4+ T-cells in the regulation of inflammatory responses in the intestine. *Res Immunol* 1997;148(8–9):576–581.
57. Sakaguchi S, Fukuma K, Kuribayashi K, Masuda T. Organ-specific autoimmune diseases induced in mice by elimination of T cell

subset. I. Evidence for the active participation of T cells in natural self-tolerance: Deficit of a T cell subset as a possible cause of autoimmune disease. *J Exp Med* 1985;161(1):72–87.

58. Salomon B, Lenschow DJ, Rhee L, et al. B7/CD28 costimulation is essential for the homeostasis of the CD4+CD25+ immunoregulatory T cells that control autoimmune diabetes. *Immunity* 2000;12(4): 431–440.
59. Morgan ME, Sutmuller RP, Witteveen HJ, et al. CD25+ cell depletion hastens the onset of severe disease in collagen-induced arthritis. *Arthritis Rheum* 2003;48(5):1452–1460.
60. Morgan ME, Flierman R, van Duivenvoorde LM, et al. Effective treatment of collagen-induced arthritis by adoptive transfer of CD25+ regulatory T cells. *Arthritis Rheum* 2005;52(7):2212–2221.
61. Cao D, Malmstrom V, Baecher-Allan C, et al. Isolation and functional characterization of regulatory CD25brightCD4+ T cells from the target organ of patients with rheumatoid arthritis. *Eur J Immunol* 2003;33(1):215–223.
62. Ehrenstein MR, Evans JG, Singh A, et al. Compromised function of regulatory T cells in rheumatoid arthritis and reversal by anti-TNFα therapy. *J Exp Med* 2004;200(3):277–285.
63. Valencia X, Stephens G, Goldbach-Mansky R, et al. TNF downmodulates the function of human CD4+CD25hi T-regulatory cells. *Blood* 2006;108(1):253–261.
64. Harrington LE, Hatton RD, Mangan PR, et al. Interleukin 17-producing CD4+ effector T cells develop via a lineage distinct from the T helper type 1 and 2 lineages. *Nat Immunol* 2005;6(11):1123–1132.
65. Afzali B, Lombardi G, Lechler RI, Lord GM. The role of T helper 17 (Th17) and regulatory T cells (Treg) in human organ transplantation and autoimmune disease. *Clin Exp Immunol* 2007;148(1):32–46.
66. Nakae S, Nambu A, Sudo K, Iwakura Y. Suppression of immune induction of collagen-induced arthritis in IL-17–deficient mice. *J Immunol* 2003;171(11):6173–6177.
67. Bush KA, Farmer KM, Walker JS, Kirkham BW. Reduction of joint inflammation and bone erosion in rat adjuvant arthritis by treatment with interleukin-17 receptor IgG1 Fc fusion protein. *Arthritis Rheum* 2002;46(3):802–805.
68. Lubberts E, Koenders MI, Oppers-Walgreen B, et al. Treatment with a neutralizing anti-murine interleukin-17 antibody after the onset of collagen-induced arthritis reduces joint inflammation, cartilage destruction, and bone erosion. *Arthritis Rheum* 2004; 50(2):650–659.
69. Lubberts E, Joosten LA, van de Loo FA, et al. Reduction of interleukin-17–induced inhibition of chondrocyte proteoglycan synthesis in intact murine articular cartilage by interleukin-4. *Arthritis Rheum* 2000;43(6):1300–1306.
70. Lubberts E, Joosten LA, van de Loo FA, et al. Overexpression of IL-17 in the knee joint of collagen type II immunized mice promotes collagen arthritis and aggravates joint destruction. *Inflamm Res* 2002;51(2):102–104.
71. Chabaud M, Durand JM, Buchs N, et al. Human interleukin-17: A T cell–derived proinflammatory cytokine produced by the rheumatoid synovium. *Arthritis Rheum* 1999;42(5):963–970.
72. Kotake S, Udagawa N, Takahashi N, et al. IL-17 in synovial fluids from patients with rheumatoid arthritis is a potent stimulator of osteoclastogenesis. *J Clin Invest* 1999;103(9):1345–1352.

The Role of B Cells in Rheumatoid Arthritis

Thomas Dörner and Peter E. Lipsky

Historically, B cells have not been thought of as playing a central role in the immunopathogenesis of inflammatory joint diseases, in particular, rheumatoid arthritis (RA). Despite this, it has been accepted that autoantibodies play an important amplifying role in joint inflammation, and serve also as diagnostic, classification, and prognostic markers. The traditional model of RA pathogenesis describes a central role for CD4$^+$ T cells and macrophages.[1] When therapeutic trials of anti-CD4 therapy in RA failed to show clinical benefit, questions were raised about the central role of CD4$^+$ T cells.[2] However, more recent success achieved by blocking T-cell costimulation with CTLA4Ig (abatacept) has again implied a role for CD4$^+$ T cells in RA pathogenesis. Similarly, the potent effect of cytokine blockade, including neutralization of TNF, IL-1, and IL-6, has confirmed the important role of macrophages and elements of the innate immune system in propagating rheumatoid inflammation and tissue damage. Finally, the success of B-cell–depleting therapy in ameliorating rheumatoid inflammation has documented a role for B cells in the pathogenesis of RA. It is clear from these clinical results that CD4$^+$ T cells, B cells, and the innate immune system all play important roles in the propagation of RA. However, their specific contributions and their unique impacts on different stages of the disease have not been clearly delineated. Particularly, the unique contribution of B cells and specific B-cell subsets in rheumatoid inflammation has not been dissected in detail.[3]

B-Cell Development in Health

B cells follow a tightly regulated life cycle (Figure 8B-1). Knowledge of the stages of B-cell development is important not only to understand potential derangements in autoimmune diseases, such as RA, but also to delineate possible points for therapeutic intervention. In the bone marrow, B cells develop from stem cells through a series of precursor stages during which they rearrange their immunoglobulin genes to generate a wide range of unique antigen binding specificities. Immature CD20$^+$ transitional B cells expressing surface IgM/IgD emigrate from the bone marrow into the peripheral blood, and then mature in the spleen into naive B cells. After encountering their cognate antigen and receiving T-cell help in follicles in secondary lymphoid organs, mature naive B cells undergo germinal center (GC) reactions, during which antigen-specific B cells clonally expand, somatically mutate their immunoglobulin genes to achieve avidity maturation, undergo Ig heavy chain class-switch recombination, and mature either into memory B cells or Ig-secreting plasma cells. GC reactions expand antigen-specific B cells, and cause them to differentiate into memory B cells with altered functional capabilities or Ig-secreting plasma cells. Because of somatic hypermutation and class-switch recombination, the avidity of the B-cell immunoglobulin receptor can be increased and the biologic function of secreted immunoglobulin altered. Important for the interaction with T cells and the generation of GC reactions are a series of ligand receptor interactions, including those mediated by CD154/CD40 and ICOS-L/ICOS. Defects in these interactions have been shown to lead to hyper-IgM syndrome, resulting in impaired plasma cell and memory B-cell generation and adult-onset common-variable hypogammaglobulinemia, respectively.[4,5]

Besides T-cell–dependent GC responses, some B cells can respond to specific antigens in a T-cell–independent manner (TI responses). TI responses largely induce production of IgM antibodies and fail to generate post-switch memory B cells. These responses are thought to be restricted to IgM^{high} marginal zone B cells residing in the spleen that recognize polysaccharide antigens in a TI response. Whether human TI responses are limited to one or another B-cell subset has been called into question recently.[6]

B cells are characteristically divided into two major lineages, B1 cells and B2 cells. It is still a matter of debate whether B1 and B2 cells are similar in mice and humans (Table 8B-1). B1 cells are considered to be self-renewing and long-lived, emerging early in development, and residing in the peritoneal and pleural cavities. In mice, B1a and B1b B cells can be differentiated, whereas it is unclear whether these also occur in humans. Most notably in mice, B1 cells produce polyreactive IgM antibodies. These natural antibodies are important for the immediate defense against encapsulated bacteria, but have also been

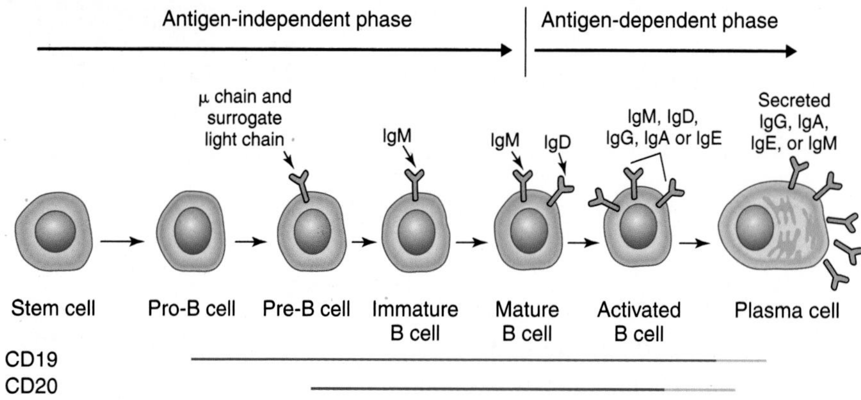

Figure 8B-1. B-cell development in humans. Early stages of B-cell development in the bone marrow are T-cell and antigen independent. Subsequently, in the periphery, the development of memory B cells and plasma cells is largely T-cell and antigen dependent. (Adapted from Sell S, Max EE. *Immunology, Immunopathology, and Immunity*, 6th ed. Washington, DC: ASM Press, 2001; Roitt I, Brostoff J, Male D, eds. *Immunology*, 6th ed. New York: Mosby 2001; and Tedder T, et al. The B cell surface molecule B1 is functionally linked with B cell activation and differentiation. *J Immunol* 1985;135(2):973-979.)

Table 8B-1. Subsets of Mature B Cells Comprising B1 and B2 Cells and Functions

B cell Subset	Function	V Gene Rearrangements	Origin	Residence
B1	Natural antibodies	Nontemplated insertions No mutations	Fetal liver Bone marrow	Peritoneal cavity and secrete Ig in the spleen
B2	Reactivity against three-dimensional structures (proteins, glycoproteins, DNA/RNA-protein structures)	Hypermutated, nontemplated insertions, diverse VH CDR3s	Fetal liver, adult bone marrow	Recirculating, spleen, blood, lymph nodes
Marginal zone (MZ) B cells	Antipolysaccharide response	Less common mutations	Adult bone marrow	Outside marginal sinus

described in increased numbers in autoimmune diseases, such as systemic lupus erythematosus (SLE)[7] and primary Sjögren's syndrome (pSS).[8] The natural autoantibodies produced by B1 cells are important in the clearance of apoptotic material, senescent red blood cells, and other cellular and subcellular debris. In mice, the subset of B1 cells has therefore been considered to be a bridge between innate with adaptive immunity.

On the other hand, B2 cells comprise the adaptive portion of humoral immune responses. B2 cells participate preferentially in GC reactions, during which they can hypermutate their IgV gene rearrangements, switch Ig classes, and differentiate into memory cells and long-lived plasma cells. However, B2 cells can also be activated during TI responses. B2 cells are generated in the bone marrow where there is a checkpoint for removal of autoreactive cells (central tolerance). The immature survivors with functional B-cell receptors leave the marrow and migrate to the spleen, where they are thought to be exposed to further selection if one extrapolates from studies in mice (peripheral tolerance). Although it has not been delineated for humans, in mice B cells at this point are routed into either a mature follicular B-cell or a marginal-zone B-cell (MZ-B) program.[9] Follicular B cells traffic throughout the secondary lymphoid organs, whereas MZ-B cells are specialized to reside in a compartment in the spleen that samples the bloodstream for pathogens. In some ways, B1 and MZ-B cells are functionally similar, being key parts of the immune system that is designed to activate and respond immediately to pathogens in the blood as well as the peritoneal and pleural cavities.[10] Both B1 and MZ B-cell responses occur independent of T-cell help, and they are thought to be excluded from undergoing GC reactions.

An important aspect is whether pathogenic autoantibodies are primarily the end products of the B1 cells or B2 cells or both lineages, which could have therapeutic consequences. Since most pathogenic autoreactive antibodies are encoded by mutated IgV gene rearrangements of the heavy- and light-chain genes,[11] they are likely generated from B2 cells, but such exclusivity has not been clearly documented yet.

Germinal Center Responses

Naive follicular B cells encounter antigens in the secondary lymphoid organs, and after they receiving T-cell help, undergo proliferation and differentiation either into plasmablasts, plasma cells, or memory B cells.[12] Newly generated plasma cells emerge after 2 to 3 days, providing immediate responses to a pathogen[13] that can be detected between days 6 and 8 in peripheral blood after secondary vaccination.[14] The initial immune response resulting in activation of antigen-specific B cells, local expansion, and the generation of short-lived plasma cells represents the extrafollicular immune response since it occurs outside the B-cell follicles. Subsequently, activated B cells migrate into the B-cell follicle where a well-organized structure or "immune unit," called GC is formed.[15] GCs consist of activated proliferating and postproliferative B cells, and follicular dendritic cells (FDCs), which are important for selection of the immune repertoire. Plasma cells derived from GC reactions appear to egress from the lymph nodes, spleen, and likely other secondary lymphoid organs, and navigate to survival niches in the bone marrow as well as other sites, such as MALT tissue. However, there is also the likelihood that a substantial number of these cells remain in tissues in which they are generated. Although the lifetime of these cells may vary considerably, there is clear evidence that plasma cells in these sites can persist for very long periods of time.[12]

Role of B Cells in Immune Responses

B cells are an essential component of normal immune responses and are responsible for the maintenance of humoral protective memory.[16–18] The nature of the serologic component of protective memory is illustrated by the persisting protective antibody titers against a variety of microorganisms. As an example, antibodies to smallpox can persist for up to 75 years without further vaccination, having a substantially longer half-life than either CD4 or CD8 memory T cells.[19] Interestingly, $CD4^+$ T cells are important in instructing memory B cells to differentiate into long-lived plasma cells, whereas these long-lived nonproliferating antibody-secreting cells survive independent of antigen and further direct interaction with antigen-specific T cells.[20] However, antigen-nonspecific interactions with T cells may contribute to the survival of human plasma cells in secondary lymphoid organs.[21]

Another important function of memory B cells is antigen presentation, which is facilitated by expression of high-avidity BCR and also MHC class II molecules on their surface. It has been shown that B cells, in particular memory B cells, are very efficient antigen-presenting cells.[3,16,22] This relates to the very efficient uptake of antigen owing to high avidity BCR.[22] Despite the efficiency of antigen uptake, memory B cells appear to be most effective at presenting antigen and stimulating memory T cells, whereas dendritic cells (DCs) are the preferred antigen-presenting cells for initiating responses of naive T cells.[23]

Antigen presentation mediated by MHC class II can be performed by cognate B cells after receiving help by autoreactive T cells that in turn have been activated by mature dendritic cells. Thus, antigen presentation by B cells, in particular by memory B cells, may be important in the amplification and maintenance of autoimmunity after it has been initiated.

B cells also produce proinflammatory cytokines, such as tumor necrosis factor (TNF) and interleukin (IL)-6, and immunoregulatory cytokines, such as IL-10. The cytokines produced by activated B cells may influence the function of antigen-presenting DCs.[16] Proinflammatory cytokines, such as TNF and IL-6, may activate macrophages, amplifying the proinflammatory signal and resulting in enhanced levels of IL-1, IL-6, and additional TNF. Although IL-6 itself is an important cytokine for B-cell growth, BAFF produced by synovial fibroblasts and regulated by TNF and IFNγ also can maintain RA synovial B cells.[24] Another important cytokine produced by B cells is IL-10, which is able to activate DCs to be more effective antigen-presenting cells, and with the help of T cells, to enhance the differentiation of B cells into plasma cells. The extent to which cytokines produced by B cells contribute to certain steps in immune activation in general as well as in particular for RA is unknown.

B cells also regulate FDC differentiation and the organization of the lymphatic architecture. For example, mice that lack B cells do not develop antigen-presenting M cells in the gut. B cells are also involved in the regulation of T-cell activation, anergy, differentiation, and the expansion of T cells. B cells play an important role in T-cell activation. *In vivo* in humans, this conclusion is supported by recent studies in patients with SLE that demonstrated a deactivation of T cells after selective B-cell depletion,[25,26] but it has not yet been shown for RA patients. However, data from experiments in which synovial tissue was transplanted into immunodeficient scid/NOD mice,[27] showing that B-cell depletion by rituximab, caused a substantial down-regulation of T-cell activation and reduction in IFNγ occurred. These data indicate that synovial B cells are necessary for T-cell activation.

B-Cell Functions and Involvement in Rheumatoid Arthritis

B cells are directly and indirectly involved in the regulation of certain parts of immune activation in RA (Figure 8B-2). They can ultimately differentiate into antibody-producing cells known to produce IgM-rheumatoid factor (IgM-RF) and IgG antibodies to citrullinated peptides (anti-CCP) in 60% to 80% of the patients. Higher RF and anti-CCP levels in synovial fluid suggest that these autoantibodies are produced in the synovial membrane. However, clear detection of autoantigen-specific cells in this inflamed site is still lacking. Ig production within the synovium also results in local formation of immune complexes and activation of the coagulation system with fibrin generation, each of which can contribute to local inflammation.

Antibodies against immunoglobulin G (IgG), IgM-RF, and antibodies against CCP are the autoantibodies most frequently found in patients with RA. IgM-RF has been shown to be a reliable marker for the disease and considered an objective diagnostic serologic marker for RA and associated with disease with a more severe erosive course.[16] The spectrum of autoantibodies in RA comprise anti-CCP antibodies with a high specificity for the diagnosis of RA, RF as well as anti-RA 33 IgG antibodies directed to the human nuclear (hn)RNP proteins A2, B1, and B2 (the "RA33 complex").[23] Enhanced production of autoantibodies[16]

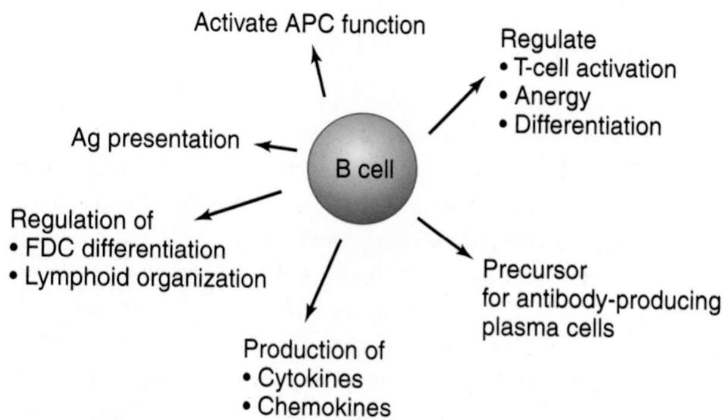

Figure 8B-2. The various functions of B cells. APC, antigen-presenting cell; FDC, follicular dendritic cell. (Adapted from Dörner T, Burmester GR. The role of B cells in RA: mechanisms and therapeutic targets. *Curr Opin Rheumatol* 2003;15:246–252; and Lipsky PE. Systemic lupus erythematosus: An autoimmune disease of B-cell hyperactivity. *Nat Immunol* 2001;2:764–766.)

has been associated with severe forms of RA, which underscores the role of activated B cells in those patients.

Although autoantibodies are usually taken as an indication of the breakdown of immune tolerance, there are interesting differences between the autoantibodies. RF is directed against IgG which is a ubiquitous antigen. By contrast, anti-CCP antibodies target postranslationally modified peptides that appear after inflammation has upregulated the enzymes PADI4 and PADI2 permitting the generation of neoantigens.[28] The mechanisms of breaking immune tolerance are very complex, since IgM-RF usually occurs nonspecifically in very active inflammatory disease and therefore may have a quantitative threshold. Anti-CCP antibodies are almost exclusively induced in patients with RA—although citrullination occurs nonspecifically in many inflamed tissues,[29] and therefore may represent a qualitative biomarker of broken immune tolerance. Moreover, anti-CCP activity is directed against an artificial autoantigen being a cyclic ring of citrullinated amino acid residues but providing cross-reactivity to antigens expressed in inflamed tissues. With regard to these citrullinated antigens in inflamed sites, a central question is whether these are real "autoantigens" that are widely expressed and to which there is no natural tolerance or whether these are neoantigens to which the subject was previously ignorant. Resolution of this question could provide important insights into the nature of the abnormalities resulting in autoantibody production in RA.

In addition, it remains unclear whether IgM-RF and IgG anti-CCP antibodies are generated using different forms of T-cell help. Notably, RA patients also produce IgG-RF and IgA-RF, which require class switch, and likely are produced from progeny of B2 cells after costimulation by T cells. A substantial number of IgM-RF are encoded by V_H gene rearrangements in the germline configuration, which frequently can be found in lymphomas.[30] By contrast, RA-associated RFs usually have somatically mutated V_H gene rearrangements, and probably have developed using T-cell help. It is interesting to note that the production of anti-CCP antibodies has been linked to certain HLA-DR alleles (shared epitope), specific PADI4 alleles as inherited factors, and smoking as an environmental factor. Whereas this was demonstrated for European populations,[29,31] it could not be confirmed by a U.S. study.[32]

Autoantibody Production before Rheumatoid Arthritis Onset

Rheumatoid factor testing is used commonly in clinical practice with a very low specificity (around 40% to 60%) since it also occurs in a wide range of other diseases and with progressing age.[33] However, markedly elevated RF titers have a high specificity for RA. The introduction of tests for anti-CCP antibodies increased the diagnostic specificity for RA, especially in combination with RF (specificity up to 98%).[28,33,34] This makes testing for the combination of autoantibodies very useful in confirming a diagnosis of RA. However, they are not sufficiently specific to be used as broad screening tests in the absence of other diagnostic criteria. Anti-CCP testing is useful for diagnosing RA in patients with early synovitis, as well as differentiating RA from other inflammatory arthritides and other connective tissue diseases.

The presence of RF and/or anti-CCP can be observed in some patients 6 to 10 years before the onset of the disease indicating that the breakdown of immune tolerance in the B-cell system can be a very early step in disease pathogenesis.[35,36] However, because of the imperfect specificity of the tests and the relative low incidence of RA, documentation of these humoral disturbances is currently insufficient for clinical decision making before the onset of clinical manifestations. This is further confounded by the finding that less than 50% of the patients will have a positive test within the year before the onset of the first symptoms.[35,36]

Besides having a poorer prognosis and a greater tendency for erosive disease, it is interesting to note that patients who produce IgM-RF and anti-CCP IgG respond better to B-cell depletion than so-called seronegative RA patients.[37] Moreover, the titer of IgM-RF decreases in about one-third of RA patients treated with B-cell–depleting therapy.[37] Anti-CCP antibodies also decrease with B-cell–depleting therapy,[38] which suggests that a portion of these specific autoantibodies derive from antibody secreting cells that express CD20 on their surface directly on those plasma cells that require continuous replenishment from $CD20^+$ B cells. It is likely that this subset of antibody secreting cells is sensitive to a variety of other therapeutics since glucocorticoids, methotrexate, gold,[17,39] and TNF blockers, as well as abatacept, have also been reported to reduce autoantibody levels. Most remarkably, some patients treated with intramuscular gold showed significant IgG reductions requiring intravenous Ig in some of the patients,[39] suggesting that a stage in the pathway of the differentiation of antibody-producing cells may also be sensitive to the action of gold salts. The mechanisms by which these agents cause decreases in autoantibodies or serum Ig have not been fully delineated, but direct effects on B cells have been reported for some.[39]

Ectopic Germinal Center

It is known that memory B cells and plasma cells reside in the RA synovium[40] in proximity to ectopic GCs in the affected tissue. Aggregates of $CD20^+$ B cells have been identified in synovial tissue in about one-third of patients with RA[40] surrounded by T cells and FDCs within these GC-like structures. The function of these FDCs has not been intensively studied in the RA synovium. Specifically, it is not known whether they have the full capacity to select antigen-reactive cells and delete autoreactive B cells appropriately as in typical GCs. Notably, ectopic GCs are detectable in only about 25% to 35% of RA patients, whereas there is only moderate infiltration or even slight infiltration in the remaining patients[41,42] (Figure 8B-3). These aggregates have been found in the affected organs in many autoimmune conditions, such as in RA synovium[40] and the kidneys of patients with SLE,[43] as well as in the salivary glands of patients with Sjögren's syndrome, in the thymus in myasthenia gravis, and in the central nervous system of patients with multiple sclerosis.[8,17,44]

Whereas plasma cells likely have been generated there, it is not clear whether synovial memory B cells have been generated locally or migrated from distant secondary lymphoid organs. Formally, it cannot be excluded that synovial plasma cells have also migrated into the site of inflammation. This implies that the presence of memory B cells and plasma cells in RA synovium may reflect local generation in ectopic GC or tissue infiltration by cells generated in secondary lymphoid organs because of inflammation. Whereas higher RF levels in the synovial fluid versus blood argue for the primary role of GCs in the synovial

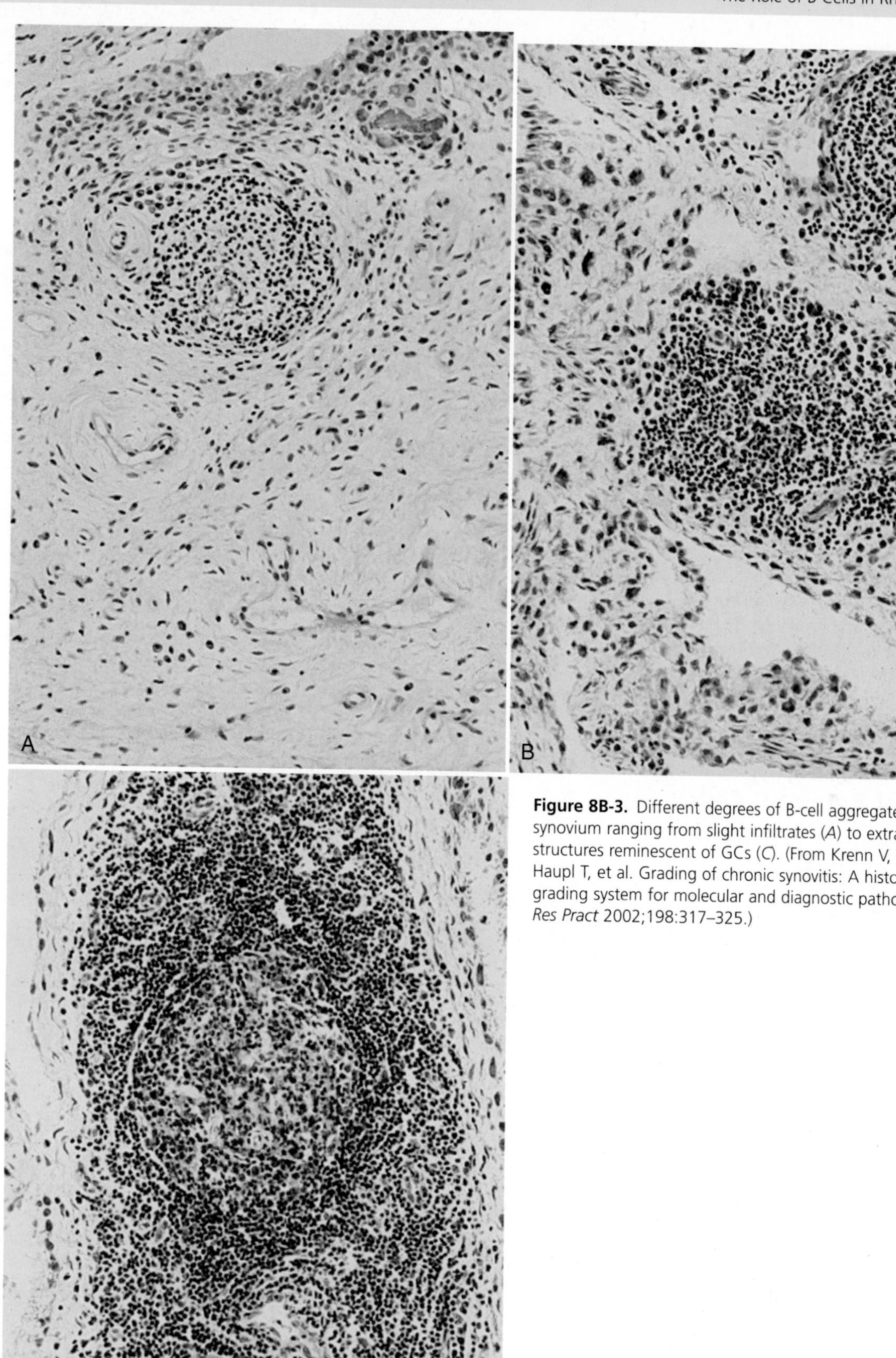

Figure 8B-3. Different degrees of B-cell aggregates in the RA synovium ranging from slight infiltrates (*A*) to extrafollicular structures reminescent of GCs (*C*). (From Krenn V, Morawietz L, Haupl T, et al. Grading of chronic synovitis: A histopathological grading system for molecular and diagnostic pathology. *Pathol Res Pract* 2002;198:317–325.)

membrane, detection of various clones of plasma cells,[40] and even the presence of antitetanus-specific plasma cells after systemic tetanus vaccination,[45] suggest that the synovial membrane may be a site for their survival after egress from a distant site of induction, possibly the lymph nodes.

In this regard, provision of CXCL13 by synovial fibroblasts and interaction with CXCR5 expressed by B cells along with follicular helper T cells are important signals to navigate B cells into GCs where they can undergo activation and differentiation.[40] These processes do not appear to be restricted to classical lymphoid organs, and are also effective in ectopic GCs as shown for the role of CXCL13 for the RA synovium.[46] Since formation of ectopic GCs in the synovium is not a unique finding in RA patients, they may not be essential for generation of plasma cells and memory B cells. An alternative explanation is that these structures develop during very active inflammation because of locally produced proinflammatory stimuli (cytokines, chemokines). Once established, lymphotoxin β produced by B cells essential for the differentiation of FDCs into secondary lymphoid organs and the organization of effective lymphoid architecture can further promote the development of these structures.

Currently available data indicate that the formation of ectopic GCs in the RA synovium is a typical but not an essential finding of autoimmunity. One possibility is that they represent exaggerated local immune reactions, but whether the presence of these structures correlates with disease activity is not known. Identification of these structures in longstanding bacterial infections[23] is consistent with the possibility that they form as a result of inflammation and not as a cause.

Evidence of Role of B Cells in Autoimmunity Provided by Animal Models

B cells can function as antigen-presenting cells as has been suggested by instructive data from animal models,[47,48] in which a lupus-like disease developed when autoimmune-prone mice were reconstituted with B cells that lacked the ability to secrete Ig but not when they were deprived of B cells completely.[47,48] Although these studies were performed in a murine lupus model, it provided data on the possible role of antigen presentation by B cells.

The K/BxN model has raised particular interest for the potential role of humoral immunity in the development of arthritis.[49,50] In this model, spontaneous arthritis occurs in mice that express both the transgene encoded KRN T-cell receptor and the IAg^7 MHC class II allele. The transgenic T cells have specificity for glucose-6-phosphate isomerase (G6PI), and are able to break tolerance in the B-cell compartment resulting in the production of autoantibodies to G6PI. Affinity-purified anti-G6PI Ig from these mice can transfer joint-specific inflammation to healthy recipient mice. A mechanism for joint-specific disease arising from autoimmunity to G6PI has been suggested recently. G6PI bound to the surface of cartilage is the target for anti-G6PI binding and subsequent complement-mediated damage.[50] In this model, the inciting event is the expression of an autoreactive T-cell receptor in the periphery, whereas the disease manifestations are subsequently induced by the autoantibody. In this context, joint destruction was strictly mediated by innate immune mechanisms since the disease could be transferred by autoantibodies to animals that lack B and T cells.[49,50] These data led to the renaissance of an immune paradigm in which adaptive immunity can activate innate mechanisms in inflammatory arthritis that finally account for the disabling joint destruction. This model was proposed initially based on data obtained in antigen-induced arthritis in rabbits.[51]

Whereas animal studies with anti-G6PI were very compelling, analyses of anti-G6PI antibodies in the serum of RA patients indicate that these autoantibodies apparently do not play a significant role and confirm clearly the limitations of animal data for understanding the details of human disease.

Further involvement of B-cell activation has also been shown for antibody-mediated arthritis[52] by co-ligation of toll-like receptors (TLR) with the BCR in collagen-induced arthritis with inflammatory joint destruction and CpG-induced TLR9 and BCR activation in adjuvant-induced arthritis.[53] Collagen-induced arthritis is also antibody-dependent and abolished in B-cell–deprived mice, which supports a central pathogenic role of B cells in arthritis.[54]

Humoral and B-Cell Memory

A primary immune response leads to release of polyreactive IgM by B1 B cells in a T-cell–independent way and provides a first line of defense. This immune reaction usually does not induce immune memory. By contrast, immunologic memory is provided by plasma cells, which secrete (auto)antibodies, and by memory T cells and B cells, with the latter having the capacity to rapidly respond to a recall antigen challenge by differentiating into plasma cells. How the two differentiation pathways of B cells relate to each other, how cells are selected into these effector populations, and how these populations are maintained in general and in particular in RA remain unresolved.

There is a possibility that (1) immune reactions lacking the induction of immune memory and T-cell interaction (TI immune activation) result in polyreactive IgM, and (2) TD B-cell activation with the induction of longer lasting immune memory (i.e., IgG autoantibodies) coexist to different degrees in RA. Although their detailed contributions have not been deciphered, the various therapeutic approaches may have a distinct impact on these two types of B-cell reactivity.

The frequency of memory B cells in RA is enhanced as compared to controls in the peripheral blood as well in the inflamed synovium[55,56] (Figure 8B-4). However, their specificity and whether they are autoreactive is unknown. It is currently unclear whether this reflects a loss in immune tolerance or selection processes, or if their enhanced number is simply the result of increased immune activation. Independent of these considerations, an enlarged pool of memory B cells poses a risk for autoimmunity since these cells have lower activation thresholds and have passed all checkpoints of the immune system for negative selection. The enhanced risk for autoimmunity is illustrated by recent data showing that some memory B cells acquire poly- and auto-reactivity induced by somatic hypermutation.[57] In this context, anti-CD20 therapy with rituximab provided new insights into B-cell biology of RA by demonstrating that depletion of nonproliferating memory B cells seems to be important for effective treatment.[58] Memory B-cell depletion is not achieved with other forms of drug therapy. Moreover, persistent loss of memory B cells was associated with longer-lasting responses after rituximab in RA.[59,60]

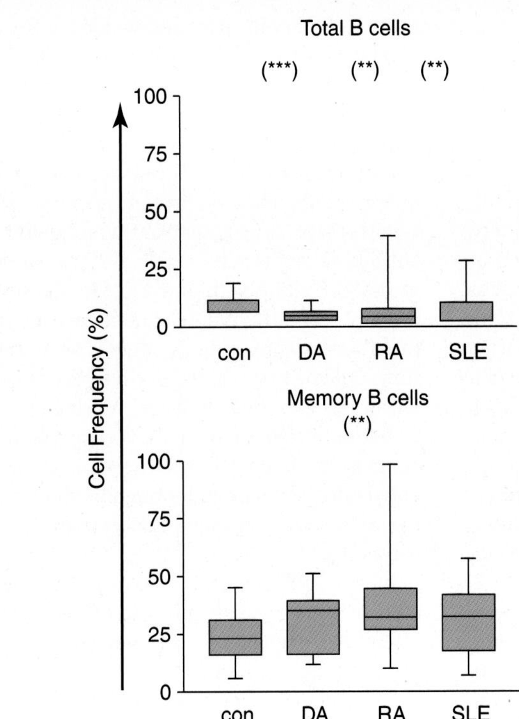

Figure 8B-4. Frequency of total and memory B cells in the peripheral blood of patients with RA (RA) patients versus controls (con), and osteoarthritis (OA) and systemic lupus erythematosus (SLE) patients. (Adapted from Henneken M, Dörner T, Burmester GR, Berek C. Differential expression of chemokine receptors on peripheral blood B cells from patients with RA and systemic lupus erythematosus. *Arthritis Res Ther* 2005;7:R1001–R1013.)

Mechanisms of T-Cell–Independent B-Cell Activation and B-Cell Survival

B-cell activating factor (BAFF)/B lymphocyte stimulator (BLyS) and possibly APRIL (a proliferation-inducing ligand), which belong to the TNF ligand family, increases survival of most B-cell subsets as well as plasma cells. Enhanced BAFF/BLyS levels could contribute to prolonged survival of autoreactive cells that otherwise would be deleted. BAFF/BLyS and APRIL, therefore, may lead to a vicious cycle of continuous antibody-mediated inflammation and tissue destruction. Fibroblast-like synoviocytes of mesenchymal origin produce functional BAFF/BLyS in response to proinflammatory cytokines (TNF, IFNγ) in the synovium of patients with RA.[24] Notably, however, BAFF transgenic mice[61] develop autoimmunity, including Sjögren's-like disease, but they do not develop arthritis.

T-cell–independent activation of B cells can occur in severe immunodeficiency and *in vitro*, which is dependent on one of the receptors for BAFF/BLyS and APRIL, the transmembrane activator and calcium modulator and cyclophilin ligand interactor (TACI).[62–67] Other studies[68] found that only a subset of memory B cells undergo BAFF/BLyS-induced activation. Currently, the degree to which BAFF/BLyS is involved in activation or survival of certain B-cell subsets is not clear, nor is it clear whether these mechanisms are operative in RA patients.

BAFF/BLyS levels in autoimmune diseases, such as Sjögren's syndrome, SLE, and RA, were found to be significantly increased, and BAFF/BLyS levels in the RA synovial fluid are higher than in the blood. Whether this increase reflects the degree of inflammation or is a primary etiologic factor in RA is not known.

Another mechanism by which B cells can be activated in the absence of T cells is by TLRs. They are also known as "pathogen-associated molecular pattern receptors" or "pattern recognition receptors," and are expressed by nearly every cell in the body. TLR-7, TLR-8, and TLR-9 are the most important of these with respect to B cells. Bacterial DNA is the natural ligand of TLR-9, and single-stranded RNA is the ligand of TLR-7 and TLR-8. All three receptor–ligand interactions lead to activation of B cells by an NF-κB–dependent mechanism.[66,70] As a result, B cells can differentiate into (auto)antibody-producing plasma cells or produce proinflammatory cytokines.[70] Similar to BAFF-dependent activation, signaling via TLRs uniquely affects memory B cells. The impact of this activation pathway is a subject of current controversy. Whereas some studies identified TLR-dependent memory B-cell activation by cPG-DNA as rather weak,[71] other studies report an even stronger activation than by CD40.[22] Some of the differences may be related to the sources of peripheral blood B cells since it could be demonstrated that B cells from autoimmune patients, that is, SLE, have apparently a different activation threshold than those from normal donors.[72]

Although there is a possibility that some of the disturbances of B cells occurring in autoimmunity, and in particular RA, may relate to T-cell independent activation of memory B cells via TLRs, thorough studies characterizing memory B cells from RA patients on the functional level are still lacking.

Proper Selection of B Cells after Differentiation and Affinity Maturation

The processes of recombination and somatic hypermutation for affinity maturation are under tight control in the bone marrow and subsequently in several lymphoid organs, respectively, under normal conditions to protect the body from autoimmunity. A number of checkpoints in B-cell development have been proposed between immature and mature naive B cells as well as those operative on IgG$^+$ memory B cells in normals.[57,73–75] With regard to RA, 35% to 52% of mature naive B cells were reported to be autoreactive including those recognizing Ig and citrullinated peptides[11,76] compared to 20% of normal B cells. Although this suggests that B-cell tolerance checkpoints are defective in RA patients, which permits the development of autoimmunity, normalization of these disturbances after TNF and MTX therapy[77] as well as after retreatment with rituximab[59,60] indicate that they may occur secondary to inflammation and are not likely to be genetic or etiologic in nature.

Several processes can delete or anergize lymphocytes with self-reactive receptors by deletion, receptor revision/editing, or anergy. The contribution of these processes in regulating B-cell homeostasis in RA or defects substantially contributing to autoimmunity in this disease are suspected but not identified so far.

Aspects by Targeting B Cells

Recent data show that deleting B cells using an anti-CD20 antibody, rituximab, provides an effective therapy with an acceptable safety profile. Interestingly, the ACR20, 50% and 70% response rates achieved when rituximab is used in combination with methotrexate were very similar to those observed with other biologics, such as TNF antagonists.[37] In contrast, blocking BAFF/BLyS with the humanized antibody belimumab did not meet the primary endpoints in a clinical study of RA patients. Studies are underway exploring whether other anti-CD20 antibodies, such as ocrelizumab, TRU015, ofatumumab, or inhibition of BAFF/BLys are effective and safe in RA treatment.[58]

The broadest data set of B-cell–directed therapy pertains to rituximab. This antibody depletes CD20$^+$ B cells by ADCC, CDC, and possibly apoptosis mechanisms, and therefore does not target CD20– pro-B cells and subsets of CD20– human plasma cells. With regard to apoptosis, it is notable that it occurs *in vitro* after binding to CD20, a molecule with a hitherto unknown function. However, anti-CD20 effects are inhibited in FcR-deficient mice,[78] which indicates that the major mechanism of B-cell depletion by rituximab involves ADCC and/or opsonic phagocytosis by macrophages.

Repletion of B cells occurs within 6 to 8 months, although there is a trend that subsequent courses lead to longer-lasting periods of B-cell depletion, that is, an increase from 7.5 months after the first cycle to 8.1 months after the second cycle of treatment.[59] Repletion of CD20$^+$ B cells is also characterized by modulation of B-cell subsets with a preferential recurrence of naive B cells and a delay in the recurrence of memory B cells.[59] In particular, the reduction of memory B cells is very striking,[58] and may reflect a "resetting of the immune system" similar to that observed after autologous stem-cell transplantation in SLE.[12,79] It has also been reported that early recurrence of CD27$^+$ memory B cells is associated with a significantly higher likelihood of an early RA flare as compared to patients maintaining predominantly naive B cells.[59]

One concern about B-cell depletion has been the consequence of depletion on protective antibody titers. A number of reports have shown that antitetanus and antipneumococcus antibody titers remain stable,[38,80–83] whereas there is a decline in IgM-RF along with anti-CCP IgG antibody with rituximab therapy.[38,80,82] The difference between the protective antibody titers versus autoantibody titers is very striking. One explanation could be that the responsible plasma cell subsets are different in terms of their half-life, survival conditions, their ability to be mobilized, or their CD20 expression density. Currently, conclusive evidence of the mechanisms underlying the differential effect of rituximab on autoantibody titers versus protective antitetanus, antipneumococcus antibody levels, and so on, is lacking.

In a study[38] following rituximab therapy, an increase of the autoantibodies was seen before to the recurrence of active RA. However, it should be noted that the declines in IgM-RF titers were initially very similar in the control group (methotrexate alone) and the patients treated with rituximab (in combination with methotrexate) likely because of the use of high-dose steroids in the first 17 days,[84] but this decrease was more long-lasting and progressively greater in the latter group. It is notable that patients treated with the combination of rituximab and methotrexate[84] had substantially longer periods of RF reductions than those treated with rituximab alone. This confirms the complexity of RA, and indicates that B-cell depletion alone is less effective than combination therapy with methotrexate.

Conclusion

Recently, interest has focused on the role of B cells in RA beyond their status as the precursors of antibody-producing plasma cells since they are also an important component of the immune system. They are involved in antigen presentation, T-cell activation, and cytokine production. Disturbances of peripheral B-cell homeostasis together with the formation of ectopic GCs in some patients appear to be a characteristic in patients with RA. As a result, enhanced generation of memory B cells and autoreactive plasma cells producing IgM-RF and anti-CCP IgG antibodies together with formation of immune complexes appear to contribute to the pathogenesis of RA. Recent data have documented the contribution of B cells to RA pathogenesis by depletion of these cells using the chimeric anti-CD20 antibody, rituximab, with response rates similar to those noted with other biologics, and thus far with an acceptable safety profile. As long as there are no direct comparisons between anti-TNF and B-cell–depletion approaches in a comparable population, a number of questions, such as whether responding patients differ in their clinical and laboratory profiles or whether the current therapeutic strategies are really sufficient to induce disease remission, and whether B-cell depletion is of greater value in early or late-stage disease remain unanswered. Upon entering the era of B-cell–directed therapy in the treatment of RA, we face the challenge of identifying the proper place of this treatment modality for patients' well-being.

References

1. Panayi GS. The immunopathogenesis of rheumatoid-arthritis. *Br J Rheumatol* 1992;32:4–14.
2. Horneff G, Burmester GR, Emmrich R, Kalden JR. Treatment of rheumatoid-arthritis with an anti-Cd4 monoclonal-antibody. *Arthritis Rheum* 1991;34:129–140.
3. Dörner T, Hiepe F, Burmester GR. Immune dominant auto-epitopes—indications for mechanisms of autoantibody induction in autoimmune diseases. *Deutsche Medizinische Wochenschrift* 1996;121:1267–1270.
4. Peter HH, Warnatz K. Molecules involved in T-B co-stimulation and B cell homeostasis: possible targets for an immunological intervention in autoimmunity. *Exp Opin Biol Ther* 2005;5:S61–S71.
5. Warnatz K, Bossaller L, Salzer U, et al. Human ICOS deficiency abrogates the germinal center reaction and provides a monogenic model for common variable immunodeficiency. *Blood* 2006;107:3045–3052.
6. Tangye SG, Good KL. Human IgM(1)CD27(1) B cells: Memory B cells or "memory" B cells? *J Immunol* 179:13–19.
7. Milner ECB, Anolik J, Cappione A, Sanz I. Human innate B cells: A link between host defense and autoimmunity? *Springer Semin Immunopathol* 2005;26:433–452.
8. Hansen A, Odendahl M, Reiter K, et al. Diminished peripheral blood memory B cells and accumulation of memory B cells in the salivary glands of patients with Sjogren's syndrome. *Arthritis Rheum* 2002;46:2160–2171.
9. Tarlinton D. B-cell memory: Are subsets necessary? *Nat Rev Immunol* 2006;6:785–790.
10. Bendelac A, Bonneville M, Kearney JF. Autoreactivity by design: Innate B and T lymphocytes. *Nat Rev Immunol* 2001;1:177–186.
11. Samuels J, Ng YS, Coupillaud C, et al. Impaired early B cell tolerance in patients with rheumatoid arthritis. *J Exp Med* 2005;201: 1659–1667.
12. Radbruch A, Muehlinghaus G, Luger EO, et al. Competence and competition: The challenge of becoming a long-lived plasma cell. *Nat Rev Immunol* 2006;6:741–750.
13. McHeyzer-Williams LJ, McHeyzer-Williams MG. Antigen-specific memory B cell development. *Annu Rev Immunol* 2005;23:487–513.
14. Odendahl M, Mei H, Hoyer BF, et al. Generation of migratory antigen-specific plasma blasts and mobilization of resident plasma cells in a secondary immune response. *Blood* 2005;105:1614–1621.
15. Manser T. Textbook germinal centers? *J Immunol* 172:3369–3375.
16. Dörner T, Burmester GR. The role of B cells in rheumatoid arthritis: Mechanisms and therapeutic targets. *Curr Opin Rheumatol* 2003;15: 246–252.
17. Dörner T. Crossroads of B cell activation in autoimmunity: Rationale of targeting B cells. *J Rheumatol* 2006;33:3–11.
18. Lipsky PE. Systemic lupus erythematosus: An autoimmune disease of B cell hyperactivity. *Nat Immunol* 2001;2:764–766.
19. Hammarlund E, Lewis MW, Hansen SG, et al. Duration of antiviral immunity after smallpox vaccination. *Nat Med* 2003;9:1131–1137.
20. Dörner T, Radbruch A. Antibodies and B cell memory in viral immunity. *Immunity* 2007;27:384–392.
21. Withers DR, Fiorini C, Fischer RT, et al. T cell-dependent survival of CD20(1) and CD20(-) plasma cells in human secondary lymphoid tissue. *Blood* 2007;109:4856–4864.
22. Bernasconi NL, Traggiai E, Lanzavecchia A. Maintenance of serological memory by polyclonal activation of human memory B cells. *Science* 2002;298:2199–2202.
23. Browning JL. B cells move to centre stage: Novel opportunities for autoimmune disease treatment. *Nat Rev Drug Discov* 2006;5:564–576.
24. Ohata J, Zvaifler NJ, Nishio M, et al. Fibroblast-like synoviocytes of mesenchymal origin express functional B cell–activating factor of the TNF family in response to proinflammatory cytokines. *J Immunol* 2005;174:864–870.
25. Tokunaga M, Fujii K, Saito K, et al. Down-regulation of CD40 and CD80 on B cells in patients with life-threatening systemic lupus erythematosus after successful treatment with rituximab. *Rheumatology* 2005;44:176–182.
26. Sfikakis PP, Boletis JN, Lionaki S, et al. Remission of proliferative lupus nephritis following anti-B cell therapy is preceded by downregulation of the T cell costimulatory molecule CD40-ligand. *Arthritis Rheum* 2004;50:S227.
27. Takemura S, Klimiuk PA, Braun A, et al. . T cell activation in rheumatoid synovium is B cell dependent. *J Immunol* 2001;167:4710–4718.
28. Schellekens GA, Visser H, De Jong BAW, et al. The diagnostic properties of rheumatoid arthritis antibodies recognizing a cyclic citrullinated peptide. *Arthritis Rheum* 2000;43:155–163.
29. Klareskog L, Padyukov L, Lorentzen J, et al. Mechanisms of disease: Genetic susceptibility and environmental triggers in the development of rheumatoid arthritis. *Nat Clin Pract Rheumatol* 2006;2:425–433.
30. Hansen A, Lipsky PE, Dörner T. B-cell lymphoproliferation in chronic inflammatory rheumatic diseases. *Nat Clin Pract Rheumatol* 2007;3:561–569.
31. Klareskog L, Padyukov L, Alfredsson L. Smoking as a trigger for inflammatory rheumatic diseases. *Curr Opin Rheumatol* 2007;19:49–54.
32. Lee HS, Irigoyen P, Kern M, et al. Interaction between smoking, the, shared epitope, and anti-cyclic citrullinated peptide—A mixed picture in three large North American rheumatoid arthritis cohorts. *Arthritis Rheum* 2007;56:1745–1753.
33. Dörner T, Egerer K, Feist E, Burmester GR. Rheumatoid factor revisited. *Curr Opin Rheumatol* 2004;16:246–253.
34. Bizzaro N, Mazzanti G, Tonutti E, et al. Diagnostic accuracy of the anti-citrulline antibody assay for rheumatoid arthritis. *Clin Chem* 2001;47:1089–1093.
35. van Gaalen FA, Linn-Rasker SP, van Venrooij WJ, et al. In undifferentiated arthritis autoantibodies to cyclic citrullinated peptides (CCP) predict progression to rheumatoid arthritis: A prospective cohort study. *Arthritis Rheum* 2003;48:S108.
36. van Gaalen FA, Linn-Rasker SP, van Venrooij WJ, et al. Autoantibodies to cyclic citrullinated peptides predict progression to rheumatoid arthritis in patients with undifferentiated arthritis—a prospective cohort study. *Arthritis Rheum* 2004;50:709–715.
37. Cohen SB, Emery P, Greenwald MW, et al. Rituximab for rheumatoid arthritis refractory to anti-tumor necrosis factor therapy—results of a multicenter, randomized, double-blind, placebo-controlled, phase III trial evaluating primary efficacy and safety at twenty-four weeks. *Arthritis Rheum* 2006;54:2793–2806.
38. Cambridge G, Leandro MJ, Edwards JCW, et al. Serologic changes following B lymphocyte depletion therapy for rheumatoid arthritis. *Arthritis Rheum* 2003;48:2146–2154.
39. Snowden N, Dietch DM, Teh LS, et al. Antibody deficiency associated with gold treatment: Natural history and management in 22 patients. *Ann Rheum Dis* 1996;55:616–621.
40. Schröder AE, Greiner A, Seyfert C, Berek C. Differentiation of B cells in the nonlymphoid tissue of the synovial membrane of patients with rheumatoid arthritis. *Proc Natl Acad Sci U S A* 1996;93: 221–225.
41. Magalhaes R, Stiehl P, Moraweitz L, et al. Morphological and molecular pathology of the B cell response in synovitis of rheumatoid arthritis. *Virchows Archiv* 2002;441:415–427.
42. Krenn V, Moraweitz L, Haupl T, et al. Grading of chronic synovitis—A histopathological grading system for molecular and diagnostic pathology. *Pathol Res Pract* 2002;198:317–325.
43. Hutloff A, Buchner K, Reiter K, et al. Involvement of inducible costimulator in the exaggerated memory B cell and plasma cell generation in systemic lupus erythematosus. *Arthritis Rheum* 2004;50: 3211–3220.

44. Stott DI, Hiepe F, Hummel M, et al. Antigen-driven clonal proliferation of a cells within the target tissue of an autoimmune disease—The salivary glands of patients with Sjogren's syndrome. *J Clin Invest* 1998;102:938–946.
45. Hoffman WL, Strucely PD, Jump AA, et al. A restricted human antitetanus clonotype shares idiotypic cross-reactivity with tetanus antibodies from most human donors and rabbits—reactivity with antibodies of widely differing electrophoretic mobility. *J Immunol* 1985;135:3802–3807.
46. Manz RA, Hauser AE, Hiepe F, Radbruch A. Maintenance of serum antibody levels. *Annu Rev Immunol* 2005;23:367–386.
47. Chan OTM, Madaio MP, Shlomchik MJ. B cells are required for lupus nephritis in the polygenic, Fas-intact MRL model of systemic autoimmunity. *J Immunol* 1999;163:3592–3596.
48. Chan OTM, Hannum LG, Haberman AM, et al. A novel mouse with B cells but lacking serum antibody reveals an antibody-independent role for B cells in murine lupus. *J Exp Med* 1999;189:1639–1647.
49. Matsumoto I, Staub A, Benoist C, et al. Arthritis provoked by linked T and B cell recognition of a glycolytic enzyme. *Science* 1999;286: 1732–1735.
50. Matsumoto I, Maccioni M, Lee DM, et al. How antibodies to a ubiquitous cytoplasmic enzyme may provoke joint-specific autoimmune disease. *Nat Immunol* 2002;3:360–365.
51. Dumonde DC, Glynn LE. Production of arthritis in rabbits by an immunological reaction to fibrin. *Br J Exp Pathol* 1962;43:373–383.
52. Lee DM, Friend DS, Gurish MF, et al. Mast cells: A cellular link between autoantibodies and inflammatory arthritis. *Science* 2002; 297:1689–1692.
53. Ronaghy A, Prakken BJ, Takabayashi K, et al. Immunostimulatory DNA sequences influence the course of adjuvant arthritis. *J Immunol* 2002;168:51–56.
54. Svensson L, Jirholt J, Holmdahl R, Jansson L. B cell–deficient mice do not develop type II collagen–induced arthritis. *Clin Exp Immunol* 1998;111:521–526.
55. Henneken M, Dorner T, Burmester GR, Berek C. Differential expression of chemokine receptors on peripheral blood B cells from patients with rheumatoid arthritis and systemic lupus erythematosus. *Arthritis Res Ther* 2005;7:R1001–R1013.
56. Kim HJ, Berek C. B cells in rheumatoid arthritis. *Arthritis Res* 2000;2:126–131.
57. Tiller T, Tsuiji M, Yurasov S et al. Autoreactivity in human IgG(1) memory B cells. *Immunity* 2007;26:205–213.
58. Dörner T, Lipsky PE. B cell targeting: A novel approach to immune intervention today and tomorrow. *Expert Opin Biol Ther* 2007;7: 1287–1299.
59. Roll P, Palanichamy A, Kneitz C, et al. Regeneration of B cell subsets after transient B cell depletion using anti-CD20 antibodies in rheumatoid arthritis. *Arthritis Rheum* 2006;54:2377–2386.
60. Rouziere A, Kneitz C, Palanichamy A, et al. Regeneration of the immunoglobulin heavy-chain repertoire after transient B-cell depletion with an anti-CD20 antibody. *Arthritis Res Ther* 2005;7: R714–R724.
61. Groom J, Kalled SL, Cutler AH, et al. Association of BAFF/BLyS overexpression and altered B cell differentiation with Sjogren's syndrome. *J Clin Invest* 2002;109:59–68.
62. Salzer U, Chapel HM, Webster ADB, et al. Mutations in TACI are associated with immunodeficient phenotypes in humans. *Clin Immunol* 2005;115:S29–S30.
63. Salzer U, Chapel HM, Webster ADB, et al. Mutations in TNFRSF13B encoding TACI are associated with common variable immunodeficiency in humans. *Nat Genet* 2005;37:820–828.
64. Salzer U, Grimbacher B. TACItly changing tunes: Farewell to a yin and yang of BAFF receptor and TACI in humoral immunity? New genetic defects in common variable immunodeficiency. *Curr Opin Allergy Clin Immunol* 2005;5:496–503.
65. Castigli E, Wilson SA, Garibyan L, et al. The TACI gene is mutated in common variable immunodeficiency and IgA deficiency. *Clin Immunol* 2005;116:282.
66. Castigli E, Wilson SA, Garibyan L, et al. TACI is mutant in common variable immunodeficiency and IgA deficiency. *Nat Genet* 2005; 37:829–834.
67. Castigli E, Wilson SA, Scott S, et al. TACI and BAFF-R mediate isotype switching in B cells. *J Exp Med* 2005;201:35–39.
68. Ettinger R, Sims GP, Robbins R, et al. IL-21 and BAFF/BLyS synergize in stimulating plasma cell differentiation from a unique population of human splenic memory B cells. *J Immunol* 2007;178:2872–2882.
69. Christensen SR, Kashgarian M, Alexopoulou L, et al. Toll-like receptor 9 controls anti-DNA autoantibody production in murine lupus. *J Exp Med* 2005;202:321–331.
70. Lau CM, Broughton C, Tabor AS, et al. RNA-associated autoantigens activate B cells by combined B cell antigen receptor/Toll-like receptor 7 engagement. *J Exp Med* 2005;202:1171–1177.
71. Liang H, Nishioka Y, Reich CF, et al. Activation of human B cells by phosphorothioate oligodeoxynucleotides. *J Clin Invest* 1996;98: 1119–1129.
72. Jacobi AM, Goldenberg DM, Hiepe FT, et al. Differential effects of epratuzumab on peripheral blood B cells of SLE patients versus normal controls. *Ann Rheum Dis* 2008;67:450–457.
73. Wardemann H, Yurasov S, Schaefer A, et al. Predominant autoantibody production by early human B cell precursors. *Science* 2003;301:1374–1377.
74. Yurasov S, Wardemann H, Hammersen J, et al. Defective B cell tolerance checkpoints in systemic lupus erythematosus. *J Exp Med* 2005;201:703–711.
75. Yurasov SV, Wardemann H, Hammersen J, et al. Autoreactive B cells and immune tolerance alterations in peripheral blood of patients with systemic autoimmunity. *Pediatr Res* 2004;55:292A.
76. Samuels J, Na YS, Coupillaud C, et al. Defective B cell tolerance in patients with rheumatoid arthritis. *Arthritis Rheum* 2005;52:4056.
77. Samuels J, Meffre E. The effect of methotrexate monotherapy on impaired B cell tolerance in rheumatoid arthritis. *Arthritis Rheum* 2005;52:4082.
78. Uchida JJ, Hamaguchi Y, Oliver JA, et al. The innate mononuclear phagocyte network depletes B lymphocytes through Fc receptor–dependent mechanisms during anti-CD20 antibody immunotherapy. *J Exp Med* 2004;199:1659–1669.
79. Hiepe F, Manz RA, Hoyer BF, et al. Impact of cellular therapies on autoreactive, long-lived plasma cells in autoimmune diseases. *Bone Marrow Transplant* 2004;33:S26.
80. Cambridge G, Leandro MJ, Edwards JCW, et al. B lymphocyte depletion in patients with rheumatoid arthritis: Serial studies of immunological parameters. *Arthritis Rheum* 2002;46:S506.
81. Emery P, Fleischmann RM, Filipowicz–Sosnowska A, et al. Rituximab in rheumatoid arthritis: A double-blind, placebo-controlled, dose-ranging trial. *Arthritis Rheum* 2005;52:S709.
82. Leandro MJ, Edwards JCW, Cambridge G. B lymphocyte depletion in rheumatoid arthritis. Early evidence for safety, efficacy, and dose response. *Arthritis Rheum* 2001;44:S370.
83. Leandro MJ, Ehrenstein MR, Cambridge G, Edwards JC. Reconstitution of peripheral blood B cells after depletion with rituximab in patients with rheumatoid arthritis. *Arthritis Rheum* 2005;52: S338–S339.
84. Edwards JC, Szczepanski L, Szechinski J, et al. Efficacy of B-cell targeted therapy with rituximab in patients with rheumatoid arthritis. *N Engl J Med* 2004;350:2572–2581.

Macrophages

Raimund W. Kinne, Bruno Stuhlmüller, and Gerd R. Burmester

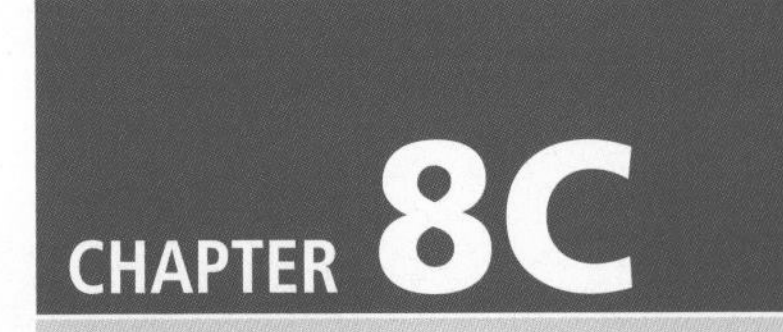

Macrophages (Mϕ) possess broad proinflammatory, destructive, scavenging, and remodeling potential, and considerably contribute to inflammation and joint destruction in acute and chronic RA (RA), as proven by the profound antirheumatic effect of macrophage-directed therapy.[1–3] In addition, activation of the macrophage lineage extends to circulating monocytes and other cells of the mononuclear phagocyte system (MPS), including bone marrow precursors of the myelomonocytic lineage and osteoclasts.[2,4,5] Although Mϕ probably do not occupy a causal pathogenetic position in RA (except for their potential antigen-presenting capacity), the findings summarized here underline their pivotal position.

Differentiation and Activation of the Mononuclear Phagocyte System

Cells of the myelomonocytic lineage differentiate into several cell types critically involved in disease, that is, monocytes/Mϕ, osteoclasts, and dendritic cells. Under the influence of an excess/imbalance of cytokines or growth factors, this marked plasticity results in altered differentiation/maturation. In RA, such imbalances are observed in inflamed joints, peripheral blood, and bone marrow.[1,2]

Cells of the MPS in RA are clearly activated in both synovial and juxta-articular compartments such as the synovial membrane or the cartilage–pannus and bone–pannus junction (including the subchondral bone), and extra-articular compartments (e.g., peripheral blood and subendothelial space—the former the site of the acute phase response and the latter the site of foam cell formation and development of atherosclerotic plaques in RA). These findings stress the systemic inflammatory component of RA and are likely linked to the occurrence of cardiovascular events and increased mortality.[2,6–8]

Stimulation/Regulation of Monocyte/Macrophage Activation

The role of monocytes/Mϕ in RA results from the integrated effects of stimulatory, effector, dually active, and autoregulatory mediators/mechanisms. At the tissue level, there is influx of preactivated monocytes, maturation into resident Mϕ, full activation, and interaction with other synovial cells. The complexity of the interaction is the result of paracrine activation mechanisms generated via sheer cell–cell contact, as well as of numerous autocrine mechanisms—in fact, nearly any soluble mediator shows abnormalities. The interactions between Mϕ and fibroblasts, T cells, endothelial cells, or NK cells are definite factors of disease, as thoroughly reviewed recently.[9–17] A simplified scheme of this integrated system and the currently known mediators is provided in Figure 8C-1.[2]

Soluble Stimuli of Macrophage Activation

Cytokine Stimuli with Proinflammatory Effects on Macrophages

Numerous cytokines with known or potential stimulatory activity on monocytes/Mϕ have been identified, as schematically shown in Figure 8C-1.[1,2] Some of these mediators are produced by monocytes/Mϕ themselves, and therefore activate Mϕ in an autocrine fashion. T-cell cytokines acting on Mϕ (e.g., IL-17) have been comprehensively reviewed elsewhere.[18,19]

Bacterial/Viral Components and Toll-Like Receptors

The ability of bacterial toxins or superantigens to initiate the secretion of Mϕ-derived cytokines is relevant in view of a possible microorganism etiology of RA and in view of side effects of anti–TNF-α therapy, particularly mycobacterial infections.[20,21] Lipopolysaccharide (LPS), for example, binds to Mϕ through the CD14/lipopolysaccharide-binding protein receptor complex and, *in vitro*, stimulates the production of IL-1β, TNF-α, and MIP-1α. Staphylococcal enterotoxin-B (SEB), a potent Mϕ activator, enhances arthritis in MRL-*lpr/lpr* mice. Anti-TNF-α therapy, in this case, reverses both the severe wasting effects of SEB and the incidence of arthritis, indicating that TNF-α is central in this system. Finally, the staphylococcal enterotoxin-A increases the expression of the toll-like receptor [TLR]-4 in human monocytes by ligation of MHC-II, with subsequent enhancement of proinflammatory cytokines by known TLR-4 ligands (e.g., LPS[22]).

TLR are part of the recently discovered cellular pattern-recognition receptors (PRRs), involved in first-line defense of the innate immune system against microbial infections. In addition to bacterial or viral components, some PPRs also recognize host-derived molecules, such as the glycoprotein gp96, nucleic acids, hyaluronic-acid oligosaccharides, heparan sulfate, fibronectin fragments, and surfactant-protein A.[23] Notably, in RA functional TLR-2 and TLR-4 are expressed on CD16^{+} synovial

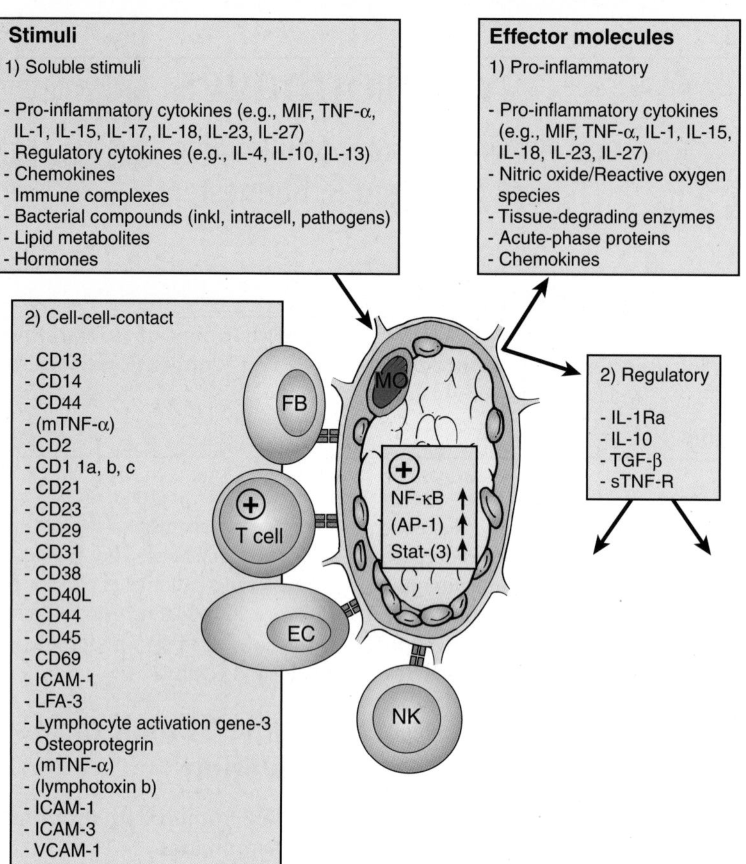

Figure 8C–1. Paracrine, juxtacrine, and autocrine stimuli (left column) and effector molecules (right column) of macrophage (Mϕ) activation in RA. Most regulatory products of activated macrophages also act on macrophages, resulting in autocrine regulatory loops with relevance for disease severity and chronicity. *FB,* fibroblasts; *EC,* endothelial cells; *NK,* natural killer cells. The (+) in the T cell indicates the necessity of preactivating T cells for effective stimulation of macrophages.

Mϕ, peripheral blood mononuclear cells, and synovial fibroblasts.[24] Also, their expression can be upregulated by cytokines present in the inflamed RA joint (e.g., IL-1β, TNF-α, M-CSF, and IL-10); this suggests that activation of synovial cells *via* TLRs may contribute to disease processes,[23] as supported by findings in experimental arthritis.[25] On the other hand, the chronic polyarthritis observed in mice with deletion of the DNase II gene—whose Mϕ are incapable of degrading mammalian DNA—appears to occur independently of the nucleic acid–specific TLR-9.[26]

Hormones

Females are affected by RA at a ratio of approximately 3:1 compared to males, and experience clinical fluctuations during menstrual cycle and pregnancy, indicating a major modulating role for sex hormones. Monocytes/Mϕ are strongly involved in hormone modulation of RA, due to their expression of sex-hormone receptors and their cytokine response upon exposure to estrogens.[27] Indeed, physiological levels of estrogens stimulate RA Mϕ to the production of the proinflammatory cytokine IL-1, whereas higher levels inhibit IL-1 production, conceivably mimicking the clinical improvement during pregnancy. Interestingly, selective estrogen-receptor ligands inhibiting NF-κB transcriptional activity (but lacking estrogenic activity) can markedly inhibit joint swelling and destruction in experimental arthritis.[28]

Cytokine Stimuli with Regulatory Effects on Macrophages

Several cytokines that downregulate monocyte/Mϕ function in RA have been described to date (summarized in Figure 8C-1[2]). Interestingly, some of these molecules are produced by Mϕ themselves (most notably IL-10), so that autocrine regulation probably plays a prominent role during the different clinical phases of RA. Other regulatory cytokines derive from other cell types present in the inflamed synovial membrane, for example T cells (e.g., IL-4, IL-13) or stromal cells (e.g., IL-11).[19,29,30]

Monocyte/Macrophage Effector Molecules

Proinflammatory Effects

Macrophages produce a number of proinflammatory cytokines, as schematically shown in Figure 8C-1 and Table 8C-1.[2]

Tumor Necrosis Factor-α

TNF-α is a pleiotropic cytokine which increases the expression of cytokines, adhesion molecules, PGE_2, collagenase, and collagen by synovial cells. TNF-α exists in membrane-bound and soluble forms, both acting as proinflammatory mediators. Transmembrane TNF-α is involved in local, cell-contact–mediated processes, and appears the prime stimulator of the R75 receptor.[31] Interestingly, the transgenic expression of this form is alone sufficient to

Table 8C-1. Main Proinflammatory Cytokines Involved in Macrophageϕ (Dys)function in Rheumatoid Arthritis

Family	Cytokine	Proinflammatory	Dual	Autocrine	Main Pathogenetic Features
IL-1	IL-1	YES	No	YES	Predominantly produced by Mϕ; critical mediator of tissue damage
	IL-18	YES	No	YES	Predominantly produced by Mϕ; critical pleiotropic mediator of disease
IL-18 inducible	IL-32	YES	No	No	Proinflammatory effects on both myeloid and nonmyeloid cells[100,107]; elevated in RA synovial tissue in correlation with synovial inflammation, TNF-α , IL-1β, and IL-18; proinflammatory in wildtype, but not in TNF-α deficient mice[102]
IL-2	IL-7	YES	No	YES	Elevated in RA, although a relative paucity is also possible[103,104]; induces osteoclastic bone loss in mice[105]; produced by stromal cells and chondrocytes, but also by Mϕ; correlation of IL-7 and TNF-α levels in RA synovial fluis and tissue.[105a]
	IL-15	YES	No	YES	Produced by Mϕ; important autocrine mediator of disease processes
IL-6	IL-6	YES	YES	No	Predominantly produced by fibroblasts under the influence of Mϕ; most strikingly elevated cytokine in acute RA, with phase-dependent differential effects
	LIF	YES	No	No	Stimulates proteoglycan resorption in cartilage[106]
	Oncostatin M	YES	No	No	Recruits leukocytes to inflammatory sites and stimulates MMP and TIMP production[106]
IFN type I/ IL-10	IL-19	YES	No	YES	Produced by Mϕ; involved in both Th_1 and Th_2 inflammatory disorders[107–110]
	IL-20	YES	No	YES	Produced by Mϕ; overexpressed in psoriasis[107]
	IL-28, IL-29	YES	No	YES	Produced by Mϕ; involved in microbial recognition by upregulation of toll-like receptors[24,111,112]
IL-12	IL-12	YES	No	No	Predominantly produced by synovial mϕ and dendritic cells, promotes Th_1 responses[113]
	IL-23	YES	No	No	Shares p40 subunit with IL-12 and possibly antagonizes IL-12; possibly involved in joint destruction in RA via interplay with IL-17, TNF-α, and IL-1β[114]
	IL-27	YES	YES	YES	Produced by Mϕ, its neutralization has antiarthritic effects,[115] but IL-27 attenuates collagen-induced arthritis at the onset of disease[116]
IL-17	IL-17	YES	No	No	Th_0-Th_1 lymphokine with pleiotropic, amplifying effects on Mϕ

induce chronic arthritis[32]; likewise, a mutant membrane–TNF-α, which utilizes both R55 and R75 receptors, can also cause arthritis. Conversely, the soluble form of TNF-α, shed via MMP cleavage from the membrane-bound form, primarily stimulates the R55 receptor, acting transiently and at a distance.[31]

In RA, TNF-α is mostly produced by Mϕ in the synovial membrane and at the cartilage–pannus junction and possibly occupies a proximal position in the RA inflammatory cascade.[33] While an average of approximately 5% of synovial cells express TNF-α mRNA/protein *in situ*,[34] the degree of TNF-α expression in the synovial tissue depends on the prevailing histological configuration, resulting in different clinical variants.[35] Different disease stages and clinical variants are also reflected in serum and synovial fluid levels of TNF-α.[36]

The critical importance of TNF-α in RA is supported by several experimental observations: (1) TNF-α, in combination with IL-1, is a potent inducer of synovitis[37]; (2) transgenic, deregulated expression of TNF-α causes the development of chronic arthritis[38]; (3) TNF-α is produced in synovial membrane and extra-articular/lymphoid organs in experimental arthritides, mimicking the systemic character of RA[2]; (4) neutralization of TNF-α suppresses experimental arthritides[33,37]; and (5) most importantly, administration of chimeric/human anti-TNF-α monoclonal antibodies or TNF-α receptor constructs has shown remarkable efficacy in human disease, both in reducing acute signs and in retarding radiographic progression of joint damage.[3,39,40] As a proof of concept, recent evidence demonstrates that the level of TNF-α expression in RA synovial tissue at baseline is associated with (and may be predictable of) the future response to anti–TNF-α therapy,[41] although there was no distinct threshold value and TNF-α expression only accounted for 10 to 20% of the variance in response to therapy.[41,42] This supports the concept that baseline levels of (bioactive) TNF-α in blood or synovial tissue may be predictive for anti–TNF-α therapy.[41,43–45]

Recently, gene expression has also been investigated in circulating monocytes of anti-TNF-α–treated RA patients to identify regulation patterns applicable for diagnosis and therapy stratification or monitoring.[46–48] Conceivably, gene analyses of monocytes easily obtainable from circulating blood may also provide means to predict which patients are future responders to anti–TNF-α therapy.

TNF-α Receptors

TNF-α receptors are found in synovial tissue and fluid of RA patients, especially in severe disease.[33] There are two known TNF receptors, the R55 (TNF-R1, high-affinity receptor) and the R75 (TNF-R2, low-affinity receptor), which are expressed by both synovial Mϕ and fibroblasts.[49,50] The two TNF receptors can operate independently of one another, cooperatively, or by "passing" TNF-α to one another,[31] a complexity that may explain the tremendous sensitivity of target cells (including Mϕ themselves) to minute concentrations of TNF-α. TNF-α receptors can also be shed, binding to soluble TNF-α and hence acting as natural inhibitors in disease. Recent studies have demonstrated that TNF-R1 may be primarily responsible for proinflammatory effects of TNF-α, whereas TNF-R2 may predominantly mediate anti-inflammatory effects of TNF-α.[51] Thus, selective blockade of TNF-R1 may suffice to attain therapeutic effects.[50,52]

Interleukin-1

In the RA synovial membrane, IL-1 is found predominantly in CD14$^+$ Mϕ[53]; also, IL-1 levels in the synovial fluid significantly correlate with joint inflammation.[54] The two existing forms of IL-1 (IL-1α and IL-1β) show some differences (e.g., low-protein homology, stronger proinflammatory regulation of the IL-1β promoter, secretion of inactive pro–IL-1β versus expression of membrane-bound IL-1α activity), but also great similarities (i.e., three-dimensional structures of the essential domains, molecular masses of propeptides and mature form, processing proteases), resulting in almost identical binding capacity to the IL-1 receptors and comparable function. In arthritis, IL-1 appears to mediate large part of the articular damage, as it profoundly influences proteoglycan synthesis and degradation.[37,55] At the same time, IL-1 induces the production of MMP-1 and MMP-3 and enhances bone resorption; this is compatible with recent evidence from arthritis models and human RA, suggesting that the tissue-destruction capacities of IL-1β may outweigh its role in joint inflammation.[55]

Interleukin-1 Receptors

The IL-1 type I receptor (IL-1R1), which mediates cell activation via IL-1R accessory protein and the IL-1 receptor–associated kinase IRAK, is found on numerous cells in the synovial tissue of RA patients.[56] In contrast, the type II receptor (IL-1R2, also found in soluble form in serum), which lacks cell-activating properties and acts exclusively as a decoy receptor, is low in synovial tissue.[57] Similarly, the IL-1 receptor antagonist (IL-1RA), a soluble protein that blocks the action of IL-1 by binding to the type I receptor without receptor activation, has only been sporadically detected in RA synovial samples. In RA, the balance between IL-1 and its physiological inhibitor IL-1RA is therefore shifted in favor of IL-1, indicating a dysregulation crucial in promoting chronicity.[55] However, therapeutic application of IL-1RA (anakinra) appears only modestly effective in RA.[58] Therefore, it remains to be clarified whether the IL-1 pathway is a less suitable therapeutic target than TNF-α (e.g., due to functional redundancy in the IL-1 receptor superfamily) or whether the biological molecule IL-1RA is suboptimal for therapy.

Chemokines and Chemokine Receptors

Chemokines (subdivided into the CXC, CC, C, and CX3C families) are small proteins specialized in differential recruitment of leukocyte populations via a number of transmembrane receptors. Chemokines do not only favor monocyte influx into inflamed tissue, but they also play a key role in activation, functional polarization, and homing of patrolling monocytes/Mϕ.[59] Notably, monocytes/Mϕ express only select types of the numerous chemokine receptors (e.g., CCR1, 2, 5, 7, and 8, as well as CX3CR1), representing a partially specific basis for prominent trafficking of monocyte/Mϕ in arthritis. In RA, synovial Mϕ produce several chemokines (e.g., CCL3 [or Mϕ inflammatory protein 1α], CCL5 [or RANTES], and CX3CL1 [or fractalkine]), and carry at the same time chemokine receptors, indicating the presence of autocrine loops in disease.[8,60] At the same time, chemokines are upregulated by the Mϕ-derived TNF-α and IL-1. Significantly, some chemokines expressed in synovial Mϕ (e.g., IL-8 and fractalkine) are powerful promoters of angiogenesis, thus providing a link between Mϕ activation and the prominent neovascularization of the RA synovium.[61] In RA, angiogenesis may be further promoted via activation of Mϕ by advanced glycation end-products, whereas thrombospondin 2 seems to downregulate angiogenesis. Because the enlargement of the vascular bed potentiates the influx of activated monocytes, downmodulation of the chemokine system represents a multipotential target of antirheumatic therapy, as indicated by the promising results of treatment with a CCR1 antagonist in RA.[8,60]

Macrophage Migration Inhibitory Factor

One of the first interleukins ever discovered, migration inhibitory factor (MIF) is an early-response cytokine abundantly released by Mϕ. MIF stimulates a number of Mϕ functions in an autocrine fashion, such as secretion of TNF-α, phagocytosis, and generation of reactive oxygen species (ROS). In addition, MIF confers resistance to apoptosis in Mϕ and synovial fibroblasts, thus prolonging the survival of activated, disease-relevant cells. In RA, MIF is overexpressed in serum and synovial tissue in correlation with disease activity. Also, polymorphisms in the promoter or coding region of the human MIF gene are associated with features of juvenile idiopathic arthritis or adult RA.[8,62]

Monocyte/Macrophage Effector Molecules with Anti-Inflammatory/Regulatory Effects

Mϕ also produce anti-inflammatory cytokines, most notably IL-RA and IL-10, both engaged in autocrine regulatory loops[2] (Figure 8C-1).

Interleukin-1–Receptor Antagonist

Differentiated Mϕ constitutively express interleukin-1–receptor antagonist (IL-1RA), which is upregulated by proinflammatory mediators, including IL-1 itself or GM-CSF, and induces strong anti-inflammatory effects. By means of this feedback mechanism, Mϕ contribute therefore to the termination of inflammatory reactions[63,64] (see also above).

Interleukin-10

IL-10, a Th_2- and Mϕ-derived cytokine with clear autocrine functions, reduces HLA-DR expression and antigen presentation in monocytes and inhibits the production of proinflammatory cytokines, GM-CSF, and Fc-γ-receptors by synovial Mϕ. Consistently with cytokine and chemokine downregulation, IL-10 clearly suppresses experimental arthritis. In spite of IL-10 elevation in serum and synovial compartments of RA patients,[65] some studies suggest a relative deficiency of IL-10.[66] A combined IL-4/IL-10 deficiency probably tilts the cytokine balance to a proinflammatory predominance. In addition, the *ex vivo* production of IL-10 by RA peripheral blood mononuclear cells is negatively correlated with radiographic joint damage and progression of joint damage, suggesting that high IL-10 production is protective in RA. Similar to IL-4, however, treatment with recombinant IL-10 does not improve RA. This may be partially explained by upregulation of the proinflammatory Fc-γ-receptors I and IIA, TNF-α receptors, and interferon-γ–inducible genes in monocytes/Mϕ.[2,8]

Monocyte/Macrophage Effector Molecules with Dual Effects

Interleukin-6

IL-6 is the most strikingly elevated cytokine in RA, especially in the synovial fluid during acute disease.[67] The acute rise is consistent with the role of IL-6 in acute-phase responses. However, while IL-6 levels in the synovial fluid correlate with the degree of radiologic joint damage, and IL-6 and soluble IL-6 receptors promote the generation of osteoclasts, this cytokine has phase-dependent effects—it protects cartilage in acute disease but promotes excessive bone formation in chronic disease. While IL-6 is mostly produced by synovial fibroblasts and only partially by Mϕ, two findings suggest that the striking IL-6 rise is a prominent outcome of Mϕ activation: (1) the morphologic vicinity of IL-6–expressing fibroblasts with $CD14^+$ Mϕ in the RA synovial tissue[2]; and (2) co-culture studies showing that IL-1 stimulates IL-6 production.[9] The role of IL-6 in experimental arthritis and the antiarthritic effects of anti-IL-6 receptor antibodies suggest a role for anti-IL-6 therapy in RA.[68,69]

Transforming Growth Factor-β

In RA, Mϕ express different TGF-β molecules and TGF-β receptors in the lining and sublining layer, at the cartilage–pannus junction, and in the synovial fluid.[70–72] The proinflammatory effects of TGF-β are substantiated by induction of Mϕ expression of Fc-γ-receptor III (which elicits the release of tissue-damaging reactive oxygen species) and promotion of monocyte adhesion and infiltration during chronic disease.[72] Interestingly, the expression of TGF-β molecules and TGF-β receptors is not limited to Mϕ, but extends to RA synovial fibroblasts, which show broad, constitutive activation/alteration of the TGF-β/activin pathway.[73,74]

At the same time, TGF-β has anti-inflammatory properties; for instance, it counteracts some IL-1 effects, including phagocytosis of collagen and possibly MMP production. A protective role of TGF-β in RA is also stressed by the association between TGF-β polymorphism and disease severity, that is, alleles associated with low TGF-β expression are correlated with stronger inflammation and poorer outcome.[75] Likewise, experimental arthritis is significantly ameliorated by activation of TGF-β via adenoviral expression of thrombospondin 1.[76]

The effects of TGF-β on TIMP are also unclear, since the regulation of MMP and TIMP may depend on different tissue domains (superficial versus deep cartilage layers) and may vary for intra- or extra-cellular digestion of collagen.[2]

Finally, some systems involved in the first-line defense of the innate immune system against microbial infections, that is, LPS-binding TLR-4 (see above), appear to be interconnected with the TGF-β/activin pathway, in that the bone morphogenetic protein and activin membrane-bound inhibitor (BAMBI) is strongly downregulated in response to LPS, thereby favoring the development of fibrosis in chronic inflammatory diseases.[77,78]

Treatment of Human Rheumatoid Arthritis with Conventional Antimacrophage Approaches

The role of Mϕ-derived cytokines in the perpetuation of RA, the pathophysiologic dichotomy between joint inflammation and cartilage destruction, and the crucial significance of activated synovial Mϕ in relationship to permanent joint damage,[1] have led to a radical re-evaluation of the conventional anti-inflammatory and disease-modifying treatments in relationship to Mϕ parameters, in order to potentiate therapeutic effects (e.g., via combination approaches) and reduce side effects (see Franz,[40] Kobayashi,[79] and Han[80] for anti-Mϕ effects of conventional anti-rheumatic therapy in RA, including methotrexate, leflunomide, antimalarials, gold compounds, corticosteroids, and non-steroidal anti-inflammatory drugs). Recent findings show that conventional and specific antirheumatic treatments predominantly target sublining rather than lining Mϕ; also, different therapeutic approaches seem to result in similar histologic changes in the inflamed synovial membrane, including significant reduction of sublining Mϕ. This, in turn, is significantly correlated with the degree of clinical improvement.[40,81] Thus, different pathogenetic mechanisms may funnel into similar disease pathway(s), leading to massive activation of (sublining) Mϕ and providing the rationale for targeted anti-Mϕ therapy.

Nonconventional/Experimental Antimacrophage Therapy

Counteraction of Monocyte/Mϕ Activation at Cellular Level

Apoptosis-Inducing Agents

Physical elimination of disease-relevant cells (e.g., activated Mϕ or osteoclasts) by apoptosis is advantageous because it circumvents secondary tissue damage by restraining cellular organelles in apoptotic vesicles. Phagocytic incorporation of liposome-encapsulated, non-aminobisphosphonates by activated monocytes, for example, induces apoptosis in these cells.[2,82] Systemic application of encapsulated bisphosphonates in experimental arthritis not only counteracts joint swelling, but also prevents local joint destruction and subchondral bone damage[83]; in addition, it shows protective effects on remote bone damage. Studies in RA show that a single intra-articular administration of clodronate liposomes leads to Mϕ depletion and decreased expression of adhesion molecules in the lining layer of RA synovial tissue.[84]

Selective targeting of activated Mϕ has also been demonstrated using either apoptosis-inducing immunotoxins coupled to anti–Fc-γ-receptor I (CD64) antibodies or folate receptor–mediated targeting.[2] In general, liposome encapsulation can also be exploited for selective delivery of Mϕ-modulating drugs[2,85–87] or gene therapy constructs.[88]

Control of Gene Transcription

The transcription of most cytokine genes in monocytes/Mϕ depends on the activation of NF-κB and NF-κM transcription factors or that of the AP-1 complex. In RA synovial Mϕ, the expression of NF-κB is more pronounced than that of AP-1, a selectivity that may bear important therapeutic implications.[89] Accordingly, the antiarthritic effects of IL-4 may be based on the selective suppression of NF-κB in Mϕ. IL-10 also downregulates the production of proinflammatory monokines, inhibiting the nuclear factors NF-κB, AP-1, or NF-IL-6. Unlike IL-4, IL-10 can also enhance degradation of the mRNA for IL-1 and TNF-α.[2] Another relevant proinflammatory target pathway that has recently evolved from studies in animal models and human RA is phosphoinositide 3-kinase signaling, presently one of the foci for the development of new therapeutics in RA based on signal-transduction pathways in Mϕ.[16,90–94]

Conclusion

The multitude and abundance of Mϕ-derived mediators in RA and their paracrine and autocrine effects (including those directed to other cells of the myeloid lineage) indicate that Mϕ are local and systemic amplifiers of disease severity and perpetuation. The main local mechanisms include (1) self-perpetuating, chemokine-mediated recruitment of inflammatory cells; (2) cytokine-mediated activation of newly immigrated inflammatory cells; (3) cell-contact–mediated activation of neighboring inflammatory cells; (4) cytokine- and cell-contact–mediated secretion of matrix-degrading enzymes; (5) activation of mature dendritic cells and cytokine-mediated differentiation of Mϕ (and possibly B cells, T cells, and mesenchymal cells) into antigen-presenting cells; (6) neovascularization, with potentiation of cellular and exudatory mechanisms; and (7) (trans)differentiation of Mϕ into osteoclasts involved in subchondral bone damage. At a systemic level, amplification of disease can proceed through the (1) acute phase response network (via IL-6, among others), (2) systemic production of TNF-γ, (3) anomalies in bone marrow differentiation, and (4) chronic activation of circulating monocytes.

Although uncovering the etiology of disease remains the ultimate goal of research in RA, the efforts aimed at understanding how activated Mϕ influence disease have led to optimization strategies to selectively target activated Mϕ, resulting in the retardation of the radiologic progression of joint destruction.[2] The anti-Mϕ approach has the advantage of striking the very cell population that mediates/amplifies most of the irreversible cartilage destruction, and of minimizing adverse effects on other cells that may have no (or marginal) effects on joint damage.

It has also become clear that the therapeutic efficacy of conventional antirheumatic therapy coincides with downregulation of MPS functions,[95] encouraging further research into selective targeting of conventional or experimental drugs to Mϕ or their different subcellular compartments[2,96] or specific inhibition of differentially activated intracellular signal transduction pathways or key metabolic enzymes.[97,98] In addition, the amplifying role of Mϕ in RA has emerged so clearly that the effects of antirheumatic therapy (whether specific or conventional) on monocytes/Mϕ may become an objective read-out of the effectiveness of treatment.[40,48,81,99]

Acknowledgments

E. Palombo-Kinne is gratefully acknowledged for critical revision of the manuscript. The study was supported by the German Federal Ministry of Education and Research (grants FKZ 01ZZ9602, 01ZZ0105, and 010405 to R.W. Kinne; Interdisciplinary Center for Clinical Research, Jena, including grants for junior researchers; grants FKZ 0312704B and 0313652B to R.W. Kinne, Jena Centre for Bioinformatics; and grant 01GS0413, NGFN-2 to R.W. Kinne), German Research Foundation (grants KI 439/7-1/3 and KI 439/6-1/3 to R.W. Kinne), Thuringian Ministry of Science, Research, and Art (grant B 311-00026), and a grant for the advancement of female scientists (LUBOM Thuringia).

References

1. Mulherin D, Fitzgerald O, Bresnihan B. Synovial tissue macrophage populations and articular damage in rheumatoid arthritis. *Arthritis Rheum* 1996;39(1):115–124.
2. Kinne RW, Stuhlmuller B, Palombo-Kinne E, Burmester GR. The role of macrophages in rheumatoid arthritis. In: Firestein GS, Panayi GS, Wollheim FA, eds. *Rheumatoid Arthritis.* New York: Oxford University Press, 2006, 55–75.
3. Smolen JS, Steiner G. Therapeutic strategies for rheumatoid arthritis. *Nat Rev Drug Discov* 2003;2(6):473–488.
4. Stuhlmuller B, Ungethüm U, Scholze S, et al. Identification of known and novel genes in activated monocytes from patients with rheumatoid arthritis. *Arthritis Rheum* 2000;43(4):775–790.
5. Maeno N, Takei S, Imanaka H, et al. Increased interleukin-18 expression in bone marrow of a patient with systemic juvenile idiopathic arthritis and unrecognized macrophage-activation syndrome. *Arthritis Rheum* 2004;50(6):1935–1938.
6. Sattar N, McCarey DW, Capell H, McInnes IB. Explaining how "high-grade" systemic inflammation accelerates vascular risk in rheumatoid arthritis. *Circulation* 2003;108(24):2957–2963.
7. Monaco C, Andreakos E, Kiriakidis S, et al. T-cell–mediated signalling in immune, inflammatory and angiogenic processes: The cascade of events leading to inflammatory diseases. *Curr Drug Targets Inflamm Allergy* 2004;3(1):35–42.
8. Szekanecz Z, Koch AE. Macrophages and their products in rheumatoid arthritis. *Curr Opin Rheumatol* 2007;19(3):289–295.
9. Chomarat P, Rissoan MC, Pin JJ, et al. Contribution of IL-1, CD14, and CD13 in the increased IL-6 production induced by in vitro monocyte-synoviocyte interactions. *J Immunol* 1995;155(7):3645–3652.
10. Scott BB, Weisbrot LM, Greenwood JD, et al. Rheumatoid arthritis synovial fibroblast and U937 macrophage/monocyte cell line interaction in cartilage degradation. *Arthritis Rheum* 1997;40(3):490–498.

11. McInnes IB, Leung BP, Liew FY. *Cell*-cell interactions in synovitis: Interactions between T lymphocytes and synovial cells. *Arthritis Res* 2000;2(5):374–378.
12. Sebbag M, Parry SL, Brennan FM, Feldmann M. Cytokine stimulation of T lymphocytes regulates their capacity to induce monocyte production of tumor necrosis factor-alpha, but not interleukin-10: possible relevance to pathophysiology of rheumatoid arthritis. *Eur J Immunol* 1997;27(3):624–632.
13. Burger D, Dayer JM. The role of human T-lymphocyte-monocyte contact in inflammation and tissue destruction. *Arthritis Res* 2002; 4(Suppl 3):S169–S176.
14. Tran CN, Lundy SK, Fox DA. Synovial biology and T cells in rheumatoid arthritis. *Pathophysiology* 2005;12(3):183–189.
15. Dalbeth N, Gundle R, Davies RJ, et al. CD56bright NK cells are enriched at inflammatory sites and can engage with monocytes in a reciprocal program of activation. *J Immunol* 2004;173(10):6418–6426.
16. Brennan FM, Foey AD, Feldmann M. The importance of T cell interactions with macrophages in rheumatoid cytokine production. *Curr Top Microbiol Immunol* 2006;305:177–194.
17. Tran CN, Thacker SG, Louie DM, et al. Interactions of T cells with fibroblast-like synoviocytes: Role of the b7 family costimulatory ligand b7-h3. *J Immunol* 2008;180(5):2989–2998.
18. Miossec P. An update on the cytokine network in rheumatoid arthritis. *Curr Opin Rheumatol* 2004;16(3):218–222.
19. Lundy SK, Sarkar S, Tesmer LA, Fox DA. Cells of the synovium in rheumatoid arthritis. T lymphocytes. *Arthritis Res Ther* 2007;9(1):202.
20. Giles JT, Bathon JM. Serious infections associated with anticytokine therapies in the rheumatic diseases. *J Intensive Care Med* 2004; 19(6):320–334.
21. Gartlehner G, Hansen RA, Jonas BL, et al. The comparative efficacy and safety of biologics for the treatment of rheumatoid arthritis: A systematic review and metaanalysis. *J Rheumatol* 2006;33(12): 2398–2408.
22. Hopkins PA, Fraser JD, Pridmore AC, et al. Superantigen recognition by HLA class II on monocytes up-regulates toll-like receptor 4 and enhances proinflammatory responses to endotoxin. *Blood* 2005;105(9):3655–3662.
23. Seibl R, Kyburz D, Lauener RP, Gay S. Pattern recognition receptors and their involvement in the pathogenesis of arthritis. *Curr Opin Rheumatol* 2004;16(4):411–418.
24. Pierer M, Rethage J, Seibl R, et al. Chemokine secretion of rheumatoid arthritis synovial fibroblasts stimulated by Toll-like receptor 2 ligands. *J Immunol* 2004;172(2):1256–1265.
25. Frasnelli ME, Tarussio D, Chobaz-Peclat V, et al. TLR2 modulates inflammation in zymosan-induced arthritis in mice. *Arthritis Res Ther* 2005;7:R370–R379.
26. Kawane K, Ohtani M, Miwa K, et al. Chronic polyarthritis caused by mammalian DNA that escapes from degradation in macrophages. *Nature* 2006;443(7114):998–1002.
27. Cutolo M, Lahita RG. Estrogens and arthritis. *Rheum Dis Clin North Am* 2005;31(1):19–27.
28. Keith JC, Albert LM, Leathurby Y, et al. The utility of pathway selective estrogen receptor ligands that inhibit nuclear factor-kB transcriptional activity in models of rheumatoid arthritis. *Arthritis Res Ther* 2005;7:R427–R438.
29. Taylor PC. Anti-cytokines and cytokines in the treatment of rheumatoid arthritis. *Curr Pharm Des* 2003;9(14):1095–1106.
30. Wong PK, Campbell IK, Robb L, Wicks IP. Endogenous IL-11 is pro-inflammatory in acute methylated bovine serum albumin/ interleukin-1-induced (mBSA/IL-1)arthritis. *Cytokine* 2005;29(2): 72–76.
31. Grell M, Douni E, Wajant H, et al. The transmembrane form of tumor necrosis factor is the prime activating ligand of the 80 kDa tumor necrosis factor receptor. *Cell* 1995;83(5):793–802.
32. Georgopoulos S, Plows D, Kollias G. Transmembrane TNF is sufficient to induce localized tissue toxicity and chronic inflammatory arthritis in transgenic mice. *J Inflamm* 1996;46(2):86–97.
33. Feldmann M, Brennan FM, Maini RN. Role of cytokines in rheumatoid arthritis. *Annu Rev Immunol* 1996;14:397–440.
34. Firestein GS, Alvaro-Gracia JM, Maki R, Alvaro-Garcia JM. Quantitative analysis of cytokine gene expression in rheumatoid arthritis. *J Immunol* 1990;144(9):3347–3353.
35. Klimiuk PA, Goronzy JJ, Bjorn J, et al. Tissue cytokine patterns distinguish variants of rheumatoid synovitis. *Am J Pathol* 1997; 151(5):1311–1319.
36. Klimiuk PA, Sierakowski S, Latosiewicz R, et al. Serum cytokines in different histological variants of rheumatoid arthritis. *J Rheumatol* 2001;28(6):1211–1217.
37. van den Berg WB, Joosten LA, Kollias G, Van De Loo FA. Role of tumour necrosis factor alpha in experimental arthritis: separate activity of interleukin 1beta in chronicity and cartilage destruction. *Ann Rheum Dis* 1999;58(Suppl 1):I40–I48.
38. Kollias G. Modeling the function of tumor necrosis factor in immune pathophysiology. *Autoimmun Rev* 2004;3(Suppl 1):S24–S25.
39. Feldmann M, Brennan FM, Foxwell BM, et al. Anti-TNF therapy: where have we got to in 2005. *J Autoimmun* 2005;25(Suppl):26–28.
40. Franz JK, Burmester GR. The needle and the damage done. *Ann Rheum Dis* 2005;64(6):798–800.
41. Wijbrandts CA, Dijkgraaf MG, Kraan MC, et al. The clinical response to infliximab in rheumatoid arthritis is in part dependent on pre-treatment TNFα expression in the synovium. *Ann Rheum Dis* 2007 (published online November 29).
42. Van der Pouw Kraan TC, Wijbrandts CA, van Baarsen LG, et al. Responsiveness to anti-TNFα therapy is related to pre-treatment tissue inflammation levels in rheumatoid arthritis patients. *Ann Rheum Dis* 2007 (published online November 27).
43. Marotte H, Maslinski W, Miossec P. Circulating tumour necrosis factor-alpha bioactivity in rheumatoid arthritis patients treated with infliximab: link to clinical response. *Arthritis Res Ther* 2005;7(1): R149–R155.
44. Lindberg J, Af KE, Catrina AI, et al. Effect of infliximab on mRNA expression profiles in synovial tissue of rheumatoid arthritis patients. *Arthritis Res Ther* 2006;8(6):R179.
45. Sugihara M, Tsutsumi A, Suzuki E, et al. Effects of infliximab therapy on gene expression levels of tumor necrosis factor alpha, tristetraprolin, T cell intracellular antigen 1, and Hu antigen R in patients with rheumatoid arthritis. *Arthritis Rheum* 2007;56(7):2160–2169.
46. Toh ML, Marotte H, Blond JL, et al. Overexpression of synoviolin in peripheral blood and synoviocytes from rheumatoid arthritis patients and continued elevation in nonresponders to infliximab treatment. *Arthritis Rheum* 2006;54(7):2109–2118.
47. Lequerre T, Gauthier-Jauneau AC, Bansard C, et al. Gene profiling in white blood cells predicts infliximab responsiveness in rheumatoid arthritis. *Arthritis Res Ther* 2006;8(4):R105.
48. Stuhlmuller B, Hernandez MM, Haeupl T, et al. Prediction of therapeutic response by genome-wide microarray analysis of peripheral blood monocytes from rheumatoid arthritis patients undergoing anti-tumor necrosis factor-alpha therapy. 2008 in revision.
49. Alsalameh S, Winter K, Al-Ward R, et al. Distribution of TNF-α, TNF-R55 and TNF-R75 in the rheumatoid synovial membrane: TNF receptors are localized preferentially in the lining layer; TNF-α is distributed mainly in the vicinity of TNF receptors in the deeper layers. *Scand J Immunol* 1999;49(3):278–285.
50. Kunisch E, Gandesiri M, Fuhrmann R, et al. Predominant activation of MAP kinases and pro-destructive/pro-inflammatory features by TNF-alpha in early-passage synovial fibroblasts via tumor necrosis factor receptor- 1: Failure of p38 inhibition to suppress matrix metalloproteinase-1 in rheumatoid arthritis. *Ann Rheum Dis* 2007; 66:1043–1051.
51. Alsalameh S, Amin RJ, Kunisch E, et al. Preferential induction of prodestructive matrix metalloproteinase-1 and proinflammatory interleukin 6 and prostaglandin E2 in rheumatoid arthritis synovial fibroblasts via tumor necrosis factor receptor-55. *J Rheumatol* 2003;30(8):1680–1690.

52. Deng GM, Zheng L, Chan FK, Lenardo M. Amelioration of inflammatory arthritis by targeting the pre-ligand assembly domain of tumor necrosis factor receptors. *Nat Med* 2005;11(10): 1066–1072.
53. Wood NC, Dickens E, Symons JA, Duff GW. In situ hybridization of interleukin-1 in CD14-positive cells in rheumatoid arthritis. *Clin Immunol Immunopathol* 1992;62(3):295–300.
54. Arend WP, Malyak M, Guthridge CJ, Gabay C. Interleukin-1 receptor antagonist: Role in biology. *Annu Rev Immunol* 1998;16:27–55.
55. Dinarello CA. The IL-1 family and inflammatory diseases. *Clin Exp Rheumatol* 2002;20(5 Suppl 27):S1–S13.
56. Deleuran BW, Chu CQ, Field M, et al. Localization of interleukin-1 alpha, type 1 interleukin-1 receptor and interleukin-1 receptor antagonist in the synovial membrane and cartilage/pannus junction in rheumatoid arthritis. *Br J Rheumatol* 1992;31(12):801–809.
57. Silvestri T, Pulsatelli L, Dolzani P, et al. In vivo expression of inflammatory cytokine receptors in the joint compartments of patients with arthritis. *Rheumatol Int* 2006;26(4):360–368.
58. McInnes IB, Liew FY. Cytokine networks-towards new therapies for rheumatoid arthritis. *Nat Clin Pract Rheumatol* 2005;1(1): 31–39.
59. Mantovani A, Sica A, Sozzani S, et al. The chemokine system in diverse forms of macrophage activation and polarization. *Trends Immunol* 2004;25(12):677–686.
60. Haringman JJ, Kraan MC, Smeets TJ, et al. Chemokine blockade and chronic inflammatory disease: proof of concept in patients with rheumatoid arthritis. *Ann Rheum Dis* 2003;62(8):715–721.
61. Koch AE. Angiogenesis as a target in rheumatoid arthritis. *Ann Rheum Dis* 2003;62(Suppl 2):ii60–ii67.
62. Morand EF, Leech M. Macrophage migration inhibitory factor in rheumatoid arthritis. *Front Biosci* 2005;10:12–22.
63. Bresnihan B. Anakinra as a new therapeutic option in rheumatoid arthritis: Clinical results and perspectives. *Clin Exp Rheumatol* 2002;20(5 Suppl 27):S32–S34.
64. Dinarello CA. Therapeutic strategies to reduce IL-1 activity in treating local and systemic inflammation. *Curr Opin Pharmacol* 2004; 4(4):378–385.
65. Isomaki P, Luukkainen R, Saario R, et al. Interleukin-10 functions as an antiinflammatory cytokine in rheumatoid synovium. *Arthritis Rheum* 1996;39(3):386–395.
66. Katsikis PD, Chu CQ, Brennan FM, et al. Immunoregulatory role of interleukin 10 in rheumatoid arthritis. *J Exp Med* 1994;179(5): 1517–1527.
67. Houssiau FA, Devogelaer JP, Van Damme J, et al. Interleukin-6 in synovial fluid and serum of patients with rheumatoid arthritis and other inflammatory arthritides. *Arthritis Rheum* 1988;31(6): 784–788.
68. Maini RN, Taylor PC, Szechinski J, et al. Double-blind randomized controlled clinical trial of the interleukin-6 receptor antagonist, tocilizumab, in European patients with rheumatoid arthritis who had an incomplete response to methotrexate. *Arthritis Rheum* 2006; 54(9):2817–2829.
69. Smolen JS, Maini RN. Interleukin-6: A new therapeutic target. *Arthritis Res Ther* 2006;8(Suppl 2):S5.
70. Chu CQ, Field M, Abney E, et al. Transforming growth factor-beta 1 in rheumatoid synovial membrane and cartilage/pannus junction. *Clin Exp Immunol* 1991;86(3):380–386.
71. Szekanecz Z, Haines GK, Harlow LA, et al. Increased synovial expression of transforming growth factor (TGF)-beta receptor endoglin and TGF-beta 1 in rheumatoid arthritis: possible interactions in the pathogenesis of the disease. *Clin Immunol Immunopathol* 1995;76(2):187–194.
72. Chen W, Wahl SM. TGF-beta: Receptors, signaling pathways and autoimmunity. *Curr Dir Autoimmun* 2002;5:62–91.
73. Pohlers D, Beyer A, Koczan D, et al. Constitutive upregulation of the transforming growth factor-beta pathway in rheumatoid arthritis synovial fibroblasts. *Arthritis Res Ther* 2007;9(3):R59.
74. Kasperkovitz PV, Timmer TC, Smeets TJ, et al. Fibroblast-like synoviocytes derived from patients with rheumatoid arthritis show the imprint of synovial tissue heterogeneity: Evidence of a link between an increased myofibroblast-like phenotype and high-inflammation synovitis. *Arthritis Rheum* 2005;52(2):430–441.
75. Mattey DL, Kerr JR, Nixon NB, Dawes PT. Association of polymorphism in the transforming growth factor {beta}1 gene with disease outcome and mortality in rheumatoid arthritis. *Ann Rheum Dis* 2005;64(8):1190–1194.
76. Jou IM, Shiau AL, Chen SY, et al. Thrombospondin 1 as an effective gene therapeutic strategy in collagen-induced arthritis. *Arthritis Rheum* 2005;52(1):339–344.
77. Friedman SL. A deer in the headlights: BAMBI meets liver fibrosis. *Nat Med* 2007;13(11):1281–1282.
78. Seki E, De Minicis S, Osterreicher CH, et al. TLR4 enhances TGF-beta signaling and hepatic fibrosis. *Nat Med* 2007;13(11): 1324–1332.
79. Kobayashi K, Suda T, Manabe H, Miki I. Administration of PDE4 inhibitors suppressed the pannus-like inflammation by inhibition of cytokine production by macrophages and synovial fibroblast proliferation. *Mediators Inflamm* 2007;2007:58901.
80. Han S, Kim K, Kim H, et al. Auranofin inhibits overproduction of pro-inflammatory cytokines, cyclooxygenase expression and PGE2 production in macrophages. *Arch Pharm Res* 2008;31(1): 67–74.
81. Haringman JJ, Gerlag DM, Zwinderman AH, et al. Synovial tissue macrophages: A sensitive biomarker for response to treatment in patients with rheumatoid arthritis. *Ann Rheum Dis* 2005;64(6): 834–838.
82. Schmidt-Weber CB, Rittig M, Buchner E, et al. Apoptotic cell death in activated monocytes following incorporation of clodronate-liposomes. *J Leukoc Biol* 1996;60(2):230–244.
83. Kinne RW, Schmidt-Weber CB, Hoppe R, et al. Long-term amelioration of rat adjuvant arthritis following systemic elimination of macrophages by clodronate-containing liposomes. *Arthritis Rheum* 1995;38(12):1777–1790.
84. Barrera P, Blom A, van Lent PL, et al. Synovial macrophage depletion with clodronate-containing liposomes in rheumatoid arthritis. *Arthritis Rheum* 2000;43(9):1951–1959.
85. Metselaar JM, van den Berg WB, Holthuysen AE, et al. Liposomal targeting of glucocorticoids to synovial lining cells strongly increases therapeutic benefit in collagen type II arthritis. *Ann Rheum Dis* 2004;63(4):348–353.
86. Avnir Y, Ulmansky R, Wasserman V, et al. Amphipathic weak acid glucocorticoid prodrugs remote-loaded into sterically stabilized nanoliposomes evaluated in arthritic rats and in a Beagle dog: A novel approach to treating autoimmune arthritis. *Arthritis Rheum* 2008;58(1):119–129.
87. Cohen IR, Klareskog L. Antiinflammatory therapy for rheumatoid arthritis? *Arthritis Rheum* 2008;58(1):2–4.
88. Evans CH, Ghivizzani SC, Lechman ER. Lessons learned from gene transfer approaches. *Arthritis Res* 1999;1(1):21–24.
89. Handel ML, Girgis L. Transcription factors. *Best Pract Res Clin Rheumatol* 2001;15(5):657–675.
90. Camps M, Ruckle T, Ji H, et al. Blockade of PI3Kgamma suppresses joint inflammation and damage in mouse models of rheumatoid arthritis. *Nat Med* 2005;11(9):936–943.
91. Rommel C, Camps M, Ji H. PI3K delta and PI3K gamma: partners in crime in inflammation in rheumatoid arthritis and beyond? *Nat Rev Immunol* 2007;7(3):191–201.
92. Reedquist KA, Ludikhuize J, Tak PP. Phosphoinositide 3-kinase signalling and FoxO transcription factors in rheumatoid arthritis. *Biochem Soc Trans* 2006;34:727–730.
93. Evans CH, Robbins PD. Gene therapy of arthritis. *Intern Med* 1999;38(3):233–239.
94. Firestein GS. NF-kappaB: Holy Grail for rheumatoid arthritis? *Arthritis Rheum* 2004;50(8):2381–2386.

95. Lavagno L, Gunella G, Bardelli C, et al. Anti-inflammatory drugs and tumor necrosis factor-alpha production from monocytes: Role of transcription factor NF-kappaB and implication for rheumatoid arthritis therapy. *Eur J Pharmacol* 2004;501(1–3):199–208.
96. van Rooijen N, Kesteren-Hendrikx E. "In vivo" depletion of macrophages by liposome-mediated "suicide." *Methods Enzymol* 2003; 373:3–16.
97. Sweeney SE, Firestein GS. Signal transduction in rheumatoid arthritis. *Curr Opin Rheumatol* 2004;16(3):231–237.
98. Westra J, Doornbos-van der Meer B, de Boer P, et al. Strong inhibition of TNF-alpha production and inhibition of IL-8 and COX–2 mRNA expression in monocyte-derived macrophages by RWJ 67657, a p38 mitogen-activated protein kinase (MAPK) inhibitor. *Arthritis Res Ther* 2004;6(4):R384–R392.
99. Gordon S, Taylor PR. Monocyte and macrophage heterogeneity. *Nat Rev Immunol* 2005;5(12):953–964.
100. Kim SH, Han SY, Azam T, et al. Interleukin-32: A cytokine and inducer of TNFalpha. *Immunity* 2005;22(1):131–142.
101. Brennan F, Beech J. Update on cytokines in rheumatoid arthritis. *Curr Opin Rheumatol* 2007;19(3):296–301.
102. Joosten LA, Netea MG, Kim SH, et al. IL-32, a proinflammatory cytokine in rheumatoid arthritis. *Proc Natl Acad Sci U S A* 2006;103(9):3298–3303.
103. Van Roon JA, Glaudemans KA, Bijlsma JW, Lafeber FP. Interleukin 7 stimulates tumour necrosis factor alpha and Th1 cytokine production in joints of patients with rheumatoid arthritis. *Ann Rheum Dis* 2003;62(2):113–119.
104. Leonard WJ. Interleukin-7 deficiency in rheumatoid arthritis. *Arthritis Res Ther* 2005;7(1):42–43.
105. Toraldo G, Roggia C, Qian WP, et al. IL-7 induces bone loss in vivo by induction of receptor activator of nuclear factor kappa B ligand and tumor necrosis factor alpha from T cells. *Proc Natl Acad Sci U S A* 2003;100(1):125–130.
105a. van Roon JA, Lafeber FPJG. Role of interleukin-7 in degenerative and inflammatory joint diseases. *Arthritis Res Ther* 2008;10: 107–108.
106. Wong PK, Campbell IK, Egan PJ, et al. The role of the interleukin-6 family of cytokines in inflammatory arthritis and bone turnover. *Arthritis Rheum* 2003;48(5):1177–1189.
107. Romer J, Hasselager E, Norby PL, et al. Epidermal overexpression of interleukin-19 and -20 mRNA in psoriatic skin disappears after short-term treatment with cyclosporine a or calcipotriol. *J Invest Dermatol* 2003;121(6):1306–1311.
108. Liao SC, Cheng YC, Wang YC, et al. IL-19 induced Th2 cytokines and was up-regulated in asthma patients. *J Immunol* 2004; 173(11):6712–6718.
109. Parrish-Novak J, Xu W, Brender T, et al. Interleukins 19, 20, and 24 signal through two distinct receptor complexes. Differences in receptor-ligand interactions mediate unique biological functions. *J Biol Chem* 2002;277(49):47517–47523.
110. Wolk K, Kunz S, Asadullah K, Sabat R. Cutting edge: Immune cells as sources and targets of the IL-10 family members? *J Immunol* 2002;168(11):5397–5402.
111. Radstake TR, Roelofs MF, Jenniskens YM, et al. Expression of toll-like receptors 2 and 4 in rheumatoid synovial tissue and regulation by proinflammatory cytokines interleukin-12 and interleukin-18 via interferon-gamma. *Arthritis Rheum* 2004;50(12):3856–3865.
112. Siren J, Pirhonen J, Julkunen I, Matikainen S. IFN-α Regulates TLR-Dependent Gene Expression of IFN-α, IFN-β, IL-28, and IL-29. *J Immunol* 2005;174(4):1932–1937.
113. Vandenbroeck K, Alloza I, Gadina M, Matthys P. Inhibiting cytokines of the interleukin-12 family: Recent advances and novel challenges. *J Pharm Pharmacol* 2004;56(2):145–160.
114. Kim HR, Kim HS, Park MK, et al. The clinical role of IL-23p19 in patients with rheumatoid arthritis. *Scand J Rheumatol* 2007; 36(4):259–264.
115. Villarino AV, Hunter CA. Biology of recently discovered cytokines: discerning the pro- and anti-inflammatory properties of interleukin-27. *Arthritis Res Ther* 2004;6(5):225–233.
116. Niedbala W, Cai B, Wei X, et al. Interleukin-27 attenuates collagen-induced arthritis. *Ann Rheum Dis* 2008 (published online January 16).

Dendritic Cells

Saparna Pai and Ranjeny Thomas

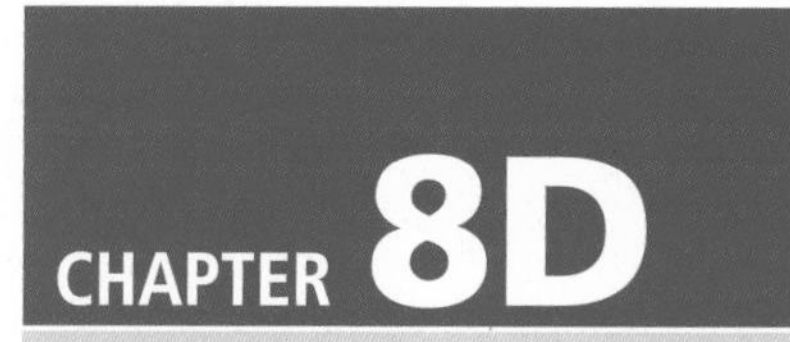

Dendritic cells (DCs) are sparsely but widely distributed cells of hematopoietic origin that are specialized for the capture, processing and presentation of antigens to T cells. They also play an important role in innate immune function. DCs are heterogeneous and differ in location, migratory pathways and immunologic function. While DCs are the major cells of the immune system that promote immune response to foreign antigens, it has become increasingly clear that these antigen-presenting cells (APCs) are also involved in promoting tolerance to self-antigens. This is because DCs that carry foreign antigens from the periphery into the lymph nodes must also carry self-antigens. Based on their role in both immunity and tolerance, and their capacity to educate the various players, or effectors, in the immune response, these critical decision making cells have been called "masterminds" of the immune system.[1] There is evidence supporting the concepts that both the intrinsic properties of various DCs, and their environmental context and cellular interactions affect the response outcome. In this chapter, we first review the functions of DCs, then summarize their contribution to RA and animal models of RA, and finally compare these contributions with those in some other organ-specific and systemic autoimmune diseases: type 1 diabetes and Sjögren's syndrome and the systemic autoimmune disease systemic lupus erythematosus (SLE). What emerges from this analysis is that DCs clearly contribute in different ways to different autoimmune diseases. This has important implications for designing immunotherapy for different autoimmune diseases.

Dendritic Cell Function

Bone marrow DC precursors migrate via the bloodstream to peripheral tissues where they reside as immature DCs. Immature DCs efficiently capture invading pathogens and other particulate and soluble antigens (Ag). After Ag uptake, DCs rapidly cross the endothelium of lymphatic vessels and migrate to the draining secondary lymphoid organs, where they are the key APCs responsible for the priming of naive T cells. Following the uptake of immunogenic Ag and lymphatic migration, DCs undergo a process of maturation, which is characterized by downregulation of the capacity to capture Ag and upregulation of Ag processing and presentation, expression of costimulatory molecules, and altered dendritic morphology.[2–4] DCs mature in response to activation through pattern recognition molecules to present Ag to rare, naive Ag-specific T cells, and induce Ag-specific T-cell clonal expansion. There is also accumulating evidence that DCs migrating to lymphoid organs also transfer membrane fragments or exosomes, including MHC molecules and peptide to other APCs, including those normally resident in the lymph node (LN).

Dendritic cells are also involved in immune tolerance. Along with thymic epithelial cells, DCs contribute to thymic central tolerance and shaping of the T-cell repertoire by self-antigen presentation, and deletion of T cells that exhibit strong autoreactivity.[5] DCs contribute to peripheral tolerance by promoting expansion of the population of regulatory T cells (Treg) and deletion of autoreactive lymphocytes. As in the thymus, lymph node epithelial cells also make a major contribution to peripheral deletion of autoreactive lymphocytes. In view of their central antigen-presenting roles, it is clear that the function of DCs impacts critically on the initiation and perpetuation of autoimmunity and autoimmune diseases, and conversely that DCs have considerable potential to be harnessed for immunotherapy.

The process of DC maturation can be stimulated by various mechanisms, including pathogen-derived molecules (LPS, DNA, RNA), proinflammatory cytokines (TNF, IL-1, IL-6), tissue factors such as hyaluronan fragments, migration of DCs across endothelial barriers between inflamed tissues and lymphatics, and T-cell–derived signals (CD154).[6–8] Within DCs, the NF-κB transcription factor family and the MAP kinases transduce these signals into cellular survival, differentiation, and activation outcomes. There are two major pathways of NF-κB—classical (comprising homo- and hetero-dimers of RelA, c-Rel and p50) and alternate (comprising RelB, and p52). In DCs, the classical pathway drives transcription of prosurvival and proinflammatory response genes, including cytokines such as IL-6, TNF, and IL-12. The alternate pathway controls DC maturation for antigen-presenting function, thymic mTEC development required for negative selection, expression of AIRE and thus thymic expression of many peripheral tissue antigens, and chemokines required for lymphoid organ development (for review see O'Sullivan et al.[9]). In B cells, signals such as TNF and TLR ligands drive classical pathway activation, and B-cell activation factor of the TNF ligand family (BAFF) and CD154 drive the alternate pathway. However TNF, TLR agonists, or CD154 signal activation of both pathways uniquely in DCs, through exchange of NF-κB dimers in the nucleus.[10] Given its role in DC function, immunohistochemical detection of nuclear RelB is an excellent marker of functionally differentiated DC in perivascular regions of synovial tissue biopsies from patients with untreated RA, and can be used to quantitate mature DCs in biopsies.[11–13]

In contrast, anti-inflammatory signals, such as IL-10, prostaglandins, and corticosteroids tend to inhibit maturation by blocking NF-κB.[14–16] Transforming growth factor (TGF)-β, while inhibiting DC maturation, promotes differentiation to epithelial Langerhans cells (LC), with specialized properties in the epithelium. Given the ease with which DCs can be modified by proinflammatory adjuvants and anti-inflammatory immune modulators, DCs have been shown to represent both attractive therapeutic targets and to have potential as therapeutic agents, to attenuate immunity for modulation of disease. Most disease-modifying or biologic therapies block at least the classical NF-κB pathway, which will lead to reduction of RelB activity in DCs. Thus, we have shown that synovial nuclear RelB$^+$ DC numbers decrease after treatment with DMARDs.[13] For immunotherapy of RA, *ex vivo* manipulation of DC maturation and activation potential, and exposure to antigen before transfer into mice has thus far been the major approach to achieve protective and therapeutic immunity.

In humans, two major subsets of DCs, known as myeloid and plasmacytoid, are described. Both subtypes have the capacity for activation, in response to particular TLR or T-cell ligands, with resulting effects on antigen presentation and cytokine production. Major subsets of myeloid DCs include those in epithelial tissues, known as Langerhans cells, and those in other tissues, known as interstitital DCs. Plasmacytoid DCs represent a distinct population of APCs with the capacity for tolerance as well as potent antigen-presenting function and production of large amounts of cytokines, including TNF and interferon (IFN)-α, particularly after stimulation by viruses, double-stranded RNA, CpG DNA motifs, and CD154.[17–22]

Rheumatoid Arthritis

Autoimmune rheumatic diseases result from a process involving three distinct but related components—a break in self-tolerance, development of chronic inflammation in one or several organs, and if ongoing, tissue destruction and its resultant detrimental effects. DCs are likely to contribute in several ways to the pathogenesis of RA. First, it is clear from autoimmune models that DCs are able to prime MHC-restricted autoimmune T- and B-lymphocyte responses in lymphoid organs.[23–25] Through this process, DCs orchestrate the development of the autoantibody and chronic inflammatory pathology on which the clinical features of RA are based. Second, DCs infiltrate synovial tissue and synovial fluid and here are able to take up, process and present antigen locally, contributing to disease perpetuation.[26,27] Furthermore DCs, along with synoviocytes and macrophages, produce innate immune inflammatory mediators, and these mediators drive inflammatory pathology in RA.[24,28]

In autoimmune diseases, when tolerance against self-determinants is impaired, activated autoreactive lymphocytes participate in the process of tissue damage. As translocation of antigens from the periphery to secondary lymphoid organs and their presentation to naive T cells are primarily mediated by DCs, these cells play an essential role in the priming of lymphocytes toward infectious antigens and in autoimmunity.[29,30] Moreover, DCs are critical APCs for the activation of CD25$^+$ regulatory T cells.[31] Therefore, abnormalities of DCs have implications not only for immune priming of infection- or self-specific effector T cells, but also for induction of regulatory T-cell function.

Genetic and Environmental Risk Factors for RA

Genetic factors contribute about two-thirds of the risk for the development of RA. Evidence for a gene–environment interaction has emerged from twin studies.[32] HLA-DR gene variation in the major histocompatibility locus (MHC) is the strongest gene region associated with RA. A second major association is the tyrosine phosphatase PTPN22 gene, in which a gain-of-function polymorphism reduces the T-cell activation response to antigen. This appears to be a general susceptibility polymorphism for a number of autoimmune diseases, which is hypothesized to reduce the capacity of thymocytes for negative selection toward self-antigen.[33] Additional polymorphisms associated with RA risk are emerging as a result of large genomewide association studies.[34] Significant environmental risk factors include cigarette smoking, parturition, and lactation, and mineral oil exposure, and protective factors include use of the oral contraceptive pill and a diet rich in fruit and vegetables.[35] Finally, EBV exposure and a greater EBV viral load is associated with RA. EBV has immunomodulatory effects, including B-cell activation, and could potentially contribute cross-reactive viral peptides or antibodies.[36,37] Anticyclic citrullinated peptide (CCP) autoantibodies and rheumatoid factor (RF) are more likely in RA patients who smoke.[32,38,39] Thus, it has been proposed, in view of evidence that smoking promotes citrullination of self-proteins, that smoking promotes anti-CCP in those with at-risk HLA genotypes.[38]

Role of DCs in Disease Initiation

"Central" tolerance defects are important contributors to spontaneous autoimmune disease. In the fetal and neonatal period, central tolerance is actively maintained in the thymus.[40] During this process, a repertoire of T cells restricted to self-MHC displayed by the thymic cortical epithelial cells (cTEC) is selected in each individual. In addition, those T cells reactive to self-antigen expressed and presented by medullary epithelial cells (mTEC) and medullary DCs are deleted by negative selection, a process that deletes T cells that have a high affinity for self-antigens.[41] An affinity threshold for thymic deletion exists, and thus affinity might vary due to polymorphisms affecting either the antigen-presenting machinery or TCR-signaling pathway, as clearly demonstrated by the ZAP70 mutation, which characterizes the skg mouse model of spontaneous autoimmune arthritis.[42] Exit of high-affinity self-reactive T cells into the periphery is inevitable, and the extent to which this occurs will vary according to the genetic background of the individual. Subsequent genetic or environmental proinflammatory events more readily trigger the priming of these T cells and the development of autoimmune disease.[43] In the skg model, for example, DCs activated by fungal beta-glucans prime autoreactive peripheral T cells that escaped deletion, which can then drive the proliferation of autoantibodies and a proinflammatory arthritogenic response.[42]

Alternatively, to initiate autoimmunity, peripheral DCs may prime the immune system to respond to modified self-antigens, potentially generated for the first time in the periphery, either circumventing central tolerance mechanisms, or compounding central defects. Presentation of viral or modified self-antigens, of which the immune system has been ignorant, represents a common theme in the initiation of autoimmunity. A variety of post-translationally modified citrullinated proteins are common autoantigens associated with RA. Citrullination replaces charged imino side-chain groups with an uncharged carbonyl group, increasing the affinity of citrullinated proteins for the "shared epitope," an MHC region highly associated with RA. Fibrin and vimentin are two citrullinated proteins identified thus far in synovial extracts from inflamed joints, and are prominent synovial candidate antigens in anti–CCP-positive RA.[44,45] Citrullinated collagen types I and II and eukaryotic translation initiation factor 4G1 are additional protein candidates.[46]

Specific HLA-DR gene variants in the MHC region known as the "shared epitope" (SE) are also highly associated with RA. This susceptibility epitope is found in multiple RA-associated DR molecules, including DRB10401, DRB10404, DRB0101, and DRB11402. The SE is positively charged and would bind proteins or peptides containing a negatively charged or nonpolar amino acid. The SE-encoding HLA alleles are particularly associated with anti–CCP-positive RA.[38,47,48] Thus, citrullinated self-proteins produced in inflamed synovial tissue are likely taken up, processed, and presented by activated synovial DC to prime populations of citrulline self–peptide-specific T cells in draining lymph nodes.[49] Effector function, including cytokine production, B-cell and monocyte help of autoantigen-specific memory T cells trafficking to joints would be boosted by local DCs presenting citrullinated peptides. Antigen-specific T cells are critical for the promotion of autoantibody production, and for driving monocyte activation and cytokine production. These T cells would promote production of anti-CCP autoantibodies in follicular areas of RA synovial tissue and lymphoid organs (Figure 8D-1).

DCs and RA Synovial Inflammation

Dendritic cells and macrophages contribute very early in the development of autoimmune inflammatory lesions in mouse models, such as autoimmune diabetes and polyarthritis, to produce local cytokines, including TNF.[50–52] DCs enter synovial tissue by means of inflamed synovial blood vessels and are chemoattracted there by virtue of specific chemokine receptor expression, in response to CX3CL1 (fractalkine), CCL19 (SLC), CCL21 (ELC), and CCL20 (MIP3α). These chemokines play an important role in driving the inflammatory disease. For example, ectopic expression of CCL19 has been shown to be sufficient for formation of lymphoid tissue similar to that seen in rheumatoid synovial tissue.[53] Inhibition of CX3CL1 has been shown to reduce clinical scores in the murine CIA model.[54] RA synovial DCs have also been shown to produce high levels of CCL18 (DCCK1), a chemotactic factor for naive T cells, and stimulator of collagen production by fibroblasts.[55] The sustained immunomodulatory effect of TNF blockade in RA relates in part to reduction of traffic of DC and other immunocytes to the inflammatory site.[56]

Increased numbers of myeloid and plasmacytoid DCs are observed in synovial fluid and perivascular regions of synovial tissues in patients with RA and other autoimmune rheumatic diseases, in which cells producing TNF are co-located.[11,27,28,57,58] A large proportion of these DCs have an activated phenotype, and produce cytokine, and thus are likely to play an important proinflammatory role, particularly after sensing immunostimulatory nucleic acid sequences. However, immature DCs and myeloid DC precursors can also be observed in RA synovial tissues. Similar cell populations reside in normal resting synovial tissue.[11] In inflamed joints, activated DCs, expressing nuclear RelB are generally found closely associated with T lymphocytes,[11,12,59] which may signal NF-κB through proinflammatory cytokines, CD154 (CD40L) and lymphotoxin-β.[60,61]

Type 1 Diabetes

A number of observations in patients with type 1 diabetes (T1DM) contribute to the view that peripheral T-cell responses to antigen presentation by DCs are dysregulated. In contrast to RA, DCs from individuals with, or at risk of T1DM, have been shown to express lower levels of costimulatory molecules after activation, than healthy control DCs, accompanied by reduced stimulation of autologous or allogeneic CD4 T cells.[62,106] As in RA, an SNP at 1858 (c>t) in the gene encoding tyrosine

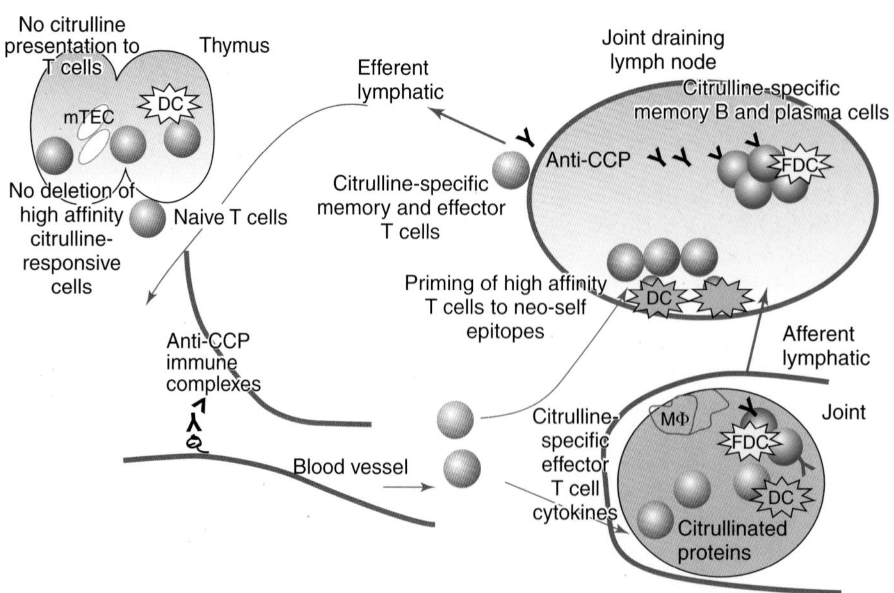

Figure 8D-1. Schema for the priming of citrulline-specific autoimmunity by dendritic cells in rheumatoid arthritis.

phosphatase PTPN22 occurs frequently in T1DM. This SNP has been associated with decreased IL-2 production by diabetic T cells.[63] These data suggest that, either through dysfunction of the APC or the T cell, an altered T-cell signaling threshold may represent a critical immune dysregulation driving disease pathogenesis. In both T1DM and RA, $CD4^+CD25^+$ regulatory T-cell numbers are normal, but their ability to suppress T-cell effector cytokines during *in vitro* cultures is reduced compared with healthy subjects.[64] At least in RA, inhibition of TNF can be sufficient to reverse this abnormality, suggesting a feedback proinflammatory loop that further promotes the capacity of the immune system to regulate inflammation. DCs play an important role in inducing Treg function. In contrast to RA, impaired DC function could impact on regulatory T-cell function in T1DM, and thus on the maintenance of peripheral tolerance.

As in RA, T1DM is characterized by cellular autoimmune infiltration of the target tissue, in this case the β cells in the islets of Langerhans. Clinically, however, joint inflammation is painful and associated with systemic disease, prompting the patient to seek medical attention. In contrast, T1DM is associated with neither of these features, and patients present only after autoimmune destruction of the pancreatic islets has occurred leading to endocrine dysfunction. Nevertheless, in rodent models, prior to end-organ destruction, TNF-producing $RelB^+$ DCs have been shown to be the first cells to arrive around the islets, followed by T cells and scavenger macrophages,[50] suggesting a role for DCs in induction of the autoimmune inflammatory process. As noted above, RelB expression is necessary for the development of secondary or ectopic lymphoid tissue, and DCs have been shown to play a critical role in the initiation of this process.

Mature DCs have a shorter life span than immature DCs.[65] TLR ligands may set a "molecular timer" to actively regulate the life span of DCs in healthy individuals. Perturbation of the "timer" can impact on the life span of DCs, and therefore their ability to induce tolerance or functions associated with immune activation, such as infection clearance. The yield *in vitro* of monocyte-derived DCs is lower in T1DM than in healthy controls.[66] Absolute blood myeloid DC and plasmacytoid DC numbers are also decreased in recent-onset and established T1DM compared to age-matched controls.[67] TLRs activate the MyD88-dependent, classical NF-κB pathway. Increased monocyte NF-κB activity has been demonstrated in T1DM patients and also in the NOD murine model of T1DM.[68,106] However, in response to LPS, T1DM monocytes or DCs secrete proinflammatory cytokines, followed by NF-κB repression, suggesting that activated T1DM monocytes and DCs became "exhausted," resulting in cell death and reduced DC numbers in the periphery. Clearly, reduced DC numbers or T-cell activation function would then impact on T-cell–mediated immune and regulatory responses.

Systemic Lupus Erythematosus

Systemic lupus erythematosus is a multiorgan autoimmune disease characterized by antibodies against a spectrum of autoantigens. Myeloid DCs from individuals with SLE display distinct phenotypic and functional proinflammatory characteristics and have been shown to promote abnormal T-cell responses. In marked contrast to T1DM, SLE monocytes show accelerated differentiation to monocyte-derived myeloid DCs as measured by increased expression of the DC differentiation marker CD1a, upregulation of various costimulatory molecules involved in T-cell priming and increased production of the proinflammatory cytokine IL-8.[69] These phenotypic differences in lupus DCs have functional relevance, as DCs from lupus patients stimulate a significantly increased allogeneic T-cell proliferation and activation response, when compared with healthy controls. Type I interferon (IFN) present within SLE patient serum promotes this spontaneous monocyte differentiation and DC maturation. Further, monocytes and monocyte-derived DCs very efficiently capture apoptotic cells and nucleosomes, present in SLE patients' blood and tissues.[70]

Initially recognized for their antiviral properties, type I IFNs play important roles in autoimmunity by promoting DC maturation, T-cell survival, and antibody production. Peripheral blood mononuclear cells from SLE patients display a typical "interferon signature" by gene microarray, which correlates with disease activity including renal and central nervous system involvement.[71] In view of the high levels of IFNα in serum, and its detrimental effects in SLE, IFNα is being developed as a potential target for therapeutic intervention in SLE.[72] IFNα, which is produced by plasmacytoid DCs,[73] activates not only myeloid cells, including monocytes and myeloid DCs, but also plasmacytoid DCs themselves, which are enriched in the inflammatory site in SLE skin lesions.[74] SLE patients also display reduced numbers of plasmacytoid DCs in blood, potentially because of migration into inflamed tissues.[75] The RNA components of the Ro 60 and Sm/RNP small ribonucleoprotein autoantigens may act as endogenous adjuvants, which stimulate plasmacytoid DC (PDC) maturation and type I IFN production.[76–78] Type I IFN production by PDCs can also be triggered in cutaneous LE by UV light, which stimulates local production of chemokines for T cells and PDCs.

Sjögren Syndrome

An activated type I interferon system is also described in salivary glands of Sjögren syndrome (SS) patients, and PDCs might play an important role in pathogenesis,[79,80] although elevated IFNα levels in serum are not observed. As in T1DM, the total number of various DC populations is reduced in peripheral blood and salivary glands of SS patients.[81] In human SS salivary glands, IL-1, IL-6, TNF, and IFNα were identified in parts of the salivary gland specimens that localize to mononuclear cell infiltrates.[82] Apoptosis appears to play an important role in the destruction of the glandular epithelial cells. Apoptotic cell death may release autoantigens that are captured by DCs and presented to T cells in draining lymph nodes, promoting induction and maintenance of autoimmunity. The follicular DCs residing within germinal centers (GCs) of salivary glands from SS patients are proposed to retain self-antigens on their surface and thus mediate B-cell clonal differentiation and activation *in situ*. Clonally differentiated antigen-specific B lymphocytes in large lymphoid follicles resembling GCs have been documented in biopsies of SS patients.[83]

Dendritic Cells and Immune Tolerance

Blocking NF-κB Function to Induce Tolerance

The ability of a myeloid DC to induce immunity or tolerance is linked to NF-κB activity.[84–87] Various drugs and cytokines, and inhibitors of NF-κB inhibit myeloid DC maturation,[16,88–92] including corticosteroids, salicylates, mycophenolate mofetil, TGF-β, and IL-10. DCs generated in the presence of these agents then alter T-cell function *in vitro* and *in vivo*, including promotion of antigen-specific tolerance.[88,93–95] RelB regulates DC and B-cell APC function through regulation of CD40 and MHC molecule expression.[96–98] Antigen-exposed DCs in which RelB function is inhibited lack cell surface CD40, prevent priming of immunity, and suppress previously primed immune responses.[98] Increasing evidence in humans and rodents strongly suggests that NF-β–deficient DC may control peripheral tolerance by inducing the differentiation of regulatory T cells.[84,85,98,99]

Generation of Regulatory DCs for Tolerance

Antirheumatic disease modifying drugs act systemically, and as a result of nonspecific immune suppressive effects, opportunistic infections may occur. Thus, it is desirable to develop a therapeutic means to modulate immune responses in an antigenic-specific manner. DCs are an attractive target for a therapeutic strategy that attenuates autoimmune responses. During the last decade, the development of techniques to generate large numbers of DCs *in vitro*, together with advances in gene transfer technology and understanding of the role of DCs in peripheral tolerance have opened up the possibility of generating DCs with regulatory properties in the laboratory. Strategies used to generate DCs with such potential include modification of tissue culture conditions, pharmacologic modification, and genetic engineering.[88,100,101] Regulatory DCs have potential utility as a platform for prevention or therapy of a range of autoimmune diseases. However, different approaches might need to be designed based on the roles of DCs in different autoimmune diseases, and not just differences in autoantigens. *In vitro*, human DCs can be directly isolated from blood, or generated in larger numbers from monocytes or bone marrow $CD34^+$ hematopoietic precursor cells.[102–104] Alternatively, regulatory DCs could be directly differentiated from embryonic stem cells.[105] This approach generates stable, long-term DC cultures, which can be manipulated subsequently by viral or nonviral gene transfer.

Conclusion

Restoration of tolerance to self-antigens is currently an exciting field. Much progress has been made in recent years in our understanding of how T-cell regulation occurs, how to control the APCs for generation of regulation, and the nature of the autoantigens driving rheumatic diseases. DCs are an attractive target to attenuate immune responses in autoimmune diseases. The plasticity of DCs provides a wide platform, enabling expansion of DCs, modification of DC function and promotion of immunity in a predicted direction. Further detailed understanding of the phenotype and function of DCs may aid the development of therapeutic strategies in future clinical applications. There are still challenges; first, to demonstrate that the principles of antigen-specific therapy using DCs already demonstrated in animal models can actually work in practice in patients with spontaneous autoimmunity, and second to develop cell-free, antigen-specific therapy to target appropriate APCs with relevant autoantigens *in vivo*.

References

1. Fazekas de St Groth B. The evolution of self-tolerance: A new cell arises to meet the challenge of self-reactivity. *Immunol Today* 1998;19:448–454.
2. Steinman RM. The dendritic cell system and its role in immunogenicity. *Ann Rev Immunol* 1991;9:271–296.
3. Cella M, Sallusto F, Lanzavecchia A. Origin, maturation and antigen presenting function of dendritic cells. *Curr Opin Immunol* 1997; 9:10–16.
4. Cella M, Scheidegger D, Palmer Lehmann K, et al. Ligation of CD40 on dendritic cells triggers production of high levels of interleukin-12 and enhances T cell stimulatory capacity: T-T help via APC activation. *J Exp Med* 1996;184:747–752.
5. Brocker T. Survival of mature CD4 T lymphocytes is dependent on major histocompatibility complex class II–expressing dendritic cells. *J Exp Med* 1997;186:1223–1232.
6. Sparwasser T, Koch ES, Vabulas RM, et al. Bacterial DNA and immunostimulatory CpG oligonucleotides trigger maturation and activation of murine dendritic cells. *Eur J Immunol* 1998;28:2045–2054.
7. Cella M, Salio M, Sakakibara Y, et al. Maturation, activation, and protection of dendritic cells induced by double-stranded RNA. *J Exp Med* 1999;189:821–829.
8. De Smedt T, Pajak B, Muraille E, et al. Regulation of dendritic cell numbers and maturation by lipopolysaccharide in vivo. *J Exp Med* 1996;184:1413–1424.
9. O'Sullivan B, Thompson AG, Thomas R. NF-kappa B as a therapeutic target in autoimmune disease. *Current Opin Ther Targets* 2007; 11:111–122.
10. Saccani S, Pantano S, Natoli G. Modulation of NF-kappaB activity by exchange of dimers. *Mol Cell* 2003;11:1563–1574.
11. Pettit AR, MacDonald KPA, O'Sullivan B, Thomas R. Differentiated dendritic cells expressing nuclear RelB are predominantly located in rheumatoid synovial tissue perivascular mononuclear cell aggregates. *Arthritis Rheum* 2000;43:791–800.
12. Pettit AR, Quinn C, MacDonald KP, et al. Nuclear localization of RelB is associated with effective antigen- presenting cell function. *J Immunol* 1997;159:3681–3691.
13. Pettit AR, Weedon H, Ahern S, et al. Association of clinical, radiological and synovial immunopathological response to antirheumatic treatment in rheumatoid arthritis. *Rheumatology* 2001; 40:1243–1255.
14. De Smedt T, Van Mechelen M, De Becker G, et al. Effect of interleukin-10 on dendritic cell maturation and function. *Eur J Immunol* 1997;27:1229–1235.
15. Geissmann F, Revy P, Regnault A, et al. TGF-beta 1 prevents the noncognate maturation of human dendritic Langerhans cells. *J Immunol* 1999;162:4567–4575.
16. de Jong EC, Vieira PL, Kalinski P, Kapsenberg ML. Corticosteroids inhibit the production of inflammatory mediators in immature monocyte-derived DC and induce the development of tolerogenic DC3. *J Leukoc Biol* 1999;66:201–204.
17. Banchereau J, Paczesny S, Blanco P, et al. Dendritic cells: Controllers of the immune system and a new promise for immunotherapy. *Ann N Y Acad Sci* 2003;987:180–187.
18. Krug A, Towarowski A, Britsch S, et al. Toll-like receptor expression reveals CpG DNA as a unique microbial stimulus for plasmacytoid dendritic cells which synergizes with CD40 ligand to induce high amounts of IL-12. *Eur J Immunol* 2001;31: 3026–3037.

19. Kadowaki N, Ho S, Antonenko S, et al. Subsets of human dendritic cell precursors express different toll-like receptors and respond to different microbial antigens. *J Exp Med* 2001;194:863–869.
20. Hochrein H, Shortman K, Vremec D, et al. Differential production of IL-12, IFN-alpha, and IFN-gamma by mouse dendritic cell subsets. *J Immunol* 2001;166:5448–5455.
21. Cella M, Facchetti F, Lanzavecchia A, Colonna M. Plasmacytoid dendritic cells activated by influenza virus and CD40L drive a potent TH1 polarization. *Nat Immunol* 2000;1:305–310.
22. Penna G, Sozzani S, Adorini L. Cutting edge: selective usage of chemokine receptors by plasmacytoid dendritic cells. *J Immunol* 2001;167:1862–1866.
23. Dittel BN, Visintin I, Merchant RM, Janeway CA Jr. Presentation of the self antigen myelin basic protein by dendritic cells leads to experimental autoimmune encephalomyelitis. *J Immunol* 1999;163:32–39.
24. Leung BP, Conacher M, Hunter D, et al. A novel dendritic cell–induced model of erosive inflammatory arthritis: distinct roles for dendritic cells in T cell activation and induction of local inflammation. *J Immunol* 2002;169:7071–7077.
25. Ludewig B, Odermatt B, Landmann S, et al. Dendritic cells induce autoimmune diabetes and maintain disease via de novo formation of local lymphoid tissue. *J Exp Med* 1998;188:1493–1501.
26. Thomas R, Davis LS, Lipsky PE. Rheumatoid synovium is enriched in mature antigen-presenting dendritic cells. *J Immunol* 1994;152: 2613–2623.
27. Thomas R, Lipsky PE. Could endogenous self-peptides presented by dendritic cells initiate rheumatoid arthritis? *Immunol Today* 1996; 17:559–564.
28. Cavanagh LL, Boyce A, Smith L, et al. Rheumatoid arthritis synovium contains plasmacytoid dendritic cells. *Arthritis Res Ther* 2005;7:R230–R240.
29. Drakesmith H, O'Neil D, Schneider SC, et al. In vivo priming of T cells against cryptic determinants by dendritic cells exposed to interleukin 6 and native antigen. *Proc Natl Acad Sci U S A* 1998; 95:14903–14908.
30. Ludewig B, Odermatt B, Ochsenbein AF, et al. Role of dendritic cells in the induction and maintenance of autoimmune diseases. *Immunol Rev* 1999;169:45–54.
31. Yamazaki S, Iyoda T, Tarbell K, et al. Direct expansion of functional CD25+ CD4+ regulatory T cells by antigen-processing dendritic cells. *J Exp Med* 2003;198:235–247.
32. Silman AJ, Newman J, MacGregor AJ. Cigarette smoking increases the risk of rheumatoid arthritis. Results from a nationwide study of disease-discordant twins. *Arthritis Rheum* 1996;39: 732–735.
33. Bottini N, Vang T, Cucca F, Mustelin T. Role of PTPN22 in type 1 diabetes and other autoimmune diseases. *Semin Immunol* 2006; 18:207–213.
34. Wellcome Trust Case Control Consortium. Genome-wide association study of 14,000 cases of seven common diseases and 3,000 shared controls. *Nature* 2007;447:661–678.
35. Oliver JE, Silman AJ. Risk factors for the development of rheumatoid arthritis. *Scand J Rheumatol* 2006;35:169–174.
36. Balandraud N, Meynard JB, Auger I, et al. Epstein-Barr virus load in the peripheral blood of patients with rheumatoid arthritis: Accurate quantification using real-time polymerase chain reaction. *Arthritis Rheum* 2003;48:1223–1228.
37. Balandraud N, Roudier J, Roudier C. Epstein-Barr virus and rheumatoid arthritis. *Autoimmun Rev* 2004;3:362–367.
38. Klareskog L, Stolt P, Lundberg K, et al. A new model for an etiology of rheumatoid arthritis: smoking may trigger HLA-DR (shared epitope)-restricted immune reactions to autoantigens modified by citrullination. *Arthritis Rheum* 2006;54:38–46.
39. Padyukov L, Silva C, Stolt P, et al. A gene-environment interaction between smoking and shared epitope genes in HLA-DR provides a high risk of seropositive rheumatoid arthritis. *Arthritis Rheum* 2004;50:3085–3092.
40. Ardavin C. Thymic dendritic cells. *Immunol Today* 1997;18:350–361.
41. Kappler JW, Roehm N, Marrack P. T cell tolerance by clonal elimination in the thymus. *Cell* 1987;49:273–280.
42. Sakaguchi N, Takahashi T, Hata H, et al. Altered thymic T-cell selection due to a mutation of the ZAP-70 gene causes autoimmune arthritis in mice. *Nature* 2003;426:454–460.
43. Yoshitomi H, Sakaguchi N, Kobayashi K, et al. A role for fungal {beta}-glucans and their receptor dectin-1 in the induction of autoimmune arthritis in genetically susceptible mice. *J Exp Med* 2005; 201:949–960.
44. Hida S, Miura NN, Adachi Y, Ohno N. Influence of arginine deimination on antigenicity of fibrinogen. *J Autoimmun* 2004;23:141–150.
45. Hill JA, Southwood S, Sette A, et al. Cutting edge: The conversion of arginine to citrulline allows for a high-affinity peptide interaction with the rheumatoid arthritis-associated HLA-DRB1*0401 MHC class II molecule. *J Immunol* 2003;171:538–541.
46. Dessen A, Lawrence CM, Cupo S, et al. X-ray crystal structure of HLA-DR4 (DRA*0101, DRB1*0401) complexed with a peptide from human collagen II. *Immunity* 1997;7:473–481.
47. van Gaalen F, Ioan-Facsinay A, Huizinga TW, Toes RE. The devil in the details: The emerging role of anticitrulline autoimmunity in rheumatoid arthritis. *J Immunol* 2005;175:5575–5580.
48. van Gaalen FA, van Aken J, Huizinga TW, et al. Association between HLA class II genes and autoantibodies to cyclic citrullinated peptides (CCPs) influences the severity of rheumatoid arthritis. *Arthritis Rheum* 2004;50:2113–2121.
49. Kuhn KA, Kulik L, Tomooka B, et al. Antibodies against citrullinated proteins enhance tissue injury in experimental autoimmune arthritis. *J Clin Invest* 2006;116:961–973.
50. Jansen A, Delarch-Homo F, Hooijkaas H, et al. Immunohistochemical characterization of monocytes-macrophages and dendritic cells involved in the initiation of the insulitis and b-cell destruction in NOD mice. *Diabetes* 1994;43:667–675.
51. Dahlen E, Dawe K, Ohlsson L, Hedlund G. Dendritic cells and macrophages are the first and major producers of TNF-alpha in pancreatic islets in the nonobese diabetic mouse. *J Immunol* 1998; 160:3585–3593.
52. Kawane K, Ohtani M, Miwa K, et al. Chronic polyarthritis caused by mammalian DNA that escapes from degradation in macrophages. *Nature* 2006;443:998–1002.
53. Fan L, Reilly CR, Luo Y, et al. Cutting edge: Ectopic expression of the chemokine TCA4/SLC is sufficient to trigger lymphoid neogenesis. *J Immunol* 2000;164:3955–3959.
54. Nanki T, Urasaki Y, Imai T, et al. Inhibition of fractalkine ameliorates murine collagen-induced arthritis. *J Immunol* 2004;173:7010–7016.
55. van Lieshout AW, van der Voort R, le Blanc LM, et al. Novel insights in the regulation of CCL18 secretion by monocytes and dendritic cells via cytokines, toll-like receptors and rheumatoid synovial fluid. *BMC Immunol* 2006;7:23.
56. Paleolog EM, Hunt M, Elliott MJ, et al. Deactivation of vascular endothelium by monoclonal anti-tumor necrosis factor alpha antibody in rheumatoid arthritis. *Arthritis Rheum* 1996;39:1082–1091.
57. Harding B, Knight SC. The distribution of dendritic cells in the synovial fluids of patients with arthritis. *Clin Exp Immunol* 1986;63: 594–600.
58. Van Krinks CH, Matyszak MK, Gaston JS. Characterization of plasmacytoid dendritic cells in inflammatory arthritis synovial fluid. *Rheumatology (Oxford)* 2004;43:453–460.
59. Thompson AG, Pettit AR, Padmanabha J, et al. Nuclear RelB+ cells are found in normal lymphoid organs and in peripheral tissue in the context of inflammation, but not under normal resting conditions. *Immunol Cell Biol* 2002;80:164–169.
60. Thomas R, MacDonald KPA, Pettit AR, et al. Dendritic cells and the pathogenesis of rheumatoid arthritis. *J Leukoc Biol* 1999;66:286–292.
61. Muller JR, Siebenlist U. Lymphotoxin beta receptor induces sequential activation of distinct NF-kappa B factors via separate signaling pathways. *Biol ChemJ Biol Chem* 2003;278:12006–12012.

62. Takahashi K, Honeyman MC, Harrison LC. Impaired yield, phenotype, and function of monocyte-derived dendritic cells in humans at risk for insulin-dependent diabetes. *J Immunol* 1998;161:2629–2635.
63. Vang T, Congia M, Macis MD, et al. Autoimmune-associated lymphoid tyrosine phosphatase is a gain-of-function variant. *Nat Genet* 2005;37:1317–1319.
64. Lindley S, Dayan CM, Bishop A, et al. Defective suppressor function in CD4(+)CD25(+) T-cells from patients with type 1 diabetes. *Diabetes* 2005;54:92–99.
65. Rescigno M, Martino M, Sutherland CL, et al. Dendritic cell survival and maturation are regulated by different signaling pathways. *J Exp Med* 1998;188:2175–2180.
66. Jansen A, van Hagen M, Drexhage HA. Defective maturation and function of antigen-presenting cells in type 1 diabetes. *Lancet* 1995; 345:491–492.
67. Vuckovic S, Withers G, Harris M, et al. Decreased blood dendritic cell counts in type 1 diabetic children. *Clin Immunol* 2007;123:281–288.
68. Devaraj S, Dasu MR, Rockwood J, et al. Increased toll-like receptor (TLR) 2 and TLR4 expression in monocytes from patients with type 1 diabetes: Further evidence of a proinflammatory state. *J Clin Endocrinol Metab* 2008;93:578–583.
69. Ding D, Mehta H, McCune WJ, Kaplan MJ. Aberrant phenotype and function of myeloid dendritic cells in systemic lupus erythematosus. *J Immunol* 2006;177:5878–5889.
70. Amoura Z, Piette JC, Chabre H, et al. Circulating plasma levels of nucleosomes in patients with systemic lupus erythematosus: Correlation with serum antinucleosome antibody titers and absence of clear association with disease activity. *Arthritis Rheum* 1997; 40:2217–2225.
71. Lee PY, Reeves WH. Type I interferon as a target of treatment in SLE. *Endocr Metab Immune Disord Drug Targets* 2006;6:323–330.
72. Vallin H, Blomberg S, Alm GV, et al. Patients with systemic lupus erythematosus (SLE) have a circulating inducer of interferon-alpha (IFN-alpha) production acting on leucocytes resembling immature dendritic cells. *Clin Exp Immunol* 1999;115:196–202.
73. Asselin-Paturel C, Boonstra A, Dalod M, et al. Mouse type I IFN-producing cells are immature APCs with plasmacytoid morphology. *Nat Immunol* 2001;2:1144–1150.
74. Farkas L, Beiske K, Lund-Johansen F, et al. Plasmacytoid dendritic cells (natural interferon-alpha/beta-producing cells) accumulate in cutaneous lupus erythematosus lesions. *Am J Pathol* 2001;159: 237–243.
75. Blanco P, Palucka AK, Gill M, et al. Induction of dendritic cell differentiation by IFN-alpha in systemic lupus erythematosus. *Science* 2001;294:1540–1543.
76. Kelly KM, Zhuang H, Nacionales DC, et al. "Endogenous adjuvant" activity of the RNA components of lupus autoantigens Sm/RNP and Ro 60. *Arthritis Rheum* 2006;54:1557–1567.
77. Savarese E, Chae OW, Trowitzsch S, et al. U1 small nuclear ribonucleoprotein immune complexes induce type I interferon in plasmacytoid dendritic cells through TLR7. *Blood* 2006;107:3229–3234.
78. Vollmer J, Tluk S, Schmitz C, et al. Immune stimulation mediated by autoantigen binding sites within small nuclear RNAs involves Toll-like receptors 7 and 8. *J Exp Med* 2005;202:1575–1585.
79. Bave U, Nordmark G, Lovgren T, et al. Activation of the type I interferon system in primary Sjogren's syndrome: A possible etiopathogenic mechanism. *Arthritis Rheum* 2005;52:1185–1195.
80. Gottenberg JE, Cagnard N, Lucchesi C, et al. Activation of IFN pathways and plasmacytoid dendritic cell recruitment in target organs of primary Sjogren's syndrome. *Proc Natl Acad Sci U S A* 2006; 103:2770–2775.
81. Ozaki Y, Amakawa R, Ito T, et al. Alteration of peripheral blood dendritic cells in patients with primary Sjogren's syndrome. *Arthritis Rheum* 2001;44:419–431.
82. Oxholm P, Daniels TE, Bendtzen K. Cytokine expression in labial salivary glands from patients with primary Sjogren's syndrome. *Autoimmunity* 1992;12:185–191.
83. Stott DI, Hiepe F, Hummel M, et al. Antigen-driven clonal proliferation of B cells within the target tissue of an autoimmune disease. The salivary glands of patients with Sjogren's syndrome. *J Clin Invest* 1998;102:938–946.
84. Dhodapkar MV, Steinman RM, Krasovsky J, et al. Antigen-specific inhibition of effector T cell function in humans after injection of immature dendritic cells. *J Exp Med* 2001;193:233–238.
85. Jonuleit H, Schmitt E, Schuler G, et al. Induction of interleukin 10-producing, non-proliferating CD4+ T cells with regulatory properties by repetitive stimulation with allogeneic immature human dendritic cells. *J Exp Med* 2000;192:1213–1222.
86. Lutz MB, Suri RM, Niimi M, et al. Immature dendritic cells generated with low doses of GM-CSF in the absence of IL-4 are maturation resistant and prolong allograft survival in vivo. *Eur J Immunol* 2000;30:1813–1822.
87. Mehling A, Grabbe S, Voskort M, et al. Mycophenolate mofetil impairs the maturation and function of murine dendritic cells. *J Immunol* 2000;165:2374–2381.
88. Griffin MD, Lutz W, Phan VA, et al. Dendritic cell modulation by 1alpha,25 dihydroxyvitamin D3 and its analogs: A vitamin D receptor-dependent pathway that promotes a persistent state of immaturity in vitro and in vivo. *Proc Natl Acad Sci U S A* 2001;98: 6800–6805.
89. Hackstein H, Morelli AE, Larregina AT, et al. Aspirin inhibits in vitro maturation and in vivo immunostimulatory function of murine myeloid dendritic cells. *J Immunol* 2001;166: 7053–7062.
90. Lee JI, Ganster RW, Geller DA, et al. Cyclosporine A inhibits the expression of costimulatory molecules on in vitro-generated dendritic cells: Association with reduced nuclear translocation of nuclear factor kappa B. *Transplantation* 1999;68:1255–1263.
91. Steinbrink K, Wolfl M, Jonuleit H, et al. Induction of tolerance by IL-10–treated dendritic cells. *J Immunol* 1997;159:4772–4780.
92. Yoshimura S, Bonderson J, Brennan F, et al. Role of NF-KappaB in antigen presentation and development of regulatory T cells elucidated by treatment of dendritic cells with protease inhibitor PSI. *Eur J Immunol* 2001;31:1883–1893.
93. Giannoukakis N, Bonham CA, Qian S, et al. Prolongation of cardiac allograft survival using dendritic cells treated with NF-kB decoy oligodeoxyribonucleotides. *Mol Ther* 2000;1:430–437.
94. Read S, Malmstrom V, Powrie F. Cytotoxic T lymphocyte-associated antigen 4 plays an essential role in the function of CD25(+)CD4(+) regulatory cells that control intestinal inflammation. *J Exp Med* 2000;192:295–302.
95. Adorini L, Penna G, Giarratana N, Uskokovic M. Tolerogenic dendritic cells induced by vitamin D receptor ligands enhance regulatory T cells inhibiting allograft rejection and autoimmune diseases. *J Cell Biochem* 2003;88:227–233.
96. O'Sullivan BJ, MacDonald KP, Pettit AR, Thomas R. RelB nuclear translocation regulates B cell MHC molecule, CD40 expression, and antigen-presenting cell function. *Proc Natl Acad Sci U S A* 2000;97:11421–11426.
97. O'Sullivan BJ, Thomas R. CD40 Ligation conditions dendritic cell antigen-presenting function through sustained activation of NF-kappaB. *J Immunol* 2002;168:5491–5498.
98. Martin E, O'Sullivan B, Low P, Thomas R. Antigen-specific suppression of a primed immune response by dendritic cells mediated by regulatory T cells secreting interleukin-10. *Immunity* 2003;18: 155–167.
99. Roncarolo M-G, Levings MK, Traversari C. Differentiation of T regulatory cells by immature dendritic cells. *J Exp Med* 2001;193: F5–F9.
100. Hara M, Kingsley CI, Niimi M, et al. IL-10 is required for regulatory T cells to mediate tolerance to alloantigens in vivo. *J Immunol* 2001;166:3789–3796.
101. Min WP, Gorczynski R, Huang XY, et al. Dendritic cells genetically engineered to express Fas ligand induce donor-specific

hyporesponsiveness and prolong allograft survival. *J Immunol* 2000;164:161–167.

102. Romani N, Gruner S, Brang D, et al. Proliferating dendritic cell progenitors in human blood. *J Exp Med* 1994;180:83–93.
103. Sallusto F, Lanzavecchia A. Efficient presentation of soluble antigen by cultured human dendritic cells is maintained by granulocyte/macrophage colony-stimulating factor plus interleukin 4 and down-regulated by tumor necrosis factor alpha. *J Exp Med* 1994;179:1109–1118.
104. Caux C, Dezutter-Dambuyant C, Schmitt D, Banchereau J. GM-CSF and TNF-a cooperate in the generation of dendritic Langerhans cells. *Nature* 1992;360:258–261.
105. Fairchild PJ, Waldmann H. Dendritic cells and prospects for transplantation tolerance. *Curr Opin Immunol* 2000;12:528–535.
106. Mollah ZUA, Pai S, Moore C, et al. Abnormal NF-κB function characterizes human type 1 diabetes dendritic cells and monocytes. *J Immunol* 2008;180:3166–3175.

Mast Cells

Hans P. Kiener, Peter A. Nigrovic, and David M. Lee

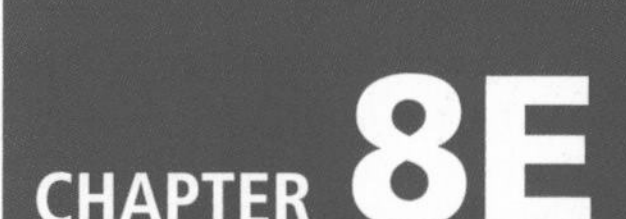

Mast Cell Development

Mast cells are long-lived, tissue-resident, myeloid-lineage cells with a distinctive histologic appearance characterized by abundant cytoplasmic granules. Indeed, their characteristic appearance led the German pathologist Paul Ehrlich to name them *Mastzellen* (*mästen*, German, to feed or fatten an animal) because they appeared to be "overfed" tissue cells[1] (Figure 8E-1). Unlike most other myeloid cells, mast cells do not terminally differentiate in the bone marrow, but rather circulate as rare committed progenitors that deposit in tissues where they complete their differentiation.[2,3] In humans, this progenitor has a surface signature of $CD34^+$/c-kit^+/$CD13^+$.[4] Further developmental details have been worked out most extensively in the mouse, where intermediate multipotent progenitors have been identified in spleen.[5]

Upon entering the tissues, murine mast cells may differentiate further into classic granulated cells or remain as ungranulated progenitors, awaiting local signals to mature fully. Since mast cell maturation is uniquely dependent on local factors, mast cell heterogeneity is extensive. Indeed, some have argued that each tissue supports development of a unique mast cell subpopulation. While this notion awaits further experimental definition, most authorities divide mast cells broadly into two categories termed either connective tissue or mucosal populations, although it is clear that there exist numerous definable subsets within these two populations. Human mast cells are conventionally divided into these two broad classes on the basis of the neutral protease content of their granules (Figure 8E-2).[6] MC_{TC}, typically found in connective tissue such as skin, muscle, intestinal submucosa and the normal synovium, display rounded granules containing the neutral proteases tryptase and chymase.[7] MC_{TC} also express other proteases, including carboxypeptidase and cathepsin G. MC_T, typically found in mucosal sites including the gut lining and the respiratory tract, feature smaller and more irregularly shaped granules that contain tryptase but not chymase. In the mouse, there exists an analogous distinction between connective tissue mast cells (CTMC) and mucosal mast cells (MMC).[8] While these generalities of expression are helpful for discussion of mast cell physiology, it is important to keep in mind that in fact both MC_{TC} and MC_T are present in many locations.[9,10] Beyond protease signatures, other differences between these subsets include their profile of cytokine elaboration as well as cell-surface receptor expression.

Interestingly, in contrast to many other bone marrow–derived lineages whose maturation is unidirectional (including lymphocytes and other myeloid lineages), mature mast cells demonstrate plasticity in their subset phenotype. In classic experiments, adoptive transfer of connective tissue mast cells into a mucosal site engenders a phenotypic switch to that present in the recipient tissue.[11,12] Thus, caution must be exercised in applying overly simplistic rules regarding mast cell behavior or participation in disease.

The mechanisms regulating tissue homing are poorly understood, but are known to involve integrin adhesion molecules and chemokines. Comparison of murine lung and intestine has demonstrated that these tissues use distinct pathways to regulate the constitutive and inducible recruitment of mast cell progenitors, illustrating that mast cell homing is a precisely controlled process.[13]

Tissue Factors

Few details regarding the tissue factors that regulate mast cell maturation and function have been elucidated. Among the factors defined thus far, one of the most important signals from tissue to local mast cells is stem cell factor (SCF).[14] SCF occurs in two alternate forms resulting from differential mRNA splicing: soluble and membrane-bound.[14] The importance of this latter form is clear from Sl/Sl^d mice, which lack only the membrane-bound isoform yet exhibit very few tissue mast cells.[15] SCF is synthesized by multiple lineages, including mast cells themselves. Expression by fibroblasts is probably especially important, given the intimate physical contacts observed between fibroblasts and mast cells in situ. Rodent mast cells co-cultured with fibroblasts demonstrate enhanced survival, connective-tissue phenotypic differentiation, and heightened capacity to elaborate proinflammatory eicosanoids, effects mediated at least in part by direct contact, including interactions between SCF and its ligand c-kit.[16,17] The extent of similar regulation in human mast cells is uncertain.[18]

The receptor for SCF, c-kit, is expressed widely on hematopoietic lineages early in differentiation, but among mature lineages only mast cells express c-kit at a high level. In addition to promoting maturation, stimulation of mast cells by SCF blocks apoptosis, induces chemotaxis and activates mast cells to release mediators. Accordingly, mice with defects in c-kit are strikingly deficient in mature tissue mast cells (examples include W/W^v and W^{sash} strains). Consistent with a central role for c-kit in regulating mast cell behavior, clonal mast cells obtained from

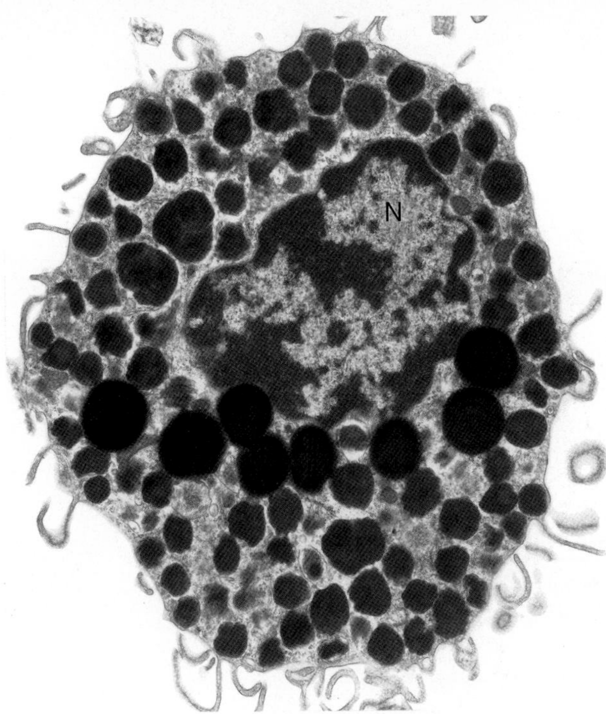

Figure 8E-1. Mast cell morphology. Intact mast cell. *N,* Nucleus. (From Galli SJ, Dvorak AM, Dvorak HF. Basophils and mast cells: Morphologic insights into their biology, secretory patterns, and function. In: Ishizaka K, ed. *Progress in Allergy: Mast Cell Activation and Mediator Release*. Basel: S. Karger, 1984, 1–141.)

patients with systemic mastocytosis commonly exhibit activating mutations in c-kit.[19]

In addition to SCF, it is also known that T-lymphocyte–derived cytokines exert a profound effect on the phenotype of the mucosal subset of tissue mast cells. SCID mice lacking T cells fail to develop mucosal mast cells, a defect that may be corrected by T-cell engraftment.[20] An analogous observation has been made in human patients deficient in T cells due to congenital immunodeficiency or AIDS. Intestinal biopsy in these patients shows that mucosal mast cells (MC_T) are strikingly reduced, while the connective tissue (MC_{TC}) mast cells are present in normal numbers.[21] The pathways by which T cells exert this striking effect are not defined, although it is clear that T-cell cytokines such as IL-3, IL-4, IL-6, and IL-9 may have profound effects on mast cells matured in culture, skewing toward either MC_T or MC_{TC} phenotype.[22,23] By contrast, IFN-γ inhibits mast cell proliferation and may induce apoptosis. These observations imply that cells recruited to an inflamed tissue may profoundly impact the phenotype and survival of local mast cells.

Tissue Distribution

The tissue distribution of mast cells is extensive. Mast cells tend to cluster around blood vessels, nerves, and near epithelial and mucosal surfaces. They are also found in the lining of vulnerable body cavities such as the peritoneum and the diarthrodial joint. Given this localization, mast cells are among the first immune cells to encounter pathogens invading into tissue from the external world or via the bloodstream.

This microanatomic localization, combined with their innate immune effector functions, support the concept that mast cells are immune sentinel cells that sense pathogen presence and rapidly mobilize the immune response.[24] Consistent with this sentinel function, mast cells are equipped to recognize pathogens or other threats both autonomously and in the context of signals from other immune lineages. Mast cells are capable of response in the absence of guidance from other lineages via their expression of a range of pathogen receptors, including multiple toll-like receptors and CD48, a surface protein recognizing the fimbrial antigen FimH.[25,26] Furthermore, mast cells may also be activated through complement, including the anaphylatoxins C3a and C5a.[27] Additionally, mast cells can respond directly to physical stimuli including trauma, temperature, and osmotic stress.[28] Together, these receptors enable autonomous mast cell involvement in a broad range of immune and nonimmune processes.

Mast cells also respond to input stimuli from a number of other members of the immune system. The canonical pathway to mast cell activation is via IgE and its receptor FcεRI. With a K_a of 10^{10}/M, this receptor is essentially constantly saturated with IgE at typical serum concentrations.[29] Cross-linking FcεRI-bound IgE by antigen induces a brisk and vigorous response. Within minutes, granules within the mast cell fuse together and with the surface membrane, creating a set of labyrinthine channels that allow rapid release of granule contents[30] in a process termed anaphylactic degranulation (Figure 8E-3). This brisk event is followed within minutes by the elaboration of eicosanoids newly synthesized from arachidonic acid cleaved from internal membrane lipids. Finally, signals transduced via FcεRI induce the transcription of new genes and elaboration of a wide range of chemokines and cytokines. However, IgE is only one among many pathways of mast cell activation. It has more recently been appreciated that IgG is a key trigger for mast cell activation in both human and mouse. The importance of this pathway was demonstrated first in mice rendered genetically deficient in IgE which surprisingly remained susceptible to mast cell–dependent anaphylaxis mediated through IgG and the low-affinity IgG receptor FcγRIII.[31,32] The human counterpart of this receptor, FcγRIIa, is equally capable of inducing activation of human mast cells.[33] Mast cells also coordinate with immune and non-immune lineages via soluble mediators and surface receptors. Examples of such signals include the cytokine TNF and the neurogenic peptide substance P, which can induce mast cell degranulation.[27,34] Physical contact with other cells can also induce mast cell activation. For example, CD30 on lymphocytes can interact with CD30L on mast cells to induce the production of a range of chemokines.[35] Interestingly, ligation of CD30L does not induce release of granule contents or lipid mediators, illustrating the selectivity of response of which mast cells are capable.

Mast Cells in the Normal Joint

Mast cells have long been recognized to reside in the normal human joint,[36–39] where they constitute almost 3% of nucleated cells residing within 70 μm of the synovial lining.[40] The contribution of synovial mast cells to normal joint physiology is unknown. Electron microscopy of normal human synovium reveals morphologic evidence of degranulation in approximately 1% to 5% of mast cells, suggesting a basal elaboration of mast cell factors with a potential contribution to joint homeostasis. However, it remains possible that this observation represents an artifact of tissue extraction and preparation.[41,42] Synovial morphology is grossly

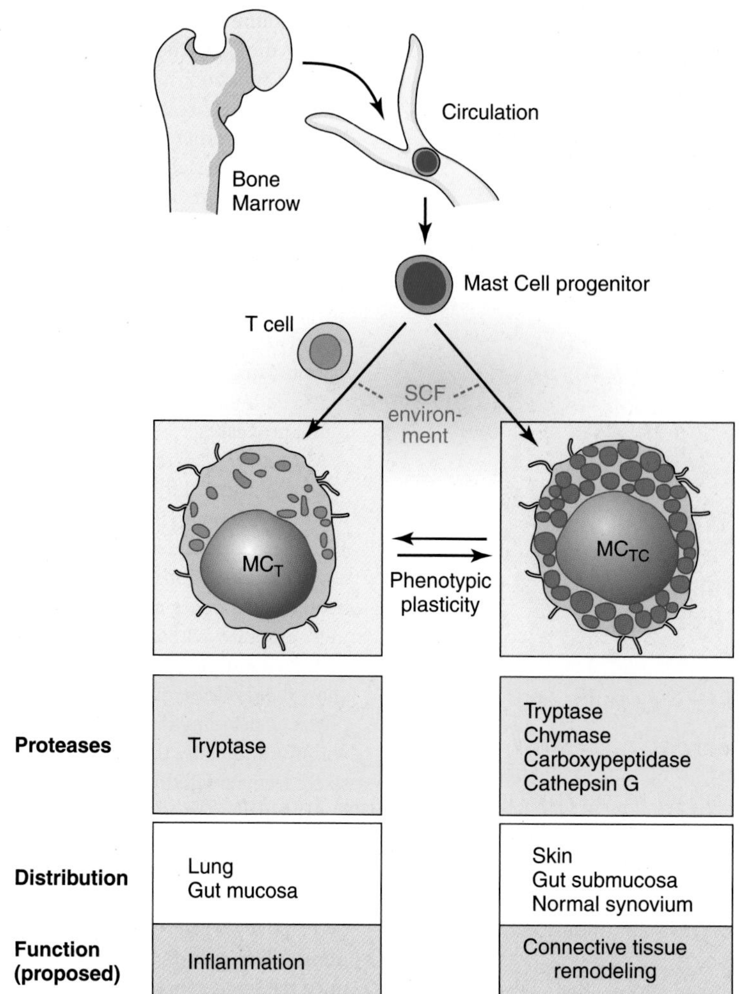

Figure 8E-2. Mast cell differentiation. Mast cells arise in the bone marrow, circulate as committed progenitors, and differentiate into mature mast cells upon entering tissue. Human mast cells may be classified on the basis of granule proteases into tryptase$^+$ mast cells (MC_T) and tryptase$^+$/chymase$^+$ mast cells (MC_{TC}), with characteristic tissue localization and mediator production. (Adapted from Gurish MF, Austen KF. The diverse roles of mast cells. *J Exp Med* 2001;194:F1–F5. Illustration by Steven Moskowitz.)

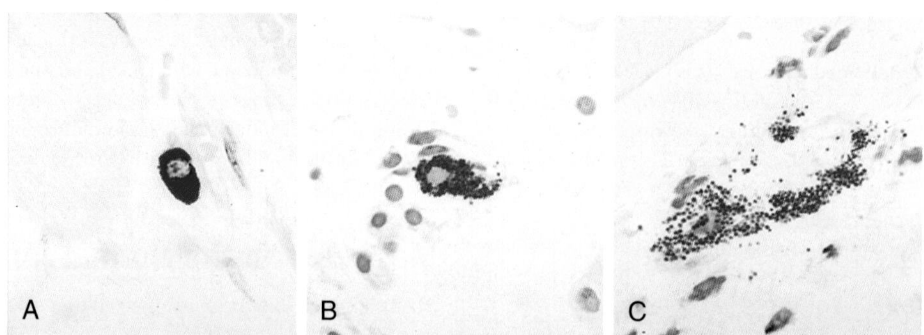

Figure 8E-3. Mast cell degranulation. Shown are murine tissue mast cells stained with chloroacetate esterase and hematoxylin to highlight granule contents. (A) Normal mast cell with tightly packed cytoplasmic granules and a central nucleus. (B) Activated mast cell displaying piecemeal degranulation. Note the loosely packed cytoplasmic granules and the presence of granules beyond the apparent cell membrane. (C) Mast cell undergoing robust "anaphylactic" degranulation with extensive extravasation of granules into the surrounding microenvironment. Magnification 630×. (Courtesy of Daniel S. Friend, MD.)

intact in mast cell–deficient W/W^v and W^{sash} mice, weighing against an obligate trophic role for this cell.

Phenotypically, the granules of most synovial mast cells contain both tryptase and chymase (MC_{TC}), though mast cells staining for tryptase alone (MC_T) are also observed in varying proportion, usually in mast cells found close to the synovial lining.[43,44] Microanatomically, they are not observed within the synovial lining layer itself but rather populate the sublining loose connective tissue and adipose tissue, where they cluster near blood vessels and nerves and may occasionally be seen at the junction of cartilage and synovium.[37,40,45] The concentration of mast cells in the immediate synovial sublining appears to be several-fold higher than in areas more distant from the joint, implying a kind of "focus" on the joint lining and articular cavity.[43] They are not seen within the cartilage and are rare in normal periarticular bone.[37,45]

Functional characterization of mast cell responses to stimulation has not been reported from healthy human synovium. Extrapolation from mast cells obtained from osteoarthritic tissue suggests that they may be activated by cross-linking of IgE and calcium ionophores as well as stem cell factor (SCF); some authors but not others identify responsiveness to the polyamine 48/80.[41,46–49] Unlike cutaneous mast cells, mast cells from osteoarthritis (OA) synovium do not respond to the anaphylatoxin C5a[41,49] or morphine.[48] In addition to histamine, synovial mast cells obtained from OA specimens are capable of elaborating approximately equivalent amounts of prostaglandin D_2 (PGD_2) and leukotriene C_4 (LTC_4) when stimulated by IgE cross-linking, unlike mast cells in skin which synthesize PGD_2 preferentially.[41,46] The interpretation of all these functional studies is limited by the presence of non-mast cell lineages in the preparations tested, resulting in the potential for activation of mast cell by bystander cells. However, in aggregate, these observations support the idea that synovial mast cells exhibit a functional profile distinct from mast cells in other tissue sites.

In the normal mouse joint, mast cells are also localized to the sublining, where they cluster around blood vessels and nerves. Recent studies demonstrate that these cells are uniformly of the connective tissue mast cell (CTMC) subtype, expressing the murine mast cell proteases (mMCP) -4, -5, -6, and -7, but not mMCP-1 and -2.[50] Unlike murine mucosal mast cells, their presence in tissue is not dependent on functional T cells. Some regional heterogeneity of phenotype is observed. Mast cells near blood vessels stain brightly for mMCP5, while mast cells near the synovial lining stain more dimly, suggesting microenvironmental regulation of the mast cell phenotype within normal synovium.[50] While isolation of these cells for functional characterization has not been performed, data in rats indicate the expected susceptibility of rodent synovial mast cells to degranulation via IgE cross-linking,[51,52] while experimental data in the mouse implicate the presence of the low-affinity IgG receptor FcγRIII on at least a subpopulation of murine synovial mast cells.[53]

Mast Cell Mediators

Mast cell effector functions encompass a broad range of biologic activities (Table 8E-1). Upon stimulation, initial events are generally a very rapid (within seconds to minutes) release of granule contents. Mature mast cells package a range of mediators in their granules, ready for immediate release through fusion with the surface membrane. Beyond preformed granules, activated mast cells elaborate a range of mediators that are generated *de novo*. These mediators are released minutes to hours after stimulation, extending the impact of activated mast cells on surrounding tissues. Among these mediators are proinflammatory lipids, which are generated rapidly (within minutes) after stimulation. Thereafter, a broad range of newly synthesized immunomodulatory proteins are elaborated over hours after stimulation. Not surprisingly, the release of these mediators is not all or none. Rather, mast cell effector responses are highly regulated and variable. For release of granule contents, in addition to anaphylactic degranulation, mast cells may release only a few granules at a time in a process termed *piecemeal degranulation*[54] (Figure 8E-3). Alternately, under other conditions mast cells may elaborate cytokines and chemokines without any release of granule contents, as illustrated by activation via CD30L.[35] Thus, while the mast cell is well equipped to release large volumes of preformed mediators, it is equally capable of responses tailored to the activating stimulus.

Granule Contents

The most abundant of these are the neutral proteases, named tryptases, chymases, and carboxypetidases for their enzymatic activity at normal extracellular (neutral) pH. In addition, vasoactive amines, proteoglycans such as heparin, and preformed cytokines play distinct roles in the biologic consequences of mast cell degranulation. Tryptase, named for its enzymatic similarity to pancreatic trypsin, is the most abundant granule protein in human mast cells[55] and is an essentially specific marker for mast cells.[56] The enzyme found in granules is the beta isomer, which becomes enzymatically active upon formation of a homotetramer that relies on the scaffolding function of the proteoglycan heparin.[57] Mast cells also synthesize α-tryptase, which is not stored in granules but constitutively released into circulation, where its function is unknown. The distinction between tryptase isomers is important for diagnostic reasons: as a marker of degranulation, systemic levels of β-tryptase constitute a marker of recent anaphylaxis.[58] By contrast, α-trypsin levels reflect total body mast cell load and serve as a useful biomarker in systemic mastocytosis.[59] Functionally, β-tryptase directly cleaves structural proteins such as fibronectin and type IV collagen, and enzymatically activates stromelysin, an enzyme responsible for activating collagenase.[60] Cleavage of protease-activated receptors such as PAR2 likely contributes to other activities such as promoting hyperplasia and activation of fibroblasts, airway smooth muscle cells, and epithelium.[61–63] Taken together, these effects point to an important role for tryptase in regulating extracellular matrix. A further contribution to the inflammatory milieu is suggested by the capacity of tryptase to promote neutrophil and eosinophil recruitment and to cleave C3 to generate the anaphylatoxin C3a.[64,65]

The chymotrypsin-like neutral protease chymase is found in the MC_{TC} subset of human mast cells, packaged within the same granules as tryptase.[7] Like tryptase, chymase can cleave matrix components and activate stromelysin, though it can also activate collagenase directly, suggesting a role in matrix remodeling.[66] Chymase can also potentially impact inflammatory responses, with capacity to inactivate proinflammatory cytokines such as IL-6 and TNF as well as to cleave pro–IL-1β to generate active cytokine.[67,68]

Other mast cell granule contents include vasoactive amines, the proteoglycans heparin and chondroitin sulfate E, and

Table 8E-1. Human Mast Cell Mediators of Potential Importance in Arthritis

	Relevant Functions
Granules	
Histamine	Vascular permeability, leukocyte recruitment, fibroblast/chondrocyte activation
Heparin	Angiogenesis, osteoclast differentiation and activation
Tryptase	Matrix degradation, leukocyte recruitment, fibroblast activation, cytokine inactivation
Chymase	
	Matrix degradation, cytokine inactivation
TNF	Leukocyte recruitment, fibroblast/chondrocyte activation
Eicosanoid mediators	
PGD_2	Vascular permeability, neutrophil recruitment
LTB_4	Vascular permeability, leukocyte recruitment and activation
Cysteinyl leukotrienes	Vascular permeability, fibroblast mitogen (LTC_4)
PAF	Leukocyte recruitment
Cytokines/chemokines	
IL-1	Leukocyte recruitment, fibroblast/chondrocyte activation, angiogenesis
IL-3	Leukocyte growth factor, mast cell growth factor
IL-4	Immunomodulatory, pro-fibrotic
IL-6	Activation of T and B lymphocytes and fibroblasts
IL-8	Neutrophil recruitment
IL-10	Immunomodulatory
IL-13	Immunomodulatory, B-cell stimulation
IL-18	Angiogenesis, lymphocyte stimulation
TNF	Leukocyte recruitment and activation, fibroblast/chondrocyte activation
TGF-β	Immunomodulatory, fibroblast mitogen
PDGF	Fibroblast mitogen
VEGF	Fibroblast mitogen, angiogenesis
bFGF	Fibroblast mitogen, angiogenesis
MCP-1	Leukocyte recruitment
MIP-1α, -1β	Leukocyte recruitment, osteoclast differentiation
RANTES	Leukocyte recruitment

Modified from Nigrovic PA, Lee DM. Mast cells in inflammatory arthritis. *Arthritis Res Ther* 2005;7:1–11.
For a comprehensive list of human and rodent mast cell mediators, see Galli SJ, Nakae S, Tsai M. Mast cells in the development of adaptive immune responses. *Nat Immunol* 2005;6:135–142.
TNF, Tumor necrosis factor; *PGD_2,* Prostaglandin D_2, *LTB_4,* Leukotriene B_4; *LTC_4,* Leukotriene C_4; *PAF,* Platelet activating factor; *IL,* Interleukin; *TGF-β,* Transforming growth factor-β; *PDGF,* Platelet-derived growth factor; *VEGF,* Vascular endothelial growth factor; *bFGF,* Basic fibroblast growth factor; *MCP-1,* Monocyte chemoattractant protein-1; *MIP,* Macrophage inflammatory protein; *RANTES,* Released upon activation, normal T-cell expressed and secreted.

preformed cytokines. Histamine is by far the most abundant vasoactive amine found in both MC_T and MC_{TC} mast cells. Synthesized by neutrophils as well as mast cells, histamine is involved in the wheal-and-flare response to cutaneous allergen challenge, via augmented vascular permeability, transendothelial vesicular transport, and neurogenic vasodilatation.[69] The large proteoglycans enable the ordered packing of mediators within human mast cell granules.[70,71] Negatively-charged carbohydrate side chains complex tightly with positively-charged proteins, allowing very high concentrations of β-tryptase and other proteases. Heparin also has a wide range of effects beyond the mast cell including stimulation of angiogenesis,[72] anticoagulation via activation of antithrombin III, and the inhibition of both classical and alternative pathways of complement activation.[73] Furthermore, mast cells store cytokines in their granules for rapid release. The first of these to be documented was TNF.[74] In the mouse, this pool of TNF is implicated in the rapid recruitment of neutrophils to the peritoneum during peritonitis.[75,76] Other cytokines that may be stored in granules include IL-4, IL-16, basic fibroblast growth factor (bFGF), and vascular endothelial growth factor (VEGF).

Mast Cells in Rheumatoid Synovitis

In rheumatoid synovitis, mast cells accumulate in the synovial membrane to such a degree that early histomorphometric studies described a "mastocytosis" within the rheumatoid synovium[43,45–47,77,78] (Figure 8E-4). Indeed, mast cells are markedly increased in number in most synovial specimens from patients with rheumatoid arthritis (RA). Averaging in excess of

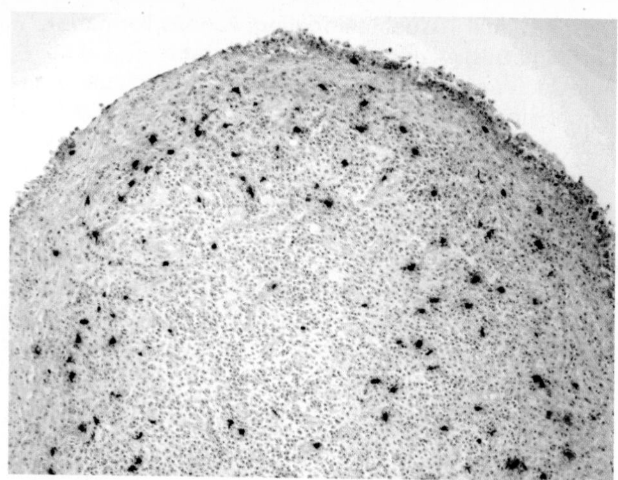

Figure 8E-4. Mast cells within the rheumatoid synovium. Fixed, paraffin-embedded synovial tissue was obtained during arthroplasty from a patient with RA. Tissue sections were labeled with an antibody against tryptase and counterstained with hematoxylin. Note the frequent tryptase positive mast cells (brown) present beneath the synovial sublining. (Section 5 μm thick, original magnification ×100.)

tenfold above normal, mast cells can make up 5% or more of the expanded population of total synovial cells. Varying directly with the intensity of joint inflammation, however, the number of accumulated mast cells differs substantially from patient to patient.[45,79] Accompanying the increased numbers of mast cells, mast cell mediators such as histamine and tryptase are also present at higher concentrations in the synovial fluid of the afflicted joints.[80–82] Levels of histamine in the synovial fluid are typically higher when compared to those in plasma, suggesting local release.[83] Mast cells are present throughout the rheumatoid synovial sublining, often accumulating in close proximity to the hyperplastic synovial lining layer and around lymphoid aggregates.[45] By contrast, they are rarely found within the thickened synovial lining layer or within lymphoid aggregates. Occasionally, mast cells populate the pannus near sites of cartilage and bone erosion.[84] Unlike the normal human synovium, rheumatoid synovium contains mast cells of both subtypes, MC_{TC} and MC_T, at various ratios.[85] MC_T tend to be found more superficially in association with lymphoid aggregates, whereas MC_{TC} are generally found in deeper, more fibrotic areas of the inflamed synovium.[43,49,86] Interestingly, although mast cells from RA and OA express a generally similar panel of surface receptors, RA but not OA mast cells have been observed to express the receptor for the anaphylatoxin complement fragment C5a (CD88).[49] Microanatomic mast cell accumulation, the various ratios of MC_{TC} and MC_T, and the altered surface receptor expression (e.g., C5a-receptor expression) associated with rheumatoid synovitis presumably reflect the heterogeneity of pathologic pathways operative in patients with RA.

Mechanisms of Mast Cell Accumulation in Rheumatoid Synovitis

Synovial mastocytosis is not limited to RA. Expansion of human synovial mast cells has been noted in a range of arthropathies, including OA, psoriatic arthritis, and traumatic arthritis.[43,46,47,49,78,87] The mechanisms underlying local mast cell accumulation at sites of inflammation are poorly defined. Based on several observations, mast cell expansion is most likely due to an enhanced influx of mast cell progenitors followed by local maturation. In fact, mast cells detectable at sites of active inflammation often display features of immature cells. Furthermore, immunostaining revealed low expression of the proliferation antigen Ki-67 in synovial mast cells, suggesting that proliferation is not a critical contributor to expansion.[78]

In the context of rheumatoid synovitis several molecular pathways may account for the recruitment of mast cell progenitors to the synovium. In contrast to mature mast cells, mast cell progenitors express β2-integrins and ligands for selectins that may facilitate transmigration through the endothelial cell layer.[13,88] Potential chemoattractants promoting recruitment of mast cells to the joint include C5a, LTB_4, TGF-β, and serotonin, mediators abundantly detectable in the synovial fluid of patients with RA.[89–91] Further, synovial mast cells express the urokinase-type plasminogen activator receptor (CD87), ligation of which induces chemotaxis in human mast cells.[49,92] More recently, RA but not OA synovial mast cells have been observed to express the chemokine receptor CXCR3. The respective ligands, CXCL9 and CXCL10, are heavily expressed in the rheumatoid synovium.[93]

Stem cell factor, the major regulator of mast cell growth, survival and differentiation may play a pivotal role in synovial mast cell accumulation in RA.[94] SCF also functions as a mast cell chemoattractant.[95] It is abundantly expressed in the inflamed synovium on various cell populations including lining and sublining fibroblast-like synoviocytes, endothelial cells, and macrophages.[78,96] Importantly, the arthritogenic cytokine TNF promotes the expression of SCF in synovial fibroblasts resulting in their increased capacity to induce mast cell chemotaxis, maturation, and survival.[96]

The distribution and retention of leukocytes in solid tissues is determined in part by adhesion molecules mediating cellular binding to components of the extracellular matrix or tissue resident cells. Mast cells isolated from the inflamed synovium express various adhesion molecules, including the β-chain of β1 integrins (CD29), the β-chain of β3 integrins (CD61), the glycoprotein CD44, leukosialin (CD43), the intercellular adhesion molecule-3 (CD50), the intercellular adhesion molecule-1 (CD54), and the leukocyte function–associated antigen-3 (CD58).[49] The functional importance of these molecules for the accumulation of mast cells in RA remains to be elucidated.

Mechanisms of Mast Cell Activation in Rheumatoid Synovitis

Consistent with their activation in the context of synovial inflammation, granule exocytosis from a significant proportion of synovial mast cells is evident in microscopic analyses of synovial tissue sections from patients with RA.[45,46,84] In fact, 10% to 15% of mast cells showed signs of degranulation in one series. By contrast, in the normal synovium less than 1% of mast cells demonstrated granule exocytosis.[42] In the context of RA, several pathways may be involved in mast cell activation. Like mast cells in other tissues, synovial mast cells express FcεRI and granule exocytosis could be initiated by cross-linking of FcεRI-bound IgE.[49] IgE antibodies against collagen, rheumatoid factor of the IgE isotype, and autoantibodies directed to IgE have been observed in some patients with RA.[97–99]

Given the abundance of IgG immune complexes in rheumatoid synovitis, activation through receptors for IgG (FcγRs) is particularly relevant. Like cutaneous mast cells, human synovial mast cells express the low affinity activating IgG Fc-receptor FcγRIIa (CD32a) (P.A. Nigrovic, unpublished observation).[33] Thus, autoantibodies commonly associated with RA, such as those against citrullinated peptides might contribute to synovial mast cell activation. Other potential agonists for synovial mast cell activation in RA include SCF and components of the complement system. SCF is elaborated by synovial fibroblasts and its expression is augmented by TNF.[96] SCF induces release of granule content via c-kit and significantly enhances FcεRI-dependent activation of synovial mast cells.[49] Likewise, complement activation in the inflammatory microenvironment, as evidenced by appreciable concentrations of C5a in the synovial fluid of patients with RA, is a plausible pathway for mast cell activation via the C5a receptor (CD88).[49,100]

It is important to keep in mind that the extent to which these stimuli mediate activation of synovial mast cells in human arthritis remains speculative. Even though potential mechanisms have been identified, other pathways including direct interaction of mast cells with infiltrating T cells (CD30L, see above) or stimulation through toll-like receptors (TLRs) could potentially be involved. Expression of TLRs by synovial mast cells has not yet been defined, but mast cells in other tissues have been noted to express TLRs.[25] Therefore, even in the absence of infection, potential endogenous TLR ligands such as degradation products of hyaluronan, fibronectin, or heat shock proteins, could be relevant for mast cell activation in inflammatory arthritis.[101]

Mast Cell Effector Functions in Rheumatoid Synovitis

Endothelial Cell Activation, Leukocyte Recruitment, and Angiogenesis

In line with the concept that mast cells serve as immune sentinels, several mast cell mediators act on the vasculature to initiate or propagate inflammation. Once activated, mast cells release preformed or newly synthesized vasoactive mediators. Histamine, prostaglandine D2, and the leukotriens increase vascular permeability, thereby contributing to edema formation and fibrin deposition.[102] TNF, IL-1, and histamine promote the expression of the adhesion molecules P-selectin, E-selectin, ICAM-1, and VCAM-1 on endothelial cells.[103] Circulating leukocytes could then be efficiently recruited to the synovium along gradients of chemotactic mast cell products such as leukotriene B_4, monocytes chemoattractant protein-1, IL-8, and RANTES.[104] Mast cell–derived proteases (tryptases, chymases, tissue plasminogen activator [tPA]) together with heparin may facilitate leukocyte locomotion within the inflamed synovium by means of matrix degradation and inhibition of fibrin deposition.[105] Further, mast cells have been shown to elaborate potent angiogenic factors including vascular endothelial growth factor (VEGF), basic fibroblast growth factor (bFGF), and platelet-derived growth factor (PDGF).[106] Thus, mast cells, in cooperation with other sources of these angiogenic factors, may contribute to the growth of blood vessels that is associated with synovial hyperplasia in RA.

Mesenchymal Tissue Remodeling, Pannus Formation, Cartilage Destruction, and Bone Erosions

In RA, a distinct mesenchymal tissue reaction yields the formation of an aggressive, condensed mass of cells (pannus) that erodes into the articular cartilage and bone. Prominent within the pannus are synovial fibroblasts which are the predominant cell type at the cartilage-pannus junction.[107] Mast cells produce an array of mediators that may direct synovial fibroblasts in the context of rheumatoid synovitis. Mast cell tryptase is a potent mitogen for fibroblasts, also inducing fibroblast chemotaxis and synthesis of collagen.[108] Other mast cell–derived products regulating fibroblast behavior may include histamine, nerve growth factor (NGF), PDGF, bFGF, and TGF-β.[109] Consistent with microanatomic accumulation of mast cells of the tryptase-chymase phenotype MC_{TC} in deep, more fibrotic areas of the hyperplastic synovial lining, these mast cells are capable of producing the cytokine IL-4,[110] an inducer of proliferation and collagen synthesis in fibroblasts.[111] Moreover, synovial mast cells may activate synovial fibroblasts through cytokines such as TNF and IL-1. Both TNF and IL-1 stimulate fibroblasts to produce matrix metalloproteinases and prostaglandin E_2. Strikingly, collagenase expression by fibroblasts has been observed to localize to the immediate environment of activated mast cells.[112] Besides acting on fibroblasts, mast cells may determine connective tissue matrix turnover through their proteases. For example, tryptase activates stromelysin (MMP3) that in turn activates collagenase, an enzyme whose substrates include collagen, fibronectin, and proteoglycans.[97,113] In rheumatoid synovitis, mast cells frequently localize to the cartilage–pannus junction and may facilitate pannus invasion into cartilage by inducing fibroblast cellular condensation, their invasive migratory behavior, and increasing their destructive potential through the abovementioned mediators.[84] Mast cells may also modulate the function of chondrocytes. Chondrocytes express receptors for mast cell mediators including histamine, IL-1, TNF, and bFGF. Indeed, chondrocytes co-cultured with mast cells exhibit increased proteoglycan synthesis. Once mast cells are activated, however, newly synthesized proteoglycans rapidly become degraded.[114] Thus, mast cells may contribute to cartilage loss of proteoglycans observed in inflammatory arthritis.

Mast cells may similarly participate in inflammatory bone resorption in RA, both focal erosions and periarticular osteopenia. Mast cells may facilitate this process through mediators such as heparin, MIP-1α, IL-6, and TNF which promote the differentiation and activation of osteoclasts, the cells ultimately mediating bone resorption.[115–118]

Resolution of Inflammation

Beyond their role in mediating inflammatory reactions, several lines of evidence now suggest that mast cells may contribute to the resolution of inflammation. Mechanisms by which mast cells counterbalance inflammation are beginning to emerge. For example, both mast cell tryptase and chymase are capable of degrading proinflammatory cytokines such as IL-6, a cytokine successfully targeted therapeutically in RA.[68] Fibrin deposition is a characteristic feature of rheumatoid synovitis. Mast cell mediators such as heparin and tPA support fibrinolysis and counteract further fibrin generation.[105] Notably, the number of mast cells is inversely related to the amount of fibrin deposits in the inflamed synovium in RA.[79] Further, recent observations suggest that mast cells may down-modulate immune-mediated inflammatory reactions by acting downstream of regulatory T cells to achieve peripheral immunologic tolerance.[119]

Lessons from Animal Models

Numerous rodent models point to a functional contribution from mast cells in the pathogenesis of inflammatory arthritis. In the rat adjuvant arthritis model (induced by intradermal injection of mycobacterial adjuvant), mast cells are the first cell to accumulate abnormally in the joint, several days prior to the onset of clinical arthritis.[120] Mast cell numbers appear to decline strikingly as arthritis begins and other lineages began to arrive, perhaps a result of the difficulty visualizing fully degranulated mast cells with standard stains ("phantom mast cells").[51,52,121] Degranulation early in arthritis has been noted in other rodent models as well. These include streptococcal cell wall arthritis (initiated by intravenous injection of Group A streptococcal polysaccharide),[122] intra-articular injection of arthritogenic factor in collagen-induced arthritis,[123] arthritis mediated by systemic administration of autoantibody-containing K/BxN serum[124] as well as antigen-induced arthritis and collagen-induced arthritis in rats.[125,126] These observations suggest that mast cell activation may be an important early event in arthritis, perhaps contributing to the initiation of joint inflammation.

More recently, experiments in mast cell–deficient animals have enabled a more detailed understanding of the contributions of the mast cell to arthritis. In the autoantibody-driven, K/BxN serum transfer model, mast cell–deficient W/W^v and Sl/Sl^d mice are resistant to arthritis induction.[124,127] This resistance is defeated in the W/W^v animal by engraftment with wildtype mast cells, implicating the mast cell as a key link in the pathogenesis of this immune complex-mediated arthritis. Subsequent analyses provide further insight into the mechanisms by which the mast cells enable arthritis. In the hyperacute phase of K/BxN serum transfer arthritis, mast cells have emerged as a key player in modulating access of arthritogenic antibodies to the joint by contributing to joint-specific vascular leak within minutes of K/BxN serum infusion.[128–130] Yet vascular leak does not appear to be the entire contribution of this lineage. Rats depleted of mast cell granules by pretreatment with compound 48/80 fail to develop limb edema, but still go on to develop arthritis following intravenous injection of streptococcal polysaccharide.[122] Similarly, mice engineered to be resistant to vascular leak remain partially susceptible to K/BxN arthritis.[128] While in both models arthritis without vascular leak tended to be mild, this phenotype does not approach the pronounced resistance of W/W^v and Sl/Sl^d mice[124] providing strong evidence that mast cells do more than mediate vascular permeability.

The K/BxN serum transfer model also affords opportunity to examine the stimuli that activate mast cells as well as the contribution of candidate mast cell effector functions to arthritis pathogenesis. Engrafting W/W^v animals with mast cells genetically deficient in expression of the low-affinity Fc gamma receptor, FcγRIII, demonstrated that mast cell expression of this receptor is required for activation through K/BxN serum.[131] This observation is consistent with the demonstrated contribution of immune complexes to K/BxN arthritis pathogenesis, and murine mast cell susceptibility to immune complex activation via FcγRIII.[132–135] Among the mast cell effector functions elicited by stimulation through FcγRIII is production of IL-1, an essential cytokine in K/BxN arthritis.[136] Engrafting W/W^v animals with mast cells unable to elaborate IL-1 demonstrates these selectively defective mast cells are incapable of restoring arthritis susceptibility to W/W^v animals, implying that mast cells are an essential source of this proinflammatory mediator.[131] These observations contrast with other candidate mast cell–effector functions. Since mast cells can robustly elaborate leukotrienes, and since K/BxN arthritis is dependent on leukotriene generation,[137] the contribution of synovial mast cells as a source of lipid mediators was assessed. These studies demonstrated that mast cells deficient in leukotriene production mediate arthritis normally.[137]

Taken together, these observations suggest the following model for a role for mast cells in initiating arthritis in this mouse model. Mast cells resident within the murine synovium are activated by immune complexes formed either in circulation or within the joint via the low affinity Fc-receptor FcγRIII. Subsequent elaboration of IL-1 by mast cells contributes to the establishment of full arthritis, with influx of inflammatory cells and activation of local synoviocytes. We have referred to this activity of the mast cell as the "jump start"—a burst of proinflammatory mediators that promotes the establishment of autoantibody-driven synovitis. Assessment of the generalizability of these observations awaits further experimental evidence.

These mechanisms will likely not apply in all causes of arthritis. One group has found that W/W^v mice remain susceptible to antigen-induced arthritis (AIA), in which immunized animals develop arthritis in joints injected directly with the immunizing antigen; a subtle contribution of mast cells was identified to the intensity of arthritis flare induced by systemic administration of antigen.[138] The pathophysiologic pathways underlying the differential requirement for mast cells in K/BxN serum transfer arthritis and AIA have not been defined.

Conclusion

Mast cells are potent immune cells present in abundance in the inflamed synovium of RA. Their contributions to murine models of arthritis is increasingly appreciated and the subject of active investigation. Since this lineage is characterized by phenotypic diversity and an extremely broad range of functions in health and disease, it is likely that their participation in arthritis pathophysiology will be multifactorial (Figure 8E-5). Further insights into the mechanisms by which they contribute to arthritis may present interesting targets for the development of novel anti-inflammatory therapies in RA.

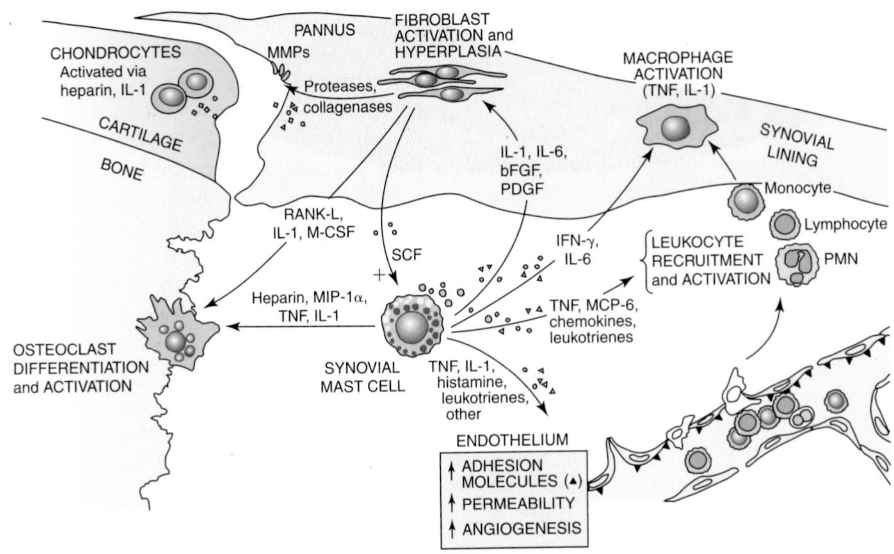

Figure 8E-5. Candidate proinflammatory functions of mast cells in rheumatoid synovitis. Mast cell effector functions suggest their participation in diverse pathogenic pathways in arthritis, including endothelial cell activation, leukocyte recruitment and activation, synovial fibroblast activation and hyperplasia, angiogenesis, and cartilage and bone destruction. Activated mast cells elaborate mediators potently capable of enhancing vasopermeability, including endothelial expression of adhesion molecules, recruiting circulating leukocytes, and activating infiltrating leukocytes as well as resident macrophages, thereby contributing to the early phases of inflammatory arthritis. In chronic synovitis, mast cells synthesize mitogens and cytokines that activate synovial fibroblasts, recruit macrophages, and promote the growth of new blood vessels, implicating them in synovial lining hyperplasia and pannus formation. Further, mast cells may participate in joint destruction by the induction of matrix metalloproteinases (MMPs) from fibroblasts, by activation of chondrocytes, and by direct and indirect promotion of osteoclast differentiation and activation. Because activated synovial fibroblasts demonstrate enhanced stem cell factor (SCF) expression, a potentially important positive feedback loop is established in which SCF promotes mast cell differentiation from progenitors and survival of mature mast cells, leading to the mastocytosis described in inflamed synovium. Note that the importance of these candidate pathways in vivo remains to be established. *bFGF,* Basic fibroblast growth factor; *IFN,* Interferon; *IL,* Interleukin; *MCP,* Monocyte chemoattractant protein; *M-CSF,* Macrophage colony–stimulating factor; *MIP,* Macrophage inflammatory protein; *PDGF,* Platelet-derived growth factor; *PMN,* Polymorphnuclear cell; *Rank-L,* Receptor activator of NF-κB ligand; *TNF,* Tumor necrosis factor. (From Nigrovic PA, Lee DM. Mast cells in inflammatory arthritis. *Arthritis Res Ther* 2005;7:1–11. Graphic design by Steve Moskowitz.)

References

1. Ehrlich P. *Beiträge zur Theorie und Praxis der Histologischen Färbung.* Thesis, Leipzig University, 1878.
2. Kitamura Y, Go S, Hatanaka K. Decrease of mast cells in W/Wv mice and their increase by bone marrow transplantation. *Blood* 1978;52:447–452.
3. Rodewald HR, Dessing M, Dvorak AM, Galli SJ. Identification of a committed precursor for the mast cell lineage. *Science* 1996;271: 818–822.
4. Rottem M, Okada T, Goff JP, Metcalfe DD. Mast cells cultured from the peripheral blood of normal donors and patients with mastocytosis originate from a CD34+/Fc epsilon RI− cell population. *Blood* 1994;84:2489–2496.
5. Arinobu Y, Iwasaki H, Gurish MF. Developmental checkpoints of the basophil/mast cell lineages in adult murine hematopoiesis. *Proc Natl Acad Sci U S A* 2005;102:18105–18110.
6. Irani AA, Schechter NM, Craig SS, et al. Two types of human mast cells that have distinct neutral protease compositions. *Proc Natl Acad Sci U S A* 1986;83:4464–4468.
7. Craig SS, Schechter NM, Schwartz LB. Ultrastructural analysis of human T and TC mast cells identified by immunoelectron microscopy. *Lab Invest* 1988;58:682–691.
8. Gurish MF, Austen KF. The diverse roles of mast cells. *J Exp Med* 2001;194:F1–F5.
9. Weidner N, Austen KF. Heterogeneity of mast cells at multiple body sites. Fluorescent determination of avidin binding and immunofluorescent determination of chymase, tryptase, and carboxypeptidase content. *Pathol Res Pract* 1993;189:156–162.
10. Irani AM, Bradford TR, Kepley CL, et al. Detection of MCT and MCTC types of human mast cells by immunohistochemistry using new monoclonal anti-tryptase and anti-chymase antibodies. *J Histochem Cytochem* 1989;37:1509–1515.
11. Sonoda S, Sonoda T, Nakano T, et al. Development of mucosal mast cells after injection of a single connective tissue-type mast cell in the stomach mucosa of genetically mast cell-deficient W/Wv mice. *J Immunol* 1986;137:1319–1322.
12. Kanakura Y, Thompson H, Nakano T, et al. Multiple bidirectional alterations of phenotype and changes in proliferative potential during the in vitro and in vivo passage of clonal mast cell populations derived from mouse peritoneal mast cells. *Blood* 1988;72:877–885.
13. Gurish MF, Tao H, Abonia JP, et al. Intestinal mast cell progenitors require CD49dbeta7 (alpha4beta7 integrin) for tissue-specific homing. *J Exp Med* 2001;194:1243–1252.
14. Galli SJ, Zsebo M, Geissler EN. The kit ligand, stem cell factor. *Adv Immunol* 1994;55:1–96.
15. Flanagan JG, Chan DC, Leder P. Transmembrane form of the kit ligand growth factor is determined by alternative splicing and is missing in the Sld mutant. *Cell* 1991;64:1025–1035.
16. Levi-Schaffer F, Austen KF, Caulfield JP, et al. Fibroblasts maintain the phenotype and viability of the rat heparin-containing mast cell in vitro. *J Immunol* 1985;135:3454–3462.

17. Fujita J, Nakayama H, Onoue H, et al. Fibroblast-dependent growth of mouse mast cells in vitro: Duplication of mast cell depletion in mutant mice of W/Wv genotype. *J Cell Physiol* 1988;134:78–84.
18. Sellge G, Lorentz A, Gebhardt T, et al. Human intestinal fibroblasts prevent apoptosis in human intestinal mast cells by a mechanism independent of stem cell factor, IL-3, IL-4, and nerve growth factor. *J Immunol* 2004;172:260–267.
19. Nagata H, Worobec AS, Oh CK, et al. Identification of a point mutation in the catalytic domain of the protooncogene c-kit in peripheral blood mononuclear cells of patients who have mastocytosis with an associated hematologic disorder. *Proc Natl Acad Sci U S A* 1995;92:10560–10564.
20. Ruitenberg EJ, Elgersma A. Absence of intestinal mast cell response in congenitally athymic mice during Trichinella spiralis infection. *Nature* 1976;264:258–260.
21. Irani AM, Craig SS, DeBlois G, et al. Deficiency of the tryptase-positive, chymase-negative mast cell type in gastrointestinal mucosa of patients with defective T lymphocyte function. *J Immunol* 1987;138:4381–4386.
22. Toru H, Eguchi M, Matsumoto R, et al. Interleukin-4 promotes the development of tryptase and chymase double-positive human mast cells accompanied by cell maturation. *Blood* 1998;91:187–195.
23. Ochi H, Hirani WM, Yuan Q, et al. T helper cell type 2 cytokine-mediated comitogenic responses and CCR3 expression during differentiation of human mast cells in vitro. *J Exp Med* 1999;190:267–280.
24. Galli SJ, Maurer M, Lantz CS. Mast cells as sentinels of innate immunity. *Curr Opin Immunol* 1999;11:53–59.
25. Marshall JS. Mast-cell responses to pathogens. *Nat Rev Immunol* 2004;4:787–799.
26. Malaviya R, Ikeda T, Abraham SN, Malaviya R. Contribution of mast cells to bacterial clearance and their proliferation during experimental cystitis induced by type 1 fimbriated E. coli. *Immunol Lett* 2004;91:103–111.
27. Lawrence ID, Warner JA, Cohan VL, et al. Purification and characterization of human skin mast cells. Evidence for human mast cell heterogeneity. *J Immunol* 1987;139:3062–3069.
28. Stokes AJ, Shimoda LM, Koblan-Huberson M. A TRPV2-PKA signaling module for transduction of physical stimuli in mast cells. *J Exp Med* 2004;200:137–147.
29. Gould HJ, Sutton BJ, Beauvil AJ, et al. The biology of IGE and the basis of allergic disease. *Annu Rev Immunol* 2003;21:579–628.
30. Dvorak AM, Schleimer RP, Schulman ES, Lichtenstein LM. Human mast cells use conservation and condensation mechanisms during recovery from degranulation. In vitro studies with mast cells purified from human lungs. *Lab Invest* 1986;54:663–678.
31. Oettgen HC, Martin TR, Wynshaw-Boris A, et al. Active anaphylaxis in IgE-deficient mice. *Nature* 1994;370:367–370.
32. Miyajima I, Dombrowicz D, Martin TR, et al. Systemic anaphylaxis in the mouse can be mediated largely through IgG1 and Fc gammaRIII. Assessment of the cardiopulmonary changes, mast cell degranulation, and death associated with active or IgE- or IgG1-dependent passive anaphylaxis. *J Clin Invest* 1997;99:901–914.
33. Zhao W, Kepley CL, Morel PA, et al. Fc gamma RIIa, not Fc gamma RIIb, is constitutively and functionally expressed on skin-derived human mast cells. *J Immunol* 2006;177:694–701.
34. van Overveld FJ, Jorens PG, Rampart M, et al. Tumour necrosis factor stimulates human skin mast cells to release histamine and tryptase. *Clin Exp Allergy* 1991;21:711–714.
35. Fischer M, Harvima IT, Carvalho RF, et al. Mast cell CD30 ligand is upregulated in cutaneous inflammation and mediates degranulation-independent chemokine secretion. *J Clin Invest* 2006;116:2748–2756.
36. Davies DV. The staining reactions of normal synovial membrane with special reference to the origin of synovial mucin. *J Anat* 1943; 77:160–169.
37. Janes J, McDonald JR. Mast cells: Their distribution in various human tissues. *Arch Pathol* 1948;45:622–634.
38. Asboe-Hansen G. The origin of synovial mucin: Ehrlich's mast cell—a secretory element of the connective tissue. *Ann Rheum Dis* 1950;9:149–157.
39. Lever JD, Ford EHR. Histological, histochemical and electron microscopic observations on synovial membrane. *Anat Record* 1958;132:525–534.
40. Castor W. The microscopic structure of normal human synovial tissue. *Arthritis Rheum* 1960;3:140–151.
41. de Paulis A, Marino I, Ciccarelli A, et al. Human synovial mast cells. I. Ultrastructural in situ and in vitro immunologic characterization. *Arthritis Rheum* 1996;39:1222–1233.
42. Dean G, Hoyland JA, Denton J, et al. Mast cells in the synovium and synovial fluid in osteoarthritis. *Br J Rheumatol* 1993;32: 671–675.
43. Gotis-Graham I, McNeil HP. Mast cell responses in rheumatoid synovium. Association of the MCTC subset with matrix turnover and clinical progression. *Arthritis Rheum* 1997;40:479–489.
44. Buckley MG, Gallagher PJ, Walls AF. Mast cell subpopulations in the synovial tissue of patients with osteoarthritis: selective increase in numbers of tryptase-positive, chymase-negative mast cells. *J Pathol* 1998;186:67–74.
45. Crisp AJ, Chapman CM, Kirkham SE, et al. Articular mastocytosis in rheumatoid arthritis. *Arthritis Rheum* 1984;27:845–851.
46. Kopicky-Burd JA, Kagey-Sobotka A, Peters SP, et al. Characterization of human synovial mast cells. *J Rheumatol* 1988;15:1326–1333.
47. Bridges AJ, Malone DG, Jicinsky J, et al. Human synovial mast cell involvement in rheumatoid arthritis and osteoarthritis. Relationship to disease type, clinical activity, and antirheumatic therapy. *Arthritis Rheum* 1991;34:1116–1124.
48. Verbsky JW, McAllister PK, Malone DG. Mast cell activation in human synovium explants by calcium ionophore A23187, compound 48/80, and rabbit IgG anti-human IgE, but not morphine sulfate. *Inflamm Res* 1996;45:35–41.
49. Kiener HP, Baghestanian M, Dominkus M, et al. Expression of the C5a receptor (CD88) on synovial mast cells in patients with rheumatoid arthritis. *Arthritis Rheum* 1998;41:233–245.
50. Shin K, Gurish MF, Friend DS, et al. Lymphocyte-independent connective tissue mast cells populate murine synovium. *Arthritis Rheum* 2006;54:2863–2871.
51. Malone DG, Metcalfe DD. Demonstration and characterization of a transient arthritis in rats following sensitization of synovial mast cells with antigen-specific IgE and parenteral challenge with specific antigen. *Arthritis Rheum* 1988;31:1063–1067.
52. de Clerck LS, Struyf NJ, Bridts CH, et al. Experimental arthritis in rats induced by intra-articular injection of IgE aggregates: Evidence for arthritogenic role of complexed IgE. *Ann Rheum Dis* 1992; 51:210–213.
53. Nigrovic PA, Binstadt BA, Monach PA, et al. Mast cells contribute to initiation of autoantibody-mediated arthritis via IL-1. *Proc Natl Acad Sci U S A* 2007;104:2325–2330.
54. Dvorak AM, Kissell S. Granule changes of human skin mast cells characteristic of piecemeal degranulation and associated with recovery during wound healing in situ. *J Leukoc Biol* 1991;49:197–210.
55. Schwartz LB, Irani AM, Roller K, et al. Quantitation of histamine, tryptase, and chymase in dispersed human T and TC mast cells. *J Immunol* 1987;138:2611–2615.
56. Castells MC, Irani AM, Schwartz LB. Evaluation of human peripheral blood leukocytes for mast cell tryptase. *J Immunol* 1987;138: 2184–2189.
57. Schwartz LB, Bradford TR. Regulation of tryptase from human lung mast cells by heparin. Stabilization of the active tetramer. *J Biol Chem* 1986;261:7372–7379.
58. Schwartz LB, Metcalfe DD, Miller JS, et al. Tryptase levels as an indicator of mast-cell activation in systemic anaphylaxis and mastocytosis. *N Engl J Med* 1987;316:1622–1626.
59. Schwartz LB, Sakai K, Bradford TR, et al. The alpha form of human tryptase is the predominant type present in blood at baseline in

normal subjects and is elevated in those with systemic mastocytosis. *J Clin Invest* 1995;96:2702–2710.

60. Gruber BL, Marchese MJ, Suzuki K, et al. Synovial procollagenase activation by human mast cell tryptase dependence upon matrix metalloproteinase 3 activation. *J Clin Invest* 1989;84:1657–1662.
61. Cairns JA, Walls AF. Mast cell tryptase stimulates the synthesis of type I collagen in human lung fibroblasts. *J Clin Invest* 1997;99: 1313–1321.
62. Berger P, Perng DW, Thabrew H, et al. Tryptase and agonists of PAR-2 induce the proliferation of human airway smooth muscle cells. *J Appl Physiol* 2001;91:1372–1379.
63. Cairns JA, Walls AF. Mast cell tryptase is a mitogen for epithelial cells. Stimulation of IL-8 production and intercellular adhesion molecule-1 expression. *J Immunol* 1996;156:275–283.
64. He S, Peng Q, Walls AF. Potent induction of a neutrophil and eosinophil-rich infiltrate in vivo by human mast cell tryptase: selective enhancement of eosinophil recruitment by histamine. *J Immunol* 1997;159:6216–6225.
65. Schwartz LB, Kawahara MS, Hugli TE, et al. Generation of C3a anaphylatoxin from human C3 by human mast cell tryptase. *J Immunol* 1983;130:1891–1895.
66. Saarinen J, Kalkkinen N, Welgus HG, et al. Activation of human interstitial procollagenase through direct cleavage of the Leu83–Thr84 bond by mast cell chymase. *Biol ChemJ Biol Chem* 1994; 269:18134–18140.
67. Mizutani H, Schechter N, Lazarus G, et al. Rapid and specific conversion of precursor interleukin 1 beta (IL-1 beta) to an active IL-1 species by human mast cell chymase. *J Exp Med* 1991;174: 821–825.
68. Zhao W, Oskeritzian CA, Pozez AL, et al. Cytokine production by skin-derived mast cells: Endogenous proteases are responsible for degradation of cytokines. *J Immunol* 2005;175:2635–2642.
69. Kushnir-Sukhov NM, Brown JK, Wu Y, et al. Human mast cells are capable of serotonin synthesis and release. *J Allergy Clin Immunol.*
70. Humphries DE, Wong GW, Friend DS, et al. Heparin is essential for the storage of specific granule proteases in mast cells. *Nature* 1999;400:769–772.
71. Forsberg E, Pejler G, Ringvall M, et al. Abnormal mast cells in mice deficient in a heparin-synthesizing enzyme. *Nature* 1999;400: 773–776.
72. Azizkhan RG, Azizkhan JC, Zetter BR, et al. Mast cell heparin stimulates migration of capillary endothelial cells in vitro. *J Exp Med* 1980;152:931–944.
73. Church MK, Holgate ST, Schute JK, et al. Mast cell–derived mediators. In: E Middleton, CE Reed, EF Ellis, NF Adkinson, JW Yunginger, and WW Busse, eds. *Allergy: Principle and Practice*, 5th ed. Mosby: St. Louis, 1998, 146–167.
74. Gordon JR, Galli SJ. Mast cells as a source of both preformed and immunologically inducible TNF-alpha/cachectin. *Nature* 1990;346: 274–276.
75. Zhang Y, Ramos BF, Jakschik BA. Neutrophil recruitment by tumor necrosis factor from mast cells in immune complex peritonitis. *Science* 1992;258:1957–1959.
76. Malaviya R, Ikeda T, Ross E, Abraham SN. Mast cell modulation of neutrophil influx and bacterial clearance at sites of infection through TNF-alpha. *Nature* 1996;381:77–80.
77. Godfrey HP, Ilardi C, Engber W, Graziano FM. Quantitation of human synovial mast cells in rheumatoid arthritis and other rheumatic diseases. *Arthritis Rheum* 1984;27:852–856.
78. Ceponis A, Konttinen YT, Takagi M, et al. Expression of stem cell factor (SCF) and SCF receptor (c-kit) in synovial membrane in arthritis: Correlation with synovial mast cell hyperplasia and inflammation. *J Rheumatol* 1998;25:2304–2314.
79. Malone DG, Wilder RL, Saavedra-Delgado AM, Metcalfe DD. Mast cell numbers in rheumatoid synovial tissues. Correlations with quantitative measures of lymphocytic infiltration and modulation by antiinflammatory therapy. *Arthritis Rheum* 1987;30:130–137.
80. Malone DG, Irani AM, Schwartz LB, et al. Mast cell numbers and histamine levels in synovial fluids from patients with diverse arthritides. *Arthritis Rheum* 1986;29:956–963.
81. Buckley MG, Walters C, Wong WM, et al. Mast cell activation in arthritis: Detection of alpha- and beta-tryptase, histamine and eosinophil cationic protein in synovial fluid. *Clin Sci (Lond)* 1997;93: 363–370.
82. Lavery JP, Lisse JR. Preliminary study of the tryptase levels in the synovial fluid of patients with inflammatory arthritis. *Ann Allergy* 1994;72:425–427.
83. Frewin DB, Cleland LG, Jonsson JR, Robertson PW. Histamine levels in human synovial fluid. *J Rheumatol* 1986;13:13–14.
84. Bromley M, Woolley DE. Histopathology of the rheumatoid lesion. Identification of cell types at sites of cartilage erosion. *Arthritis Rheum* 1984;27:857–863.
85. Tetlow LC, Woolley DE. Distribution, activation and tryptase/chymase phenotype of mast cells in the rheumatoid lesion. *Ann Rheum Dis* 1995;54:549–555.
86. Gotis-Graham I, Smith MD, Parker A, McNeil HP. Synovial mast cell responses during clinical improvement in early rheumatoid arthritis. *Ann Rheum Dis* 1998;57:664–671.
87. Yamamoto T, Matsuuchi M, Watanabe K, et al. Mast cells in the synovium of patients with psoriasis arthropathy. *Dermatology* 1997;195:73–74.
88. Tachimoto H, Hudson SA, Bochner BS. Acquisition and alteration of adhesion molecules during cultured human mast cell differentiation. *J Allergy Clin Immunol* 2001;107:302–309.
89. Olsson N, Ulfgren AK, Nilsson G. Demonstration of mast cell chemotactic activity in synovial fluid from rheumatoid patients. *Ann Rheum Dis* 2001;60:187–193.
90. Weller CL, Collington SJ, Brown JK, et al. Leukotriene B4, an activation product of mast cells, is a chemoattractant for their progenitors. *J Exp Med* 2005;201:1961–1971.
91. Kushnir-Sukhov NM, Gilfillan AM, Coleman JW, et al. 5-hydroxytryptamine induces mast cell adhesion and migration. *J Immunol* 2006;177:6422–6432.
92. Sillaber C, Baghestanian M, Hofbauer I, et al. Molecular and functional characterization of the urokinase receptor on human mast cells. *Biol ChemJ Biol Chem* 1997;272:7824–7832.
93. Ruschpler P, Lorenz P, Eichler W, et al. High CXCR3 expression in synovial mast cells associated with CXCL9 and CXCL10 expression in inflammatory synovial tissues of patients with rheumatoid arthritis. *Arthritis Res Ther* 2003;5:R241–R252.
94. Valent P. The riddle of the mast cell: Kit(CD117)-ligand as the missing link? *Immunol Today* 1994;15:111–114.
95. Nilsson G, Butterfield JH, Nilsson K, Siegbahn A. Stem cell factor is a chemotactic factor for human mast cells. *J Immunol* 1994; 153:3717–3723.
96. Kiener HP, Hofbauer R, Tohidast-Akrad M, et al. Tumor necrosis factor alpha promotes the expression of stem cell factor in synovial fibroblasts and their capacity to induce mast cell chemotaxis. *Arthritis Rheum* 2000;43:164–174.
97. Gruber B, Ballan D, Gorevic PD. IgE rheumatoid factors: quantification in synovial fluid and ability to induce synovial mast cell histamine release. *Clin Exp Immunol* 1988;71:289–294.
98. Bartholomew JS, Evanson JM, Woolley DE. Serum IgE anti-cartilage collagen antibodies in rheumatoid patients. *Rheumatol Int* 1991;11: 37–40.
99. Zuraw BL, O'Hair CH, Vaughan JH, et al. Immunoglobulin E–rheumatoid factor in the serum of patients with rheumatoid arthritis, asthma, and other diseases. *J Clin Invest* 1981;68: 1610–1613.
100. Ward PA, Zvaifler NJ. Complement-derived leukotactic factors in inflammatory synovial fluids of humans. *J Clin Invest* 1971;50:606–616.
101. Johnson GB, Brunn GJ, Platt JL. Activation of mammalian Toll-like receptors by endogenous agonists. *Crit Rev Immunol* 2003;23: 15–44.

102. Kubes P, Gaboury JP. Rapid mast cell activation causes leukocyte-dependent and -independent permeability alterations. *Am J Physiol* 1996;271:H2438–2446.
103. Gaboury JP, Johnson B, Niu XF, Kubes P. Mechanisms underlying acute mast cell-induced leukocyte rolling and adhesion in vivo. *J Immunol* 1995;154:804–813.
104. Metcalfe DD, Baram D, Mekori YA. Mast cells. *Physiol Rev* 1997; 77:1033–1079.
105. Sillaber C, Baghestanian M, Bevec D, et al. The mast cell as site of tissue-type plasminogen activator expression and fibrinolysis. *J Immunol* 1999;162:1032–1041.
106. Grutzkau A, Kruger-Krasagakes S, Baumeister H, et al. Synthesis, storage, and release of vascular endothelial growth factor/vascular permeability factor (VEGF/VPF) by human mast cells: Implications for the biological significance of VEGF206. *Mol Biol Cell* 1998;9:875–884.
107. Pap T, Muller-Ladner U, Gay RE, Gay S. Fibroblast biology. Role of synovial fibroblasts in the pathogenesis of rheumatoid arthritis. *Arthritis Res* 2000;2:361–367.
108. Gruber BL, Kew RR, Jelaska A, et al. Human mast cells activate fibroblasts: tryptase is a fibrogenic factor stimulating collagen messenger ribonucleic acid synthesis and fibroblast chemotaxis. *J Immunol* 1997;158:2310–2317.
109. Li CY, Baek JY. Mastocytosis and fibrosis: Role of cytokines. *Int Arch Allergy Immunol* 2002;127:123–126.
110. Bradding P, Okayama Y, Howarth PH, et al. Heterogeneity of human mast cells based on cytokine content. *J Immunol* 1995;155: 297–307.
111. Sempowski GD, Beckmann MP, Derdak S, Phipps RP. Subsets of murine lung fibroblasts express membrane-bound and soluble IL-4 receptors. Role of IL-4 in enhancing fibroblast proliferation and collagen synthesis. *J Immunol* 1994;152:3606–3614.
112. Tetlow LC, Woolley DE. Mast cells, cytokines, and metalloproteinases at the rheumatoid lesion: dual immunolocalisation studies. *Ann Rheum Dis* 1995;54:896–903.
113. Birkedal-Hansen H, Cobb CM, Taylor RE, Fullmer HM. Activation of fibroblast procollagenase by mast cell proteases. *Biochim Biophys Acta* 1976;438:273–286.
114. Stevens RL, Somerville LL, Sewell D, et al. Serosal mast cells maintain their viability and promote the metabolism of cartilage proteoglycans when cocultured with chondrocytes. *Arthritis Rheum* 1992;35:325–335.
115. Goldhaber P. Heparin enhancement of factors stimulating bone resorption in tissue culture. *Science* 1965;147:407–408.
116. Kotake S, Sato K, Kim KJ, et al. Interleukin-6 and soluble interleukin-6 receptors in the synovial fluids from rheumatoid arthritis patients are responsible for osteoclast-like cell formation. *J Bone Miner Res* 1996;11:88–95.
117. Scheven BA, Milne JS, Hunter I, Robins SP. Macrophage-inflammatory protein-1alpha regulates preosteoclast differentiation in vitro. *Biochem Biophys Res Commun* 1999;254:773–778.
118. Kitaura H, Zhou P, Kim HJ, et al. M-CSF mediates TNF-induced inflammatory osteolysis. *J Clin Invest* 2005;115:3418–3427.
119. Lu LF, Lind EF, Gondek DC, et al. Mast cells are essential intermediaries in regulatory T-cell tolerance. *Nature* 2006;442:997–1002.
120. Gryfe A, Sanders PM, Gardner DL. The mast cell in early rat adjuvant arthritis. *Ann Rheum Dis* 1971;30:24–30.
121. Claman HN, Choi KL, Sujansky W, Vatter AE. Mast cell "disappearance" in chronic murine graft-vs-host disease (GVHD)-ultrastructural demonstration of "phantom mast cells." *J Immunol* 1986;137:2009–2013.
122. Dalldorf FG, Anderle SK, Brown RR, Schwab JH. Mast cell activation by group A streptococcal polysaccharide in the rat and its role in experimental arthritis. *Am J Pathol* 1988;132:258–264.
123. Caulfield JP, Hein A, Helfgott SM, et al. Intraarticular injection of arthritogenic factor causes mast cell degranulation, inflammation, fat necrosis, and synovial hyperplasia. *Lab Invest* 1988;59:82–95.
124. Lee DM, Friend DS, Gurish MF, et al. Mast cells: A cellular link between autoantibodies and inflammatory arthritis. *Science* 2002; 297:1689–1692.
125. Tiggelman AM, Van Noorden CJ. Mast cells in early stages of antigen-induced arthritis in rat knee joints. *Int J Exp Pathol* 1990; 71:455–464.
126. Morgan K, Reeve-Stephenson JO, Denton J, Freemont AJ. Type II collagen induced arthritis: Comparison of histological changes in arthritis-susceptible and arthritis-resistant rats. *Clin Exp Rheumatol* 1992;10:109–116.
127. Corr M, Crain B. The role of FcgammaR signaling in the K/B x N serum transfer model of arthritis. *J Immunol* 2002;169: 6604–6609.
128. Binstadt BA, Patel PR, Alencar H, et al. Particularities of the vasculature can promote the organ specificity of autoimmune attack. *Nat Immunol* 2006;7:284–292.
129. Wipke BT, Wang Z, Kim J, et al. Dynamic visualization of a joint-specific autoimmune response through positron emission tomography. *Nat Immunol* 2002;3:366–372.
130. Wipke BT, Wang Z, Nagengast W, et al. Staging the initiation of autoantibody-induced arthritis: A critical role for immune complexes. *J Immunol* 2004;172:7694–7702.
131. Nigrovic PA, Binstadt BA, Monach PA, et al. Mast cells contribute to initiation of autoantibody-mediated arthritis via IL-1. *Proc Natl Acad Sci U S A* 2007 (published online February 2).
132. Maccioni M, Zeder-Lutz G, Huang H, et al. Arthritogenic monoclonal antibodies from K/BxN mice. *J Exp Med* 2002;195: 1071–1077.
133. Takai T, Ono M, Hikida M, et al. Augmented humoral and anaphylactic responses in Fc gamma RII–deficient mice. *Nature* 1996;379: 346–349.
134. Ji H, Ohmura K, Mahmood U, et al. Arthritis critically dependent on innate immune system players. *Immunity* 2002;16:157–168.
135. Matsumoto I, Maccioni M, Lee DM, et al. How antibodies to a ubiquitous cytoplasmic enzyme may provoke joint-specific autoimmune disease. *Nat Immunol* 2002;3:360–365.
136. Ji H, Pettit A, Ohmura K, et al. Critical roles for interleukin 1 and tumor necrosis factor alpha in antibody-induced arthritis. *J Exp Med* 2002;196:77–85.
137. Chen M, Lam BK, Kanaoka Y, et al. Neutrophil-derived leukotriene B4 is required for inflammatory arthritis. *J Exp Med* 2006;203: 837–842.
138. van den Broek MF, van den Berg WB, van de Putte LB. The role of mast cells in antigen induced arthritis in mice. *J Rheumatol* 1988; 15:544–551.

Synovial Fibroblasts: Important Players in the Induction of Inflammation and Joint Destruction

CHAPTER 8F

Caroline Ospelt, Thomas Pap, and Steffen Gay

Fibroblasts are mesenchymal cells that constitute the primary resident cell type of connective tissues. In synovial tissues of articular capsules, resident cells are divided into macrophage-like synoviocytes and fibroblast-like synoviocytes (synovial fibroblasts [SF]). About one-third of the cells in the most superficial "lining" layer of the synovial tissue are fibroblast-like cells. They have a typical appearance and lack specific surface markers but in the context of the synovium can be identified by antibodies recognizing prolyl-4-hydroxylase[1,2] or antibodies against Thy-1/CD90.[3] As one peculiarity, the synovial tissue lacks a basement membrane, and thus, the classical architecture of an epithelium. Consequently, the lining layer has to fulfill this function. Accordingly, synovial fibroblasts have a barrier function and provide the joint cavity and the adjacent cartilage with lubricating molecules such as hyaluronic acid and nutritive plasma. However, in the synovial tissue and elsewhere, fibroblasts are more than merely structural cells. They react very specifically to environmental triggers, which include soluble factors, components of the extracellular matrix (ECM), and a variety of other stimuli such as oxygen tension and pH. Under disease conditions such as synovial inflammation, fibroblasts become even more important as they are critically involved in regulating the response to tissue injury. Within joints, synovial fibroblasts contribute to the resolution or chronification of inflammation, and thereby determine the consequences of disease. They are not only involved in the production and resorption of matrix components, but synovial fibroblasts also mediate neoangiogenesis and the accumulation of inflammatory cells. To this end, fibroblasts secrete chemokines[4–6] and mediate the subsequent recruitment of inflammatory cells to sites of tissue injury. In addition, they can inhibit programmed cell death in inflammatory cells[7] and modulate the activity and behavior of inflammatory cells through direct cell-to-cell interactions.[8] All these findings have changed our view on fibroblasts significantly in recent years. Not too long ago it was thought that fibroblasts are more or less passively responding cells, which upon stimulation purely react by changing the deposition or resorption of ECM. But a great number of studies have demonstrated that fibroblasts are a key part of the immune system and integrate signals from different sources into a coordinated tissue response.[9,10] This is particularly true for synovial fibroblasts in rheumatoid arthritis (RA), the most frequent chronic inflammatory joint disease.

Stable Activation of Fibroblasts in Rheumatoid Synovium

Synovial fibroblasts contribute to all aspects of RA synovial pathology, namely hyperplasia, particularly of the lining layer, perpetuation of chronic inflammation, and joint destruction.[11,12] They differ significantly from normal fibroblast-like synoviocytes, and are therefore called RA synovial fibroblasts (RASFs). Being part of a complex cellular network, RASFs contribute to chronic inflammation and joint destruction by direct mechanisms as well as through interaction with neighboring cells.[13] It has been understood that RASFs show features of stable activation that provides the basis for both their direct and indirect effects on RA joint pathology.[14]

The hypothesis that activated synovial fibroblasts are critically involved in the rheumatoid joint destruction is based on observations that date back to the 1970s.[15] By analyzing large numbers of synovial specimens from RA patients, Fassbender found that invasion of cartilage and subchondral bone by synovial lining cells does not require the presence of inflammatory infiltrates. It was demonstrated that RASFs exhibit considerable morphologic alterations. They have abundant cytoplasm, a dense rough endoplasmatic reticulum and large pale nuclei with several prominent nucleoli.[14,15] Based on these morphologic analyses in humans, arthritis in a spontaneous RA-like mouse model (MRL-lpr/lpr) was analyzed.[16] Also in this mouse model, synovial cells appeared activated and invaded joint structures even before the presence of inflammatory cells. Thus, in addition to activation of fibroblasts by inflammatory mediators, an inflammatory-independent pathway for the activation of RASFs was suggested.[16] To further investigate this transformed appearing phenotype of RASFs severe combined immunodeficient (SCID) mice were used. In this model, RASFs or normal synovial fibroblasts are co-implanted with normal human cartilage. Due to a defective immune system, SCID mice do not reject the implants and allow the study of aggressive behavior of RASFs in the absence of human inflammatory cells and their soluble factors. In this model, it was confirmed that RASFs exhibit an invasive phenotype but even more intriguingly it was shown that RASFs are able to maintain this phenotype over prolonged periods of time in the absence of continuous stimulation by an inflammatory environment[17] (Figure 8F-1). This observation provided the first clear evidence that the major parts of RASFs are constitutively, endogenously activated. Since then, a number of groups have set out to better characterize the specific phenotype of RASFs, and interest has mainly been focused on the characteristics of these cells at a cellular and molecular level as well as at the mechanisms of activation with respect to their destructive properties. Since it was shown that fibroblasts that have undergone this activation exhibit some features of tumor cells such as anchorage-independent growth, alterations in their response to apoptotic stimuli, firm attachment to ECM molecules of the cartilage, and finally invasiveness toward articular cartilage and bone, this activation is sometimes also referred to as "tumor-like" transformation (Figure 8F-2). The underlying mechanisms for this "transformation" are not clear, because these cells neither proliferate faster nor grow unlimited. However, there is evidence that the chronic exposure of fibroblast-like cells to a combination of inflammatory cytokines, growth factors and ECM components in the synovial lining together with less clearly defined environmental triggers such as hypoxia[18] and potentially also bacterial or viral products[19,20] and microparticles[21] result in the activation of these cells into an aggressive phenotype. As a consequence of this stable activation, the disease process is perpetuated and even progresses when inflammation ameliorates or becomes controlled through anti-inflammatory treatment.

Altered Expression of Proto-Oncogenes

Expression of proto-oncogenes and transcriptional factors in RASFs has been described as a major feature indicating the activated nature of these cells.[22–24]

The *c-fos* proto-oncogene for instance has been found increased in RA synovium.[25–27] It encodes for a basic leucine zipper transcription factor and is part of the transcriptional

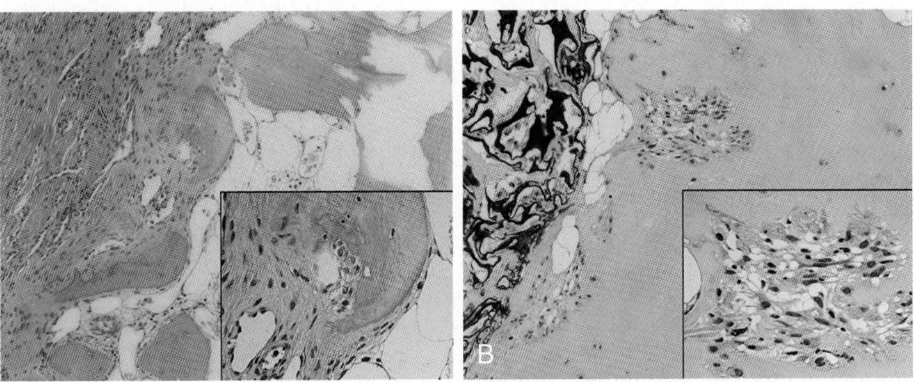

Figure 8F-1. (A) Synovial invasion into bone in RA synovium. (B) RASFs invading co-implanted human cartilage in the SCID mouse model of cartilage invasion. Magnification 100×, insert 400×.

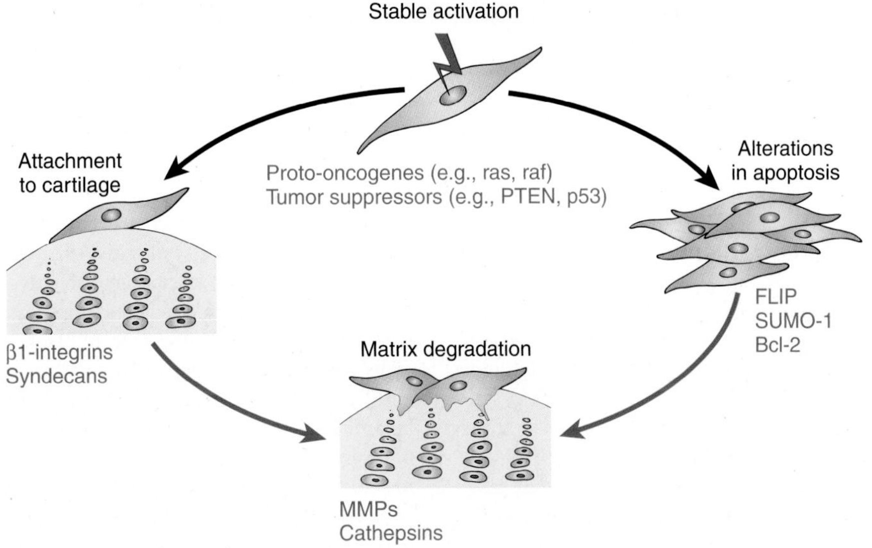

Figure 8F-2. The stable activation of synovial fibroblasts in RA is reflected by the altered expression of proto-oncogenes and tumor suppressors, and results in distinct changes that comprise an increased attachment to the extracellular matrix of the cartilage and alterations in apoptosis, as well as increased expression of matrix-degrading enzymes such as MMPs and cathepsins, ultimately leading to progressive cartilage destruction.

activator AP-1 (jun/fos). The promoters of several of the matrix metalloproteinases (MMPs) not only contain consensus binding sites for the transcription factor AP-1, but the AP-1 site has also been shown to be involved in tissue-specific expression of MMPs.[28,29] More than 15 years ago the proto-oncogene *fos* has already been identified in this context in MMP-1 producing RASFs[27] and together with additional data pointing to the same conclusion,[30] it has been suggested that *fos* related proto-oncogenes play an important role in cell activation via the formation of AP-1.

Other oncogenes such as *ras, raf, sis, myb,* and *myc* have also been detected at elevated levels in RA patients and were found predominantly upregulated in synovial cells attaching to cartilage and bone.[22,24] About 70% of RA patients exhibit high expression of Ras and Myc proteins in synovial lining cells and in the promoters of the oncogenes sis and ras, binding sites for early response genes such as *egr-1* could be identified.[27] Some of these proto-oncogenes appear to be directly involved in the regulation of different MMPs. c-Ras, for instance, plays a critical role in the increased expression and proteolytic activation of MMPs in fibroblasts. In particular, gelatinases (MMP-2 and MMP-9) together with MT1-MMP are likely regulated by growth factors that mediate their effects through the *ras* proto-oncogene.[31,32] In addition, gene transfer with dominant negative (dn) mutants of Raf-1 and c-Myc demonstrated the relevance of the Ras-Raf-MAPK pathway for the activation and invasive behavior of RASFs.[33] In this study, nontreated RASFs most prominently invaded into the cartilage in the SCID mouse model, while RASFs transduced with dn-Raf-1 or with dn-c-Myc exhibited a marked reduction of invasion. This was accompanied by a decreased expression of MMP-1 and MMP-13 in dn-Raf-1 transduced fibroblasts both *in vitro* and *in vivo*. No significant changes in apoptosis were seen in the dn-Raf-1 or dn-c-Myc–transduced cells. However, RASFs that were transduced with both dn-Raf-1 and dn-c-Myc rapidly underwent apoptosis. These results demonstrated that both Raf-1 and c-Myc contribute to the activation of synovial cells in RA. The clear effect of dn-Raf-1 and dn-c-Myc on the invasiveness of RASFs in the SCID mouse model is in line with the concept that upregulation of relevant signaling pathways is maintained in RASFs even in the absence of human inflammatory cells.

Taken together, different lines of evidence suggest that pathologic expression of proto-oncogenes constitutes an important step leading to the expression of matrix-degrading enzymes in RA and consecutive joint destruction.

Altered Expression of Tumor Suppressor Genes in RASFs

Alterations in different tumor suppressor genes have become of growing interest in explaining some features of fibroblast activation and survival in RA. Thus, somatic mutations of the tumor suppressor gene p53 have been described in rheumatoid synoviocytes.[34] Based on additional evidence that some of these mutations can exert dominant negative effects, it has been hypothesized that the accumulation of p53 mutations may contribute to the activation of rheumatoid fibroblast-like synoviocytes. Although mutations in the p53 gene apparently show a great variability, such mutations may nonetheless constitute one mechanism that imprints the aggressive behavior into RASFs. This notion is supported by data showing that inhibition of p53 in normal synovial fibroblasts results in an invasive, RA like phenotype.[35] Consequently, RA specific expression of p53 in the synovial tissue in both earliest and late stage of RA has been studied. It was found that synovial expression of p53 is specific for RA and can be found in cells at sites of cartilage invasion.[36] Integrating all these data, it may be hypothesized that already at an early time point the local environment in the rheumatoid joint results in an altered expression and function of p53 at least in a subset of RASFs, which in turn contributes to the stable activation of these cells.[37] With respect to the stability of p53, one has also to note that the ubiquitin ligase synoviolin which resides in the endoplasmatic reticulum destroys cytoplasmic p53.[38] Future research is designed to explore the comprehensive role of synoviolin in more detail.

Another strong modulator of apoptosis is the metastasis-inducing protein S100A4 (Mts-1), which is strongly overexpressed in synovial tissues of RA patients and thereby stabilizes the p53 tumor suppressor in RASFs and changes the regulation of p53 target genes.[39]

Regarding the tumor suppressor PTEN, it could be shown that aggressive RASFs lack the expression of mRNA for PTEN. PTEN is a tyrosine phosphatase that shows homology to the cytoskeletal proteins tensin and auxillin. Mutations in PTEN have been described in different malignancies and associated with their invasiveness and metastatic properties.[40–42] In RA, no mutations of PTEN have been found, but RA synovium showed a distinct pattern of PTEN expression with negligible staining in the lining but very strong expression in the sublining.[43] It can be assumed that the lack of PTEN expression, especially at sites of invasion is an intrinsic feature of RASFs. This is of special interest, since PTEN is involved in the regulation of the focal adhesion kinase (FAK),[44,45] a key molecule for the activation of signaling cascades after cell contact, as further described below. Some data also indicate that PTEN is an essential mediator of FasL-mediated apoptosis through regulation of the PI 3-kinase/Akt/NF-κB pathway.[46]

Interaction of Synovial Fibroblasts with ECM

In search for joint-specific factors that trigger and maintain the activation of synovial fibroblasts in RA, the specific composition of the ECM in the joints and the interaction of RASFs with joint-specific matrix components has become of special interest in recent years.

In this context, integrins are of particular importance. Integrins represent a complex family of adhesion molecules that contain heterodimers of alpha and beta chains. So far, at least 16 alpha and eight beta chains have been described that can combine into at least 24 integrins.[47] For the attachment of fibroblasts to ECM components of connective tissue and cartilage, $beta_1$ integrins are of particular importance. Different studies have demonstrated that apart from being expressed on lymphocytes, several $beta_1$ integrins are highly expressed on RASFs,[48,49] and the binding of RASFs to ECM is inhibited, at least in part, by anti-$beta_1$ integrin antibodies with the blocking efficacy being significantly higher in RASFs compared to normal synovial fibroblasts.[49] $Alpha_1beta_1$ and $alpha_2beta_1$ integrins are the main adhesion molecules responsible for the attachment of fibroblasts to collagen, but novel data suggest that the recently described $alpha_{10}beta_1$ and $alpha_{11}beta_1$ integrins may also be involved. Other $beta_1$ integrins such as $alpha_4beta_1$ and $alpha_5beta_1$ integrins mediate the attachment of fibroblasts to fibronectin and its spliced variants, while $alpha_v$ integrins are responsible additionally for the attachment to vitronectin. Of note, various integrins function as fibronectin receptors, which is why the fibronectin-rich environment of RA cartilage surface might facilitate the adhesion of RASFs to the cartilage. In this context it will be important to determine how the loss of cartilage components during disease progression affects the adhesion of RASFs to the articular cartilage.

Integrins might be crucial in the pathogenesis of RA not only because of their function as receptor molecules but also because of their interaction with several signaling pathways and cellular proto-oncogenes.[50] For example, the expression of early cell cycle genes such as *c-fos* and *c-myc* is stimulated by integrin-mediated cell adhesion, and gene expression driven by the *fos* promoter shows synergistic activation by integrin-mediated adhesion.[51,52]

Furthermore, integrin signals are important molecules for the growth of fibroblasts. It has been demonstrated that RASFs require integrin co-signaling for proliferation after stimulation with platelet-derived growth factor (PDGF).[53] Upon PDGF binding, integrins contribute to Ras-dependent pathways,[54] involving extracellular signal-regulated kinase (ERK), c-Jun N-terminal kinase (JNK), and Akt, and modulate the activation of mitogen-activated protein kinases (MAPKs).[55]

Importantly, the activation of beta$_1$ integrins has also been demonstrated to induce the expression of proteases contributing to ECM degradation,[56] and their inhibition by antibodies reduced the invasive capacity of RASFs.[57] How integrins mediate this response both under normal conditions and in RASFs has been studied intensively in recent years. Engagement of integrin receptors on the surface of fibroblasts results in the formation of focal adhesion complexes. These focal adhesion complexes regulate gene transcription through activation of a variety of intracellular signaling cascades. The activated genes then control cell proliferation and survival and secretion of certain cytokines and chemokines, as well as matrix deposition and resorption. Among the signaling molecules that transmit the signals from integrins to the cell interior, the focal adhesion kinase (FAK) plays a central role.[58,59] FAK is a tyrosine kinase that is recruited into newly established focal contacts and in turn recruits adaptor proteins such as p130Cas and Grb2. These adaptor proteins then lead to the activation of PI3-kinase and Src-kinase and promote the initiation of a variety of signaling cascades, such as the Raf-MEK-Erk pathway. It is important to note though that these signaling pathways can be activated also through FAK-independent signaling events, such as growth factors. The exact mechanisms by which different signals cooperate to mediate the specific response of synovial fibroblasts and how this translates into the distinct pathologic reaction pattern of RASFs will need further investigation.

The picture of how binding of RASFs to ECM components triggers synovial activation is further complicated by the fact that in addition to integrins, other cell surface molecules are involved in this attachment as well as in the response of RASFs to growth factors. Among those, transmembrane heparan sulfate proteoglycans have recently gained special interest. Syndecans are a family of such transmembrane heparan sulfate proteoglycans that possess highly conserved cytoplasmic and transmembrane domains, but have highly variable extracellular domains. The extracellular parts of syndecans contain different numbers of glycosaminoglycan (GAG) side chains through which they interact with factors released at tissue injury like growth factors and interleukins, but also with a great number of ECM components and adhesion molecules.[60] Syndecans are expressed on fibroblasts in a tissue-specific and development-dependent manner. Data from syndecan knock out mice have taught us important lessons on their functional role in tissue remodeling. They indicate that in particular syndecan-4 is important for the response of fibroblasts to tissue injury. Syndecan-4–deficient mice show no gross abnormalities and are viable. It is only under certain stress conditions that these mice show differences compared to their wildtype controls. They exhibit alterations in wound healing, and the response of syndecan-4 deficient fibroblasts to fibronectin attachment is significantly altered.[61] Also, syndecan-4 deficient fibroblasts are compromised in their ability to differentiate into alpha-smooth muscle actin (a-SMA) expressing myofibroblasts. The exact mechanisms by which syndecans are involved in the specific functions of different fibroblast populations remain to be determined, but it appears that syndecans are important cell surface receptors that due to their unique properties integrate signals from ECM components and soluble factors.

Also, RASFs tend to bind easier to the cartilage oligomeric protein (COMP) compared to SF from patients with osteoarthritis (OA). Most interestingly, the adherence to COMP induces the production of galectin-3 in synovial fibroblasts.[62] Galectin-3, a soluble galactoside-binding protein that has been shown to be elevated in neoplastic cells induces angiogenesis, and is a chemoattractant for monocytes and macrophages.[63]

Resistance against Apoptosis

Regarding fibroblast proliferation, it was shown that even though synovial cells from patients with RA are activated, they do not proliferate faster than those from OA patients.[64] Using thymidine incorporation, only 1% to 5% of synovial cells have been found to proliferate,[65] and immunohistochemistry for specific proliferation markers such as Ki-67 revealed only a very low number of positive cells.[66] Also, only 1% of fibroblast-like cells expressing proto-oncogenes such as *jun-B* and *c-fos* were positive for Ki-67, indicating that the majority of RASFs do not show accelerated proliferation.[67] In contrast, more recent data have provided growing evidence for changes of apoptotic pathways in RA synovium, particularly within the lining layer (for review see Baier et al.[68]). When examined by ultrastructural methods, less than 1% of lining cells exhibit morphological features of apoptosis.[69,70]

Generally, apoptosis can be triggered through cell-surface death receptors, or induced by intrinsic, mitochondrial pathways that can also be modulated by hypoxia.[68,71,72] Members of the Bcl-family have been identified as important regulators of mitochondrial pathways of apoptosis. Specifically, Bcl-2 has been demonstrated to exert strong antiapoptotic effects and to contribute to the pathogenesis of experimental arthritis.[73] *In-situ* analysis showed increased presence of Bcl-2 in human RASFs,[69] and this enhanced expression of Bcl-2 in RASFs was found to correlate with synovial lining thickening and inflammation.[74] Of interest, it was demonstrated that stimulation of RASFs with IL-15 suppresses Bcl-2 and Bcl-x(L) mRNA.[75] In this study it was found that apoptosis could be increased when the autocrine stimulation of RASFs with IL-15 is inhibited, strengthening the role of Bcl-family members in the regulation of fibroblast apoptosis and providing a link between cytokine-mediated stimulation of RASFs and their resistance to cell-death. As mentioned above, somatic mutations of p53 tumor suppressor gene in RA synovial cells may also contribute to reduced apoptosis in these cells.[34]

In addition to the changes in the mitochondrial pathway of apoptosis, there is evidence that RASFs are also resistant to receptor-induced apoptosis. These receptors include members of the TNF-receptor family, specifically the TNF-receptor 1, TNF-related apoptosis-inducing ligand (TRAIL) receptors 1 and 2, and the Fas receptor. They all possess conserved intracellular motifs, termed death domains, which upon receptor activation induce the formation of a signaling complex that initiates the apoptotic cascade. There are several factors that have been suggested to be involved in this resistance of RASFs against death receptor–induced cell death but the ultimate mechanisms are still not completely understood. It is currently estimated that only about 15% of RASFs are susceptible to Fas.[14] It has been conjectured that the extensive resistance to Fas-induced apoptosis despite the surface expression of Fas is conveyed by inflammatory cytokines present in the synovial fluid, such as TNFα and TGFβ. But the involvement of soluble Fas (sFas) has been suggested, since elevated levels of sFas have been found in the synovial fluids of patients with RA.[76] However, the resistance of RASFs against Fas-induced apoptosis is maintained *in vitro* indicating that also intrinsic factors are responsible for this specific feature. Some evidence points to a role for the PI3-Kinase/Akt pathway in resistance to Fas. In endothelial cells, Fas activates Akt without inducing apoptosis,[77] and in a gastric carcinoma cell lines, inhibition of this pathway made the cells susceptible to Fas-induced apoptosis.[78]

Also the antiapoptotic FLICE inhibitory protein (Flip) is elevated in the rheumatoid synovium,[79] and correlates with low levels of apoptosis in early RA.[80] Most interestingly, the strongest expression of Flip is detected at sites of invasion.[81] Flip expression can also be induced by TNFα and prevents the interaction of caspase-8 with the Fas-associated death domain (FADD) adapter protein. It was shown that its downregulation sensitizes RASFs to Fas-induced apoptosis.[82]

Another molecule that modulates downstream mechanisms of Fas is SUMO-1. This small ubiquitin-like protein in contrast to ubiquitination does not lead to the degradation of proteins. Rather, SUMOylation results in altered binding of modified proteins to subsequent substrates, and significantly affects the signaling of SUMOylated proteins.[83] In the rheumatoid synovium, there is a marked expression of SUMO-1, predominantly in fibroblasts of the lining layer and at sites of cartilage invasion, whereas normal synovial tissues and synovial tissues of OA patients do not show prominent expression of SUMO-1.[84] Intriguingly, RASFs maintain the high expression of SUMO-1 when analyzed in the SCID mouse model, and most recent data demonstrate that SUMO-1 is prominently involved in the resistance of RASFs to Fas-induced apoptosis. Although SUMO-1 has been demonstrated to interact with the Fas- and TNFRI-associated death domain,[85] direct SUMOylation of FADD does not appear to constitute the main mechanism of action. Rather, as we have shown recently SUMO-1 indirectly contributes to the resistance of RASFs against Fas-induced apoptosis by creating nuclear depots of proteins that under physiologic conditions are involved in the dynamic balancing of death signals[86] (Figure 8F-3). One of these molecules is the transcriptional repressor DAXX. It was shown that increased expression of SUMO-1 in RASFs through increased SUMOylation of the nuclear PML protein results in an increased recruitment of DAXX to PML-nuclear bodies. The nuclear SUMO-protease SENP1, which is found at lower levels in RASFs, can revert the apoptosis-inhibiting effects of SUMO-1 by releasing DAXX from PML nuclear bodies. The importance of these data lies in the fact that not only altered expression of proteins regulating apoptosis, but also trapping of pro-apoptotic regulators after increased SUMOylation of PML may be an important pathologic factor for the resistance of RASFs against apoptotic death.

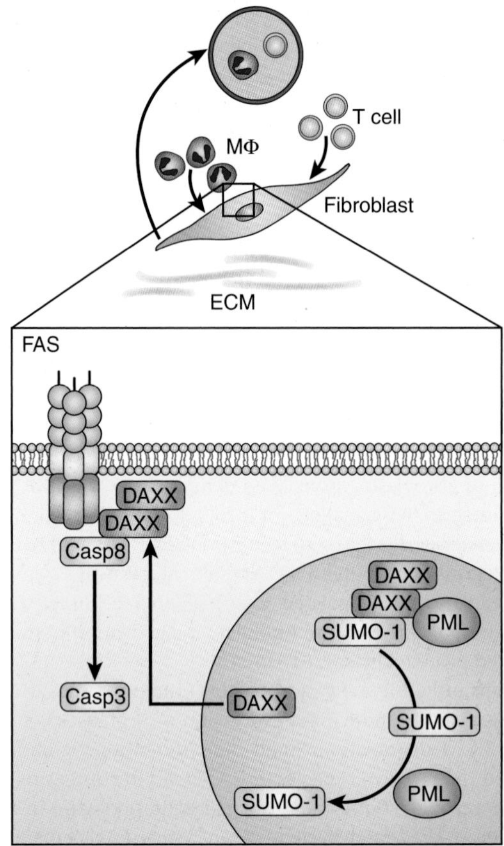

Figure 8F-3. Post-translational modification of apoptotic regulators constitute an important mechanism by which RA synovial fibroblasts are protected from apoptosis. Specifically, increased expression of SUMO-1 results in an enhanced SUMOylation of the nuclear PML protein, as a result of which the apoptotic modulator DAXX is bound at increased levels in the PML nuclear bodies. Inhibition of SUMO-1 or overexpression of the nuclear SUMO–specific protease SENP1 results in deSUMOylation of PML and the release of DAXX, resulting in sensitization of RA fibroblasts to programmed cell death.

TNFα can activate the apoptotic pathway through the caspases 3 and 8. But TNFα can also initiate pathways diverging downstream of the TNF receptor-binding protein TRADD, leading to the activation of nuclear factor kappa B (NF-κB),[87] which in turn promotes cell survival, as well as the production of proinflammatory factors.[88] In RASFs, TNFα thus inhibits apoptosis and induces cell death only after inhibition of NF-κB.[89] Furthermore, TNFα has been demonstrated to rapidly and potently activate the Akt kinase via phosphatidylinositide 3-kinase (PI3K) and inhibition of PI3K similar to inhibition to NF-κB strongly potentiates TNFα-induced apoptosis.[90] Apparently, however, not all antiapoptotic effects of TNFα through the Akt pathway depend on NF-κB. According to some studies, TNFα interferes with Fas-mediated apoptosis at physiologic levels, and induces apoptosis only at 100-fold higher levels.[91] Of note, stimulation of RASFs with TNFα also significantly increases the production of soluble Fas.[92] In this context, it was most recently shown that the tissue inhibitor of metalloproteinases (TIMP)-3 can sensitize RASFs to Fas-ligand–induced apoptosis when expressed through adenoviral gene transfer.[92] In addition, adenoviral delivery of TIMP-3 completely reverses the apoptosis-inhibiting effects of TNFα in these cells. These findings provide a link between matrix degradation and the resistance of RASFs against apoptosis and indicate that overexpression of TIMP-3 in such cells may have beneficial effects both by inhibiting matrix degradation and by facilitating cell death.

Taken together, it is suggested that apoptosis-suppressing signals outweigh proapoptotic signaling in RA causing an imbalance of pro- and anti-apoptotic pathways. This subsequently might lead to an extended life span of synovial lining cells and results in a prolonged expression of matrix-degrading enzymes at sites of joint destruction. In addition, it appears that similar mechanisms that regulate the altered apoptotic response also regulate the invasive behavior of RASFs.[93]

Epigenetic Changes in RASFs

Recent advancements in the study of gene expression revealed that numerous regulative mechanisms hereditarily change gene expression without changing the DNA sequence itself. These mechanisms are summarized under the term "epigenetics," and became of special interest for RA researchers, since complex diseases like RA often exhibit a heritable component, but do not strictly follow Mendel's laws of inheritance.[94] It is most feasible to assume that a combination of various heritable and environmental factors leads to the development of RA. The impact of environmental factors might thereby be mediated by epigenetic changes. Epigenetic changes comprise histone modifications (acetylation, methylation, ubiquitination, phosphorylation), RNA-associated silencing (micro-RNA) and DNA methylation. In RA synovium, the balance of histone acetylation and deacetylation was shown to be shifted toward hyperacetylation with a lack of expression of histone deactylases (HDACs).[95] Since acetylation is in general associated with active transcription, this hyperacetylated state in RA might reflect general activation of the diseased tissue. Despite the fact that HDACs seem to be downregulated in RA patients, the use of HDAC inhibitors positively modulated disease activity in mouse models of arthritis.[96,97] This discrepancy might stem from the fact that currently used HDAC inhibitors lack selectivity and their actual mechanisms of action are not fully elucidated. Their anti-inflammatory properties might stem from non–histone-mediated effects. Furthermore, HDAC inhibitors were shown to induce cell-cycle arrest and apoptosis, which also could account for their beneficial effects in arthritis models.[98] As such, it was shown that treatment of RASFs with the HDAC inhibitor trichostatin A could increase their apoptotic response to the tumor necrosis factor–related apoptosis-inducing ligand (TRAIL).[99]

In accordance to the transcriptionally active state of RA synovium suggested by hyperacetylation of histones, global hypomethylation of DNA could be shown in RA synovial tissues.[100] Most interestingly, previous work showed that LINE1 retrotransposable elements are transcribed in RA patients and that at least one of their products, p40, is found in RA synovial fluids as well as in RA tissues.[101] The transcription of retrotransposons is usually silenced by DNA methylation. Accordingly, *in vitro* treatment of RASFs with demethylating agents induced the expression of p40. The impact of the expression of LINE1 elements in RASFs has prompted us to study the induction of novel molecules in these cells such as galectin-3 and its binding protein as discussed above.[62,102,103]

In addition to epigenetic modifications, microRNAs (miRNAs) have recently emerged as a new class of modulators of gene expression. These molecules are 18 to 24 nucleotides long, evolutionarily conserved, noncoding RNAs that function as post-transcriptional repressors of gene expression. MiRNAs bind to 3' untranslated regions of their target mRNA and mediate cleavage and/or inhibition of translation of the targeted mRNA. More than 800 different miRNAs have thus far been estimated in humans, but it is predicted that miRNAs may actually constitute 2% to 3% of the human genome. Growing evidence suggests a crucial role of miRNAs in a number of human physiologic and pathologic conditions, since they have been found to regulate a wide variety of biologic processes such as proliferation, apoptosis, differentiation, and developmental timing.[104] In RA, RASFs and monocytes derived from synovial fluid revealed altered levels of miRNAs as shown by increased expression of miR-155 and miR-146a. In addition, TNF-α, IL-1β, and toll-like receptor (TLR) ligands upregulated these specific miRNAs in RASFs, indicating the possibility that the proinflammatory milieu in RA joints influences the expression patterns or miRNAs in resident cells of the joint. Moreover, a regulatory function of miR-155 for the control of expression of MMP3 and MMP1 in RASFs has been proposed.[105]

Matrix Degradation

Fibroblasts are not only responsible for the deposition and assembly of ECM molecules, but they are also critically involved in the destruction and removal of ECM. In RA, this aspect becomes of particular importance as the progressive destruction of articular cartilage is one of the very prominent features of disease and RASFs are involved most critically in this process. To this end, RASFs produce a great variety of matrix-degrading enzyme, including matrix metalloproteinases (MMPs) and cysteine proteinases (cathepsins), which can cleave ECM components (for detailed review, see Pap, et al.[106]).

The MMP family of matrix-degrading enzymes consists of more than 20 structurally related members.[107] MMPs are characterized by a zinc molecule at the active site and include collagenases (MMP-1, MMP-13), gelatinases (MMP-2 and MMP-9), stromelysin (MMP-3), and membrane-type MMPs (MT-MMP). The latter are characterized by a transmembrane domain and act on the surface of fibroblasts and other cells. Two types of enzyme families are structurally related to MMPs: the ADAMs (a disintegrin and a metalloproteinase)[108] and the ADAMTS (a disintegrin and a metalloproteinase with thrombospondin motifs).[109]

Regulation of MMP Production in Fibroblasts

Matrix metalloproteinases are secreted as inactive proenzymes and activated proteolytically by various enzymes such as trypsin, plasmin, and other proteases. MMPs differ with respect to their substrate specificities.[110] While MMP-1 degrades collagen types I, II, III, VII, and X, but only when they are arranged in a triple helical structure, MMP-2 can also cleave denatured collagen. MMP-3 is able to activate MMP-1 as well as to degrade proteoglycans. With the exception of MMP-2 and the MT-MMPs, which are constitutively expressed in fibroblasts, MMP expression is regulated by extracellular signals via transcriptional activation. Three major groups of inducers can be differentiated: (1) proinflammatory cytokines, (2) growth factors, and (3) matrix molecules. Among the cytokines, IL-1 is a central inducer of a variety of MMPs, including MMP-1, -3, -8, -13, and -14. The growth factors fibroblast growth factor (FGF) and PDGF are also known inducers of MMPs in fibroblasts, as they potentiate the effect of IL-1 on the expression of MMPs. Vascular endothelial growth factor (VEGF) was shown to induce MMP-13, and macrophage inflammatory protein (MIP) acts on MMP-9 and -13. In addition, matrix proteins and their degradation products can activate expression of MMPs in fibroblasts, providing the possibility of site-specific MMP activation at places of matrix breakdown.[111,112]

In fibroblasts, signaling for transcriptional activation of MMPs is mediated by several pathways. The activator protein-1 (AP-1)–binding site is present in the promotor region of all MMPs (except MMP-2), suggesting a central role of jun/fos transcription factor binding. Indeed, much experimental evidence demonstrates that all three mitogen/stress-activated protein-kinase (MAPK/SAPK) families—ERK, JNK and p38 kinase—that integrate extracellular signals upstream from jun/fos, are involved in the regulation of MMP expression. In particular, the induction of MMP-1, -9, and -13 is mediated through MAPK/SAPK signaling.[113–115] Aside from AP-1, the promotor regions of some MMPs contain NF-κB-,[113–115] STAT-,[116] and Ets[117]-binding sites. Activation of these transcription factors has been demonstrated to occur during the induction of MMP-1, -3, and -13, all of which are thought to be essential for joint damage in RA. Interesting data have come from studies of the transcriptional factor NF-κB in RASFs. NF-κB is a dimeric (p65, p50), regulatory, DNA-binding protein that interacts with a number of different signal cascades. Several studies have confirmed that NF-κB is highly activated in the synovial tissues of RA patients, and constitutes a key integrating factor for intracellular as well as cytokine-mediated activation pathways.[118,119] Thus, NF-κB, a key molecule that mediates the resistance of RASFs against apoptosis,[120–122] regulates the production of inflammatory cytokines,[120,121] adhesion molecules,[120,121,123] and matrix-degrading enzymes.[120,124] The activation of NF-κB in RASFs appears to constitute an important link between synovial inflammation, hyperplasia, and matrix degeneration.[119,120]

Recently, regulation of MMPs by the Ets-1 transcription factor has received some attention. In addition to the well-established role of Ets-1 in regulating the expression of MMPs in vascular endothelial cells, novel data from the Ets-1 knockout mouse indicate that Ets-1 is also involved in the expression of MMPs in fibroblasts.[125,126] In this study, it was found that Ets-1 is prominently involved in the fast induction of MMP-2, -3, and -13 by FGF-2.

Activation of these various transcription factors and MAPK/SAPK, all of which are not tissue-specific signaling molecules, occurs at distinct subcompartments of the rheumatoid joint, thus determining a specific pattern of MMP expression in the synovium.[126,127]

Expression of MMPs in RASFs

The unbalanced expression of MMPs has been described as a principal characteristic of RASFs, and the progressive destruction of the ECM of joints in RA has been attributed largely to this feature. MMP-1 is found in the synovial tissues of all RA patients but only in about 55% to 80% of synovial samples from trauma patients.[128] The expression of MMP-1 in the diseased synovium is mostly located in synovial lining cells, which release MMP-1 immediately after its production (for review, see Sorsa et al.[129]). As a result, expression of MMP-1 in the synovial fluid correlates with the degree of synovial inflammation.[130] However, serum concentrations of MMP-1 do not appear to reflect synovial fluid levels, and therefore, measuring serum MMP-1 has not been established as a marker for disease activity.

MMP-3 has been assigned a key role in the destruction of rheumatoid joints because MMP-3 not only degrades matrix molecules, but is also involved in the conversion of pro-MMPs into their active forms. RASFs in the lining layer are a major source of MMP-3,[131] and MMP-3 is abundantly produced by RASFs when stimulated with macrophage-conditioned medium.[132] Synovial fluids from patients with RA contain about 100-fold higher concentrations of active MMP-3 than control samples,[133] and increased levels of MMP-3 have also been found in the sera of patients with RA.[134–137] These increased serum levels correlate with systemic inflammation at clinical[134,138] and serologic levels,[135,136,138] but it is not clear whether the levels of circulating MMP-3 reflect radiologic damage. No correlation between serum MMP-3 and radiologic or functional scores was found,[135] and it was reported that no differences in the serum levels of MMP-3 between low or high erosion scores in RA patients with long-standing RA exist.[136] In contrast, other data indicate that serum MMP-3 might predict joint damage possibly only at early stages of disease.[139]

MMP-13 is found expressed at the mRNA[140] and protein level,[141] especially in the lining layer of rheumatoid synovium. Due to its localization, its substrate specificity for collagen type II and its relative resistance to known MMP inhibitors, MMP-13 has been suggested to play an important role in joint destruction. Of interest, expression of MMP-13 correlates with elevated levels of systemic inflammation markers,[142] but studies in OA demonstrated clearly that the expression of MMP-13 is not specific for RA. Rather, it appears that MMP-13 is associated closely with degeneration of cartilage in various pathologies.

MT-MMPs are abundantly detected in cells aggressively destroying cartilage and bone in RA.[143] MT1-MMP is produced constitutively by RASFs, and elevated levels have been found in RA. This is of importance, because MT1-MMP degrades ECM components as well as activates other disease-relevant MMPs such as MMP-2 and MMP-13. In addition, a recent study comparing the expressions of MT-MMPs in RA suggested that MT1-MMP was of particular relevance to RA.[143] In this analysis, the expression of MT3-MMP mRNA was seen in fibroblasts and some macrophages, particularly in the lining layer, but expression of MT2- and MT4-MMP was characterized by a scattered staining of only few CD68 negative fibroblasts.

Upregulation of MMPs in RASFs

The expression of MMPs in RA synovial cells is regulated by several extracellular signals. These include inflammatory cytokines, growth factors and molecules of the extracellular matrix. Some interesting data have come from studies showing that microparticles derived from immune cells can also directly stimulate the expression of both inflammatory cytokines and disease-relevant MMPs in synovial fibroblasts.[21] These results further highlight the emerging important role of microparticles in cellular communication.[144]

Among the inflammatory cytokines IL-1 and TNFα are important inducers of MMPs. IL-1 induces the expression of a variety of MMPs, including MMP-1, -3, -8, -13, and -14 (see Pap, et al.[106]). As demonstrated in several studies using antigen-induced arthritis in animals, IL-1 not only enhanced the production of MMPs but also suppressed the synthesis of proteoglycans (PGs).[145] In some of these studies, anti–IL-1 treatment was able to normalize chondrocyte synthetic function and reduce the activation of MMPs.[146] These data go along with observations showing that overexpression of the IL-1 receptor antagonist (IL-1ra) using retroviral gene transfer significantly reduces perichondrocytic matrix degradation in the SCID mouse model.[147] However, the mechanisms by which cytokines such as IL-1 induce MMPs appear to be variable and dependent on the cell type. Thus, in chondrocytes, IL-1 upregulates MMP-13 via JNK and p38 protein kinase signaling,[148] but MMP-1 upregulates via STAT transcription factors.[149]

Other macrophage-derived inflammatory cytokines such as TNFα have been shown to amplify the destructive processes by stimulating the expression of some MMPs. Thus, TNFα can stimulate the production of MMP-1 in cultured synovial cells.[150,151] However, animal models of arthritis have suggested a difference in the relative importance of TNFα and IL-1 with respect to inflammation and joint destruction. In this regard, it was concluded that TNFα primarily appears responsible for the extent of the synovitis, while IL-1 was predicted to have a greater impact on the destruction of cartilage.[152] However, the clinical success of anti-TNF therapies has clearly proven otherwise.

Other cytokines that regulate the expression of MMP in the RA synovium include IL-17 (MMP-1 and -9)[153] and TGFβ (MMP-13).[56] Growth factors such as FGF and PDGF are also potent inducers of MMPs and potentiate the effect of IL-1.[154] The expression of MMP can further be induced by various matrix proteins such as collagen and fibronectin. In particular, their degradation products can activate the expression of MMPs in chondrocytes and fibroblasts, which provides the possibility for specific activation of MMPs at sites of matrix degradation.[111,155] As a consequence, the synthesis of matrix-degrading enzymes in the inflamed joint is not only regulated by inflammatory cytokines and growth factors, but also by cleavage products of the destroyed matrix itself in an amplifying fashion. In this respect, it is of interest that cleavage products of ECM molecules have been described as endogenous ligands for TLRs.[156,157] Consequently, it is suggested that TLRs not only induce activation of the innate immune system after recognition of microbial fragments, but that they also function as sensors of general tissue damage. In accordance with this "surveillance" hypothesis, it could be shown that RASFs highly express TLR3 and that incubation with dsRNA from necrotic cells leads to the production of MMPs by RASFs in a TLR3-dependent manner.[158] Similarly, stimulation of RASFs with fibrin, an endogenous ligand for TLR4, leads to upregulation of proinflammatory cytokines and MMPs.[159,160]

Although some studies have shown a close correlation between the expression of the MMPs -1, -3, and -10 with the invasive growth of RASFs,[161] the specific contribution of individual members of the MMP family to matrix degradation remains poorly understood. Using gene transfer of ribozymes to MMP-1, we observed that the specific inhibition of MMP-1 significantly reduces the production of this enzyme in RASFs and inhibits the invasiveness of the cells in the SCID mouse model.[162] In a similar study, it was shown that gene transfer of antisense RNA-expression constructs against MT1-MMP, a membrane-anchored MMP, also inhibits the invasiveness of RASFs.[163]

Tissue Inhibitors of Metalloproteinase in RASFs

The activity of MMPs is balanced by the naturally occurring tissue inhibitors of metalloproteinase (TIMPs). They interact irreversibly with MMPs and are synthesized and secreted by chondrocytes, synovial fibroblasts, and endothelial cells.[164–166] *In situ* hybridization studies revealed striking amounts of TIMP-1 mRNA in the synovial lining of patients with RA.[166] However, the molar ratio of MMPs to TIMP, rather than the absolute levels of TIMP, are crucial for joint destruction. In RA, the amount of MMPs produced far outweighs that of TIMPs, which allows destruction to take place. This notion has been supported by data demonstrating that overexpression of TIMP-1 and TIMP-3 by gene transfer results in a marked reduction of the invasiveness of RASFs.[167] Of interest, TIMP-3 not only inhibits ECM degradation, but also has been associated with a number of features that are distinct from other TIMPs. Thus, TIMP-3 has the ability to prevent shedding of cell membrane proteins such as the TNF receptor,[168] the IL-6 receptor,[169] and of TACE.[170] As mentioned above, another interesting feature of TIMP-3 is its ability to induce apoptosis in different cell types.[171–174] In this context, it was most recently shown that in addition to its general proapoptotic function, TIMP-3 can sensitize RASFs to Fas-ligand–induced apoptosis when expressed through adenoviral gene transfer (see above).[92]

When all of these data are considered, it can be concluded that TIMP-3 by itself or a drug with a TIMP-3–like structure and function might be extremely beneficial in inhibiting both the *cytokine-driven pathway* by blocking TNF-α and IL-6 as well as the *cytokine-independent pathway* mediated by RASFs by blocking MMPs.[16,22]

Cathepsins in RASFs

Cathepsins are the second major group of proteases involved in joint destruction.[175] They are classified by their catalytic mechanism and cleave cartilage types II, IX, and XI, as well as proteoglycans. Although their main function has been attributed to the regulation of ECM remodeling, more recent research revealed that cathepsins are also major regulators of the immune response.[176] The cysteine proteases cathepsin B and L are upregulated in RA synovium, especially at sites of cartilage invasion.[177–179] Similar to MMPs, cathepsins are activated by proto-oncogenes. Transfection of fibroblasts with the *ras* proto-oncogene leads to cellular transformation and the induction of cathepsin L.[180] This is supported by the *in vivo* finding of associated *ras* and cathepsin L expression in rheumatoid synovium.[179] Several studies have shown that inflammatory cytokines such as IL-1 and TNF-α can also stimulate the production of cathepsins B and L by RASFs.[181,182] Most recently, it was demonstrated that gene transfer of ribozymes targeting cathepsin L can significantly inhibit cartilage degradation mediated by fibroblasts both *in vitro* and *in vivo*.[183]

Cathepsin K is a cysteine proteinase that has been reported to play an important role in osteoclast-mediated bone resorption. In the context of RA, cathepsin K expression by RASFs and macrophages has been reported, especially at sites of synovial invasion into articular bone. This suggests that in RA, cathepsin K mainly participates in bone destruction.[184]

Interactions of Rheumatoid Arthritis Synovial Fibroblasts with Inflammatory Cells

As outlined above, RASFs not simply react to stimulation from neighboring cells, but exhibit features of stable activation. The specific activation of these cells contributes to the chronification of disease by regulating the accumulation of inflammatory and immune cells, particularly macrophages, B cells, and T cells. Of course, these inflammatory cells release a variety of cytokines that result in the stimulation of neighboring cells and contribute to the specific environment in the rheumatoid joint. It has been well established that cytokines derived from inflammatory cells, such as TNF-α, IL-1, and IFN-γ, among others, contribute to the stimulation and hence to the aggressive behavior of RASFs. However, it is now evident that the inflammatory cells not only affect fibroblasts but that, in turn, RASFs contribute significantly to the accumulation and survival of inflammatory cells. RASFs interact with and regulate important functions of T cells, B cells, and macrophages.

RASFs as Cells of Innate Immune System

Expression of TLRs, which are pattern recognition receptors and activators of the innate immune system, was found to be highly elevated in synovial tissues of RA patients.[158,185] As resident cells of the synovium, synovial fibroblasts are predestined to serve as sensors for invading pathogens and tissue damage. A selective panel of TLRs, namely TLR2, TLR3, and TLR4, are expressed and functionally active in RASFs.[158,186] TLR activation upon binding of conserved microbial patterns or endogenous ligands in RASFs leads to the expression of proinflammatory cytokines, matrix-degrading enzymes, and most interestingly, a wide panel of chemokines.[20,158,159,186] Thus, it is feasible to assume that activation of TLRs in the synovium is an initial event that leads to attraction of inflammatory cells and to a boost of adaptive immune mechanisms. A recently found new factor contributing to joint inflammation and destruction after activation of TLRs on RASFs is pre–B-cell enhancing factor (PBEF), also referred to as an adipokine called Visfatin.[187] The expression of PBEF/Visfatin in RASFs is induced by stimulation of TLR3 and TLR4, and leads to the expression of proinflammatory mediators (IL-6, TNF) and matrix-degrading enzymes (MMPs). Furthermore, higher levels of PBEF/Visfatin were found in the synovium, synovial fluid, and serum of patients with RA compared to patients with OA. Interestingly, levels of PBEF/Visfatin in the sera positively correlated with levels of C-reactive protein and the disease activity score (DAS). Thus, future therapeutics targeting PBEF might not only attenuate joint inflammation but also joint destruction.

Recruitment of T Cells by RASFs in RA

Interactions between RASFs and T cells appear to be of importance for the specific composition of the rheumatoid synovium. In this context, it has been shown that RASFs contribute to impaired apoptosis and anergy of synovial lymphocytes.[7]

It is mainly through the regulation of local cytokine levels that RASFs play a key role in modulating the transition from acute resolving inflammation to a persistent immune response that is accompanied by chronic inflammation.[11] Several inflammatory cytokines have been implicated in the interaction of RASFs and T cells. Prominent examples include IL-8,[188] IL-16,[189,190] IL-7, and IL-15,[191] all activators of T cells. In addition, the stromal cell–derived factor (SDF) 1, and particularly IL-6, have been associated with the maintenance of the inflammatory milieu. SDF1 stimulates the migration and inhibits the activation-induced apoptosis of T cells,[192] while IL-6, a highly abundant cytokine in the RA synovial fluid supports antigen-independent inflammation. Monocyte chemoattractant proteins (MCP) have been implicated in various diseases characterized by monocyte-rich infiltrates, including RA.[6,20,21] In addition, interesting data for IL-16 have been obtained. Levels of IL-16 in the synovial fluid positively correlate with the chemotactic activity toward $CD4^+$ T cells, and are highest in early RA.[189] In fibroblasts, expression of IL-16 is strongly induced by IL-1β,[193] a key inflammatory cytokine implicated in RA. Most interestingly, IL-16 has also been demonstrated to be induced by immunoglobulin G (IgG) targeting the insulin-like growth factor 1 receptor (IGF-1R) in RA, but not in OA. This mechanism may provide a link between B-cell activity and T-cell infiltration, and potentially constitutes a novel therapeutic target.[190]

Interactions between RASFs and T cells appear to be of importance for the specific composition of the rheumatoid synovium. Thus, it was found that human thymocytes and mitogen-activated peripheral blood T cells bind to RASFs, whereas fresh peripheral blood T cells do not show this behavior. Of note, antibodies against CD2 and synovial cell lymphocyte-function–associated antigen-3 inhibited this binding.[194]

Most recently, it was also shown that the T-cell–derived molecule LIGHT contributes to the resistance of apoptosis in RASFs, further highlighting the cellular interaction between T cells and RASFs.[195]

RASFs Interact with B Cells

RASFs have been implicated in the direct attraction and accumulation of B lymphocytes in the inflamed joints of RA patients. It was shown that RASFs act as follicular dendritic cells and bind B cells.[196] It appears that this function is intrinsic to RASFs and quite specific for these cells when compared to non-RA fibroblasts. Also, B cells co-cultured with RASFs show reduced apoptosis with an increase of mitochondrial apoptosis inhibitors such as Bcl-X(L).[197] In this study, it was proven that RASFs promote the survival of B cells, mainly through upregulation of Bcl-X(L), and block their apoptosis through VLA-4 (CD49d/CD29)–VCAM (CD106) interactions. Also other studies showed that B cells co-cultured with RASFs are protected from cell death in a cell contact– and VCAM-1–dependent mechanism,[198] but the significance of these findings is less clear, as similar effects have been seen with synovial fibroblasts from non-RA patients.

Interaction of RASFs with Synovial Macrophages Leading to Osteoclastogenesis

A number of research efforts support the notion that RASFs play a significant role in the activation of macrophages and their differentiation into multinucleated, bone-resorbing cells. Specifically, the osteoclast differentiating factor, the "receptor activator of NF-κB" (RANKL), has been identified as major factor promoting osteoclastogenesis in the RA synovium. It was demonstrated that RASFs produce large amounts of the osteoclast differentiation factor (ODF) now called RANKL *in vivo*, and that the levels of this factor correlate with the ability of RASFs to generate osteoclasts from PBMCs *in vitro*.[199] These data indicate that RASFs contribute to the degradation of ECM, not only directly by releasing matrix-degrading enzymes, but also indirectly by effecting the differentiation and activation of osteoclasts. The interaction of macrophages and fibroblasts in the RA synovium is also highlighted by studies indicating that the cooperation of synovial macrophages and fibroblasts is mediated through direct cell–cell interactions via ligation of CD55 on RASFs with CD97 on macrophages.[200] Interestingly, these interactions appear to take place predominantly in the synovial lining, which mediates the progressive destruction of cartilage and bone.

Outlook

In recent years, substantial progress was achieved in the elucidation of fibroblast biology in the context of RA. The picture of fibroblasts as passively reacting cells of the connective tissue has been corrected; currently it is widely accepted that synovial fibroblasts are actively embedded in the intricate network of cells and soluble factors contributing to chronic inflammation and joint destruction in RA. By their expression of toll-like receptors and their ability to react to changing environmental parameters such as oxygen tension and pH, synovial fibroblasts can be described as sentinel cells in the joints.[201] They are capable of producing a wide range of cytokines, chemokines, and growth factors, and thereby modulate and regulate immune responses in the joint. In the case of RA, however, synovial fibroblasts have changed to a stably activated phenotype, which is characterized by resistance to apoptotic stimuli and excessive production of proinflammatory cytokines and matrix-degrading enzymes. This aggressive behavior is aggravated by but not dependent on the inflammatory environment, and remains stable even in the absence of inflammatory cells. Since current therapies are targeting the inflammatory pathway mediated by cytokines, but not the RASFs mediated part of the pathogenesis, it is not surprising that ACR70 has not been higher than 60%. The successful depletion of B cells, T cells, and macrophages from the RA joint by current therapies does not result in a cure of the disease, and as soon as the therapy is ceased, inflammatory cells move back into the joint, most likely attracted by the powerful chemokines produced by RASFs upon continuous TLR stimulation.[20,158,185] Based on these results, future therapeutic strategies should include activated RASFs. Thus far, the initiating mechanisms of this activation are not known yet, but most recent data point to epigenetic mechanisms as mediators of this specific RA phenotype.[202]

Future therapeutic interventions that are designed to normalize fibroblast function in RA might have a critical advantage to currently used disease-modifying drugs that dampen inflammation via immunosuppression, but not specifically inhibit activated RASFs. Modulation of fibroblast activity might have an anti-inflammatory as well as an antidestructive effect, and thereby might control disease mechanisms on a wide scale.

References

1. Firestein GS. Rheumatoid synovitis and pannus. In: Klippel JH, Dieppe PA, eds. *Rheumatology*. 2nd ed. London: Mosby, 1998, 5.13.1–5.13.24.
2. Hoyhtya M, Myllyla R, Piuva J, et al. Monoclonal antibodies to human prolyl 4-hydroxylase. *Eur J Biochem* 1984;141(3):472–482.
3. Zimmermann T, Kunisch E, Pfeiffer R, et al. Isolation and characterization of rheumatoid arthritis synovial fibroblasts from primary culture—primary culture cells markedly differ from fourth-passage cells. *Arthritis Res* 2001;3(1):72–76.
4. Franz JK, Kolb SA, Hummel KM, et al. Interleukin-16, produced by synovial fibroblasts, mediates chemoattraction for CD4+ T lymphocytes in rheumatoid arthritis. *Eur J Immunol* 1998;28(9): 2661–2671.
5. Yaszay B, Trindade MC, Lind M, et al. Fibroblast expression of C-C chemokines in response to orthopaedic biomaterial particle challenge in vitro. *J Orthop Res* 2001;19(5):970–976.
6. Koch AE, Kunkel SL, Harlow LA, et al. Enhanced production of monocyte chemoattractant protein-1 in rheumatoid arthritis. *J Clin Invest* 1992;90(3):772–779.
7. Salmon M, Scheel Toellner D, Huissoon AP, et al. Inhibition of T cell apoptosis in the rheumatoid synovium. *J Clin Invest* 1997;99(3): 439–446.
8. Burger JA, Zvaifler NJ, Tsukada N, et al. Fibroblast-like synoviocytes support B-cell pseudoemperipolesis via a stromal cell-derived factor-1- and CD106 (VCAM-1)-dependent mechanism. *J Clin Invest* 2001;107(3):305–315.
9. Buckley CD. Why does chronic inflammatory joint disease persist? *Clin Med* 2003;3(4):361–366.
10. Meyer LH, Franssen L, Pap T. The role of mesenchymal cells in the pathophysiology of inflammatory arthritis. *Best Pract Res Clin Rheumatol* 2006;20(5):969–981.
11. Buckley CD, Pilling D, Lord JM, et al. Fibroblasts regulate the switch from acute resolving to chronic persistent inflammation. *Trends Immunol* 2001;22(4):199–204.
12. Qu Z, Garcia CH, O'Rourke LM, et al. Local proliferation of fibroblast-like synoviocytes contributes to synovial hyperplasia. Results of proliferating cell nuclear antigen/cyclin, c-myc, and nucleolar organizer region staining [see comments]. *Arthritis Rheum* 1994;37(2):212–220.
13. Firestein GS. Evolving concepts of rheumatoid arthritis. *Nature* 2003;423(6937):356–361.
14. Pap T, Muller-Ladner U, Gay RE, Gay S. Fibroblast biology. Role of synovial fibroblasts in the pathogenesis of rheumatoid arthritis. *Arthritis Res* 2000;2(5):361–367.
15. Fassbender HG. Histomorphological basis of articular cartilage destruction in rheumatoid arthritis. *Coll Relat Res* 1983;3(2):141–155.
16. Gay S, Gay RE, Koopman WJ. Molecular and cellular mechanisms of joint destruction in rheumatoid arthritis: Two cellular mechanisms explain joint destruction? *Ann Rheum Dis* 1993;52(Suppl 1): S39–S47.
17. Muller-Ladner U, Kriegsmann J, Franklin BN, et al. Synovial fibroblasts of patients with rheumatoid arthritis attach to and invade normal human cartilage when engrafted into SCID mice. *Am J Pathol* 1996;149(5):1607–1615.
18. Distler JH, Wenger RH, Gassmann M, et al. Physiologic responses to hypoxia and implications for hypoxia-inducible factors in the pathogenesis of rheumatoid arthritis. *Arthritis Rheum* 2004;50(1):10–23.
19. Ospelt C, Kyburz D, Pierer M, et al. Toll-like receptors in rheumatoid arthritis joint destruction mediated by two distinct pathways. *Ann Rheum Dis* 2004;63(Suppl 2):ii90–ii91.
20. Pierer M, Rethage J, Seibl R, et al. Chemokine secretion of rheumatoid arthritis synovial fibroblasts stimulated by Toll-like receptor 2 ligands. *J Immunol* 2004;172(2):1256–1265.

21. Distler JH, Jungel A, Huber LC, et al. The induction of matrix metalloproteinase and cytokine expression in synovial fibroblasts stimulated with immune cell microparticles. *Proc Natl Acad Sci U S A* 2005;102(8):2892–2897.
22. Muller-Ladner U, Gay RE, Gay S. Activation of synoviocytes. *Curr Opin Rheumatol* 2000;12(3):186–194.
23. Trabandt A, Gay RE, Gay S. Oncogene activation in rheumatoid synovium. *APMIS* 1992;100(10):861–875.
24. Muller-Ladner U, Kriegsmann J, Gay RE, Gay S. Oncoges in rheumatoid synovium. *Rheum Dis Clin North Am* 1995;21:675–690.
25. Asahara H, Hasunuma T, Kobata T, et al. In situ expression of protooncogenes and Fas/Fas ligand in rheumatoid arthritis synovium. *J Rheumatol* 1997;24(3):430–435.
26. Dooley S, Herlitzka I, Hanselmann R, et al. Constitutive expression of c-fos and c-jun, overexpression of ets-2, and reduced expression of metastasis suppressor gene nm23-H1 in rheumatoid arthritis. *Ann Rheum Dis* 1996;55(5):298–304.
27. Trabandt A, Aicher WK, Gay RE, et al. Spontaneous expression of immediately-early response genes c-fos and egr-1 in collagenase-producing rheumatoid synovial fibroblasts. *Rheumatol Int* 1992; 12(2):53–59.
28. Benbow U, Brinckerhoff CE. The AP-1 site and MMP gene regulation: What is all the fuss about? *Matrix Biol* 1997;15(8–9): 519–526.
29. Himelstein BP, Koch CJ. Studies of type IV collagenase regulation by hypoxia. *Cancer Lett* 1998;124(2):127–133.
30. Asahara H, Fujisawa K, Kobata T, et al. Direct evidence of high DNA binding activity of transcription factor AP-1 in rheumatoid arthritis synovium. *Arthritis Rheum* 1997;40(5):912–918.
31. Gum R, Wang H, Lengyel E, et al. Regulation of 92 kDa type IV collagenase expression by the jun aminoterminal kinase- and the extracellular signal–regulated kinase-dependent signaling cascades. *Oncogene* 1997;14(12):1481–1493.
32. Korzus E, Nagase H, Rydell R, Travis J. The mitogen-activated protein kinase and JAK-STAT signaling pathways are required for an oncostatin M-responsive element–mediated activation of matrix metalloproteinase 1 gene expression. *Biol ChemJ Biol Chem* 1997; 272(2):1188–1196.
33. Pap T, Nawrath M, Heinrich J, et al. Cooperation of Ras- and c-Myc-dependent pathways in regulating the growth and invasiveness of synovial fibroblasts in rheumatoid arthritis. *Arthritis Rheum* 2004;50(9):2794–2802.
34. Firestein GS, Echeverri F, Yeo M, et al. Somatic mutations in the p53 tumor suppressor gene in rheumatoid arthritis synovium. *Proc Natl Acad Sci U S A* 1997;94(20):10895–10900.
35. Pap T, Aupperle KR, Gay S, et al. Invasiveness of synovial fibroblasts is regulated by p53 in the SCID mouse in vivo model of cartilage invasion. *Arthritis Rheum* 2001;44(3):676–681.
36. Seemayer CA, Kuchen S, Neidhart M, et al. p53 in rheumatoid arthritis synovial fibroblasts at sites of invasion. *Ann Rheum Dis* 2003; 62(12):1139–1144.
37. Muller-Ladner U, Nishioka K. p53 in rheumatoid arthritis: Friend or foe? *Arthritis Res* 2000;2(3):175–178.
38. Yamasaki S, Yagishita N, Sasaki T, et al. Cytoplasmic destruction of p53 by the endoplasmic reticulum-resident ubiquitin ligase 'Synoviolin'. *EMBO J* 2007;26(1):113–122.
39. Klingelhofer J, Senolt L, Baslund B, et al. Up-regulation of metastasis-promoting S100A4 (Mts-1) in rheumatoid arthritis: Putative involvement in the pathogenesis of rheumatoid arthritis. *Arthritis Rheum* 2007;56(3):779–789.
40. Li J, Yen C, Liaw D, et al. PTEN, a putative protein tyrosine phosphatase gene mutated in human brain, breast, and prostate cancer [see comments]. *Science* 1997;275(5308):1943–1947.
41. Steck PA, Pershouse MA, Jasser SA, et al. Identification of a candidate tumour suppressor gene, MMAC1, at chromosome 10q23.3 that is mutated in multiple advanced cancers. *Nat Genet* 1997;15(4): 356–362.
42. Teng DH, Hu R, Lin H, et al. MMAC1/PTEN mutations in primary tumor specimens and tumor cell lines. *Cancer Res* 1997;57(23): 5221–5225.
43. Pap T, Franz JK, Hummel KM, et al. Activation of synovial fibroblasts in rheumatoid arthritis: Lack of expression of the tumour suppressor PTEN at sites of invasive growth and destruction. *Arthritis Res* 2000; 2(1):59–64.
44. Tamura M, Gu J, Danen EH, et al. PTEN interactions with focal adhesion kinase and suppression of the extracellular matrix–dependent phosphatidylinositol 3-kinase/Akt cell survival pathway. *Biol ChemJ Biol Chem* 1999;274(29):20693–20703.
45. Tamura M, Gu J, Matsumoto K, et al. Inhibition of cell migration, spreading, and focal adhesions by tumor suppressor PTEN. *Science* 1998;280(5369):1614–1617.
46. Di Cristofano A, Kotsi P, Peng YF, et al. Impaired Fas response and autoimmunity in Pten+/− mice. *Science* 1999;285(5436):2122–2125.
47. Mojcik CF, Shevach EM. Adhesion molecules: A rheumatologic perspective. *Arthritis Rheum* 1997;40(6):991–1004.
48. Ishikawa H, Hirata S, Andoh Y, et al. An immunohistochemical and immunoelectron microscopic study of adhesion molecules in synovial pannus formation in rheumatoid arthritis. *Rheumatol Int* 1996;16(2):53–60.
49. Rinaldi N, Schwarz EM, Weis D, et al. Increased expression of integrins on fibroblast-like synoviocytes from rheumatoid arthritis in vitro correlates with enhanced binding to extracellular matrix proteins. *Ann Rheum Dis* 1997;56(1):45–51.
50. Schwartz MA. Integrins, oncogenes, and anchorage independence. *J Cell Biol* 1997;139(3):575–578.
51. Dike LE, Farmer SR. *Cell* adhesion induces expression of growth-associated genes in suspension-arrested fibroblasts. *Proc Natl Acad Sci U S A* 1988;85:6792–6796.
52. Dike LE, Ingber DE. Integrin-dependent induction of early growth response genes in capillary endothelial cells. *J Cell Sci* 1996;109: 2855–2863.
53. Sarkissian M, Lafyatis R. Integrin engagement regulates proliferation and collagenase expression of rheumatoid synovial fibroblasts. *J Immunol* 1999;162(3):1772–1779.
54. Lin TH, Chen Q, Howe A, Juliano RL. *Cell* anchorage permits efficient signal transduction between ras and its downstream kinases. *Biol ChemJ Biol Chem* 1997;272(14):8849–8852.
55. Inoue H, Yamashita A, Hakura A. Adhesion-dependency of serum-induced p42/p44 MAP kinase activation is released by retroviral oncogenes. *Virology* 1996;225(1):223–226.
56. Ravanti L, Heino J, Lopez-Otin C, Kahari VM. Induction of collagenase-3 (MMP-13) expression in human skin fibroblasts by three-dimensional collagen is mediated by p38 mitogen-activated protein kinase. *Biol ChemJ Biol Chem* 1999;274(4):2446–2455.
57. Wang AZ, Wang JC, Fisher GW, Diamond HS. Interleukin-1beta-stimulated invasion of articular cartilage by rheumatoid synovial fibroblasts is inhibited by antibodies to specific integrin receptors and by collagenase inhibitors. *Arthritis Rheum* 1997;40(7):1298–1307.
58. Mitra SK, Hanson DA, Schlaepfer DD. Focal adhesion kinase: In command and control of cell motility. *Nat Rev Mol Cell Biol* 2005; 6(1):56–68.
59. Yamada KM, Miyamoto S. Integrin transmembrane signaling and cytoskeletal control. *Curr Opin Cell Biol* 1995;7(5):681–689.
60. Echtermeyer F, Baciu PC, Saoncella S, et al. Syndecan-4 core protein is sufficient for the assembly of focal adhesions and actin stress fibers. *J Cell Sci* 1999;112:3433–3441.
61. Echtermeyer F, Streit M, Wilcox-Adelman S, et al. Delayed wound repair and impaired angiogenesis in mice lacking syndecan-4. *J Clin Invest* 2001;107(2):R9–R14.
62. Neidhart M, Zaucke F, von Knoch R, et al. Galectin-3 is induced in rheumatoid arthritis synovial fibroblasts after adhesion to cartilage oligomeric matrix protein. *Ann Rheum Dis* 2005;64(3):419–424.
63. Liu FT, Hsu DK. The role of galectin-3 in promotion of the inflammatory response. *Drug News Perspect* 2007;20(7):455–460.

64. Aicher WK, Heer AH, Trabandt A, et al. Overexpression of zinc-finger transcription factor Z-225/Egr-1 in synoviocytes from rheumatoid arthritis patients. *J Immunol* 1994;152(12): 5940–5948.
65. Nykanen P, Bergroth V, Raunio P, et al. Phenotypic characterization of 3H-thymidine incorporating cells in rheumatoid arthritis synovial membrane. *Rheumatol Int* 1986;6(6):269–271.
66. Petrow P, Theis B, Eckard A, et al. Determination of proliferating cells at sites of cartilage invasion in patients with rheumatoid arthritis. *Arthritis Rheum* 1997;40(Suppl):S251.
67. Kinne RW, Palombo Kinne E, Emmrich F. Activation of synovial fibroblasts in rheumatoid arthritis. *Ann Rheum Dis* 1995;54(6):501–504.
68. Baier A, Meineckel I, Gay S, Pap T. Apoptosis in rheumatoid arthritis. *Curr Opin Rheumatol* 2003;15(3):274–279.
69. Matsumoto S, Muller Ladner U, Gay RE, et al. Multistage apoptosis and Fas antigen expression of synovial fibroblasts derived from patients with rheumatoid arthritis. *J Rheumatol* 1996;23: 1345–1352.
70. Nakajima T, Aono H, Hasunuma T, et al. Apoptosis and functional Fas antigen in rheumatoid arthritis synoviocytes. *Arthritis Rheum* 1995;38:485–491.
71. Pope RM. Apoptosis as a therapeutic tool in rheumatoid arthritis. *Nat Rev Immunol* 2002;2(7):527–535.
72. Kammouni W, Wong K, Ma G, et al. Regulation of apoptosis in fibroblast-like synoviocytes by the hypoxia-induced Bcl-2 family member Bcl-2/adenovirus E1B 19-kd protein-interacting protein 3. *Arthritis Rheum* 2007;56(9):2854–2863.
73. Perlman H, Liu H, Georganas C, et al. Differential expression pattern of the antiapoptotic proteins, Bcl-2 and FLIP, in experimental arthritis. *Arthritis Rheum* 2001;44(12):2899–2908.
74. Perlman H, Georganas C, Pagliari LJ, et al. Bcl-2 expression in synovial fibroblasts is essential for maintaining mitochondrial homeostasis and cell viability. *J Immunol* 2000;164(10):5227–5235.
75. Kurowska M, Rudnicka W, Kontny E, et al. Fibroblast-like synoviocytes from rheumatoid arthritis patients express functional IL-15 receptor complex: Endogenous IL-15 in autocrine fashion enhances cell proliferation and expression of Bcl-x(L) and Bcl-2. *J Immunol* 2002;169(4):1760–1767.
76. Hasunuma T, Kayagaki N, Asahara H, et al. Accumulation of soluble Fas in inflamed joints of patients with rheumatoid arthritis. *Arthritis Rheum* 1997;40(1):80–86.
77. Takemura Y, Fukuo K, Yasuda O, et al. Fas signaling induces Akt activation and upregulation of endothelial nitric oxide synthase expression. *Hypertension* 2004;43(4):880–884.
78. Osaki M, Kase S, Adachi K, et al. Inhibition of the PI3K-Akt signaling pathway enhances the sensitivity of Fas-mediated apoptosis in human gastric carcinoma cell line, MKN–45. *J Cancer Res Clin Oncol* 2004;130(1):8–14.
79. Perlman H, Pagliari LJ, Liu H, et al. Rheumatoid arthritis synovial macrophages express the Fas-associated death domain-like interleukin-1–beta-converting enzyme-inhibitory protein and are refractory to Fas-mediated apoptosis. *Arthritis Rheum* 2001;44(1):21–30.
80. Catrina AI, Ulfgren AK, Lindblad S, et al. Low levels of apoptosis and high FLIP expression in early rheumatoid arthritis synovium. *Ann Rheum Dis* 2002;61(10):934–936.
81. Schedel J, Gay RE, Kuenzler P, et al. FLICE-inhibitory protein expression in synovial fibroblasts and at sites of cartilage and bone erosion in rheumatoid arthritis. *Arthritis Rheum* 2002;46(6): 1512–1518.
82. Palao G, Santiago B, Galindo M, et al. Down-regulation of FLIP sensitizes rheumatoid synovial fibroblasts to Fas-mediated apoptosis. *Arthritis Rheum* 2004;50(9):2803–2810.
83. Melchior F. SUMO—nonclassical ubiquitin. *Annu Rev Cell Dev Biol* 2000;16:591–626.
84. Franz JK, Pap T, Hummel KM, et al. Expression of sentrin, a novel antiapoptotic molecule, at sites of synovial invasion in rheumatoid arthritis. *Arthritis Rheum* 2000;43(3):599–607.
85. Okura T, Gong L, Kamitani T, et al. Protection against Fas/APO-1- and tumor necrosis factor-mediated cell death by a novel protein, sentrin. *J Immunol* 1996;157(10):4277–4281.
86. Meinecke I, Cinski A, Baier A, et al. Modification of nuclear PML protein by SUMO-1 regulates Fas-induced apoptosis in rheumatoid arthritis synovial fibroblasts. *Proc Natl Acad Sci U S A* 2007;104(12): 5073–5078.
87. Hsu H, Shu HB, Pan MG, Goeddel DV. TRADD-TRAF2 and TRADD-FADD interactions define two distinct TNF receptor 1 signal transduction pathways. *Cell* 1996;84(2):299–308.
88. Mountz JD, Hsu HC, Matsuki Y, Zhang HG. Apoptosis and rheumatoid arthritis: Past, present, and future directions. *Curr Rheumatol Rep* 2001;3(1):70–78.
89. Liu H, Pope RM. The role of apoptosis in rheumatoid arthritis. *Curr Opin Pharmacol* 2003;3(3):317–322.
90. Reddy SA, Huang JH, Liao WS. Phosphatidylinositol 3-kinase as a mediator of TNF-induced NF-kappa B activation. *J Immunol* 2000; 164(3):1355–1363.
91. Ohshima S, Mima T, Sasai M, et al. Tumour necrosis factor alpha (TNF-alpha) interferes with Fas-mediated apoptotic cell death on rheumatoid arthritis (RA) synovial cells: A possible mechanism of rheumatoid synovial hyperplasia and a clinical benefit of anti–TNF-alpha therapy for RA. *Cytokine* 2000;12(3):281–288.
92. Drynda A, Quax PH, Neumann M, et al. Gene transfer of tissue inhibitor of metalloproteinases-3 reverses the inhibitory effects of TNF-alpha on Fas-induced apoptosis in rheumatoid arthritis synovial fibroblasts. *J Immunol* 2005;174(10):6524–6531.
93. Pap T, Cinski A, Baier A, et al. Modulation of pathways regulating both the invasiveness and apoptosis in rheumatoid arthritis synovial fibroblasts. *Joint Bone Spine* 2003;70(6):477–479.
94. van Vliet J, Oates NA, Whitelaw E. Epigenetic mechanisms in the context of complex diseases. *Cell Mol Life Sci* 2007;64(12):1531–1538.
95. Huber LC, Brock M, Hemmatazad H, et al. Histone deacetylase/acetylase activity in total synovial tissue derived from rheumatoid arthritis and osteoarthritis patients. *Arthritis Rheum* 2007;56(4): 1087–1093.
96. Chung YL, Lee MY, Wang AJ, Yao LF. A therapeutic strategy uses histone deacetylase inhibitors to modulate the expression of genes involved in the pathogenesis of rheumatoid arthritis. *Mol Ther* 2003;8(5):707–717.
97. Lin HS, Hu CY, Chan HY, et al. Anti-rheumatic activities of histone deacetylase (HDAC) inhibitors in vivo in collagen-induced arthritis in rodents. *Br J Pharmacol* 2007;150(7):862–872.
98. Marks PA, Richon VM, Miller T, Kelly WK. Histone deacetylase inhibitors. Adv *Cancer Res* 2004;91:137–168.
99. Jungel A, Baresova V, Ospelt C, et al. Trichostatin A sensitises rheumatoid arthritis synovial fibroblasts for TRAIL-induced apoptosis. *Ann Rheum Dis* 2006;65(7):910–912.
100. Karouzakis E, Ospelt C, Schumann G, et al. Genomic hypomethylation of rheumatoid arthritis synovial fibroblasts. *Arthritis Rheum* 2007;56:S317.
101. Neidhart M, Rethage J, Kuchen S, et al. Retrotransposable L1 elements expressed in rheumatoid arthritis synovial tissue: Association with genomic DNA hypomethylation and influence on gene expression. *Arthritis Rheum* 2000;43(12):2634–2647.
102. Neidhart M, Rethage J, Kuchen S, et al. Retrotransposable L1 elements expressed in rheumatoid arthritis synovial tissue: Association with genomic DNA hypomethylation and influence on gene expression. *Arthritis Rheum* 2000;43(12):2634–2647.
103. Ohshima S, Kuchen S, Seemayer CA, et al. Galectin 3 and its binding protein in rheumatoid arthritis. *Arthritis Rheum* 2003;48(10): 2788–2795.
104. Esquela-Kerscher A, Slack FJ. Oncomirs—microRNAs with a role in cancer. *Nat Rev Cancer* 2006;6(4):259–269.
105. Stanczyk J, Leslie Pedrioli D, Brentano F, et al. Altered expression of microRNA in synovial fibroblasts and synovial tissue in rheumatoid arthritis. *Arthritis Rheum* 2008;58(4):1001–1009.

106. Pap T, Gay S, Schett. Matrix metalloproteinases. In: Smolen JS, Lipsky PE, eds. *Contemporary Targeted Therapies in Rheumatology,* London: Informa Healthcare, 2007, 353–366.
107. Nagase H, Woessner JF Jr. Matrix metalloproteinases. *Biol ChemJ Biol Chem* 1999;274(31):21491–21494.
108. Wolfsberg TG, Primakoff P, Myles DG, White JM. ADAM, a novel family of membrane proteins containing A Disintegrin And Metalloprotease domain: Multipotential functions in cell-cell and cell-matrix interactions. *J Cell Biol* 1995;131(2):275–278.
109. Kaushal GP, Shah SV. The new kids on the block: ADAMTSs, potentially multifunctional metalloproteinases of the ADAM family. *J Clin Invest* 2000;105(10):1335–1337.
110. Krane SM, Conca W, Stephenson ML, et al. Mechanisms of matrix degradation in rheumatoid arthritis. *Am N Y Acad Sci* 1990;580: 340–354.
111. Loeser RF, Forsyth CB, Samarel AM, Im HJ. Fibronectin fragment activation of proline-rich tyrosine kinase PYK2 mediates integrin signals regulating collagenase-3 expression by human chondrocytes through a protein kinase C-dependent pathway. *Biol ChemJ Biol Chem* 2003;278(27):24577–24585.
112. Yasuda T, Shimizu M, Nakagawa T, et al. Matrix metalloproteinase production by COOH-terminal heparin-binding fibronectin fragment in rheumatoid synovial cells. *Lab Invest* 2003;83(2): 153–162.
113. Barchowsky A, Frleta D, Vincenti MP. Integration of the NF-kappaB and mitogen-activated protein kinase/AP-1 pathways at the collagenase-1 promoter: Divergence of IL-1 and TNF-dependent signal transduction in rabbit primary synovial fibroblasts. *Cytokine* 2000;12(10):1469–1479.
114. Brauchle M, Gluck D, Di Padova F, et al. Independent role of p38 and ERK1/2 mitogen-activated kinases in the upregulation of matrix metalloproteinase-1. *Exp Cell Res* 2000;258(1):135–144.
115. Mengshol JA, Vincenti MP, Coon CI, et al. Interleukin-1 induction of collagenase 3 (matrix metalloproteinase 13) gene expression in chondrocytes requires p38, c-Jun N-terminal kinase, and nuclear factor kappaB: Differential regulation of collagenase 1 and collagenase 3. *Arthritis Rheum* 2000;43(4):801–811.
116. Li WQ, Dehnade F, Zafarullah M. Oncostatin M-induced matrix metalloproteinase and tissue inhibitor of metalloproteinase-3 genes expression in chondrocytes requires Janus kinase/STAT signaling pathway. *J Immunol* 2001;166(5):3491–3498.
117. Westermarck J, Seth A, Kahari VM. Differential regulation of interstitial collagenase (MMP-1) gene expression by ETS transcription factors. *Oncogene* 1997;14(22):2651–2660.
118. Marok R, Winyard PG, Coumbe A, et al. Activation of the transcription factor nuclear factor-kappaB in human inflamed synovial tissue. *Arthritis Rheum* 1996;39(4):583–591.
119. Miagkov AV, Kovalenko DV, Brown CE, et al. NF-kappaB activation provides the potential link between inflammation and hyperplasia in the arthritic joint. *Proc Natl Acad Sci U S A* 1998; 95(23):13859–13864.
120. Georganas C, Liu H, Perlman H, et al. Regulation of IL-6 and IL-8 expression in rheumatoid arthritis synovial fibroblasts: The dominant role for NF-kappa B but not C/EBP beta or c- Jun. *J Immunol* 2000;165(12):7199–7206.
121. Karin M, Lin A. NF-kappaB at the crossroads of life and death. *ImmunolNat Immunol* 2002;3(3):221–227.
122. Makarov SS. NF-kappaB in rheumatoid arthritis: A pivotal regulator of inflammation, hyperplasia, and tissue destruction. *Arthritis Res* 2001;3(4):200–206.
123. Li P, Sanz I, O'Keefe RJ, Schwarz EM. NF-kappa B regulates VCAM-1 expression on fibroblast-like synoviocytes. *J Immunol* 2000;164(11):5990–5997.
124. Vincenti MP, Coon CI, Brinckerhoff CE. Nuclear factor kappaB/ p50 activates an element in the distal matrix metalloproteinase 1 promoter in interleukin-1beta-stimulated synovial fibroblasts. *Arthritis Rheum* 1998;41(11):1987–1994.
125. Hahne JC, Fuchs T, El Mustapha H, et al. Expression pattern of matrix metalloproteinase and TIMP genes in fibroblasts derived from Ets-1 knock-out mice compared to wild-type mouse fibroblasts. *Int J Mol Med* 2006;18(1):153–159.
126. Redlich K, Kiener HP, Schett G, et al. Overexpression of transcription factor Ets-1 in rheumatoid arthritis synovial membrane: Regulation of expression and activation by interleukin-1 and tumor necrosis factor alpha. *Arthritis Rheum* 2001;44(2):266–274.
127. Schett G, Tohidast-Akrad M, Smolen JS, et al. Activation, differential localization, and regulation of the stress-activated protein kinases, extracellular signal-regulated kinase, c-JUN N-terminal kinase, and p38 mitogen-activated protein kinase, in synovial tissue and cells in rheumatoid arthritis. *Arthritis Rheum* 2000;43(11):2501–2512.
128. Konttinen YT, Ainola M, Valleala H, et al. Analysis of 16 different matrix metalloproteinases (MMP-1 to MMP-20) in the synovial membrane: Different profiles in trauma and rheumatoid arthritis. *Ann Rheum Dis* 1999;58(11):691–697.
129. Sorsa T, Konttinen YT, Lindy O, et al. Collagenase in synovitis of rheumatoid arthritis. *Semin Arthritis Rheum* 1992;22(1):44–53.
130. Maeda S, Sawai T, Uzuki M, et al. Determination of interstitial collagenase (MMP-1) in patients with rheumatoid arthritis. *Ann Rheum Dis* 1995;54(12):970–975.
131. Tetlow LC, Lees M, Ogata Y, et al. Differential expression of gelatinase B (MMP-9) and stromelysin-1 (MMP-3) by rheumatoid synovial cells in vitro and in vivo. *Rheumatol Int* 1993;13(2):53–59.
132. Okada Y, Takeuchi N, Tomita K, et al. Immunolocalization of matrix metalloproteinase 3 (stromelysin) in rheumatoid synovioblasts (B cells): Correlation with rheumatoid arthritis. *Ann Rheum Dis.* 1989;48(8):645–653.
133. Beekman B, van El B, Drijfhout JW, et al. Highly increased levels of active stromelysin in rheumatoid synovial fluid determined by a selective fluorogenic assay. *FEBS Lett* 1997;418(3):305–309.
134. Ichikawa Y, Yamada C, Horiki T, et al. Serum matrix metalloproteinase-3 and fibrin degradation product levels correlate with clinical disease activity in rheumatoid arthritis. *Clin Exp Rheumatol* 1998;16(5):533–540.
135. Manicourt DH, Fujimoto N, Obata K, Thonar EJ. Levels of circulating collagenase, stromelysin-1, and tissue inhibitor of matrix metalloproteinases 1 in patients with rheumatoid arthritis. Relationship to serum levels of antigenic keratan sulfate and systemic parameters of inflammation. *Arthritis Rheum* 1995;38(8):1031–1039.
136. So A, Chamot AM, Peclat V, Gerster JC. Serum MMP-3 in rheumatoid arthritis: Correlation with systemic inflammation but not with erosive status. *Rheumatol (Oxford)* 1999;38(5):407–410.
137. Taylor DJ, Cheung NT, Dawes PT. Increased serum proMMP-3 in inflammatory arthritides: A potential indicator of synovial inflammatory monokine activity. *Ann Rheum Dis* 1994;53(11): 768–772.
138. Yoshihara Y, Obata K, Fujimoto N, et al. Increased levels of stromelysin-1 and tissue inhibitor of metalloproteinases-1 in sera from patients with rheumatoid arthritis. *Arthritis Rheum* 1995; 38(7):969–975.
139. Yamanaka H, Matsuda Y, Tanaka M, et al. Serum matrix metalloproteinase 3 as a predictor of the degree of joint destruction during the six months after measurement, in patients with early rheumatoid arthritis. *Arthritis Rheum* 2000;43(4):852–858.
140. Petrow P, Hummel KM, Franz JK, et al. In-situ detection of MMP-13 mRNA in the synovial membrane and cartilage-pannus junction in rheumatoid arthritis. *Arthritis Rheum* 1997;40:S336.
141. Lindy O, Konttinen YT, Sorsa T, et al. Matrix-metalloproteinase 13 (collagenase 3) in human rheumatoid synovium. *Arthritis Rheum* 1997;40:1391–1399.
142. Westhoff CS, Freudiger D, Petrow P, et al. Characterization of collagenase 3 (matrix metalloproteinase 13) messenger RNA expression in the synovial membrane and synovial fibroblasts of patients with rheumatoid arthritis. *Arthritis Rheum* 1999;42(7): 1517–1527.

143. Pap T, Shigeyama Y, Kuchen S, et al. Differential expression pattern of membrane-type matrix metalloproteinases in rheumatoid arthritis. *Arthritis Rheum* 2000;43(6):1226–1232.
144. Distler JH, Pisetsky DS, Huber LC, et al. Microparticles as regulators of inflammation: Novel players of cellular crosstalk in the rheumatic diseases. *Arthritis Rheum* 2005;52(11):3337–3348.
145. van de Loo FA, Joosten LA, van Lent PL, et al. Role of interleukin-1, tumor necrosis factor alpha, and interleukin-6 in cartilage proteoglycan metabolism and destruction. Effect of in situ blocking in murine antigen- and zymosan-induced arthritis. *Arthritis Rheum* 1995;38(2):164–172.
146. van den Berg WB, Joosten LA, Helsen M, van de Loo FA. Amelioration of established murine collagen-induced arthritis with anti–IL-1 treatment. *Clin Exp Immunol* 1994;95(2):237–243.
147. Muller-Ladner U, Roberts CR, Franklin BN, et al. Human IL-1Ra gene transfer into human synovial fibroblasts is chondroprotective. *J Immunol* 1997;158(7):3492–3498.
148. Mengshol JA, Vincenti MP, Brinckerhoff CE. IL-1 induces collagenase-3 (MMP-13) promoter activity in stably transfected chondrocytic cells: Requirement for Runx–2 and activation by p38 MAPK and JNK pathways. *Nucleic Acids Res* 2001;29(21):4361–4372.
149. Catterall JB, Carrere S, Koshy PJ, et al. Synergistic induction of matrix metalloproteinase 1 by interleukin-1alpha and oncostatin M in human chondrocytes involves signal transducer and activator of transcription and activator protein 1 transcription factors via a novel mechanism. *Arthritis Rheum* 2001;44(10):2296–2310.
150. Brinckerhoff CE, Auble DT. Regulation of collagenase gene expression in synovial fibroblasts. *Ann N Y Acad Sci* 1990;580:355–374.
151. Dayer JM, Beutler B, Cerami A. Cachectin/tumor necrosis factor stimulates collagenase and prostaglandin E2 production by human synovial cells and dermal fibroblasts. *J Exp Med* 1985;162(6): 2163–2168.
152. Kuiper S, Joosten LA, Bendele AM, et al. Different roles of TNFα and IL-1 in murine streptococcal wall arthritis. *Cytokine* 1998;10: 690–702.
153. Jovanovic DV, Martel-Pelletier J, Di Battista JA, et al. Stimulation of 92-kd gelatinase (matrix metalloproteinase 9) production by interleukin-17 in human monocyte/macrophages: A possible role in rheumatoid arthritis. *Arthritis Rheum* 2000;43(5):1134–1144.
154. Bond M, Fabunmi RP, Baker AH, Newby AC. Synergistic upregulation of metalloproteinase-9 by growth factors and inflammatory cytokines: An absolute requirement for transcription factor NF-kappa B. *FEBS Lett* 1998;435(1):29–34.
155. Forsyth CB, Pulai J, Loeser RF. Fibronectin fragments and blocking antibodies to alpha2beta1 and alpha5beta1 integrins stimulate mitogen-activated protein kinase signaling and increase collagenase 3 (matrix metalloproteinase 13) production by human articular chondrocytes. *Arthritis Rheum* 2002;46(9):2368–2376.
156. Johnson GB, Brunn GJ, Tang AH, Platt JL. Evolutionary clues to the functions of the Toll-like family as surveillance receptors. *Trends Immunol* 2003;24(1):19–24.
157. Okamura Y, Watari M, Jerud ES, et al. The extra domain A of fibronectin activates Toll-like receptor 4. *Biol ChemJ Biol Chem* 2001; 276(13):10229–10233.
158. Brentano F, Schorr O, Gay RE, et al. RNA released from necrotic synovial fluid cells activates rheumatoid arthritis synovial fibroblasts via Toll-like receptor 3. *Arthritis Rheum* 2005;52(9):2656–2665.
159. Sanchez-Pernaute O, Brentano F, Ospelt C, et al. Fibrin triggers an innate immune response in rheumatoid arthritis synovial fibroblasts acting as endogenous ligand of toll-like receptor. *Arthritis Rheum* 2007;56:S626.
160. Sanchez-Pernaute O, Karouzakis E, Jungel A, et al. Fibrin promotes invasivness of rheumatoid arthritis synovial fibroblasts by the induction of matrix metalloproteinases 1 and 3. *Arthritis Rheum* 2007;56:S429.
161. Tolboom TC, Pieterman E, van der Laan WH, et al. Invasive properties of fibroblast-like synoviocytes: Correlation with growth characteristics and expression of MMP-1, MMP-3, and MMP-10. *Ann Rheum Dis* 2002;61(11):975–980.
162. Rutkauskaite E, Zacharias W, Schedel J, et al. Ribozymes that inhibit the production of matrix metalloproteinase 1 reduce the invasiveness of rheumatoid arthritis synovial fibroblasts. *Arthritis Rheum* 2004;50(5):1448–1456.
163. Rutkauskaite E, Volkmer D, Shigeyama Y, et al. Retroviral gene transfer of an antisense construct against membrane type 1 matrix metalloproteinase reduces the invasiveness of rheumatoid arthritis synovial fibroblasts. *Arthritis Rheum* 2005;52(7):2010–2014.
164. Clark IM, Powell LK, Ramsey S, et al. The measurement of collagenase, TIMP and collagenase-TIMP complex in synovial fluids from patients with osteoarthritis and rheumatoid arthritis. *Arthritis Rheum* 1993;36:372–380.
165. DiBattista JA, Pelletier JP, Zafarullah M, et al. Coordinate regulation of matrix metalloproteases and tissue inhibitor of metalloproteinase expression in human synovial fibroblasts. *J Rheumatol* Suppl 1995;43:123–128.
166. Firestein GS, Paine MM. Stromelysin and tissue inhibitor of metalloproteinases gene expression in rheumatoid arthritis synovium. *Am J Pathol* 1992;140(6):1309–1314.
167. van der Laan WH, Quax PH, Seemayer CA, et al. Cartilage degradation and invasion by rheumatoid synovial fibroblasts is inhibited by gene transfer of TIMP-1 and TIMP-3. *Gene Ther* 2003;10: 234–242.
168. Smith MR, Kung H, Durum SK, et al. TIMP-3 induces cell death by stabilizing TNF-alpha receptors on the surface of human colon carcinoma cells. *Cytokine* 1997;9(10):770–780.
169. Hargreaves PG, Wang F, Antcliff J, et al. Human myeloma cells shed the interleukin-6 receptor: Inhibition by tissue inhibitor of metalloproteinase-3 and a hydroxamate-based metalloproteinase inhibitor. *Br J Haematol* 1998;101(4):694–702.
170. Amour A, Slocombe PM, Webster A, et al. TNF-alpha converting enzyme (TACE) is inhibited by TIMP-3. *FEBS Lett* 1998;435(1): 39–44.
171. Ahonen M, Baker AH, Kahari VM. Adenovirus-mediated gene delivery of tissue inhibitor of metalloproteinases-3 inhibits invasion and induces apoptosis in melanoma cells. *Cancer Res* 1998; 58(11):2310–2315.
172. Baker AH, George SJ, Zaltsman AB, et al. Inhibition of invasion and induction of apoptotic cell death of cancer cell lines by overexpression of TIMP-3. *Br J Cancer* 1999;79(9–10):1347–1355.
173. Baker AH, Zaltsman AB, George SJ, Newby AC. Divergent effects of tissue inhibitor of metalloproteinase-1, -2, or -3 overexpression on rat vascular smooth muscle cell invasion, proliferation, and death in vitro. TIMP-3 promotes apoptosis. *J Clin Invest* 1998; 101(6):1478–1487.
174. Majid MA, Smith VA, Easty DL, et al. Adenovirus mediated gene delivery of tissue inhibitor of metalloproteinases-3 induces death in retinal pigment epithelial cells. *Br J Ophthalmol* 2002;86(1): 97–101.
175. Muller-Ladner U, Gay RE, Gay S. Cysteine proteinases in arthritis and inflammation. *Perspectives Drug Discov Des* 1996;6:87–98.
176. Zavasnik-Bergant T, Turk B. Cysteine proteases: Destruction ability versus immunomodulation capacity in immune cells. *Biol Chem* 2007;388(11):1141–1149.
177. Keyszer G, Redlich A, Haupl T, et al. Differential expression of cathepsins B and L compared with matrix metalloproteinases and their respective inhibitors in rheumatoid arthritis and osteoarthritis: A parallel investigation by semiquantitative reverse transcriptase-polymerase chain reaction and immunohistochemistry. *Arthritis Rheum* 1998;41(8):1378–1387.
178. Keyszer GM, Heer AH, Kriegsmann J, et al. Comparative analysis of cathepsin L, cathepsin D, and collagenase messenger RNA expression in synovial tissues of patients with rheumatoid arthritis and osteoarthritis, by in situ hybridization. *Arthritis Rheum* 1995;38(7):976–984.

179. Trabandt A, Aicher WK, Gay RE, et al. Expression of the collagenolytic and Ras-induced cysteine proteinase cathepsin L and proliferation-associated oncogenes in synovial cells of MRL/I mice and patients with rheumatoid arthritis. *Matrix* 1990;10(6): 349–361.
180. Joseph L, Lapid S, Sukhatme V. The major ras induced protein in NIH3T3 cells is cathepsin L. *Nucleic Acids Res* 1987;15(7):3186.
181. Huet G, Flipo RM, Colin C, et al. Stimulation of the secretion of latent cysteine proteinase activity by tumor necrosis factor alpha and interleukin-1. *Arthritis Rheum* 1993;36(6):772–780.
182. Lemaire R, Huet G, Zerimech F, et al. Selective induction of the secretion of cathepsins B and L by cytokines in synovial fibroblast-like cells. *Br J Rheumatol* 1997;36(7):735–743.
183. Schedel J, Seemayer CA, Pap T, et al. Targeting cathepsin L (CL) by specific ribozymes decreases CL protein synthesis and cartilage destruction in rheumatoid arthritis. *Gene Ther* 2004;11(13): 1040–1047.
184. Hummel KM, Petrow PK, Franz JK, et al. Cysteine proteinase cathepsin K mRNA is expressed in synovium of patients with rheumatoid arthritis and is detected at sites of synovial bone destruction. *J Rheumatol* 1998;25(10):1887–1894.
185. Seibl R, Birchler T, Loeliger S, et al. Expression and regulation of Toll-like receptor 2 in rheumatoid arthritis synovium. *Am J Pathol* 2003;162(4):1221–1227.
186. Kyburz D, Rethage J, Seibl R, et al. Bacterial peptidoglycans but not CpG oligonucleotides activate synovial fibroblasts by Toll-like receptor signaling. *Arthritis Rheum* 2003;48(3):590–593.
187. Brentano F, Schorr O, Ospelt C, et al. Pre-B cell colony-enhancing factor/visfatin, a new marker of inflammation in rheumatoid arthritis with proinflammatory and matrix-degrading activities. *Arthritis Rheum* 2007;56(9):2829–2839.
188. Min DJ, Cho ML, Lee SH, et al. Augmented production of chemokines by the interaction of type II collagen–reactive T cells with rheumatoid synovial fibroblasts. *Arthritis Rheum* 2004;50(4): 1146–1155.
189. Franz JK, Kolb SA, Hummel KM, et al. Interleukin-16, produced by synovial fibroblasts, mediates chemoattraction for CD4+ T lymphocytes in rheumatoid arthritis. *Eur J Immunol* 1998;28(9):2661–2671.
190. Pritchard J, Tsui S, Horst N, et al. Synovial fibroblasts from patients with rheumatoid arthritis, like fibroblasts from Graves' disease, express high levels of IL-16 when treated with Igs against insulin-like growth factor-1 receptor. *J Immunol* 2004;173(5):3564–3569.
191. McInnes IB, al Mughales J, Field M, et al. The role of interleukin-15 in T-cell migration and activation in rheumatoid arthritis. *Nat Med* 1996;2(2):175–182.
192. Nanki T, Hayashida K, El Gabalawy HS, et al. Stromal cell–derived factor-1–CXC chemokine receptor 4 interactions play a central role in CD4+ T cell accumulation in rheumatoid arthritis synovium. *J Immunol* 2000;165(11):6590–6598.
193. Sciaky D, Brazer W, Center DM, et al. Cultured human fibroblasts express constitutive IL-16 mRNA: Cytokine induction of active IL-16 protein synthesis through a caspase-3-dependent mechanism. *J Immunol* 2000;164(7):3806–3814.
194. Haynes BF, Grover BJ, Whichard LP, et al. Synovial microenvironment-T cell interactions. Human T cells bind to fibroblast-like synovial cells in vitro. *Arthritis Rheum* 1988;31(8):947–955.
195. Pierer M, Brentano F, Rethage J, et al. The TNF superfamily member LIGHT contributes to survival and activation of synovial fibroblasts in rheumatoid arthritis. *Rheumatology (Oxford)* 2007;46(7): 1063–1070.
196. Lindhout E, van Eijk M, van Pel M, et al. Fibroblast-like synoviocytes from rheumatoid arthritis patients have intrinsic properties of follicular dendritic cells. *J Immunol* 1999;162(10):5949–5956.
197. Hayashida K, Shimaoka Y, Ochi T, Lipsky PE. Rheumatoid arthritis synovial stromal cells inhibit apoptosis and up-regulate Bcl-xL expression by B cells in a CD49/CD29-CD106–dependent mechanism. *J Immunol* 2000;164(2):1110–1116.
198. Reparon-Schuijt CC, van Esch WJ, van Kooten C, et al. Regulation of synovial B cell survival in rheumatoid arthritis by vascular cell adhesion molecule 1 (CD106) expressed on fibroblast-like synoviocytes. *Arthritis Rheum* 2000;43(5):1115–1121.
199. Shigeyama Y, Pap T, Kunzler P, et al. Expression of osteoclast differentiation factor in rheumatoid arthritis. *Arthritis Rheum* 2000; 43(11):2523–2530.
200. Hamann J, Wishaupt JO, van Lier RA, et al. Expression of the activation antigen CD97 and its ligand CD55 in rheumatoid synovial tissue. *Arthritis Rheum* 1999;42(4):650–658.
201. Smith RS, Smith TJ, Blieden TM, Phipps RP. Fibroblasts as sentinel cells. Synthesis of chemokines and regulation of inflammation. *Am J Pathol* 1997;151(2):317–322.
202. Sanchez-Pernaute O, Ospelt C, Neidhart M, Gay S. Epigenetic clues to rheumatoid arthritis. *J Autoimmun* 2008;(1–2):12–20.

Chondrocytes: Pathogenesis of Rheumatoid Arthritis

CHAPTER 8G

Mary B. Goldring

The chondrocyte, the unique cell type in mature cartilage, maintains a stable equilibrium between the synthesis and the degradation of matrix components. During aging and joint disease, this equilibrium is disrupted, and the rate of loss of collagens and proteoglycans from the matrix may exceed the rate of deposition of newly synthesized molecules. Cartilage destruction in rheumatoid arthritis (RA) occurs primarily in areas contiguous with the proliferating synovial pannus due to the release and activation of proteinases from the synovial cells and, to some extent, at the cartilage surface exposed to matrix-degrading enzymes from polymorphonuclear leukocytes in the synovial fluids. In addition to the direct action of proteinases, the RA synovial tissues contribute indirectly to cartilage loss by releasing cytokines and other mediators that act on the chondrocytes to produce dysregulation of chondrocyte function.[1] Our understanding of basic cellular mechanisms regulating chondrocyte responses to inflammatory cytokines has been inferred from numerous studies *in vitro* using cultures of cartilage explants or isolated chondrocytes, and is supported by studies in experimental models of inflammatory arthritis such as collagen-induced arthritis (CIA) and antigen-induced arthritis (AIA) in mice.[2,3] Direct analysis of cartilage or chondrocytes from RA patients undergoing joint replacement has yielded less information, since cartilage damage is extensive and may not reflect early disease. The impact of cytokines on chondrocyte function, particularly with respect to their various roles in cartilage destruction, has been reviewed extensively.[4–7] This chapter will cover current knowledge about the cellular and biochemical mechanisms that account for the destruction of the cartilage matrix in RA.

The Chondrocyte in Adult Articular Cartilage

The cartilage of diarthrodial joints is a specialized hyaline tissue that covers the two opposing bone surfaces, providing a low-friction, articulating interface. Adult human articular cartilage is populated exclusively by chondrocytes, specialized mesenchymal cells, which are somewhat unique to this tissue. In homeostasis, the chondrocyte is a resting cell with no detectable mitotic activity and a very low rate of synthetic activity. Penetration of other cell types from the joint space or subchondral bone is restricted. Because articular cartilage is not vascularized, the chondrocyte must rely upon diffusion from the articular surface or subchondral bone for the exchange of nutrients and metabolites. Chondrocytes maintain active membrane transport systems for exchange of cations, including Na+, K+, Ca2+, and H+, whose intracellular concentrations fluctuate with charge, mechanical loading, and alterations in the composition of the cartilage matrix.[8] Chondrocytes do not normally contain abundant mitochondria, glucose serves as the major energy source for the chondrocytes and as an essential precursor for glycosaminoglycan synthesis, and the energy requirements may be modulated by mechanical stress.[9,10] Facilitated glucose transport in chondrocytes is mediated by several distinct glucose transporter proteins (GLUTs) that are either constitutively expressed (GLUT3 and GLUT8) or cytokine-inducible (GLUT1 and GLUT6).[11,12] Chondrocyte metabolism operates at low oxygen tension, ranging from 10% at the surface to less than 1% in the deep zones of the cartilage. Chondrocytes adapt to low oxygen tensions by upregulating hypoxia-inducible factor-1α (HIF-1α), which can stimulate expression of GLUTs[11] and angiogenic factors such as VEGF,[13,14] as well as ascorbate transport[15] and a number of genes associated with cartilage anabolism and chondrocyte differentiation, including Sox9 and type II collagen.[16] Findings that catabolic stress and inflammatory cytokines upregulate HIF-1α also suggest that it may serve as a survival factor in RA cartilage.[17–19] The chondrocyte cytoskeleton, composed of actin, tubulin, and vimentin filaments, may also respond to external stimuli.[20,21] A proteomic study of chondrocytes identified 93 different intracellular proteins known to be involved in cell organization (26%), energy (16%), protein fate (14%), metabolism (12%), and cell stress (12%).[22] Thus, by modulating the intracellular expression of a unique set of genes, chondrocytes have a high capacity to survive in the avascular cartilage matrix and to maintain homeostasis in response to the environmental changes.

The collagen network of the interterritorial cartilage matrix is composed of types II, IX, and XI collagens, which provide tensile strength and promote the retention of proteoglycans. Type XI collagen is part of the type II collagen fibril, and type IX integrates with the surface of the fibril with the noncollagen domain projecting outward, permitting association with other matrix components. The other major component, the large aggregating proteoglycan aggrecan, which is attached to hyaluronic acid (HA) polymers via link protein, bestows compressive resistance. Under physiological conditions, studies on the turnover of collagen estimate a half-life of over 100 years.[23] In contrast, the glycosaminoglycan constituents on the aggrecan core protein are more readily replaced, and the half-life of aggrecan subfractions has been estimated in the range of 3 to 24 years.[24] A large number of other noncollagen molecules in the interterritorial matrix, including biglycan, decorin, fibromodulin, the matrilins, and cartilage oligomeric matrix protein (COMP), incorporated previously into the matrix during development, may also be synthesized by chondrocytes under low turnover conditions. The chondrocytes are surrounded by a pericellular matrix composed of type VI collagen microfibrils that interact with HA, biglycan, and decorin, and maintain chondrocyte attachment, but little or no fibrillar collagen. Observations on regional differences in the remodeling activities of chondrocytes indicate that matrix turnover is more rapid in the immediate pericellular zones.[25]

Cartilage in Rheumatoid Arthritis

In RA, the underlying disturbance in immune regulation that is responsible for the localized joint pathology results in the release of inflammatory mediators in the synovial fluid and synovium that directly and indirectly influence cartilage homeostasis. In normal conditions, synovium lines the joint cavity and produces synovial fluid that provides the nutrition and lubrication for the articular cartilage. In contrast, rheumatoid synovium is characterized by proliferation of the synovial lining cells, increased vascularization, and infiltration of the tissue by inflammatory cells, including lymphocytes, plasma cells, and activated macrophages.[26,27] With the growth and expansion of the synovial lining, the adjacent articular cartilage is progressively overgrown by the synovial pannus, which penetrates the cartilage surface and is associated with erosion of the extracellular matrix of the cartilage. RA synovium produces a broad spectrum of factors possessing the capacity to stimulate cartilage matrix destruction, as well as bone erosion.[28–30] Among these are cadherin-11,[31] a cell–cell adhesion molecule, and DKK-1,[32] an inhibitor of Wnt/β-catenin signaling, which are expressed at the cartilage–pannus junction and associated with increased synovial invasion into cartilage during RA.

The role of the chondrocyte itself in cartilage destruction in the human rheumatoid joint has been difficult to address, but has been inferred from studies *in vitro* and in animal models. Although there is an association between inflammation and the development of joint damage, the destruction may progress in spite of attenuated inflammatory activity, and cartilage erosions may develop in the absence of overt clinical signs of inflammation.[33–35] Evidence from human and animal studies indicates that although the specific cellular mechanisms of cartilage and bone destruction are different, tumor necrosis factor (TNF)-α, interleukin (IL)-1, and additional proinflammatory cytokines and mediators can drive elements of both processes.[3,36]

Joint Inflammation and Cartilage Destruction in Rheumatoid Arthritis

Cartilage destruction in RA occurs primarily in areas contiguous with the proliferating synovial pannus.[37,38] In the cartilage–pannus junction, there is evidence of attachment of both fibroblast-like and macrophage-like synovial cell types, which release proteinases capable of digesting the cartilage matrix components.[39] Nevertheless, there is evidence of loss of proteoglycan throughout the cartilage matrix, particularly in the superficial zone in contact with the synovial fluid at sites not directly associated with the pannus.[40,41] This has been attributed to the release of inflammatory mediators and degradative enzymes released by polymorphonuclear leukocytes and other inflammatory cells in the synovial fluid. In early RA, however, the loss of proteoglycan occurs throughout the cartilage matrix and selective damage to type II collagen fibrils can be observed in middle and deep zones,[42,43] suggesting that the chondrocyte may also participate in degrading its own matrix by releasing autocrine-paracrine factors. Interestingly, there is evidence of a distinctive fibroblast-like cell type, the so-called "pannocyte," in RA synovium that exhibits anchorage-independent growth and cartilage invasion in the absence of an inflammatory environment.[26]

Proteinases and Inhibitors in Cartilage Destruction

Of the enzymes involved in the degradation of cartilage collagens and proteoglycans in RA, the metalloproteinase (MMP) and adamalysin families have been given greatest attention because they degrade native collagens and proteoglycans.[44] Chondrocytes synthesize and secrete MMPs in latent forms, which are activated outside the cells via activation cascades. An important cascade in cartilage is initiated by plasmin, the product of plasminogen activator activity, which may be produced by the chondrocyte; plasmin, in turn, activates latent stromelysin (MMP-3), an activator of latent collagenases.[45] MMPs are localized at sites of degradation in cartilage derived from RA patients.[46] Collagenases-1, -2, and -3 (MMP-1, MMP-8, MMP-13, respectively), gelatinases (MMP-2 and MMP-9), stromelysin-1 (MMP-3), and membrane type I MMP (MT1)-MMP (MMP-14) are present in active RA synovium.[47,48] Although elevated levels of MMPs in the synovial fluid likely originate from the synovium, intrinsic chondrocyte-derived chondrolytic activity may be present at the cartilage–pannus junction as well as in deeper zones of cartilage matrix.[49] For example, MMP-1 does not derive from the RA synovial pannus, but is produced by chondrocytes.[50] MMP-10, similar to MMP-3, activates procollagenases and is produced by both the synovium and chondrocytes in response to inflammatory cytokines.[51] On the other hand, MMP-14, produced principally by the synovial tissue, is important for synovial invasiveness, and antisense mRNA inhibition of this membrane proteinase has been shown to reduce cartilage destruction.[52]

Other MMPs, including MMP-16 and MMP-28,[53,54] and a large number of members of the reprolysin-related proteinases of the ADAM (a disintegrin and metalloproteinase) family, including ADAM-17/TACE (TNF-α converting enzyme),[55] are expressed in cartilage, but their roles in cartilage damage in RA have yet to be defined.[45,56,57] Although several of the MMPs, including MMP-3, MMP-8, and MMP-14, are capable of degrading proteoglycans, ADAMTS (ADAM with thrombospondin-1 domains) –4 and –5, are now regarded as the principal mediators of aggrecan degradation.[58,59] ADAMTS-4 is prominently regulated by inflammatory cytokines, whereas ADAMTS-5 is constitutively expressed and is most strongly associated with increased susceptibility to cartilage degradation due to surgical osteoarthritis (OA), as shown in Adamts5-deficient mice.[60,61] The activities of MMPs and aggrecanases are complementary, however.[62]

In early studies, chondrocytes were among the first identified sources of tissue inhibitor of MMP (TIMP)-1, and they are now known to synthesize additional TIMPs. Chondrocytes, therefore, are assumed to be a major source of the TIMPs detected in synovial fluids, where they may reflect an adaptive response to the local imbalance due to increased production of active MMPs by chondrocytes and other joint tissues. TIMP-3, but not TIMP-1, -2, or -4, is a potent inhibitor of ADAMTS-4 and -5 *in vitro*.[63] The capacity of TGF-β to increase TIMP gene expression may account partially for its protective effects against MMP- and ADAMTS-mediated cartilage breakdown.[64,65]

Other proteinases, including the cathepsins B, L, and D, which degrade various cartilage matrix components and may be produced by the chondrocytes themselves, also contribute to breakdown of the cartilage matrix.[66,67] Cathepsin K is expressed in synovial fibroblasts on the cartilage surface at the pannus–cartilage junction, and is upregulated by inflammatory cytokines.[68] Among the known cathepsins, cathepsin K is the only proteinase that is capable of hydrolyzing types I and II collagens at multiple sites within the triple-helical regions, and its requirement for acidic pH may be provided by the microenvironment between the synovial pannus and the cartilage.[69]

Cartilage Biomarkers in RA

Degraded cartilage matrix components are considered both as diagnostic markers of cartilage damage and as potential autoantigens in the induction and maintenance of RA synovial inflammation.[6,70,71] Markers originating from the articular cartilage, including aggrecan fragments, which contain chondroitin sulfate and keratan sulfate, type II collagen fragments, and collagen pyridinoline cross-links are considered to be products of catabolic processes. Specific antibodies that detect either synthetic or cleavage epitopes have been developed to study biological markers of cartilage metabolism in RA body fluids (reviewed in Goldring and Goldring[6]). These include the C2C antibody (previously known as COL2-3/4$C_{Long\ mono}$), which has been used to detect cleavage of the triple helix of type II collagen in experimental models of RA and in RA cartilage.[72] Similarly, the degradation of aggrecan in cartilage has been characterized using antibodies 846, 3B3(−) and 7D4 that detect chondroitin sulfate neoepitopes, 5D4 that detects keratan sulfate epitopes, and the VIDIPEN and NITEGE antibodies that recognize aggrecanase and MMP cleavage sites, respectively, within the interglobular G1 domain of aggrecan.[58,66]

Additional markers include COMP, which is considered a general indicator of cartilage turnover that reflects processes distinct from inflammatory aspects of RA.[73] YKL-40/HC-gp39, also known as chitinase 3-like protein 1 (CH3L1) is a specific histological marker in inflamed RA synovium that forms immune complexes with HLA-DR4.[74] The immune response to YKL-40, which is biased toward the regulatory, suppressor T-cell phenotype in healthy individuals, is shifted from an anti-inflammatory to a proinflammatory phenotype in RA patients.[75] In cartilage, CH3L1 is induced by inflammatory cytokines. It inhibits cytokine-induced cellular responses and may function as a feed back regulator.[76,77] A related member of the chitinase family, YKL-39, may be a more specific serum marker as a cartilage-derived autoantigen.[78,79] Another novel molecule is the cartilage-derived, retinoic-acid–sensitive protein (CD-RAP), also known as melanoma inhibitory activity, which is found at high levels in synovial fluids from patients with mild RA and decreases with disease progression.[80]

The Balance of Cytokines in Cartilage Destruction in Rheumatoid Arthritis

Of the cytokines that affect cartilage metabolism, most are pleiotropic factors that were identified originally as immunomodulators, but were found to regulate cellular functions in cells of mesenchymal origin. For example, interleukin-1 (IL-1) and tumor necrosis factor (TNF)-α not only stimulate chondrocytes to synthesize cartilage matrix-degrading proteinases, but they also regulate matrix protein synthesis and cell proliferation. Considerable redundancy and overlap in biologic activities exist among the individual cytokines, and they do not act alone, but rather in synergy or partnership with or in opposition to other cytokines via cytokine networks. In addition to IL-1 and TNF-α, IL-17 and IL-18 have been characterized as catabolic cytokines and their actions may be modulated by inhibitory or anabolic cytokines produced by the chondrocytes themselves or by other cells in joint tissues. Investigations *in vitro* and *in vivo* have begun to sort out the complexities of the cytokine networks and to determine how the balance in normal homeostasis can be restored once it is disrupted (Figure 8G-1). Examination of type II collagen–induced arthritis (CIA) and other types of inflammatory arthritis in transgenic animals with overexpressed or deleted genes encoding cytokines, their receptors, or activators has provided further insights into the roles of these factors in cartilage destruction.

Interleukin-1 and Tumor Necrosis Factor-α

Numerous studies *in vitro* and *in vivo* indicate that IL-1 and TNF-α are the predominant catabolic cytokines involved in the destruction of the articular cartilage in RA.[1–3] The first recognition of IL-1 as a regulator of chondrocyte function stems largely from studies in culture models showing that activities derived from synovium or monocyte-macrophages induce the production of cartilage-degrading proteinases (reviewed in Dayer[1] and Arend and Goldring[81]). There is evidence that the chondrocytes participate in this destructive process not only by responding to the cytokines released from other joint tissues, but also by synthesizing them.[5,82] Thus, they may be exposed continuously to the autocrine and paracrine effects of IL-1 and other inflammatory mediators at high local concentrations. IL-1 has the capacity to stimulate the production of most, if not all, of the proteinases involved in cartilage destruction, and it colocalizes with TNF-α, MMP-1, 3, 8, and 13, and type II collagen cleavage epitopes in regions of matrix depletion in RA cartilage.[47,72] Originally known as cachectin, TNF-α produces many effects on chondrocytes *in vitro* that are similar to those of IL-1, including stimulation of the production of matrix-degrading proteinases and suppression of cartilage matrix synthesis. Interleukin-1 is 100-fold to 1000-fold more potent on a molar basis than TNF-α, but strong synergistic effects occur at low concentrations of the two cytokines together.[3]

The concept that TNF-α drives acute inflammation, while IL-1 has a pivotal role in sustaining both inflammation and cartilage erosion, has been derived from work in animal models of RA using cytokine-specific neutralizing antibodies, soluble receptors, or receptor antagonists and in transgenic or knockout mouse models. For example, the spontaneous development of a chronic destructive arthritis in IL-1Ra–deficient mice established the importance of IL-1 in arthritis.[83] In a surgically induced OA model, for example, IL-1 knockout mice are protected against cartilage damage.[84] Earlier studies showing that blockade of IL-1 is more effective than TNF-α neutralization in CIA mice,[85] and that IL-1 is a secondary mediator in TNFα transgenic mice[86] supported the higher potency of IL-1 compared to TNF-α in driving cartilage erosion. Later studies in the human RA/SCID mouse chimera indicated that TNF-α is a key

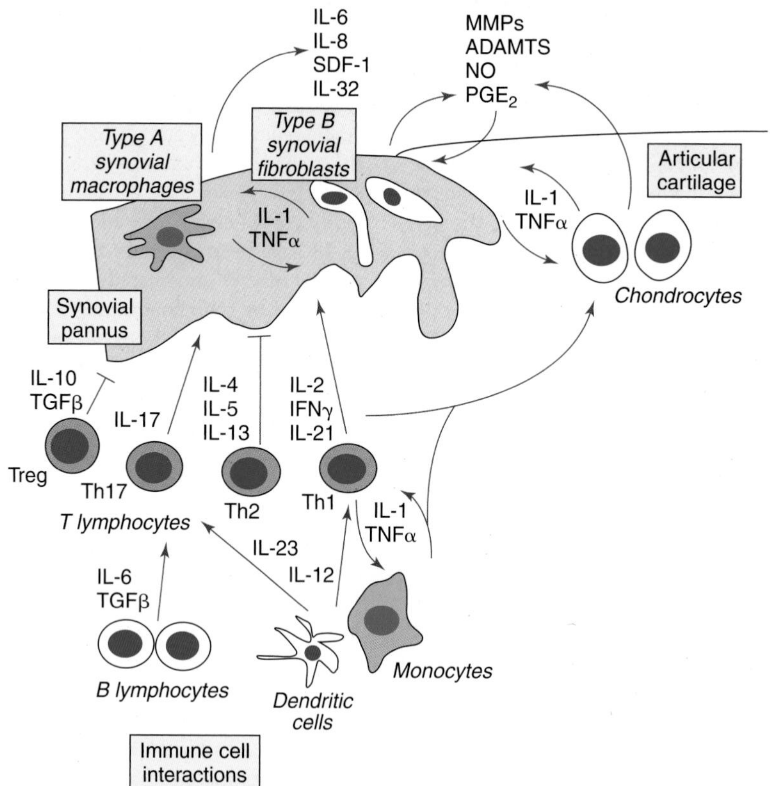

Figure 8G-1. Cytokine networks and cellular interactions in cartilage destruction in rheumatoid arthritis. This scheme represents the progressive destruction of the cartilage associated with the invading synovial pannus in RA. As a result of immune cell interactions involving T and B lymphocytes, monocyte/macrophages, and dendritic cells, a number of different cytokines are produced in the inflamed synovium due to the influx of inflammatory cells from the circulation and synovial cell hyperplasia. The upregulation of proinflammatory cytokines produced primarily in the synovium, but also by chondrocytes, result in the upregulation of cartilage-degrading enzymes, of the MMP and ADAMTS families, at the cartilage–pannus junction. Chemokines, nitric oxide, and prostaglandins also contribute to the inflammation and tissue catabolism. (Adapted from Otero M, Goldring MB. Cells of the synovium in rheumatoid arthritis. Chondrocytes. *Arthritis Res Ther* 2007;9:220.)

molecule in the inflammatory changes that occur in the rheumatoid synovium, whereas cartilage damage occurs independently of this cytokine.[87] Furthermore, a recent study showed that crossing the arthritic human TNF transgenic (hTNFtg) mice with IL-1α– and -β–deficient mice protects against cartilage erosion without affecting synovial inflammation.[88] Despite these findings in animal models, anti-TNF therapy has been more successful than anti–IL-1 therapy in RA patients, possibly related to the poor pharmacokinetic properties of IL-1Ra. Alternative approaches for targeting IL-1, including the use of soluble receptors and neutralizing antibodies, need to be tested.[3,89]

IL-1 and TNF-α also induce the production of a number of inflammatory mediators that can modulate chondrocyte responses, including nitric oxide (NO) via inducible nitric oxide synthetase (iNOS, or NOS2), and prostaglandin E2 (PGE2) by stimulating the expression or activities of cyclooxygenase (COX)-2, microsomal PGE synthase-1 (mPGES-1), and soluble phospholipase A2 (sPLA2).[82,90,91] Although PGE2 and NO have been well characterized as proinflammatory mediators, there is evidence that they may also be protective and play roles in chondrocyte survival and responses to mechanical stress. For example, COX-2 is involved in the chondrocyte response to high shear stress, associated with reduced antioxidant capacity and increased apoptosis.[92]

Roles for NO as a mediator of other IL-1–induced responses, including the inhibition of aggrecan synthesis, enhancement of MMP activity, and reduction in IL-1Ra synthesis, have also been suggested.[93] NO has also been implicated as an important mediator in chondrocyte apoptosis, but the role of endogenous, IL-1–induced NO has not been proven conclusively.[94] Indeed, IL-1 appears to protect chondrocytes from Fas ligand–induced apoptosis by a mechanism that is independent of IL-1–induced NO, and whether NO donors induce apoptosis is dependent on the levels of other mediators such as reactive oxygen species (ROS).[95] Overproduction of NO may also contribute to IGF-I resistance in chondrocytes through disruption of integrin signaling, reducing phosphorylation of the IGF-1 receptor, stimulation of cGMP production or suppression of mitochondrial oxidative metabolism.[96–100]

Cytokine Networks

In addition to IL-1 and TNF-α, networks of a number of other cytokines involved in the immune response and inflammatory responses in the rheumatoid joint contribute to the destruction of cartilage.[101] These include IL-6, leukemia inhibitory factor (LIF), IL-17, and IL-18, all of which are induced in chondrocytes by IL-1 and TNF-α.[5,82,102] IL-6 is an example of a pleiotropic cytokine, since it plays a dual role by increasing IL-1ra, soluble

TNF receptor (sTNFR), and TIMPs, while also enhancing immune cell function and inflammation.[54,103] Although IL-1 induces IL-6 synthesis and release and antisense IL-6 blocks the IL-1–induced inhibition of proteoglycan synthesis, direct effects of IL-6 on chondrocyte responses *in vitro* are difficult to observe in the absence of the soluble IL-6 receptor (sIL-6R), which is required for the full response to IL-6 in chondrocytes *in vitro*. Interaction of IL-6 with sIL-6R permits synergistic stimulation of MMPs by IL-1 and IL-6,[104] as well as direct IL-6–induced upregulation of MMP and ADAMTS and downregulation of COL2A1 and aggrecan in cultured chondrocytes via the JAK/STAT pathway.[105] However, IL-6 knockout mice are more susceptible to the development of OA during aging,[106] suggesting that this cytokine may play a protective role in normal physiology. IL-6 blockade is under current investigation in clinical trials.[107,108]

Other members of the IL-6 family that act via gp130-associated receptors may also serve modulatory roles. IL-11 shares several actions of IL-6, including stimulation of TIMP production without affecting MMP production by chondrocytes[104] and may actually inhibit cartilage destruction.[109] LIF, which is induced by IL-6, participates in a positive feedback loop by increasing the production of IL-6 by chondrocytes. Oncostatin M (OSM), a product of macrophages and activated T cells that acts via the JAK/STAT pathway, is a potent stimulator of chondrocyte production of MMPs and aggrecanases in synergism with IL-1 or TNF-α.[51,104,110] Direct evidence supporting a role for OSM in contributing to cartilage loss in inflammatory arthritis is provided by studies in animal models.[111,112]

Two additional cytokines, IL-17 and IL-18, are potent inducers of catabolic responses in chondrocytes. IL-18 is produced by macrophages, and IL-17 is produced by activated T helper type 1 (Th1), or CD4, lymphocytes in RA synovial fluid and tissue. Interleukin-17 is unique among the proinflammatory cytokines in that it mediates its effects through a receptor that is not related to any known cytokine receptor family. In contrast, the IL-18 receptor shares homology with type I IL-1R. IL-18 has effects similar to IL-1 in human chondrocytes, but stimulates chondrocyte apoptosis, although studies do not suggest a pivotal role in cartilage destruction in RA.[113,114] Both IL-17 and IL-18 increase the expression of IL-1α by human chondrocytes, as well as stimulating the production of MMPs, IL-6, iNOS, COX-2, and mPGES-1,[115] and are proven mediators of the autoimmune and inflammatory processes in the CIA model.[116,117] IL-17A, one of at least six family members, is primarily a product of Th17 cells, a newly described subset of T cells, which is a potent inducer of catabolic responses in chondrocytes by itself or in synergy with other cytokines.[116] IL-17 can drive T-cell–dependent erosive arthritis in TNF-α–deficient or IL-1Ra knockout mice, and treatment of CIA or AIA mice with neutralizing IL-17 antibody effectively inhibits cartilage destruction in those models of RA.[118] A role for IL-17 in the promotion of angiogenesis through induction of VEGF in OA chondrocytes and synovial fibroblasts has been proposed.[119] IL-18 deficiency and/or blockade with IL-18-neutralizing antibody or IL-18–binding protein reduces cartilage destruction, as well as inflammation, and IL-18 gene transfer promotes IL-1–driven cartilage destruction in a TNF-α–independent manner.[120] IL-32, a recently discovered cytokine induces TNF-α, IL-1β, IL-6, and chemokines, is expressed in the synovia of patients with RA, and contributes to TNFα-dependent inflammation and cartilage proteoglycan loss.[121]

Of the other members of the IL-1 family recently identified by DNA database searches, IL-1F8 appears to be capable of stimulating IL-6, IL-8, and NO production by human chondrocytes, but at 100- to 1000-fold higher concentrations than IL-1.[122] The IL-1R/toll-like receptor (TLR) superfamily of receptors, in addition to playing key roles in innate immunity and inflammation, also modulates cartilage metabolism. Studies in streptococcal cell wall (SCW)–induced arthritis showed that joint inflammation and cartilage proteoglycan loss are predominantly dependent on TLR-2 signaling.[123] Human articular chondrocytes are capable of expressing TLR1, 2, and 4, and activation of TLR2 by IL-1, TNF-α, peptidoglycans, LPS, or FN fragments increases the production of MMPs, NO, PGE, and VEGF.[124–126] In immune complex–mediated arthritis, TLR4 regulates early onset inflammation and cartilage destruction by IL-10-mediated upregulation of IL-1γ receptor expression and enhanced cytokine production.[127] Since the IL-18 receptor shares homology with IL-1RI and has a TLR signaling domain, therapeutic strategies similar to those for targeting IL-1 signaling have been explored.[103,128] In animal models, IL-18 via TLR2 promotes joint inflammation in a partially TNF-α–dependent manner and induces IL-1–driven cartilage destruction.[120] Recent findings indicate that TLR4 is critical for the catabolic and antianabolic responses of chondrocytes to IL-1 *in vitro* and for cartilage destruction in inflammatory arthritis models.[129–131]

IL-4, IL-10, and IL-13, as well as the naturally occurring IL-1Ra, are classified as inhibitory cytokines, because they decrease the production and activities of the catabolic and proinflammatory cytokines in chondrocytes *in vitro* and suppress cartilage destruction *in vivo*.[3,4,132,133] IL-4 and IL-10 inhibit cartilage-degrading proteinases and reverse some effects of the catabolic cytokines *in vitro*, and together they produce a synergistic suppression of cartilage destruction *in vivo*. The efficacy of IL-4, IL-10, and IL-13 in retarding cartilage damage may be related, in part, to their stimulatory effects on IL-1Ra production,[132,134] and their therapeutic application has been proposed as a means of restoring the cytokine balance in RA.[135] IL-1Ra is capable of blocking the actions of IL-1 if added at sufficiently high concentrations *in vitro*, and is among the first agents to be developed for anticytokine therapy.[1,81] IL-1Ra, which can be produced by the same cells that secrete IL-1, exists as at least three isoforms, including intracellular forms.

Despite the capacity of IL-4 to inhibit the effects of proinflammatory cytokines on chondrocyte function,[136,137] differential effects have been observed in mice depending on the model.[138,139] IL-10 is part of the response induced by immunomodulatory neuropeptides that have been shown recently to inhibit inflammation and cartilage and bone destruction by downregulating the Th1-driven immune response and upregulating IL-10/TGF-β–producing T-regulatory (Treg) lymphocytes.[140] Gene transfer of IL-10 in combination with IL-1Ra inhibits cartilage destruction by a mechanism involving activin, a TNF-β family member.[141] IL-13 decreases the breakdown of collagen and proteoglycans by inhibiting IL-1- and OSM-induced MMP-3 and MMP-13 expression,[142] and is a potent antiangiogenic factor *in vivo*.[143] Local gene transfer of IL-13 inhibits chondrocyte death and MMP-mediated cartilage degradation despite enhanced inflammation in the immune-complex arthritis model.[144] Thus, the inhibitory cytokines may have both direct effects on cartilage metabolism and indirect effects by mediating the production and actions of catabolic cytokines and inhibitors.

Novel Mediators of Chondrocyte Metabolism

The identification of novel mediators affecting chondrocyte function during inflammation has led to the reexamination of the regulation of cytokine networks and elucidation of potential therapeutic targets. Peroxisome proliferator-activated receptor γ (PPAR-γ), following activation by the endogenous ligand 15-deoxy-$\Delta^{12,14}$ prostaglandin J_2 (PGJ_2), opposes the induction of COX-2, iNOS, MMPs, and mPGES-1, and the suppression of aggrecan synthesis by IL-1.[115,145] Recent evidence indicates that PPAR-α agonists, however, may protect chondrocytes against IL-1–induced responses by increasing the expression of IL-1Ra.[146]

The IL-1–induced suppressor of cytokine signaling 3 (SOCS3) acts as a negative feedback regulator during IGF-1 desensitization in the absence of NO by inhibiting insulin receptor substrate (IRS)-1 phosphorylation.[147] Recent evidence indicates that RAGE, the receptor for advanced glycation end products (AGEs), interacts preferentially with S100A4, a member of the S100 family of calcium-binding proteins, in chondrocytes and stimulates MMP-13 production via phosphorylation of Pyk2, MAP kinases, and NF-κB.[148] The fibroblast activation protein α (FAP-α), a membrane serine proteinase, which colocalizes in synovium with MMP-1 and MMP-13, and is induced by IL-1 and OSM in chondrocytes, may play a role in collagen degradation.[149,150] Many of these proteins may be activated during the chondrocyte response to abnormal stimuli and may serve as endogenous mediators of cellular responses to stress and inflammation.

Adipokines, which were identified originally as products of adipocytes, also have roles in cartilage metabolism.[151] White adipose tissue has been proposed as a major source of both pro- and anti-inflammatory cytokines, including IL-Ra and IL-10.[152] Leptin has been proposed to serve as a link between the neuroendocrine and immune systems.[153] Leptin synergizes with IL-1 or IFN-γ to increase NO production in chondrocytes,[154] and leptin deficiency attenuates inflammatory processes in experimental arthritis.[155] Although leptin expression is enhanced during acute inflammation, it correlates negatively with inflammatory markers in chronic RA sera.[156] Thus, it has been proposed that a dysregulated balance between leptin and the anti-inflammatory adipokine, adiponectin, promotes destructive inflammatory processes.[157] Furthermore, the elevated expression of leptin in OA cartilage and in osteophytes, and its capacity to stimulate IGF-1 and TGF-α1 synthesis suggests a role for this adipokine in anabolic responses of chondrocytes.[158]

Chemokines, which are small heparin-binding cytokines identified originally as chemotactic factors, are classified as C, CX3C, or CC molecules the presence of distinct N-terminal cysteine (C) residues. The role of chemokines in RA synovium, where their induction by proinflammatory cytokines, including IL-1, TNF-α, IL-17, IL-18, and OSM, is associated with neutrophil activation, chemotaxis, and angiogenesis, is well established.[159–162] IL-8, probably the most potent and abundant chemotactic agent in RA synovial fluids, and other chemokines, such as monocyte chemoattractant protein (MCP)-1 and regulated-on-activation normal T-cell expressed and secreted (RANTES), are produced primarily by the synovium and serve as indicators of synovitis. Chondrocytes, when activated by IL-1 and TNF-α, also express several chemokines, including IL-8, MCP-1 and 4, RANTES, macrophage inflammatory protein (MIP-1)α, MIP-1β, and gro-related oncogene (GRO)-α, as well as the receptors CCR1, CCR2, CCR3, CCR5, and CXCR1, which enable responses to some of these chemokines.[163,164] For example, MCP-1, RANTES, and GRO-α upregulate expression of MMP-3 and RANTES induces the expression of iNOS, IL-6, and MMP-1 in chondrocytes. The RANTES receptors CCR3 and CCR5, but not CCR1, are expressed in normal cartilage, whereas all three receptors are expressed after stimulation by IL-1α. High levels of stromal cell–derived factor 1 (SDF-1) are detected in RA synovial fluids, and its receptor, CXCR4, is expressed by chondrocytes, but not synovial fibroblasts, suggesting a direct influence of this chemokine on cartilage damage.[165] Microarray studies have elucidated a number of chemokines that are inducible in chondrocytes by FN fragments and cytokines.[166] SDF-1 and several other cytokines also increase the synthesis of S100A, N-acetyl-b-D-glucuronidase, cathepsin B, and several MMPs by chondrocytes, as well as DNA synthesis, cell proliferation, and PGE_2 production.[167,168] When placed in contact with autologous T lymphocytes, chondrocytes produce enhanced levels of MMP-1, 3, and 13, and RANTES.[169] Thus, in addition to recruiting leukocytes to sites of inflammation in arthritic joints and mediating synovial fibroblast responses and actions, chemokines are capable of modulating chondrocyte functions that are associated with cartilage degradation.

Cytokine Signaling Pathways and Transcription Factors in Cartilage

Signal transduction molecules and transcription factors activated by inflammatory mediators in chondrocytes and synovial cells have been studied to identify potential therapeutic targets.[170,171] Although the receptors for IL-1 and TNF-α and associated adaptor molecules are distinct, they share the capacity to activate similar signaling pathways in chondrocytes.[4,172,173] The major pathways induced by catabolic cytokines involve signal transduction by the stress-activated protein kinases c-Jun N-terminal kinases (JNKs) and p38 kinases and the nuclear factor (NF)-κB, and phosphatidylinositol-3-kinase (PI-3K) pathways. The JAK/STAT signaling pathway is important for signaling by gp130 cytokines, including IL-6 and OSM.[174] Specific adaptor molecules involved in the pathways induced by TNF-α receptors, which are members of the TNF receptor (TNFR) superfamily, are different from those used by IL-1 signaling pathways. The TNFR pathway uses TNFR-associated factor (TRAF2), TRAF6, and the receptor interacting protein (RIP) kinase, whereas the IL-1R pathway uses TRAF6, IL-1R–associated kinase (IRAK), and evolutionarily conserved signaling intermediate in toll pathways (ECSIT) as adaptor molecules. Signaling through TNFRI associated with TNFR-associated death domain receptor (TRADD) activates apoptosis, whereas TNFRII signaling through TRAF2 activates JNK and NF-κB.

The p38 and JNK cascades mediate the induction of many IL-1- and TNF-α–inducible genes associated with catabolic and inflammatory responses in chondrocytes *in vitro* and *in vivo* (see Goldring[4] for review). These pathways may also be activated in chondrocytes by mechanical stress and cartilage matrix products via integrins and other receptor-mediated events.[175–178] The upregulation of IL-1 and TNF-α expression via these pathways also suggests a their involvement as secondary mediators in a feedback mechanism. At least four isoforms of p38 MAPK exist with different substrate specificities and potentially distinct effects on essential chondrocyte functions.[179] For example, a selective p38α inhibitor reverses cartilage and bone destruction in the CIA mouse.[180]

JNKs are serine threonine protein kinases that phosphorylate Jun family members, components of AP-1 transcription factors, and they exist as three isoforms in humans, JNK1, -2, and -3. A potent JNK1/2 inhibitor, SP600125, which blocks inflammation and joint damage in animal models of RA, and other JNK isoform-specific inhibitors, are useful tools for analyzing chondrocyte function *in vitro* and *in vivo*.[181] JNK is regulated by mechanical stimulation and JNK inhibition attenuates cytokine-induced chondrocyte responses.[182–185] NF-κB is a "master switch" of the inflammatory cascade.[186] NF-κB is activated when the IκB kinases, IKK-1 and IKK-2, phosphorylate IκB, dissociating it from NF-κB and permitting translocation of active NF-κB to the nucleus. NF-κB mediates the expression of cytokines and chemokines induced by FN fragments,[166] and inhibition of DNA-binding activity of NF-κB by agents that deplete polyamine blocks IL-1 and TNF-α without promoting chondrocyte apoptosis.[187]

In addition to NF-κB, transcription factors of the C/EBP, ETS, and AP-1 families have been localized in rheumatoid tissues[188,189] and are important for the regulation of cytokine-induced gene expression in chondrocytes[57,190–193] (for review, see Goldring and Sandell[194]). These transcription factors also mediate suppression of a number of genes associated with the differentiated chondrocyte phenotype, including type II collagen (COL2A1), aggrecan, and CD-RAP.[195–198] Chondrocyte-specific transcription factors that regulate cartilage formation during development such as Sox9.[191] have not been studied in the context of cartilage metabolism in RA. Genomic and proteomic analyses that have been performed in cytokine-treated chondrocytes, in cartilage from patients with osteoarthritis, and in rheumatoid synovium have provided some insights into novel mechanisms that might govern chondrocyte responses in RA.[166,199–204]

Conclusion

In RA, an inflammatory joint disease that results in destruction of the articular cartilage, the underlying disturbance in immune regulation results in the release of inflammatory mediators in the synovial fluid and synovium that directly and indirectly influence cartilage homeostasis. Significant advances in recent years have contributed to our understanding of the cellular interactions in the RA joint involving macrophages, T and B lymphocytes, and synovial fibroblasts. The mediators involved in immunomodulation and synovial cell function, including cytokines, chemokines, and adhesion molecules may also, directly or indirectly, promote cartilage damage. Laboratory investigations *in vitro* and *in vivo* have provided new findings regarding the role of the chondrocyte in remodeling the cartilage matrix in the RA joint. Available evidence indicates that chondrocytes produce and respond to proinflammatory cytokines, as well as inhibitory and anabolic cytokines that modulate the responses. Despite the clinical success of anti-TNF therapy for RA, there is still a need for therapeutic strategies that prevent the extensive cartilage and bone loss. Recent work that has identified novel molecules and mechanisms, as well as providing new understanding of the contributions of known mediators, offers the possibility of developing new therapies for targeting cartilage destruction in inflammatory joint disease.

References

1. Dayer JM. The process of identifying and understanding cytokines: From basic studies to treating rheumatic diseases. *Best Pract Res Clin Rheumatol* 2004;18:31–45.
2. van den Berg WB. Animal models of arthritis. What have we learned? *J Rheumatol Suppl* 2005;72:7–9.
3. van den Berg WB, van Riel PL. Uncoupling of inflammation and destruction in rheumatoid arthritis: Myth or reality? *Arthritis Rheum* 2005;52:995–999.
4. Goldring MB. Update on the biology of the chondrocyte and new approaches to treating cartilage diseases. *Best Pract Res Clin Rheumatol* 2006;20:1003–1025.
5. Goldring SR, Goldring MB. The role of cytokines in cartilage matrix degeneration in osteoarthritis. *Clin Orthop* 2004;427:S27–S36.
6. Goldring SR, Goldring MB. Rheumatoid arthritis and other inflammatory joint pathologies. In: Seibel MJ, Robins SP, Bilezikian JP, eds. *Dynamics of Bone and Cartilage Metabolism Principles and Clinical Applications*. 2nd ed. San Diego: Academic Press 2006, 843–869.
7. Otero M, Goldring MB. Cells of the synovium in rheumatoid arthritis. Chondrocytes. *Arthritis Res Ther* 2007;9:220.
8. Wilkins RJ, Browning JA, Ellory JC. Surviving in a matrix: Membrane transport in articular chondrocytes. *J Membr Biol* 2000; 177:95–108.
9. Lee RB, Wilkins RJ, Razaq S, et al. The effect of mechanical stress on cartilage energy metabolism. *Biorheology* 2002;39:133–143.
10. Sengers BG, Heywood HK, Lee DA, et al. Nutrient utilization by bovine articular chondrocytes: A combined experimental and theoretical approach. *J Biomech Eng* 2005;127:758–766.
11. Mobasheri A, Richardson S, Mobasheri R, et al. Hypoxia inducible factor-1 and facilitative glucose transporters GLUT1 and GLUT3: Putative molecular components of the oxygen and glucose sensing apparatus in articular chondrocytes. *Histol Histopathol* 2005;20: 1327–1338.
12. Shikhman AR, Brinson DC, Lotz MK. Distinct pathways regulate facilitated glucose transport in human articular chondrocytes during anabolic and catabolic responses. *Am J Physiol Endocrinol Metab* 2004;286:E980–E985.
13. Lin C, McGough R, Aswad B, et al. Hypoxia induces HIF-1α and VEGF expression in chondrosarcoma cells and chondrocytes. *J Orthop Res* 2004;22:1175–1181.
14. Pufe T, Kurz B, Petersen W, et al. The influence of biomechanical parameters on the expression of VEGF and endostatin in the bone and joint system. *Ann Anat* 2005;187:461–472.
15. McNulty AL, Stabler TV, Vail TP, et al. Dehydroascorbate transport in human chondrocytes is regulated by hypoxia and is a physiologically relevant source of ascorbic acid in the joint. *Arthritis Rheum* 2005;52:2676–2685.
16. Robins JC, Akeno N, Mukherjee A, et al. Hypoxia induces chondrocyte-specific gene expression in mesenchymal cells in association with transcriptional activation of Sox9. *Bone* 2005;37:313–322.
17. Coimbra IB, Jimenez SA, Hawkins DF, et al. Hypoxia inducible factor-1α expression in human normal and osteoarthritic chondrocytes. *Osteoarthritis Cartilage* 2004;12:336–345.
18. Martin G, Andriamanalijaona R, Grassel S, et al. Effect of hypoxia and reoxygenation on gene expression and response to interleukin-1

in cultured articular chondrocytes. *Arthritis Rheum* 2004;50: 3549–3560.

19. Yudoh K, Nakamura H, Masuko-Hongo K, et al. Catabolic stress induces expression of hypoxia-inducible factor (HIF)-1α in articular chondrocytes: Involvement of HIF-1α in the pathogenesis of osteoarthritis. *Arthritis Res Ther* 2005;7:R904–R914.
20. Langelier E, Suetterlin R, Hoemann CD, et al. The chondrocyte cytoskeleton in mature articular cartilage: Structure and distribution of actin, tubulin, and vimentin filaments. *J Histochem Cytochem* 2000; 48:1307–1320.
21. Woods A, Wang G, Beier F. Regulation of chondrocyte differentiation by the actin cytoskeleton and adhesive interactions. *J Cell Physiol* 2007;213:1–8.
22. Ruiz-Romero C, Lopez-Armada MJ, Blanco FJ. Proteomic characterization of human normal articular chondrocytes: A novel tool for the study of osteoarthritis and other rheumatic diseases. *Proteomics* 2005;5:3048–3059.
23. Verzijl N, DeGroot J, Thorpe SR, et al. Effect of collagen turnover on the accumulation of advanced glycation end products. *J Biol Chem* 2000;275:39027–39031.
24. Maroudas A, Bayliss MT, Uchitel-Kaushansky N, et al. Aggrecan turnover in human articular cartilage: Use of aspartic acid racemization as a marker of molecular age. *Arch Biochem Biophys* 1998; 350:61–71.
25. Wu W, Billinghurst RC, Pidoux I, et al. Sites of collagenase cleavage and denaturation of type II collagen in aging and osteoarthritic articular cartilage and their relationship to the distribution of matrix metalloproteinase 1 and matrix metalloproteinase 13. *Arthritis Rheum* 2002;46:2087–2094.
26. Firestein GS. Evolving concepts of rheumatoid arthritis. *Nature* 2003;423:356–361.
27. Tak PP, Bresnihan B. The pathogenesis and prevention of joint damage in rheumatoid arthritis: Advances from synovial biopsy and tissue analysis. *Arthritis Rheum* 2000;43:2619–2633.
28. Knedla A, Neumann E, Muller-Ladner U. Developments in the synovial biology field 2006. *Arthritis Res Ther* 2007;9:209.
29. Meyer LH, Franssen L, Pap T. The role of mesenchymal cells in the pathophysiology of inflammatory arthritis. *Best Pract Res Clin Rheumatol* 2006;20:969–981.
30. Szekanecz Z, Koch AE. Macrophages and their products in rheumatoid arthritis. *Curr Opin Rheumatol* 2007;19:289–295.
31. Lee DM, Kiener HP, Agarwal SK, et al. Cadherin-11 in synovial lining formation and pathology in arthritis. *Science* 2007;315: 1006–1010.
32. Diarra D, Stolina M, Polzer K, et al. Dickkopf-1 is a master regulator of joint remodeling. *Nat Med* 2007;13:156–163.
33. Mulherin D, Fitzgerald O, Bresnihan B. Clinical improvement and radiological deterioration in rheumatoid arthritis: Evidence that the pathogenesis of synovial inflammation and articular erosion may differ. *J Rheumatol Br J Rheumatol* 1996;35:1263–1268.
34. Kirwan J, Byron M, Watt I. The relationship between soft tissue swelling, joint space narrowing and erosive damage in hand x-rays of patients with rheumatoid arthritis. *Rheumatology (Oxford)* 2001; 40:297–301.
35. Graudal N. The natural history and prognosis of rheumatoid arthritis: Association of radiographic outcome with process variables, joint motion and immune proteins. *Scand J Rheumatol Suppl* 2004:1–38.
36. van Lent PL, Grevers L, Lubberts E, et al. Fcγ receptors directly mediate cartilage, but not bone, destruction in murine antigen-induced arthritis: Uncoupling of cartilage damage from bone erosion and joint inflammation. *Arthritis Rheum* 2006;54:3868–3877.
37. Kobayashi I, Ziff M. Electron microscopic studies of the cartilage-pannus junction in rheumatoid arthritis. *Arthritis Rheum* 1975;18: 475–483.
38. Woolley DE, Crossley MJ, Evanson JM. Collagenase at sites of cartilage erosion in the rheumatoid joint. *Arthritis Rheum* 1977;20: 1231–1239.
39. Edwards JCW. Fibroblast biology. Development and differentiation of synovial fibroblasts in arthritis. *Arthritis Res* 2000;2:344–347.
40. Kimura H, Tateishi HJ, Ziff M. Surface ultrastructure of rheumatoid articular cartilage. *Arthritis Rheum* 1977;20:1085–1098.
41. Dodge GR, Poole AR. Immunohistochemical detection and immunochemical analysis of type II collagen degradation in human normal, rheumatoid, and osteoarthritic articular cartilages and in explants of bovine articular cartilage cultured with interleukin 1. *J Clin Invest* 1989;83:647–661.
42. Mitchell NS, Shepard N. Changes in proteoglycan and collagen in cartilage in rheumatoid arthritis. *J Bone Joint Surg* 1978;60A: 349–354.
43. Dodge GR, Pidoux I, Poole AR. The degradation of type II collagen in rheumatoid arthritis: An immunoelectron microscopic study. *Matrix* 1991;11:330–338.
44. Rengel Y, Ospelt C, Gay S. Proteinases in the joint: Clinical relevance of proteinases in joint destruction. *Arthritis Res Ther* 2007;9:221.
45. Murphy G, Lee MH. What are the roles of metalloproteinases in cartilage and bone damage? *Ann Rheum Dis* 2005;64(Suppl 4):iv44–47.
46. Hembry RM, Bagga MR, Reynolds JJ, et al. Immunolocalisation studies on six matrix metalloproteinases and their inhibitors, TIMp-1 and TIMp-2, in synovia from patients with osteo- and rheumatoid arthritis. *Ann Rheum Dis* 1995;54:25–32.
47. Tetlow LC, Woolley DE. Comparative immunolocalization studies of collagenase 1 and collagenase 3 production in the rheumatoid lesion, and by human chondrocytes and synoviocytes in vitro. *Br J Rheumatol* 1998;37:64–70.
48. Cunnane G, FitzGerald O, Hummel KM, et al. Synovial tissue protease gene expression and joint erosions in early rheumatoid arthritis. *Arthritis Rheum* 2001;44:1744–1753.
49. Woolley DE, Tetlow LC. Observations on the microenvironmental nature of cartilage degradation in rheumatoid arthritis. *Ann Rheum Dis* 1997;56:151–161.
50. Ainola MM, Mandelin JA, Liljestrom MP, et al. Pannus invasion and cartilage degradation in rheumatoid arthritis: Involvement of MMP-3 and interleukin-1β. *Clin Exp Rheumatol* 2005;23:644–650.
51. Barksby HE, Milner JM, Patterson AM, et al. Matrix metalloproteinase 10 promotion of collagenolysis via procollagenase activation: Implications for cartilage degradation in arthritis. *Arthritis Rheum* 2006;54:3244–3253.
52. Rutkauskaite E, Volkmer D, Shigeyama Y, et al. Retroviral gene transfer of an antisense construct against membrane type 1 matrix metalloproteinase reduces the invasiveness of rheumatoid arthritis synovial fibroblasts. *Arthritis Rheum* 2005;52:2010–2014.
53. Kevorkian L, Young DA, Darrah C, et al. Expression profiling of metalloproteinases and their inhibitors in cartilage. *Arthritis Rheum* 2004;50:131–141.
54. Cawston TE, Wilson AJ. Understanding the role of tissue degrading enzymes and their inhibitors in development and disease. *Best Pract Res Clin Rheumatol* 2006;20:983–1002.
55. Patel IR, Attur MG, Patel RN, et al. TNF-α convertase enzyme from human arthritis–affected cartilage: Isolation of cDNA by differential display, expression of the active enzyme, and regulation of TNF-α. *J Immunol* 1998;160:4570–4579.
56. Overall CM, Blobel CP. In search of partners: Linking extracellular proteases to substrates. *Nat Rev Mol Cell Biol* 2007;8:245–257.
57. Burrage PS, Huntington JT, Sporn MB, et al. Regulation of matrix metalloproteinase gene expression by a retinoid X receptor–specific ligand. *Arthritis Rheum* 2007;56:892–904.
58. Arner EC. Aggrecanase-mediated cartilage degradation. *Curr Opin Pharmacol* 2002;2:322–329.
59. Plaas A, Osborn B, Yoshihara Y, et al. Aggrecanolysis in human osteoarthritis: Confocal localization and biochemical characterization of ADAMTS5-hyaluronan complexes in articular cartilages. *Osteoarthritis Cartilage* 2007;15:719–734.
60. Sandy JD. A contentious issue finds some clarity: On the independent and complementary roles of aggrecanase activity and MMP

activity in human joint aggrecanolysis. *Osteoarthritis Cartilage* 2006;14:95–100.

61. Glasson SS, Askew R, Sheppard B, Carito B, Blanchet T, Ma HL, Flannery CR, Peluso D, Kanki K, Yang Z, et al: Deletion of active ADAMTS5 prevents cartilage degradation in a murine model of osteoarthritis. *Nature* 2005;434:644–648.
62. Stanton H, Rogerson FM, East CJ, Golub SB, Lawlor KE, Meeker CT, Little CB, Last K, Farmer PJ, Campbell IK, et al: ADAMTS5 is the major aggrecanase in mouse cartilage in vivo and in vitro. *Nature* 2005;434:648–652.
63. Kashiwagi M, Tortorella M, Nagase H, et al. TIMP-3 is a potent inhibitor of aggrecanase 1 (ADAM-TS4) and aggrecanase 2 (ADAM-TS5). *J Biol Chem* 2001;276:12501–12504.
64. Hui W, Cawston T, Rowan AD. Transforming growth factor β 1 and insulin-like growth factor 1 block collagen degradation induced by oncostatin M in combination with tumour necrosis factor α from bovine cartilage. *Ann Rheum Dis* 2003;62:172–174.
65. El Mabrouk M, Qureshi HY, Li WQ, et al. Interleukin-4 antagonizes oncostatin M and transforming growth factor β–induced responses in articular chondrocytes. *J Cell Biochem* 2007;103:588–597.
66. Nagase H, Kashiwagi M. Aggrecanases and cartilage matrix degradation. *Arthritis Res Ther* 2003;5:94–103.
67. Yamanishi Y, Firestein GS. Pathogenesis of rheumatoid arthritis: The role of synoviocytes. *Rheum Dis Clin North Am* 2001;27:355–371.
68. Hou WS, Li W, Keyszer G, et al. Comparison of cathepsins K and S expression within the rheumatoid and osteoarthritic synovium. *Arthritis Rheum* 2002;46:663–674.
69. Salminen-Mankonen HJ, Morko J, Vuorio E. Role of cathepsin K in normal joints and in the development of arthritis. *Curr Drug Targets* 2007;8:315–323.
70. Charni-Ben Tabassi N, Garnero P. Monitoring cartilage turnover. *Curr Rheumatol Rep* 2007;9:16–24.
71. Verstappen SM, Poole AR, Ionescu M, et al. Radiographic joint damage in rheumatoid arthritis is associated with differences in cartilage turnover and can be predicted by serum biomarkers: An evaluation from 1 to 4 years after diagnosis. *Arthritis Res Ther* 2006;8:R31.
72. Fraser A, Fearon U, Billinghurst RC, et al. Turnover of type II collagen and aggrecan in cartilage matrix at the onset of inflammatory arthritis in humans: Relationship to mediators of systemic and local inflammation. *Arthritis Rheum* 2003;48:3085–3095.
73. Lindqvist E, Eberhardt K, Bendtzen K, et al. Prognostic laboratory markers of joint damage in rheumatoid arthritis. *Ann Rheum Dis* 2005;64:196–201.
74. Baeten D, Steenbakkers PG, Rijnders AM, et al. Detection of major histocompatibility complex/human cartilage gp-39 complexes in rheumatoid arthritis synovitis as a specific and independent histologic marker. *Arthritis Rheum* 2004;50:444–451.
75. van Bilsen JH, van Dongen H, Lard LR, et al. Functional regulatory immune responses against human cartilage glycoprotein-39 in health vs. proinflammatory responses in rheumatoid arthritis. *Proc Natl Acad Sci U S A* 2004;101:17180–17185.
76. Recklies AD, White C, Ling H. The chitinase 3-like protein human cartilage glycoprotein 39 (HC-gp39) stimulates proliferation of human connective-tissue cells and activates both extracellular signal-regulated kinase- and protein kinase B–mediated signalling pathways. *Biochem J* 2002;365:119–126.
77. Ling H, Recklies AD. The chitinase 3-like protein human cartilage glycoprotein 39 inhibits cellular responses to the inflammatory cytokines interleukin-1 and tumour necrosis factor-α. *Biochem J* 2004; 380:651–659.
78. Sekine T, Masuko-Hongo K, Matsui T, et al. Recognition of YKL-39, a human cartilage related protein, as a target antigen in patients with rheumatoid arthritis. *Ann Rheum Dis* 2001;60:49–54.
79. Knorr T, Obermayr F, Bartnik E, et al. YKL-39 (chitinase 3-like protein 2), but not YKL-40 (chitinase 3-like protein 1), is up regulated in osteoarthritic chondrocytes. *Ann Rheum Dis* 2003;62: 995–998.
80. Saito S, Kondo S, Mishima S, et al. Analysis of cartilage-derived retinoic-acid-sensitive protein (CD-RAP) in synovial fluid from patients with osteoarthritis and rheumatoid arthritis. *J Bone Joint Surg Br* 2002;84:1066–1069.
81. Arend WP, Goldring MB. The development of anti-cytokine therapeutics for rheumatic diseases. *Arthritis Rheum* 2008;58: S102–S109.
82. Goldring MB, Berenbaum F. The regulation of chondrocyte function by proinflammatory mediators: Prostaglandins and nitric oxide. *Clin Orthop* 2004:S37–S46.
83. Horai R, Saijo S, Tanioka J, et al. Development of chronic inflammatory arthropathy resembling rheumatoid arthritis in interleukin 1 receptor antagonist-deficient mice. *J Exp Med* 2000;191:313–320.
84. Glasson SS. In vivo osteoarthritis target validation utilizing genetically-modified mice. *Curr Drug Targets* 2007;8:367–376.
85. Joosten LA, Helsen MM, van de Loo FA, et al. Anticytokine treatment of established type II collagen-induced arthritis in DBA/1 mice. A comparative study using anti-TNF α, anti-IL-1 α/β, and IL-1Ra. *Arthritis Rheum* 1996;39:797–809.
86. Probert L, Plows D, Kontogeorgos G, et al. The type I interleukin-1 receptor acts in series with tumor necrosis factor (TNF) to induce arthritis in TNF-transgenic mice. *Eur J Immunol* 1995;25:1794–1797.
87. Matsuno H, Yudoh K, Katayama R, et al. The role of TNF-α in the pathogenesis of inflammation and joint destruction in rheumatoid arthritis (RA): A study using a human RA/SCID mouse chimera. *Rheumatology (Oxford)* 2002;41:329–337.
88. Zwerina J, Redlich K, Polzer K, et al. TNF-induced structural joint damage is mediated by IL-1. *Proc Natl Acad Sci U S A* 2007;104(28): 11742–11747.
89. Burger D, Dayer JM, Palmer G, et al. Is IL-1 a good therapeutic target in the treatment of arthritis? *Best Pract Res Clin Rheumatol* 2006;20:879–896.
90. Masuko-Hongo K, Berenbaum F, Humbert L, et al. Up-regulation of microsomal prostaglandin E synthase 1 in osteoarthritic human cartilage: Critical roles of the ERK-1/2 and p38 signaling pathways. *Arthritis Rheum* 2004;50:2829–2838.
91. Whiteman M, Spencer JP, Zhu YZ, et al. Peroxynitrite-modified collagen-II induces p38/ERK and NF-κB–dependent synthesis of prostaglandin E2 and nitric oxide in chondrogenically differentiated mesenchymal progenitor cells. *Osteoarthritis Cartilage* 2006; 14:460–470.
92. Healy ZR, Lee NH, Gao X, et al. Divergent responses of chondrocytes and endothelial cells to shear stress: Cross-talk among COX-2, the phase 2 response, and apoptosis. *Proc Natl Acad Sci U S A* 2005.
93. Abramson SB, Attur M, Amin AR, et al. Nitric oxide and inflammatory mediators in the perpetuation of osteoarthritis. *Curr Rheumatol Rep* 2001;3:535–541.
94. Kuhn K, D'Lima DD, Hashimoto S, et al. Cell death in cartilage. *Osteoarthritis Cartilage* 2004;12:1–16.
95. Clancy RM, Gomez PF, Abramson SB. Nitric oxide sustains nuclear factor κB activation in cytokine-stimulated chondrocytes. *Osteoarthritis Cartilage* 2004;12:552–558.
96. Clancy R. Nitric oxide alters chondrocyte function by disrupting cytoskeletal signaling complexes. *Osteoarthritis Cartilage* 1999;7: 399–400.
97. Johnson K, Jung A, Murphy A, et al. Mitochondrial oxidative phosphorylation is a downstream regulator of nitric oxide effects on chondrocyte matrix synthesis and mineralization. *Arthritis Rheum* 2000;43:1560–1570.
98. Loeser RF, Carlson CS, Del Carlo M, et al. Detection of nitrotyrosine in aging and osteoarthritic cartilage: Correlation of oxidative damage with the presence of interleukin-1β and with chondrocyte resistance to insulin-like growth factor 1. *Arthritis Rheum* 2002; 46:2349–2357.
99. Studer RK, Decker K, Melhem S, et al. Nitric oxide inhibition of IGF-1 stimulated proteoglycan synthesis: Role of cGMP. *J Orthop Res* 2003;21:914–921.

100. van den Berg WB, van de Loo F, Joosten LA, et al. Animal models of arthritis in NOS2-deficient mice. *Osteoarthritis Cartilage* 1999; 7:413–415.
101. McInnes IB, Schett G. Cytokines in the pathogenesis of rheumatoid arthritis. *Nat Rev Immunol* 2007;7:429–442.
102. Aida Y, Maeno M, Suzuki N, et al. The effect of IL-1β on the expression of inflammatory cytokines and their receptors in human chondrocytes. *Life Sci* 2006;79:764–771.
103. Connell L, McInnes IB. New cytokine targets in inflammatory rheumatic diseases. *Best Pract Res Clin Rheumatol* 2006;20: 865–878.
104. Rowan AD, Koshy PJ, Shingleton WD, et al. Synergistic effects of glycoprotein 130 binding cytokines in combination with interleukin-1 on cartilage collagen breakdown. *Arthritis Rheum* 2001;44:1620–1632.
105. Legendre F, Dudhia J, Pujol JP, et al. JAK/STAT but not ERK1/ERK2 pathway mediates interleukin (IL)-6/soluble IL-6R down-regulation of type II collagen, aggrecan core, and link protein transcription in articular chondrocytes. Association with a down-regulation of SOX9 expression. *J Biol Chem* 2003;278: 2903–2912.
106. de Hooge AS, van de Loo FA, Bennink MB, et al. Male IL-6 gene knock out mice developed more advanced osteoarthritis upon aging. *Osteoarthritis Cartilage* 2005;13:66–73.
107. Gabay C. Interleukin-6 and chronic inflammation. *Arthritis Res Ther* 2006;8(Suppl 2):S3.
108. Nishimoto N, Kishimoto T. Interleukin 6: From bench to bedside. *Nat Clin Pract Rheumatol* 2006;2:619–626.
109. Sack U, Sehm B, Kahlenberg F, et al. Investigation of arthritic joint destruction by a novel fibroblast-based model. *Ann N Y Acad SciAnn N Y Acad Sci* 2005;1051:291–298.
110. Hui W, Barksby HE, Young DA, et al. Oncostatin M in combination with tumour necrosis factor α induces a chondrocyte membrane associated aggrecanase that is distinct from ADAMTS aggrecanase-1 or -2. *Ann Rheum Dis* 2005;64:1624–1632.
111. van de Loo FA, de Hooge AS, Smeets RL, Bakker AC, Bennink MB, Arntz OJ, Joosten LA, van Beuningen HM, van der Kraan PK, Varley AW, van den Berg WB: An inflammation-inducible adenoviral expression system for local treatment of the arthritic joint. *Gene Ther* 2004;11:581–590.
112. Rowan AD, Hui W, Cawston TE, Richards CD: Adenoviral gene transfer of interleukin-1 in combination with oncostatin M induces significant joint damage in a murine model. *Am J Pathol* 2003;162: 1975–1984.
113. John T, Kohl B, Mobasheri A, et al. Interleukin-18 induces apoptosis in human articular chondrocytes. *Histol Histopathol* 2007;22: 469–482.
114. Dai SM, Shan ZZ, Nishioka K, et al. Implication of interleukin 18 in production of matrix metalloproteinases in articular chondrocytes in arthritis: Direct effect on chondrocytes may not be pivotal. *Ann Rheum Dis* 2005;64:735–742.
115. Li X, Afif H, Cheng S, et al. Expression and regulation of microsomal prostaglandin E synthase-1 in human osteoarthritic cartilage and chondrocytes. *J Rheumatol* 2005;32:887–895.
116. Lubberts E, Koenders MI, van den Berg WB. The role of T cell interleukin-17 in conducting destructive arthritis: Lessons from animal models. *Arthritis Res Ther* 2005;7:29–37.
117. Smeets RL, van de Loo FA, Arntz OJ, et al. Adenoviral delivery of IL-18 binding protein C ameliorates collagen-induced arthritis in mice. *Gene Ther* 2003;10:1004–1011.
118. Koenders MI, Joosten LA, van den Berg WB. Potential new targets in arthritis therapy: Interleukin (IL)-17 and its relation to tumour necrosis factor and IL-1 in experimental arthritis. *Ann Rheum Dis* 2006;65(Suppl 3):iii29–iii33.
119. Honorati MC, Neri S, Cattini L, et al. Interleukin-17, a regulator of angiogenic factor release by synovial fibroblasts. *Osteoarthritis Cartilage* 2006;14:345–352.
120. Joosten LA, Smeets RL, Koenders MI, et al. Interleukin-18 promotes joint inflammation and induces interleukin-1–driven cartilage destruction. *Am J Pathol* 2004;165:959–967.
121. Joosten LA, Netea MG, Kim SH, et al. IL-32, a proinflammatory cytokine in rheumatoid arthritis. *Proc Natl Acad Sci U S A* 2006; 103:3298–3303.
122. Magne D, Palmer G, Barton JL, et al. The new IL-1 family member IL-1F8 stimulates production of inflammatory mediators by synovial fibroblasts and articular chondrocytes. *Arthritis Res Ther* 2006;8:R80.
123. Joosten LA, Koenders MI, Smeets RL, et al. Toll-like receptor 2 pathway drives streptococcal cell wall-induced joint inflammation: Critical role of myeloid differentiation factor 88. *J Immunol* 2003;171:6145–6153.
124. Varoga D, Paulsen F, Mentlein R, et al. TLR–2-mediated induction of vascular endothelial growth factor (VEGF) in cartilage in septic joint disease. *J Pathol* 2006;210:315–324.
125. Su SL, Tsai CD, Lee CH, et al. Expression and regulation of toll-like receptor 2 by IL-1β and fibronectin fragments in human articular chondrocytes. *Osteoarthritis Cartilage* 2005;13:879–886.
126. Kim HA, Cho ML, Choi HY, et al. The catabolic pathway mediated by toll-like receptors in human osteoarthritic chondrocytes. *Arthritis Rheum* 2006;54:2152–2163.
127. van Lent PL, Blom AB, Grevers L, et al. Toll-like receptor 4 induced FcγR expression potentiates early onset of joint inflammation and cartilage destruction during immune complex arthritis: Toll-like receptor 4 largely regulates FcγR expression by interleukin 10. *Ann Rheum Dis* 2007;66:334–340.
128. Asquith DL, McInnes IB. Emerging cytokine targets in rheumatoid arthritis. *Curr Opin Rheumatol* 2007;19:246–251.
129. Haglund L, Bernier SM, Onnerfjord P, et al. Proteomic analysis of the LPS-induced stress response in rat chondrocytes reveals induction of innate immune response components in articular cartilage. *Matrix Biol* 2008;27:107–118.
130. Abdollahi-Roodsaz S, Joosten LA, Roelofs MF, et al. Inhibition of toll-like receptor 4 breaks the inflammatory loop in autoimmune destructive arthritis. *Arthritis Rheum* 2007;56:2957–2967.
131. Bobacz K, Sunk IG, Hofstaetter JG, et al. Toll-like receptors and chondrocytes: The lipopolysaccharide-induced decrease in cartilage matrix synthesis is dependent on the presence of toll-like receptor 4 and antagonized by bone morphogenetic protein 7. *Arthritis Rheum* 2007;56:1880–1893.
132. Fernandes JC, Martel-Pelletier J, Pelletier JP. The role of cytokines in osteoarthritis pathophysiology. *Biorheology* 2002;39:237–246.
133. Bessis N, Boissier MC. Novel pro-inflammatory interleukins: Potential therapeutic targets in rheumatoid arthritis. *Joint Bone Spine* 2001;68:477–481.
134. Palmer G, Guerne PA, Mezin F, et al. Production of interleukin-1 receptor antagonist by human articular chondrocytes. *Arthritis Res* 2002;4:226–231.
135. van de Loo FA, Geurts J, van den Berg WB. Gene therapy works in animal models of rheumatoid arthritis... So what! *Curr Rheumatol Rep* 2006;8:386–393.
136. Chowdhury TT, Bader DL, Lee DA. Anti-inflammatory effects of IL-4 and dynamic compression in IL-1β stimulated chondrocytes. *Biochem Biophys Res Commun* 2006;339:241–247.
137. Schuerwegh AJ, Dombrecht EJ, Stevens WJ, et al. Influence of pro-inflammatory (IL-1 β, IL-6, TNF-α, IFN-γ) and anti-inflammatory (IL-4) cytokines on chondrocyte function. *Osteoarthritis Cartilage* 2003;11:681–687.
138. Ho SH, Hahn W, Lee HJ, et al. Protection against collagen-induced arthritis by electrotransfer of an expression plasmid for the interleukin-4. *Biochem Biophys Res Commun* 2004;321: 759–766.
139. Nandakumar KS, Holmdahl R. Arthritis induced with cartilage-specific antibodiesis IL-4–dependent. *Eur J Immunol* 2006;36: 1608–1618.

140. Gonzalez-Rey E, Chorny A, Varela N, et al. Therapeutic effect of urocortin on collagen-induced arthritis by down-regulation of inflammatory and Th1 responses and induction of regulatory T cells. *Arthritis Rheum* 2007;56:531–543.
141. Neumann E, Judex M, Kullmann F, Grifka J, et al. Inhibition of cartilage destruction by double gene transfer of IL-1Ra and IL-10 involves the activin pathway. *Gene Ther* 2002;9:1508–1519.
142. Cleaver CS, Rowan AD, Cawston TE. Interleukin 13 blocks the release of collagen from bovine nasal cartilage treated with proinflammatory cytokines. *Ann Rheum Dis* 2001;60:150–157.
143. Haas CS, Amin MA, Ruth JH, et al. In vivo inhibition of angiogenesis by interleukin-13 gene therapy in a rat model of rheumatoid arthritis. *Arthritis Rheum* 2007;56:2535–2548.
144. Nabbe KC, van Lent PL, Holthuysen AE, et al. Local IL-13 gene transfer prior to immune-complex arthritis inhibits chondrocyte death and matrix-metalloproteinase-mediated cartilage matrix degradation despite enhanced joint inflammation. *Arthritis Res Ther* 2005;7:R392–R401.
145. Cheng S, Afif H, Martel-Pelletier J, et al. Activation of peroxisome proliferator-activated receptor γ inhibits interleukin-1β-induced membrane-associated prostaglandin E2 synthase-1 expression in human synovial fibroblasts by interfering with Egr-1. *J Biol Chem* 2004;279:22057–22065.
146. Francois M, Richette P, Tsagris L, et al. Activation of the peroxisome proliferator-activated receptor α pathway potentiates interleukin-1 receptor antagonist production in cytokine-treated chondrocytes. *Arthritis Rheum* 2006;54:1233–1245.
147. Smeets RL, Veenbergen S, Arntz OJ, et al. A novel role for SOCS3 in cartilage destruction via induction of chondrocyte desensitization towards IGF-1. *Arthritis Rheum* 2006;54:1518–1528.
148. Yammani RR, Carlson CS, Bresnick AR, et al. S100A4 activates receptor for advanced glycation end-products (RAGE) signaling and stimulates matrix metalloproteinase-13 production in human articular chondrocytes. *Arthritis Rheum* 2006;54:2901–2911.
149. Bauer S, Jendro MC, Wadle A, et al. Fibroblast activation protein is expressed by rheumatoid myofibroblast-like synoviocytes. *Arthritis Res Ther* 2006;8:R171.
150. Milner JM, Kevorkian L, Young DA, et al. Fibroblast activation protein α is expressed by chondrocytes following a pro-inflammatory stimulus and is elevated in osteoarthritis. *Arthritis Res Ther* 2006; 8:R23.
151. Loeser RF. Systemic and local regulation of articular cartilage metabolism: where does leptin fit in the puzzle? *Arthritis Rheum* 2003;48:3009–3012.
152. Dayer JM, Chicheportiche R, Juge-Aubry C, et al. Adipose tissue has anti-inflammatory properties: Focus on IL-1 receptor antagonist (IL-1Ra). *Ann N Y Acad Sci* 2006;1069:444–453.
153. Otero M, Lago R, Gomez R, et al. Towards a pro-inflammatory and immunomodulatory emerging role of leptin. *Rheumatology (Oxford)* 2006;45:944–950.
154. Otero M, Lago R, Lago F, et al. Leptin, from fat to inflammation: Old questions and new insights. *FEBS Lett* 2005;579:295–301.
155. Palmer G, Aurrand-Lions M, Contassot E, et al. Indirect effects of leptin receptor deficiency on lymphocyte populations and immune response in db/db mice. *J Immunol* 2006;177: 2899–2907.
156. Popa C, Netea MG, Radstake TR, et al. Markers of inflammation are negatively correlated with serum leptin in rheumatoid arthritis. *Ann Rheum Dis* 2005;64:1195–1198.
157. Lago F, Dieguez C, Gomez-Reino J, et al. Adipokines as emerging mediators of immune response and inflammation. *Nat Clin Pract Rheumatol* 2007;3:716–724.
158. Dumond H, Presle N, Terlain B, et al. Evidence for a key role of leptin in osteoarthritis. *Arthritis Rheum* 2003;48:3118–3129.
159. Goldring MB, Goldring SR. Role of cytokines and chemokines in cartilage and bone destruction in arthritis. *Curr Opin Orthopaed* 2002;13:351–362.
160. Koch AE. Chemokines and their receptors in rheumatoid arthritis: Future targets? *Arthritis Rheum* 2005;52:710–721.
161. Nakamura H, Masuko K, Yudoh K, et al. Effects of celecoxib on human chondrocytes—enhanced production of chemokines. *Clin Exp Rheumatol* 2007;25:11–16.
162. Vergunst CE, van de Sande MG, Lebre MC, et al. The role of chemokines in rheumatoid arthritis and osteoarthritis. *Scand J Rheumatol* 2005;34:415–425.
163. Borzi RM, Mazzetti I, Marcu KB, et al. Chemokines in cartilage degradation. *Clin Orthop Relat Res* 2004:S53–S61.
164. Iwamoto T, Okamoto H, Iikuni N, et al. Monocyte chemoattractant protein-4 (MCp-4)/CCL13 is highly expressed in cartilage from patients with rheumatoid arthritis. *Rheumatology (Oxford)* 2006;45:421–424.
165. Kanbe K, Takemura T, Takeuchi K, et al. Synovectomy reduces stromal-cell–derived factor-1 (SDF-1) which is involved in the destruction of cartilage in osteoarthritis and rheumatoid arthritis. *J Bone Joint Surg Br* 2004;86:296–300.
166. Pulai JI, Chen H, Im HJ, et al. NF-κB mediates the stimulation of cytokine and chemokine expression by human articular chondrocytes in response to fibronectin fragments. *J Immunol* 2005;174: 5781–5788.
167. Mazzetti I, Magagnoli G, Paoletti S, et al. A role for chemokines in the induction of chondrocyte phenotype modulation. *Arthritis Rheum* 2004;50:112–122.
168. Masuko-Hongo K, Sato T, et al. Chemokines differentially induce matrix metalloproteinase-3 and prostaglandin E2 in human articular chondrocytes. *Clin Exp Rheumatol* 2005;23:57–62.
169. Nakamura H, Tanaka M, Masuko-Hongo K, et al. Enhanced production of MMp-1, MMp-3, MMp-13, and RANTES by interaction of chondrocytes with autologous T cells. *Rheumatol Int* 2006:1–7.
170. Sweeney SE, Firestein GS. Primer: Signal transduction in rheumatic disease—a clinician's guide. *Nat Clin Pract Rheumatol* 2007; 3:651–660.
171. Schett G, Zwerina J, Firestein G. The p38 mitogen activated protein kinase (MAPK) pathway in rheumatoid arthritis. *Ann Rheum Dis* 2007.
172. Berenbaum F. Signaling transduction: Target in osteoarthritis. *Curr Opin Rheumatol* 2004;16:616–622.
173. Malemud CJ. Protein kinases in chondrocyte signaling and osteoarthritis. *Clin Orthop Relat Res* 2004:S145–151.
174. Katoh M. STAT3-induced WNT5A signaling loop in embryonic stem cells, adult normal tissues, chronic persistent inflammation, rheumatoid arthritis and cancer. [Review.] *Int J Mol Med* 2007; 19:273–278.
175. Agarwal S, Deschner J, Long P, et al. Role of NF-κB transcription factors in antiinflammatory and proinflammatory actions of mechanical signals. *Arthritis Rheum* 2004;50:3541–3548.
176. Fanning PJ, Emkey G, Smith RJ, et al. Mechanical regulation of mitogen-activated protein kinase signaling in articular cartilage. *J Biol Chem* 2003;278:50940–50948.
177. Fitzgerald JB, Jin M, Dean D, et al. Mechanical compression of cartilage explants induces multiple time-dependent gene expression patterns and involves intracellular calcium and cyclic AMP. *J Biol Chem* 2004;279:19502–19511.
178. Xu L, Peng H, Glasson S, Lee PL, Hu K, Ijiri K, Olsen BR, Goldring MB, Li Y: Increased expression of the collagen receptor discoidin domain receptor 2 in articular cartilage as a key event in the pathogenesis of osteoarthritis. *Arthritis Rheum* 2007;56:2663–2673.
179. Korb A, Tohidast-Akrad M, Cetin E, et al. Differential tissue expression and activation of p38 MAPK α, β, γ, and δ isoforms in rheumatoid arthritis. *Arthritis Rheum* 2006;54:2745–2756.
180. Medicherla S, Ma JY, Mangadu R, et al. A selective p38 α mitogen-activated protein kinase inhibitor reverses cartilage and bone destruction in mice with collagen-induced arthritis. *J Pharmacol Exp Ther* 2006;318:132–141.

181. Hammaker DR, Boyle DL, Chabaud-Riou M, et al. Regulation of c-Jun N-terminal kinase by MEKK-2 and mitogen-activated protein kinase kinase kinases in rheumatoid arthritis. *J Immunol* 2004; 172:1612–1618.
182. Ahmed S, Rahman A, Hasnain A, et al. Phenyl N-tert-butylnitrone down-regulates interleukin-1 β-stimulated matrix metalloproteinase-13 gene expression in human chondrocytes: Suppression of c-Jun NH2-terminal kinase, p38-mitogen-activated protein kinase and activating protein-1. *J Pharmacol Exp Ther* 2003;305:981–988.
183. Loeser RF, Forsyth CB, Samarel AM, et al. Fibronectin fragment activation of proline-rich tyrosine kinase PYK2 mediates integrin signals regulating collagenase-3 expression by human chondrocytes through a protein kinase C-dependent pathway. *J Biol Chem* 2003;278:24577–24585.
184. Nieminen R, Leinonen S, Lahti A, et al. Inhibitors of mitogen-activated protein kinases downregulate COX-2 expression in human chondrocytes. *Mediators Inflamm* 2005;2005:249–255.
185. Zhou Y, Millward-Sadler SJ, Lin H, et al. Evidence for JNK-dependent up-regulation of proteoglycan synthesis and for activation of JNK1 following cyclical mechanical stimulation in a human chondrocyte culture model. *Osteoarthritis Cartilage* 2007;15:884–893.
186. Firestein GS. NF-κB: Holy grail for rheumatoid arthritis? *Arthritis Rheum* 2004;50:2381–2386.
187. Facchini A, Borzi RM, Marcu KB, et al. Polyamine depletion inhibits NF-κB binding to DNA and interleukin-8 production in human chondrocytes stimulated by tumor necrosis factor-a. *J Cell Physiol* 2005;204:956–963.
188. Benito MJ, Murphy E, Murphy EP, et al. Increased synovial tissue NF-κ B1 expression at sites adjacent to the cartilage-pannus junction in rheumatoid arthritis. *Arthritis Rheum* 2004;50:1781–1787.
189. Grall F, Gu X, Tan L, et al. Responses to the pro-inflammatory cytokines interleukin-1 and tumor necrosis factor a in cells derived from rheumatoid synovium and other joint tissues involve NF κB-mediated induction of the Ets transcription factor ESE-1. *Arthritis Rheum* 2003;48:1249–1260.
190. Grall FT, Prall WC, Wei W, et al. The Ets transcription factor ESE-1 mediates induction of the COX-2 gene by LPS in monocytes. *FEBS J* 2005;272:1676–1687.
191. Imamura T, Imamura C, Iwamoto Y, et al. Transcriptional co-activators CREB-binding protein/p300 increase chondrocyte CD-RAP gene expression by multiple mechanisms including sequestration of the repressor CCAAT/enhancer-binding protein. *J Biol Chem* 2005;280:16625–16634.
192. Rannou F, Francois M, Corvol MT, et al. Cartilage breakdown in rheumatoid arthritis. *Joint Bone Spine* 2006;73:29–36.
193. Raymond L, Eck S, Mollmark J, et al. Interleukin-1β induction of matrix metalloproteinase-1 transcription in chondrocytes requires ERK-dependent activation of CCAAT enhancer–binding protein-β. *J Cell Physiol* 2006;207:683–688.
194. Goldring MB, Sandell LJ. Transcriptional control of chondrocyte gene expression. In: Buckwalter J, Lotz M, Stoltz JF, eds. *OA, Inflammation and Degradation: A Continuum*. Amsterdam: IOS Press, 2007, pp. 118–142.
195. Seguin CA, Bernier SM. TNFα suppresses link protein and type II collagen expression in chondrocytes: Role of MEK1/2 and NF-κB signaling pathways. *J Cell Physiol* 2003;197:356–369.
196. Okazaki K, Li J, Yu H, et al. CCAAT/Enhancer-binding proteins β and δ mediate the repression of gene transcription of cartilage-derived retinoic acid–sensitive protein induced by interleukin-1β. *J Biol Chem* 2002;277:31526–31533.
197. Tan L, Peng H, Osaki M, et al. Egr-1 mediates transcriptional repression of COL2A1 promoter activity by interleukin-1β. *J Biol Chem* 2003;278:17688–17700.
198. Peng H, Tan L, Osaki M, et al. ESE-1 is a potent repressor of type II collagen gene (COL2A1) transcription in human chondrocytes. *J Cell Physiol* 2008;215:562–573.
199. Heller RA, Schena M, Chai A, et al. Discovery and analysis of inflammatory disease-related genes using cDNA microarrays. *Proc Natl Acad Sci U S A* 1997;94:2150–2155.
200. Vincenti MP, Brinckerhoff CE. Early response genes induced in chondrocytes stimulated with the inflammatory cytokine interleukin-1β. *Arthritis Res* 2001;3:381–388.
201. Barksby HE, Hui W, Wappler I, et al. Interleukin-1 in combination with oncostatin M up-regulates multiple genes in chondrocytes: Implications for cartilage destruction and repair. *Arthritis Rheum* 2006;54:540–550.
202. Aigner T, Fundel K, Saas J, et al. Large-scale gene expression profiling reveals major pathogenetic pathways of cartilage degeneration in osteoarthritis. *Arthritis Rheum* 2006;54:3533–3544.
203. Sato T, Konomi K, Yamasaki S, et al. Comparative analysis of gene expression profiles in intact and damaged regions of human osteoarthritic cartilage. *Arthritis Rheum* 2006;54:808–817.
204. Attur MG, Dave MN, Akamatsu M, et al. A system biology approach to bioinformatics and functional genomics in complex human diseases: Arthritis. *Curr Issues Mol Biol* 2002;4:129–146.

Osteoclasts and Osteoblasts

Georg Schett and Kurt Redlich

The cells that allow the body to resorb bone are called osteoclasts. Resorption of bone is part of a remodeling process that enables bone growth, repair of damage, and adaptation of the skeletal architecture to individual demands. Generation of osteoclasts and bone resorption are part of a physiological process that is the basis of plasticity of the skeletal system. Osteoclasts are multinucleated cells stemming from the hematopoietic cell lineage, and are closely related to monocytes/macrophages and dendritic cells (see Figure 8H-1). The cells responsible for bone formation are called osteoblasts and, in contrast to osteoclasts, stem from mesenchymal cell lineage. Osteoblasts produce the bone matrix, which then calcifies. Osteoblasts are functionally linked to osteoclasts, enabling a balance between bone formation and bone resorption, and overall bone mass remains constant.

Inflammatory Bone Damage

Chronic inflammation perturbs bone homeostasis and precipitates bone loss. Virtually all inflammatory diseases, including rheumatic diseases, connective tissue diseases, inflammatory bowel diseases, and chronic infections lead to premature osteoporosis. Even small elevations of C-reactive protein lead to enhanced fracture risk in humans.[1] In chronic arthritis, such as rheumatoid arthritis (RA) and psoriatic arthritis, bone loss is a common finding, which is closely linked to disease duration and inflammatory disease activity, and most prominently affects the skeletal regions close to the inflamed joint.[2] This tight link between inflammation and bone destruction in inflammatory arthritis can only be explained by an imbalance between bone resorption and bone formation. These clinical findings focus attention on the link between inflammation and osteoclast, and potentially also osteoblast function, to explain the profound architectural changes of bone during inflammatory arthritis.

Osteoclasts in Inflamed Joints

Multinucleated cells have been identified in inflamed joint as early as over 120 years ago. Theodor Billroth established his reputation by introducing new surgery techniques to effectively treat serious ulcers of the stomach and rescue patients from lethal gastrointestinal bleeding. As typical of doctors at the time, Billroth was not specialized in surgery but he was also interested in other fields in medicine, especially in anatomy and pathology. When reading the slides of tissue sections derived from joint surgery of patients with inflammatory arthritis, he observed giant cells at the interphase between inflammatory tissue and bone. He termed these cells "bone breakers," based on the appearance of microscopic sites of bone resorption (lacunae) adjacent to these cells.[3] His contemporary Anton Weichselbaum first described the appearance of local bone erosions in RA (at this time termed fungus synovitis because of the fungus-like appearance of the synovial inflammatory tissue) and characterized these lesions as caries of the joint ends.[4] These two findings actually represented a very detailed and informative description of structural damage in RA: A special giant-like cell type populates chronically inflamed joints, appears to resorb the bone, and creates localized skeletal defects within the inflamed joint.

The presence of multinucleated cells in the inflamed synovial membrane of patients with rheumatoid arthritis with the phenotype of osteoclasts has been virtually "forgotten" for almost 100 years before their rediscovery. Refinement of immunological methods to selectively specify various cell types and to visualize them in normal and diseased tissue, together with clinical observations that structural damage of joints is a main contributor to the disease burden of patients with RA and PsA, has stimulated research on the cellular and molecular basis of inflammatory bone erosion. In the 1980s, Bromley and Woolley described multinucleated cells at the interface between bone and synovial inflammatory tissue and called them "osteoclasts" when attached to bone, and "chondroclasts" when attached to cartilage.[5] In the 1990s, Gravallese and Goldring reported that the multinucleated cells present in the inflamed synovial tissue of RA patients showed the specific marker profile of osteoclasts, suggesting that bone-resorbing cells are indeed an integral part of the inflamed synovial membrane.[6] Late-stage differentiation markers of osteoclasts such as the calcitonin receptor are also present, as well as earlier differentiation markers such as cathepsin K and tartrate-resistant acid phosphatase. Fully differentiated osteoclasts, appearing as multinucleated cells expressing late-stage differentiation markers, are only observed in direct contact or at least in close proximity to the bone surface. In contrast, mononuclear cells expressing early osteoclast differentiation markers and resembling osteoclast precursors are also found at more distant sites within the inflamed synovium. These precursor cells serve as a pool for the recruitment of further osteoclasts. It has not been fully clarified, however, whether these cells have already undergone differentiation into the osteoclast lineage before entering the synovium or emerge from monocyte/macrophages recruited to the inflamed joint. Some data in fact indicate that the proportion of cells capable of differentiating into the osteoclast lineage, such as CD11b-positive

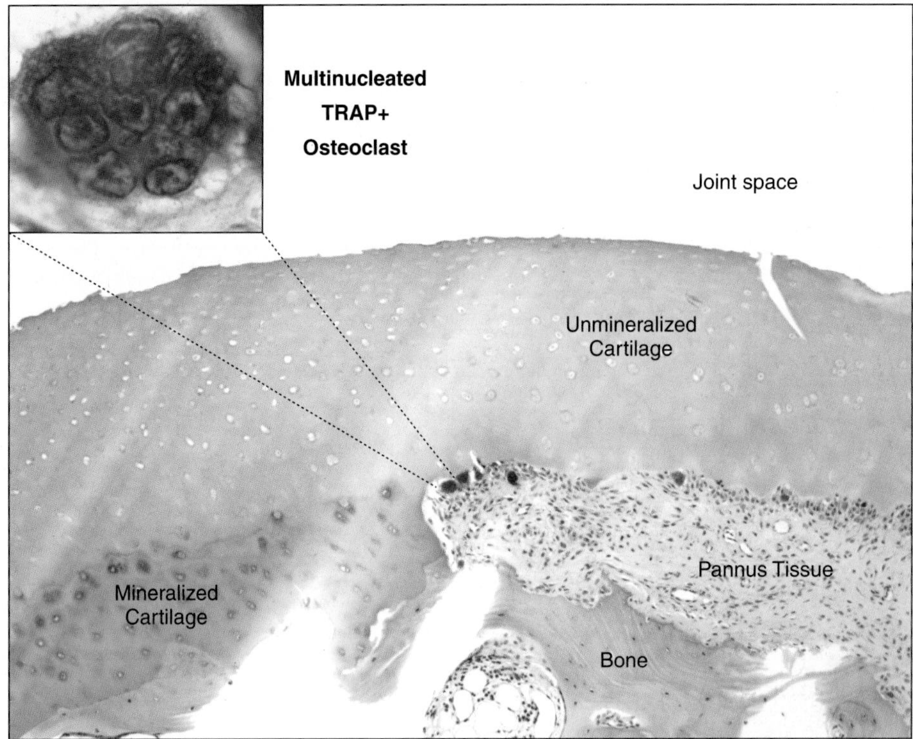

Figure 8H-1. Osteoclasts at sites of inflammatory bone erosion. Section through a metacarpal head of a patient with RA. Osteoclasts appear as purple-stained multinucleated cells at the erosion front between pannus and mineralized tissue.

monocytes, is elevated in the peripheral blood of patients with inflammatory arthritis, suggesting that systemic inflammation per se facilitates osteoclast recruitment.[7,8]

Osteoclasts are specialized to resorb bone.[9] They can create an acidic milieu, which is necessary to solubilize calcium and extract it from bone. As one of the few regions in the body with a low pH, resorption pits are acidified by the proton pump of the osteoclast, which carries H+ ions into a small compartment between the osteoclast and the bone surface. This compartment is sealed from the rest of the extracellular tissue by tight junctions, which are part of a ring-like structure (F-actin ring), which allows tight attachment of the osteoclast to the bone. This ring-like structure is part of a polarization process of osteoclasts during maturation, which allows targeting the bone resorption machinery of the cell to the bone surface. Thus the membrane of the osteoclast next to bone is termed the ruffled membrane because if its large surface, which is also the metabolically most active part of the cell. Osteoclasts also carry a battery of proteolytic enzymes, which cleave bone matrix proteins. One of the most specific matrix-degrading enzymes of osteoclasts is cathepsin K.

Molecular Regulation of Osteoclastogenesis in Joints

What are the factors that allow the formation of osteoclasts within the inflamed synovium? Osteoclasts require two essential growth and differentiation factors for their full development from monocytic precursors: macrophage colony–stimulating factor (MCSF), and the receptor antagonist of NF-κB ligand (RANKL) (Figure 8H-2). Both factors are expressed in the inflamed synovium and affect immigrating mononuclear cells expressing their receptors, c-Fms and RANK, respectively.[10–12] The expression of MCSF and RANKL is crucial for understanding osteoclast formation in the diseased joint. Each on their own is absolutely required to generate osteoclasts, and only the combination of both allows a full differentiation process. The cells expressing MSCF and RANKL are T lymphocytes as well as synovial fibroblasts, suggesting that these are the primary cell types responsible for osteoclast formation in the joint. The interaction between synovial fibroblasts and osteoclast resembles the close interaction of (pre-) osteoblasts (as mesenchymal cells) with osteoclasts as typically seen during physiological bone remodeling, whereas the interaction between T lymphocytes and osteoclasts is the hallmark for the cross-talk interaction between the immune system and bone, commonly known as osteoimmunology. The current model suggests that TH17 cells are of key importance in driving osteoclast formation due to production of IL-17, which is a potent stimulator of RANKL.[13] TH1 cells may also support osteoclast formation in the joint, since TH1 cells produce not only pro-osteoclastogenic mediators such as MCSF and RANKL. However, they also express potent repressors of osteoclast differentiation, such as IFN-γ and GM-CSF, which makes it less clear whether their net effect on osteoclast formation *in vivo* is positive or negative. Regulatory T cells (Treg), in fact, suppress osteoclast formation through contact-dependent inhibition of osteoclastogenesis, which is mediated by CTLA-4 binding to the osteoclast precursor.[14]

Increased osteoclast formation in inflamed joints appears to be fueled by an imbalance between factors that support osteoclast formation and those inhibiting it. RANKL, for instance, is upregulated in arthritis.[15] High RANKL expression

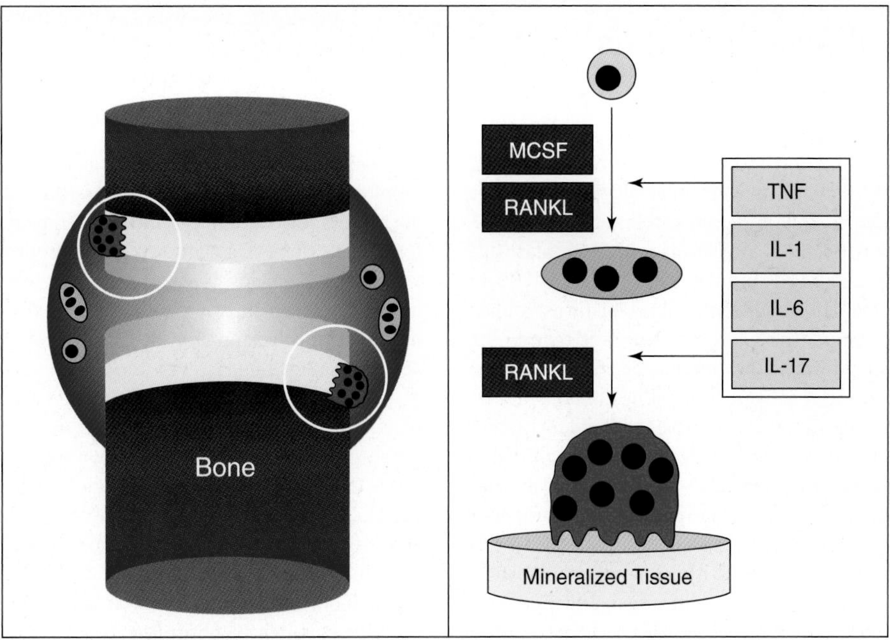

Figure 8H-2. Cytokines driving osteoclast differentiation in the inflamed joint. Macrophage-colony stimulating factor (MCSF) and receptor activator of NF-κB ligand (RANKL) are essential cytokines for osteoclastogenesis, which allow differentiation of monocytes entering the joint space to multinucleated osteoclasts. Proinflammatory cytokines like tumor necrosis factor (TNF and interleukin [IL]-1, -6, and -17 support osteoclast formation through influencing RANKL expression.

outweighs the function of osteoprotegerin (OPG), which is a natural inhibitor of RANKL, and prevents receptor binding of RANKL.[16] Supplementation of OPG, for instance, completely blocks RANKL-induced osteoclast formation and bone erosion in murine models of chronic destructive arthritis.[17–19] This highlights the role of RANKL in synovial osteoclast formation and also the role of osteoclast in bone erosion in general. The key role of osteoclasts in structural remodeling of joints during arthritis is supported by studies on experimental arthritis in mice that lack osteoclasts.[20,21] These mice do not develop erosive disease despite the formation of chronic inflammatory infiltrates in the synovium in close proximity to bone. Proinflammatory cytokines also support a change in the micromilieu of the synovium, shifting it to a more pro-osteoclastogenic pattern. Tumor necrosis factor (TNF) as well as interleukins (IL)-1, -6, and -17 induce RANKL expression, and therefore support osteoclast formation. In addition to regulating RANKL, TNF engages the TNFR1 on osteoclast precursors, which adds to the pro-osteoclastogenic potential of this cytokine.[22] IL-1 is additionally involved in the regulation of RANK, and thus susceptibility of osteoclast to RANKL.[23,24] IL-6 enhances the differentiation of plasma cells, which are producers of RANKL and stimulate bone loss.[25] IL-17 has been already described in the context of TH17 cells, but it also increases the expression of TNF and IL-1, which indirectly support osteoclast formation.[27] All of these inflammatory mediators speed up the differentiation process of osteoclast in the inflamed synovium. In fact, it takes only a few days for osteoclasts to form in experimental arthritis, and it can be assumed that similar circumstances are found in RA as well.[27]

Imbalance of Bone Metabolism in Inflamed Joints

Under physiological conditions, only a few osteoclasts and osteoblasts populate periarticular bone to ensure basal bone remodeling. In arthritis, however, the number and activity of osteoclasts increase and seem to outweigh bone formation. Generation of bone erosion always requires a negative net balance of bone metabolism, where bone resorption dominates over bone formation. The inability of osteoblasts to counteract increased bone formation is stunning, and does not follow the standard coupling process, which links bone resorption and bone formation. Indeed, histopathologic investigations of RA joints have shown that osteoblasts are virtually absent in inflammatory bone erosions, suggesting the absence of effective repair process in RA.[6,28] Whereas a periosteal bone response is missing, which is reflected by the absence of osteophytes in RA, osteoblasts can be observed in endosteal regions close to inflamed joints. These osteoblasts are closely linked to inflammatory bone marrow infiltrates, which consist of B and T lymphocytes, and emerge at sites where cortical bone has been destroyed by the invading synovial membrane.[28] These endosteal osteoblasts are metabolically active and appear as cuboid-shaped cells producing matrix molecules such as osteocalcin and osteopontin. Osteoblast activity at the endosteum is also reflected by osteoid seams underneath these cells, which indicate a skeletal response to inflammation in RA. This response, however, emerges from endosteal sites within the bone marrow, and is a reaction to the exposure of bone marrow sites to synovial inflammatory tissue after breaking the cortical bone barriers.[29]

Suppression of Bone Formation in Joints

These observations suggest that synovial inflammation may actively suppress bone formation and prevent a bone response at sites of inflammatory damage, in particular at periosteal sites where bone erosion starts. Inflammatory cytokines such as TNF can suppress bone formation by interfering with osteoblast differentiation. For instance, TNF induces Dickkopf (DKK)-1 in synovial fibroblasts, which is a potent suppressor of osteoblast formation.[30] DKK-1 competitively binds to a plasma membrane receptor LRP5/6, and prevents the binding of wingless (Wnt) proteins, which then cannot activate a signaling cascade involving beta-catenin, which is necessary to drive the bone formation process (see Figure 8H-3). Similar interactions between inflammation and bone formation might also hold true for another protein family involved in bone formation, the bone morphogenic protein (BMP), transforming growth factor beta (TGFβ) family. These proteins play a role in the formation of osteophytes, bony spurs that form along joint edges and insertion sites of tendons, where they trigger osteoblast differentiation and the formation of new bone.[31,32] Noggin, an inhibitor of BMP/TGF proteins, blocks osteophyte formation and may thus also act as an inhibitor of repair responses in RA, where osteophytes are consistently absent.[33] Thus, proteins such as DKK-1 and noggin prevent bone formation in RA by blocking molecules that are essentially involved in osteoblast formation, such as Wnt and BMP/TGF. On the other hand, these pathways are active in diseases with a prominent periosteal bone response such as ankylosing spondylitis, where they support the formation of osteophytes.

Therapeutic Implications

Osteoclasts as well as osteoblasts contribute to the remodeling of joints during inflammation. Therefore, both cells are interesting targets for current and future therapeutic agents. As a matter of fact, there is a tight link between proinflammatory cytokines and osteoclast formation, which explains that cytokine inhibitors show an effect on joint structure, particularly in inhibiting bone erosion as well. The pivotal role of TNF-blocking agents in retarding or even blocking joint damage can be explained by the function of TNF in osteoclast formation. Similar results might also be expected for IL-6 blockade, since IL-6 is a potent inducer of RANKL, and thus supports osteoclast formation. Thus far, there is only limited evidence that direct and specific blockade of osteoclasts inhibits bone erosion in human arthritis. In all experimental animal models of arthritis, however, interference with osteoclast differentiation and activation through blocking RANKL as well as interference with osteoclast function through bisphosphonates was effective to block bone erosion.[17–21,34] Whether potent bisphosphonates can retard structural damage in inflamed joints of humans is less clear, although a recent study suggests a beneficial role of zolendronic acid, a new amino-bisphosphonate.[35,36] In addition, RANKL blockade might have structural preserving effects in human RA, but further studies are needed to more clearly define the role of RANKL blockade in human RA. Since in all animal models of arthritis, the selective blockade of osteoclasts effectively

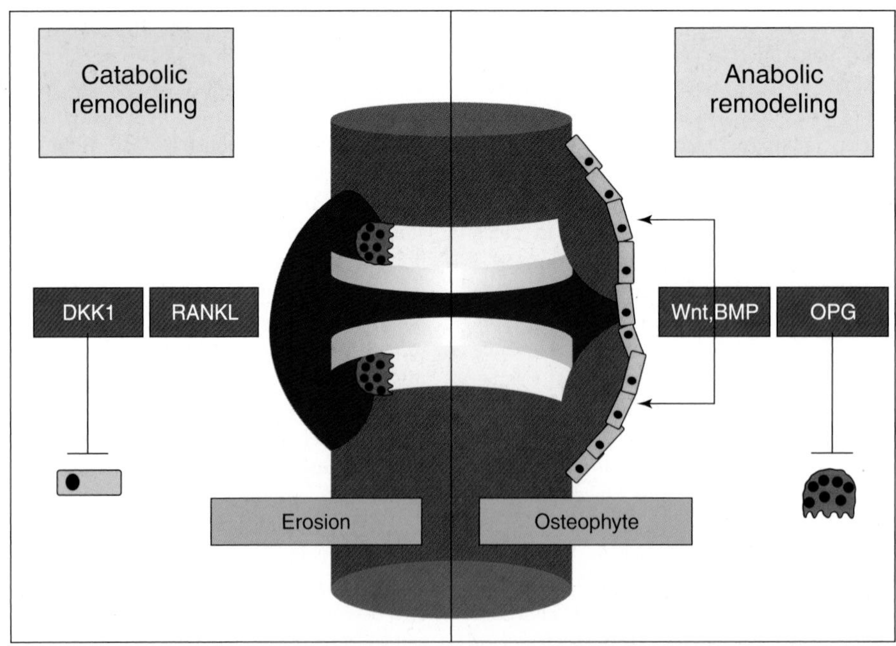

Figure 8H-3. Joint remodeling pathways in inflammatory disease. Catabolic joint remodeling is a direct effect of inflammation with induction of RANKL leading to osteoclastogenesis and bone resorption and Dickkopf (DKK)-1 inhibiting osteoblast differentiation and preventing bone repair. Anabolic joint remodeling is driven by a periosteal bone response leading to formation of bony spurs (osteophytes) by increased osteoblast activity and new bone formation. This is driven by wingless (Wnt) proteins and bone morphogenic proteins (BMPs). At the same time, they induce osteoprotegerin (OPG), which blocks bone resorption.

retarded joint damage but not inflammation, an effect on signs and symptoms of RA cannot be expected by such interventions. Therefore, a combination of such agents with anti-inflammatory drugs is most likely warranted. Stimulation of osteoblasts might be another interesting strategy for overcoming bone damage in RA. Strategies that stimulate bone formation such as parathyroid hormone have not yet been applied in RA, although they are able to induce repair of bone erosion in animal models of arthritis.[37] However, the use of parathyroid hormone is limited due to cost and mode of application, suggesting that more innovative bone anabolic approaches might fill this therapeutic gap in the future.

References

1. Schett G, Kiechl S, Weger S, et al. High-sensitivity C-reactive protein and risk of nontraumatic fractures in the Bruneck study. *Arch Intern Med* 2006;166:2495–2501.
2. McInnes I, Schett G. Cytokines in the pathogenesis of rheumatoid arthritis. *Nat Immunol* 2007;7:429–442.
3. Billroth T, Von Winiwarter A. *Die allgemeine chirurgische Pathologie und Therapie in fünfzig Vorlesungen: Ein Handbuch f. Studierende u. Ärzte*. 10th ed. Berlin: Reimer, 1882.
4. Weichselbaum A. Die feineren Veränderungen des Gelenkknorpels bei fungöser Synovitis und Karies der Gelenkenden. *Archiv Pathol Anat Physiol Klin Med* 1878;73:461–475.
5. Bromley M, Woolley DE. Chondroclasts and osteoclasts at subchondral sites of erosion in the rheumatoid joint. *Arthritis Rheum* 1984;27:968–975.
6. Gravallese EM, Harada Y, Wang JT, et al. Identification of cell types responsible for bone resorption in rheumatoid arthritis and juvenile rheumatoid arthritis. *Am J Pathol* 1998;152:943–951.
7. Li P, Schwarz EM, O'Keefe Ma L, et al. RANK signaling is not required for TNF-mediated increase in CD11(hi) osteoclast precursors but is essential for mature osteoclast formation in TNFα-mediated inflammatory arthritis. *J Bone Miner Res* 2004;19:207–213.
8. Ritchlin CT, Haas-Smith SA, Li P, et al. Mechanisms of TNF-alpha– and RANKL-mediated osteoclastogenesis and bone resorption in psoriatic arthritis. *J Clin Invest* 2003;111:821–831.
9. Teitelbaum SL. Bone resorption by osteoclasts. *Science* 2000;289: 1504–1508.
10. Seitz M, Loetscher P, Fey MF, et al. Constitutive mRNA and protein production of macrophage colony-stimulating factor but not of other cytokines by synovial fibroblasts from rheumatoid arthritis and osteoarthritis patients. *Br J Rheumatol* 1994;33: 613–619.
11. Gravallese EM, Manning C, Tsay A, et al. Synovial tissue in rheumatoid arthritis is a source of osteoclast differentiation factor. *Arthritis Rheum* 2000;43:250–258.
12. Shigeyama Y, Pap T, Kunzler P, et al. Expression of osteoclast differentiation factor in rheumatoid arthritis. *Arthritis Rheum* 2000; 43:2523–2530.
13. Sato K, Suematsu A, Okamoto K, et al. Th17 functions as an osteoclastogenic T helper cell subset that links T cell activation and bone destruction. *J Exp Med* 2006, 203:2673–2682.
14. Zaiss M, Axmann R, Zwerina J, et al. Regulatory T cells suppress osteoclast formation: A new link between the immune system and bone. *Arthritis Rheum* 2007;56:4104–4112.
15. Stolina M, Adamu S, Ominsky M, et al. RANKL is a marker and mediator of local and systemic bone loss in two rat models of inflammatory arthritis. *J Bone Miner Res* 2005;20:1756–1765.
16. Catrina AI, af Klint E, Ernestam S, et al. Anti-tumor necrosis factor therapy increases synovial osteoprotegerin expression in rheumatoid arthritis. *Arthritis Rheum* 2006;54:76–81.
17. Redlich K, Hayer S, Maier A, et al. Tumor necrosis factor a–mediated joint destruction is inhibited by targeting osteoclasts with osteoprotegerin. *Arthritis Rheum* 2002;46:785–792.
18. Kong YY, Feige U, Sarosi I, et al. Activated T cells regulate bone loss and joint destruction in adjuvant arthritis through osteoprotegerin ligand. *Nature* 1999;402:304–309.
19. Romas E, Gillespie MT, Martin TJ. Involvement of receptor activator of NFκB ligand and tumor necrosis factor-β in bone destruction in rheumatoid arthritis. *Bone* 2002;30:340–346.
20. Redlich K, Hayer S, Ricci R, et al. Osteoclasts are essential for TNF-α–mediated joint destruction. *J Clin Invest* 2002;110:1419–1427.
21. Pettit AR, Ji H, von Stechow D, et al. TRANCE/RANKL knockout mice are protected from bone erosion in a serum transfer model of arthritis. *Am J Pathol* 2001;159:1689–1699.
22. Lam J, Takeshita S, Barker JE, et al. TNF-alpha induces osteoclastogenesis by direct stimulation of macrophages exposed to permissive levels of RANK ligand. *J Clin Invest* 2000;106:1481–1488.
23. Zwerina J, Redlich K, Polzer K, et al. TNF-induced structural joint damage is mediated by interleukin-1. *Proc Natl Acad Sci U S A* 2007;104:11742–11747.
24. Wei S, Kitaura H, Zhou P, et al. IL-1 mediates TNF-induced osteoclastogenesis. *J Clin Invest* 2005;115:282–290.
25. Dai J, Lin D, Zhang J, et al. Chronic alcohol ingestion induces osteoclastogenesis and bone loss through IL-6 in mice. *J Clin Invest* 2000;106:887–895.
26. Lubberts E, van den Bersselaar L, Oppers-Walgreen B, et al. IL-17 promotes bone erosion in murine collagen-induced arthritis through loss of the receptor activator of NF-kappa B ligand/osteoprotegerin balance. *J Immunol* 2003;170:2655–2662.
27. Schett G, Stolina M, Bolon B, et al. Analysis of the kinetics of osteoclastogenesis in arthritic rats. *Arthritis Rheum* 2005;52:3192–3201.
28. Jimenez-Boj E, Redlich K, Turk B, et al. Interaction between synovial inflammatory tissue and bone marrow in rheumatoid arthritis. *J Immunol* 2005;175:2579–2588.
29. Hayer S, Polzer K, Brandl A, et al. B cell infiltrates induce endosteal bone formation in inflammatory arthritis. *J Bone Miner Res* 2008; in press.
30. Diarra D, Stolina M, Polzer K, et al. Dickkopf-1 is a master regulator of joint remodeling. *Nat Med* 2007;13:156–163.
31. Lories RJ, Derese I, de Bari C, et al. Evidence for uncoupling of inflammation and joint remodeling in a mouse model of spondylarthritis. *Arthritis Rheum* 2007;56:489–497.
32. Benjamin M, McGonagle D. The anatomical basis for disease localization in seronegative spondylarthropathy at entheses and related sites. *J Anat* 2001;199:503–526.
33. Lories RJ, Derese I, Luyten FP. Modulation of bone morphogenetic protein signaling inhibits the onset and progression of ankylosing enthesitis. *J Clin Invest* 2005;115:1571–1579.
34. Herrak P, Gortz B, Hayer S, et al. Zoledronic acid protects against local and systemic bone loss in tumor necrosis factor–mediated arthritis. *Arthritis Rheum* 2004;50:2327–2337.
35. Goldring SR, Gravallese EM. Bisphosphonates: Environmental protection for the joint? *Arthritis Rheum* 2004;50:2044–2047.
36. Conaghan PG, Sloan VS, Papanstasiou P, et al. Preliminary evidence for a structural benefit of the new bisphosphonate zoledronic acid in early rheumatoid arthritis. *Arthritis Rheum* 2004;50:265–276.
37. Redlich K, Gortz B, Hayer S, et al. Repair of local bone erosions and reversal of systemic bone loss upon therapy with anti-tumor necrosis factor in combination with osteoprotegerin or parathyroid hormone in tumor necrosis factor-mediated arthritis. *Am J Pathol* 2004;164:543–555.

Endothelial Cells and Angiogenesis

CHAPTER 81

Zoltán Szekanecz and Alisa E. Koch

In rheumatoid arthritis (RA), inflammatory cells migrate into the synovium through the vascular endothelium. Endothelial cells (ECs) are active players in this process as they undergo morphological changes and secrete numerous inflammatory mediators, including various cytokines, chemokines, and growth factors. The formation of blood vessels, termed *angiogenesis*, is a key event underlying RA. As the perpetuation of synovial neovascularization in RA leads to increased number of blood vessels and total endothelial surface, anigogenesis may enhance the recruitment of leukocytes into the inflamed synovium.[1–18]

ECs line the lumina of blood vessels; thus they both separate and connect the bloodstream and the extravascular synovial matrix. ECs respond to inflammatory stimuli and, on the other hand, produce various mediators.[9,10,13]

Angiogenesis is involved in both physiological states, such as reproduction and tissue development and repair, as well as in malignant and inflammatory diseases. By accepting this concept, for example, RA, psoriasis, proliferative diabetic retinopathy, and numerous other inflammatory conditions may be termed as "angiogenic diseases." The angiogenic process, its *in vitro* and *in vivo* models, the most important angiogenic mediators and angiogenesis inhibitors, and the prognostic and therapeutic relevance of RA-associated neovascularization have been recently reviewed.[1,2,5,6,8,11] Several growth factors, cytokines, chemokines, cellular adhesion molecules (CAMs), extracellular matrix (ECM) components, and other factors involved in neovascularization have been detected in abundance in the RA synovium.[1–3,6–8,15–18]

While *angiogenesis* encompasses new vessel formation from pre-existing vessels, the term *vasculogenesis* refers to capillary formation from endothelial precursor cells (EPCs). EPCs are a subpopulation of circulating CD34^{+} cells expressing the vascular endothelial growth factor 2 (VEGF-2) receptor. These functional EPCs are involved in vasculogenesis.[19–21]

In this chapter, we review the role of blood vessels, ECs, angiogenesis, and, very briefly, vasculogenesis in the pathogenesis of RA. Leukocyte–endothelial adhesion and adhesion receptors will be reviewed. The most important angiogenic pathways will be described in more detail. Regarding vasculogenesis, the role of EPCs in RA will be discussed. The regulation of leukocyte recruitment through synovial endothelia and that of neovascularization will be reviewed. Finally, the clinical relevance of these important issues will also be presented.

Endothelial Functions in Rheumatoid Synovitis

Endothelial Injury

Vascular injury has been associated with inflammatory diseases, including RA.[9,10,13] Vasodilation, as well as EC contraction and retraction result in increased vascular permeability and leakage.[9,10,13] Numerous inflammatory mediators, such as histamine, serotonin, C3a, C5a, bradykinin, prostacyclin (PGI_2), nitric oxide (NO), platelet-activating factor (PAF), and antiendothelial antibodies (AECA) have been implicated in these processes.[13,22–24] Among cytokines, tumor necrosis factor-α (TNF-α), interleukin-1 (IL-1), and interferon-γ (IFN-γ) induce cytoskeletal reorganization and thus retraction in ECs.[25]

As described above, leukocytes interact with the vascular endothelium during their diapedesis into the inflamed synovium. Migrating leukocytes themselves cause EC injury by producing reactive oxygen intermediates and some matrix metalloproteinases (MMPs).[26] Resting leukocytes extravasate without causing vascular leakage; however, activated white blood cells trigger endothelial injury.[9,10,27]

Early Endothelial Dysfunction in RA

Cardiovascular disease is a leading cause of mortality in RA. Early endothelial dysfunction often precedes overt atherosclerosis. Endothelial function may be assessed by the determination of flow-mediated vasodilation (FMD) using ultrasound imaging of brachial arteries. FMD is an indicator of EC-dependent vasodilation. We and others found significantly lower FMD in RA patients in comparison to controls matched for sex, age, and traditional cardiovascular risk factors.[28,29] RA patients with normal versus impaired FMD significantly differed in age and disease duration. Thus, an early endothelial dysfunction was demonstrated in RA patients.[28] Endothelial dysfunction in RA assessed by endothelium-dependent vasodilatation has been associated with a reduced number and impaired function of circulating EPCs.[30]

Role of Endothelium in Leukocyte Ingress into Synovium

Adhesion of peripheral blood leukocytes to ECs is a key event during leukocyte transendothelial emigration into inflammatory sites.[3,31–33] Specialized, fenestrated high endothelial venule (HEV)–like microvessels, similar to HEV involved in physiological "lymphocyte homing," are present in the synovial tissue.[3] Leukocytes adhere to these ECs and transmigrate through the vessel wall into the synovium.[3,33]

CAMs are involved in EC adhesion to leukocytes, as well as in angiogenesis. CAMs have been classified into several distinct supergene families. However, CAMs, which are the most relevant for synovial inflammation, belong to three families: the integrins, selectins, and the immunoglobulin supergene family.[3,17,31–33] Integrins mediate EC adhesion to ECM macromolecules, while members of the immunoglobulin superfamily and selectins play a role in EC adhesion to other cells.[31–33]

As described later, in the multistep paradigm of leukocyte–EC adhesion, selectins mediate leukocyte tethering and rolling, while integrins and their ligands are involved in firm adhesion and transendothelial migration.[34,35]

Among *selectins*, E- and P-selectin are present on ECs, while L-selectin is expressed by leukocytes.[31–33] Proinflammatory cytokines abundantly produced in RA induce E-selectin expression on ECs.[36] Cytokine-activated ECs shed E-selectin, and soluble E-selectin is a measurable marker for EC activation.[3,37] Abundant expression of E-selectin in RA synovial tissues and increased production of soluble E-selectin in RA synovial fluids have been described.[37,38] P-selectin is constitutively expressed in EC membrane Weibel-Palade bodies.[3,39] Proinflammatory cytokines also upregulate P-selectin expression[40] and there is significant P-selectin shedding in RA.[41] P-selectin is expressed on RA synovial endothelium,[3,42] and this CAM is involved in the very early phases of adhesion.[40] L-selectin serves as a lymphocyte homing receptor, when these cells recirculate through HEVs expressing the MadCAM-1 and GlyCAM-1 L-selectin ligand addressins.[31–33] L-selectin may also be involved in leukocyte–EC interactions underlying arthritis.[3,17,33]

Integrins are $\alpha\beta$ heterodimers, and each of the common β chains is associated with one or more α subunits.[31–33] Among these CAMs, β_1 and β_3 integrins are expressed on ECs. The $\alpha_1\beta_1$-$\alpha_9\beta_1$ and $\alpha_V\beta_3$ integrins mediate cell adhesion to ECM components, including various types of collagen, fibronectin, laminin, vitronectin, and tenascin. However, the $\alpha_4\beta_1$ integrin also binds to vascular cell adhesion molecule 1 (VCAM-1), a member of the immunoglobulin supergene family.[31–33,43] A number of β_1 integrins, as well as $\alpha_V\beta_3$, are involved in EC migration, angiogenesis, and are required for the maturation of new blood vessels.[43,44] Integrins have been implicated in leukocyte transendothelial migration underlying inflammatory diseases, such as RA.[3,17,42]

Among members of the *immunoglobulin supergene family*, VCAM-1, a ligand for $\alpha_4\beta_1$ and $\alpha_4\beta_7$ integrins, is expressed on both resting and cytokine-activated ECs.[3,31–33,45] ICAM-1 is a ligand for β_2 integrins, and its expression of ICAM-1 on ECs can be induced by proinflammatory cytokines.[31–33,46] VCAM-1 and ICAM-1 are expressed on ECs in inflammatory sites including RA synovial tissues.[3,38] LFA-3 and its counterreceptor CD2 are expressed on ECs and T cells, respectively.[3,17] Platelet-endothelial cell adhesion molecule 1 (PECAM-1; CD31) homotypically binds to another PECAM-1 molecule, and heterotypically to the $\alpha_V\beta_3$ integrin.[3,31–33] LFA-3, CD2, and PECAM-1 have been implicated in RA-associated, leukocyte–EC adhesion.[3,17,42]

Other CAMs mediating leukocyte–EC adhesion during synovitis include L-selectin–ligand vascular addressins, junctional CAMs (JAMs), CD44, vascular adhesion protein-1 (VAP-1), endoglin, VE-cadherin, certain glycoconjugates, CD99, and possibly ICAM-3.[3,17,31–33,35,43,47–58] Addressins recognized by L-selectin, such as CD34, MadCAM-1, and GlyCAM-1 are expressed by HEV-like vessels in the RA synovium, and they are involved in the transendothelial migration of inflammatory leukocytes ("inflammatory homing").[31–33,43] JAM-1, JAM-2, and JAM-3 are ligands for β_2 and $\alpha_4\beta_1$ integrins. All of these JAMs may be involved in leukocyte migration during synovial inflammation.[47,48] CD44 is a receptor for hyaluronate.[31–33] CD44 is present on activated ECs in inflammatory synovitis.[3,17,42,52,53] VAP-1 was originally isolated from synovial ECs. There is abundant expression of VAP-1 in the inflamed synovium.[3,49] Endoglin, a receptor for transforming growth factor-β_1 (TGF-β_1) and TGF-β_3, is expressed by most ECs in the RA synovium.[51] VE-cadherin, a major constituent of EC junctions, mediates homophilic binding between ECs and is involved in EC migration and polarization.[54] Among glycoconjugates, MUC18 (CD146), Lewis^y/H, and CD99 are involved in leukocyte migration to the joint.[55–57] ICAM-3 is generally absent from resting ECs; however, it has been detected on some RA synovial ECs.[3,50,58]

Leukocyte ingress into the synovium through vascular endothelia occurs through HEV-like vessels.[3,31,32,59] This process is a sequence of events. An early, weak adhesion of leukocytes to ECs, termed *tethering* and *rolling*, occurs first mediated primarily by selectins and their ligands. This is followed by leukocyte activation, which involves interactions between leukocyte chemokine receptors and endothelial proteoglycans, as well as PECAM-1. Cell activation leads to firm adhesion, which involves the $\alpha_4\beta_1$ integrin/VCAM-1, LFA-1/ICAM-1, and JAM/integrin adhesion pathways. Leukocyte–EC adhesion is associated with abundant production of chemokines. When these secreted chemokines bind to the EC matrix, diapedesis of leukocytes through the EC layer occurs.[33–35]

Synovial Angiogenesis

In Vitro and *In Vivo* Models of Angiogenic Process

Angiogenesis, the formation of new blood vessels, is pathologically enhanced in RA.[1,2,5,8,10] New vessels are generated following a program of distinct steps. First, ECs are activated by different angiogenic stimuli including soluble mediators or cell surface–bound molecules. In response, ECs secrete proteases, which degrade the underlying basement membrane and ECM. This enables the emigration of loose ECs, resulting in the formation of primary capillary sprouts. ECs then further proliferate, migrate, and synthesize new basement membrane. This process is followed by lumen formation within the sprouts. Two sprouts may link to form capillary loops. Further escape of ECs out of these sprouts results in the development of further generation sprouts.[1,2,8,10,60]

A number of *in vitro* and *in vivo* models are available to study angiogenesis.[1,61] *In vitro* systems include EC cultures grown on ECM substrata, such as the laminin-containing Matrigel, tissue culture systems, or EC chemotaxis assays.[1,2,6,8,10,61] *In vivo* capillary formation has been investigated using the rat, murine, rabbit, or guinea pig corneal micropocket, the chick embryo chorioallantoic membrane, the hamster cheek pouch, the mesenteric, the aortic ring, the implanted matrix assays, or sponge models.[1,2,6,8,10,61] All of these models are suitable to investigate the role of neovascularization in the pathogenesis of RA. Antiangiogenic therapeutic strategies may also be tested in these systems[1,2,61] (Figure 8I-1, Figure 8I-2).

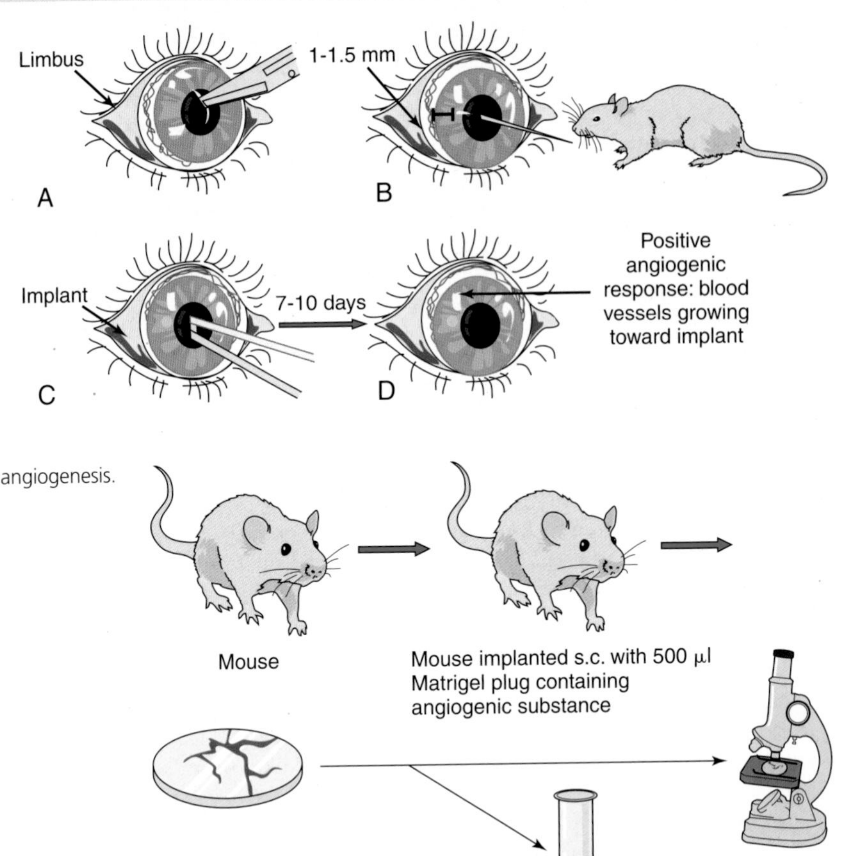

Figure 8I-1. Rodent cornea bioassay, an *in vivo* model for angiogenesis.

Figure 8I-2. The *in vitro* Matrigel assay for angiogenesis.

There are hundreds of soluble or cellular factors that may promote neovascularization (Table 8I-1). First, the most well-known cellular and molecular pathways will be discussed. These include the hypoxia-vascular endothelial growth factor (VEGF)-angiopoietin (Ang)-survivin system and angiogenic chemokines.

Hypoxia-VEGF-Angiopoietin-Survivin System in Angiogenesis

Some growth factors are bound to heparin in the synovial ECM and are released by heparanase and plasmin during angiogenesis. VEGF is a heparin-binding growth factor, which is possibly the most widely characterized angiogenic mediator. VEGF is essential for early vascular morphogenesis, EC proliferation, and migration.[7] VEGF is abundantly produced in the RA synovium.[62] Hypoxia, as well as proinflammatory cytokines including TNF-α, IL-1, and TGF-β, enhance the synovial release of VEGF.[6,7,63] Some other inflammatory mediators, such as hepatocyte growth factor (HGF), epidermal growth factor (EGF), hypoxia-inducible factor 1α (HIF-1α), nitric oxide (NO), or prostaglandins, may indirectly stimulate angiogenesis by stimulating VEGF production.[6,7,64]

Hypoxia is a crucial trigger of synovial neovascularization. Hypoxia stimulates the formation and stabilization of the heterodimer HIF-1α/HIF-1β. HIF heterodimers then further stimulate VEGF production.[65,66] Hypoxia has been detected within the RA joint.[67] There is abundant HIF-1α and HIF-2α expression in the RA synovium.[68]

There is a downstream interaction between VEGF and the Ang1-Tie2 system.[7,69] Ang1 and Ang2 regulate EC growth and functions upon stimulation by VEGF. Both Ang1 and Ang2 interact with Tie2, an endothelial tyrosine kinase receptor.[7,70] The interaction of Ang1 and Tie2 results in the stabilization of newly formed blood vessels.[71] On the other hand, the interaction of Ang2 with Tie2 antagonizes the effects of Ang1, and thus stimulates vascular invasion and suppresses vessel maturation.[7,69] Interactions among VEGF, angiopoietins, and TNF-α may transduce signals, resulting in EC plasticity and survival. Survivin is an inhibitor of apoptosis, which is also involved in EC survival and VEGF-mediated angiogenesis.[7,72] Survivin, as well as VEGF, Ang1, and Tie2 have been detected in the RA synovium.[7,62,73,74]

Angiogenic Chemokines and Chemokine Receptors

Chemokines are chemotactic inflammatory mediators that have been classified as CXC, CC, C, and CX$_3$C chemokines according to the position of cysteine residues in their structure.[2,4,18] These chemokines bind to their respective receptors abbreviated as CXCR, CCR, CR, and CX$_3$CR.

Among CXC chemokines, those containing the ELR amino-acid motif promote synovial neovascularization. These ELR$^+$ CXC chemokines include interleukin-8 (IL-8)/CXCL8, epithelial-neutrophil activating protein 78 (ENA-78)/CXCL5, growth-related oncogene α (groα)/CXCL1, and connective tissue activating protein III (CTAP-III)/CXCL7. In contrast, ELR$^-$ CXC chemokines, such as platelet factor 4 (PF4)/CXCL4, IFN-γ-inducible protein 10 (IP-10)/CXCL10, and monokine induced

Table 8I-1. Some Mediators and Inhibitors of Angiogenesis in Rheumatoid Arthritis[a]

	Mediators	Inhibitors
Growth factors	VEGF, HGF, EGF, HIF-1, PDGF, aFGF, bFGF, IGF-I, TGF-β	—
Proinflammatory cytokines	TNF-α, IL-1, IL-6, IL-15, IL-17, IL-18, G-CSF, GM-CSF, oncostatin M, MIF	IFN-α, IFN-γ, IL-4, IL-12, IL-13, LIF
Chemokines	ELR$^+$ CXC chemokines, SDF-1/CXCL12, MCP-1/CCL2, fractalkine/CXC3CL1	ELR$^-$ CXC chemokines
Extracellular matrix components	Collagen, laminin, fibronectin, vitronectin tenascin	Thrombospondin 1, thrombospondin 2
Cell-adhesion molecules	$\alpha_V\beta_3$ integrin, E-selectin, VCAM-1, endoglin, MUC18, Lewis^y/H, PECAM-1	—
Proteases	MMPs, plasminogen activators	TIMPs, PAIs
Environmental factors	Hypoxia	
Vessel stabilizers, apoptosis inhibitors	Ang1-Tie2, survivin	
Others	Prostaglandin E2, angiogenin, angiotropin, PAF, prolactin, substance P	DMARDs, antibiotics, angiostatin, endostatin, paclitaxel, troponin, osteonectin, chondromodulin, kallistatin

[a]See text for abbreviations.

by IFN-γ (Mig)/CXCL9, inhibit angiogenesis (for reviews, see Szekanecz and Koch,[2] Walz et al.,[75] and Strieter et al.[76]). As an exception to the rule, stromal cell–derived factor 1 (SDF-1)/CXCL12 lacks the ELR sequence, yet this chemokine stimulates neovascularization.[2,76]

IL-8/CXCL8, ENA-78/CXCL5, CTAP-III/CXCL7, and groα/CXCL1 all bind to their endothelial receptor, CXCR2, and are chemotactic and mitogenic for vascular ECs.[2,18,75–77] All of these chemokines are abundantly produced in the RA synovium.[2,4,6,18]

IP-10/CXCL10 VEGF–induced EC migration and angiogenesis; however, VEGF induces the expression of IP-10/CXCL10 on ECs.[78] Thus, IP-10/CXCL10 may be an autocrine inhibitory regulator of VEGF-mediated angiogenesis.[78] Mig/CXCL9 and PF4/CXCL4 are also angiostatic.[2,76,79] All of these ELR$^-$ chemokines have been detected in RA synovial tissues.[2,4,18] A nonallelic variant of PF4/CXCL4 termed *PF4var/CXCL4L1* is also a potent inhibitor of angiogenesis.[80]

SDF-1/CXCL12 lacks the ELR sequence, yet the SDF-1/CXCL12-CXCR4 pathway may be a key regulator of angiogenesis and, as described later, vasculogenesis.[81–83] SDF-1/XCXL12 binds to heparin and heparan sulfate proteoglycans on the endothelial surface, induces EC chemotaxis and angiogenesis.[81,82,84] This chemokine also acts in concert with the hypoxia-VEGF system discussed above. Hypoxia induces the release of SDF-1/CXCL12 by RA synovial fibroblasts.[81] Furthermore, the interaction of SDF-1/CXCL12 with its receptor CXCR4 induces Akt phosphorylation, resulting in the stimulation of VEGF production via the phosphatidyl inositol 3 kinase (PI3K)/Akt pathway.[85,86] SDF-1/CXCL4–mediated angiogenesis also involves the activation of heme oxygenase 1.[87] This chemokine also synergizes with granulocyte colony–stimulating factor (G-CSF) during neovascularization.[88] *In vivo*, SDF-1/CXCL12 expression has been associated with the growth of gliomas; thus, it may serve as an indicator of neovascularization and as a prognostic marker.[89]

Very little information is available with respect to CC chemokines. MCP-1/CCL2 stimulates angiogenesis via its endothelial receptor, CCR2.[2,18,77,90] MCP-1/CCL2–induced angiogenesis involves integrins, ERK-1/2 activation, and the upregulation of the Ets-1 transcription factor.[90] MCP-1/CCL2 acts in concert with TGF-β and fibroblast growth factor 2 (FGF-2) during angiogenesis and vasculogenesis.[91,92] Myeloid progenitor inhibitory factor 1 (MPIF-1)/CCL23 has been implicated in EC migration and matrix metalloproteinase (MMP) secretion.[93]

Fractalkine/CX_3CL1 has also been implicated in RA-associated angiogenesis.[94,95] This chemokine produced by ECs stimulated with TNF-α, IL-1, and IFN-γ,[96] and is abundantly produced in RA.[94,95]

Among chemokine receptors, as discussed above, CXCR2 recognizes the most important proinflammatory and proangiogenic, ELR$^+$ CXC chemokines.[2,18] CXCR2 exerts abundant expression on ECs during inflammation.[2,18,97] CXCR4 has been implicated in SDF-1/CXCL12–induced synovial angiogenesis.[98,99] Hypoxia induces CXCR4 expression via HIF-1 and VEGF production.[100] Recently, an alternative receptor for SDF-1/CXCL12, different from CXCR4, has been identified and implicated in chemokine-induced angiogenesis.[101] CCR2, a receptor for MCP-1/CCL2 and some other CC chemokines, has been implicated in synovial angiogenesis.[77] In a recent study, CCR2-deficient animals exerted delayed muscular angiogenesis and decreased VEGF production.[102] Thus, CCR2 may be important in VEGF-mediated neovascularization. DARC, originally described on erythrocytes, binds the Duffy–blood group antigen and some chemokines.[103] DARC, which is expressed by synovial ECs, has been implicated in tumor-associated neovascularization.[103,104]

Other Angiogenic Pathways

Growth factors other than VEGF and HIFs implicated in neovascularization include FGF-1, FGF-2, HGF, platelet-derived growth factor (PDGF), EGF, insulin-like growth factor-I (IGF-I), and TGF-β.[2,6,8,11] Among proinflammatory cytokines, TNF-α, IL-1, IL-6, IL-15, IL-18, and possibly IL-17 are also involved in angiogenesis[2,6,11,15,16,105–108] (Figure 8I-3). TNF-α may also regulate capillary formation via the Ang1-Tie2 system described above.[109] IL-18 acts via the upregulation of SDF-1/CXCL12, MCP-1/CCL2,

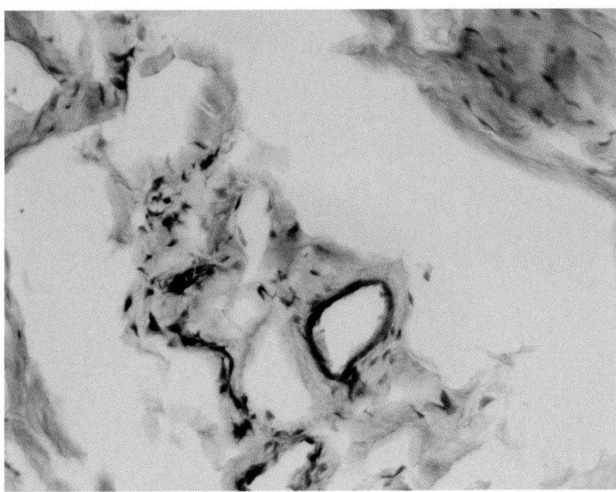

Figure 8I-3. IL-18 expression in the rheumatoid synovium (hematoxylin-eosin, magnification: 400×).

and VEGF production by synovial fibroblasts[108] (Figure 8I-3). Other angiogenic cytokines include G-CSF, granulocyte–macrophage colony-stimulating factor (GM-CSF), oncostatin M and macrophage migration inhibitory factor (MIF).[6,11,110–112] Oncostatin M induced ICAM-1 expression on RA synovial fibroblasts and ECs. This cytokine also induced EC migration and tubule formation.[110] MIF upregulates the production of angiogenic factors including VEGF and IL-8/CXCL8, and thus indirectly promotes neovascularization.[111,113] MIF-induced angiogenesis involves MAP kinase and PI3K activation.[111]

ECM macromolecules, CAMs, and proteases are also involved in EC adhesion, emigration, and angiogenesis. Type I collagen, fibronectin, laminin, vitronectin, tenascin, and proteoglycans, as well as cell β_1 integrins, $\alpha_V\beta_3$, E-selectin, selectin-related glycoconjugates including Lewis^y/H and melanoma cell adhesion molecule (MUC18), VCAM-1, PECAM-1, and endoglin are involved in EC adhesion and migration during angiogenesis.[1,6,11,114] Among CAMs, the $\alpha_V\beta_3$ integrin is of outstanding importance. This mediates synovial angiogenesis and osteoclast-mediated bone resorption in RA.[42] The α_V subunit of this integrin is encoded by the ITGAV gene. A significant association has been found between the ITGAV rs3738919-C allele and RA in the European Caucasian population.[115] Mast cells may be highly involved in integrin-dependent angiogenesis and joint destruction, as mast cell silencing with salbutamol or cromolyn prevented $\alpha_V\beta_3$ integrin activation and angiogenesis in mice. Mast cell reconstitution restored susceptibility to integrin activation, neovascularization, and joint destruction.[116] Synovial mast cells are involved in leukocyte recruitment into the synovium, fibrosis, angiogenesis, matrix remodeling, and bone destruction.[117] Some proteolytic enzymes, such as MMPs and plasminogen activators are involved in ECM degradation during the perpetuation of angiogenesis.[6,8,11,12,118]

Endothelin 1 (ET-1) is secreted by ECs. ET-1 exerts a number of effects on the vasculature including VEGF production, EC proliferation, and angiogenesis.[5,119] There is increased levels of ET-1 in the synovial fluids and sera of RA patients.[5,119]

Serum amyloid A (SAA) is a major acute-phase reactant, which has been implicated in the pathogenesis of arthritis. The effects of SAA are mediated by the formyl peptide receptor–like 1 (FPRL1). The binding of SAA to FPRL1 stimulated synovial hyperplasia, EC proliferation, migration, enhanced EC sprouting activity, and neovascularization.[120]

Other angiogenic factors not mentioned above include prostaglandin E_2, angiogenin, angiotropin, pleiotrophin, platelet-activating factor (PAF), histamine, substance P, erythropoietin, adenosine, prolactin, thrombin, and many others[6,8,11] (Table 8I-1).

Angiogenesis Inhibition

There are numerous mediators and compounds that counterbalance neovascularization (Table 8I-1). Many of them may be theoretically used as therapeutic strategies targeting tumor- or inflammation-associated angiogenesis (Table 8I-2). Some examples for antiangiogenesis therapy will be discussed later.

Among cytokines, interferon-α (IFN-α), IFN-γ, IL-4, IL-12, IL-13, and leukemia inhibitory factor (LIF) inhibit angiogenesis by inhibiting the production of VEGF and some other angiogenic mediators described above.[6,63,121,122] Tissue inhibitors of metalloproteinases (TIMPs) and plasminogen activator inhibitors (PAIs) antagonize the effects of angiogenic proteases.[2,6–8,12,118] Thrombospondin-1 and the PF4/CXCL4 chemokine block the action of heparin-binding growth factors.[2,6,11] Other ELR$^-$ chemokines, such as Mig/CXCL9 and IP-10/CXCL10, also inhibit angiogenesis.[2,11,76] Among CC chemokines, secondary lymphoid tissue chemokine (SLC)/CCL21 exerts angiostatic effects and inhibits tumor progression.[123] While some chemokine receptors described above are involved in chemokine-induced angiogenesis, CXCR3, which binds the angiostatic chemokines IP-10/CXCL10 and Mig/CXCL9, may rather be involved in chemokine-mediated angiogenesis inhibition.[2]

Several anti-inflammatory drugs, DMARDs, and biologics used in the treatment of RA, such as dexamethasone, gold salts, chloroquine, sulfasalazine, methotrexate (MTX), cyclosporine A, azathioprine, cyclophosphamide, leflunomide, thalidomide, minocycline, and some anti-TNF agents may also inhibit neovascularization.[2,6–8,11] There are some conflicting results regarding MTX, as it suppressed cancer-related angiogenesis; however, no such effect was observed in psoriatic arthritis.[7] Some antibiotics and their derivatives, such as minocycline, fumagillin, deoxyspergualin and clarithromycin suppress neovascularization via the inhibition of VEGF and other angiogenic mediators.[2,6,8]

Other known angiostatic compounds include angiostatin (a fragment of plasminogen), endostatin (a fragment of type XIII collagen), kallistatin, paclitaxel, osteonectin, opioids, troponin I, and chondromodulin-1[2,6,11,63,124] (Table 8I-1).

Endothelial Progenitor Cells and Vasculogenesis

The process of new vessel formation from EPCs is termed vasculogenesis.[19,20] Vasculogenesis is involved in both prenatal and postnatal tissue development. It is also involved in vascular repair and atherosclerosis.[21,125–127] EPCs have been described within the population of blood stem cells. These cells express both hematopoietic markers, such as CD34 and CD133, as well as EC markers including CD31 and type 2 VEGF receptor (Flk-1).[20,21] EPCs may develop into mature ECs.[20,21,128,129] EPCs have been detected in the RA synovium in apposition to RA synovial vessels.[21,130]

EPCs may be mobilized from the bone marrow to differentiate into ECs in RA.[131] Yet, there is a relative deficiency of EPCs in vascular diseases, as well as in RA and scleroderma.[19,126,127,132–135] In RA, there is an $\alpha_4\beta_1$ integrin/VCAM-1–mediated recruitment of EPCs from the blood into the synovium resulting in the depletion of these stem cells from the circulation.[21,126,136] A decreased number of EPCs in the circulation leads to impaired vasculogenesis in RA.[126] EPCs show reduced migration in RA in response to VEGF.[21,30] EPC depletion in RA may be associated with depressed NO-dependent EPC mobilization as serum levels of asymmetric dimethyl-L-arginine, an endogenous inhibitor of NO synthesis, are elevated in RA, and are associated with impaired EPC function.[137] In addition, the amount of EPCs in patients with active RA was significantly lower than that in patients with inactive disease.[126,127] Thus, the number of circulating EPCs in RA may correlate inversely with disease activity. Anti-TNF therapy in RA resulted in the restoration of circulating EPC levels and function.[127,138]

Among chemokines, SDF-1/CXCL12 plays a significant role in EPC recruitment to developing tissues or injured vessels.[21,83,86,125,139] Most EPCs also express CXCR4 and migrate in response to SDF-1/CXCL12.[20] This chemokine induces tissue vascularization by recruiting CXCR4$^+$ EPCs.[140] Thus, SDF-1/CXCL4 induces the revascularization of ischemic organs.[83] Hypoxia and HIF-1 act in part via SDF-1/CXCL4–mediated pathway during EPC recruitment to injured vessels.[139] SDF-1/CXCL4-CXCR4–mediated EPC recruitment involves the PI3K/Akt/eNOS signal transduction pathway.[86] In conclusion, SDF-1/CXCL4 may serve as a "molecular hub" that modulates vasculogenesis, as well as angiogenesis.[83]

Among other regulators of vasculogenesis, IL-6 stimulates EPC migration and Matrigel tube formation.[141] CCN1, an angiogenic factor promotes the adhesion and migration of EPCs. This involves numerous integrins including $\alpha_V\beta_3$.[142] E-selectin is involved in EPC recruitment, and soluble E-selectin rescued impaired vasculogenesis in an ischemic limb model.[143]

Accelerated atherosclerosis and increased cardiovascular morbidity and mortality have been associated with RA.[28,144] Some studies also suggest that the depletion of circulating EPCs may be linked to increased cardiovascular morbidity in RA.[21,145] Reduced numbers and migratory activity of EPCs in RA may result in a poorer response of circulating EPCs to ischemia leading to stroke or myocardial infarction.[21,126,127] Carotid atherosclerosis in RA has been associated with impaired NO-dependent EPC mobilization.[137] Thus, the loss of EPCs in the circulation of RA patients may link synovial inflammation and increased cardiovascular morbidity and mortality.

EPCs may be used for the induction of neovascularization in therapeutic trials in certain vascular and inflammatory diseases associated with insufficient EPC number or function.[19,132,133] Indeed, peripheral blood–derived EPCs integrate into newly formed vessels in animal models of limb ischemia, as well as in human obliterative atherosclerosis.[19,21,146]

Regulation of Endothelial Function and Angiogenesis

Most angiogenic mediators described above, including growth factors, proinflammatory cytokines, chemokines, and proteases are abundantly produced in the RA synovial tissue.[2,6,15,16] In contrast, although numerous angiogenesis inhibitors are released in the synovium, there may be a relative deficiency of angiostatic factors in RA. For example, there is a low production of IFN-γ and PF4/CXCL4 in RA.[2,15,16]

In addition, the following intermolecular interactions and feedback loops exist in the RA synovial tissue, which regulate endothelial function and the outcome of angiogenesis[1,60,63] (Table 8I-1):

Balance between antagonistic angiogenic and angiostatic couples. Such antagonistic couples include MMPs and TIMPs, ELR$^+$ and ELR$^-$ CXC chemokines, and proinflammatory angiogenic (TNF-α, IL-1) and anti-inflammatory, angiostatic (IL-4, IFNs) cytokines.[1,2,8,10,11,18,63]

Direct or indirect interactions between soluble and cell-bound angiogenic factors. For example, VEGF, at least in part, acts via integrin-dependent pathways.[147] The regulation of angiogenesis also involves toll-like receptors (TLRs): the stimulation of TLR-2 by its ligands resulted in increased production of VEGF and IL-8/CXCL8 by RA synovial fibroblasts.[148]

Stimulation of angiostatic factor production by angiogenic mediators. As described above, an autocrine loop between VEGF and IP-10/CXCL10 has been described.[149,150]

Angiogenesis inhibition by externally administered drugs or other compounds. Numerous DMARDs, as well as corticosteroids and TNF blockers may block synovial neovascularization.[2,6,11]

In conclusion, the regulatory network of synovial angiogenesis includes inflammatory leukocytes and ECs, as well as growth factors, cytokines, chemokines, CAMs, and other factors. Endogenous regulatory loops or externally administered angiostatic compounds may interfere with pathologically enhanced synovial neovascularization and leukocyte recruitment, indicating potentially new strategies in antirheumatic therapy.

Targeting of Synovial Angiogenesis in Rheumatoid Arthritis

There are two major approaches for controlling angiogenesis in RA.[6,8,11,63,65] First, there are endogenous inhibitors including cytokines, chemokines, protease inhibitors, and others that are naturally produced in the RA synovium; however, their quantities are not enough to counterbalance the excessive neovascularization observed in arthritis. On the other hand, externally administered angiostatic compounds, including corticosteroids, disease-modifying antirheumatic drugs (DMARDs), and antibiotic derivatives, may also be used to inhibit RA-associated neovascularization[2,6,11,63] (Table 8I-2).

Most endogenous inhibitors act via $\alpha_V\beta_3$ integrin-dependent mechanisms.[7,64] Angiostatin and endostatin seem to be of importance. Both molecules inhibited the course of arthritis in animal models.[2,6,63,151,152] For example, gene transfer of angiostatin, a plasminogen fragment, reduced synovial inflammation and pannus formation in mice with collagen-induced arthritis (CIA).[65,152] An angiostatin-related angiogenesis inhibitor, protease-activated kringles 1-5 (K1-5), suppressed CIA more potently than angiostatin itself.[153] Endostatin, a fragment of collagen, interferes with type 2 VEGF receptor signaling.[7,151,154] Endostatin improved murine and rat arthritis, suppressed pannus formation and bone destruction.[65,151,155] Kallistatin is an endogenous inhibitor of angiogenesis exerting increased expression in RA joints. Local injection of the kallistatin gene attenuated rat ankle arthritis.[124] Type IV collagen

Table 8I-2. Potential Antiangiogenic Targets[a]

Endogenous inhibitors	Angiostatin
	Endostatin
	Thrombospondin 2
	Cytokines (e.g., IL-4, IL-13)
	Chemokines (e.g., PF4/CXCL4)
	Fumagillin and its analogues
	2-methoxyestradiol
Exogenous inhibitors	Most classical DMARDs
	Anti-TNF agents (e.g., infliximab)
	Thalidomide
	VEGF inhibitors
	HIF inhibitors
	Ang1/Tie2 inhibitors
	$\alpha_V\beta_3$ integrin inhibitors
	Microtubule destabilizers (e.g., paclitaxel)
	Others (soluble FasL, PPARγ agonists)

[a]See text for abbreviations.

fragments, such as arresten, canstatin, and tumstatin also inhibit neovascularization.[156]

Thrombospondin 1 (TSP1) and TSP2 are angiostatic matrix components produced by RA synovial macrophages and fibroblasts. A TSP1-derived peptide ameliorated inflammation and angiogenesis in peptidoglycan-polysaccharide–induced rat arthritis.[157] TSP2 inhibited synovial vascularization in the SCID mouse model of arthritis.[158] In gene transfer studies, IL-4 and IL-13, two endogenously produced cytokines in RA, blocked neovascularization in rat adjuvant–induced arthritis (AIA).[121,159] PF4/CXCL4 has also been tested in rodent models of arthritis.[2,11]

TNP-470 and PPI2458 are two angiostatic analogues of fumagillin, a naturally occurring product of *Aspergillus fumigatus*. These compounds inhibit methionine aminopeptidase-2, an enzyme involved in EC migration and angiogenesis.[160] They also lower serum levels of VEGF and inhibit capillary formation.[6,65] TNP-470 was able to prevent rodent arthritis before the onset of the disease, and it also successfully improved the disease.[65,161] In animal models of arthritis, PPI2458 also suppressed arthritis and the development of joint erosions.[162] 2-methoxyestradiol, a natural metabolite of estrogen, blocks angiogenesis by disrupting microtubules and by suppressing HIF-1α activity.[163]

Among externally administered angiogenesis inhibitors, both classical DMARDs and biologics may inhibit neovascularization.[2,7,11] Infliximab treatment in combination with methotrexate resulted in decreased VEGF production and synovial VEGF expression, as well as attenuated synovial vascularization.[7,11,164] Anti-TNF therapy in arthritic patients reduced Ang1-Tie2 and stimulated Ang2 expression.[7,109] Anti-TNF treatment also downregulated survivin expression.[7] Thalidomide, used in the therapy of multiple myeloma, is a potent TNF-α antagonist and angiogenesis inhibitor.[65,165] The effects of thalidomide on neovascularization is controversial, as in one study it suppressed VEGF production,[166] while in rat CIA thalidomide did not affect VEGF or TNF-α release.[167] Nevertheless, thalidomide suppressed capillary formation and synovitis.[65,166] CC1069, a thalidomide analogue, even more potently inhibited rat AIA.[65] Thalidomide has been tried in numerous RA studies but it demonstrated only little efficacy.[65] HMG-CoA reductase inhibitors or statins modify EC function, CAM expression and they may be used in the long-term therapy of RA.[168]

VEGF is a crucial pathogenic factor in RA-associated angiogenesis; thus, it is a primary therapeutic target. VEGF has been targeted by using synthetic VEGF and VEGF receptor inhibitors and anti-VEGF antibodies, as well as inhibitors of VEGF and VEGF receptor signaling.[6,11,149] There are several small molecular VEGF receptor tyrosine kinase inhibitors under development including vatalanib, sunitinib malate, sorafenib, vandetanib, and AG013736.[65,149] These small molecules are administered orally and generally exert favorable safety profiles. Among these small molecules, vatalanib inhibited knee swelling in rabbit arthritis.[65,169] The VEGF-Trap construct is a composite decoy receptor based on the fusion of VEGFR1 and VEGFR2 with IgG1-Fc.[170] Bevacizumab, a human monoclonal antibody to VEGF has been approved for the treatment of colon cancer.[65] However, to date there have been no completed studies with either bevacizumab or VEGF-Trap in arthritis. Semaphorin-3A blocks the function of the 165 amino-acid form of VEGF (VEGF165). It also suppressed EC survival and neovascularization.[171]

Hypoxia-HIF–mediated neovascularization may also be targeted. For example, YC-1, a superoxide-sensitive stimulator of soluble guanylyl cyclase developed for the therapy of hypertension and thrombosis, also inhibits HIF-1.[65,172] Microtubule destabilizers, such as 2-methoxyestradiol mentioned above, as well as paclitaxel, a drug already used in human cancer, also downregulate HIF-1α expression and activity.[65] In a phase I study, paclitaxel was effective and safe in RA patients.[65]

Regarding the Ang-Tie system, a soluble Tie2 receptor transcript was delivered via an adenoviral vector to mice with CIA. Inhibition of Tie2 resulted in attenuated onset, incidence, and severity of arthritis.[173]

Among other external blockade strategies, inhibition of CXCR2 suppressed tumor–induced angiogenesis.[174] Mig/CXCL9 gene therapy improved the effects of cytotoxic agents in cancer.[175] AMD3100, a highly selective antagonist of SDF-1/CXCL4, inhibits the proliferation and migration of EPCs and induces EPC apoptosis.[176] IL-4 gene therapy reduced synovial angiogenesis in the rat AIA model.[159]

Among adhesion molecules, the $\alpha_V\beta_3$ integrin exerts an important role in EC migration and neovascularization. Vitaxin, a humanized antibody to this integrin, inhibited synovial angiogenesis in animal models of arthritis.[6,11,65] However, in a phase-II human RA trial it showed little efficacy and thus the study was interrupted.[65] Numerous MMP inhibitors have been tried in angiogenesis models.[118] Soluble Fas ligand (CD178) inhibited VEGF165 production by RA synovial fibroblasts, as well as neovascularization.[177] Pioglitazone, a PPARγ agonist developed for the treatment of diabetes, is antiangiogenic. It showed some efficacy in controlling psoriatic arthritis in 10 patients.[178] Endothelin-1 antagonists currently used in the therapy of pulmonary hypertension and scleroderma may also exert antiangiogenic effects.[5]

In general, most endogenous and externally administered angiogenesis inhibitors may have therapeutic relevance for RA-associated neovascularization. Most inhibitors act through the modification of VEGF- and $\alpha_V\beta_3$-mediated pathways. Many of these compounds are already in preclinical or clinical trials. However, as there is an immensely complex regulatory network of angiogenesis in the inflamed synovium, antiangiogenic agents against one specific target may only have limited efficacy, while compounds with several modes of action may be more effective.[2,8]

Conclusion

Endothelial cells are involved in a number of mechanisms underlying synovial inflammation. Several factors lead to increased vascular permeability. ECs play a central role in leukocyte extravasation, a key feature of inflammation. A number of adhesion receptors termed integrins, selectins, immunoglobulins and others act in concert and regulate the sequence of distinct steps. The action of various CAM pairs and the existence of distinct steps of rolling, activation, adhesion, and migration account for the diversity and specificity of leukocyte–endothelial interactions.

ECs are active participants in new vessel formation termed angiogenesis. A number of soluble and cell-bound factors may stimulate neovascularization. The perpetuation of angiogenesis involving numerous soluble and cell surface–bound mediators has been associated with RA. There are numerous potential endogenous or exogenously administered compounds that inhibit neovascularization. Theoretically, all of these agents may be used to control synovial inflammation. Among the several potential angiogenesis inhibitors, targeting of VEGF, HIF-1, angiopoietin, and the $\alpha_V\beta_3$ integrin, as well as some endogenous or synthetic compounds including angiostatin, endostatin, paclitaxel, fumagillin analogues, and thalidomide seem to be promising for the management of synovial inflammation.

Acknowledgments

This work was supported by National Institutes of Health grants AR-048267 and AI-40987 (A.E.K.), the William D. Robinson, M.D., and Frederick G.L. Huetwell Endowed Professorship (A.E.K.), funds from the Veterans Administration (A.E.K.); and grant T048541 from the National Scientific Research Fund (OTKA) (Z.S.).

References

1. Szekanecz Z, Szegedi G, Koch AE. Angiogenesis in rheumatoid arthritis: Pathogenic and clinical significance. *J Invest Med* 1998;46: 27–41.
2. Szekanecz Z, Koch AE. Chemokines and angiogenesis. *Curr Opin Rheumatol* 2001;13:202–208.
3. Szekanecz Z, Szegedi G, Koch AE. Cellular adhesion molecules in rheumatoid arthritis. Regulation by cytokines and possible clinical importance. *J Invest Med* 1996;44:124–135.
4. Szekanecz Z, Kunkel SL, Strieter RM, et al. Chemokines in rheumatoid arthritis. *Springer Semin Immunopathol* 1998;20:115–132.
5. Koch AE, Distler O. Vasculopathy and disordered angiogenesis in selected rheumatic diseases: Rheumatoid arthritis and systemic sclerosis. *Arthritis Res Ther* 2007;9(Suppl 2):S3.
6. Koch AE. Angiogenesis: Implications for rheumatoid arthritis. *Arthritis Rheum* 1998;41:951–962.
7. Veale DJ, Fearon U. Inhibition of angiogenic pathways in rheumatoid arthritis: Potential for therapeutic targeting. *Best Pract Res Clin Rheumatol* 2006;20:941–947.
8. Walsh DA. Angiogenesis and arthritis. *Rheumatology* 1999;38: 103–112.
9. Szekanecz Z, Koch AE. Endothelial cells in inflammation and angiogenesis. *Curr Drug Targets* 2005;4:319–323.
10. Szekanecz Z, Koch AE. Vascular endothelium and immune responses: Implications for inflammation and angiogenesis. *Rheum Dis Clin N Am* 2004;30:97–114.
11. Szekanecz Z, Gáspár L, Koch AE. Angiogenesis in rheumatoid arthritis. *Front Biosci* 2005;10:1739–1753.
12. Szekanecz Z, Koch AE. Macrophages and their products in rheumatoid arthritis. *Curr Opin Rheumatol* 2007;19:289–295.
13. Pober JS, Cotran RS. Cytokines and endothelial cell biology. *Physiol Rev* 1990;70:427–434.
14. Brenchley PE. Angiogenesis in inflammatory joint disease: A target for therapeutic intervention. [Editorial.] *Clin Exp Immunol* 2000;121: 426–429.
15. Szekanecz Z, Strieter RM, Koch AE. Cytokines in rheumatoid arthritis: Potential targets for pharmacological intervention. *Drugs Aging* 1998;12:377–390.
16. Brennan F, Beech J. Update on cytokines in rheumatoid arthritis. *Curr Opin Rheumatol* 2007;19:296–301.
17. Agarwal SK, Brenner MB. Role of adhesion molecules in synovial inflammation. *Curr Opin Rheumatol* 2006;18:268–276.
18. Szekanecz Z, Kim J, Koch AE. Chemokines and chemokine receptors in rheumatoid arthritis. *Semin Immunol* 2002;399:1–7.
19. Freedman SB, Isner JM. Therapeutic angiogenesis for ischemic cardiovascular disease. *J Mol Cell Cardiol* 2001;33:379–393.
20. Peichev M, Naiyer AJ, Pereira D, et al. Expression of VEGFR-2 and AC133 by circulating human CD34(+) cells identifies a population of functional endothelial precursors. *Blood* 2000;95: 952–958.
21. Paleolog E. It's all in the blood: Circulating endothelial progenitor cells link synovial vascularity with cardiovascular mortality in rheumatoid arthritis? *Arthritis Res Ther* 2005;7:270–272.
22. Brenner BM, Troy JL, Ballermann BJ. Endothelium-dependent vascular responses. Mediators and mechanisms. *J Clin Invest* 1989;84: 1373–1378.
23. Joris I, Majno G, Corey EJ, et al. The mechanism of vascular leakage induced by leukotriene E4. Endothelial contraction. *Am J Pathol* 1987;126:19–24.
24. Editorial. Antibodies to endothelial cells. *Lancet* 1991;337:649–650.
25. Brett J, Gerlach H, Nawroth P, et al. Tumor necrosis factor/cachectin increases permeability of endothelial cell monolayers by a mechanism involving regulatory G proteins. *J Exp Med* 1989;169: 1977–1991.
26. Varani J, Ginsburg I, Schuger L, et al. Endothelial cell killing by neutrophils. Synergistic interaction of oxygen products and proteases. *Am J Pathol* 1989;135:435–438.
27. Mulligan MS, Varani J, Dame MK, et al. Role of endothelial–leukocyte adhesion molecule 1 (ELAM-1) in neutrophil-mediated lung injury in rats. *J Clin Invest* 1991;88:1396–1406.
28. Szekanecz Z, Kerekes G, Dér H, et al. Accelerated atherosclerosis in rheumatoid arthritis. *Ann N Y Acad Sci* 2007;1108:349–358.
29. Bergholm R, Leirisalo-Repo M, Vehkavaara S, et al. Impaired responsiveness to NO in newly diagnosed patients with rheumatoid arthritis. *Arterioscler Thromb Vasc Biol* 2002;22:1637–1641.
30. Herbrig K, Haensel S, Oelschlaegel U, et al. Endothelial dysfunction in patients with rheumatoid arthritis is associated with a reduced number and impaired function of endothelial progenitor cells. *Ann Rheum Dis* 2006;65:157–163.

31. Albelda SM, Buck CA. Integrins and other cell adhesion molecules. *FASEB J* 1990;4:2868–2880.
32. Springer TA. Adhesion receptors of the immune system. *Nature* 1990;346:425–433.
33. Carlos TM, Harlan JM. Leukocyte-endothelial adhesion molecules. *Blood* 1994;84:2068–2101.
34. Butcher EC. Leukocyte–endothelial cell recognition: Three (or more) steps to specificity and diversity. *Cell* 1991;67:1033–1036.
35. Imhof BA, Aurrand-Lions M. Adhesion mechanisms regulating the migration of monocytes. *Nat Rev Immunol* 2004;4:432–444.
36. Bevilacqua MP, Pober JS, Mendrick DL, et al. Identification of an inducible endothelial–leukocyte adhesion molecule. *Proc Natl Acad Sci U S A* 1987;84:9238–9242.
37. Koch AE, Turkiewicz W, Harlow LA, et al. Soluble E-selectin in arthritis. *Clin Immunol Immunopathol* 1993;69:29–35.
38. Koch AE, Burrows JC, Haines GK, et al. Immunolocalization of leukocyte and endothelial adhesion molecules in human rheumatoid and osteoarthritic synovial tissue. *Lab Invest* 1991;64:313–320.
39. McEver RP, Beckstead JH, Moore KL, et al. GMp-140, a platelet alpha-granule membrane protein, is also synthesized by vascular endothelial cells and is localized in Weibel-Palade bodies. *J Clin Invest* 1989;84:92–99.
40. Lawrence MB, Springer TA. Leukocytes roll on a selectin at physiologic flow rates: Distinction from and prerequisite for adhesion through integrins. *Cell* 1991;65:859–873.
41. Hosaka S, Shah MR, Pope RM, et al. Soluble forms of P-selectin and intercellular adhesion molecule-3 in synovial fluids. *Clin Immunol Immunopathol* 1996;78:276–282.
42. Johnson B, Haines GK, Harlow LA, et al. Adhesion molecule expression in human synovial tissues. *Arthritis Rheum* 1993;36:137–146.
43. Bischoff J. Approaches to studying cell adhesion molecules in angiogenesis. *Trends Cell Biol* 1995;5:69–75.
44. Brooks PC, Clark RA, Cheresh DA. Requirement of vascular integrin alpha v beta 3 for angiogenesis. *Science* 1994;264:569–571.
45. Thornhill MH, Haskard DO. IL-4 regulates endothelial cell activation by IL-1, tumor necrosis factor, or IFN-gamma. *J Immunol* 1990; 145:865–872.
46. Pober JS, Gimbrone MA Jr, Lapierre LA, et al. Overlapping patterns of activation of human endothelial cells by interleukin 1, tumor necrosis factor, and immune interferon. *J Immunol* 1986;137:1893–1896.
47. Ostermann G, Weber KS, Zernecke A, et al. JAM-1 is a ligand of the beta-2 integrin LFA-1 involved in transendothelial migration of leukocytes. *Nat Immunol* 2002;3:151–158.
48. Cunningham SA, Rodriguez JM, Arrate MP, et al. JAM2 interacts with ?4?1. Facilitation by JAM3. *J Biol Chem* 2002;277:27589–27595.
49. Salmi M, Kalimo K, Jalkanen S. Induction and function of vascular adhesion protein-1 at sites of inflammation. *J Exp Med* 1993;178: 2255–2260.
50. Szekanecz Z, Haines GK, Lin TR, et al. Differential distribution of ICAM-1, ICAM-2 and ICAM-3, and the MS-1 antigen in normal and diseased human synovia. *Arthritis Rheum* 1994;37:221–231.
51. Szekanecz Z, Haines GK, Harlow LA, et al. Increased synovial expression of transforming growth factor (TGF)-β receptor endoglin and TGF-β1 in rheumatoid arthritis: Possible interactions in the pathogenesis of the disease. *Clin ImmunolClin Immunol Immunopathol* 1995;76:187–194.
52. Haynes BF, Hale LP, Patton KL, et al. Measurement of an adhesion molecule as an indicator of inflammatory disease activity. Upregulation of the receptor for hyaluronate (CD44) in rheumatoid arthritis. *Arthritis Rheum* 1991;34:1434–1443.
53. Brennan FR, Mikecz K, Glant TT, et al. CD44 expression by leucocytes in rheumatoid arthritis and modulation by specific antibody: Implications for lymphocyte adhesion to endothelial cells and synoviocytes in vitro. *Scand J Immunol* 1997;45:213–220.
54. Dejana E. Endothelial adherens junctions: Implications in the control of vascular permeability and angiogenesis. *J Clin Invest* 1996;98: 1949–1953.
55. Halloran MM, Carley WW, Polverini PJ, et al. Ley/H: An endothelial-selective, cytokine-inducible, angiogenic mediator. *J Immunol* 2000; 164:4868–4877.
56. Neidhart M, Wehrli R, Bruhlmann P, et al. Synovial fluid CD146 (MUC18), a marker for synovial membrane angiogenesis in rheumatoid arthritis. *Arthritis Rheum* 1999;42:622–630.
57. Schenkel AR, Mamdouh Z, Chen X, et al. CD99 plays a major role in the migration of monocytes through endothelial junctions. *Nat Immunol* 2002;3:143–150.
58. Szekanecz Z, Koch AE. Intercellular adhesion molecule (ICAM)-3 expression on endothelial cells. *Am J Pathol* 1997;151:313–314.
59. van Dinther-Janssen ACHM, Pals ST, Scheper R, et al. Dendritic cells and high endothelial venules in the rheumatoid synovial membrane. *J Rheumatol* 1990;17:11–17.
60. Folkman J, Klagsbrun M. Angiogenic factors. *Science* 1987;235: 442–447.
61. Fearon U, Veale DJ. Angiogenesis in arthritis: Methodological and analytical details. *Methods Mol Med* 2007;135:343–358.
62. Koch AE, Harlow LA, Haines GK, et al. Vascular endothelial growth factor. A cytokine modulating endothelial function in rheumatoid arthritis. *J Immunol* 1994;152:4149–4156.
63. Auerbach W, Auerbach R. Angiogenesis inhibition: A review. *Pharmacol Ther* 1994;63:265–311.
64. Milkiewicz M, Ispanovic E, Doyle JL, et al. Regulators of angiogenesis and strategies for their respective manipulation. *Int J Biochem Cell Biol* 2006;38:333–357.
65. Lainer-Carr D, Brahn E. Angiogenesis inhibition as a therapeutic approach for inflammatory synovitis. *Nat Clin Pract Rheumatol* 2007;3:434–442.
66. Liu LX, Lu H, Luo Y, et al. Stabilization of vascular endothelial growth factor mRNA by hypoxia-inducible factor 1. *Biochem Biophys Res Commun* 2002;291:908–914.
67. Taylor PC, Sivakumar B, Hypoxia and angiogenesis in rheumatoid arthritis. *Curr Opin Rheumatol* 2005;17:293–298.
68. Giatromanolaki A, Sivridis E, Maltezos E, et al. Upregulated hypoxia inducible factor-1α and -2α pathway in rheumatoid arthritis and osteoarthritis. *Arthritis Res Ther* 2003;5:R193–R201.
69. Holash J, Maisonpierre PC, Compton D, et al. Vessel cooption, regression and growth in tumors mediated by angiopoietins and VEGF. *Science* 1999;284:1994–1998.
70. Suri C, Jones PF, Patan S, et al. Requisite role of angiopoietin-1 a ligand for the TIE2 receptor, during embryonic angiogenesis. *Cell* 1996;87:1171–1180.
71. Davis S, Aldrich TH, Jones PF, et al. Isolation of angiopoietin-1, a ligand for the TIE2 receptor, by secretion-trap expression cloning. *Cell* 1996;87:1161–1169.
72. Tran J, Master Z, Yu JL, et al. A role for survivin in chemoresistance of endothelial cells mediated by VEGF. *Proc Natl Acad Sci U S A* 2002;99:4349–4354.
73. Gravallese EM, Pettit AR, Lee R, et al. Angiopoietin-1 is expressed in the synovium of patients with rheumatoid arthritis and is induced by tumour necrosis factor alpha. *Ann Rheum Dis* 2003;62:100–107.
74. Shahrara S, Volin MV, Connors MA, et al. Differential expression of the angiogenic Tie receptor family in arthritic and normal synovial tissue. *Arthritis Res* 2002;4:201–208.
75. Walz A, Kunkel SL, Strieter RM. C-X-C chemokines—an overview. In: Koch AE, Strieter RM, eds. *Chemokines in Disease*. Austin, TX: RG Landes Company, 1996, 1–25.
76. Strieter RM, Polverini PJ, Kunkel SL, et al. The functional role of the ELR motif in CXC chemokine-mediated angiogenesis. *J Biol Chem* 1995;270:27348–27357.
77. Salcedo R, Ponce ML, Young HA, et al. Human endothelial cells express CCR2 and respond to MCp-1: Direct role of MCp-1 in angiogenesis and tumor progression. *Blood* 2000;96:34–40.
78. Bodnar RJ, Yates CC, Wells A. Ip-10 blocks vascular endothelial growth factor-induced endothelial cell motility and tube formation via inhibition of calpain. *Circ Res* 2006;98:617–625.

79. Maurer AM, Zhou B, Han ZC. Roles of platelet factor 4 in hematopoiesis and angiogenesis. *Growth Factors* 2006;24:242–252.
80. Vandercappellen J, Noppen S, Verbeke H, et al. Stimulation of angiostatic platelet factor-4 variant (CXCL4L1/PF-4var) versus inhibition of angiogenic granulocyte chemotactic protein-2 (CXCL6/GCp-2) in normal and tumoral mesenchymal cells. *J Leukoc Biol* 2007 (published online before print September 7).
81. Pablos JL, Santiago B, Galindo M, et al. Synoviocyte-derived CXCL12 is displayed on endothelium and induces angiogenesis in rheumatoid arthritis. *J Immunol* 2003;170:2147–2152.
82. Salcedo R, Wasserman K, Young HA, et al. Vascular endothelial growth factor and basic fibroblast growth factor induce expression of CXCR4 on human endothelial cells: In vivo neovascularization induced by stromal-derived factor-1alpha. *Am J Pathol* 1999;154: 1125–1135.
83. Petit I, Jin D, Rafii S. The SDF-1-CXCR4 signaling pathway: A molecular hub modulating neo-angiogenesis. *Trends Immunol* 2007;28: 299–307.
84. Santiago B, Baleux F, Palao G, et al. CXCL12 is displayed by rheumatoid endothelial cells through its basic amino-terminal motif on heparan sulfate proteoglycans. *Arthritis Res Ther* 2006;8:R43.
85. Liang Z, Brooks J, Willard M, et al. CXCR4/CXCL12 axis promotes VEGF-mediated tumor angiogenesis through Akt signaling pathway. *Biochem Biophys Res Commun* 2007;359:716–722.
86. Zheng H, Fu G, Dai T, et al. Migration of endothelial progenitor cells mediated by stromal cell–derived factor-1α/CXCR4 via PI3K/Akt/eNOS signal transduction pathway. *J Cardiovasc Pharmacol* 2007;50:274–280.
87. Deshane J, Chen S, Caballero S, et al. Stromal cell-derived factor 1 promotes angiogenesis via a heme oxygenase 1–dependent mechanism. *J Exp Med* 2007;204:605–618.
88. Tan Y, Shao H, Eton D, et al. Stromal cell–derived factor-1 enhances pro-angiogenic efft of granulocyte colony stimulating factor. *Cardiovasc Res* 2007;73:823–832.
89. Calatozzolo C, Maderna E, Pollo B, et al. Prognostic value of CXCL12 expression in 40 low-grade oligodendrogliomas and oligoastrocytomas. *Cancer Biol Ther* 2006;5:827–832.
90. Stamatovic SM, Keep RF, Mostarica-Stojkovic M, et al. CCL2 regulates angiogenesis via activation of Ets-1 transcription factor. *J Immunol* 2006;177:2651–2661.
91. Ma J, Wang Q, Fei T, et al. MCP-1 mediates TGF-β–induced angiogenesis by stimulating vascular smooth muscle cell migration. *Blood* 2007;109:987–994.
92. Fujii T, Yonemitsu Y, Onimaru M, et al. Nonendothelial mesenchymal cell–derived MCp-1 is required for FGF-2 mediated therapeutic neovascularization. *Arterioscler Thromb Vasc Biol* 2006;26:2483–2489.
93. Son KN, Hwang J, Kwon BS, et al. Human CC chemokine CCL23 enhances expression of matrix metalloproteinase-2 and invasion of vascular endothelial cells. *Biochem Biophys Res Commun* 2006;340: 498–504.
94. Ruth JH, Volin MV, Haines III GK, et al. Fractalkine, a novel chemokine in rheumatoid arthritis and rat adjuvant–induced arthritis. *Arthritis Rheum* 2001;44:1568–1581.
95. Volin MV, Woods JM, Amin MA, et al. Fractalkine: A novel angiogenic chemokine in rheumatoid arthritis. *Am J Pathol* 2001;159: 1521–1526.
96. Imaizumi T, Yoshida H, Satoh K. Regulation of CX3CL1/fractalkine expression in endothelial cells. *J Atheroscler Thromb* 2004;11: 15–21.
97. Borzi RM, Mazzetti I, Cattini L. Human chondrocytes express functional chemokine receptors and release matrix-degrading enzymes in response to C-X-C and C-C chemokines. *Arthritis Rheum* 2000;43:1734–1741.
98. Buckley CD, Amft N, Bradfield PF, et al. Persistent induction of the chemokine receptor CXCR4 by TGF-beta 1 on synovial T cells contributes to their accumulation within the rheumatoid synovium. *J Immunol* 2000;165:3423–3429.
99. Nanki T, Hayashida K, El-Gabalawy HS, et al. Stromal cell–derived factor-1-CXC chemokine receptor 4 interactions play a central role in CD4+ T-cell accumulation in rheumatoid arthritis synovium. *J Immunol* 2000;165:6590–6598.
100. Zagzag D, Lukyanov Y, Lan L, et al. Hypoxia-inducible factor 1 an VEGF upregulate CXCR4 in glioblastoma: Implications for angiogenesis and glioma cell invasion. *Lab Invest* 2006;86:1221–1232.
101. Burns JM, Summers BC, Wang Y, et al. A novel chemokine receptor for SDF-1 and I-TAC involved in cell survival, cell adhesion and tumor development. *J Exp Med* 2006;203:2201–2213.
102. Ochoa O, Sun D, Reyes-Reyna SM, et al. Delayed angiogenesis and VEGF production in CCR2-/- mice during impaired skeletal muscle regeneration. *Am J Physiol Regul Integr Comp Physiol* 2007;293: R651–R661.
103. Patterson AM, Siddall H, Chamberlain G. Expression of the Duffy antigen/receptor for chemokines (DARC) by the inflamed synovial endothelium. *J Pathol* 2002;197:108–116.
104. Wang J, Ou ZL, Hou YF, et al. Enhanced expression of Duffy antigen receptor for chemokines by breast cancer cells attenuates growth and metastasis potential. *Oncogene* 2006;25:7201–7211.
105. Park CC, Morel JC, Amin MA, et al. Evidence of IL-18 as a novel angiogenic mediator. *J Immunol* 2001;167:1644–1653.
106. Angiolillo AL, Kanegane H, Sgadari C, et al. Interleukin-15 promotes angiogenesis in vivo. *Biochem Biophys Res Commun* 1997; 233:231–237.
107. Numasaki M, Watanabe M, Suzuki T, et al. IL-17 enhances the net angiogenic activity and in vivo growth of human non–small cell lung cancer in SCID mice through promoting CXCR2-dependent angiogenesis. *J Immunol* 2005;175:6177–6189.
108. Amin MA, Mansfield PJ, Pakozdi A, et al. Interleukin-18 induces angiogenic factors in rheumatoid arthritis synovial tissue fibroblasts via distinct signaling pathways. *Arthritis Rheum* 2007;56: 1787–1797.
109. Markham T, Mullan R, Golden-Mason L, et al. Resolution of endothelial activation and down-regulation of Tie2 receptor in psoriatic skin after infliximab therapy. *J Am Acad Dermatol* 2006;54: 1003–1012.
110. Fearon U, Mullan R, Markham T, et al. Oncostatin M induces angiogenesis and cartilage degradation in rheumatoid arthritis synovial tissue and human cartilage cocultures. *Arthritis Rheum* 2006; 54:3152–3162.
111. Amin MA, Volpert OV, Woods JM, et al. Migration inhibitory factor mediates angiogenesis via mitogen-activated protein kinase and phosphatidylinositol kinase. *Circ Res* 2003;93:321–329.
112. Morand EF, Leech M, Bernhagen J. MIF: A new cytokine link between rheumatoid arthritis and atherosclerosis. *Nat Rev Drug Discov* 2006;5:399–410.
113. Kim HR, Park MK, Cho ML, et al. Macrophage migration inhibitory factor upregulates angiogenic factors and correlates with clinical measures in rheumatoid arthritis. *J Rheumatol* 2007;34:927–936.
114. Madri JA, Williams KS. Capillary endothelial cell cultures: Phenotypic modulation by matrix components. *J Cell Biol* 1983;97: 153–165.
115. Jacq L, Garnier S, Dieudé P, et al. The ITGAV rs3738919-C allele is associated with rheumatoid arthritis in the European Caucasian population: A family-based study. *Arthritis Res Ther* 2007;9:R63.
116. Kneilling M, Hültner L, Pichler BJ, et al. Targeted mast cell silencing protects against joint destruction and angiogenesis in experimental arthritis in mice. *Arthritis Rheum* 2007;56:1806–1816.
117. Nigrovic PA, Lee DM. Synovial mast cells: Role in acute and chronic arthritis. *Immunol Rev* 2007;217:19–37.
118. Skotnicki JS, Zask A, Nelson FC, et al. Design and synthetic considerations of matrix metalloproteinase inhibitors. *Ann N Y Acad Sci* 1999;878:61–72.
119. Haq A, El-Ramahi K, Al-Dalaan A, et al. Serum and synovial fluid concentrations of endothelin-1 in patients with inflammatory arthritides. *J Med* 1999;30:51–60.

120. Lee MS, Yoo SA, Cho CS, et al. Serum amyloid A binding to formyl peptide receptor-like 1 induces synovial hyperplasia and angiogenesis. *J Immunol* 2006;177:5585–5594.
121. Haas CS, Amin MA, Ruth JH, et al. In vivo inhibition of angiogenesis by interleukin-13 gene therapy in a rat model of rheumatoid arthritis. *Arthritis Rheum* 2007;56:2535–2548.
122. Hong KH, Cho ML, Min SY, et al. Effect of interleukin-4 on vascular endothelial growth factor production in rheumatoid synovial fibroblasts. *Clin Exp Immunol* 2007;147:573–579.
123. Vicari AP, Ait-Yahia S, Chemin K, et al. Antitumor effects of the mouse chemokine 6Ckine/SLC through angiostatic and immunological mechanisms. *J Immunol* 2000;165:1992–2000.
124. Wang CR, Chen SY, Shiau AL, et al. Upregulation of kallistatin expression in rheumatoid joints. *J Rheumatol* 2007 (published online before print October 15).
125. Stellos K, Gawaz M. Platelets and stromal cell-derived factor-1 in progenitor cell recruitment. *Semin Thromb Hemost* 2007;33:159–164.
126. Grisar J, Aletaha D, Steiner CW, et al. Depletion of endothelial progenitor cells in the peripheral blood of patients with rheumatoid arthritis. *Circulation* 2005;111:204–211.
127. Grisar J, Aletaha D, Steiner CW, et al. Endothelial progenitor cells in active rheumatoid arthritis: Effects of tumour necrosis factor and glucocorticoid therapy. *Ann Rheum Dis* 2007;66:1284–1288.
128. Gehling UM, Ergun S, Schumacher U, et al. In vitro differentiation of endothelial cells from AC133-positive progenitor cells. *Blood* 2000;95:3106–3112.
129. Eichmann A, Corbel C, Nataf V, et al. Ligand-dependent development of the endothelial and hemopoetic lineages from embryonic mesodermal cells expressing vascular endothelial growth factor receptor 2. *Proc Natl Acad Sci U S A* 1997;94:5141–5146.
130. Rüger B, Giurea A, Wanivenhaus AH, et al. Endothelial precursor cells in the synovial tissue of patients with rheumatoid arthritis and osteoarthritis. *Arthritis Rheum* 2004;50:2157–2166.
131. Hirohata S, Yanagida T, Nampei A, et al. Enhanced generation of endothelial cells from CD34+ cells of the bone marrow in rheumatoid arthritis: Possible role in synovial neovascularization. *Arthritis Rheum* 2004;50:3888–3896.
132. Shyu KG, Manor O, Magner M, et al. Direct intramuscular injection of plasmid DNA encoding angiopoietin-1 but not angiopoietin-2 augments revascularization in the rabbit ischemic hindlimb. *Circulation* 1998;98:2081–2087.
133. Isner JM, Baumgartner I, Rauh G, et al. Treatment of thromboangiitis obliterans (Buerger's disease) by intramuscular gene transfer of vascular endothelial growth factor: Preliminary clinical results. *J Vasc Surg* 1998;28:964–973.
134. Distler JHW, Gay S, Distler O. Angiogenesis and vasculogenesis in systemic sclerosis. *Rheumatology* 2006;45:iii26–iii27.
135. Allanore Y, Batteux F, Avouac J, et al. Levels of circulating endothelial progenitor cells in systemic sclerosis. *Clin Exp Rheumatol* 2007;25:60–66.
136. Silverman MD, Haas CS, Rad AM, et al. The role of vascular cell adhesion molecule 1/very late activation antigen 4 in endothelial progenitor cell recruitment to rheumatoid arthritis synovium. *Arthritis Rheum* 2007;56:1817–1826.
137. Surdacki A, Martens-Lobenhoffer J, Wloch A, et al. Elevated plasma asymmetric dimethyl-L-arginine levels are linked to endothelial progenitor cell depletion and carotid atherosclerosis in rheumatoid arthritis. *Arthritis Rheum* 2007;56:809–819.
138. Ablin JN, Boguslavski V, Aloush V, et al. Effect of anti-TNFα treatment on circulating endothelial progenitor cells (EPCs) in rheumatoid arthritis. *Life Sci* 2006;79:2364–2369.
139. Ceradini DJ, Gurtner GC. Homing to hypoxia: HIF-1 as a mediator of progenitor cell recruitment to injured tissue. *Trends Cardiovasc Med* 2005;15:57–63.
140. DK Jin, K Shido, HG Kopp, et al. Cytokine-mediated deployment of SDF-1 induces revascularization through recruitment of CXCR4+ hemangiocytes. *Nat Med* 2006;12:557–567.
141. Fan Y, Ye J, Shen F, et al. Interleukin-6 stimulates circulating blood-derived endothelial progenitor cell angiogenesis in vitro. *J Cereb Blood Flow Metab* 2007 (published online before print May 16).
142. Grote K, Salguero G, Ballmaier M, et al. The angiogenic factor CCN1 promotes adhesion and migration of circulating CD34+ progenitor cells: Potential role in angiogenesis and endothelial regeneration. *Blood* 2007;110:877–885.
143. Oh IY, Yoon CH, Hur J, et al. Involvement of E-selectin in recruitment of endothelial progenitor cells and angiogenesis in ischemic muscle. *Blood* 2007 (published online before print August 15).
144. Shoenfeld Y, Gerli R, Doria A, et al. Accelerated atherosclerosis in autoimmune rheumatic diseases. *Circulation* 2005;112:3337–3347.
145. Akhavani MA, Larsen H, Paleolog E. Circulating endothelial progenitor cells link between synovial vascularity and cardiovascular mortality in rheumatoid arthritis. *Scand J Rheumatol* 2007;36:83–90.
146. Asahara T, Murohara T, Sullivan A, et al. Isolation of putative progenitor endothelial cells for angiogenesis. *Science* 1997;275:964–967.
147. Senger DR, Claffey IKP, Benes JE, et al. Angiogenesis promoted by vascular endothelial growth factor: Regulation through α1β1 and α2β1 integrins. *Proc Natl Acad Sci U S A* 1997;94:13612–13617.
148. Cho ML, Ju JH, Kim HR, et al. Toll-like receptor 2 ligand mediates the upregulation of angiogenic factor, vascular endothelial growth factor and interleukin-8/CXCL8 in human rheumatoid synovial fibroblasts. *Immunol Lett* 2007;108:121–128.
149. Kiselyov A, Balakin KV, Tkachenko SE. VEGF/VEGFR signaling as a target for inhibiting angiogenesis. *Expert Opin Invest Drugs* 2007;16:83–107.
150. Boulday G, Haskova Z, Reinders ME, et al. Vascular endothelial growth factor-induced signaling pathways in endothelial cells that mediate overexpression of the chemokine IFN-γ–inducible protein of 10 kDa in vitro and in vivo. *J Immunol* 2006;176:3098–3107.
151. Yin G, Liu W, An P, et al. Endostatin gene transfer inhibits joint angiogenesis and pannus formation in inflammatory arthritis. *Mol Ther* 2002;5:547–554.
152. Takahashi H, Kato K, Miyake K, et al. Adeno-associated virus vector-mediated anti-angiogenic gene therapy for collagen-induced arthritis in mice. *Clin Exp Rheumatol* 2005;23:455–461.
153. Sumariwalla PF, Cao Y, Wu HL, et al. The angiogenesis inhibitor protease-activated kringles 1–5 reduces the severity of murine collagen-induced arthritis. *Arthritis Res Ther* 2003;5:R32–R39.
154. O'Reilly MS, Boehm T, Shing Y, et al. Endostatin: An endogenous inhibitor of angiogenesis and tumor growth. *Cell* 1997;88:277–285.
155. Yue L, Shen YX, Feng LJ, et al. Blockage of the formation of new blood vessels by recombinant human endostatin contributes to the regression of rat adjuvant arthritis. *Eur J Pharmacol* 2007;567:166–170.
156. Mundel TM, Kalluri R. Type IV collagen-derived angiogenesis inhibitors. *Microvasc Res* 2007 (published online before print May 25).
157. Rico MC, Castaneda JL, Manns JM, et al. Amelioration of inflammation, angiogenesis and CTGF expression in an arthritis model by a TSp-1–derived peptide treatment. *J Cell Physiol* 2007;211:504–512.
158. Park YW, Kang YM, Butterfield J, et al. Thrombospondin 2 functions as an endogenous regulator of angiogenesis and inflammation in rheumatoid arthritis. *Am J Pathol* 2004;165:2087–2098.
159. Haas CS, Amin MA, Allen BB, et al. Inhibition of angiogenesis by interleukin-4 gene therapy in rat adjuvant-induced arthritis. *Arthritis Rheum* 2006;54:2402–2414.
160. Ingber D, Fujita T, Kishimoto S, et al. Synthetic analogues of fumagillin that inhibit angiogenesis and suppress tumour growth. *Nature* 1990;348:555–557.
161. Peacock DJ, Banquerigo ML, Brahn E. Angiogenesis inhibition suppresses collagen arthritis. *J Exp Med* 1992;175:1135–1138.

162. Hannig G, Bernier SG, Hoyt JG, et al. Suppression of inflammation and structural damage in experimental arthritis through molecular targeted therapy with PPI–2458. *Arthritis Rheum* 2007;56:850–860.
163. Mabjeesh NJ, Escuin D, LaVallee TM, et al. 2ME2 inhibits tumor growth and angiogenesis by disrupting microtubules and dysregulating HIF. *Cancer Cell* 2003;3:363–375.
164. Goedkoop AY, Kraan MC, Picavet DI, et al. Deactivation of endothelium and reduction in angiogenesis in psoriatic skin and synovium by low dose infliximab therapy in combination with stable methotrexate therapy. *Arthritis Res Ther* 2004;6:R326–R334.
165. D'Amato RJ, Loughnan MS, Flynn E, et al. Thalidomide is an inhibitor of angiogenesis. *Proc Natl Acad Sci U S A* 1994;91: 4082–4085.
166. Komorowski J, Jerczynska H, Siejka A, et al. Effect of thalidomide affecting VEGF secretion, cell migration, adhesion and capillary tube formation of human endothelial EA.hy926 cells. *Life Sci* 2006; 78:2558–2663.
167. Oliver SJ, Cheng TP, Banquerigo ML, et al. The effect of thalidomide and two analogs on collagen induced arthritis. *J Rheumatol* 1998;25:964–969.
168. McCarey DW, Sattar N, McInnes IB. Do the pleiotropic effects of statins in the vasculature predict a role in inflammatory diseases? *Arthritis Res Ther* 2005;7:55–61.
169. Grosios K, Wood J, Esser R, et al. Angiogenesis inhibition by the novel VEGF tyrosine kinase inhibitor, PTK787/ZK222584, causes significant anti-arthritic effects in models of rheumatoid arthritis. *Inflamm Res* 2004;53:133–142.
170. Holash J, Davis S, Papadopoulos N, et al. VEGF-Trap: A VEGF blocker with potent antitumor effects. *Proc Natl Acad Sci U S A* 2002;99:11393–11398.
171. Guttmann-Raviv N, Shraga-Heled N, Varshavsky A, et al. Semaphorin-3A and semaphorin-3F work together to repel endothelial cells and to inhibit their survival by induction of apoptosis. *J Biol Chem* 2007;282:26294–26305.
172. Yeo EJ, Chun YS, Cho YS, et al. YC-1: A potential anticancer drug targeting hypoxia-inducible factor 1. *J Natl Cancer Inst* 2003; 95:516–525.
173. Chen Y, Donnelly E, Kobayashi H, et al. Gene therapy targeting the Tie2 function ameliorates collagen-induced arthritis and protects against bone destruction. *Arthritis Rheum* 2005;52:1585–1594.
174. Wente MN, Keane MP, Burdick MD, et al. Blockade of the chemokine receptor CXCR2 inhibits pancreatic cancer cell-induced angiogenesis. *Cancer Lett* 2006;241:221–227.
175. Zhang R, Tian L, Chen LJ, et al. Combination of MIG (CXCL9) chemokine gene therapy with low-dose cisplatin improves therapeutic efficacy against murine carcinoma. *Gene Ther* 2006;13: 1263–1271.
176. Yin Y, Huang L, Zhao X, et al. AMD3100 mobilizes endothelial progenitor cells in mice, but inhibits its biological functions by blocking an autocrine/paracrine regulatory loop of stromal cell derived factor-1 in vitro. *J Cardiovasc Pharmacol* 2007;50: 61–67.
177. Kim WU, Kwok SK, Hong KH, et al. Soluble Fas ligand inhibits angiogenesis in rheumatoid arthritis. *Arthritis Res Ther* 2007; 26:9:R42.
178. Bongartz T, Coras B, Vogt T, et al. Treatment of active psoriatic arthritis with the PPARγ ligand pioglitazone: An open-label pilot study. *Rheumatology* 2005;44:126–129.

Autoantibodies: Diagnostic Helpers and Pathogenetic Players

CHAPTER 8J

Günter Steiner

Autoimmunity, that is, the presence of autoantibodies and autoreactive T cells in blood and joint fluid, is a characteristic feature of rheumatoid arthritis (RA) that distinguishes this disease from other inflammatory or degenerative joint disorders, such as psoriatic arthritis, reactive arthritis, or osteoarthritis, where autoimmune phenomena are rarely observed. As in other systemic autoimmune diseases, most autoantibodies of patients with RA are not directed to joint-specific structures, but rather target antigens that are more or less ubiquitously expressed. However, antibodies to nuclear antigens (i.e., antinuclear antibodies), which are a typical feature of connective tissue diseases (e.g., systemic lupus erythematosus, systemic sclerosis or primary Sjögren's syndrome), are infrequently seen in RA. Thus, the hallmark autoantibody of RA, rheumatoid factor (RF), is directed against immunoglobulin G (IgG), a major serum component, while autoantibodies to cartilage proteins, particularly collagen II, occur much less frequently, and are also not specific for RA. Antigens described as targets of autoimmune responses in RA include quite diverse structures such as heat-shock proteins, enzymes, cytoskeleton proteins, nuclear proteins, and, most importantly, citrullinated proteins (Table 8J-1). Antibodies to the latter proteins show rather high disease specificity, while all other antibodies including RF may occur in other diseases and even in healthy individuals. Even though most antibodies are not used as diagnostic markers, they may contribute to the pathological processes characteristic of RA such as chronic synovitis and erosiveness. In the following, the major antibodies are described and their value as diagnostic tools as well as their potential role in the pathogenesis of RA are discussed.

Rheumatoid Factors

General Properties

Rheumatoid factors are a family of autoantibodies that recognize antigenic determinants on the Fc portion of IgG. This part of the molecule is essential for complement fixation and interaction with the Fc receptor, and thus for uptake of immune complexes. In contrast to most other autoAb, the major RF species is the IgM isotype, while IgG- and IgA-RF occur less frequently. RF can be measured by various methods including agglutination techniques such as the classical Waaler-Rose test, and turbidometric techniques such as laser nephelometry and ELISA, the latter method being particularly useful for the determination of RF subtypes.

Transient increases of IgM-RF are part of the normal immunoregulatory process occurring during bacterial and viral infections, probably in response to immune complexes containing microbial antigens. Thus, low-titered IgM-RF can be found in 10% to 15% of healthy individuals, whereas chronic persistence of high-titer and high-affinity IgM-RF as well as the presence of IgG and IgA subtypes is a characteristic feature of RA. Interestingly, genes encoding RF from RA patients are often somatically mutated, while RF from healthy individuals are predominantly germ-line encoded and polyreactive. Somatic mutation of immunoglobulin genes and class switch from IgM to other subtypes is an indicator of a T-cell–driven process which, however, is still poorly understood.[1,2]

Pathogenetic Involvement

The physiological role of RF during a normal immune response is to enhance the avidity and size of immune complexes, thereby improving immune complex clearance. Immune complexes are present in the joint, and complement fixation by IgG-containing immune complexes is enhanced by IgM-RF binding. This may be particularly important for immune complexes containing antibodies to cartilage antigens and other proteins expressed in the joint, including antigens that are not joint specific such as stress proteins, citrullinated proteins, or nuclear antigens. Therefore, it is conceivable that RFs may contribute to the activity and chronicity of the disease via complement-mediated pathways (Figure 8J-1). Furthermore, RF-bearing B cells may act as antigen-presenting cells and efficiently present (foreign or self) antigens to T cells via uptake of immune complexes. Thus, RF in serum and especially the RF-producing B cells in synovial tissue of RA patients may exert such functions, and thereby contribute to the pathophysiology of RA. Finally, the association of high-titer RF with more severe disease, particularly with bone erosion and extra-articular manifestations, may be considered further, albeit indirect, evidence for a pathogenetic role of RFs.[1–3]

Rheumatoid Factors as Diagnostic and Prognostic Markers

IgM-RF can be detected in 60% to 80% of RA patients with established disease, while prevalence in patients with early RA is usually not higher than 50%. IgM-RF is present in high titers also in the majority of patients with primary Sjögren's syndrome or mixed cryoglobulinemia and can be found in lower titers in all other rheumatic autoimmune diseases. Thus, at the commonly

Table 8J-1. Targets of Autoantibodies in Rheumatoid Arthritis

Antigen	Antibody	Diagnostic Specificity	T-Cell Reactivity to Target Antigen
Immunoglobulin G	Rheumatoid factors	Moderate-High[a]	Unknown
Citrullinated proteins	ACPA	High	Yes
HnRNP-A2	Anti-RA33	Moderate	Yes
Collagen II	Anticollagen	Low	Yes
Stress proteins	Anti-BiP, anti-hsp90	Low	Yes
Glucose-6 phosphate isomerase	Anti-GPI	Low	Unknown
Calpastatin	Anticalpastatin	Low-high[b]	Unknown

[a]Dependent on cut-off value.
[b]Dependent on the ethnic background.

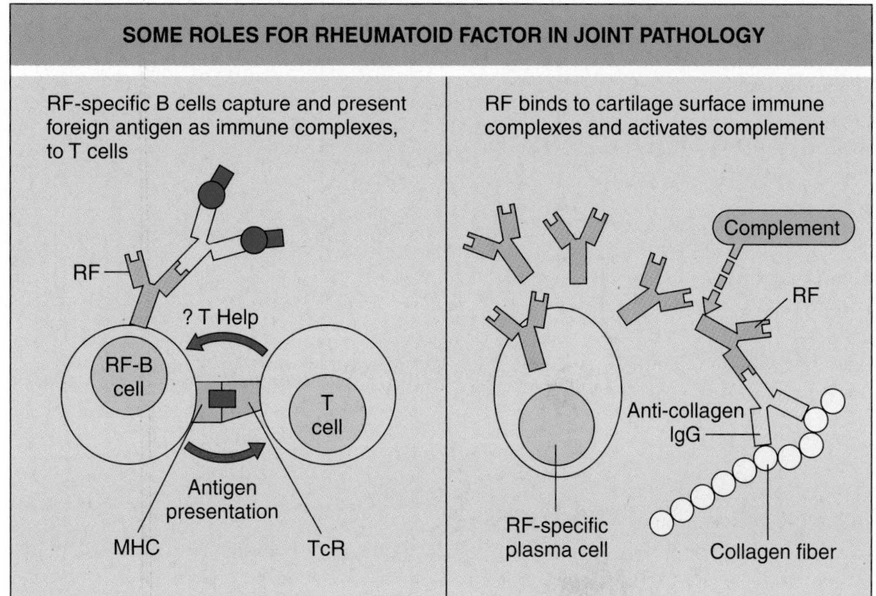

Figure 8J-1. Some roles for rheumatoid factor in joint pathology. (From Hochberg MC, Silman AJ, Smolen JS, et al. *Rheumatology*, 4th ed. London: Mosby, 2008, fig. 78.3, 821.)

used cut-off value of 15 or 20 IU/ml, IgM-RF shows only moderate specificity for RA. However, specificity is considerably increased at higher titers, and several studies have found RF above 40 or 50 IU/ml (high-titer RF) to be rather specific for RA.[4–8] However, high-titer RF is present in only 50% to 60% of RA patients with established disease and is even less frequent in patients with early RA (Table 8J-2).

RFs of all subtypes may be present already in the earliest stages of the disease and can precede the onset of RA by several years.[9,10] Interestingly, IgA-RF appears to be a more specific marker antibody for RA than IgM- or IgG-RF that may precede disease onset similar to IgM-RF.[9,11–13] Importantly, high-titer IgM-RF as well as IgA-RF also have considerable prognostic value because they are associated with severity of RA, such as greater erosion (Figure 8J-2), more rapid disease progression, worse outcome, and extra-articular manifestations.[7,12,14–16]

Taken together, IgM-RF is an indispensable tool that helps the clinician in making a diagnosis as well as in decisions concerning therapeutic measures. Therefore, RF is still the most widely used serological marker of RA, and one of the seven criteria of the American College of Rheumatology for classification of RA.

Autoantibodies to Citrullinated Antigens

General Properties

The identification of autoantibodies in sera of patients with RA directed to epitopes containing the unusual amino acid citrulline was one of the most exciting contributions to the field of RA research of the past decade.[17,18] Arginyl residues are post-translationally deiminated by the enzyme peptidyl arginine deiminase leading to generation of citrullinated proteins (Figure 8J-3). Therefore, autoantibodies recognizing citrullinated epitopes are now generally named anticitrullinated protein antibodies (ACPAs).[18] Citrullinated epitopes were first identified in filaggrin, a protein that is highly expressed in squamous epithelial cells where it promotes aggregation of intermediate filaments.[19] Citrullinated filaggrin forms the target of antikeratin antibodies that were first described in 1979 and shown to be highly specific

Table 8J-2. Sensitivity and Specificity of IgM-RF for Rheumatoid Arthritis

Diagnosis	RF > 20 U/ml (%)	RF > 50 U/ml (%)
Rheumatoid arthritis	66	46
Sjögren's syndrome	62	52
Systemic lupus erythematosus	27	10
Scleroderma	44	8
Poly/dermatomyositis	18	0
Reactive arthritis	10	4
Osteoarthritis	25	4
Healthy controls	13	0
Sensitivity for established RA (%)	66	46
Specificity for established RA (%)	78	88
Sensitivity for early RA⁺ (%)	56	46
Specificity for early RA⁺ (%)	89	96

Data are derived from a prospective early arthritis study including arthritis patients with less than 3 months disease duration. (Data from Nell V, Machold KP, Stamm TA, et al. Autoantibody profiling as early diagnostic and prognostic tool for rheumatoid arthritis. *Ann Rheum Dis* 2005;64(12): 1731–1736.)

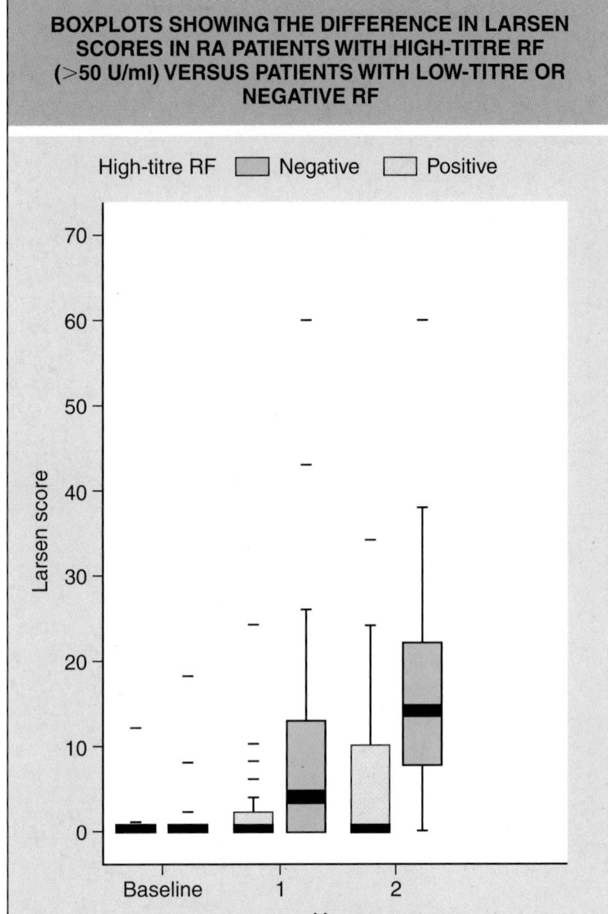

Figure 8J-2. High-titer RF is predicitive of rapid radiographic progression. Box plots showing the difference in Larsen scores in RA patients with high-titer RF (>50 U/ml) versus patients with low-titer or negative RF. The boxes show median values and 25th/75th percentiles. Baseline values were similar in both groups, but Larsen score progression was significantly higher in patients with high-titer RF, and this both in the overall RA population ($p<0.0001$), and also in the subpopulation of anti-CCP negative patients ($p=0.0014$, not shown). (Adapted from Nell V, Machold KP, Stamm TA, et al. Autoantibody profiling as early diagnostic and prognostic tool for rheumatoid arthritis. *Ann Rheum Dis* 2005;64(12):1731–1736.)

for RA.[20] Antifilaggrin antibodies were found to bind to short citrulline-containing peptide epitopes,[21–23] which may also be derived from other proteins or be even of synthetic origin such as a cyclic citrullinated peptide (CCP), which is commonly employed as antigen in most commercial assays for determination of ACPAs.[24–26]

Since filaggrin is only expressed in (terminally differentiated) epithelial cells and not at all in the joint, it is presumably not the primary target of ACPAs but rather seems to represent a cross-reacting antigen. One candidate antigen that might be involved in the initiation of the ACPAs response is fibrin and its precursor fibrinogen, since citrullinated forms of these proteins are abundantly present in synovial tissue of patients with RA[27] (Figure 8J-4). Although deimination of fibrin is not specific for RA and can be generally observed in inflamed joints,[28,29] citrullinated fibrin was shown to be recognized almost exclusively by sera of RA patients and also by affinity-purified antifilaggrin antibodies.[5,27,30,31] Accumulation of fibrin on synovial and cartilage surfaces is a well-known feature of RA, and therefore it is conceivable that deiminated fibrin deposited in the synovial membrane may form a preferred target structure of ACPAs.

Another attractive antigen is the intermediate filament protein vimentin, which has recently been identified as target of ACPAs.[32,33] Vimentin is an ubiquitously expressed cytoskeleton protein that occurs in various citrullinated isoforms, and thus might indeed be one of the primary targets of the ACPA response. Interestingly, cDNAs encoding somatically mutated forms of vimentin were recently isolated from the joint of patients with RA and shown to be recognized by the majority of RA patients when citrullinated.[34]

Additional investigations on citrullinated antigens have been performed with alpha enolase,[35] Epstein-Barr virus nuclear antigen 1,[36] and collagen I and II.[37,38] However, the relevance of these antigens is unclear since it has not been demonstrated until now that their citrullinated isoforms occur also *in vivo*.

Pathogenetic Involvement

Anticitrullinated protein antibodies are locally produced by synovial B cells, and may therefore together with RFs contribute to the inflammatory and destructive processes in the

DEIMINATION (CITRULLINATION) OF ARGININE BY PEPTIDYLARGININE DEIMINASE (PAD)

Arginine	PAD	Citrulline
$NH_2-\overset{+}{C}=NH_2$ / NH / CH_2 / CH_2 / CH_2 / $-NH-CH-C(=O)-$	⟹	$O=C-NH_2$ / NH / CH_2 / CH_2 / CH_2 / $-NH-CH-C(=O)-$

Figure 8J-3. Deimination (citrullination) of an argininyl residue by peptidylarginine deiminase (PAD). Enzymatic arginyl to citrullyl conversion is a post-translational modification that changes the charge and biochemical properties of proteins. Citrullination is predominantly observed in proteins of the cytoskeleton such as cytokeratin, vimentin or filaggrin, but also in other proteins, and seems to represent a general regulatory mechanism that particularly occurs during apoptosis. (From Hochberg MC, Silman AJ, Smolen JS, et al. *Rheumatology*, 4th ed. London: Mosby, 2008, fig. 78.4, 822.)

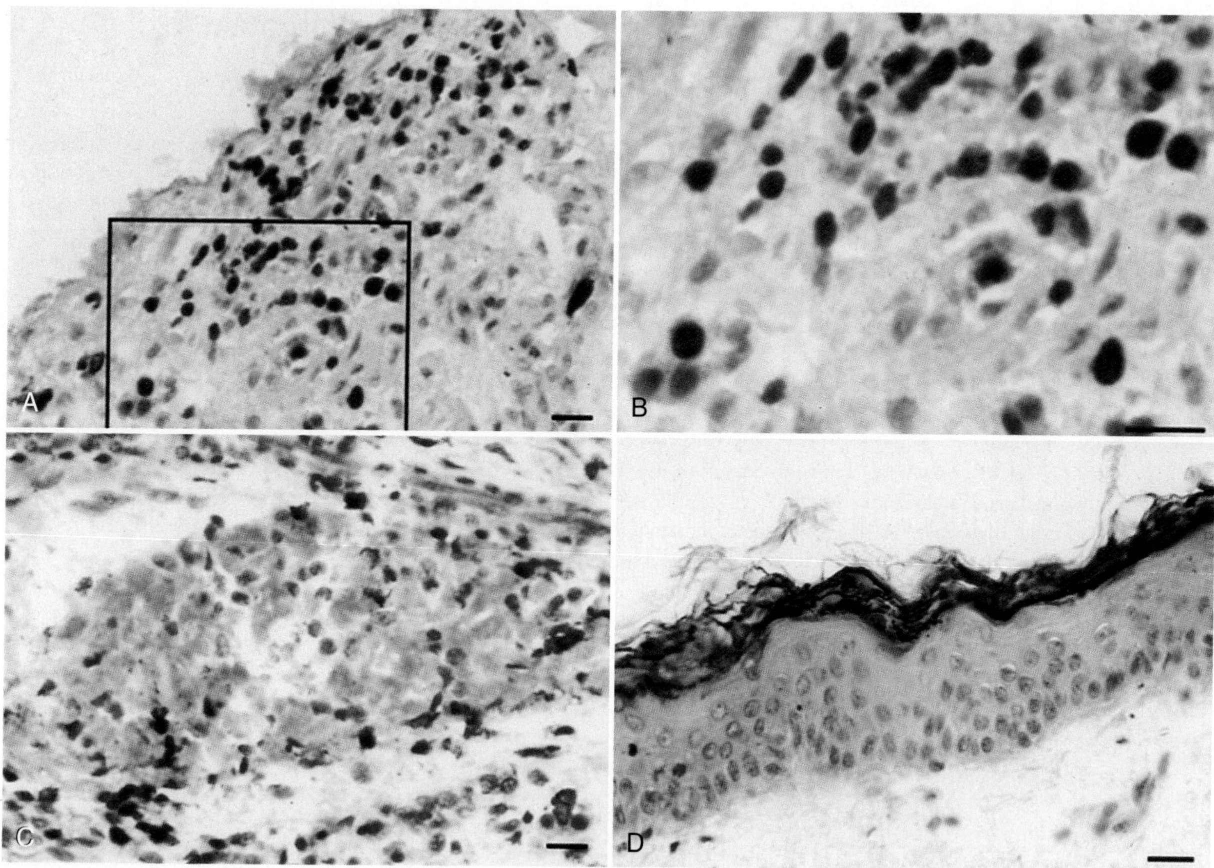

Figure 8J-4. Detection of deiminated (i.e., citrullinated) proteins in RA synovial tissue as demonstrated by immunoperoxidase staining with an antibody to modified citrulline. (A, B) In positive synovial membranes, the cytoplasm of numerous macrophage-like or fibroblast-like mononuclear cells, located in the lining or in the deep synovium, is intensely stained. (C) In addition, the staining of interstitial amorphous deposits located in the vicinity or close periphery of labeled mononuclear cells is observed in the deep synovium. (D) For comparison, a section of human skin is shown, where the whole cornified layer of the epidermis (containing deiminated filaggrin) is stained. Scale bars, 50 mm. (With permission of the American Association of Immunologists, from Masson-Bessiere C, Sebbag M, Girbal-Neuhauser E, et al. The major synovial targets of the rheumatoid arthritis-specific antifilaggrin autoantibodies are deiminated forms of the alpha- and beta-chains of fibrin. *J Immunol* 2001;166(6):4177–4184.)

rheumatoid joint.[39] Their occurrence shows a strong association with the immunogenetic background, that is, with HLA-DR alleles carrying the "shared epitope,"[40–43] but little is known about autoreactive T cells driving the ACPA response.[44,45] Thus far, direct experimental evidence for pathogenetic involvement of ACPAs is scarce, and induction of arthritis in experimental animals by citrullinated fibrinogen or vimentin has not been achieved.[46] Interestingly, however, ACPAs have recently been described in collagen-induced arthritis in mice, which is surprising because the collagen used for immunization is not known to be citrullinated. Remarkably, induction of tolerance to a citrullinated peptide led to a significant reduction in disease susceptibility and administration of monoclonal antibodies against citrullinated fibrinogen enhanced arthritis.[47] These results, which need to be confirmed in other experimental settings, seem to provide direct evidence for the first time of involvement of the anticitrullinated protein autoimmune response in the pathogenesis of erosive arthritis.

ACPAs as Diagnostic and Prognostic Markers

For the detection of ACPAs, several commercial assays are available, most of which use second-generation CCP (CCP2) as the antigen. Other assays use third-generation CCP (CCP3), MCV, or filaggrin, while thus far no assay employing citrullinated fibrinogen has appeared on the market. Assays employing CCP2 show similar performance, while assays employing citrullinated proteins appear to be somewhat less specific.[26,48] However, antibodies to MCV seem to better correlate with RA disease activity than anti-CCP antibodies,[34,49] and may therefore provide additional information. Moreover, even though anti-CCP and anti-MCV antibodies are largely overlapping, anti-MCV antibodies may also occur in anti-CCP (and RF)–negative patients.[49–51] It is not known whether patients recognizing solely MCV differ clinically from patients recognizing both CCP and MCV, but this question will certainly be addressed in future studies.

Similar to RF, ACPAs are present early in the course of the disease and may also precede clinical onset.[4,5,7,9,10,52–55] ACPAs have a specificity for RA of at least 95% and a diagnostic sensitivity of approximately 75% in established RA. However, their sensitivity at disease onset was found to be below 50% in patients with very short disease duration and between 55% and 64% in patients with less than 1 year of disease duration (Table 8J-3). The positive predictive value of ACPAs is greater than 90%, which is comparable or even superior to high-titer IgM-RF.[7,55,56] In all studies, ACPAs and IgM-RF were found to be highly associated with each other, particularly in early RA where two-thirds or even more of ACPA-positive patients are usually also positive for IgM-RF (Table 8J-3).

Significant correlations between the presence of ACPAs and radiographic disease progression (i.e., erosiveness) have been established in several retrospective and longitudinal studies (Figure 8J-5). Most of these studies demonstrated the prognostic value of ACPAs, particularly the correlation with bone damage.[7,12,15,52,55,57,58] Furthermore, ACPAs were found to be significantly associated with the presence of RA-associated HLA-DR alleles ("the shared epitope"), and ACPA-positive carriers of the shared epitope appear to be at particularly high risk for developing severe forms of RA.[41,59,60] Thus, ACPAs are extremely valuable marker antibodies whose determination is particularly useful in RF-negative patients with early arthritis who do not yet fulfill the diagnostic criteria for RA.

Autoantibodies to Heterogeneous Nuclear Ribonucleoprotein A2 (Anti-RA33)

General Properties

In contrast to most other systemic autoimmune diseases, nuclear antigens do not form common target structures in RA. Thus, the incidence of antinuclear antibodies as detected by indirect immunofluorescence is only 20% to 30% and antibodies are usually directed to antigens that are also targeted in other disease, and therefore they are of little if any relevance for diagnostic purposes. An exception is the heterogeneous nuclear ribonucleoprotein (hnRNP) A2, which appears to have some relevance both for pathogenesis and diagnosis of RA. The antigen, which was initially termed RA33, is a 36 kDa protein that is associated with mRNA and involved in regulation of pre-mRNA splicing, mRNA transport, and translation. HnRNP-A2 is more or less ubiquitously expressed, with the highest expression levels observed in skin, lymphoid tissue, the brain, and reproductive organs.[61]

Autoantibodies to hnRNP A2, which are commonly known as anti-RA33 antibodies, occur in approximately one-third of RA patients and with similar frequency in patients with SLE or

Table 8J-3. ACPA and RF in Patients with Early Rheumatoid Arthritis

Author, Year	Disease Duration (months)	Sensitivity (%)	Specificity (%)	RF in ACPA+ Patients (%)
Meyer, 2003[57]	<12	59	—	65
Kastbom, 2004[58]	<12	64	—	78
Forslind, 2004[54]	<12	55	—	90
Nielen, 2005[5]	<10	58	94	75
Soderlin, 2004[56]	<3	44	96	82
Nell, 2005[7]	<3	41	98	67

Notes: In all studies, ACPAs were measured by anti-CCP ELISAs. In patients with very early RA with a disease duration of less than 3 months, ACPAs were detected in less than 50% of the samples, while prevalence was between 55% and 64% in patients with disease duration of less than 12 months.

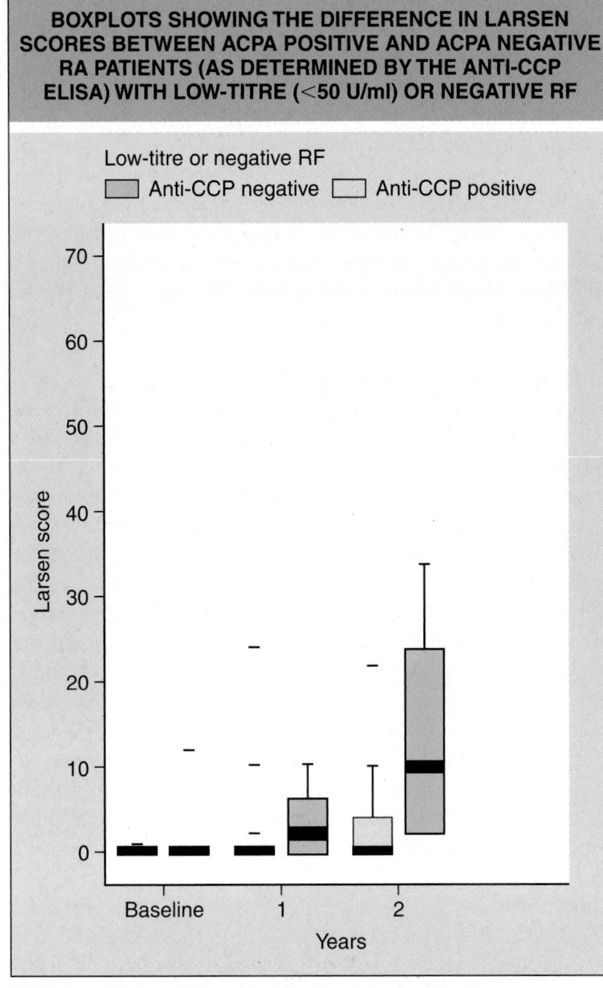

Figure 8J-5. ACPAs are predictive of rapid radiographic progression. Box plots showing the difference in Larsen scores between ACPA-positive and -negative RA patients (as determined by the anti-CCP ELISA) with low-titer (<50 U/ml) or negative RF. The boxes show median values and 25th/75th percentiles. Baseline values were similar in both groups, but Larsen score progression was significantly higher in ACPA-positive patients ($p=0.038$). (Adapted from Nell V, Machold KP, Stamm TA, et al. Autoantibody profiling as early diagnostic and prognostic tool for rheumatoid arthritis. *Ann Rheum Dis* 2005;64(12):1731–1736.)

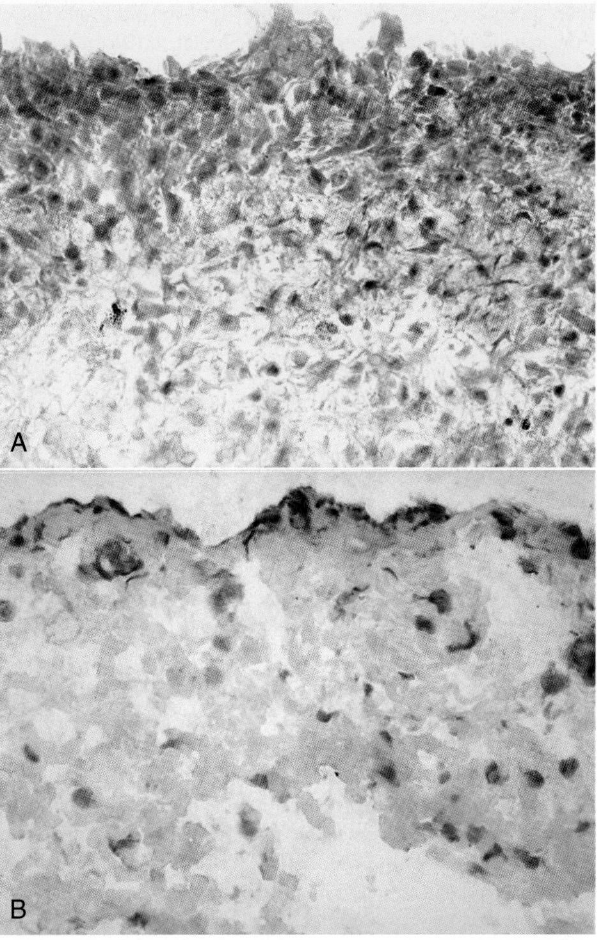

Figure 8J-6. Expression of hnRNP-A2 (RA33) in human synovial tissue as demonstrated by immunoperoxidase staining with a monoclonal antibody to hnRNP-A2. Pronounced staining of macrophage-like and fibroblast-like cells overexpressing hnRNP-A2 is seen in the lining layer and the sublining area of RA synovial tissue, whereas expression is barely detectable in osteoarthritis synovial tissue. (From Hochberg MC, Silman AJ, Smolen JS, et al. *Rheumatology*, 4th ed. London: Mosby, 2008, fig. 78.9, 825.)

mixed connective tissue disease, while they are rare in other rheumatic disorders.[62] In patients with SLE, their occurrence is significantly associated with the presence of antibodies to spliceosomal antigens (such as Sm and U1 snRNP), which are virtually never targeted in RA.[63]

Pathogenetic Involvement

Pronounced T-cell reactivity to hnRNP-A2 has been observed in patients with RA, but not in patients with osteoarthritis or psoriatic arthritis, and the antigen was found to be highly overexpressed in inflamed synovial tissue, while expression was low in normal joints (Figure 8J-6).[44] Remarkably, antibodies to hnRNP-A2 were also found to spontaneously occur in animal models of arthritis, namely in TNF-α transgenic mice,[64] and most recently in rats with pristane-induced arthritis that also showed pronounced T-cell reactivity.[65] Similar to RA, joint-specific overexpression was seen in both models. Importantly, and of great relevance for possible pathogenetic involvement, immunization of TNF transgenic mice with a peptide corresponding to a major B-cell epitope significantly enhanced arthritis.[64] Taken together, these findings point to a role of hnRNP-A2 in the pathogenesis of erosive arthritis that remains to be proven.

Anti-RA33 (hnRNP-A2) Antibodies as Diagnostic and Prognostic Markers

Since anti-RA33 antibodies occur in about one-third of RA patients, but are rare in arthritides with a nonautoimmune pathogenesis (such as osteoarthritis, reactive arthritis, ankylosing spondylitis, or psoriatic arthritis), they can be helpful for differential diagnosis, particularly in patients with early arthritis who are negative for RF and/or ACPAs. Anti-RA33 antibodies have a specificity of approximately 90% for RA, which is lower than specificity of ACPAs or high-titer IgM-RF, but much better than specificity of low-titer IgM-RF.[7] Similar to RF and ACPAs, anti-RA33 antibodies may be present already in the earliest stages of the disease. Importantly, they do not correlate with IgM-RF or ACPAs, and are also not associated with radiographic progression, but rather seem to characterize patients with a more favorable prognosis.[7]

Autoantibodies to Other Proteins

In recent decades, several antigens have been described to be targeted by autoantibodies from patients with RA. These include collagen and other cartilage proteins, various stress or heat-shock proteins, and proteins with enzymatic properties. However, so far none of these antigens has proven useful for diagnostic or prognostic purposes.

Collagen

Among the 14 different collagens, type II collagen is the major collagen species in the joint and also the major collagen antigen. Antibodies can be directed to both native and denatured forms of collagen II. They are found in numerous pathologic conditions, and are therefore not specific for RA. Antibodies to collagen II are present in RA synovial fluids and are presumably locally produced in the joint as indicated by higher antibody levels in synovial fluid than in serum. Furthermore, anticollagen antibodies as well as other autoantibodies and immune complexes may be contained within the cartilage that is ready to absorb and bind these molecules. It is therefore conceivable that immobilized IgG within the cartilage matrix may contribute to local macrophage activation and inflammation in RA. Even though pathogenicity of anticollagen autoimmunity is obvious in collagen-induced arthritis, there is not much evidence that anticollagen autoantibodies play a major role in the pathogenesis of human RA. However, recent observations that ACPAs may recognize *in vitro* deiminated collagens may shed some new light on a role for collagen as autoantigen in the pathogenesis of RA.[37,38]

The prevalence of anticollagen II antibodies in RA has been reported at between 10% and 50%, and titers may be particularly high in early disease and decline as the disease progresses,[66,67] but the published data are sometimes contradictory and presumably at least partially reflect differences in the assays used for determination of anticollagen II antibodies. High levels of serum antibodies to native collagen II are restricted to a subset of patients with RA, leprosy and relapsing polychondritis, whereas low-titer antibodies and those to denatured collagen II are found more generally. Most studies do not find a significant correlation between autoantibodies to collagen II and disease duration, activity, and severity of RA. Because of this and due to their apparent lack of disease specificity, anticollagen antibodies are generally not considered as useful diagnostic markers.

Stress or Heat-Shock Proteins

Stress or heat-shock proteins are required for correct folding and transport of newly synthesized proteins between cellular compartments. They are upregulated under conditions of cellular stress and protect cells from severe damage and premature death. Stress proteins are evolutionarily highly conserved from bacteria to humans and are among the most immunodominant microbial antigens. This has led to speculations about potentially pathogenetic cross-reactivities that might arise in the course of infections.[68] Antibodies to stress proteins can be found in many pathologic conditions, including rheumatic diseases, and may also occur in healthy individuals but do in general not show specificity for any disease,[69] even though they may be elevated in sera of RA patients as compared to patients with osteoarthritis, as recently demonstrated for the 78-kDa stress protein BiP.[70] Therefore, antibodies to stress proteins are of little if any diagnostic value. However, cellular autoimmunity to heat shock proteins seems to play a beneficial role in RA involving mostly Th2 and Treg responses and may have therapeutic implications.[71]

Glucose-6 Phosphate Isomerase

Glucose-6 phosphate isomerase (GPI) is a highly conserved glycolytic enzyme that catalyzes the interconversion of glucose-6 phosphate and fructose-6 phosphate. GPI was identified as the arthritogenic autoantigen in the KRNxNOD mouse model of RA in which a transgenic T-cell receptor induces arthritis closely resembling human RA. In this model, arthritis is dependent on both T and B cells, and disease can be transferred by anti-GPI autoantibodies in a complement-dependent manner.[72] Moreover, immunization with GPI has been shown to induce arthritis in susceptible mouse strains.[73] Although anti-GPI antibodies may be present in sera and synovial fluids of RA patients, their incidence is low and they are by no means specific for RA.[74,75] Interestingly, however, they were found with increased frequency in RA patients suffering from extra-articular manifestations (Felty's syndrome), which may be indicative of a potential pathogenetic role in human RA.[76]

Calpastatin

Calpastatin is a natural inhibitor of the protease calpain, and both proteins can be found in elevated concentrations in RA synovial fluid. Antibodies to calpastatin have been described to occur in 40% to 60% of RA patients but also in other autoimmune diseases, and it has been suggested that anticalpastatin antibodies may contribute to RA pathology by inhibiting calpastatin function thereby aggravating disease.[77] In contrast to Caucasian patients, anticalpastatin antibodies showed high sensitivity and specificity for RA in Japanese patients and thus might be diagnostically useful at least in the Japanese population.[78] It is noteworthy that their occurrence in Caucasian RA patients has recently been found to be significantly associated with the shared epitope containing allele HLA-DR*0404 allele.[79]

Discussion: Role of Autoantibodies in Pathogenesis of Rheumatoid Arthritis

Despite many years of intensive research, the role of autoimmune reactions in the pathogenesis of RA is still incompletely understood. The search for antigens that might induce or modulate the disease has led to the identification of novel autoantigens and characterization of the autoimmune responses directed to them. Similar to RF, the majority of these responses are not particularly specific for RA at the B-cell or T-cell level. A most remarkable exception are ACPAs, that is, antibodies targeting citrullinated proteins, which are almost exclusively present in RA patients showing the highest disease specificity for RA of all autoantibodies identified thus far. However, as with other autoimmune responses in RA, the pathogenetic role of ACPAs is not fully understood.[17,18] The immunologic conflict they induce when binding their targets in the synovial tissue probably has proinflammatory effects, leading to B- and T-cell stimulation, inducing fibrinogen extravasation, fibrin formation, and then deimination. This is most likely a self-maintained process that is presumably at least partly responsible for the chronicity of the disease (Figure 8J-7). The immune complex ACPA-citrullinated fibrin may represent the main target for RF, which would also explain the close association of these two antibodies that has been observed in numerous studies. Since fibrin deposition occurs after the onset of joint inflammation, ACPAs might be initially induced by another antigen and subsequently cross-react with deiminated fibrin. Thus, ACPAs may be primarily directed to vimentin or another citrullinated antigen yet to be identified and later spread to citrullinated fibrin and other deiminated proteins deposited in the joint. Subsequently, novel ACPAs may arise as a consequence of the pathologic alterations in the joint, which may be also true for other autoimmune reactions in RA.

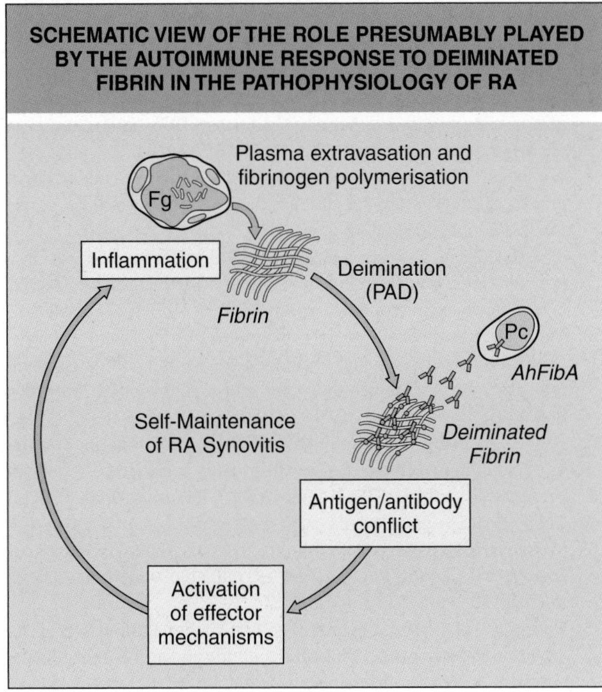

Figure 8J-7. Schematic view of the role presumably played by the autoimmune response to deiminated fibrin in the pathophysiology of RA. In the rheumatoid synovial tissue fibrin is deiminated by PAD isoforms PAD2 and PAD4 which are abundantly expressed by synovial monocytes/macrophages and granulocytes, and becomes the target of the disease-specific antibodies (AhFibA), locally produced by synovial plasmocytes (Pc). This leads to an antigen/antibody conflict that, via activation of effector mechanisms probably involving complement and/or Fc receptors, has proinflammatory effects. In turn, these effects lead to plasma extravasation and fibrinogen polymerization, and therefore provoke the formation of new fibrin deposits in the tissue, which become the substrate of one or several locally expressed PAD. This closes a vicious circle that could account for the self-maintenance of rheumatoid inflammation. In the synovial tissue of nonRA patients, even if deiminated fibrin is present, the absence of AhFibA prevents establishment of this self-maintenance loop. Fg, fibrinogen. (From Hochberg MC, Silman AJ, Smolen JS, et al. *Rheumatology*, 4th ed. London: Mosby, 2008, fig. 78.10, 826.)

Concerning joint-specific antigens such as collagen II, the inflammatory and destructive processes lead to abundant release of materials, which may give rise to autoimmunization of the patient via phagocytosing macrophages and dendritic cells, and subsequent immune complex formation, which may also involve RFs.[80] Autoimmune reactions to ubiquitously expressed proteins may arise due to overexpression, post-translational modification, and aberrant processing of the antigens induced and maintained by the proinflammatory milieu within the joint as observed for stress proteins or hnRNP-A2. Thus, based on a susceptible genetic background (particularly HLA-DR) and environmental factors (particularly tobacco consumption), an increasing number of autoimmune reactions may be generated in the course of disease, all of which may somehow contribute to the pathophysiology of RA.[81,82]

The lack of disease specificity of autoantibodies other than ACPAs does not necessarily exclude a pathogenetic role for them. In other systemic autoimmune diseases as well, only a few antibodies are truly disease specific, while several diagnostically useful marker antibodies may show only a preponderance for a certain disease. For example, antiphospholipid antibodies are not specific for the antiphospholipid syndrome, but are nevertheless among the pathogenetic key players of this condition. Moreover, even if the antibodies may represent only epiphenomena, the underlying T-cellular autoimmune responses may be essentially involved in the pathogenesis of systemic autoimmune disorders by virtue of production of proinflammatory cytokines and/or by exerting cytotoxic functions. Thus, histone-specific T cells are known to drive the autoantibody response to dsDNA in SLE, which is both disease-specific and of pathogenetic relevance, while antihistone antibodies are not specific for SLE and can be found in both rheumatic and nonrheumatic diseases. Therefore, it is conceivable that autoreactive T cells directed to a large number of antigens are presumably operative in the joint and may initiate, perpetuate, but also downmodulate, the disease process.[44,45,65,71,83–86]

Due to the exciting observations made in recent years, autoantibodies are no longer regarded as epiphenomena and may be quite useful as diagnostic markers. Identification of new autoantigens and the characterization of the cellular and molecular processes underlying the pathologic autoimmune reactions against them has provided new insights into the pathogenesis of RA. A better understanding of the disease process will finally make possible the development of novel therapeutic concepts that may allow treatment of the disease in its initial stages in an antigen-specific manner, bearing in mind that this may be the only way to definitely cure RA and other autoimmune diseases.

Acknowledgments

This work was supported by CeMM, the Center for Molecular Medicine of the Austrian Academy of Sciences, and by funding from a European Union Framework 6 Integrated Project (Autocure).

References

1. Sutton B, Corper A, Bonagura V, et al. The structure and origin of rheumatoid factors. *Immunol Today* 2000;21(4):177–183.
2. Westwood OM, Nelson PN, Hay FC. Rheumatoid factors: What's new? *Rheumatology* 2006;45(4):379–385.
3. Dorner T, Egerer K, Feist E, et al. Rheumatoid factor revisited. *Curr Opin Rheum* 2004;16(3):246–253.
4. Jansen AL, van der Horst-Bruinsma I, van Schaardenburg D, et al. Rheumatoid factor and antibodies to cyclic citrullinated peptide differentiate rheumatoid arthritis from undifferentiated polyarthritis in patients with early arthritis. *J Rheumatol* 2002;29(10):2074–2076.
5. Nielen MM, van der Horst AR, van Schaardenburg D, et al. Antibodies to citrullinated human fibrinogen (ACF) have diagnostic and prognostic value in early arthritis. *Ann Rheum Dis* 2005;64(8):1199–1204.
6. Sinclair D, Hull RG. Why do general practitioners request rheumatoid factor? A study of symptoms, requesting patterns and patient outcome. *Ann Clin Biochem* 2003;40(Pt 2):131–137.
7. Nell V, Machold KP, Stamm TA, et al. Autoantibody profiling as early diagnostic and prognostic tool for rheumatoid arthritis. *Ann Rheum Dis* 2005;64(12):1731–1736.
8. Symmons DP. Classification criteria for rheumatoid arthritis—time to abandon rheumatoid factor? *Rheumatology* 2007;46(5):725–726.
9. Rantapaa-Dahlqvist S, de Jong BA, et al. Antibodies against cyclic citrullinated peptide and IgA rheumatoid factor predict the development of rheumatoid arthritis. *Arthritis Rheum* 2003;48(10):2741–2749.
10. Nielen MMJ, van Schaardenburg D, Reesink HWR, et al. Specific autoantibodies precede the symptoms of rheumatoid arthritis: A study of serial measurements in blood donors. *Arthritis Rheum* 2004;50(2):380–386.
11. Jonsson T, Steinsson K, Jonsson H, et al. Combined elevation of IgM and IgA rheumatoid factor has high diagnostic specificity for rheumatoid arthritis. *Rheumatol Int* 1998;18(3):119–122.
12. Bas S, Genevay S, Meyer O, et al. Anti-cyclic citrullinated peptide antibodies, IgM and IgA rheumatoid factors in the diagnosis and prognosis of rheumatoid arthritis. *Rheumatology* 2003;42(5):677–680.
13. Greiner A, Plischke H, Kellner H, et al. Association of anti-cyclic citrullinated peptide antibodies, anti-citrullin antibodies, and IgM and IgA rheumatoid factors with serological parameters of disease activity in rheumatoid arthritis. *Ann N Y Acad Sci* 2005;1050:295–303.
14. Scott DL. Prognostic factors in early rheumatoid arthritis. *Rheumatology* 2000(39):124–129.
15. Lindqvist E, Eberhardt K, Bendtzen K, et al. Prognostic laboratory markers of joint damage in rheumatoid arthritis. *Ann Rheum Dis* 2005;64(2):196–201.
16. Turesson C, Jacobsson LT, Sturfelt G, et al. Rheumatoid factor and antibodies to cyclic citrullinated peptides are associated with severe extra-articular manifestations in rheumatoid arthritis. *Ann Rheum Dis* 2007;66(1):59–64.
17. Vossenaar ER, van Venrooij WJ. Citrullinated proteins: Sparks that may ignite the fire in rheumatoid arthritis. *Arthritis Res Ther* 2004;6(3):107–111.
18. Vincent C, Nogueira L, Clavel C, et al. Autoantibodies to citrullinated proteins: ACPA. *Autoimmunity* 2005;38(1):17–24.
19. Simon M, Girbal E, Sebbag M, et al. The cytokeratin filament-aggregating protein filaggrin is the target of the so-called "antikeratin antibodies," autoantibodies specific for rheumatoid arthritis. *J Clin Invest* 1993;92(3):1387–1393.
20. Youinou P, Serre G. The antiperinuclear factor and antikeratin antibody systems. *Int Arch Allergy Immunol* 1995;107(4):508–518.
21. Schellekens GA, de Jong BA, van den Hoogen FH, et al. Citrulline is an essential constituent of antigenic determinants recognized by rheumatoid arthritis–specific autoantibodies. *J Clin Invest* 1998;101(1):273–281.
22. Girbal Neuhauser E, Durieux JJ, et al. The epitopes targeted by the rheumatoid arthritis-associated antifilaggrin autoantibodies are posttranslationally generated on various sites of (pro)filaggrin by deimination of arginine residues. *J Immunol* 1999;162(1):585–594.
23. Union A, Meheus L, Humbel RL, et al. Identification of citrullinated rheumatoid arthritis–specific epitopes in natural filaggrin relevant for antifilaggrin autoantibody detection by LINE immunoassay. *Arthritis Rheum* 2002;46(5):1185–1195.
24. Schellekens GA, Visser H, de Jong BA, et al. The diagnostic properties of rheumatoid arthritis antibodies recognizing a cyclic citrullinated peptide. *Arthritis Rheum* 2000;43(1):155–163.
25. Zendman AJ, van Venrooij WJ, Pruijn GJ. Use and significance of anti-CCP autoantibodies in rheumatoid arthritis. *Rheumatology* 2006;45(1):20–25.
26. Bizzaro N, Tonutti E, Tozzoli R, et al. Analytical and diagnostic characteristics of 11 2nd- and 3rd-generation immunoenzymatic methods for the detection of antibodies to citrullinated proteins. *Clin Chem* 2007;53(8):1527–1533.
27. Masson-Bessiere C, Sebbag M, Girbal-Neuhauser E, et al. The major synovial targets of the rheumatoid arthritis–specific antifilaggrin autoantibodies are deiminated forms of the alpha- and beta-chains of fibrin. *J Immunol* 2001;166(6):4177–4184.
28. Vossenaar ER, Smeets TJ, Kraan MC, et al. The presence of citrullinated proteins is not specific for rheumatoid synovial tissue. *Arthritis Rheum* 2004;50(11):3485–3494.
29. Chapuy-Regaud S, Sebbag M, Baeten D, et al. Fibrin deimination in synovial tissue is not specific for rheumatoid arthritis but commonly occurs during synovitides. *J Immunol* 2005;174(8):5057–5064.
30. Vander Cruyssen B, Cantaert T, Nogueira L, et al. Diagnostic value of anti-human citrullinated fibrinogen ELISA and comparison with four other anti-citrullinated protein assays. *Arthritis Res Ther* 2006;8(4):R122.
31. Hill JA, Al-Bishri J, Gladman DD, et al. Serum autoantibodies that bind citrullinated fibrinogen are frequently found in patients with rheumatoid arthritis. [See comment.] *J Rheumatol* 2006;33(11):2115–2119.
32. Vossenaar ER, Despres N, Lapointe E, et al. Rheumatoid arthritis specific anti-Sa antibodies target citrullinated vimentin. *Arthritis Res Ther* 2004;6(2):R142–R150.
33. Rodriguez-Mahou M, Lopez-Longo FJ, Sanchez-Ramon S, et al. Association of anti-cyclic citrullinated peptide and anti-Sa/citrullinated vimentin autoantibodies in rheumatoid arthritis. *Arthritis Rheum* 2006;55(4):657–661.
34. Bang H, Egerer K, Gauliard A, et al. Mutation and citrullination modifies vimentin to a novel autoantigen for rheumatoid arthritis. *Arthritis Rheum* 2007;56(8):2503–2511.
35. Kinloch A, Tatzer V, Wait R, et al. Identification of citrullinated alpha-enolase as a candidate autoantigen in rheumatoid arthritis. *Arthritis Res Ther* 2005;7(6):R1421–R1429.
36. Pratesi F, Tommasi C, Anzilotti C, et al. Deiminated Epstein-Barr virus nuclear antigen 1 is a target of anti-citrullinated protein antibodies in rheumatoid arthritis. *Arthritis Rheum* 2006;54(3):733–741.
37. Burkhardt H, Sehnert B, Bockermann R, et al. Humoral immune response to citrullinated collagen type II determinants in early rheumatoid arthritis. European *J Immunol* 2005;35(5):1643–1652.
38. Suzuki A, Yamada R, Ohtake-Yamanaka M, et al. Anti-citrullinated collagen type I antibody is a target of autoimmunity in rheumatoid arthritis. *Biochem Biophys Res Commun* 2005;333(2):418–426.
39. Masson Bessiere C, Sebbag M, Durieux JJ, et al. In the rheumatoid pannus, anti-filaggrin autoantibodies are produced by local plasma cells and constitute a higher proportion of IgG than in synovial fluid and serum. *Clin Exp Immunol* 2000;119(3):544–552.

40. Klareskog L, Padyukov L, Ronnelid J, et al. Genes, environment and immunity in the development of rheumatoid arthritis. *Curr Opin Immunol* 2006;18(6):650–655.
41. van der Helm-van Mil AH, Verpoort KN, Breedveld FC, et al. The HLA-DRB1 shared epitope alleles are primarily a risk factor for anti-cyclic citrullinated peptide antibodies and are not an independent risk factor for development of rheumatoid arthritis. *Arthritis Rheum* 2006;54(4):1117–1121.
42. Gourraud PA, Dieude P, Boyer JF, et al. A new classification of HLA-DRB1 alleles differentiates predisposing and protective alleles for autoantibody production in rheumatoid arthritis. *Arthritis Res Ther* 2007;9(2):R27.
43. Verpoort KN, Cheung K, Ioan-Facsinay A, et al. Fine specificity of the anti-citrullinated protein antibody response is influenced by the shared epitope alleles. *Arthritis Rheum* 2007;56(12):3949–3952.
44. Fritsch R, Eselböck D, Skriner K, Jahn-Schmid B, et al. Characterization of autoreactive T cells to the autoantigens RA33 (hnRNP A2) and filaggrin in patients with rheumatoid arthritis. *J Immunol* 2002; 169:1068–1076.
45. Auger I, Sebbag M, Vincent C, et al. Influence of HLA-DR genes on the production of rheumatoid arthritis–specific autoantibodies to citrullinated fibrinogen. *Arthritis Rheum* 2005;52(11):3424–3432.
46. Duplan V, Foulquier C, Clavel C, et al. In the rat, citrullinated autologous fibrinogen is immunogenic but the induced autoimmune response is not arthritogenic. *Clin Exp Immunol* 2006;145(3):502–512.
47. Kuhn KA, Kulik L, Tomooka B, et al. Antibodies against citrullinated proteins enhance tissue injury in experimental autoimmune arthritis. *J Clin Invest* 2006;116(4):961–973.
48. Coenen D, Verschueren P, Westhovens R, et al. Technical and diagnostic performance of 6 assays for the measurement of citrullinated protein/peptide antibodies in the diagnosis of rheumatoid arthritis. *Clin Chem* 2007;53(3):498–504.
49. Poulsom H, Charles P. Antibodies to citrullinated vimentin are a specific and sensitive marker for the diagnosis of rheumatoid arthritis. *Clin Rev Allergy Immunol* 2008;34:4–10.
50. Dejaco C, Klotz W, Larcher H, et al. Diagnostic value of antibodies against a modified citrullinated vimentin in rheumatoid arthritis. *Arthritis Res Ther* 2006;8(4):R119.
51. Soos L, Szekanecz Z, Szabo Z, et al. Clinical evaluation of anti-mutated citrullinated vimentin by ELISA in rheumatoid arthritis. *J Rheumatol* 2007;34(8):1658–1663.
52. Visser H, le Cessie S, Vos K, et al. How to diagnose rheumatoid arthritis early: A prediction model for persistent (erosive) arthritis. *Arthritis Rheum* 2002;46(2):357–365.
53. Jansen LM, van Schaardenburg D, van der Horst-Bruinsma I, et al. The predictive value of anti-cyclic citrullinated peptide antibodies in early arthritis. *J Rheumatol* 2003;30(8):1691–1695.
54. Forslind K, Ahlmen M, Eberhardt K, et al. Prediction of radiological outcome in early rheumatoid arthritis in clinical practice: Role of antibodies to citrullinated peptides (anti-CCP). *Ann Rheum Dis* 2004;63(9):1090–1095.
55. van Gaalen FA, Linn-Rasker SP, van Venrooij WJ, et al. Autoantibodies to cyclic citrullinated peptides predict progression to rheumatoid arthritis in patients with undifferentiated arthritis: A prospective cohort study. *Arthritis Rheum* 2004;50(3):709–715.
56. Soderlin MK, Kastbom A, Kautiainen H, et al. Antibodies against cyclic citrullinated peptide (CCP) and levels of cartilage oligomeric matrix protein (COMP) in very early arthritis: Relation to diagnosis and disease activity. Scandinavian *J Rheumatol* 2004;33(3):185–188.
57. Meyer O, Labarre C, Dougados M, et al. Anticitrullinated protein/peptide antibody assays in early rheumatoid arthritis for predicting five year radiographic damage. *Ann Rheum Dis* 2003;62(2):120–126.
58. Kastbom A, Strandberg G, Lindroos A, et al. Anti-CCP antibody test predicts the disease course during 3 years in early rheumatoid arthritis (the Swedish TIRA project). *Ann Rheum Dis* 2004;63(9):1085–1089.
59. van Gaalen FA, van Aken J, Huizinga TW, et al. Association between HLA class II genes and autoantibodies to cyclic citrullinated peptides (CCPs) influences the severity of rheumatoid arthritis. *Arthritis Rheum* 2004;50(7):2113–2121.
60. Berglin E, Padyukov L, Sundin U, et al. A combination of autoantibodies to cyclic citrullinated peptide (CCP) and HLA-DRB1 locus antigens is strongly associated with future onset of rheumatoid arthritis. *Arthritis Res Ther* 2004;6(4):R303–R308.
61. Kamma H, Horiguchi H, Wan L, et al. Molecular characterization of the hnRNP A2/B1 proteins: Tissue-specific expression and novel isoforms. *Exp Cell Res* 1999;246(2):399–411.
62. Steiner G, Skriner K, Smolen JS. Autoantibodies to the A/B proteins of the heterogeneous nuclear ribonucleoprotein complex: Novel tools for the diagnosis of rheumatic diseases. *Int Arch Allergy Immunol* 1996;111(4):314–319.
63. Hassfeld W, Steiner G, Studnicka Benke A, et al. Autoimmune response to the spliceosome. An immunologic link between rheumatoid arthritis, mixed connective tissue disease, and systemic lupus erythematosus. *Arthritis Rheum* 1995;38(6):777–785.
64. Hayer S, Tohidast-Akrad M, Haralambous S, et al. Aberrant expression of the autoantigen heterogeneous nuclear ribonucleoprotein-A2 (RA33) and spontaneous formation of rheumatoid arthritis-associated anti-RA33 autoantibodies in TNF-alpha transgenic mice. *J Immunol* 2005;175(12):8327–8336.
65. Hoffmann MH, Tuncel J, Skriner K, et al. The rheumatoid arthritis–associated autoantigen hnRNP-A2 (RA33) is a major stimulator of autoimmunity in rats with pristane-induced arthritis. *J Immunol* 2007;179(11):7568–7576.
66. Cook AD, Rowley MJ, Mackay IR, et al. Antibodies to type II collagen in early rheumatoid arthritis. Correlation with disease progression. *Arthritis Rheum* 1996;39(10):1720–1727.
67. Mullazehi M, Mathsson L, Lampa J, et al. High anti-collagen type-II antibody levels and induction of proinflammatory cytokines by anti-collagen antibody-containing immune complexes in vitro characterise a distinct rheumatoid arthritis phenotype associated with acute inflammation at the time of disease onset. *Ann Rheum Dis* 2007;66(4):537–541.
68. Zugel U, Kaufmann SH. Role of heat shock proteins in protection from and pathogenesis of infectious diseases. *Clin Microbiol Rev* 1999;12(1):19–39.
69. Tishler M, Shoenfeld Y. Anti-heat-shock protein antibodies in rheumatic and autoimmune diseases. Semin *Arthritis Rheum* 1996;26(2): 558–563.
70. Bodman-Smith MD, Corrigall VM, Berglin E, et al. Antibody response to the human stress protein BiP in rheumatoid arthritis. *Rheumatology* 2004;43(10):1283–1287.
71. van Eden W, van der Zee R, Prakken B. Heat-shock proteins induce T-cell regulation of chronic inflammation. *Nat Rev Immunol* 2005; 5(4):318–330.
72. Ditzel HJ. The K/BxN mouse: A model of human inflammatory arthritis. *Trends Mol Med* 2004;10(1):40–45.
73. Kamradt T, Schubert D. The role and clinical implications of G6PI in experimental models of rheumatoid arthritis. *Arthritis Res Ther* 2005;7(1):20–28.
74. Kassahn D, Kolb C, Solomon S, et al. Few human autoimmune sera detect GPI. *Nat Immunol* 2002;3(5):411–412.
75. Matsumoto I, Lee DM, Goldbach-Mansky R, et al. Low prevalence of antibodies to glucose-6-phosphate isomerase in patients with rheumatoid arthritis and a spectrum of other chronic autoimmune disorders. *Arthritis Rheum* 2003;48(4):944–954.
76. van Gaalen FA, Toes RE, Ditzel HJ, et al. Association of autoantibodies to glucose-6-phosphate isomerase with extraarticular complications in rheumatoid arthritis. *Arthritis Rheum* 2004;50(2):395–399.
77. Menard HA, el Amine M. The calpain-calpastatin system in rheumatoid arthritis. *Immunol Today* 1996;17(12):545–547.
78. Iwaki-Egawa S, Matsuno H, Yudoh K, et al. High diagnostic value of anticalpastatin autoantibodies in rheumatoid arthritis detected by ELISA using human erythrocyte calpastatin as antigen. *J Rheumatol* 2004;31(1):17–22.

79. Auger I, Roudier C, Guis S, et al. HLA-DRB1*0404 is strongly associated with anticalpastatin antibodies in rheumatoid arthritis. *Ann Rheum Dis* 2007;66(12):1588–1593.
80. Mullazehi M, Mathsson L, Lampa J, et al. Surface-bound anti-type II collagen-containing immune complexes induce production of tumor necrosis factor alpha, interleukin-1beta, and interleukin-8 from peripheral blood monocytes via Fc gamma receptor IIA: A potential pathophysiologic mechanism for humoral anti-type II collagen immunity in arthritis. *Arthritis Rheum* 2006;54(6):1759–1771.
81. Klareskog L, Padyukov L, Lorentzen J, et al. Mechanisms of disease: Genetic susceptibility and environmental triggers in the development of rheumatoid arthritis. *Nat Clin Pract Rheumatol* 2006;2(8): 425–433.
82. Klareskog L, Padyukov L, Alfredsson L. Smoking as a trigger for inflammatory rheumatic diseases. *Curr Opin Rheumatol* 2007;19(1): 49–54.
83. Panayi GS. Targeting of cells involved in the pathogenesis of rheumatoid arthritis. *Rheumatology* 1999;38:10–28.
84. Cope AP, Schulze-Koops H, Aringer M. The central role of T cells in rheumatoid arthritis. *Clin Exp Rheumatol* 2007;25(5 Suppl 46): S4–S11.
85. Toh ML, Miossec P. The role of T cells in rheumatoid arthritis: New subsets and new targets. *Curr Opin Rheumatol* 2007;19(3):284–288.
86. Lutzky S, Hannawi S, Thomas R. Cells of the synovium in rheumatoid arthritis: Dendritic cells. *Arthritis Res Ther* 2007;9:R116–R127.

Complement in Rheumatoid Arthritis

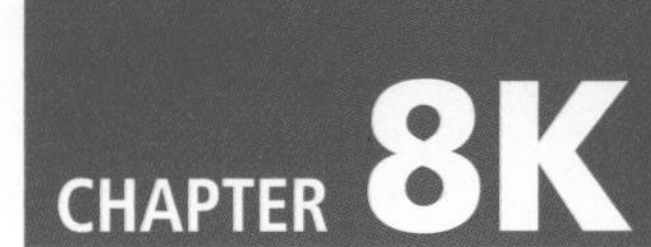

V. Michael Holers

Many lines of evidence support the conclusion that the complement system is intimately involved in the pathogenesis of rheumatoid arthritis (RA). As outlined below, the complement system is an important component of the innate immune system. Innate immune mechanisms are increasingly recognized as the primary means by which the structural components of the joint (synovium, cartilage, bone) become initially inflamed and then ultimately severely damaged. Complement can play several roles in the pathogenesis of RA using both its effector arm, which serves to promote inflammation and recruit neutrophils into the joint, as well as its B-lymphocyte receptors for complement C3 activation fragments. These lymphocyte C3 receptors link the covalent attachment of complement C3 fragments to antigens (Ags) with the subsequent amplification of autoantibody responses to the linked Ags that at the same time also bind their specific cognate B-cell receptors. Because of these many interactions, certain components of the complement system are emerging as potential therapeutic targets for RA, both from the standpoint of modulation of complement effector functions as well as through the regulation of autoreactive B cells. These findings, coupled with the recent development of both small molecule and biologic complement inhibitors that can be used in patients, provide hope that this class of therapeutics may soon join the ranks of useful drugs for this debilitating disease.

Innate and Adaptive Immune Mechanisms, Complement, and Pathogenesis of Rheumatoid Arthritis

The pathogenesis of RA can be divided into three phases: initiation, perpetuation, and chronic inflammation. Innate immune, complement-related mechanisms may be involved in all three stages.[1,2] Whether RA is primarily a disease of the cartilage with secondary extension into the synovium, or a synovial disease that can affect the cartilage, is actively debated. It is likely, though, that both sites (cartilage and synovium) are targets of immune dysregulation.

One initiating mechanism for synovitis may be the local presentation of specific antigenic epitopes to T cells with primary activation of the adaptive immune system. The association of RA with HLA-DR4 and other HLA-DRB1 alleles containing the "shared epitope"[3] has made this concept attractive, although exhaustive efforts to identify the involved antigen(s) in the synovium have largely been negative. A more likely possibility, therefore, is that RA is initiated by nonantigen-specific mechanisms involving innate immune cells and mediators.

The major cells and molecules of the innate immune system, including complement activation fragments and receptors, are all present in the rheumatoid synovium.[4] The role of infectious agents that might activate complement in initiating rheumatoid synovitis remains unknown, although dendritic cells (DCs) and macrophages may transport bacterial or viral fragments from the mucosa of the gastrointestinal tract to the synovium. These materials can stimulate cells through binding to pattern recognition receptors of the toll system, and can also activate the complement system.[5] These early events may all occur before RA becomes clinically evident, and may greatly influence how the autoimmune response develops in the adaptive immune system through interactions with complement receptors on B cells. As the disease process progresses into the second and third phases of perpetuation and chronic inflammation, all remnants of infectious agents might be gone. However, complement may still serve an important role in the episodic promotion of inflammation and activation of T cells through the recognition and activation by molecules formed by enzymatic degradation of endogenous collagen, proteoglycans, and other constituents of the matrix.[6]

Finally, it is also known that autoantibodies such as anti*c*yclic *c*itrullinated *p*eptide (CCP) antibodies (Abs) and rheumatoid factors (RFs) are present in the serum of patients with severe RA, such as patients with bone erosions and in patients whose disease progresses more rapidly despite treatment.[7] These RA-related Abs can also be present for several years prior to clinical disease onset.[8] Recent successful efficacy studies with the B-cell–depleting agent Rituxan (anti-CD20) in RA[9] have focused attention on B lymphocytes, and clearly demonstrated that B cells are pathogenic in the chronic disease phase of RA.[10] As outlined below, complement may also act to mediate the proinflammatory activities of Abs.

Complement Is Key Component of Innate Immune System and Major Link to Adaptive Immunity

The complement pathway is one of the major means by which the body senses that foreign Ags and pathogens have invaded or that cell injury, ischemia, apoptosis, and necrosis have occurred at tissue sites.[11,12] Because of this capacity, complement participates in the regulation of the immune system in response to foreign and potentially self Ags. Consistent with this concept, in addition to playing major roles in the recognition and elimination of pathogens through direct killing[13] or stimulation of phagocytosis,[14] complement has also been shown to play a central role in enhancing humoral immunity to T-dependent and -independent foreign Ags.[15–18] Complement activation also modifies cellular immunity,[19,20] influences the development of the natural Ab repertoire,[21,22] directly recognizes injured self tissues,[23] and regulates tolerance to certain nuclear and other self Ags.[17,24–27]

In addition to important roles in normal host responses to self and foreign Ags, the complement system is increasingly recognized to be causally involved in tissue injury during ischemic, inflammatory, and autoimmune diseases,[28] and major efforts are underway in many laboratories to identify within the more than 30 proteins, activation fragments and receptors that are the key mediators and optimal therapeutic targets. Even though complement is an attractive therapeutic target for a wide range of diseases, much more work in preclinical models is necessary to better understand the roles of this system in inflammatory and autoimmune processes such as RA.

Multiple Recognition Mechanisms Resulting in Complement Activation

The complement system can be activated by each of three distinct pathways: the classical (CP), alternative (AP), and lectin (LP) pathways (Figure 8K-1). Although the CP is typically thought of as activated only by pathogens or immune complexes that contain Ag and IgM or complement-fixing isotypes of IgG, many additional situations have been described in which this complement pathway is initiated (Table 8K-1). For example, the CP can be initiated in the absence of immune complexes directly through the actions of the pentraxin family proteins C-reactive protein (CRP) and serum amyloid P (SAP) protein.[29] Activation occurs in this setting when either of these two proteins bind microbial pathogens or intracellular constituents such as chromatin that are released from necrotic or dying cells, which then allows C1 to be directly bound and the pathway activated. As part of this process, CRP also binds factor H, which likely helps to control excess complement activation. The CP is also activated when C1q binds apoptotic bodies,[30] or when C1q interacts with beta amyloid fibrils or the tau protein.[31,32]

The LP is initiated by the binding of mannose binding lectin (MBL) to repeating simple carbohydrate moieties that are found primarily on the surface of viral and microbial pathogens.[33] In addition, the LP can be activated when it binds to cytokeratin-1 that is exposed on ischemic endothelial cells.[34] MBL is physically associated with proteins designated as mannose-binding, lectin-associated serum protease (MASP)-1, MASP-2, and MASP-3.[35,36] Once MBL is bound to its target, MASPs are activated in a similar fashion as C1r and C1s, resulting in the cleavage of C4 and C2, which is then followed by the assembly of the remainder of the complement pathway. MASP-2 has been

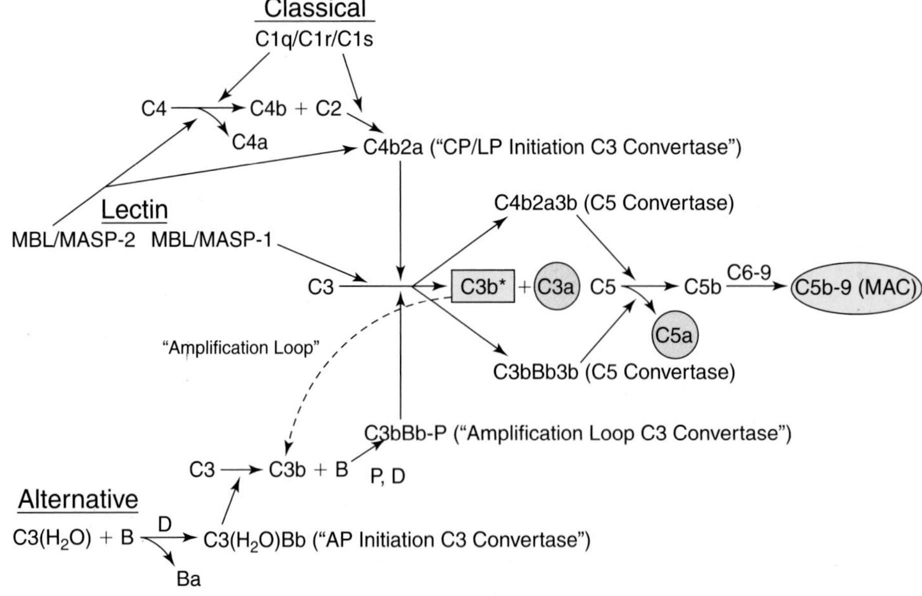

Figure 8K-1. Detailed description of complement activation pathways. Note the distinct functions and locations within the cascade of the "initiation" C3 convertases as compared to the "amplification loop" C3 convertase, which is engaged by target-bound C3b* (center, boxed) that can be generated by any of the three initiation mechanisms, as further described in the text.

Table 8K-1. Mechanisms by Which Three Complement Pathways (CP, AP, and LP) are Proposed to be Initiated and/or Activation Is Promoted *In Vivo*

Classical	Alternative	Lectin
Immune complexes (IgM, IgG)	"Tickover"	Repeating carbohydrates
C-reactive protein (CRP) (chromatin complexes)	Polysaccharides	Ficolins
Endothelial neoepitopes in ischemic tissue	Endotoxin IgA I.C.	Cytokeratin
Beta amyloid fibrils	C3 nephritic factor IgG I.C.	
Apoptotic bodies	Properdin	
Serum amyloid P (SAP)		
Mitochondrial membranes		

shown to directly cleave and activate C4 and C2, while MASP-1 has been shown to be able to cleave C3 directly in a manner that bypasses C4/C2 and is likely to be relevant *in vivo*.[37]

The AP is primarily activated on surfaces that do not express intrinsic membrane complement inhibitors, and/or have neutral or positive charge characteristics that in general restrict the ability of the soluble complement inhibitor factor H to bind to this site. Activation *in vitro* can be due to the process termed "tickover" (Figure 8K-2).[5] Tickover occurs when C3 spontaneously undergoes a conformationally alteration to generate a form called C3(H_2O), which then allows factor B to interact with this new form and be subsequently cleaved to Ba and Bb by the protease factor D. This process generates a C3 convertase that results in the generation of C3b and covalent attachment of C3b to target surfaces. Tickover is likely to be the major mechanism by which the AP activates spontaneously *in vivo*. In addition to tickover, activation of the AP can also be promoted when certain Abs impair endogenous regulatory mechanisms,[38] when expression of complement regulatory proteins is decreased or otherwise altered in a manner that restricts their local activities,[39,40] or by IgA-containing immune complexes.[41]

Importantly, another function of the AP is to greatly increase complement activation through the AP amplification loop, which is engaged when C3b that is generated by any of the three activation-pathway C3 convertases, and is thus found on target surfaces, then serves to bind factor B and also propagate activation of the pathway by this mechanism (Figure 8K-1). The alternative pathway amplification loop can be promoted at sites of local injury when inflammatory cells are recruited, either through a mechanism that involves the additional generation of necrotic cells that fix complement, or more likely because these infiltrating cells bring in C3 and properdin that increase activation specifically at that site.[42]

"Nontraditional" Mechanisms in Complement System May Be Activated *In Vivo*

Table 8K-1 includes a list of commonly accepted mechanisms whereby each of the three complement pathways may be activated. In addition to these means, however, it has been known for several decades that both C3 and C5 can be "activated" *in vitro* by proteases, most commonly those found in the clotting pathway.[43] What has been unknown is whether any of these mechanisms have biologic relevance. However, recent studies have established that C3 in some circumstances, specifically in pulmonary immune complex injury, is not absolutely necessary to activate C5 and generate C5a and cause injury.[44] Thrombin was found to be the apparent mechanism of C5 convertase activity *in vivo*. Potential relevance of this finding to RA is provided by the finding that mice are protected from the development of CIA by treatment with the thrombin inhibitor PEG-hirudin.[45] In addition, thrombin has long been known to be able to cleave C3,[46] and one of the well-known ways to convert purified whole C3 into C3b that is covalently attached to targets *in vitro* is to treat it with low doses of trypsin. Although the C3-cleaving activities have been studied almost exclusively *in vitro*, it is known that thrombin injection into rabbits will activate C3.[47]

Endogenous Complement Control Mechanisms Necessary to Keep System in Check *In Vivo*

Because of the nature of the activation mechanisms, especially tickover-generated autoactivation of the AP that allows for a rapid enzymatic amplification of complement, the complement pathway is tightly controlled at each step by a series of regulatory proteins. These proteins are found in the blood, on cell membranes, in biologic fluids such as tears, and in the interstitial spaces.[48]

There are four main types of intrinsic membrane inhibitors that differ in their target site of activation. One type is illustrated by CD59, a glycolipid-anchored protein that acts to block both the initial insertion of C9 into the MAC as well as the subsequent polymerization of C9.[49] CD59 is a widely distributed protein that is found on the vast majority of cells. A second class of intrinsic inhibitors is directed at the centrally important steps of C3 and C5 activation. These proteins include decay-accelerating factor (DAF, CD55) and membrane cofactor protein (MCP, CD46) in humans, and Crry,[50] two forms of DAF,[51,52] and MCP[53] in mice. These proteins act to either dissociate the alternative and classical pathway C3 and C5 convertases or to act as a cofactor for serum factor I–mediated cleavage and inactivation of C3b and C4b. A third class of cell membrane proteins is exemplified by complement C2 receptor inhibitor trispanning (CRIT).[54] This protein binds to C2 and blocks C2 cleavage, and thus effective classical pathway

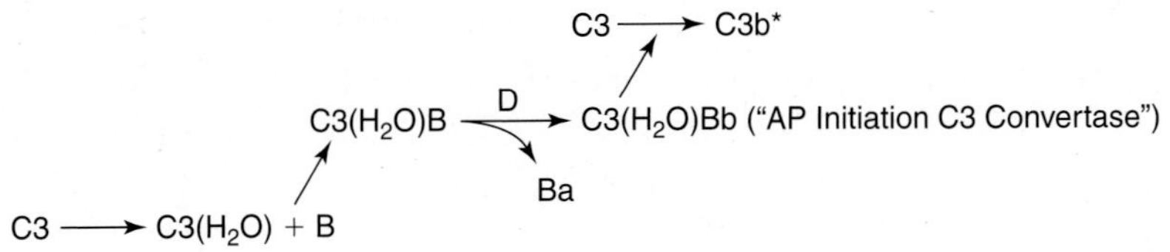

Figure 8K-2. Steps in the initiation of the AP through the tickover mechanism, which then generates tissue-bound, or fluid-phase, C3b (designated as C3b*) in a form that is identical to that generated through the classical and lectin pathways.

convertase formation. Consequently, CRIT apparently functions like other membrane regulatory proteins to block complement activation and cell injury. A fourth type of intrinsic inhibitor proteins is CR-Ig, which blocks the alternative pathway in addition to serving as a circulating immune complex receptor.[55]

The relative importance of the membrane and fluid-phase C3 inhibitors has been increasingly clarified by the use of gene-targeted mice. For instance Crry-/- mice are destroyed at the early fetal stage because of the uncontrolled activation of C3 through the AP in a fashion independent of C5.[40,56] In addition, the use of heterozygous Crry-deficient mice increases local C3 activation and subsequent tissue injury during ischemia-reperfusion injury.[57] Likewise, generation of DAF-deficient mice has shown an increase *in vivo* in autoimmune damage in a model of systemic lupus erythematosus.[58] With regard to MCP, this protein is expressed in a very tissue restricted manner mice, which is markedly different than humans. Apparently, Crry has evolved to take the functional role of this protein in murine tissues such as the kidney and joint.[59]

With regard to fluid-phase control proteins, C4b-binding protein (C4-bp) is the major inhibitor of the classical pathway, while factor H is the major inhibitor of the AP and the alternative pathway amplification loop. Importantly, factor H can function in both the fluid phase and on surfaces, and a major factor that controls its surface inhibitory capacity is its relative ability to bind to polyamines such as sialic acid on the target surface.[60] Factor H has both cofactor activity for factor I–mediated cleavage of C3b as well as decay-accelerating activity for the AP initiation and amplification C3 convertases. A diagram of the factor H molecule is shown in Figure 8K-3, and is illustrative of the structure of the short consensus repeat (SCR) family of proteins (DAF, MCP, factor H, C4-bp) designated the regulators of complement activation (RCA).[61] Factor H has a modular structure with the C3 regulatory sites in the first 4-5 short consensus repeats (SCRs), and a series of binding sites for ligands, primarily polyanions, in the carboxy-terminal 15 SCRs. It is uncertain exactly how factor H binds to target cells and tissues, but this is believed to be primarily controlled by initial contact by SCRs 19-20 with the tissue, followed by the elaboration of protective complement C3 function on the tissue itself.[62,63]

The importance of factor H in the control of complement activation has been demonstrated by studies of human diseases, where mutations or dysfunctional polymorphisms are highly associated with the diseases atypical hemolytic uremic syndrome (aHUS), membranoproliferative glomerulonephritis type II (MPGN type II), and age-related macular degeneration (AMD).[64–66] In addition, factor H gene–targeted mice have been created, and consistent with the expected role of this protein in controlling C3 activation, C3 levels are extremely low, and these mice develop proliferative glomerulonephritis that is dependent on AP activation.[67]

The AP is unique among the three pathways in that it is also affected by a positive regulator designated properdin.[42] Properdin is a polymeric protein that can bind to both C3b and factor B in the C3 convertase, thus keeping these proteins together and active with regard to additional C3 cleavage, in large part by physically blocking the effects of factor H. In addition, although properdin has been traditionally viewed as a molecule that only binds to complement convertase proteins and stabilizes them once the complex has formed, recent studies by Spitzer et al.[68] have suggested that properdin can also initially bind to a target, such as a bacterial membrane, and then "direct" the C3 convertase proteins to assemble on that site secondarily. Conceptually then, the relative rate of C3 cleavage through the AP C3 convertases is dependent on the inter-relationships and/or opposing effects of tick-over, factor H inhibition, and properdin stabilization.

Finally, with regard to the anaphylatoxins C5a and C3a, these proteins undergo a rapid loss of activity following releases in serum that is primarily caused by C-terminal cleavage of Arg to make the desArg form.[69] Serum carboxypeptidase-N performs this cleavage, which results in C3a and C5a derivatives with two to three orders of magnitude less activity.

Complement Receptors and CD19 Signal Transduction Complex

Activation of C3 by any of the three complement initiation pathways leads to cleavage of C3 into the fragments C3a and C3b. C3a is a small anaphylotoxin that binds to its receptor (C3aR) on leukocytes and other cells, resulting in activation and release of additional soluble inflammatory mediators.[70,71] C3b and its further sequential cleavage fragments, iC3b and C3dg/C3d, remain physically attached to the target in this setting and are ligands for complement receptors 1 and 2 (CR1 and CR2) and the α2 integrins, CD11b/CD18 (CR3), and CD11c/CD18 (CR4), receptors that are present on a variety of phagocytic and immune accessory cells.[12,14,72–74]

One receptor that plays a particularly important role in RA is CR2, which primarily acts as a B-cell coreceptor for antigen receptor–mediated signal transduction (Figure 8K-4). On B-cell lines or primary B lymphocytes, coligation of CR2 with surface IgM with mAbs,[75–79] covalently linked complexes of antigen with C3d ligand,[80] or biotin-conjugated C3dg complexed with biotinylated anti-IgM,[81] results in enhanced intracellular calcium release and activation of tyrosine and MAP kinases. This activity is primarily due to the association of CR2 with CD19 and CD81 in a B-cell–specific signal transduction complex,[82,83] and to the exclusion of inhibitory phosphatases during coligation of CR2 with the B-cell receptor.[81] CD19, in contrast to CR2, has a long intracytoplasmic tail that is tyrosine phosphorylated following antigen receptor ligation and then itself activates other signaling molecules.[84–88]

Support for a critical role of CR2 in the immune response has been provided by results in mice that are deficient in CR2, designated *Cr2-/-*, which demonstrate substantial defects in Ag-specific, T-dependent and -independent humoral immune

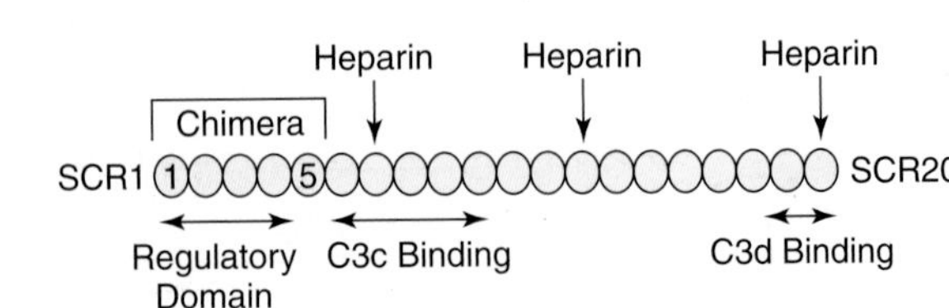

Figure 8K-3. Schematic drawing of factor H with SCR numbers in addition to domains containing polyanion (heparin) as well as C3-binding and AP regulatory functions.

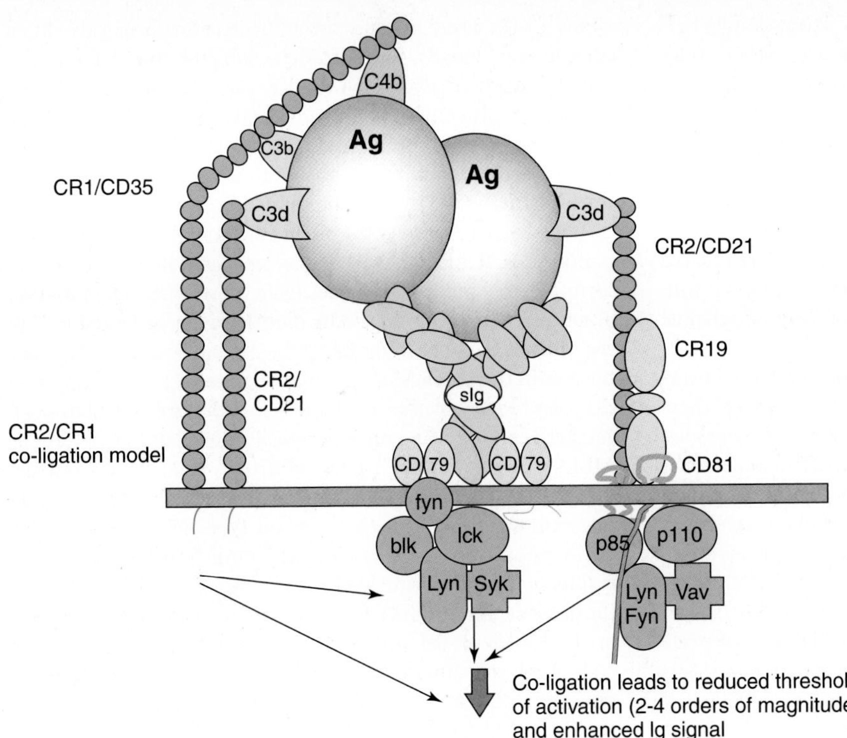

Figure 8K-4. Model of the amplification of B-cell activation through coligation of CR2 with the B-cell receptor through the interaction of C3d-bound Ag. This subsequently activates CD19-mediated signaling cascades. This action of CR2 is likely relevant to the binding of both self and foreign Ags.

responses,[15,16,89] and defects in B-cell memory.[90,91] The defects are due to a lack of receptor on both B cells and follicular dendritic cells (FDCs).[92,93] Additional studies have shown that CR2 can help to regulate T-cell responses.[19,94]

CR2 has also been shown to play key roles in the pathogenesis of organ-specific autoimmunity. In addition to studies in RA and CIA discussed below, in the experimental myocarditis model the absence of CR2 leads to the protection of mice from the development of T-cell autoimmunity as well as autoantibodies and subsequent Ab- and cytokine-mediated injury.[19]

Relevance of Collagen-Induced Arthritis and Collagen Antibody–Induced Arthritis Models to Human Rheumatoid Arthritis

The collagen-induced arthritis (CIA) model of human RA is induced by the immunization of mice with type II collagen, usually bovine or chicken in derivation, in a strong adjuvant consisting of incomplete Freund's adjuvant supplemented with *Mycobacteria*.[95] The disease is inducible in several strains, one of the most susceptible being DBA1/j.[96] Humoral autoimmunity is measured by the development of IgG antibodies to type II collagen that react with both bovine and murine collagen, with the major pathogenic Ab isotype being IgG2a.[97] T-cell autoimmunity to type II collagen develops, and the major immunodominant peptides have been previously identified.[98] The effector phase is mimicked by the transfer of anti-CII monoclonal antibodies, and C57BL/6 mice, which we have primarily used in our own passive-transfer collagen antibody–induced arthritis (CAIA) studies,[99–101] are susceptible to joint injury in this model.

Rheumatoid Arthritis and the Complement System

There is a long-standing literature supporting the involvement of complement in the pathogenesis of arthritis and joint destruction in patients with RA.[102] For example, although systemic complement C3 and total hemolytic complement (THC) levels are typically increased, reflecting the acute-phase response, complement activity of joint fluid from patients is significantly lower than in joint fluid from control noninflammatory subjects. In addition, significant increases in soluble complement activation fragments (C3d, C3a, C5a, sC5b-9) are found in the synovial cavity joint fluid, as well as enhanced local production of complement proteins in synovial tissue itself.[4] C3 and C4 activation fragments are found in the great majority of synovial tissues and on the cartilage in patients with RA. In rheumatoid nodules, a common systemic feature of the disease, C3 and the C5b-9 have been demonstrated both in the central necrotic area and in blood vessels walls of the granulomatous tissue.

Of note, RA has also long been known to be associated with an increased proportion of IgG molecules that lack terminal sialic acid or galactose and are termed G0-IgG.[103,104] The major structural feature that defines this form of IgG is the presence or absence of the so-called "G0" carbohydrate in the IgG Fc domain at Asn-297, which is generated in a regulated process that results in the trimming back of terminal galactose moieties to leave exposed N-acetyl glucosamine (GlcNAc). The functional effect of this particular structural change is that this invariant Fc-domain carbohydrate no longer makes extensive contacts with the contralateral Fc chain. The "burying" of carbohydrate side chains from this invariant position with the contralateral chain, a feature of fully glycosylated IgG, which is so stable that it is readily detected in the crystal structure of IgG molecules, typically restricts the ability of MBL to bind IgG. However, when the carbohydrate is trimmed back to the G0 form, it is no longer held in place by the contralateral chain and can move freely in solution. In addition, while MBL does not effectively bind terminal galactose, it is thought to be able to readily bind the terminal GlcNAc and then activate complement C3 through engagement of the MBL-associated MASP-1/MASP-2 proteases.[105,106] Indeed, manipulation of G0 content *in vivo* has previously been shown to influence the ability of IgG to cause joint inflammation and destruction in a passive serum transfer model of rheumatoid arthritis (RA).[107] High serum levels of G0-IgG in patients with RA have also been associated with the development of ischemic heart disease.[108]

The relative roles of C3 or C5 in CIA have been explored using therapeutic interventions that interfere with one or both of these complement components. For example, inhibition of complement with soluble complement receptor 1 (sCR1), a potent inactivator of both C3 and C5 convertases, inhibited the development and progression of CIA in mice; both anti-CII antibody levels and T-cell responses to collagen *in vitro* were reduced by this treatment.[109] Mice deficient in C3 demonstrated a much diminished development of CIA and also decreased levels of anticollagen antibodies.[110,111] Additional studies have explored the specific role of C5, C5a, and the C5b-9 MAC in CIA. Treatment of DBA/1j mice with a monoclonal antibody to murine C5 both prevented the onset of and ameliorated established CIA, and DBA/1j mice congenic for C5 deficiency also exhibited resistance to induction of CIA despite demonstrating normal humoral and cellular immune responses to collagen.[112,113] Finally, a key role for C5a and the C5a receptor has been suggested by the finding that C5aR gene–targeted mice are protected from CAIA.[114]

Other models of inflammatory arthritis, such as the passive Ab transfer model using IgG that reacts with glucose-6-phosphate isomerase, have also shown that complement, especially factor B, C3, and C5, plays a central pathogenic role.[115] The demonstration that mast cells are critically important in this particular disease model is consistent with the presence of receptors for complement activation fragments on these cells, and an attractive hypothesis is that complement activation fragments mediate activation of these cells.[116] In addition to these models, by using a nonpeptide antagonist of the C3aR, a role in adjuvant-induced arthritis has also been identified.[117] Finally, initial studies using a humanized mouse anti-C5 mAb in patients with RA have led to encouraging levels of improvement.[118] In sum, many lines of evidence support a key role for complement in the pathogenesis of inflammatory arthritis, although the optimal therapeutic strategy for human disease is yet to be established.

With regard to the roles of specific complement activation pathways (CP, LP, and AP) in the pathogenesis of RA, results from recently published studies have shown that inflammation and tissue damage in the CAIA model are markedly reduced in the absence of factor B (disabling the AP and amplification loop) but not in the absence of C4 (disabling the CP), suggesting mediation of injury by the AP alone.[99] The role of the AP has been further explored using mice genetically deficient in C3, C1q, or MBL-A/C, or in both C1q and MBL-A/C (thus having only an intact AP).[119] C3 activation has also been examined *in vitro* using immune complexes that contain type II collagen and the same mAbs used for the *in vivo* passive Ab-transfer studies. The results of these experiments have revealed that the AP alone, in the absence of both the CP and LP, can mediate arthritis *in vivo* in the CAIA model, and consistent with this effect, immune complexes can initiate C3 activation *in vitro*, again in the absence of a functional CP and LP. Thus, despite the findings that the CP and LP can lead to initial C3 deposition in the synovium and cartilage *in vivo*, the AP, likely through the amplification loop, appears to play the essential complement-related role in arthritis induction in this model.

The mechanism whereby the AP is able to initiate complement activation in the absence of the CP or LP is unclear. As noted above in Figure 8K-2, though, the AP is thought to exhibit continuous low-grade activity *in vivo* through hydrolysis of the thioester bond by interaction with water, the "tickover" mechanism. In the presence of IgG in IC, either in solution or on a solid surface, the short-lived C3b can also bind to the Fd portion of IgG to become a more stable and potent C3 convertase. This likely promotes complement activation on the cartilage surface, which is followed by unregulated activation in the synovium. Figure 8K-5 illustrates one model that would account for the findings in the CAIA model of passive transfer arthritis.

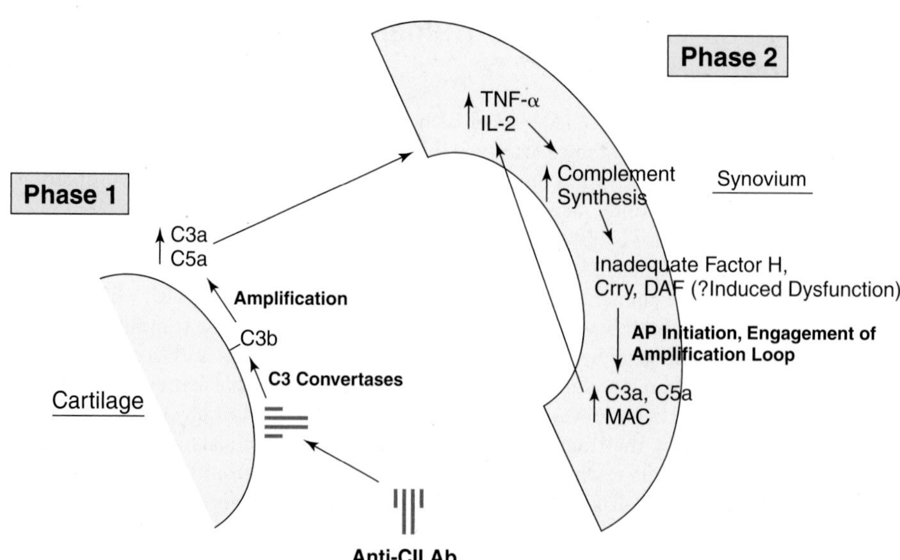

Figure 8K-5. "Two-phase" model of initiation of joint inflammation and damage following the formation of immune complexes on the cartilage surface (Phase 1) in the CAIA model and engagement of complement, specifically the AP and the amplification loop. In this model, secondary injury is initiated in the adjacent synovium through the unregulated activation at that site of the AP (Phase 2).

Finally, the role of CR2 as a B-cell activating receptor has been explored in the CIA model. In those studies, the absence of this receptor led to a markedly decreased level of arthritis and a decrease in the humoral immune response to foreign and self antigen, in this instance type II collagen.[27] Thus, CR2 is emerging as a potential B-cell target for therapeutics that attempt to modulate autoantibody production.

Conclusion

In sum, complement activation is important in the induction of experimental arthritis, both with regard to the generation of pathogenic autoantibodies as well as the effects of these antibodies in the joint. Like many effector and regulatory pathways in RA, the relative effects of this pathway on the clinical phenotypes found in patients likely depends on whether the disease is in the early or later phases of evolution. Perhaps most importantly with regard to the potential for impacting the disease in patients, though, is the recent expanded interest in the development of use of complement-targeted therapeutics.[120] It is likely that these tools will allow the formal analysis of the questions addressed above with regard to the relative roles of complement, and its individual components, in RA pathogenesis.

References

1. Arend WP. The innate immune system in rheumatoid arthritis. *Arthritis Rheum* 2001;44:2224–2234.
2. Firestein GS. Evolving concepts of rheumatoid arthritis. *Nature* 2003;423:356–361.
3. Gregersen PK, Silver J, Winchester RJ. The shared epitope hypothesis. An approach to understanding the molecular genetics of susceptibility to rheumatoid arthritis. *Arthritis Rheum* 1987;30: 1205–1213.
4. Neumann E, Barnum SR, Tarner IH, et al. Local production of complement proteins in rheumatoid arthritis synovium. *Arthritis Rheum* 2002;46:934–945.
5. Muller-Eberhard HJ. Molecular organization and function of the complement system. *Annu Rev Biochem* 1988;57:321–347.
6. Sjoberg A, Onnerfjord P, Morgelin M, et al. The extracellular matrix and inflammation: Fibromodulin activates the classical pathway of complement by directly binding C1q. *J Biol Chem* 2006;280: 32301–32308.
7. Machold KP, Stamm TA, Nell VP, et al. Very recent onset rheumatoid arthritis: Clinical and serological patient characteristics associated with radiographic progression over the first years of disease. *Rheumatology* 2007;46:185–187.
8. Rantapaa Dahlqvist S, de Jong BAW, Hallmans G, et al. Antibodies against citrullinated peptides (CCP) predict the development of rheumatoid arthritis. *Arthritis Rheum* 2002;46:S200.
9. Edwards JCW, Szczepanski L, Szechinski J, et al. Efficacy of B-cell–targeted therapy with rituximab in patients with rheumatoid arthritis. *N Engl J Med* 2004;350:2572–2581.
10. Edwards JCW, Cambridge G, Leandro MJ. B cell depletion therapy in rheumatic disease. *Best Pract Res Clin Rheum* 2006;20:915–928.
11. Fearon DT, Locksley RM. The instructive role of innate immunity in the acquired immune response. *Science* 1996;272:50–54.
12. Holers VM. Complement. In: Rich R, ed. *Principles and Practices of Clinical Immunology*. St. Louis, MO: Mosby, 2001, 21.1–21.8.
13. Frank MM, Moffitt MC, Frank MM. Complement resistance in microbes. *Springer Semin Immunopathol* 1994;15:327–344.
14. Brown EJ. Complement receptors and phagocytosis. *Curr Opin Immunol* 1991;3:76–82.
15. Ahearn JM, Fischer MB, Croix DA, et al. Disruption of the Cr2 locus results in a reduction in B-1a cells and in an impaired B cell response to T-dependent antigen. *Immunity* 1996;4:251–262.
16. Molina H, Holers VM, Li B, et al. Markedly impaired humoral immune response in mice deficient in complement receptors 1 and 2. *Proc Natl Acad Sci U S A* 1996;93:3357–3361.
17. Carroll MC. The role of complement in B cell activation and tolerance. *Adv Immunol* 2000;74:61–88.
18. Haas KM, Hasegawa M, Steeber DA, et al. Complement receptors CD21/35 link innate and protective immunity during Streptococcus phenumoniae infection by regulating IgG3 antibody responses. *Immunity* 2002;17:713–723.
19. Kaya Z, Afanasyeva M, Wang Y, et al. Contribution of the innate immune system to autoimmune myocarditis: A role for complement. *Nat Immunol* 2001;2:739–745.
20. Pratt JR, Abe K, Miyazaki M, et al. In situ localization of C3 synthesis in experimental acute renal allograft rejection. *Am J Pathol* 2000; 157:825–831.
21. Fleming SD, Shea-Donohue T, Guthridge JM, et al. Mice deficient in complement receptors 1 and 2 lack a tissue injury-inducing subset of the natural antibody repertoire. *J Immunol* 2002;169:2126–2133.
22. Reid RR, Woodstock S, Shimabukuro-Vornhagen A, et al. Functional activity of natural antibody is altered in Cr2-deficient mice. *J Immunol* 2002;169:5433–5440.
23. Thurman JM, Ljubanovic D, Edelstein CL, et al. Lack of a functional alternative pathway ameliorates ischemic acute renal failure in mice. *J Immunol* 2003;170:1517–1523.
24. Boackle SA, Holers VM, Chen X, et al. Cr2, a candidate gene in the murine Sle1c lupus susceptibility locus, encodes a dysfunctional protein. *Immunity* 2001;15:775–785.
25. Prodeus A, Goerg S, Shen L-M, et al. A critical role for complement in maintenance of self-tolerance. *Immunity* 1998;9:721–731.
26. Wu X, Jiang N, Deppong C, et al. A role for the Cr2 gene in modifying autoantibody production in systemic lupus erythematosus. *J Immunol* 2002;169:1587–1592.
27. Del Nagro CJ, Kolla RV, Rickert RC. A critical role for complement C3d and the B cell coreceptor (CD19/CD21) complex in the initiation of inflammatory arthritis. *J Immunol* 2005;175:5379–5389.
28. Holers VM. The complement system as a therapeutic target in autoimmunity. *Clin Immunol* 2003;107:140–151.
29. Gewurz H, Zhang X-H, Lint TF. Structure and function of the pentraxins. *Curr Opin Immunol* 1996;7:54–64.
30. Navratil JS, Watkins SC, Wisnieski JJ, et al. The globular heads of C1q specifically recognize surface blebs of apoptotic vascular endothelial cells. *J Immunol* 2001;166:3231–3239.
31. Bradt BM, Kolb WP, Cooper NR. Complement-dependent proinflammatory properties of the Alzheimer's disease beta-peptide. *J Exp Med* 1998;188:431–438.
32. Shen Y, Lue L, Yang L, et al. Complement activation by neurofibrillary tangles in Alzheimer's disease. *Neurosci Lett* 2001;305: 165–168.
33. Reid KBM, Turner MW. Mammalian lectins in activation and clearance mechanisms involving the complement system. *Springer Semin Immunopathol* 1994;15:307–325.
34. Collard CD, Montalto MC, Reenstra WR, et al. Endothelial oxidative stress activates the lectin complement pathway: Role of cytokeratin 1. *Am J Pathol* 2001;159:1045–1054.

35. Wong NK, Kojima M, Dobo J, et al. Activities of the MBL-associated serine proteases (MASPs) and their regulation by natural inhibitors. *Mol Immunol* 1999;36:853–861.
36. Turner MW, Hamvas RM. Mannose-binding lectin: Targeting the microbial world for complement attack and opsonophagocytosis. *Rev Immunogenet* 2000;2:303–322.
37. Takahashi M, Mori S, Shigeta S, et al. Role of MBL-associated serine protease (MASP) on activation of the lectin complement pathway. *Adv Exp Med Biol* 2007;598:93–104.
38. Ratnoff WD, Fearon DT, Austen KF. The role of antibody in the activation of the alternative complement pathway. *Springer Semin Immunopathol* 1983;6:361–371.
39. Mizuno M, Nishikawa K, Spiller OB, et al. Membrane complement regulators protect against the development of type II collagen–induced arthritis in rats. *Arthritis Rheum* 2001;44:2425–2434.
40. Xu C, Mao D, Holers VM, et al. A critical role for murine complement regulator Crry in fetomaternal tolerance. *Science* 2000;498–501.
41. Schaapherder AF, Gooszen HG, Te Bulte MT, et al. Human complement activation via the alternative pathway on porcine endothelium initiated by IgA antibodies. *Transplantation* 1995;60:287–291.
42. Schwaeble WJ, Reid KBM. Does properdin crosstalk the cellular and the humoral immune response? *Immunol Today* 1999;20:17–21.
43. Markiewski MM, Nilsson B, Ekdahl KN, et al. Complement and coagulation: Strangers or partners in crime? *Trends Immunol* 2007; 28:184–192.
44. Huber-Lang M, Sarma JV, Zetoune FS, et al. Generation of C5a in the absence of C3: A new complement activation pathway. *Nat Med* 2006;12:682–687.
45. Marty I, Peclat V, Kerdaite G, et al. Amelioration of collagen-induced arthritis by thrombin inhibition. *J Clin Invest* 2001;107:631–640.
46. Spath P, Gabl F. Critical role of the conversion of the third complement component C3 (Beta1C/Beta1A) for its immunochemical quantitation. *Clin Chim Acta* 1976;73:171–175.
47. Kalowski S, Howe EL, Margaretten W, et al. Effects of intravascular clotting on the activation of the complement system: The role of the platelet. *Am J Pathol* 1976;78:525–536.
48. Liszewski MK, Farries TC, Lublin DM, et al. Control of the complement system. *Adv Immunol* 1996;61:201–283.
49. Morgan BP, Meri S. Membrane proteins that protect against complement lysis. *Springer Semin Immunopathol* 1994;15:369–396.
50. Molina H, Wong W, Kinoshita T, et al. Distinct receptor and regulatory properties of recombinant mouse complement receptor 1 (CR1) and Crry, the two genetic homologs of human CR1. *J Exp Med* 1992;175:121–129.
51. Miwa T, Sun X, Ohta R, et al. Characterization of glycosylphosphatidylinositol-anchored decay accelerating factor (GPI-DAF) and transmembrane DAF gene expression in wild-type and GPI-DAF gene knockout mice using polyclonal and monoclonal antibodies with dual or single specificity. *Immunology* 2001;104:207–214.
52. Lin F, Fukuoka Y, Spicer A, et al. Tissue distribution of products of the mouse decay-accelerating factor (DAF) genes. Exploitation of a Daf1 knock-out mouse and site-specific monoclonal antibodies. *Immunology* 2001;104:215–225.
53. Nomura M, Tsujimura A, Shida K, et al. Membrane and secretory forms of mouse membrane cofactor protein (CD46) generated from a single gene through alternative splicing. *Immunogenetics* 1999;50: 245–254
54. Inal JM, Hui KM, Miot S, et al. Complement C2 receptor inhibitor trispanning: A novel human complement inhibitory receptor. *J Immunol* 2005;174:356–366.
55. Helmy KY, Katschke KJ, Gorgani NN, et al. CRIg: A macrophage complement receptor required for phagocytosis and circulating pathogens. *Cell* 2006;124:915–927.
56. Mao D, Wu X, Deppong C, et al. Negligible role of antibodies and C5 in pregnancy loss associated exclusively with C3-dependent mechanisms through complement alternative pathway. *Immunity* 2003;19:813–822.
57. Thurman JM, Ljubanovic D, Royer PA, et al. Altered renal tubular expression of the complement inhibitor Crry permits complement activation after ischemia/reperfusion. *J Clin Invest* 2006;116: 357–368.
58. Miwa T, Maldonado MA, Zhou L, et al. Deletion of decay-accelerating factor (CD55) exacerbates autoimmune disease development in MRL/ lpr mice. *Am J Pathol* 2002;161:1077–1086.
59. Molina H. The murine complement regulator Crry: New insights into the immunobiology of complement regulation. Cell Mol *Life Sci* 2002;59:220–229.
60. Zipfel PF, Skerka C, Hellwage J, et al. Factor H family proteins: On complement, microbes and human diseases. *Biochem Soc Trans* 2002;30:971–978.
61. Hourcade D, Holers VM, Atkinson JP. The regulators of complement activation (RCA) gene cluster. *Adv Immunol* 1989;45:381–416.
62. Jozsi M, Opperman M, Lambris JD, et al. The C-terminus of complement factor H is essential for host cell protection. *Mol Immunol* 2007;44:2697–2706.
63. Jozsi M, Manuelian T, Heinen S, et al. Attachment of the soluble complement regulator factor H to cell and tissue surfaces: Relevance for pathology. *Histol Histopathol* 2004;19:251–258.
64. Kavanaugh D, Goodship THJ, Richards A. Atypical haemolytic uraemic syndrome. *Br Med Bull* 2006;77:5–22.
65. Jha P, Bora PS, Bora NS. The role of the complement system in ocular diseases including uveitis and macular degeneration. *Mol Immunol* 2007;44:3901–3908.
66. Jokiranta ST, Zipfel PF, Fremeaux-Bacchi V, et al. Where next with atypical hemolytic uremic syndrome? *Mol Immunol* 2007;44: 3889–3900.
67. Pickering MC, Cook HT, Warren J, et al. Uncontrolled C3 activation causes membranoproliferative glomerulonephritis in mice deficient in complement factor H. *Nat Genet* 2002;31:424–428.
68. Spitzer D, Mitchell LM, Atkinson JP, et al. Properdin can initiate complement activation by binding specific target surfaces and providing a platform for de novo convertase assembly. *J Immunol* 2007;179:2600–2608.
69. Matthews KW, Mueller-Ortiz SL, Wetsel RA. Carboxypeptidase N: A pleiotropic regulator of inflammation. *Mol Immunol* 2004;40: 785–793.
70. Wetsel RA. Structure, function and cellular expression of complement anaphylatoxin receptors. *Curr Opin Immunol* 1995;7:48–53.
71. Hugli TE. Structure and function of C3a anaphylatoxin. *Curr Top Microbiol Immunol* 1989;153:181–208.
72. Ahearn JM, Fearon DT. Structure and function of the complement receptors, CR1 (CD35) and CR2 (CD21). *Adv Immunol* 1989;46: 183–219.
73. Cooper NR, Moore MD, Nemerow GR. Immunobiology of CR2, the B lymphocyte receptor for Epstein-Barr virus and the C3d complement fragment. *Ann Rev Immunol* 1988;6:85–113.
74. Ross GD. Complement receptor type 1. *Curr Top Microbiol Immunol* 1992;178:31–44.
75. Bohnsack JF, Cooper NR. CR2 ligands modulate human B cell activation. *J Immunol* 1988;141:2569–2576.
76. Carter RH, Fearon DT. Polymeric C3dg primes human B lymphocytes for proliferation induced by anti-IgM. *J Immunol* 1989;143: 1755–1760.
77. Carter RH, Spycher MO, Ng YC, et al. Synergistic interaction between complement receptor type 2 and membrane IgM on B lymphocytes. *J Immunol* 1998;141:457–463.
78. Carter RH, Fearon DT. CD19: Lowering the threshold for antigen receptor stimulation of B lymphocytes. *Science* 1992;256:105–107.
79. Luxembourg AT, Cooper NR. Modulation of signaling via the B cell antigen receptor by CD21, the receptor for C3dg and EBV. *J Immunol* 1994;153:4448–4457.
80. Dempsey PW, Allison ME, Akkaraju S, et al. C3d of complement as a molecular adjuvant: Bridging innate and acquired immunity. *Science* 1996;271:348–350.

81. Lyubchenko T, dal Porto J, Cambier JC, et al. Co-ligation of the B cell receptor with complement receptor type 2 (CR2/CD21) using its natural ligand C3dg: Activation without engagement of an inhibitory signaling pathway. *J Immunol* 2005;174:3264–3272.
82. Bradbury LE, Kansas GS, Levy S, et al. The CD19/CD21 signal transducing complex of human B lymphocytes includes the target of antiproliferative antibody-1 and Leu-13 molecules. *J Immunol* 1992;149:2841–2850.
83. Matsumoto AK, Kopicky-Burd J, Carter RH, et al. Intersection of the complement and immune systems: A signal transduction complex of the B lymphocyte–containing complement receptor type 2 and CD19. *J Exp Med* 1991;173:55–64.
84. Cambier JC, Pleiman CM, Clark MR. Signal transduction by the B cell antigen receptor and its coreceptors. *Ann Rev Immunol* 1994;12:457–486.
85. Fearon DT, Carter RH. The CD19/CR2/TAPA-1 complex of B lymphocytes: Linking natural to acquired immunity. *Ann Rev Immunol* 1995;13:127–149.
86. Tedder TF, Zhou LJ, Engel P. The CD19/CD21 signal transduction complex of B lymphocytes. *Immunol Today* 1994;15:437–442.
87. Li X, Carter RH. Systematic analysis of the role of CD19 cytoplasmic tyrosines in enhancement of activation in Daudi human B cells: Clustering of phospholipase C and Vav and of Grb2 and Sos with different CD19 tyrosines. *J Immunol* 2000;164:3123–3131.
88. Hasegawa M, Fujimoto M, Poe JC, et al. CD19 can regulate B lymphocyte signal transduction independent of complement activation. *J Immunol* 2001;167:3190–3200.
89. Croix DA, Ahearn JM, Rosengard AM, et al. Antibody response to a T-dependent antigen requires B cell expression of complement receptors. *J Exp Med* 1996;183:1857–1864.
90. Wu X, Jiang N, Fang YF, et al. Impaired affinity maturation in Cr2-/- mice is rescued by adjuvants without improvement in germinal center development. *J Immunol* 2000;165:3119–3127.
91. Chen ZM, Koralev SB, Gendelman M, et al. Humoral immune responses in Cr2-/- mice: Enhanced affinity maturation but impaired antibody persistence. *J Immunol* 2000;164:4522–4532.
92. Fang Y, Xu C, Holers VM, et al. Expression of complement receptors 1 and 2 on follicular dendritic cells is necessary for the generation of a normal antigen-specific IgG response. *J Immunol* 1998;160:5273–5279.
93. Fischer MB, Goerg S, Shen L, et al. Dependence of germinal center B cells on expression of CD21/CD35 for survival. *Science* 1998;280: 582–585.
94. Pratt JR, Basheer SA, Sacks SH. Local synthesis of complement component C3 regulates acute renal transplant rejection. *Nat Med* 2002;8:582–587.
95. Luross JA, Williams NA. The genetic and immunopathological processes underlying collagen-induced arthritis. *Immunology* 2001;103: 407–416.
96. Wooley PH. Collagen-induced arthritis in the mouse. *Methods Enzymol* 1988;162:361–373.
97. Brand DD, Marion TN, Myers LK, et al. Autoantibodies to murine type II collagen in collagen-induced arthritis: A comparison of susceptible and nonsusceptible strains. *J Immunol* 1996;157: 5178–5184.
98. Wooley PH, Luthra HS, Stuart JM, et al. Type II collagen induced arthritis in mice. I. Major histocompatibility complex (I-region) linkage and antibody production. *J Exp Med* 1981;154:688–700.
99. Banda N, Thurman JM, Kraus D, et al. Alternative complement pathway activation is essential for inflammation and joint destruction in the passive transfer model of collagen-induced arthritis. *J Immunol* 2006;177:1904–1912.
100. Banda NK, Kraus D, Vondracek A, et al. Mechanisms of effects of complement inhibition in murine collagen-induced arthritis. *Arthritis Rheum* 2002;46:3065–3075.
101. Banda NK, Kraus DM, Muggli M, et al. Prevention of collagen-induced arthritis in mice transgenic for the complement inhibitor complement receptor 1–related gene/protein y. *J Immunol* 2003;171: 2109–2115.
102. Nandakumar KS, Holmdahl R. Antibody-induced arthritis: Disease mechanisms and genes involved at the effector phase of arthritis. *Arthritis Res Ther* 2007;8:223–233.
103. Malhotra R, Wormald MR, Rudd PM, et al. Glycosylation changes of IgG associated with rheumatoid arthritis can activate complement via the mannose-binding protein. *Nat Med* 1995;1:237–243.
104. Parekh RB, Dwek RA, Sutton BJ, et al. Association of rheumatoid arthritis and primary osteoarthritis with changes in the glycosylation pattern of total serum IgG. *Nature* 1985;316:452–457.
105. Fujita T, Matsushita M, Endo Y. The lectin-complement pathway—its role in innate immunity and evolution. *Immunol Rev* 2004;198: 185–202.
106. Gadjeva M, Takahashi K, Thiel S. Mannan-binding lectin—a soluble pattern recognition molecule. *Mol Immunol* 2004;41:113–121.
107. Rademacher TW, Williams P, Dwek RA. Agalactosyl glycoforms of IgG autoantibodies are pathogenic. *Proc Natl Acad Sci U S A* 1994; 91:6123–6127.
108. Troelsen LN, Garred P, Madsen HO, et al. Genetically determined high serum levels of mannose-binding lectin and agalactosyl IgG are associated with ischemic heart disease in rheumatoid arthritis. *Arthritis Rheum* 2007;56:21–29.
109. Dreja H, Annenkov A, Chernajovsky Y. Soluble complement receptor 1 (CD35) delivered by retrovirally infected syngeneic cells or by naked DNA injection prevents the progression of collagen-induced arthritis. *Arthritis Rheum* 2000;43:1698–1709.
110. Hietala MA, Jonsson I-M, Tarkowski A, et al. Complement deficiency ameliorates collagen-induced arthritis in mice. *J Immunol* 2002;169:454–459.
111. Hietala MA, Nandakumar KS, Persson L, et al. Complement activation by both classical and alternative pathways is critical for the effector phase of arthritis. Europ *J Immunol* 2004;34:1208–1216.
112. Wang Y, Kristan J, Hao L, et al. A role for complement in antibody-mediated inflammation: C5-deficient DBA/1 mice are resistant to collagen-induced arthritis. *J Immunol* 2000;164:4370–4377.
113. Wang Y, Rollins SA, Madri JA, et al. Anti-C5 monoclonal antibody therapy prevents collagen-induced arthritis and ameliorates established disease. *Proc Natl Acad Sci U S A* 1995;92:8955–8959.
114. Grant EP, Picarella D, Burwell T, et al. Essential role for the C5a receptor in regulating the effector phase of synovial infiltration and joint destruction in experimental arthritis. *J Exp Med* 2002;196: 1461–1471.
115. Ji H, Ohmura J, Mahmood U, et al. Arthritis critically dependent on innate immune system players. *Immunity* 2002;16:157–168.
116. Lee DM, Friend DS, Gurish MF, et al. Mast cells: A cellular link between autoantibodies and inflammatory arthritis. *Science* 2002;197:1689–1692.
117. Ames RS, Lee D, Foley JJ, et al. Identification of a selective nonpeptide antagonist of the anaphylatoxin C3a receptor that demonstrates antiinflammatory activity in animal models. *J Immunol* 2001;166:6341–6348.
118. Kaplan M. Eculizumab (Alexion). *Curr Opin Invest Drugs* 2002;3: 1017–1023.
119. Banda NK, Takahashi K, Wood AK, et al. Pathogenic complement activation in collagen antibody-induced arthritis in mice requires amplification by the alternative pathway. *J Immunol* 2007;179: 4101–4109.
120. Ricklin D, Lambris JD. Complement-targeted therapeutics. *Nat Biotechnol* 2007;25:1265–1275.

Pathogenesis in Rheumatoid Arthritis: Cytokines

CHAPTER 8L

Axel J. Hueber and Iain B. McInnes

The pathogenesis of rheumatoid arthritis (RA) is complex and multifactorial. Recent genetic analyses implicate a variety of known and novel genetic loci in disease susceptibility and severity and increasingly recognize environmental interactions—particularly smoking—that influence outcome. Moreover, there is evidence that immune perturbation occurs long before clinical presentation, and as such, studies of pathogenetic mechanism are required to explain not only ongoing disease but also its early immunologic origins. Importantly, the majority of the genes associated with disease by hypothesis-free methodologies implicate genes that are implicated in immune function, such as HLA class II, PTPN22, CTLA4, and STAT4. Consequently, there is now a very persuasive basis for defining the underlying causes of the disease in immunologic terms, as opposed to connective tissue or biomechanical origins. Cytokines are critical mediators of every stage of the development and regulation of an immune response. As such they are increasingly recognized as vitally important mediators in the pathogenesis of RA. They are abundantly present in the synovial microenvironment, and increasingly their presence is detected in tissues distant from the joint, such as the bone marrow and vasculature. They have proven tractable therapeutic targets not only in RA, but also in a variety of rheumatic and immune disorders, and thus they command considerable attention to define their expression, regulation, and effector function. This chapter describes the key cytokine activities reported in RA.

General Principles of Cytokines and Cytokine Receptor Systems in Arthritis

Cytokines are mediators that signal between cells in an autocrine or paracrine manner acting either as soluble or membrane moieties. A small number of cytokines may also exhibit endocrine-like activity linking tissues via plasma expression and distribution. Historically, families of cytokines were named for their origin—for example, lymphokines, monokines, and interleukins. However, as many of these molecules also influence nonlymphoid cells, the term *cytokine* is more appropriate. Cytokines may be usefully divided into families reflecting either their core functional domains and/or shared structural homology, including, for example, chemokines, hematopoietins, interferons, TNF superfamily, IL-6 superfamily, IL-10 superfamily, and the IL-12 superfamily. Cytokines may exist as monomers, homo- or heterodimers, trimers, or tetramers.

Receptors mainly comprise heterodimers; cytokine receptor families often utilize common receptor subunits (e.g., common γ chain receptor) such that functional redundancy/overlap may arise if subunits are targeted for inhibition or agonism as a surrogate for specific cytokine targeting itself. Receptors, like cytokines, can exist as membrane-signaling molecules, or may be released as soluble entities as a result of enzymatic cleavage from the cell membrane, or through the generation of alternatively spliced mRNA species. Soluble receptors may act as inhibitors of their target ligand cytokine, or may act to facilitate signaling, whereby the receptor can bind cytokine in the fluid phase prior to binding to the complementary receptor chain on the cell membrane. This is best exemplified in RA by the biology of IL-6 that acts by binding a heterodimeric receptor containing IL-6Rα chain and gp130 coreceptor. IL-6 can thus bind to the preformed heterodimer on a target cell (cis signaling) and induce signals. However, it can also bind soluble IL-6R, forming a functional complex that is capable of binding in turn to cells expressing gp130. By this means, cells without IL-6R a priori may "become susceptible" to the effector activities of IL-6 (trans-signaling). Rather complex networks of cytokines and targets can arise since receptors may also be assembled on adjacent cells. IL-15, for example, can bind its heterodimeric receptor βγ chain on a single cell while recruiting the α chain receptor either from the same cell (cis) or from an adjacent cell (trans). Finally, there is increasing evidence in the growth factor families of cytokines that cells may transiently recruit assemblies of receptors from several cytokines simultaneously depending on the microenvironment to facilitate coordinated signaling. This makes physiologic sense in that cells can adapt to complex external stimuli in real time, but may exert a pathologic price in terms of immune dysfunction should abnormal stimuli emerge for targeted cells.

Cytokine-secreting cells may produce cytokines at a constant level, but more commonly enhance their release in response to stimuli. The effector function is mediated through the formation of receptor ligand complexes as described above to drive signal transduction (Figure 8L-1). Cytokine-receptor complexes may thereafter be internalized by endocytosis, fused with a lysosome where the cytokine will be destroyed. The receptor itself may either shuttle back to the cell surface or undergo degradation.[1] Thus, a cell will only react to a certain amount of ligand-mediated

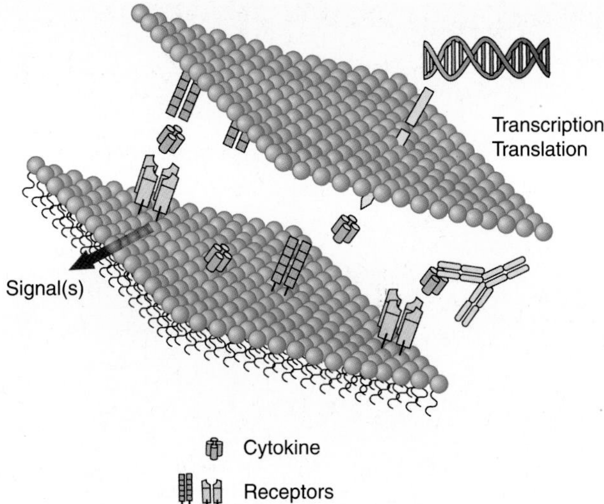

Figure 8L-1. The cell membrane orientation of cytokines and their respective receptors.

stimulation, and then dampen its response by regulating the amount of cytokine expression and/or the receptor expression, respectively. Complex intracellular signaling cascades also closely regulate and integrate signals delivered by the cytokine to achieve a concerted change in target cell behaviour. The consequence of cytokine-mediated effector function may be broad for the target cell including cell activation, division/proliferation, migration, apoptosis, differentiation, matrix synthesis/degradation, cytokine synthesis, and thereby regulatory feedback loops are often generated. This amplificatory and closely regulated functional matrix is intrinsic to cytokine biology, and lies at the heart of the potential they have as therapeutic targets. In particular, it is becoming clear that some cytokines occupy critical or pivotal checkpoints in these cascades such that their inhibition may exert disproportionate inhibitory effects on a physiological or pathologic cascade.

Cytokines Regulate Broad Systemic Effects in Rheumatoid Arthritis Patients

The tissue origins of cytokine synthesis in RA are rather widespread, and it is now recognized that they mediate both systemic effects—such as on cachexia, mood state, cognitive function, vascular risk, and fatigue—and with local effects when produced in the synovial microenvironment. Although the local effects of cytokine production have appropriately dominated research efforts over recent years (and will achieve focused attention below), there is now increasing activity to define their roles in RA processes in the lymphatic system, bone marrow, liver, and spleen, in which they drive immune dysregulation, and even beyond to the vasculature and brain where their activities may go some way to explaining the complex comorbidities associated with RA.

It is difficult to formally define the contribution of cytokines in the lymphatic tissues outwith the synovium in humans with RA, and as such recourse has been made to extensive rodent model studies, especially mouse models. It is clear that organized cellular structures in lymph node, namely germinal centers, are essential for the propagation and perpetuation of inflammatory arthritis in mice. The formation of germinal centers is critically dependent on particular chemokines and cytokines of the TNF superfamily.[2] Recently there has been renewed interest in the formation of such structures in human synovial membrane where they may have prognostic and functional significance. Several studies show the presence of competent germinal centers in synovium[3–5]; these ectopic lymphoid neogenesis formations are organized by T, B, and dendritic cells, are associated with high endothelial venules (HEVs), and result from ectopic expression of homing chemokines. Around 25% of RA patients have such local lymphoid structures. Homeostatic chemokines, such as CXCL13, CCL19, and CCL21, as well as their receptors CCR5 and CCR7, are expressed.[6] A murine model of antigen-induced arthritis in CCR5 or CCR7 knockout mice demonstrated that this lymphoid neogenesis is dependent on these specific chemokine receptors with consequent reduced inflammatory parameters.[7] Thus, these cytokine-mediated events may be of fundamental significance, and prevention of ectopic germinal center formation might be a future target for therapy. Parallel studies are now also examining human lymph-node biopsies and indeed RA-derived lymph nodes, although such work is in its infancy. Future work in this area will be of considerable importance.

The wider effects of cytokines on effector tissues in RA patients beyond the joint rely mainly on proof-of-concept clinical studies in which cytokine-blocking agents (described below in principle and elsewhere in detail) are introduced, and measures of tissue function are measured in patients. This approach has been particularly helpful in defining a potential role for TNF in the accelerated vascular disease that is prevalent in RA.[8] The overall effect of TNF inhibition on mortality as assessed in registries and other phase IV vehicles for data collection appear generally favorable. Recent relevant studies are documented in Table 8L-1, which shows that on balance TNF inhibition leads to improved endothelial dysfunction. There are also some data to suggest enhanced endothelial repair mechanisms. Effects on lipid subparticles, however, remain rather uncertain; data both support and refute significant effects on the atherogenic properties of lipids on TNF blockade. Similar analyses are ongoing to investigate the properties of other cytokines in vascular risk modification. For example, striking alterations in HDL, LDL, and other cholesterol-containing particles have been observed on inhibition of IL-6R in RA patients.[9] The clinical and functional significance of such changes remains unclear at this time, although this moiety offers fascinating potential to probe the detailed cytokine regulation of cholesterol transport and lipid particle assembly and trafficking. By inference from other disease studies, it is likely that some of the other metabolic phenomena observed in RA patients may reside in cytokine biology. Thus, IL-1 inhibition with IL-1Ra in noninsulin diabetes mellitus leads to improvement in metabolic function[10]; IL-1α and IL-1β are widely upregulated in RA, and RA patients exhibit increased incidence of metabolic syndrome. Future studies will extend beyond the cardiovascular and metabolic syndrome to include other comorbidities. Thus, there is increasing interest in the role of cytokines in regulating hippocampal function, and thus cognitive function and mood state.[11] In general, proinflammatory cytokines such as TNF and IL-1 are considered to depress mood state through direct effects on serotonin biology, and as such they represent intriguing agents to explain the fatigue and

Table 8L-1. Summary of TNF Blocking Studies That Elucidate Effects on Vascular Function in Rheumatoid Arthritis

Author	*n*=	Agent	Method	Effect
Hansel (2003)	8	Eta ~4 weeks	FMD	No change (low DAS)
Irace (2004)	10	Inf 0,2,6 weeks	FMD	Transient improvement vasoconstriction, HDL
Van Doornum (2005)	14	Inf/Ada/Eta 6 weeks	PWA	No change
Hurlimann (2002)	11	Inf 12 weeks	FMD	Transient improvement
Gonzalez-Juanatey (2004)	7	Inf 4 weeks	FMD	Transient improvement
Gonzalez-Juanatey (2006)	8	Inf 2 weeks	Carotid IMT	No difference
Maki-Petaja (2006)	9	Eta 12 weeks	aPWV	Improvement

FMD, flow-mediated dilatation; *PWA,* pulse wave analysis; *IMT,* intima media thickness; *aPWV,* aortic pulse wave velocity.

depression that is strongly associated with RA. Clinical trials in which TNF has been inhibited in seronegative inflammatory arthropathies has led to substantial improvements in depression scales, although the primary causality of this to cytokine blockade centrally has not yet been proven.[12] Finally, the systemic effects of cytokines have been attributed to the increased prevalence of osteoporosis in RA, together with a variety of other risk factors including smoking, immobility, and altered dietary habit. Emerging evidence points to improvement in bone density over time in patients in which TNF has been blocked, although again the direct causality of cytokine blockade to bone biology is patients. Nevertheless, the potent bone regulatory effects of cytokines such as TNF, IL-1, IL-17, M-CSF, and particularly RANKL, render plausible the idea that cytokines regulate not only local bone destructive pathways in the joint, but also to some extent systemic loss of bone quality and integrity.

Taken together, therefore, there is now much evidence to support a role for cytokines in the systemic presentation of RA in the clinic—the corollary to this is that we can expect improvement in such comorbidities on specific cytokine inhibition, and as such clinical benefits to be obtained may extend beyond measures only of articular function and related disability to include the totality of the clinical presentation. This in turn will have important clinical effectiveness implications that will impinge on measures of utility in due course.

Articular Effects of Cytokines in Rheumatoid Arthritis

Multiple studies have revealed an orchestrated network of proinflammatory and anti-inflammatory cytokines within the synovial microenvironment. Together such cytokine activities regulate the generation, perpetuation, and modulation of synovial inflammation, tissue remodeling, and ultimately cartilage and bone destruction. Adjacent tissues to the joint are also influential, including tendon and ligament structures and adipose tissues. The precise effects in the former may be further modified by complex biomechanical factors such as articular destruction advances. Figure 8L-2 illustrates a prioritization of proinflammatory cytokines implicated in the RA pathogenesis. It is not comprehensive, but attempts to define key activities and their major local role in disease pathogenesis. In practice, dozens of cytokines are now described in RA synovial tissues and adjacent structures. They comprise proinflammatory and anti-inflammatory activities, but may play either role dependent on disease kinetics, cytokine milieu, and target-cell differentiation status. In general, it is unwise to ascribe an entirely polarized role to any given cytokine, although clearly predominant effects are manifest when inhibition is achieved in clinic. We hereafter consider the activities of a variety of cytokines in the context of specific cellular lineages that are described in detail in other chapters to which the reader is referred for a comprehensive evaluation of these cell lineages. In this chapter, we provide a summary of key and relevant activities.

Monocytes/Macrophages: The Cytokine Factory?

Synovial macrophages can produce a variety of cytokines reflecting a central perceived role in pathogenesis. Of these, TNF release is considered of paramount importance, and although TNF is not only produced by macrophages but also from a variety of other cells (Figure 8L-2), it is the former that is considered the primary source in synovium. TNF is bioactive, both as a transmembrane protein and as a homotrimeric secreted molecule.[13] In inflammation, it mediates its effects through two distinct TNF receptors, p55TNFR (TNFRI) and p75TNFR (TNFRII).[14] Surface localization may serve to restrict activity to specific microenvironments, whereas release may lead to more broad effects. TNF is synthesized as a 26-kDa, type II transmembrane molecule, which can be processed by a TNF-α converting enzyme (TACE or ADAM17), to generate secreted 17-kDa monomers that form biologically active homotrimers.[15] TNF activates monocytes and induces cytokine and prostaglandin release. Further, it induces changes in vascular endothelium that increase vascular permeability. This leads to tissue ingress of IgG/IgM/immune complexes, complement, and cells into the tissue, as TNF is also a potent chemoattractant for neutrophils and other leukocytes. Together with IL-1 and IL-6, as noted above TNF can mediate systemic effects driving the acute-phase response. The effects of TNF are summarized in Figure 8L-3. TNF inhibition in a variety of murine models of arthritis

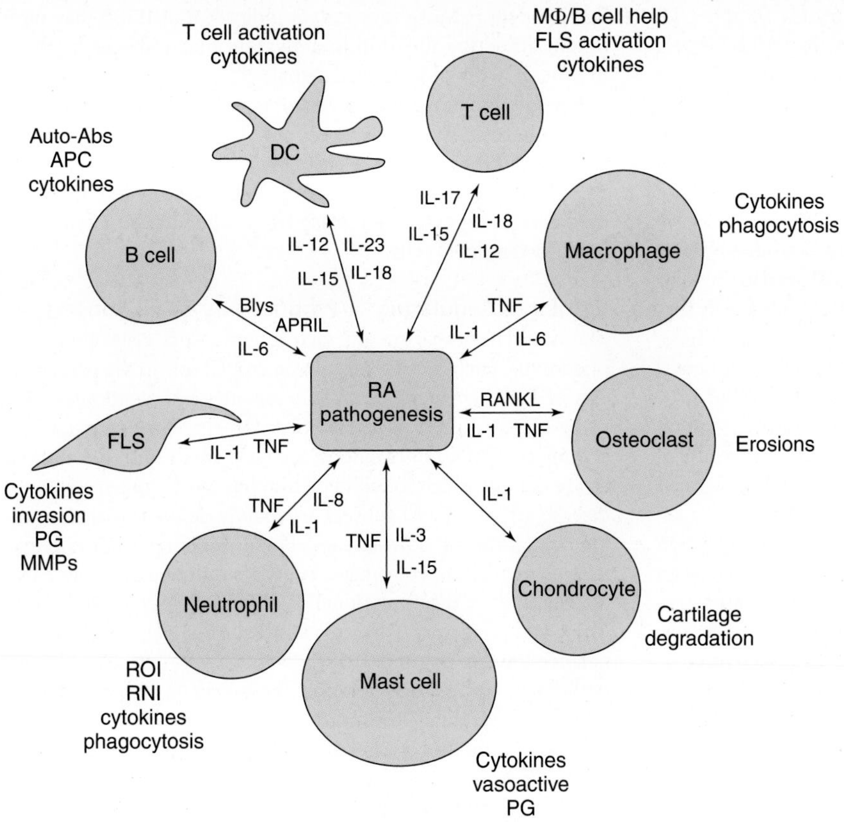

Figure 8L-2. A notional idea of the key cytokine effects in RA synovitis.

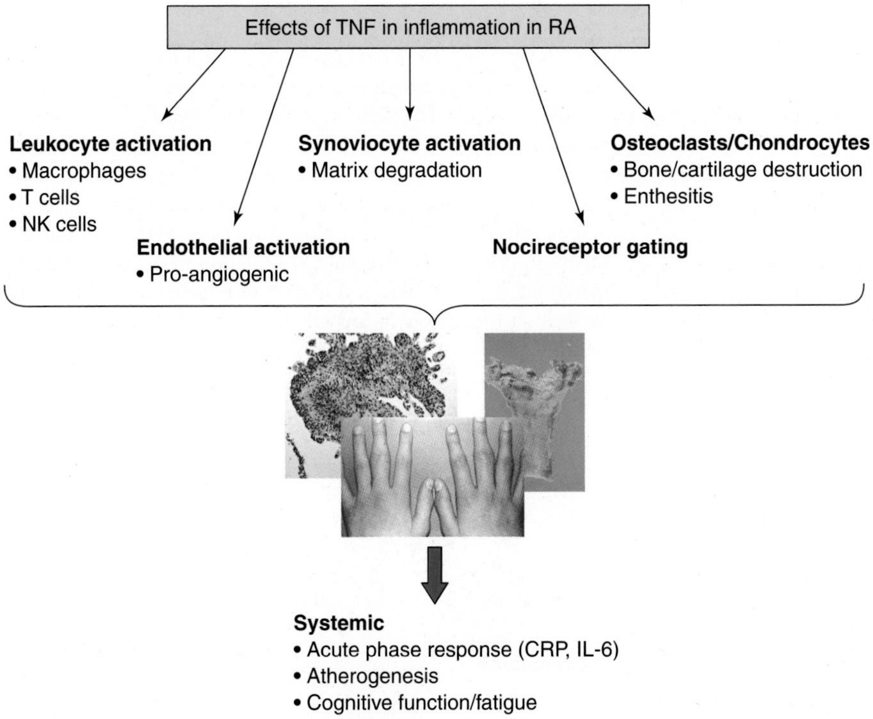

Figure 8L-3. Summary of the effects of TNF of relevance to rheumatoid arthritis.

leads to suppression of disease. TNF transgenic overexpression leads to an aggressive erosive inflammatory arthritis in mice.

IL-6, an important effector cytokine of monocytes, is also expressed by articular fibroblasts, neutrophils, and T and B cells. It is elevated in RA synovial tissues and plasma, and is related to a systemic inflammation by triggering the acute-phase response; it is highly correlated to serum CRP levels. IL-6 is involved in specific cellular and humoral immune responses, including end-stage B-cell differentiation, immunoglobulin secretion and T-cell activation. Maintenance of inflammation is provided by further recruitment of monocytes. In the CIA model, IL-6 knockout mice are protected against arthritis and IL-6 neutralization suppresses disease progression and articular destruction.[16,17] The IL-6 receptor complex is expressed on a variety of cells in synovium (gp130 and IL-6Rα together with soluble IL-6R). As noted above this provides a novel targeting modality whereby anti–IL-6R antibody is capable of inhibiting not only cis but also trans signaling *in vivo*.[16]

IL-1α and IL-1β are distinct structural entities from TNF and IL-6, although they share approximately 95% overlap in their effector function. They belong to the IL-1 superfamily family that includes 11 structurally related cytokines and IL-18 and IL-33, both of which are also implicated in RA pathology. Monocytes and activated macrophages are the main source of IL-1; but stromal cells, T and B cells and osteoclasts can produce IL-1 upon activation. IL-1α and IL-1β are expressed in the synovium of patients with RA, and mice deficient in IL-1 receptor antagonist (IL-1RA, an endogenous inhibitor of IL-1) develop erosive arthritis that is TNF dependent and associated with the induction of Th17 cells.[18,19] The capacity to drive Th17 responses may be an increasingly important component of the proinflammatory activities of IL-1 in RA. In IL-1 dependent autoimmune diseases, administration of recombinant IL-1RA is effective (such as cold-associated acute inflammation syndrome).[20] However, in RA only modest clinical results were achieved thus far with existing targeting strategies including IL-1Ra, anti–IL-1R, anti–IL-1α, and IL-1TRAP. IL-18 shares structural homology with IL-1 and is also highly upregulated in RA synovial tissues. IL-18 is generally proinflammatory by virtue of pleiotropic effector activities in activating macrophages, T cells, neutrophils NK cells, and fibroblasts. IL-18 may also expand T regulatory cells, however, and as such it is less clear what overall effect it mediates in tissues. *In vivo* inhibition of IL-18 leads to reduction in CIA in DBA/1 mice, whereas addition of IL-18 is capable of exacerbating the incidence and severity of murine arthritis. IL-18–deficient mice are unable to generate articular immune responses in the DBA/1 CIA model. Phase I clinical targeting approaches are underway in RA patients.

Granulocyte macrophage–stimulating factor (GM-CSF) is secreted by synovial macrophages, tissue cells (fibroblasts, endothelial cells), and T cells after LPS or cytokine (IL-1, TNF) stimulation. In contrast to its bone marrow–localized myelopoietic growth function, in an inflammatory environment GM-CSF acts mainly as survival and proliferation and differentiation factor. Interestingly, arthritis worsens after administration of GM-CSF in the CIA model and blockade reduces inflammation.[21] In RA patients treated with chemotherapy, disease can flare after GM-CSF administration; similarly in Felty's syndrome, flares occur after treatment for neutropenia with GM-CSF.[22] In summary, GM-CSF might be a possible target in inflammation; results of preclinical trials are awaited.

A final interesting macrophage-derived cytokine is attracting interest, namely IL-32. Originally discovered as a product of IL-18–induced stimulation in effector cells, IL-32 is produced by synovial macrophages and was detected in higher levels in RA synovial biopsies compared to osteoarthritis controls. Expression of IL-32 correlates to severity of disease measured by inflammatory synovial infiltration and markers of systemic inflammation. After injection of human IL-32-γ into mouse joints, TNF-dependent inflammation was observed; however, proteoglycan loss as a sign of matrix degradation was TNF independent.[23] More recent data indicate that IL-32 may have potent autocrine function in activating macrophages, perhaps in synergy with TLR-derived signals.[24]

Beyond the foregoing pleiotropic inflammatory cytokines, macrophages also have a direct role in moderating T-cell differentiation by cytokine release, including IL-23, IL-12, IL-27, TGF-β–this will be considered in detail below together with data describing cytokine release from other relevant cells, particularly dendritic cells.

Cytokines Regulating or Produced by T-Cell Subsets

The synovial compartment is rich in activated T cells of memory phenotype. Such T cells likely play a crucial role in the pathogenesis of RA. Recent successful therapeutic interventions in RA using CTLA-4Ig (abatacept), which targets T-cell–antigen presenting cell (APC) interactions, are compatible with this notion, as are data in which T-cell depletion has led to improvement in disease activity. T-cell subsets are mainly defined by their cytokine secretion and downstream effector function, such as cytoxicity or regulation. Four major subtypes differentiate from naive T cells into mature functional T cells: T helper 1 (Th1), Th2, Th17, and regulatory T (Treg) cells (Figure 8L-4). In RA, an imbalance toward Th1 and Th17 cells is suggested to drive disease pathology. The differentiation of these cells is cytokine dependent, produced by APCs and/or tissue resident cells.

In rodent models of arthritis, proinflammatory Th1 cells were considered critical to articular autoimmunity by production of interferon-γ (IFN-γ), lymphotoxin-β (LT-β), and TNF. This was also supported by high expression of IL-12, a cytokine responsible for Th1 development, in blood and synovial fluid of RA patients.[25] However, recent studies favor the principle that IL-17-producing Th17 cells may be pre-eminent. First, IFN-γ is only expressed at low levels in synovial fluid, suggesting only a minor role for Th1 cells in local inflammation.[26] Further, in collagen-induced arthritis (CIA, a rodent arthritis model), deficiency of the IFN-γ receptor accelerates disease, and predicts that Th1 cells could possess a protective role.[27] Th17 cells are characterized by their production of IL-17, a cytokine important for recruitment of neutrophils, stimulation of proinflammatory cytokines by epithelial and endothelial cells and fibroblasts, as well as regulation of growth factor production. IL-1, IL-6,

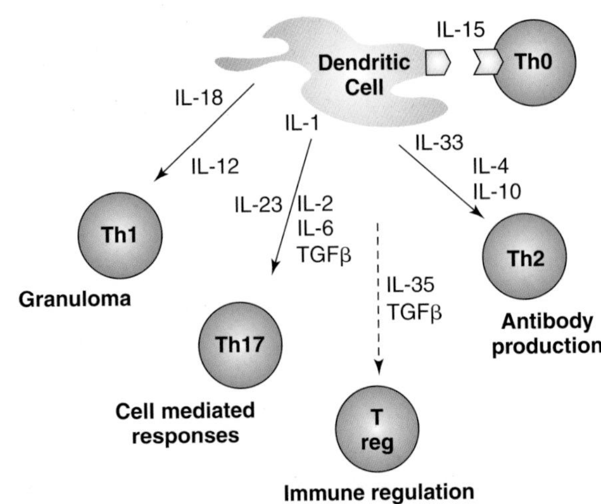

Figure 8L-4. Regulation of T cells by cytokines.

TGF-β, and IL-23, are considered to be the main drivers of differentiation and development of Th17 cells. Such cytokines are produced by macrophages, but also by myeloid and to a lesser extent plasmacytoid dendritic cells in synovial membrane. Interestingly, by inhibiting the development of Th17 cells or inhibition of IL-17, arthritis is reduced in CIA.[28,29] However, *in vitro* data between rodent and human Th17 differentiation regarding cytokine dependency is inconsistent. Nevertheless, IL-17 and IL-22, another Th17 cell cytokine, are highly expressed in RA synovial fluid compared to osteoarthritis fluid controls.[30,31] IL-17 is already targeted in clinical trials and results are awaited. The exact details concerning imbalance in the Th1-Th17-Treg cell axis, however, needs to be defined. An important clue may come from better definition of the effector profile of Th17 cells, which in some systems are now recognized to release not only IL-17 and IL-22, but also IL-26, CCL20, and TNF. Osteopontin, a pleiotropic extracellular matrix protein, is expressed by synovial T cells and has proinflammatory potential. It binds to several integrins and CD44, inducing IL-12 and IFN-γ production in macrophages.[32] Osteopontin is highly expressed in rheumatoid synovium,[33,34] especially in synovial T cells, and induced the expression of proinflammatory cytokines (e.g., IL-1) and various chemokines.[35] Further studies are awaited.

IL-15 is the main cytokine growth factor for synovial T cells. It is upregulated in inflammatory conditions, recruits and activates T cells and other inflammatory cells, and can induce TNF-α, IFN-γ, and IL-17 production by virtue of driving a downstream cascade. IL-15 inhibition suppresses CIA in DBA/1 mice, and IL-15 in turn exacerbates disease. IL-15 expression is elevated in serum and synovial fluid of RA patients and has been successfully targeted in clinical trials.[36,37] IL-2, a cytokine expressed by activated T cells, functions as a growth factor for T cells by supporting proliferation and clonal expansion. Recently, a critical role in the generation of Treg cells has been described.[38] The frequency of Treg cells is higher in synovial fluid of RA patients than in peripheral blood.[39] Despite increased numbers, Treg cells are not capable of controlling disease—the reason for this is unclear perhaps reflecting endogenous alteration in functional capability, or due to an excess of IL-2 detected in early rheumatoid synovial fluid.[40]

Cytokines and B Cells

Rituximab, a B-cell–depleting chimeric anti-CD20 antibody, has unequivocally demonstrated an important role for B-cell lineages in RA pathogenesis; rituximab elicits efficacy and meaningful improvements in disease activity in patients with active, longstanding disease.[41] In the synovium B cells likely act at least via three routes including antibody production, antigen presentation, and cytokine production. The latter (including production of TNF, IL-6, IL-10, and LT-β) contributes to the regulation of follicular dendritic cells (DCs) and influences T-cell–macrophage and T-cell–B-cell interaction, thereby driving not only general inflammation, but also the conditions in which autoreactivity may emerge or be sustained. The exact fraction and location, or indeed subpopulation of B cells contributing cytokine production in the RA synovium, needs to be determined. Cytokines also regulate B-cell maintenance in the joint. B-cell survival is regulated by bystander DCs producing APRIL,[42] and macrophages, as well as synovial fibroblasts that produce BLYS (also called BAFF, B-cell–activating factor).[43] BLYS is expressed in the RA synovial tissue, especially in the lining layer; after stimulation of synovial fibroblasts with TNF or IFN-γ, a significant increase in the production of BLYS is detected, suggesting that paracrine regulatory loops may provide a survival niche for B cells in the inflamed synovial environment.

Neutrophils

Neutrophils are present in high numbers in synovial fluid and traffic there through the synovial membrane. Studies in the K/BxN mouse RA model (a serum transfer model) demonstrate that neutrophils are crucial in the initiation of arthritis,[44] and *in vitro* studies show that synovial fibroblasts can recruit neutrophils in an IL-6–dependent manner.[45] Neutrophils are responsible for production of a variety of cytokines, including TNF, IL-1, IL-18, IL-15, IL-6, and BAFF, and a vast array of inflammatory chemokines. In response to a variety of stimuli, including those delivered by cytokines, neutrophils also produce reactive oxygen intermediates, reactive nitrogen intermediates, serine proteases, metalloproteinases, and antimicrobial products (e.g., defensins, S100 proteins). Since neutrophils may not be short-lived *in vivo* in an inflammatory environment, and since they are present in very high numbers in the RA synovial compartment, it is increasingly recognized that they may play an important pathophysiologic role in disease, at least at the level of amplification and damage perpetuation.

Mast Cells

Mast cells are found principally in mucosa and in connective tissues, generally clustered at epithelial surfaces and around nerves and blood vessels. When triggered by immune complexes, complement, TLR ligands, or microbial antigens, mast cells release granule contents such as histamine, heparin, and proteinases, as well as cytoplasmic products such as cytokines and leukotrienes. Similar to monocytes, mast cells can produce multiple cytokines. In septic peritoneal models, mast cells act as sentinels at the barrier of outer surfaces, initiating TNF production and cellular recruitment cells during early infection.[46] Mast cells are present in the inflamed synovium in RA. In the K/BxN mice arthritis model, mast cell–deficient mice are resistant to disease, indicating a major role for mast cells in arthritis.[47] In contrast, Zhou et al.[48] showed in a collagen/LPS arthritis model, that mast cell deficiency is not crucial but can be replaced by neutrophil-dependent inflammation. Mast cells exhibit plausible cytokine-mediated pathology in the context of synovitis. Histamine and TNF production stimulate proliferation of mast cells; tryptase and chymase, the two main mast-cell proteases, activate precursor forms of matrix metalloproteinases and can induce degradation of cartilage.[49,50] Serine protease release also allows for protease activated receptor 2 (PAR2)–mediated amplification of cytokine release,[51] and inhibition of PAR2 in RA synovial cultures suppresses TNF and IL-1 release. The variety of cytokines produced by mast cells are able to stimulate T and B cells, macrophages, and fibroblasts, and therefore it is likely that mast cells play an important amplificatory role in disease.

Articular Structure, Damage, and Repair

In RA, a hallmark of disease is the destruction of cartilage and bone structure adjacent to the inflamed synovial membrane. Chondrocytes, normally in anabolic status, are switched to a catabolic bias associated with matrix degradation. This fundamental metabolic shift is mediated primarily by cytokines such as IL-1 and IL-17. IL-17 and IL-1β also promote the local release and activation of metalloproteinases.[52] Further, chondrocytes themselves produce IL-1β leading to autocrine amplification of the lesion. Local cytokines provided by synovial fibroblasts, neutrophils, and mast cells enhance this process, and in turn drive invasion particularly by fibroblasts into cartilage. Via these proinflammatory stimuli, production of vascular endothelial growth factor (VEGF) by chondrocytes can be induced leading to neovascularization with further recruitment of cells. Finally, overexpression of IL-1 or IL-17 in mouse arthritis models can promote chondrocyte apoptosis.[53] Thus, cytokines play a pivotal role in the endogenous and invasive events that subserve cartilage damage in RA.

Bone erosions in RA are caused by pro-osteoclastogenic imbalance, which is cytokine driven. Key factors regulating osteoclastogenesis comprise macrophage colony–stimulating factor (M-CSF) and receptor activator of nuclear factor κB ligand (RANKL) expressed by synovial fibroblasts and T cells. M-CSF, together with RANKL, promotes maturation of osteoclast progenitors. RANKL directly expands this population to mature osteoclasts by activation via receptor activator of nuclear factor κB (RANK). TNF, IL-17, and IL-1β exert amplification activity in this cascade. TNF not only induces osteoclasts, but also inhibits osteoblast differentiation.[54] Osteoblasts can again prevent osteoclastogenesis via IL-18.[55] Osteoprotegerin (OPG), acting as a decoy receptor, may also inhibit via binding RANKL. IL-4 and IL-13 can similarly influence this network by decreasing RANKL and RANK, and increasing the expression of OPG.[56,57] In Th1- and Th17-driven inflammation, cytokines are more likely to exert a proerosive influence. However, osteoclastogenesis can be inhibited by IFN-γ–producing T cells[58] depicting a dual role for Th1 cells in bone metabolism. Thus, repair mechanisms are unlikely to operate in an inflammatory environment; a corollary is that effective treatment of RA may stabilize the local microenvironment and provide the possibility for recovery. This is not yet proven in disease, although provocative data in the TEMPO study and other early intervention trials of TNF blockade raise the possibility of "healing erosions." Such lesions have not yet been accurately correlated with the histopathologic lesion described here as cytokine driven, but it is likely that sufficiently early intervention may facilitate some healing and repair responses in articular tissues.

Synovium-specific fibroblasts (synoviocytes) play an important role as endogenous regulators of tissue remodeling but also as immunoregulatory cells that can mount and influence immune responses by being able to secrete chemokines and cytokines. Similarly to monocytes, fibroblasts have the potential to produce a large variety of different cytokines dependent on the stimulus. In RA, synoviocytes act at several levels to promote disease. By increased proliferation and loss of contact inhibition, formation of cadherin-11–dependent hyperplasia and invasion of the cartilage is promoted.[56] This involves high levels of production of proteases, such as MMPs, aggrecanases, and cathepsins. Synovial fibroblasts are activated in turn by TNF and IL-1β to produce high levels of proinflammatory cytokines, and thereby drive a broad array of proinflammatory activities. Thus, synovial fibroblasts have been shown to enhance T- and B-cell migration, in part via chemokine synthesis and survival cytokines secreted (IL-7, IL-15, IL-16, and BAFF), and to activate macrophages via autocrine regulatory loops. Moreover, osteoclasts together with fibroblasts support angiogenesis by production of VEGF, bFGF, oncostatin M, and IL-18.[60,61] In summary, the multifaceted competency of fibroblasts suggests a central role in maintenance of synovitis.

Chemokines and Synovitis

The RA synovial membrane contains a large number of inflammatory and regulatory chemokine species. Their detailed biology is beyond the scope of this chapter, but they should be considered as essential initiator and amplificatory contributors to the synovitis process. They are implicated in every stage of lesion development from early activation of endothelial cells, leukocyte recruitment, and subtissue cellular organization, cellular activation, and immediate cross-talk, and finally by promoting the invasive activities of fibroblasts and activation of chondrocytes and osteoclasts.

Conclusion

The production of cytokines is critical to the pathogenesis of RA. Whereas they exhibit functional pleiotropy and are apparently widely expressed, they in fact comprise a highly sophisticated network that drives the perpetual inflammation that is the hallmark of disease. Critical checkpoints have been identified that have yielded useful clinical therapeutic benefits (described in Chapters 10F through K). Future studies will certainly determine the presence of novel activities, but more importantly will define the functional hierarchies that exist and define disease subsets and kinetics to better derive optimization of therapeutic intervention in due course.

References

1. Pastan IH, Willingham MC. Journey to the center of the cell: Role of the receptosome. *Science* 1981;214:504–509.
2. Weyand CM, Goronzy JJ. Ectopic germinal center formation in rheumatoid synovitis. *Ann N Y Acad Sci* 2003;987:140–149.
3. Manzo A, Paoletti S, Carulli M, et al. Systematic microanatomical analysis of CXCL13 and CCL21 in situ production and progressive lymphoid organization in rheumatoid synovitis. *Eur J Immunol* 2005;35:1347–1359.
4. Kang YM, Zhang X, Wagner UG, et al. CD8 T cells are required for the formation of ectopic germinal centers in rheumatoid synovitis. *J Exp Med* 2002;195:1325–1336.
5. Takemura S, Braun A, Crowson C, et al. Lymphoid neogenesis in rheumatoid synovitis. *J Immunol* 2001;167:1072–1080.
6. Manzo A, Bugatti S, Caporali R, et al. CCL21 Expression pattern of human secondary lymphoid organ stroma is conserved in inflammatory lesions with lymphoid neogenesis. *Am J Pathol* 2007;171: 1549–1562.
7. Wengner AM, Hopken UE, Petrow PK, et al. CXCR5- and CCR7-dependent lymphoid neogenesis in a murine model of chronic antigen-induced arthritis. *Arthritis Rheum* 2007;56:3271–3283.
8. Maki-Petaja KM, Hall FC, Booth AD, et al. Rheumatoid arthritis is associated with increased aortic pulse-wave velocity, which is

reduced by anti-tumor necrosis factor-alpha therapy. *Circulation* 2006;114:1185–1192.

9. Nishimoto N, Hashimoto J, Miyasaka N, et al. Study of active controlled monotherapy used for rheumatoid arthritis, an IL-6 inhibitor (SAMURAI): Evidence of clinical and radiographic benefit from an x ray reader-blinded randomised controlled trial of tocilizumab. *Ann Rheum Dis* 2007;66:1162–1167.
10. Larsen CM, Faulenbach M, Vaag A, et al. Interleukin-1-receptor antagonist in type 2 diabetes mellitus. N Engl *J Med* 2007;356: 1517–1526.
11. Raison CL, Capuron L, Miller AH. Cytokines sing the blues: Inflammation and the pathogenesis of depression. *Trends Immunol* 2006;27: 24–31.
12. Tyring S, Gottlieb A, Papp K, et al. Etanercept and clinical outcomes, fatigue, and depression in psoriasis: Double-blind placebo-controlled randomised phase III trial. *Lancet* 2006;367:29–35.
13. Kriegler M, Perez C, DeFay K, et al. A novel form of TNF/cachectin is a cell surface cytotoxic transmembrane protein: Ramifications for the complex physiology of TNF. *Cell* 1988;53:45–53.
14. Vandenabeele P, Declercq W, Beyaert R, et al. Two tumour necrosis factor receptors: Structure and function. *Trends Cell Biol* 1995;5: 392–399.
15. Black RA, Rauch CT, Kozlosky CJ, et al. A metalloproteinase disintegrin that releases tumour-necrosis factor-alpha from cells. *Nature* 1997;385:729–733.
16. Nishimoto N, Kishimoto T. Inhibition of IL-6 for the treatment of inflammatory diseases. *Curr Opin Pharmacol* 2004;4:386–391.
17. Alonzi T, Fattori E, Lazzaro D, et al. Interleukin 6 is required for the development of collagen-induced arthritis. *J Exp Med* 1998;187: 461–468.
18. Dayer JM, Bresnihan B. Targeting interleukin-1 in the treatment of rheumatoid arthritis. *Arthritis Rheum* 2002;46:574–578.
19. Horai R, Saijo S, Tanioka H, et al. Development of chronic inflammatory arthropathy resembling rheumatoid arthritis in interleukin 1 receptor antagonist–deficient mice. *J Exp Med* 2000;191:313–320.
20. Hoffman HM, Rosengren S, Boyle DL, et al. Prevention of cold-associated acute inflammation in familial cold autoinflammatory syndrome by interleukin-1 receptor antagonist. *Lancet* 2004;364: 1779–1785.
21. Campbell IK, Bendele A, Smith DA, et al. Granulocyte-macrophage colony stimulating factor exacerbates collagen induced arthritis in mice. *Ann Rheum Dis* 1997;56:364–368.
22. Hazenberg BP, Van Leeuwen MA, Van Rijswijk MH, et al. Correction of granulocytopenia in Felty's syndrome by granulocyte-macrophage colony–stimulating factor. Simultaneous induction of interleukin-6 release and flare-up of the arthritis. *Blood* 1989;74: 2769–2770.
23. Joosten LA, Netea MG, Kim SH, et al. IL-32, a proinflammatory cytokine in rheumatoid arthritis. *Proc Natl Acad Sci U S A* 2006; 103:3298–3303.
24. Netea MG, Azam T, Lewis EC, et al. Mycobacterium tuberculosis induces interleukin-32 production through a caspase- 1/IL-18/ interferon-gamma-dependent mechanism. *PLoS Med* 2006;3:e277.
25. Kim W, Min S, Cho M, et al. The role of IL-12 in inflammatory activity of patients with rheumatoid arthritis (RA). *Clin Exp Immunol* 2000;119:175–181.
26. Firestein GS, Zvaifler NJ. Peripheral blood and synovial fluid monocyte activation in inflammatory arthritis. II. Low levels of synovial fluid and synovial tissue interferon suggest that gamma-interferon is not the primary macrophage activating factor. *Arthritis Rheum* 1987;30:864–871.
27. Vermeire K, Heremans H, Vandeputte M, et al. Accelerated collagen-induced arthritis in IFN-gamma receptor–deficient mice. *J Immunol* 1997;158:5507–5513.
28. Alonzi T, Fattori E, Cappelletti M, et al. Impaired Stat3 activation following localized inflammatory stimulus in IL-6–deficient mice. *Cytokine* 1998;10:13–18.
29. Murphy CA, Langrish CL, Chen Y, et al. Divergent pro- and anti-inflammatory roles for IL-23 and IL-12 in joint autoimmune inflammation. *J Exp Med* 2003;198:1951–1957.
30. Chabaud M, Durand JM, Buchs N, et al. Human interleukin-17: A T cell-derived proinflammatory cytokine produced by the rheumatoid synovium. *Arthritis Rheum* 1999;42:963–970.
31. Ikeuchi H, Kuroiwa T, Hiramatsu N, et al. Expression of interleukin-22 in rheumatoid arthritis: Potential role as a proinflammatory cytokine. *Arthritis Rheum* 2005;52:1037–1046.
32. Ashkar S, Weber GF, Panoutsakopoulou V, et al. Eta-1 (osteopontin): An early component of type-1 (cell-mediated) immunity. *Science* 2000;287:860–864.
33. Ohshima S, Yamaguchi N, Nishioka K, et al. Enhanced local production of osteopontin in rheumatoid joints. *J Rheumatol* 2002;29: 2061–2067.
34. Petrow PK, Hummel KM, Schedel J, et al. Expression of osteopontin messenger RNA and protein in rheumatoid arthritis: Effects of osteopontin on the release of collagenase 1 from articular chondrocytes and synovial fibroblasts. *Arthritis Rheum* 2000;43:1597–1605.
35. Xu G, Nie H, Li N, et al. Role of osteopontin in amplification and perpetuation of rheumatoid synovitis. *J Clin Invest* 2005;115: 1060–1067.
36. McInnes IB, al-Mughales J, Field M, et al. The role of interleukin-15 in T-cell migration and activation in rheumatoid arthritis. *Nat Med* 1996;2:175–182.
37. Baslund B, Tvede N, Danneskiold-Samsoe B, et al. Targeting interleukin-15 in patients with rheumatoid arthritis: A proof-of-concept study. *Arthritis Rheum* 2005;52:2686–2692.
38. Pandiyan P, Zheng L, Ishihara S, et al. CD4(+)CD25(+)Foxp3(+) regulatory T cells induce cytokine deprivation-mediated apoptosis of effector CD4(+) T cells. *Nat Immunol* 2007;8:1353–1362.
39. Mottonen M, Heikkinen J, Mustonen L, et al. CD4+ CD25+ T cells with the phenotypic and functional characteristics of regulatory T cells are enriched in the synovial fluid of patients with rheumatoid arthritis. *Clin Exp Immunol* 2005;140:360–367.
40. Raza K, Falciani F, Curnow SJ, et al. Early rheumatoid arthritis is characterized by a distinct and transient synovial fluid cytokine profile of T cell and stromal cell origin. *Arthritis Res Ther* 2005;7:R784–R795.
41. Cohen SB, Emery P, Greenwald MW, et al. Rituximab for rheumatoid arthritis refractory to anti-tumor necrosis factor therapy: Results of a multicenter, randomized, double-blind, placebo-controlled, phase III trial evaluating primary efficacy and safety at twenty-four weeks. *Arthritis Rheum* 2006;54:2793–2806.
42. Seyler TM, Park YW, Takemura S, et al. BLyS and APRIL in rheumatoid arthritis. *J Clin Invest* 2005;115:3083–3092.
43. Ohata J, Zvaifler NJ, Nishio M, et al. Fibroblast-like synoviocytes of mesenchymal origin express functional B cell–activating factor of the TNF family in response to proinflammatory cytokines. *J Immunol* 2005;174:864–870.
44. Wipke BT, Allen PM. Essential role of neutrophils in the initiation and progression of a murine model of rheumatoid arthritis. *J Immunol* 2001;167:1601–1608.
45. Lally F, Smith E, Filer A, et al. A novel mechanism of neutrophil recruitment in a coculture model of the rheumatoid synovium. *Arthritis Rheum* 2005;52:3460–3469.
46. Malaviya R, Ikeda T, Ross E, et al. Mast cell modulation of neutrophil influx and bacterial clearance at sites of infection through TNF-alpha. *Nature* 1996;381:77–80.
47. Lee DM, Friend DS, Gurish MF, et al. Mast cells: A cellular link between autoantibodies and inflammatory arthritis. *Science* 2002;297:1689–1692.
48. Zhou JS, Xing W, Friend DS, et al. Mast cell deficiency in KitW-sh mice does not impair antibody-mediated arthritis. *J Exp Med* 2007; 204:2797–2802.
49. Tetlow LC, Woolley DE. Mast cells, cytokines, and metalloproteinases at the rheumatoid lesion: Dual immunolocalisation studies. *Ann Rheum Dis* 1995;54:896–903.

50. Tetlow LC, Woolley DE. Distribution, activation and tryptase/chymase phenotype of mast cells in the rheumatoid lesion. *Ann Rheum Dis* 1995;54:549–555.
51. Kelso EB, Ferrell WR, Lockhart JC, et al. Expression and proinflammatory role of proteinase-activated receptor 2 in rheumatoid synovium: Ex vivo studies using a novel proteinase-activated receptor 2 antagonist. *Arthritis Rheum* 2007;56:765–771.
52. Honorati MC, Bovara M, Cattini L, et al. Contribution of interleukin 17 to human cartilage degradation and synovial inflammation in osteoarthritis. *Osteoarthritis Cartilage* 2002;10:799–807.
53. Lubberts E, Joosten LA, van de Loo FA, et al. Overexpression of IL-17 in the knee joint of collagen type II immunized mice promotes collagen arthritis and aggravates joint destruction. *Inflamm Res* 2002;51:102–104.
54. Bertolini DR, Nedwin GE, Bringman TS, et al. Stimulation of bone resorption and inhibition of bone formation in vitro by human tumour necrosis factors. *Nature* 1986;319:516–518.
55. Udagawa N, Horwood NJ, Elliott J, et al. Interleukin-18 (interferon-gamma-inducing factor) is produced by osteoblasts and acts via granulocyte/macrophage colony–stimulating factor and not via interferon-gamma to inhibit osteoclast formation. *J Exp Med* 1997; 185:1005–1012.
56. Mirosavljevic D, Quinn JM, Elliott J, et al. T-cells mediate an inhibitory effect of interleukin-4 on osteoclastogenesis. *J Bone Miner Res* 2003;18:984–993.
57. Palmqvist P, Lundberg P, Persson E, et al. Inhibition of hormone and cytokine-stimulated osteoclastogenesis and bone resorption by interleukin-4 and interleukin-13 is associated with increased osteoprotegerin and decreased RANKL and RANK in a STAT6-dependent pathway. *J Biol Chem* 2006;281:2414–2429.
58. Takayanagi H, Ogasawara K, Hida S, et al. T-cell-mediated regulation of osteoclastogenesis by signalling cross-talk between RANKL and IFN-gamma. *Nature* 2000;408:600–605.
59. Lee DM, Kiener HP, Agarwal SK, et al. Cadherin-11 in synovial lining formation and pathology in arthritis. *Science* 2007;315: 1006–1010.
60. Meyer LH, Franssen L, Pap T. The role of mesenchymal cells in the pathophysiology of inflammatory arthritis. *Best Pract Res Clin Rheumatol* 2006;20:969–981.
61. Pap T, Muller-Ladner U, Gay RE, et al. Fibroblast biology. Role of synovial fibroblasts in the pathogenesis of rheumatoid arthritis. *Arthritis Res* 2000;2:361–367.

Signal Transduction

Francesca I. Okoye, Nicholas D. Bushar, and Donna L. Farber

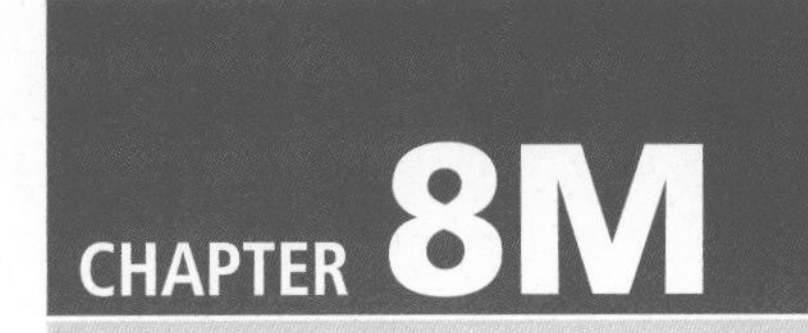

The pathogenesis of rheumatic diseases involves both inflammatory and immune-mediated processes mediated by multiple cell types, including T and B lymphocytes, monocytes/macrophages, neutrophils, and mast cells. These cells all bear surface receptors that bind to soluble factors, antigens, or other cellular components that cause these cells to become activated. When activated, lymphocytes, monocytes, neutrophils, and mast cells produce a myriad of soluble factors to recruit and activate additional immune and inflammatory cells, mediate inflammatory processes, and promote activation and cellular changes in epithelial tissue and vasculature. Activation of lymphocytes and cellular components of the inflammatory response requires engagement of a cell surface receptor, which in turn, triggers a cascade of intracellular biochemical events that couple the receptor signals from the cell surface to the nucleus for modulation of gene transcription via a process called signal transduction.

Receptor-mediated signal transduction is a fundamental cellular process essential for communicating events at the cell surface and interactions with the extracellular environment into changes of gene expression that occur in the nucleus. These events proceed from membrane to nucleus via a series of protein modifications mediated by specific enzymes such as protein kinases, the subsequent triggers the recruitment and activation of linker or scaffolding proteins, the modification of GTP-coupled intermediates serving as second messengers, an increase in the concentration of intracellular calcium, and ultimately, to the mobilization of transcription factors for gene activation in the nucleus. The identity of specific proteins kinases, G-proteins, and accessory intermediates involved in each signaling pathway depends on the specific receptor and cell type involved. In this chapter, we present some of the key receptors and their associated signaling pathways that are of importance to the pathogenesis of rheumatoid diseases, including activation of T lymphocytes through the T-cell antigen receptor (TCR), B-lymphocyte activation through the B-cell–antigen receptor (BCR) or immunoglobulin, lymphocyte and monocyte activation through cytokine receptors, and activation of monocytes, neutrophils, and mast cells through cell-surface antibody-binding Fc receptors.

T-Lymphocyte Signal Transduction

Activation of T lymphocytes is the critical event for the initiation and orchestration of adaptive immune responses. T lymphocytes mediate antipathogen immunity and are the key initiators for autoimmune diseases such as rheumatoid arthritis (RA) and systemic lupus erythematosus (SLE). At the molecular level, T-cell activation is mediated by a number of receptor-ligand and receptor–coreceptor interactions. On the T-cell surface, three main receptor–ligand interactions coordinate to initiate the signals involved in T-cell activation: (1) the T-cell antigen receptor (TCR) interacts with antigenic peptide presented by major histocompatibility molecule (pMHC) class I or class II; (2) T-cell coreceptors CD8 or CD4 bind their ligand pMHC class I and class II, respectively; and (3) the costimulatory receptor CD28 on T cells binds to its ligand B7-1/B7-2 (CD80/CD86) expressed on the surface of antigen-presenting cells (APCs).[1] While the TCR is the primary trigger for the clonal expansion of antigen-specific cells from a polyclonal population of T cells with numerous antigen specificities, the CD4 and CD8 coreceptors enhance the TCR–pMHC interaction but do not affect specificity.[2,3] Ligation of the TCR and coreceptor leads to a cascade of intracellular events resulting in the proliferation and differentiation of resting T cells into several types of effector T cells that can synthesize all the effector molecules required for their specialized functions.

The T-cell receptor complex is made up of antigen-recognition proteins and invariant signaling proteins. The peptide–MHC binding portion of the TCR consists of highly variable TCRα and β chains forming heterodimers that lack intrinsic intracellular signaling capabilities. In the functional receptor complex, α/β heterodimers are associated with a complex of four other signaling chains (two ε, one δ, and one γ) collectively called CD3, and a homodimer of TCRζ chains that are required for TCRαβ cell-surface expression and for signaling (Figure 8M-1A). The cytoplasmic portion of each CD3 and TCRζ chain contains one to three immunoreceptor tyrosine-based activation motifs (ITAMs). Each ITAM comprises a 16– to 18–amino-acid sequence containing two tyrosine residues that are substrates for cytoplasmic protein tyrosine kinases (PTKs) once the TCR is effectively engaged by antigen/MHC. The phosphorylated CD3 and TCRζ chains then serve as sites of recruitment and binding of other protein tyrosine kinases and downstream mediators.[4,5]

Tyrosine kinases associated with the TCR include members of the Src and Syk family tyrosine kinases. The initial events in TCR signaling are implemented by two Src-family kinases—p56Lck, a protein of 56 kDa constitutively associated with the cytoplasmic domain of the coreceptor molecules CD4 and CD8, and p59Fyn, which associates with the cytoplasmic domains of the ζ and CD3ε chains upon receptor clustering (Figure 8M-2). Upon TCR ligation by antigen/MHC, both Fyn and Lck phosphorylate tyrosines in the ITAMs of the TCR-associated CD3

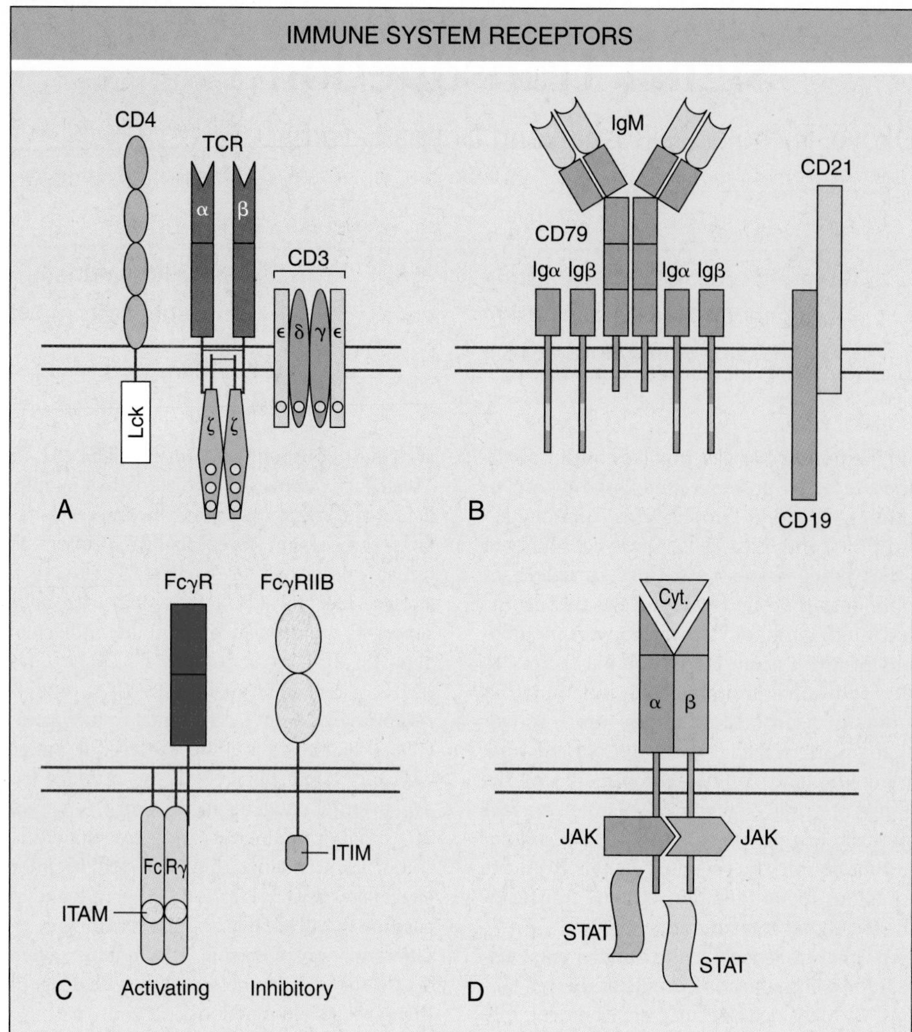

Figure 8M-1. Immune system receptors. (A) The T-cell receptor (TCR) complex is made up of antigen-recognition proteins and invariant signaling proteins. (B) The B-cell receptor complex is made up of cell surface immunoglobulin with each of the invariant proteins Iga and Igb. (C) Fc receptors. Activating-type FcRs associate with the FcR common g-chain, which contains an ITAM, and FcγRIIB is a single-chain molecule that contains an immunoreceptor tyrosine-based inhibitory motif (ITIM) for inhibition of the ITAM-induced activation cascade. (D) Cytokine receptors consist of at least two chains, the cytoplasmic domains of which bind Janus kinases (JAKs). (From Hochberg M, Silman A, Weinblatt M, et al. *Rheumatology*, 4th ed. London: Mosby, 2008, Fig. 12.1.)

signaling subunits (ϵ,δ,γ) and TCRζ. Phosphorylated ITAMs serve as docking sites for zeta-associated protein of 70kDa (ZAP-70), a member of the Syk tyrosine kinase family. The ZAP-70 kinase associated to TCRζ becomes phosphorylated by Lck which enhances the kinase activity of ZAP-70, leading to the phosphorylation of several key linker/adapter molecules including a 36-kDa protein designated linker of activated T cells (LAT) and an SH2-domain containing leukocyte protein of 76 kDa referred to as SLP-76 (Figure 8M-2). Phosphorylated LAT and SLP-76 serve to couple proximal phosphorylated events to downstream targets, including activation of phospholipase C-γ1 (PLCγ1), release of Ca^{2+} stores, and mitogen-activated protein kinase (MAPK) activation (Figure 8M-2). There are a number of MAP kinases that serve critical roles in cellular signaling pathways of many receptors involved in growth and development. In T cells, the MAP kinases involved are p42/44 (Erk1/2), p38 MAP kinase, and the JNK kinase, which each serve distinct roles in initiating T-cell proliferation and differentiation. Activation of these distal signaling intermediates result in numerous downstream events such as activation of the small G proteins Ras and Rac, which lead to actin reorganization enabling maximal contact of the T cell with the APC. Importantly, the signaling events coupled to the TCR ultimately culminate in mobilization of transcription factors NFκB, NFAT, and AP-1 that activate IL-2 gene transcription—a primary growth and differentiation factor for T lymphocytes.[5–8]

TCR Signaling in Disease

Given their critical roles in both inflammation and the progression of the immune response, the role of T cells has been the focus of numerous studies attempting to characterize the progression of disease in cases of SLE and RA. Interestingly, T cells associated with SLE and RA exhibit abnormalities in the expression and/or phosphorylation of TCR-coupled

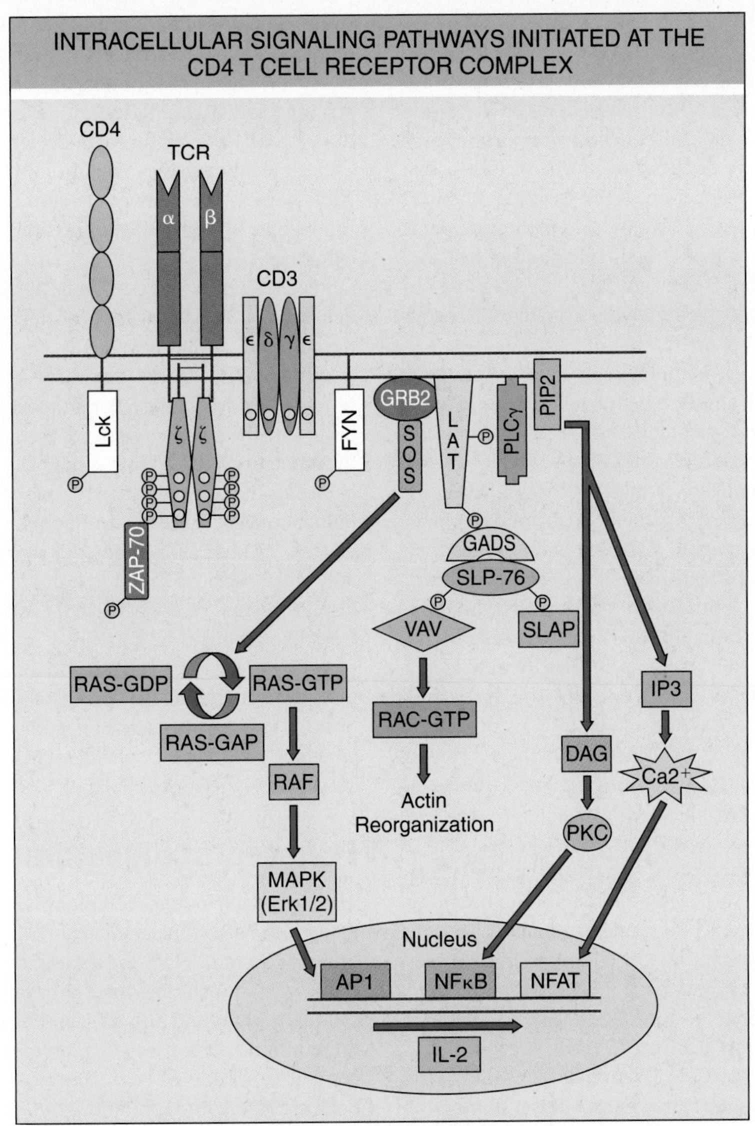

Figure 8M-2. Intracellular signaling pathways initiated at the CD4 T-cell receptor complex. The TCR and coreceptor (in this example the CD4 molecule), associated signaling molecules, their coupling to downstream biochemical events and culmination in nuclear gene transcription are shown. Upon antigen:MHC ligand binding to the TCR and coreceptor, the proximal kinases Lck and Fyn phosphorylate tyrosine residues on the ITAM regions in the intracytoplasmic domains of CD3ϵ and TCRζ, recruiting ZAP-70 to bind to phosphorylated tyrosine residues on the TCRζ chains. The bound ZAP-70 becomes phosphorylated, activating the kinase to phosphorylate the adapter proteins LAT and SLP-76, which in turn leads to the activation of PLC-γ by Tec kinases and the activation of Ras by guanine-nucleotide exchange factors (GEFs). Activated PLC-γ and Ras initiate three important pathways that culminate in the activation of transcription factors in the nucleus. Together NFκB, NFAT, and AP-1 act on the T-cell chromosomes, initiating new gene transcription. (From Hochberg M, Silman A, Weinblatt M, et al. *Rheumatology*, 4th ed. London: Mosby, 2008, Fig. 12.2.)

signaling components, which are believed to contribute to the pathology of the autoimmune process. For example, T cells from SLE and RA exhibit low-level expression of the TCRζ subunit of the TCR complex. In cases of RA, downregulation of TCRζ also appears to abrogate downstream T-cell signaling events, as these cells display a weakened pattern of intracellular tyrosine phosphorylations upon restimulation.[9,10] Furthermore, the binding capacity of p56lck in RA T cells appears disrupted and may play a role in the aberrant function of T cells during progression of this disease.[11] Lupus T cells are likewise characterized by altered tyrosine phosphorylation.[12] Whether these signaling abnormalities directly promote disease pathogenesis or result from global immune changes remains to be established.

B-Lymphocyte Signal Transduction

B cells are the central mediators of the humoral branch of the adaptive immune response. Upon activation by a particular antigen, B cells are stimulated to differentiate into plasma cells which secrete antibody molecules. The process of B-cell activation occurs in a manner analogous to that of T cells discussed above; activation signals received at the cell surface are transduced intracellularly via a series of phosphorylation events catalyzed by tyrosine kinases leading to recruitment of linker molecules, MAP kinase activation and culminating in the activation of transcription factors such as NFκB, NFAT, and AP-1 to initiate B-cell proliferation and differentiation. This process of B-cell activation must be tightly regulated, as the consequences of improper production of antibody can have devastating effects. In the case of autoimmune diseases, the production of self-reacting autoantibodies by improperly activated B cells results in pathologic damage to the host tissues as seen in the rheumatic diseases SLE and RA. Therefore, the process of B-cell activation operates in a coordinated signaling cascade, which includes a system of checks and balances to ensure proper activation.

The B-cell receptor (BCR) complex is composed of three primary elements located at the plasma membrane (Figure 8M-1B). The central receptor element consists of a membrane bound immunoglobulin (Ig) molecule which serves as the external binding site for antigen. Similar to the TCR (Figure 8M-1A), the antigen-binding membrane Ig does not contain an intracellular signaling domain, and signaling is transduced via noncovalently bound heterodimeric signaling complex (Iga and Igb, also designated CD79a and CD79b, respectively). Like the subunits of the CD3 complex in T cells, both Iga and Igb have a single ITAM in their cytosolic tails that enables them to signal when the B-cell receptor is ligated with antigen. The third component of the BCR complex is the CD19/CD21 coreceptor complex that serves an analogous function to the CD4 and CD8 coreceptors of T cells. Coligation of CD19 and the B-cell antigen receptor complex amplifies the intracellular effects of signaling through the antigen receptor.[13,14]

When a B cell receives an activation signal through the recognition of antigen at the cell surface by the membrane bound Ig molecule, ITAM motifs of the CD79 signaling complex become phosphorylated by and bound by protein tyrosine kinases (PTKs) such as Lyn, Fyn, Lck, and Blk.[13,15] The phosphorylated CD79 chains serve as binding sites for linker/adapter molecules such as SLP-65 (analogous to SLP-76 in T cells) to coordinate the downstream signaling cascade (Figure 8M-3). SLP-65 in B cells lacks intrinsic enzymatic activity and binds a number of signaling intermediates, including the Tec family kinase Btk (Bruton's tyrosine kinase) and PLCγ2 (phospholipase Cγ2) and mediates their translocation to membrane microdomains of the B cells called lipid rafts, where they are associated with the BCR components and activated by tyrosine kinases. This activation results in the subsequent release of Ca^{2+} stores within the cell, leading to mobilization of downstream effectors of B-cell activation including protein kinase C (PKC), calcineurin, and the MAP kinase cascade (Figure 8M-3). Similar to their role in T-cell activation, these signaling effectors in B cells result in the stimulation of transcription factors NFκB, NFAT, and AP-1. In the B cell, however, these transcription factors result ultimately in B-cell proliferation and differentiation into fully activated antibody-secreting plasma cells.[16,17]

BCR Signaling in Disease

Autoantibody production is a hallmark of SLE and RA pathogenesis and other rheumatic diseases. Over 100 autoantibody specificities have been described in SLE patients, several of which are associated with disease activity. The abnormal production of autoantibodies to nuclear antigens including double-stranded DNA (dsDNA), nucleosomes, and histones have been shown to contribute to the pathogenesis of SLE. Anti-dsDNA serum levels have been correlated with SLE activity and are often used clinically as predictive and/or representative of disease activity. These autoantibodies are of the IgG isotype and have acquired somatic mutations, indicating that the B cells that produce them have matured under the influence of T-cell help. Other mechanisms involved in lupus B-cell hyperactivation include defects in negative regulators of BCR signaling, defective Fcg receptor–mediated suppression, and increased responses to cytokines.[18]

Recent studies suggest that BCR signaling may be intrinsically defective in SLE. Activation of normal B cells with antigens or monoclonal antibodies results in a cascade of intracellular events that lead to cell activation and proliferation. In the absence of Lyn, receptor Syk complexes are retained in the membrane, resulting in enhanced activation of NFAT and B-cell hyperactivity. B cells from a majority of patients with SLE have been shown to have reduced levels of the Lyn kinase which may influence BCR signaling and hyperactivity characteristic of the disease.[19] Other BCR-mediated signaling abnormalities in SLE are similar to those found in lupus T cells. Activated SLE B cells display higher BCR-mediated Ca^{2+} release (mainly released from intracellular Ca^{2+} stores), increased production of the second messenger P3 and enhanced production of tyrosine phosphorylated cellular proteins compared to B cells from healthy individuals.[9] Further studies are needed to determine whether targeting of specific signaling events in B cells may ameliorate symptoms of SLE.

Fc Receptor Signal Transduction

The receptors for the Fc component of immunoglobulins, Fc receptors (FcRs), link the humoral and cellular branches of the immune system. FcRs are expressed by many cells of the immune system including macrophages, neutrophils, B cells, mast cells, basophils, and NK cells, and have a central role in controlling immune responses after interaction with antigen-antibody complexes (Table 8M-1). The biologic functions of FcRs are both activating and inhibitory and depend on the type of signal transducing molecules associated with the FcR. The activating-type of FcRs are distinguished by their association with the Fc receptor common g-chain (FcRg) which contains an ITAM (Figure 8M-1C, left) and is associated with FcγRI, FcγRIII, FcεRI, FcαRI, and other receptors, including collagen receptor glycoprotein IV, and paired immunoglobulin-like receptor-A (PIR-A). Signaling mediated by FcRγ-associated FcRs result in activation of numerous cellular processes including phagocytosis and superoxide generation in macrophages and neutrophils, antibody-dependent cellular cytotoxicity in NK cells, the production and release of cytokines and proinflammatory mediators by granulocytes, and the degranulation of mast cells. By contrast, the inhibitory Fc receptor FcγRIIB is a single-chain molecule that contains an immunoreceptor tyrosine–based inhibitory motif (ITIM) in its cytoplasmic domain for regulating ITAM-induced processes (Figure 8M-1C, right). FcγRIIB is expressed ubiquitously on immune cells, including B cells, macrophages and mast cells, and it can inhibit processes such as B-cell activation/proliferation and mast cell degranulation.[20]

FcRs function through the binding and uptake of immune complexes (ICs). FcRs can trigger the internalization of captured ICs and thereby induce the efficient processing of antigens into peptides that are presented by MHC class I or class II

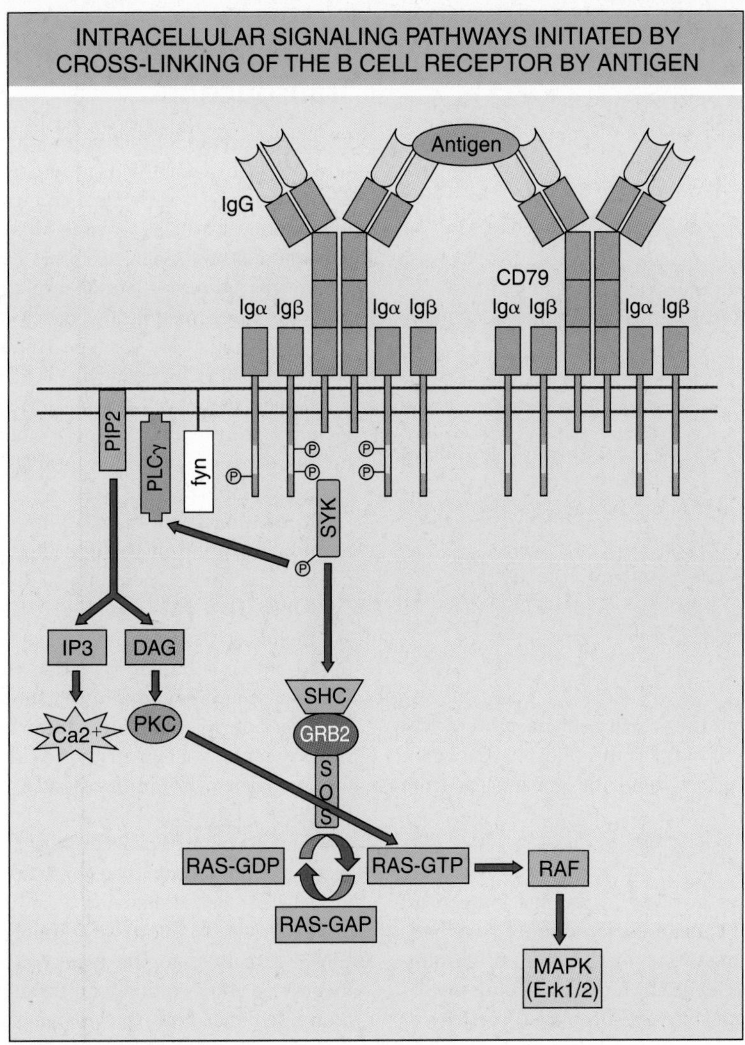

Figure 8M-3. Intracellular signaling pathways initiated by cross-linking of the B-cell receptor by antigen. The surface BCR, associated signaling molecules, and the signaling processes leading to nuclear gene transcription are shown. Cross-linking of the surface immunoglobulin molecules activates the receptor-associated Src-family protein tyrosine kinases Blk, Fyn (shown), and Lyn which in turn phosphorylate the ITAMs in the receptor complex. Phosphorylated ITAMs bind and activate the cytosolic protein kinase Syk. Syk then phosphorylates other targets, including PLC-γ, GEFs and Tec kinases. PLC-γ cleaves the membrane phospholipids PIP_2 into IP_3 and DAG, thus initiating two of the three main pathways to the nucleus. IP_3 releases Ca^{2+} from intracellular and extracellular sources, and Ca^{2+}-dependent enzymes are activated, whereas DAG activates protein kinase C with the help of Ca^{2+}. The third main pathway is initiated by GEFs that become associated with the receptor and activate small GTP-binding proteins such as Ras. Ras triggers protein kinase cascades (MAP kinase cascades) that lead to the activation of MAP kinases to translocate into the nucleus and phosphorylate proteins to regulate gene transcription. (From Hochberg M, Silman A, Weinblatt M, et al. *Rheumatology*, 4th ed. London: Mosby, 2008, Fig. 12.3.)

antigen–presentation pathways. FcRs enhance the antigen presentation of IgG—containing ICs by dendritic cells and epidermal Langerhans' cells leading to the activation of antigen specific T cells. The elimination of antigen by macrophage and the efficient presentation of antigen by dendritic cells to T lymphocytes are equally mediated by FcRs. Defects in IC clearance have been linked to development of autoimmune diseases such as SLE.[20] FcR-coupled signaling events are initiated by the Src family protein kinases such as Src, Fyn, Fgr, Hck, and Lyn upon ligation of activating FcγRs by immune complexes and they phosphorylate tyrosine residues in the ITAM. In turn, the phosphorylated ITAM then serves as a docking sight for Syk, which is also phosphorylated by Src-family kinases. Activation of Syk results in downstream events similar to the Syk-mediated pathways in BCR signaling, including the activation of PLCγ, PI3K, and the Erk1/2 MAP kinases. In macrophages, Syk activation also results in the stimulation of the cytoskeletal protein paxillin, and GTPases of the Rho and Rac families that mediate the downstream signaling events resulting in reorganization of the actin cytoskeleton similar to B and T cells (Figure 8M-4A). By contrast, FcγRIIB acts physiologically as a negative regulator of IC-triggered activation. The inhibitory function of FcγRIIB is best characterized in B cells in which coaggregation of the BCR with FcγRIIB results in the phosphorylation of the ITIM tyrosine found in the FcγRIIB cytoplasmic tail. This modification recruits the SH2-domain-containing inositol polyphosphate

Table 8M-1. Fc Receptor Expression

Fc Receptor	Expression
FcgRIA	Macrophage, monocyte, neutrophil, eosinophil, DC
FcgRIIA	Macrophage, neutrophil, eosinophil, platelet, DC, LC
FcgRIIB	B cell, mast cells, basophil, macrophage, eosinophil, DC, LC
FcgRIIIA	Macrophage, monocyte, NK cells, mast cell, eosinophil, DC, LC, neutrophil (mouse)
FcgRIIIB	Neutrophil, eosinophil
FceRI	Mast cell, basophil, eosinophil, LC (human), DC (human)
FceRII	Ubiquitous, platelet
FcaRI	Macrophage, neutrophil, eosinophil
FcRn	Placenta, small intestine, monocyte, DC
Fca/uR	B cell, macrophage
Poly-IgR	Epithelium, liver, small intestine, lung
FcRH1-5	B cell

5 phosphatase (SHIP) which is the primary effector of FcγRIIB-mediated inhibition (Figure 8M-4B), as this phosphatase counteracts the action of kinases by removing phosphates from phosphorylated residues.[20]

FcR Signaling in Disease

Due to the diverse processes involved in the development of autoimmune diseases, genetic manipulation of mice have been useful for elucidating the molecular mechanisms of autoimmune diseases. Mice that are deficient for the signaling mediator FcRγ are unable to phagocytose IgG-opsonized particles or to mediate antibody-dependent cellular cytotoxicity (ADCC) by natural killer cells, and they respond poorly to IgE-mediated mast-cell activation. Moreover, FcRγ-deficient mice are resistant to the induction or spontaneous onset of various autoimmune diseases suggesting that this signaling molecule may serve as a therapeutic target in the treatment for autoimmune diseases. In addition, disruption of the FcγRIIB gene in mice results in enhanced responses including elevated immunoglobulin levels in response to stimulation, enhanced anaphylaxis, and enhanced IC-mediated inflammatory responses. In humans, FcR polymorphisms have been linked to the development of autoimmune diseases such as SLE and RA.[20]

More recent studies have revealed that FcRg subunit can be expressed in certain activated T cells and in T cells from patients with SLE. Unlike TCRζ which mediates signaling through the tyrosine kinase ZAP-70, FcRγ mediates signaling by associating with phosphorylated protein kinase Syk. It has been shown that Syk kinase is 100-fold more potent than ZAP-70, and is preferentially recruited to the FcRg. High-level expression of FcRγ has been observed in both CD4$^+$ and CD8$^+$ T cells of SLE patients. The upregulation of FcRg in TCRζ deficient T cells appears to be disease-specific and independent of disease activity and treatment. These changes in the proximal signaling intermediates contribute to the abnormal T-cell functions found in SLE patients and other autoimmune conditions.[12]

Cytokine Receptor Signal Transduction

Cytokine receptors function in a manner similar to that previously described for the TCR and BCR—short extracellular receptor domains that mediate an intracellular signal through the interaction of crucial tyrosine kinases recruited to their cytoplasmic tails. Cytokine receptors can be classified into superfamilies based on structural similarities and subunit composition. The three main groups of relevance to rheumatic diseases include receptors for the type 1 family of cytokines, which includes receptors for many growth factors and nearly all of the interleukin family of cytokines, the type 2 cytokine receptors, including those for interferon and IL-10 signaling, and the tumor necrosis family of receptors (TNFR), which mediate TNF signaling (Table 8M-2).

As mentioned above, most Interleukin signaling, with the notable exception of IL-10, occurs through the type 1 family cytokine receptors, including all members of the IL-2 family of cytokines (IL-2, IL-4, IL-7, IL-9, IL-15, and IL-21). Receptors for members of this family of cytokines are generally composed of two subunits: a unique a chain that confers binding specificity, and a common g_c subunit that is utilized by all members of this cytokine family. In the case of the IL-2 and IL-15 receptor, a heterotrimeric complex is formed, composed of the unique α, common γ, and a third β subunit (designated IL-2Rb).[21]

Members of the type 2 family of cytokines comprise heterodimeric receptor complexes, consisting of one long and one short intracellular tail, designated a and b, respectively. In the case of IFN, these subunits are simply designated IFNGR1 and IFNGR2. Similar to the type 1 cytokine receptor complexes mentioned above, redundancy in subunit composition is a common theme in type 2 cytokine signaling. For example, the IL-10Rb is a common subunit for transducing signals through receptors for IL-10, IL-22, IL-28, and IL-29. In addition, multiple class 2 cytokines have been shown to be capable of binding more than one receptor complex, and single type 2 receptor complexes have been shown to bind more than one cytokine within the class.[22]

Despite the redundancy of subunits associated with receptors for diverse cytokines, engagement of cytokine receptors with specific cytokines leads to distinct functional outcomes, due to the signaling molecules associated with each cytokine receptor. These key signaling molecules include members of the Janus family of kinases (JAKs) and "signal transducers and activators of transcription" (STATs), which act as intracellular mediators of the cytokine signaling cascade (Figure 8M-1D). In order to initiate a signal within the cell, receptors for the type 1 and type 2 families of cytokine receptors rely primarily on the recruitment of JAKs and STATs to their cytoplasmic domains. Cytokine-induced receptor oligomerization at the cell surface results in JAK activation via a series of auto- and cross-phosphorylation events that serve to recruit downstream signaling molecules, including STATs, to the signaling complex. STATs bind the phosphorylated JAKs via their SH2 domain and are subsequently phosphorylated. Phosphorylated STATs are then released from the signaling complex and form active homodimers, which migrate to the nucleus to mediate transcription. The function of JAKs and STATs is regulated by specific

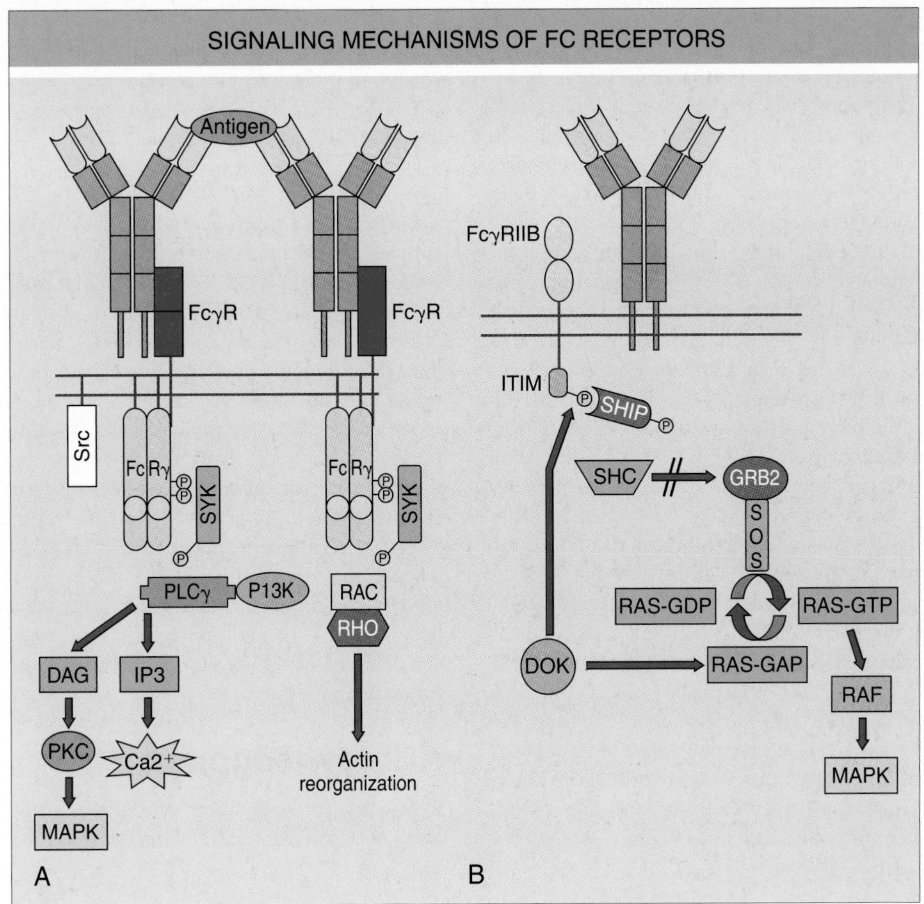

Figure 8M-4. Signaling mechanisms of Fc receptors. (A) Signaling by ITAM-containing activating FcγRs. Tyrosine residues in the ITAM become phosphorylated by Src-family protein kinases such as Src, Fyn, Fgr, Hck, and Lyn after cross-linking of cell surface FcγRs by immunoglobulin-G-containing immune complexes. The downstream effects of Syk activation include activation of PLCγ, PI3K, MAP kinases , and GTPases of the Rho and Rac families which are involved in reorganization of the actin cytoskeleton. (B) Inhibition of the activation pathway by co-aggregation of FcγRIIB. Cross-linking of FcγRIIB and the BCR results in the phosphorylation of the ITIM located on the cytoplasmic tail of FcγRIIB. The phosphorylated ITIM recruits and phosphorylates SHIP (SH2-domain-containing inositol polyphosphate 5′phosphatase), creating a binding site for SHC and DOK. SHC inhibits GRB2 whereas DOK recruits Ras-GAP, which catalyzes the conversion of Ras-GTP to Ras-GDP, leading to inhibition of the ERK-MAP kinase pathway. (From Hochberg M, Silman A, Weinblatt M, et al. *Rheumatology*, 4th ed. London: Mosby, 2008, Fig. 12.4.)

Table 8M-2. Cytokine Receptor Superfamilies

Cytokine Receptor Superfamily	Cytokines
Type 1	IL-2, IL-4, IL-7, IL-9, IL-15, IL-21
Type 2	IL-10, IL-19, IL-20, IL-22, IL-28, IL-29, IFNα, IFNβ, IFNγ
TNF-RI/TNF-RII	TNF

inhibitory proteins including members of the SOCS (suppressors of cytokine signaling) family. These proteins help to fine-tune the signal through the cytokine receptors, preventing overactivation and downregulating the signal at the cessation of the response.[23]

Signaling mediated by members of the proinflammatory tumor necrosis factor family occurs in a manner different to that proposed for type 1 and type 2 cytokines. The receptors for this family are subgrouped into TNF-R1 and TNF-R2, based on differential intracellular associated molecules. For TNF-R1, the intracellular portions of the receptors are considered "death domains" (DD), which upon ligand binding, function to recruit other DD proteins within the cell, ultimately leading to downstream caspase activation and initiation of the apoptotic pathway. TNF-R2, by contrast, associates intracellularly with TRAF (TNF receptor–associated factor) proteins, which results ultimately in the activation of the transcription factor NF-κB and AP-1. NF-κB enhances cell survival through the transcriptional regulation of a number of antiapoptotic proteins and AP-1 is involved in a number of survival and proliferation-dependent pathways.[24]

Lipid Rafts in Cellular Signaling

Cell signaling is tightly regulated and requires the organization of individual signaling molecules into discrete complexes. Rafts are cholesterol- and glycosphingolipid-rich regions of the cell membrane that are distinguished by their insolubility in detergents such as Triton-X-100, and are enriched in phosphatidylinositol (PI)-anchored membrane proteins. These ordered structures serve as molecular platforms that concentrate signaling molecules and facilitate specific protein-protein interactions allowing for efficient propagation of intracellular signals. In lymphocytes, several key signaling molecules are enriched in rafts, and upon receptor engagement by ligands, the TCR, BCR, and many FcR become raft associated.[25]

On the surface of the T lymphocyte, lipid rafts are important for the formation and stabilization of the TCR signaling complexes. TCR ligation resulting in the clustering of signaling molecules and enrichment of the lipid rafts occurs at the area of contact between APCs and T cells known as the immunologic synapse. Upon the engagement of the TCR with MHC-peptide complexes, there is rapid mobilization of p56lck, CD3ζ, Grb2, PLC-γ1, phosphorylated ZAP-70, and LAT signaling molecules to the rafts, effectively concentrating the primary signal transducers and facilitating their interactions. Another function of rafts is to exclude larger molecules such as the tyrosine phosphatase CD45 from associating with the TCR, as these molecules may sterically hinder T-APC contact.[25]

Similarly, during B-cell cross-linking, the BCR rapidly translocates into lipid rafts that contain the protein tyrosine kinase Lyn and Igα. ZAP-70, Syk, Vav, phosphatase (SHIP), PLCγ1, and protein kinase C θ (PKC θ) are also recruited into the expanding rafts whereas CD45 is excluded. Lipid raft pool size, membrane distribution pattern, protein content, and the kinetics of cytoskeletal rearrangements following T-cell or B-cell stimulation are all features that can influence the strength of signals controlled by lipid rafts. It is not known whether differential signaling may be mediated by specific recruitment or exclusion of molecules into membrane rafts.[14]

Conclusion

The complex pathogenesis of rheumatic diseases involves the participation of immune and inflammatory cells that become activated and produce soluble mediators that coordinate pathogenic processes. The primary molecular events involved in this process are the intracellular signals that are propagated and initiate cellular proliferation and activation. In this chapter, we have described the key signaling processes which occur in immune and inflammatory cells and are of central importance to understanding rheumatic diseases, including signals coupled to the TCR, BCR, FcR, and cytokine receptors. Signaling through each of these receptors involves common processes such as protein phosphorylation, recruitment, MAP kinase activation, the involvement of small GTP-binding proteins—all leading to transcription factor mobilization in the nucleus. Understanding what components are involved in each disease process such as identifying aberrant signaling mechanisms can serve as novel targets for therapeutic manipulation at the fundamental level.

Acknowledgment

Reprinted from Hochberg M, Silman A, Weinblatt M, et al. *Rheumatology*, 4th ed. (London: Mosby, 2008).

References

1. Gao GF, Jakobsen BK. Molecular interactions of coreceptor CD8 and MHC class I: The molecular basis for functional coordination with the T-cell receptor. *Immunol Today* 2000;21:630–636.
2. Luescher IF, Vivier E, Layer A, et al. CD8 modulation of T-cell antigen receptor-ligand interactions on living cytotoxic T lymphocytes. *Nature* 1995;373:353–356.
3. Hampl J, Chien YH, Davis MM. CD4 augments the response of a T cell to agonist but not to antagonist ligands. *Immunity* 1997;7:379–385.
4. Kane LP, Lin J, Weiss A. Signal transduction by the TCR for antigen. *Curr Opin Immunol* 2000;12:242–249.
5. Baniyash M. TCR zeta-chain downregulation: Curtailing an excessive inflammatory immune response. *Nat Rev Immunol* 2004;4:675–687.
6. Chu DH, Morita CT, Weiss A. The Syk family of protein tyrosine kinases in T-cell activation and development. *Immunol Rev* 1998;165:167–180.
7. Turner M, Schweighoffer E, Colucci F, et al. Tyrosine kinase SYK: Essential functions for immunoreceptor signalling. *Immunol Today* 2000;21:148–154.
8. Hatada MH, Lu X, Laird ER, et al. Molecular basis for interaction of the protein tyrosine kinase ZAp-70 with the T-cell receptor. *Nature* 1995;377:32–38.
9. Tsokos GC, Liossis SN. Immune cell signaling defects in lupus: Activation, anergy and death. *Immunol Today* 1999;20:119–124.
10. Maurice MM, Lankester AC, Bezemer AC, et al. Defective TCRmediated signaling in synovial T cells in rheumatoid arthritis. *J Immunol* 1997;159:2973–2978.
11. Romagnoli P, Strahan D, Pelosi M, et al. A potential role for protein tyrosine kinase p56(lck) in rheumatoid arthritis synovial fluid T lymphocyte hyporesponsiveness. *Int Immunol* 2001;13:305–312.
12. Tsokos GC, Nambiar MP, Tenbrock K, et al. Rewiring the T cell: Signaling defects and novel prospects for the treatment of SLE. *Trends Immunol* 2003;24:259–263.
13. Hasler P, Zouali M. B cell receptor signaling and autoimmunity. *FASEB J* 2001;15:2085–2098.
14. Cherukuri A, Cheng PC, Sohn HW, et al. The CD19/CD21 complex functions to prolong B cell antigen receptor signaling from lipid rafts. *Immunity* 2001;14:169–179.
15. Gold MR. To make antibodies or not: Signaling by the B-cell antigen receptor. *Trends Pharmacol Sci* 2002;23:316–324.
16. Leo A, Wienands J, Baier G, et al. Adapters in lymphocyte signaling. *J Clin Invest* 2002;109:301–309.
17. Koretzky GA, Abtahian F, Silverman MA. SLP76 and SLP65: Complex regulation of signalling in lymphocytes and beyond. *Nat Rev Immunol* 2006;6:67–78.
18. Lipsky PE. Systemic lupus erythematosus: An autoimmune disease of B cell hyperactivity. *Nat Immunol* 2001;2:764–766.
19. Flores-Borja F, Kabouridis PS, Jury EC, et al. Decreased Lyn expression and translocation to lipid raft signaling domains in B lymphocytes

from patients with systemic lupus erythematosus. *Arthritis Rheum* 2005;52:3955–3965.

20. Takai T. Roles of Fc receptors in autoimmunity. *Nat Rev Immunol* 2002;2:580–592.
21. Uddin S, Platanias LC. Mechanisms of type-I interferon signal transduction. *J Biochem Mol Biol* 2004;37:635–641.
22. Renauld JC. Class II cytokine receptors and their ligands: Key antiviral and inflammatory modulators. *Nat Rev Immunol* 2003;3:667–676.
23. Aringer M, Cheng A, Nelson JW, et al. Janus kinases and their role in growth and disease. *Life Sci* 1999;64:2173–2186.
24. Wajant H, Pfizenmaier K, Scheurich P. Tumor necrosis factor signaling. *Cell Death Differ* 2003;10:45–65.
25. Pizzo P, Viola A. Lymphocyte lipid rafts: Structure and function. *Curr Opin Immunol* 2003;15:255–260.

Animal Models

Rajesh Rajaiah and Kamal D. Moudgil

Experimentally Induced Arthritis Models
Spontaneously Induced Arthritis Models
Practical Utility of Animal Models of Arthritis

Several animal models are available for conducting experimental studies pertaining to the pathogenesis and treatment of autoimmune arthritis. These models share many clinical, histologic, and immunologic characteristics with human rheumatoid arthritis (RA), although no single animal model fully replicates all the features of RA. Nevertheless, these models are an invaluable resource to both academia and industry. In this chapter, we have discussed the commonly used rodent models of arthritis that belong to two distinct categories: experimentally induced and spontaneously induced disease. Arthritis can be induced in susceptible mouse or rat strains by using microbial products, joint-specific antigens, routinely used test antigens, or nonantigenic compounds (Table 8N-1). Alternatively, certain mouse strains that develop arthritis spontaneously can serve as experimental models (Table 8N-2). Overall, most of these arthritis models display similarities among themselves in disease characteristics and histologic features of synovial hyperplasia, mononuclear cell infiltration, and cartilage and bone erosions, albeit of varying extent and severity. However, they show differences in sex predilection, the presence of rheumatoid factors (RFs), and the predominant effector mechanisms involved in arthritis.

Experimentally Induced Arthritis Models

Arthritis Induced by Microbial Products

Adjuvant Arthritis

Adjuvant arthritis (AA) is a polyarthritis unique to rats.[1–3] Lewis (RT.1^l) rats are highly susceptible to AA. These rats develop AA within 10 to 12 days of subcutaneous (s.c.) immunization with complete Freund's adjuvant (CFA) containing high concentration (10 to 20 mg/ml) of heat-killed *Mycobacterium tuberculosis* (Mtb) in oil. The disease is characterized by swelling, erythema, and tenderness in distal joints of hindpaws and forepaws, with the hindpaws generally affected more than the forepaws (Figure 8N-1). Maximum severity of the disease occurs between days 16 to 18 after Mtb injection. Rats that are 6 to 8 weeks old display an optimal disease course. The frequency of arthritis is 90% to 100%. There is no significant sex difference in regard to either the incidence or the severity of the disease.[3] The most commonly used methods for grading the severity of AA are clinical evaluation and measurements of paw thickness or volume. In clinical scoring based on the extent of erythema and swelling of the paws, each paw is given a score between 0 to 4 with the maximum arthritic score of 16 per rat. For quantitative measurements, the paw thickness can be measured by using a caliper, or the paw volume can be determined by employing a plethysmometer. The clinical disease can be further validated and analyzed by histologic and radiologic examination of the paws. Histologic sections of affected joints demonstrate synovial inflammation, pannus formation with mononuclear cell infiltrate, cartilage and bone erosions, and subsequently ankylosis. Granuloma formation in periarticular tissue is a characteristic feature of AA.[3] Unlike Lewis rats, Wistar Kyoto (WKY) (RT.1^l) and Fisher F344 (RT.1^{lvl}) rats are relatively resistant to AA.[4,5] AA is a cell-mediated autoimmune disease, and it can be transferred to naive syngeneic rats via lymphoid cells (T cells) harvested from an arthritic rat in the early phase of the disease,[3] or via arthritogenic T-cell lines.[6] There is limited information on the role of antibodies in disease induction. However, antibodies from arthritic Lewis rats can induce protection against AA.[4,5] Mycobacterial heat-shock protein 65 (Bhsp65) is the most well-studied antigen regarding the pathogenesis of AA.[4–7]

Streptococcal Cell Wall–Induced Arthritis

This disease can be induced in Lewis rats by a single intraperitoneal (i.p.) injection of sonicated cell wall preparation of group A (or group B/C) streptococci in aqueous suspension.[8,9] An acute inflammation of peripheral joints occurs within 24 to 72 hours, and it is associated with activation of the alternative complement (C') pathway by the cell wall components.[10] Furthermore, it is T-cell–independent as the disease can be induced in athymic-inbred Lewis rats.[11] The acute phase of arthritis resolves within a week, and it is followed by a chronic phase that begins about 10 to 21 days after streptococcal cell wall (SCW) injection and lasts for about 4 months. The chronic phase of the disease is T-cell dependent.[11] Chronic arthritis is characterized by a remitting and relapsing disease course, and histology of the hindpaw joints reveals pannus formation, synovial T-cell infiltrates, and erosion of bone/cartilage.[11] The assessment of arthritic inflammation and joint damage at about 5 weeks after disease induction offers a reliable parameter for evaluation of the effects of disease-modifying interventions using the SCW–induced arthritis (SCWIA) model. As in AA, rats with SCWIA also raise T-cell response to Bhsp65, but the precise role of this antigen in disease pathogenesis is not yet clear. Passive arthritis can be induced in naive syngeneic recipients by lymphoid cells of rats with SCWIA or via T-cell lines reactive against SCW antigens.[12] Female rats are more susceptible to SCWIA than male rats.[11] SCWIA can be induced in mice, but repeated intra-articular (i.a.) injections of SCW fragments into the knee joint are required for inducing chronic disease.

Table 8N-1. Experimentally Induced Arthritis Models

Model	Representative Strains Used	Arthritogenic Challenge	Sex Bias (+/−)	RF (+/−)	Adoptive Transfer of Disease via	Special Features	Reference #
Adjuvant-induced arthritis (AA)	Rat: Lewis, DA	Mtb in oil (s.c./i.d.)	−	−	T cells	Unique to rats; granuloma formation in the synovial tissue	1–7
Streptococcal cell wall-induced arthritis (SCWIA)	Rat: Lewis	Cell wall of group A (or B/C) streptococci (i.p.)	+	−	T cells	Acute phase is C′-dependent, whereas chronic phase is T-cell driven	8–12
Collagen-induced arthritis (CIA)	Rat: Lewis Mouse: DBA1 DR4.Ab^0	CII in CFA/IFA (i.d.); primary and booster injection	− − +	− − +	Rat: T cells Ab Mouse: Ab	T cells and Ab play a crucial role in disease induction	19–22 13–18
Proteoglycan-induced arthritis (PGIA)	Mouse: BALB/c	Cartilage proteoglycan (aggrecan) (i.p.)	+	−	T cells	Th1-mediated disease, high ratio of IFN-γ to IL-4	23, 24
Antigen-induced arthritis (AIA)	Mouse: C57BL/6 Rat: Lewis	MBSA/CFA (i.d.) with *B. pertussis* (i.p.), and soluble mBSA into the knee joint (i.a.)	− −	− −	T cells	IL-6 and IL-17 play an important role in disease pathogenesis	25–27 28
Immune complex-mediated arthritis (ICA)	Mouse: C57BL/6	Ab injection i.v. followed by Ag challenge into the knee joint (i.a.)	−	−	−	Macrophages and FcγRs play an important role in disease initiation	29–31
Pristane-induced arthritis (PIA)	Rat: Lewis, DA Mouse: CBA/Ig^b, BALB/c	Pristane (i.d./i.p.)	+ +	− +	T cells	Noninfectious and nonantigenic mineral oil that primes autoreactive T cells	32 33–35
Avridine-induced arthritis (AvIA)	Rat: Lewis, DA	CP20961 (avridine) in IFA (s.c)	−	−	T cells	Nonantigenic compound that induces autoreactive T cells	36

Table 8N-2. Spontaneously Induced Arthritis Models

Mouse Strain	Arthritogenic Process	Sex bias (+/−)	RF (+/−)	Adoptive Transfer via T Cells/ Serum Ab	Major Effector Mechanism	Special Features	Reference #
K/BxN	Antibodies against glucose-6-phosphate isomerase (GPI)	−	−	Antibodies	Antibodies	Arthritogenic anti-GPI antibodies bind to GPI-enriched joint cartilage, and the immune complexes formed locally lead to tissue damage via effector mechanisms of innate immunity.	37,38
BALB/cA IL-1Ra$^{-/-}$	Deficiency of IL-1 receptor antagonist (IL-1Ra)	−	+	T cells	T cells	T cells and IL-17 play an important role in the induction of disease.	39–41
SKG	Mutation in SH2 domain of ZAP 70 leading to defective thymic selection	+	+	T cells	T cells	The altered activation threshold of developing thymocytes leads to positive selection of autoreactive T cells that would have otherwise been deleted via negative selection.	42
C57BL/6 × CBA TNF-α-Tg	Dysregulated TNF-α production	−	−	−	TNF-α	Chronic progressive arthritis; TNF-α induces proliferation of synoviocytes, collagenase production, and bone resoption	43

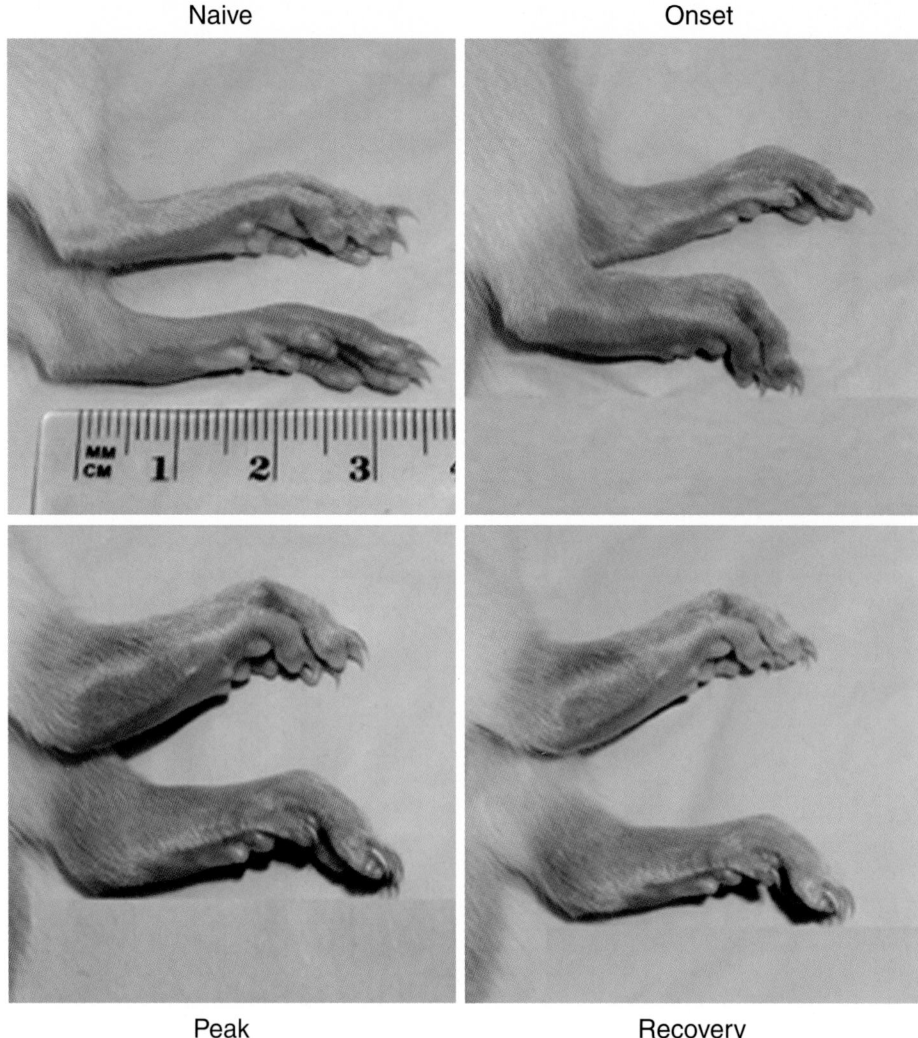

Figure 8N-1. Adjuvant arthritis can be induced in the Lewis (RT.1[l]) rat by subcutaneous immunization with heat-killed *M. tuberculosis* (H37Ra). The disease appears in 10 to 12 days (Onset), attains maximum severity from 16 to 18 days (Peak), followed by gradual regression (Recovery) over the next 10 to 14 days. Arthritis in each paw is graded on a scale from 0 to 4 for the level of erythema and swelling, and the maximum total arthritic score is 16 per rat. (Each major division on the ruler equals 1 cm, and each minor division equals 1 mm.) The arthritic paws can be further subjected to histologic and radiologic examination and graded quantitatively.

Arthritis Induced by Joint Cartilage Components

Collagen-Induced Arthritis

CIA in mice

Collagen-induced arthritis (CIA) can be induced in susceptible mouse strains by immunization with type II collagen (CII).[13] A typical arthritogenic regimen includes a primary injection of CII emulsified in CFA administered i.d. at the base of the tail, followed by a booster injection i.d. of CII in incomplete Freund's adjuvant (IFA) given 7 days (or even 14 to 21 days) later.[14,15] The onset of arthritis takes 3 to 5 weeks and the incidence of the disease varies from 50% to 100%, depending on the mouse strain and the CII type. (In the commonly used DBA/1 (H-2^q) mice, the onset of arthritis is at about 3 to 4 weeks, and the incidence is as high as 80% to 100%.) The onset of the disease is earlier in male mice than in female mice, but there is no significant difference in the overall disease incidence. Peak swelling of the affected limbs occurs within a week after disease onset. Forepaws and hindpaws are affected with equal frequency. The knee joints are involved but generally not observed or graded because of fur in that area. The majority of the affected limbs progress to joint deformities.

Strain differences in susceptibility to CIA are observed even within the same major histocompatibility complex (MHC) haplotype[14,15]: In the H-2^q group, DBA/1 Lac, B10.Q, and BUB mice develop CIA, but SWR/J mice do not; similarly, in the H-2^r group, B10.RIII mice are susceptible, whereas RIII/J mice are resistant. The species of origin of CII (e.g., chicken, bovine, or porcine CII) used for disease induction is also an important variable in influencing the incidence and severity of CIA in different mouse strains.

Arthritic mice develop anti-CII antibodies along with T-cell response to CII. The antibody response is characterized by high levels of the complement (C')-fixing isotype (IgG1 and IgG2a). The T-cell response to CII is generally less marked than that to other immunogens. However, mice may develop immune response to CII without arthritis development.

Passive CIA can be induced by intravenous (i.v.) or intra-articular (i.a.) injection of polyclonal anti-CII antibodies obtained from sera of mice with CIA, or by monoclonal anti-CII antibodies. Passive arthritis follows a course that is quite different from that of active arthritis. The onset of the passive disease is in 2 to 3 days and the inflammation resolves within 2 days without progressing onto chronic arthritis. Unlike antibody transfer, the T-cell adoptive transfer generally fails to induce passive arthritis in mice.

CIA also can be induced in HLA-transgenic ("humanized") mice expressing either the DR4 or the DR1 allele, or in those expressing the DQ8 allele.[16,17] For example, in DQ8-transgenic mice, the incidence of arthritis is in the range of 67% to 71% and the disease appears about 25 to 39 days after CII immunization. Unlike the DQ8 mice, the DQ6 mice are resistant to CIA. The recently generated line of DR4.AE(0) mice exhibits both the sex bias (females predominant over males) of arthritis susceptibility and the positivity for RF as observed in RA.[18]

CIA in Rats

This disease can be induced in susceptible rat strains by i.d./s.c. administration of native CII in IFA, followed by a booster injection i.d./s.c. of CII/IFA on day 7.[19–21] Rats develop arthritis with about 40% to 60% incidence. The evaluation (grading) of arthritis in hindpaws can be performed using the same approaches as those used for AA. On an average, the onset of arthritis is at 2 weeks, the disease peaks at 3 weeks, with maximal joint damage occurring at 5 weeks after the primary injection. Among the various rat strains used, Lewis, DA, and Louvain rats are susceptible to CIA induction, whereas Buffalo and AUG rats are resistant. Both cell-mediated and humoral immune responses against CII are involved in the pathogenesis of arthritis.[19,21,22] Passive arthritis can be transferred either via the *in vitro* restimulated lymphoid cells of rats with CIA or with sera-containing anti-CII IgG antibodies of arthritic rats. The CII-induced disease is chronic in nature, whereas the passive disease is transient and may even lack pannus formation in the joints.

Rats and mice reveal important differences in the disease characteristics in regard to CIA.[14] These include (1) earlier onset of arthritis in rats (2 weeks) than in mice (3 to 6 weeks); (2) faster progression of arthritis to new joints after disease onset in rats (1 week) than in mice (9 weeks); and (3) ready induction of passive arthritis in rats but not in mice via the adoptive transfer of T cells. Murine CIA also differs from AA in that the latter disease has a higher incidence (90% to 100%) than that of CIA, and hindpaws are affected more than forepaws in AA but equally in CIA.

Proteoglycan-Induced Arthritis

Proteoglycan-induced arthritis (PGIA) is a progressive polyarthritis with features of remissions and exacerbations, and it can be induced in BALB/c (H-2^d) mice by i.p. immunization with human cartilage proteoglycan (PG; aggrecan).[23] A total of four injections of PG are given at weekly intervals.[23,24] The first and fourth injections are of PG/CFA, whereas the second and third injections are of PG/IFA. Arthritis develops on about day 11 and reaches peak severity in 2 to 4 weeks after the last PG injection. The incidence of arthritis is approximately 100%. Mice with PGIA develop a predominantly Th1 type of $CD4^+$ T-cell response along with antibody response to PG. However, the levels of IgG1 antibodies are much higher than that of IgG2a antibodies, and the disease severity correlates with the levels of IgG2a antibodies. PGIA also can be induced in humanized mice expressing DR4 or DQ8, but on the susceptible BALB/c background.

AA, CIA, and PGIA are predominantly Th1 type of arthritis models. However, IL-4 deficiency enhances the severity of PGIA and AA, but decreases the severity of CIA. On the other hand, IFN-γ deficiency exacerbates CIA, but suppresses PGIA.[24] Furthermore, the IL-4 treatment of mice suppresses arthritis severity in PGIA.

Arthritis Induced by Nominal Antigens/ Antigen-Antibody Complexes

Antigen-Induced Arthritis

Antigen-induced arthritis (AIA) is an immune-mediated, T-cell–dependent monoarthritis.[25] Both mice (e.g., C57BL/6 [H-2^b]) and rats (e.g., Lewis) are susceptible to AIA.[25–28] The remarkable consistency of clinical and histologic changes among animals within a group, the close resemblance in the histopathologic features of AIA and RA, and the feasibility of inducing an antigen-specific flare reaction at a desired time point during the course of arthritis are the major advantages of this experimental model. Male mice/rats of 10 to 12 weeks of age are optimal for the induction of AIA.[26] The primary immunization consists of i.d. or s.c. injection of methylated bovine serum albumin (mBSA) in CFA at the base of the tail coupled with i.p. injection of heat-inactivated *Bordetella pertussis* as an additional adjuvant.[26,27] Another injection of these arthritogenic components is given after 7 days. On day 21 after the first injection, a sterile solution of mBSA in saline is injected into one of the knees, whereas saline only is injected in the other knee (control).

The incidence of arthritis is 100%. Inflammation is evident in the knee 1 day after injection of antigen, and it reaches peak phase on day 3, followed by a chronic inflammatory phase lasting for about 12 weeks. The acute phase (0 to 9 days) of AIA is comprised of vigorous swelling of the joints with infiltration of granulocytes into the synovium and the joint space. The chronic phase (10 to 85 days) of AIA involves persistent inflammation characterized by synovial hypertrophy, mononuclear cell infiltration of the synovium, and erosion of cartilage and bone. IL-6 and IL-17 play a critical role in the disease process in AIA.

Immune Complex–Mediated Arthritis

The induction of immune complex–mediated arthritis (ICA) is dependent on the *in vivo* formation of immune (antigen-antibody) complexes.[29,30] Mice (e.g., C57BL/6) are first injected i.v. with complement-free antigen-specific antibodies (e.g., antilysozyme antibodies). Then, the corresponding antigen (e.g., lysozyme coupled to poly-L-lysine) in saline is injected into one of the knee joints a day later.[29,30] The control knee is injected with saline only. This immunization regimen leads to the formation and deposition of IC locally within the joints. These IC bind to Fcγ-receptors (FcγR) on synovial macrophages (type A cells) leading to their activation and increased influx of polymorphonuclear (PMN) leukocytes and other inflammation-mediating cells.

Arthritic inflammation in the knee joint begins in about 6 h and reaches peak severity within 2 to 3 days. The severity of arthritis can be assessed on day 3 after disease induction by histologic examination of the knee joints. ICA is characterized by the loss of cartilage proteoglycans, chondrocyte death, and cartilage destruction mediated by FcγR, IL-1, and matrix metalloproteinases (MMPs). Cytokines (e.g., IFN-γ and IL-13) can influence inflammation and cartilage damage in ICA by altering the expression levels of FcγR on macrophages.[30,31]

Mice (e.g., DBA/1) that are highly susceptible to CIA are also similarly susceptible to ICA, whereas mice (e.g., C57BL/6) that are resistant to CIA develop relatively milder ICA. Furthermore, FcγR-deficient ($Fc\gamma R^{-/-}$) mice are protected against the development of ICA. However, the above three mouse strains show comparable level of susceptibility to SCWIA.

Arthritis Induced by Nonantigenic Mineral Oils

Pristane-Induced Arthritis

PIA in Rats

Pristane-induced arthritis (PIA) represents a unique model of arthritis in that an immune-based disease can be induced by a noninfectious, nonantigenic stimulus.[32] It is a chronic relapsing and progressive disease that involves the peripheral joints in a symmetrical fashion. It can be induced in DA or Lewis rats by a single injection of pristane (2,6,10,14-tetramethylpentadecane) i.d. at the base of the tail.[32] The onset of PIA occurs on about day 14 to 23 after pristane injection. The frequency of arthritis is much higher in DA rats (about 100%) than that in Lewis rats (about 80%). Female rats are more susceptible to PIA than male rats. PIA shares histologic characteristics with CIA[22] and avridine-induced arthritis (AvIA) in rats, and with RA. Unlike DA and Lewis rats, E3 rats are resistant to PIA induction. Both MHC and non MHC genes significantly influence susceptibility to PIA.[32] Although pristane is a nonantigenic lipid, immunization with pristane generates autoreactive T cells that include MHC class II-restricted Th1 cells, which are capable of adoptively transferring disease to naive recipients. This attribute of PIA makes it an ideal model system for conducting studies on genetic aspects of autoimmune arthritis.

PIA in Mice

Pristane-induced arthritis can be induced in susceptible mouse strains (e.g., CBA/Ig^b, DBA/1, and BALB/c) by i.p. injection of pristane.[33] CBA/Ig^b mice given two i.p. injections of pristane at a 50-day interval develop an inflammatory disease of the ankle and wrist joints between 3 to 6 months after the primary immunization.[34] This delayed onset of PIA in mice is a striking contrast to the short incubation period of 14-23 days in rats. Unlike BALB/c (H-2^d) mice, DBA/2 (H-2^d) mice are resistant to PIA. Susceptibility to PIA can also be influenced by the animal housing environment with higher incidence of disease in a conventional facility than that in a germ-free facility. PIA is accompanied by the generation of RF as well as antibodies to Bhsp65 and CII.[33,35] PIA is a CD4$^+$ T cell–dependent disease as the athymic homozygous BALB/c nu/nu mice fail to develop PIA.[33] Mice with PIA raise T-cell response to Bhsp65,[35] which has also been invoked in the pathogenesis of AA, SCWIA, and RA.

Avridine-Induced Arthritis

Lewis rats immunized s.c. with N,N-dioctadecyl-N',N'-bis (2-hydroxyethyl) propanediamine (CP20961, or Avridine) develop chronic arthritis with a frequency of 90% to 100%.[36] The disease starts at about 11 to 13 days and persists for about 4 months. DA rats also are susceptible to AvIA, but E3 rats are resistant. The disease is T-cell dependent, and it is influenced significantly by both MHC and non MHC genes.

Spontaneously Induced Arthritis Models

K/BXN Mouse

K/BXN mice spontaneously develop a polyarthritis that shares many features with human RA.[37,38] These mice bear a transgenic T-cell receptor (TCR) directed against an A^k-restricted epitope of bovine pancreatic ribonuclease, which is fortuitously crossreactive with an A^{g7}-restricted epitope within glucose-6-phosphate isomerase (GPI), a ubiquitous protein involved in the glycolytic pathway. The disease that develops spontaneously at about 4 to 5 weeks of age in TCR-transgenic mice of the NOD background is symmetrical in distribution and chronic progressive in nature leading to bone erosions.

The GPI-reactive CD4$^+$ T cells play a critical role in the initiation of the disease, but are dispensable thereafter. The T-cell–B-cell interaction via the CD40–CD40L pair leads to the production of arthritogenic anti-GPI antibodies. The induction of arthritis is primarily dependent on innate immune effector mechanisms initiated by GPI–anti-GPI antibody immune complexes. These pathogenic mechanisms involve the alternative complement (C') pathway, FcγR, macrophages, neutrophils and mast cells. The disease can be transferred to naive recipients via sera of arthritic mice. However, this passive arthritis is transient, and the disease undergoes regression in 2 to 4 weeks. Unlike the spontaneously induced arthritis, the serum transfer passive arthritis can be induced in mice of diverse MHC haplotypes.

GPI is neither overexpressed within the synovial tissue nor modified post-translationally. The organ specificity of the tissue damage has been attributed to the GPI-enrichment on the cartilage surface, the local physiologic milieu within the joint cavity, and the unique characteristics of the joint vasculature.

BALB/cA IL-1Ra–Deficient Mouse

IL-1R–deficient BALB/cA (H-2^d) mice develop spontaneous arthritis by 12 weeks of age with 100% incidence.[39] IL-1 receptor antagonist (IL-1Ra) is an endogenous inhibitor of IL-1 that prevents the binding of IL-1 to IL-1 receptor (IL-1R). Therefore, the deficiency of IL-1Ra permits uncontrolled proinflammatory activity of IL-1, which leads to arthritis development. Histopathologically, the lesions in these mice closely resemble that of RA. Although arthritic BALB/cA-IL-1Ra$^{-/-}$ mice develop RF, anti-CII, and anti-DNA autoantibodies, the anti-CII antibodies remain at low levels and there is little anti-CII T-cell reactivity.[39,40] The T cells of these mice can adoptively transfer disease to nu/nu mice. Furthermore, TNF-α, IL-17, and IL-23 have been shown to contribute to arthritis induction in BALB/c-IL-1Ra$^{-/-}$ mice.[40,41] The IL-1–induced IL-17 production is dependent on IL-23. The disease is genetically regulated (by the nonMHC genes) as the disease manifests in BALB/cA mice, but not in mice of DBA/1, C57BL/6, or B10.DR1 (HLA-transgenic B10 mice) background.[39,40] However, these mouse strains that do not develop spontaneous disease are highly susceptible to CII-induced disease and show an earlier and more severe CIA than controls. Anti-CII antibodies play a critical role in arthritis induction in these strains.

SKG Mouse

BALB/c (H-2^d) mice bearing a mutation of the zeta-chain–associated protein, 70-kD (ZAP-70) gene spontaneously develop autoimmune arthritis with clinical, histologic, and serologic features resembling human RA.[42] The disease manifests in homozygous mice at about 2 months of age. It is a symmetric chronic polyarthritis. Arthritic SKG mice also exhibit extra-articular features such as subcutaneous nodules and interstitial pneumonitis. Female SKG mice show more severe arthritis than male mice. The disease can be adoptively transferred to naive syngeneic recipients via $CD4^{+}$ T cells but not via serum of arthritic SKG mice.

The T cells of SKG mice have a tryptophan to cysteine change at codon 163 of the SH2 domain of ZAP70 that apparently influences the interaction of ZAP70 with TCR-ζ, CD3 and other specific signaling intermediates. These ZAP70-defective T cells have higher activation threshold than normal T cells. Consequently, potentially autoreactive T cells of SKG mice escape thymic negative selection and make it into the periphery. These autoreactive T cells possessing high avidity for self-ligands play a critical role in the initiation and propagation of autoimmune arthritis. The precise reasons for the organ specificity of the disease mediated by a general defect in thymic selection are not yet fully clear.

TNF-α Transgenic Mouse, and Mouse Lacking TNF ARE

Transgenic (Tg) mice expressing human TNF-α spontaneously develop chronic inflammatory polyarthritis at about 3 to 4 weeks of age.[43] The frequency of arthritis in the transgene positive mice is 100%. The disease is evident at the ankles and other joints. The histopathology of the joints of TNF-α transgenic mice resembles that of RA joints, but these mice lack RF in their sera. The significance of the dysregulated TNF-α in arthritis induction is validated by the observation that neutralization of TNF-α using the appropriate antibody prevents arthritis development. Similarly, impaired regulation of TNF-α biosynthesis by deletion of the regulatory TNF AU-rich elements (ARE) induces an increased production of TNF-α, which is associated with the spontaneous development of chronic inflammatory arthritis along with inflammatory bowel disease.[44]

Practical Utility of Animal Models of Arthritis

Studies in different animal models of arthritis have contributed not only to the advancements in our understanding of the pathogenesis of autoimmune arthritis, but also to the intricate processes of initial screening and follow-up testing of new therapeutic agents for their antiarthritic activity.

Explorations into the immunopathogenesis of arthritis include, but are not limited to, the influence of genetic and environmental factors on the incidence and severity of arthritis; the role of defined subsets of lymphoid and myeloid lineage cells in the initiation, propagation and regression of arthritis; the study of intracellular signaling defects in arthritis; and the interplay between innate and adaptive immune effector mechanisms in arthritis development. These studies have benefited immensely from the availability of a large collection of gene knockout and transgenic mice that can be bred onto the arthritis-susceptible/resistant backgrounds. Included among these are the new and improved versions of HLA-transgenic (humanized) mice.

An equally rewarding contribution of animal models of arthritis has been in the area of therapeutics and related translational research. Experimentally induced arthritis models have been the mainstay of preliminary screening and toxicity studies of putative antiarthritic agents. Animal testing of new compounds/products in rodents and/or subhuman primates is an essential prerequisite for conducting preclinical and clinical trials in RA patients, and it is mandated by the Food and Drug Administration (FDA). For the testing of new pharmacologic or immunotherapeutic compounds, the readout parameters in animal models consist of the clinical, histologic, and radiologic characteristics of the disease, and the immunologic and biochemical parameters associated with arthritis. For example, the incidence of arthritis and a delay in the onset of arthritis serve as useful parameters in disease-preventive protocols, whereas changes in the progression of arthritis (count of affected joints and arthritic scores) and histologic grading are useful indices in therapeutic protocols. In addition, changes in serum levels of antigen-specific antibodies, cartilage matrix-associated protein (COMP, which is released following cartilage damage and loss), and IL-1Ra represent some of the useful reference parameters in both preventive and therapeutic test regimen. For toxicity studies, new compounds are tested in animal models for changes in behavioral and physiologic indicators, as well as any alterations in hematologic, biochemical, and immunologic parameters.

With the resurgence of interest in gene therapy combined with the vast potential of the stem cell-based therapeutic regimens to follow in the near future, the optimization and further refinement of animal models has gained a new momentum. In this context, it is hoped that the recently reported[45] success in the generation of a gene knockout rat would exponentially enlarge the scope and impact of the existing diversity of animal models of arthritis.

Acknowledgment

This work was supported by grants from the National Institutes of Health, Bethesda, MD, and the Arthritis Foundation (National Office, Atlanta, Goergia, and Maryland Chapter, Baltimore, Maryland).

References

1. Stoerk H, Bielinski TC, Budzilovich T. Chronic polyarthritis in rats injected with spleen in adjuvants. *Am J Pathol* 1954;30:616.
2. Pearson CM. Development of arthritis, periarthritis and periostitis in rats given adjuvants. *Proc Soc Exp Biol Med* 1956;91:95–101.
3. Taurog JD, Argentieri DC, McReynolds RA. Adjuvant arthritis. *Methods Enzymol* 1988;162:339–355.
4. Moudgil KD. Diversification of response to hsp65 during the course of autoimmune arthritis is regulatory rather than pathogenic. *Immunol Rev* 1998;164:175–184.
5. Ulmansky R, Cohen CJ, Szafer F, et al. Resistance to adjuvant arthritis is due to protective antibodies against heat shock protein surface epitopes and the induction of IL-10 secretion. *J Immunol* 2002;168:6463–6469.
6. van Eden W, Thole JE, van der Zee R, et al. Cloning of the mycobacterial epitope recognized by T lymphocytes in adjuvant arthritis. *Nature* 1988;331:171–173.
7. Cohen IR. Autoimmunity to chaperonins in the pathogenesis of arthritis and diabetes. *Annu Rev Immunol* 1991;9:567–589.

8. Cromartie WJ, Craddock JG, Schwab JH, et al. Arthritis in rats after systemic injection of streptococcal cells or cell walls. *J Exp Med* 1977;46:1585–1602.
9. Ridge SC, Zabriskie JB, Oronsky AL, et al. Streptococcal cell wall–induced arthritis in rats. *Methods Enzymol* 1988;162:373–379.
10. Schwab JH, Allen JB, Anderle SK, et al. Relationship of complement to experimental arthritis induced in rats with streptococcal cell walls. *Immunology* 1982;46:83–88.
11. Allen JB, Malone DG, Wahl SM, et al. Role of the thymus in streptococcal cell wall-induced arthritis and hepatic granuloma formation. Comparative studies of pathology and cell wall distribution in athymic and euthymic rats. *J Clin Invest* 1985;76:1042–1056.
12. DeJoy SQ, Ferguson KM, Sapp TM, et al. Streptococcal cell wall arthritis. Passive transfer of disease with a T cell line and crossreactivity of streptococcal cell wall antigens with Mycobacterium tuberculosis. *J Exp Med* 1989;170:369–382.
13. Courtenay JS, Dallman MJ, Dayan AD, et al. Immunisation against heterologous type II collagen induces arthritis in mice. *Nature* 1980;283:666–668.
14. Wooley PH. Collagen-induced arthritis in the mouse. *Methods Enzymol* 1988;162:361–373.
15. Brand DD, Latham KA, Rosloniec EF. Collagen-induced arthritis. *Nat Protoc* 2007;2:1269–1275.
16. Nabozny GH, Baisch JM, Cheng S, et al. HLA-DQ8 transgenic mice are highly susceptible to collagen-induced arthritis: A novel model for human polyarthritis. *J Exp Med* 1996;183:27–37.
17. Rosloniec EF, Brand DD, Myers LK, et al. Induction of autoimmune arthritis in HLA-DR4 (DRB1*0401) transgenic mice by immunization with human and bovine type II collagen. *J Immunol* 1998; 160:2573–2578.
18. Taneja V, Behrens M, Mangalam A, et al. New humanized HLA-DR4-transgenic mice that mimic the sex bias of rheumatoid arthritis. *Arthritis Rheum* 2007;56:69–78.
19. Trentham DE, Townes AS, Kang AH. Autoimmunity to type II collagen an experimental model of arthritis. *J Exp Med* 1977;146:857–868.
20. Ridge SC, Oronsky AL, Kerwar SS. Type II collagen-induced arthritis in rats. *Methods Enzymol* 1988;162:355–360.
21. Brahn E, Peacock DJ, Banquerigo ML. Suppression of collagen-induced arthritis by combination cyclosporin A and methotrexate therapy. *Arthritis Rheum* 1991;34:1282–1288.
22. Holmdahl R, Rubin K, Klareskog L, et al. Appearance of different lymphoid cells in synovial tissue and in peripheral blood during the course of collagen II–induced arthritis in rats. *Scand J Immunol* 1985;21:197–204.
23. Glant TT, Mikecz K, Arzoumanian A, et al. Proteoglycan-induced arthritis in BALB/c mice. Clinical features and histopathology. *Arthritis Rheum* 1987;30:201–212.
24. Finnegan A, Mikecz K, Tao P, et al. Proteoglycan (aggrecan)-induced arthritis in BALB/c mice is a Th1-type disease regulated by Th2 cytokines. *J Immunol* 1999;163:5383–5390.
25. Brackertz D, Mitchell GF, Mackay IR. Antigen-induced arthritis in mice. I. Induction of arthritis in various strains of mice. *Arthritis Rheum* 1977;20:841–850.
26. Ohshima S, Saeki Y, Mima T, et al. Interleukin 6 plays a key role in the development of antigen-induced arthritis. *Proc Natl Acad Sci U S A* 1998;95:8222–8226.
27. Koenders MI, Lubberts E, Oppers-Walgreen B, et al. Blocking of interleukin-17 during reactivation of experimental arthritis prevents joint inflammation and bone erosion by decreasing RANKL and interleukin-1. *Am J Pathol* 2005;167:141–149.
28. von Banchet GS, Petrow PK, Brauer R, et al. Monoarticular antigen-induced arthritis leads to pronounced bilateral upregulation of the expression of neurokinin 1 and bradykinin 2 receptors in dorsal root ganglion neurons of rats. *Arthritis Res* 2000;2:424–427.
29. van Lent PL, van den Bersselaar LA, van den Hoek AE, et al. Cationic immune complex arthritis in mice—a new model. Synergistic effect of complement and interleukin-1. *Am J Pathol* 1992;140: 1451–1461.
30. Blom AB, van Lent PL, van Vuuren H, et al. Fc gamma R expression on macrophages is related to severity and chronicity of synovial inflammation and cartilage destruction during experimental immune-complex-mediated arthritis (ICA). *Arthritis Res* 2000;2: 489–503.
31. Nabbe KC, van Lent PL, Holthuysen AE, et al. Local IL-13 gene transfer prior to immune-complex arthritis inhibits chondrocyte death and matrix-metalloproteinase–mediated cartilage matrix degradation despite enhanced joint inflammation. *Arthritis Res Ther* 2005;7:R392–R401.
32. Vingsbo C, Sahlstrand P, Brun JG, et al. Pristane-induced arthritis in rats: A new model for rheumatoid arthritis with a chronic disease course influenced by both major histocompatibility complex and non–major histocompatibility complex genes. *Am J Pathol* 1996;149: 1675–1683.
33. Wooley PH, Seibold JR, Whalen JD, et al. Pristane-induced arthritis. The immunologic and genetic features of an experimental murine model of autoimmune disease. *Arthritis Rheum* 1989;32:1022–1030.
34. Beech JT, Siew LK, Ghoraishian M, et al. $CD4^+$ Th2 cells specific for mycobacterial 65-kilodalton heat shock protein protect against pristane-induced arthritis. *J Immunol* 1997;159:3692–3697.
35. Thompson SJ, Rook GA, Brealey RJ, et al. Autoimmune reactions to heat-shock proteins in pristane-induced arthritis. *Eur J Immunol* 1990;20:2479–2484.
36. Vingsbo C, Jonsson R, Holmdahl R. Avridine-induced arthritis in rats; a T cell–dependent chronic disease influenced both by MHC genes and by non-MHC genes. *Clin Exp Immunol* 1995;99:359–363.
37. Korganow AS, Ji H, Mangialaio S, Duchatelle V, et al. From systemic T cell self-reactivity to organ-specific autoimmune disease via immunoglobulins. *Immunity* 1999;10:451–461.
38. Kouskoff V, Korganow AS, Duchatelle V, et al. Organ-specific disease provoked by systemic autoimmunity. *Cell* 1996;87:811–822.
39. Horai R, Saijo S, Tanioka H, et al. Development of chronic inflammatory arthropathy resembling rheumatoid arthritis in interleukin 1 receptor antagonist–deficient mice. *J Exp Med* 2000;191:313–320.
40. Zhou F, He X, Iwakura Y, et al. Arthritis in mice that are deficient in interleukin-1 receptor antagonist is dependent on genetic background. *Arthritis Rheum* 2005;52:3731–3738.
41. Cho ML, Kang JW, Moon YM, et al. STAT3 and NF-kappaB signal pathway is required for IL-23–mediated IL-17 production in spontaneous arthritis animal model IL-1 receptor antagonist–deficient mice. *J Immunol* 2006;176:5652–5661.
42. Sakaguchi N, Takahashi T, Hata H, et al. Altered thymic T-cell selection due to a mutation of the ZAp-70 gene causes autoimmune arthritis in mice. *Nature* 2003;426:454–460.
43. Keffer J, Probert L, Cazlaris H, et al. Transgenic mice expressing human tumour necrosis factor: A predictive genetic model of arthritis. *EMBO J* 1991;10:4025–4031.
44. Kontoyiannis D, Pasparakis M, Pizarro TT, et al. Impaired on/off regulation of TNF biosynthesis in mice lacking TNF AU-rich elements: Implications for joint and gut-associated immunopathologies. *Immunity* 1999;10:387–398.
45. Zan Y, Haag JD, Chen KS, et al. Production of knockout rats using ENU mutagenesis and a yeast-based screening assay. *Nat Biotechnol* 2003;21:645–651.

Outcome Measurement of Rheumatoid Arthritis

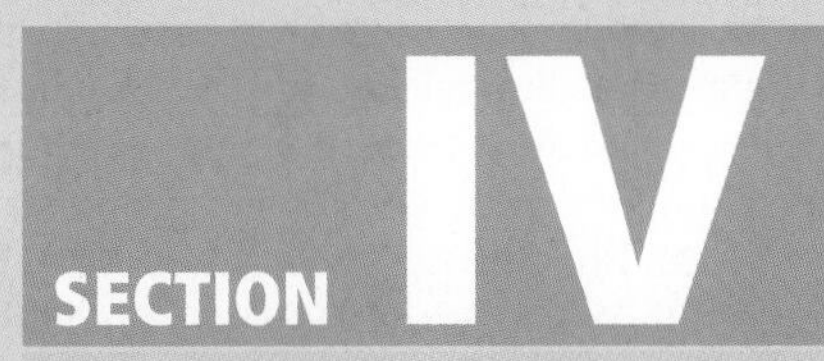

Outcome Measurement in Rheumatoid Arthritis: Disease Activity

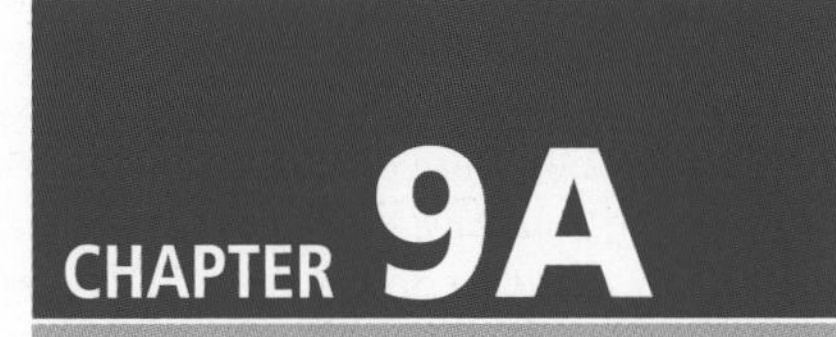

Daniel Aletaha and Josef S. Smolen

Disease activity is a central aspect in the evaluation of a patient with rheumatoid arthritis (RA). It takes center stage because it comprises signs and symptoms of the disease (such as inflammatory pain, swelling, and stiffness)—fundamental triggers of functional disability—and because it is responsible for progression of joint damage (currently the most relevant "long-term" outcome in RA). Therefore, reduction of disease activity is the major target of therapeutic interventions. From the patient's perspective, functional capacity is the most relevant outcome—and because disease activity is reversible, so must physical impairment be reversible (at least conceptually). This chapter reviews the domains or attributes relevant to RA disease activity evaluation, and provides an overview of tools and instruments used to adequately assess these. The instruments used to assess functional capacity and radiographic damage are discussed in other chapters.

Consensus on Reporting Disease Activity

One term closely associated with the assessment of disease activity is *core set*. This term was introduced by international societies in an effort to create consistency in the use and presentation of trial results.[1–3] The core set consists of counts of swollen and tender joints, patient assessment of pain, patient and evaluator global assessment of disease activity, a measure of the acute-phase response, and (according to some societies) a functional element. These variables are the minimal ("core") set that ought to be evaluated in clinical trials. Moreover, composite indices (see text following) make use of the majority of these core set variables. As the field has moved forward since the development of these variables and indices more than a decade ago, the European League Against Rheumatism (EULAR) and the American College of Rheumatology (ACR) have recently collaborated on an evidence-based consensus paper to recommend how to report trial results in RA (publication anticipated in early 2008).

Although the original core set definition and recent efforts regarding facilitating trial reporting have primarily dealt with the situation of a clinical trial, it is reasonable that the mentioned measures, reporting techniques, and standards should also be used for disease activity evaluation and response in clinical practice.

Joint Counts

Counting the number of affected joints is a logical way of assessing disease activity in an articular disease, such as RA. Joint involvement is typically evaluated for soft-tissue swelling and effusion (swollen joint count) and tenderness upon pressure or motion (tender joint count). There is evidence of some usefulness of counting deformed joints,[4,5] but this is not commonly done. Several joint indices and counts have been developed over the past 50 years,[6] which for the most part differ simply by the number of joints assessed. However, there are exceptions, which include the joint counts "weighted" for their surface area or "graded" by the severity of swelling or tenderness.

The first joint index, the Lansbury Index,[7] graded (minimal, slight, moderate, or maximal) swelling and tenderness and weighted for joint surface area in 86 joints. Two later indices were also based on evaluation of an extensive number of joints: the comprehensive 66/68-joint count, as suggested by the American Rheumatism Association (ARA; now American College of Rheumatology, ACR) in 1965[8] and the Cooperative Systemic Studies of Rheumatic Diseases (CSSRD) joint count.[9] Both are time consuming and therefore limited in their use in clinical practice. Another early index, the Ritchie Articular Index, assesses graded tenderness in 26 joint areas.[10] This index was later simplified by Hart to exclude the grading by severity, which is a major cause of inter-rater disagreement.[11] Simplifications of the extensive ACR joint count have been developed over time, reducing the number of assessed joints to 36 in 1985[12] and to 28 in 1989.[13] They are easy to evaluate in clinical practice and show similar validity and reliability compared to comprehensive joint counts.[14,15] Among other regions, the 28 joint counts exclude assessment of the foot and ankle joints because swelling and tenderness in these joints are frequently confounded by disorders other than RA.[13,15] The feet can be included using a 32-joint count, although this is no more reliable than the 28-joint count—even for the assessment of remission.[16] The 28-joint count became widely accepted.[17] Later, Wolfe and colleagues suggested an 18- and a 16-joint assessment to account for the time constraints in clinical practice.[18] At the present time, it seems most sensible to use the 28-joint count as a simple and validated measure unless the more comprehensive joint counts are easily obtainable from a logistical and cost perspective in trials and practice. Importantly, however, the 28-joint count has been reliably employed in clinical trials[19,20] and is a reliable tool in assessing remission when using composite scores.[16]

Pain Levels

The patient perspective of disease has become increasingly important over past years because it has been recognized that outcome measurement should be oriented by what patients deem important. In this regard, pain is clearly the predominant symptom, and assessment of pain is therefore important in understanding the disease impact on a patient—although pain is also captured in global assessments.

There are a number of reliable methods for the assessment of pain,[21–23] but most commonly pain is measured on 100-mm horizontal visual analogue scales (VASs).[24–26] Although it has been reported that patients might differ considerably in their applicability to the VAS,[24] it is still the predominant instrument for the evaluation of pain in rheumatic diseases. Because pain has the tendency to fluctuate, usually the past week is evaluated. Horizontal and vertical VASs are well correlated, but vertical scales tend to produce systematically higher values.[26]

Global Assessment Scales

Similar to pain, the global level of disease activity can be directly rated by a patient ("patient global assessment," PGA). In contrast to pain, it is often valuable to use the rating of a physician and/or an evaluator on the global assessment of disease activity (MD global, EGA). Typically, both attributes are presented together and are measured by using 100-mm VASs. The result can be expressed in centimeters or millimeters. The PGA has an intrinsic colinearity with the patient's assessment of pain because (as previously mentioned) pain is the attribute most important to the patient. EGA is a more integrative measure, principally considering all disease activity attributes available to the evaluator. Patients frequently rate their disease activity higher than evaluators (PGA < EGA).

Patient-Centered Disease Activity Questionnaires

Two additional patient-centered measures are the Rapid Assessment of Disease Activity in Rheumatology (RADAR)[27] questionnaire and the Rheumatoid Arthritis Disease Activity Index (RADAI)[28] questionnaire (Table 9A-1). The RADAR is a brief two-page self-administered questionnaire that includes six items scored individually. The scores of the individual RADAR items are interpreted using expert opinion or other studies as references, and there is no "overall" RADAR score. The RADAI includes five items and has been proposed for use in clinical practice. Completion and scoring of both questionnaires usually takes no more than 10 minutes, although the RADAI requires the use of a calculator.[29] The RADAI and the RADAR have been shown to be reliable and valid compared to other disease activity measures or measures of function.[30,31]

It is important to mention that these symptom questionnaires are different from clinical indices, which constitute an integration of various quantified disease attributes. The RADAR and the RADAI are tools used to obtain a patient-based assessment of disease activity without taking actual ("objective") measurements. Thus, in a way they can be regarded as a more detailed assessment of a PGA. Both questionnaires are rarely used in clinical practice and clinical trials.

Biomarkers

There are a variety of biomarkers that reflect disease activity and/or joint damage. The most frequently used biomarkers are acute phase reactants (APRs), such as C-reactive protein (CRP) and erythrocyte sedimentation rate (ESR). These markers are universally employed in studies and clinical practice. The APR correlates well with clinical disease activity, and the time-integrated APR also correlates well with disease outcomes such as radiographic progression.[32–35] However, if clinical information from joint counts, PGA and EGA are available, APR, especially CRP, tend to add little information to composite scores.[36] Although APR levels are prone to elevations due to other reasons, such as infection, they are normal in many patients with RA at their first presentation.[37] Therefore, some clinical trials of early RA allowed inclusion of patients with normal CRP and ESR.[38] Other biomarkers that reflect the immunoinflammatory cascades of active RA may more directly reflect the disease process and response to treatment. These include IL-1beta, IL-6, IL-8, and tumor necrosis factor (TNF)-alpha, matrix metalloproteinases, receptor activator for nuclear factor κB ligand (RANKL), and others. However, given their costs and more tedious methodology involved in their determination they will have to prove superiority to the easily available and inexpensive APR measures.

Table 9A-1. Indices for Evaluation of Rheumatoid Arthritis Activity

	Steinbrocker Therapeutic Scorecard[43]	Lansbury Systemic Manifestations[44]	Mallya – Mace[45]	Paulus Criteria[52]	ACR Response Criteria[53]	DAS/DAS 28 (4 items)[47,48]	SDAI[49]	CDAI[36]	RADAR[27]	RADAI[28]
Year published	1946	1956	1981[a]	1990	1995	1990[b]	2003	2005	1992	1995
Number of swollen joints	X			X	X	X	X	X	X[1]	X[1]
Number of tender joints	X		X	X	X	X	X	X	X[1,2]	X[1,2]
Joint motion/Pain on motion	X	X								
Morning stiffness		X	X	X						X
ESR/CRP	ESR	ESR	ESR	ESR	Either	ESR	CRP			
Hemoglobin (Hb)/anemia (An)	Hb	An	Hb							
Weight	X									
Fever		X								
Pain	X	X	X		X				X	X
Global health	X					X[3]				
Patient global disease activity				X	X		X	X	X[4]	X[4]
Evaluator global disease activity				X	X		X	X		
Function	X				X				X	
Grip strength			X							
Muscle weakness		X								
Fatigue		X								

[a]The index was later modified by van Riel et al. to only include the number of tender joints, morning stiffness, Hb, and ESR.[46]
[b]The DAS28 is currently the basis for the EULAR response criteria.
[1]Overall swelling and tenderness in joints is graded by patient.
[2]List of joint regions, graded for tenderness from 0 to 3.
[3]Global health excluded in the three-variable DAS/DAS28.
[4]Global disease activity over the past 6 months.
Adapted from Aletaha D, Smolen JS. The definition and measurement of disease modification in inflammatory rheumatic diseases. *Rheum Dis Clin North Am* 2006;32:9–44.

Pooled Indices

RA is a prototype of a multifaceted disease in which the evaluation of any one of the available measures does not allow us to reliably identify a patient's disease activity or response to therapy. Evaluating all possible variables independently from one another in clinical trials is linked with methodologic problems.[39] Pooled indices combine a number of disease activity measures and have been developed to overcome the previously cited limitations.[39–41] Pooled indices were developed for application in clinical trials, but have been shown to be very beneficial in following patients in clinical practice.[42] The compositions of various pooled indices are outlined in Table 9A-1. Whereas the newer indices are based on the core set of variables, the older indices of Steinbrocker[43] and Lansbury[44] included additional characteristics of disease activity (such as anemia or fever). The Mallya index (developed in 1981) included tender joints, morning stiffness, ESR, hemoglobin, pain, and grip strength.[45] The latter two items were later excluded by van Riel in a trial.[46]

The Disease Activity Score (DAS) was developed in 1990.[47] Its complex formula is a consequence of the statistical procedures behind its derivation:

$$\text{DAS} = 0.54 \times \sqrt{(\text{Ritchie})} + 0.065 \times \text{SJC44} + 0.33 \times \log_{\text{nat}}(\text{ESR}) + 0.0072 \times \text{GH},$$

where *Ritchie* is the Ritchie articular index, *SJC44* is the swollen joint count based on 44 joints, *ESR* is the erythrocyte sedimentation rate, and *GH* is global health (*not* equal to PGA).

However, the complex Ritchie Index for tenderness and the 44 swollen-joint count are rarely used in clinical practice and trials. Therefore, the joint assessment in the DAS was simplified in 1993 to include the condensed 28-joint counts for both tenderness and swelling (TJC28, SJC28). This index, the DAS28,[48] has been extensively used and is calculated based on the following formula:

$$\text{DAS28} = 0.56 \times \sqrt{(\text{TJC28})} + 0.28 \times \sqrt{(\text{SJC28})} + 0.70 \times \log_{\text{nat}}(\text{ESR}) + 0.014 \times \text{GH}.$$

Currently, there are several modifications of the DAS and the DAS28 available that have not yet been validated. One modification is the use of CRP instead of ESR (DAS-CRP and DAS28-CRP). Another modification is the exclusion of the assessment of global health (DAS-3 and DAS28-3).

Simpler indices have been developed to overcome the major practical limitations of the DAS-based indices, the requirement of a pocket calculator or computer program, and poor transparency for patients. The Simplified Disease Activity Index (SDAI)[49] was the first index to employ a linear sum of variables that were untransformed and unweighted:

$$\text{SDAI} = \text{SJC28} + \text{TJC28} + \text{PGA (cm)} + \text{EGA (cm)} + \text{CRP (mg/dL)}.$$

The SDAI has been widely validated using clinical trial data, as well as in daily settings in different ethnic groups.

The SDAI, DAS, and DAS28 all require laboratory measures (CRP or ESR), which might constitute a limitation in clinical practice because it frequently prevents the immediate assessment due to waiting time for lab results (if available at all). Whereas the DAS28 has not been tested using clinical variables only, the SDAI has been shown to convey similar results even when CRP was eliminated from the formula.[49] This simplified index, based solely on clinical measures, was further analyzed in 2005 and then termed the Clinical Disease Activity Index (CDAI).[36] It has been validated using several different cohorts of patients and has been proven to highly correlate with the DAS28 and the ACR response as well as with HAQ and radiographic changes.[36] The CDAI is calculated as follows:

$$\text{CDAI} = \text{SJC28} + \text{TJC28} + \text{PGA (cm)} + \text{EGA (cm)}.$$

The CDAI allows making prompt assessment of disease activity, facilitates immediate treatment decisions, and makes it easier to comply with the quest for improvement of patient outcomes by regular disease activity assessment.[42]

The DAS, DAS28, SDAI, and CDAI not only allow us to determine the level of a patient's disease activity but to categorize disease activity states as high, moderate, and low disease activity and remission. Although they are more similar in patients with severe disease activity, the remission criteria of the SDAI and CDAI are more stringent than those of the DAS28.[50,51]

Response Criteria

The primary purpose of response criteria is to compare disease activity changes to a reference measurement. Usually this is important in clinical trials, whereas in daily life it is often unpractical to look up previous measurements to calculate a response or relative response. The Paulus response criteria,[52] developed in 1990, required four of six selected measures for improvement. Improvement was defined as greater than or equal to 20% for morning stiffness, ESR, joint pain/tenderness score, and joint swelling score, and as two or more grades on a 5-grade scale (or from grade 2 to grade 1) for PGA and EGA. This index discriminated well between placebo- and (DMARD)-treated patients.

The ACR response criteria[53] require 20% improvement (ACR20) in swollen and tender joint counts and three of the five remaining core set variables (Table 9A-1). These criteria seek to integrate best discrimination of the rheumatologist's impression of improvement with best discrimination of active drug from placebo in clinical trials. The criteria were subsequently expanded to reflect clinically more substantial improvement, but the 50% (ACR50) and 70% (ACR70) responses did not perform better than the ACR20 in discriminating active drug from placebo.[54]

The ACR-N response, based on the original ACR criteria, provides a more quantitative (rather than categorical) readout[55,56] by grading a 0% to 100% improvement according to the smallest relative improvement seen in the following three measures: swollen joint count, tender joint count, and median of the five remaining core set variables. This transposition of the ACR criteria into a continuous rather than dichotomous scale may still not be fully mature, as deterioration from baseline may be calculated as a negative value or as zero. Importantly, its time-integrated use as ACR-N area under the curve does not provide valid discrimination between regimens.[57]

Recently, a revision of the ACR20 has been proposed by a committee of the ACR.[58] The product, the ACR-Hybrid score, is calculated by a complex algorithm. First, the average percentage change in core set measures is evaluated and limited to a range of 100% (complete improvement) to −100% (any worsening beyond 100%). However, if this percent change score is not within the respective range of the traditional ACR response (i.e., ACR nonresponder, ACR20 but not ACR50, ACR50 but not ACR70, and ACR70 or above) the percentage of change is discarded and a value of 19.99, 49.99, or 69.99 is attributed.

The response criteria of the EULAR are based on the DAS28[59] and require patients to experience a certain amount of improvement as well as to achieve a particular disease activity state at the time of evaluation (Figure 9A-1).[60] The proportion of patients achieving any EULAR response (good response and moderate response) tends to be somewhat higher than for those achieving an ACR20 response, whereas good EULAR response is usually seen in more patients than in an ACR50 response.

In clinical practice, rather than using response criteria it is advisable to regularly (every three months) evaluate disease activity by composite scores such as the CDAI, SDAI, or DAS28—aiming to reach the low disease activity range and ideally remission, which is the therapeutic goal. Disease activity states have been defined for all three indices (Table 9A-2).[50,61] In line with this, disease activity levels reached within 3 to 6 months from the start of therapy predict longer-term outcome.[62] Moreover, the disease activity category attained after 1 year of therapy determines radiographic and functional outcome irrespective of the response level reached.[63] Thus, determining the disease activity status is of equal importance with determining therapeutic response.

Achieved DAS28	DAS28 improvement		
	>1.2	0.6–1.2	<0.6
<3.2	Good	Moderate	No
3.2–5.1	Moderate	Moderate	No
>5,1	Moderate	No	No

Figure 9A-1. EULAR response criteria.

Table 9A-2. Definition of Treatment Response and Disease Activity States

	Response		**Disease Activity States**			
	Moderate	Major	Remission	Low Disease Activity	Moderate Disease Activity	High Disease Activity
DAS28	—[a]	—[a]	<2.6	<3.2	<5.1	≥5.1
SDAI	≥7	≥17	≤3.3	≤11	≤26	>26
CDAI	≥6	≥14	≤2.8	≤10	≤22	>22

[a]Part of the EULAR response criteria (see Figure 9A-1).

Summary

Disease activity is a central measurement in the follow-up of patients with RA. The nature of RA makes disease activity assessment more complicated than in many other diseases, such as diabetes or hypertension. The efforts of the past decades have shown that disease activity assessment in patients with RA is not trivial, that single aspects of disease activity are not sufficient in acquiring a sense of the severity of RA, and that pooling of attributes is the most reliable way of conducting disease activity assessment. The value of composite indices has been supported by many studies, and targeting treatments around desirable disease activity levels based on these indices has been shown to improve patient outcomes in RA. The patient's perspective and potential impact on disease activity must not be underestimated. Here, an attempt to bring patients and physicians closer would certainly be warranted. This would include listening to patients' needs on the part of the physician (and the outcomes researcher) and educating patients on the (ideally simple) tools of assessment and the meaning of our measurements in clinical practice.

References

1. Felson DT, Anderson JJ, Boers M, et al. The American College of Rheumatology preliminary core set of disease activity measures for rheumatoid arthritis clinical trials: The Committee on Outcome Measures in Rheumatoid Arthritis Clinical Trials. *Arthritis Rheum* 1993;36:729–740.
2. Smolen JS. The work of the EULAR Standing Committee on International Clinical Studies Including Therapeutic Trials (ESCISIT). *Br J Rheumatol* 1992;31:219–220.
3. Boers M, Tugwell P, Felson DT, et al. World Health Organization and International League of Associations for Rheumatology core endpoints for symptom modifying antirheumatic drugs in rheumatoid arthritis clinical trials. *J Rheumatol Suppl* 1994;41:86–89.
4. Pincus T, Brooks RH, Callahan LF. A proposed 30–45 minute 4 page standard protocol to evaluate rheumatoid arthritis (SPERA) that includes measures of inflammatory activity, joint damage, and long-term outcomes. *J Rheumatol* 1999;26:473–480.
5. Escalante A, del Rincon I. The disablement process in rheumatoid arthritis. *Arthritis Rheum* 2002;47:333–342.
6. Ward MM. Clinical and laboratory measures. In St Clair EW, Pisetsky DS, Haynes BF (eds.) *Rheumatoid Arthritis*. Philadelphia: Lippincott Williams & Wilkins 2004:51–63.
7. Lansbury J. Quantitation of the manifestations of rheumatoid arthritis. 4. Area of joint surfaces as an index to total joint inflammation and deformity. *Am J Med Sci* 1956;232:150–155.
8. deAndrade JR, Casagrgande PA. A seven-day variability study of 499 patients with peripheral rheumatoid arthritis. *Arthritis Rheum* 1965;19:302–334.
9. Williams HJ, Ward JR, Reading JC, et al. Low-dose D-penicillamine therapy in rheumatoid arthritis: A controlled, double-blind clinical trial. *Arthritis Rheum* 1983;26:581–592.
10. Ritchie DM, Boyle JA, McInnes JM, et al. Clinical studies with an articular index for the assessment of joint tenderness in patients with rheumatoid arthritis. *Q J Med* 1968;37:393–406.
11. Hart LE, Tugwell P, Buchanan WW, et al. Grading of tenderness as a source of interrater error in the Ritchie articular index. *J Rheumatol* 1985;12:716–717.
12. Egger MJ, Huth DA, Ward JR, et al. Reduced joint count indices in the evaluation of rheumatoid arthritis. *Arthritis Rheum* 1985;28:613–619.
13. Fuchs HA, Brooks RH, Callahan LF, et al. A simplified twenty-eight-joint quantitative articular index in rheumatoid arthritis. *Arthritis Rheum* 1989;32:531–537.
14. Prevoo ML, van Riel PL, van't Hof MA, et al. Validity and reliability of joint indices: A longitudinal study in patients with recent onset rheumatoid arthritis. *Br J Rheumatol* 1993;32:589–594.
15. Smolen JS, Breedveld FC, Eberl G, et al. Validity and reliability of the twenty-eight-joint count for the assessment of rheumatoid arthritis activity. *Arthritis Rheum* 1995;38:38–43.
16. Kapral T, Dernoschnig F, Machold KP, et al. Remission by composite scores in rheumatoid arthritis: Are ankles and feet important? *Arthritis Res Ther* 2007;9:R72.
17. Felson DT, Anderson JJ, Boers M, et al. for the ACR Committee on Outcome Measures. Reduced joint count in rheumatoid arthritis clinical trials. *Arthritis Rheum* 1994;37:463–464.
18. Wolfe F, O'Dell JR, Kavanaugh A, et al. Evaluating severity and status in rheumatoid arthritis. *J Rheumatol* 2001;28:1453–1462.
19. Smolen JS, Kalden JR, Scott DL, et al. Efficacy and safety of leflunomide compared with placebo and sulphasalazine in active rheumatoid arthritis: A double-blind, randomised, multicentre trial. European Leflunomide Study Group. *Lancet* 1999;353:259–266.
20. Emery P, Breedveld FC, Lemmel EM, et al. A comparison of the efficacy and safety of leflunomide and methotrexate for the treatment of rheumatoid arthritis. *Rheumatology* (Oxford) 2000;39:655–665.
21. Williamson A, Hoggart B. Pain: A review of three commonly used pain rating scales. *J Clin Nurs* 2005;14:798–804.
22. Meenan RF, Gertman PM, Mason JH. Measuring health status in arthritis: The arthritis impact measurement scales. *Arthritis Rheum* 1980;23:146–152.
23. Melzack R. The short-form McGill Pain Questionnaire. *Pain* 1987; 30:191–197.
24. Carlsson AM. Assessment of chronic pain. I. Aspects of the reliability and validity of the visual analogue scale. *Pain* 1983;16: 87–101.

25. Huskisson EC. Measurement of pain. *Lancet* 1974;2:1127–1131.
26. Scott J, Huskisson EC. Vertical or horizontal visual analogue scales. *Ann Rheum Dis* 1979;38:560.
27. Mason JH, Anderson JJ, Meenan RF, et al. The rapid assessment of disease activity in rheumatology (radar) questionnaire: Validity and sensitivity to change of a patient self-report measure of joint count and clinical status. *Arthritis Rheum* 1992;35:156–162.
28. Stucki G, Liang MH, Stucki S, et al. A self-administered rheumatoid arthritis disease activity index (RADAI) for epidemiologic research: Psychometric properties and correlation with parameters of disease activity. *Arthritis Rheum* 1995;38:795–798.
29. Fransen J, Stucki G, Van Riel PC. Rheumatoid arthritis measures. *Arthritis Care Res* 2001;49:S214–S224.
30. Mason JH, Meenan RF, Anderson JJ. Do self-reported arthritis symptom (RADAR) and health status (AIMS2) data provide duplicative or complementary information? *Arthritis Care Res* 1992;5: 163–172.
31. Fransen J, Hauselmann H, Michel BA, et al. Responsiveness of the self-assessed rheumatoid arthritis disease activity index to a flare of disease activity. *Arthritis Rheum* 2001;44:53–60.
32. Dawes PT, Fowler PD, Clarke S, et al. Rheumatoid arthritis: Treatment which controls the C-reactive protein and erythrocyte sedimentation rate reduces radiological progression. *Br J Rheumatol* 1986;25:44–49.
33. van Leeuwen MA, van Rijswijk MH, van der Heijde DM, et al. The acute-phase response in relation to radiographic progression in early rheumatoid arthritis: A prospective study during the first three years of the disease. *Br J Rheumatol* 1993;32(Suppl 3):9–13.
34. Plant MJ, Williams AL, O'Sullivan MM, et al. Relationship between time-integrated C-reactive protein levels and radiologic progression in patients with rheumatoid arthritis. *Arthritis Rheum* 2000; 43:1473–1477.
35. Combe B, Dougados M, Goupille P, et al. Prognostic factors for radiographic damage in early rheumatoid arthritis: A multiparameter prospective study. *Arthritis Rheum* 2001;44:1736–1743.
36. Aletaha D, Nell VP, Stamm T, et al. Acute phase reactants add little to composite disease activity indices for rheumatoid arthritis: Validation of a clinical activity score. *Arthritis Res Ther* 2005;7: R796–R806.
37. Wolfe F, Michaud K. The clinical and research significance of the erythrocyte sedimentation rate. *J Rheumatol* 1994;21:1227–1237.
38. St Clair EW, van der Heijde DM, Smolen JS, et al. Combination of infliximab and methotrexate therapy for early rheumatoid arthritis: A randomized, controlled trial. *Arthritis Rheum* 2004;50:3432–3443.
39. Tugwell P, Bombardier C. A methodologic framework for developing and selecting endpoints in clinical trials. *J Rheumatol* 1982;9: 758–762.
40. Goldsmith CH, Smythe HA, Helewa A. Interpretation and power of a pooled index. *J Rheumatol* 1993;20:575–578.
41. Schulz KF, Grimes DA. Multiplicity in randomised trials I: Endpoints and treatments. *Lancet* 2005;365:1591–1595.
42. Grigor C, Capell H, Stirling A, et al. Effect of a treatment strategy of tight control for rheumatoid arthritis (the TICORA study): A single-blind randomised controlled trial. *Lancet* 2004;364:263–269.
43. Steinbrocker O, Bloch DA. A therapeutic score card for rheumatoid arthritis. *N Engl J Med* 1946;14:501–506.
44. Lansbury J. Quantitation of the activity of rheumatoid arthritis. 5. A method for summation of the systemic indices of rheumatoid activity. *Am J Med Sci* 1956;232:300–310.
45. Mallya RK, Mace BE. The assessment of disease activity in rheumatoid arthritis using a multivariate analysis. *Rheumatol Rehabil* 1981; 20:14–17.
46. van Riel PL, Reekers P, van de Putte LB, et al. Association of HLA antigens, toxic reactions and therapeutic response to auranofin and aurothioglucose in patients with rheumatoid arthritis. *Tissue Antigens* 1983;22:194–199.
47. van der Heijde DM, van't Hof MA, van Riel PL, et al. Judging disease activity in clinical practice in rheumatoid arthritis: First step in the development of a disease activity score. *Ann Rheum Dis* 1990; 49:916–920.
48. Prevoo ML, van't Hof MA, Kuper HH, et al. Modified disease activity scores that include twenty-eight-joint counts: Development and validation in a prospective longitudinal study of patients with rheumatoid arthritis. *Arthritis Rheum* 1995;38:44–48.
49. Smolen JS, Breedveld FC, Schiff MH, et al. A simplified disease activity index for rheumatoid arthritis for use in clinical practice. *Rheumatology* (Oxford) 2003;42:244–257.
50. Aletaha D, Ward MM, Machold KP, et al. Remission and active disease in rheumatoid arthritis: Defining criteria for disease activity states. *Arthritis Rheum* 2005;52:2625–2636.
51. Mierau M, Schoels M, Gonda G, et al. Assessing remission in clinical practice. *Rheumatology (Oxford)* 2007;46:975–979.
52. Paulus HE, Egger MJ, Ward JR, et al. Analysis of improvement in individual rheumatoid arthritis patients treated with disease-modifying antirheumatic drugs, based on the findings in patients treated with placebo: The Cooperative Systematic Studies of Rheumatic Diseases Group. *Arthritis Rheum* 1990;33:477–484.
53. Felson DT, Anderson JJ, Boers M, et al. American College of Rheumatology: Preliminary definition of improvement in rheumatoid arthritis. *Arthritis Rheum* 1995;38:727–735.
54. Felson DT, Anderson JJ, Lange ML, et al. Should improvement in rheumatoid arthritis clinical trials be defined as fifty percent or seventy percent improvement in core set measures, rather than twenty percent? *Arthritis Rheum* 1998;41:1564–1570.
55. Schiff M, Waever A, Keystone E, Moreland L, Spencer-Gree G. Comparison of ACR response, numeric ACR, ACR AUC as measures of clinical improvement in RA clinical trials. *Arthritis Rheum* 1999;42:S81.
56. Siegel JN, Zhen BG. Use of the American College of Rheumatology N (ACR-N) index of improvement in rheumatoid arthritis: Argument in favor. *Arthritis Rheum* 2005;52:1637–1641.
57. Boers M. Use of the American College of Rheumatology N (ACR-N) index of improvement in rheumatoid arthritis: Argument in opposition. *Arthritis Rheum* 2005;52:1642–1645.
58. A proposed revision to the ACR20: The hybrid measure of American College of Rheumatology response. *Arthritis Rheum* 2007;57: 193–202.
59. van Gestel AM, Prevoo ML, van't Hof MA, et al. Development and validation of the European League Against Rheumatism response criteria for rheumatoid arthritis: Comparison with the preliminary American College of Rheumatology and the World Health Organization/International League Against Rheumatism Criteria. *Arthritis Rheum* 1996;39:34–40.
60. Scott D, Van Riel PC, van der Heijde DM, et al. on behalf of the EULAR Standing Committee for International Clinical Studies Including Therapeutic Trials (ESCISIT). *Assessing Disease Activity in Rheumatoid Arthritis: The EULAR Handbook of Standard Methods.* Zürich: EULAR, 1993.
61. Aletaha D, Smolen JS. The American College of Rheumatology N (ACR-N) debate: Going back into the middle of the tunnel? Comment on the articles by Siegel and Zhen and by Boers. *Arthritis Rheum* 2006;54:377–378.
62. Aletaha D, Funovits J, Keystone EC, et al. Disease activity early in the course of treatment predicts response to therapy after one year in rheumatoid arthritis patients. *Arthritis Rheum* 2007;56:3226–3235.
63. Aletaha D, Funovits J, Smolen JS. The importance of reporting disease activity states in clinical trials of rheumatoid arthritis. *Arthritis Rheum* 2008 (in press).

Physical Function

Michael M. Ward

CHAPTER 9B

Physical function refers to the ability to move one's body purposefully to accomplish a task. These tasks include self-care, such as dressing, eating and hygiene, transferring, ambulation, moving objects, and household chores. Accomplishing these tasks requires some measure of strength, flexibility, and endurance—and functional limitations can result from any process that compromises strength, flexibility, or endurance. Rheumatoid arthritis (RA) can have a profound impact on physical functioning, given the widespread polyarthritis that is often present—and in particular the frequent involvement of hand joints. Joint pain, swelling, and stiffness due to active synovitis can cause functional limitations by decreasing strength and flexibility. Pain and fatigue can also decrease endurance. Joint deformities and instability, muscle wasting, and deconditioning that may occur as a consequence of longstanding synovitis can also decrease strength, flexibility, and endurance to result in functional limitations. Psychologic status, mood, and comorbid conditions may also directly or indirectly affect physical function.[1]

With active synovitis, symptoms, and joint damage as potential causes, functional limitation is a risk throughout the course of RA. Functional limitations are often present at the onset of RA, may decrease in response to initial treatment, and subsequently increase as synovitis recurs and joint damage accrues.[2–4] Functional limitation is the major clinical predictor of mortality, work disability, and health care costs in RA.[5–8] Given its importance as a health outcome, physical function has been endorsed as a core endpoint in RA clinical trials and is a component of the American College of Rheumatology response criteria.[9–11]

Concepts and Models

Health outcomes are an interrelated set of attributes that describe the consequences of disease for an individual. These include impairments, symptoms, functioning, participation in activities and social roles, and health-related quality of life. Impairments are alterations in normal body structures or function.[12] These anatomic or physiologic changes may cause symptoms, which represent the somatic sensation of the abnormality. Impairments or symptoms may result in functional limitations or disability. Physical function is one category of functional ability, the others being mental function (mood, and ability to perform tasks requiring memory, thought, or concentration), role function (ability to perform a job or to do housework or schoolwork), and social function (ability to form and maintain social relationships). For example, a large knee effusion is an impairment that may cause pain and contracture, resulting in the inability to walk (a physical functional limitation) and to go to work (a role functional limitation). Health status is the term used to describe how a person feels and functions overall, and includes symptoms and the four categories of functioning. In turn, health-related quality of life is a subjective appraisal of one's health status and satisfaction with it viewed in the context of one's expectations and values.

The World Health Organization's current model of health outcomes replaces the former impairment-disability-handicap model with a simplified scheme of the relationships among a health condition, body structure and function, and activity and participation[12] (Figure 9B-1). This model emphasizes the interrelationships among these domains and uses neutral language (body structure instead of impairment; activity instead of disability) to recognize the importance of processes that promote health in addition to those that decrease health. Using this framework, a comprehensive list of the activities and participation areas impacted by RA has been developed.[13] This list can serve as a reference against which to compare the activities assessed in currently used measures of physical function, to identify functions missing from current measures (e.g., writing, driving), and to serve as a starting point for new measures.

In judging the types of physical functions to be assessed, one consideration is the standard used to define "normal" function. Most measures limit the functions assessed to those of activities of daily living (ADL) or instrumental activities of daily living (IADL, such as shopping and preparing meals). For these measures, normal physical function denotes no difficulty doing these activities. However, some measures include more rigorous activities (running 2 miles) in an attempt to differentiate functional ability among those who have no problems in functions related to ADLs or IADLs.[14,15] These measures use fitness as the standard, rather than using the level of functioning needed for successful independent living as the standard. Most measures also use an absolute standard against which functioning is compared (e.g., no difficulty in ADLs and IADLs). Other measures, such as the Human Activity Profile, use a person's prior abilities as a relative standard against which to judge changes in function.[15] This approach may permit identification of more subtle changes in physical function than measures that use an absolute standard, particularly among more vigorous activities. Measures of physical function may also be designed to assess performance (reported difficulty at tasks actually undertaken) or capability (estimated ability to accomplish a task). Performance emphasizes the person's usual experience, and is usually preferred for measures of ADLs and IADLs. Measures of performance require that

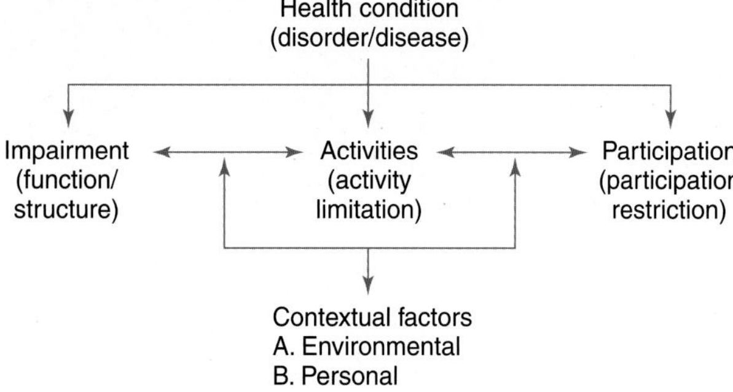

Figure 9B-1. World Health Organization model of health outcomes. (Adapted from World Health Organization. *ICF: International Classification of Functioning, Disability, and Health. Introduction*. 2001. http://www3.who.int/icf/icftemplate.cfm.)

the opportunity to perform the task existed, whereas measures of capability do not depend on this opportunity.

Measures of physical function describe the state of the individual, but do not identify the cause of any functional limitation. For example, a person who reports difficulty walking may be limited due to a large knee effusion, a fractured tibia, mechanical low back pain, or hemiplegia. Limitations due to some of these processes are completely reversible, whereas others are not. In patients with RA, identical degrees of functional limitation may be due to active polyarthritis, chronic joint damage, or some combination of the two. Knowing the degree of limitation alone does not allow distinction between these causes[16] (Figure 9B-2). Identifying the causes of functional limitations requires additional information about symptoms, impairments, or the time course of changes in function. Improvement with treatment can help establish the degree to which functional limitations are reversible and therefore likely due to acute inflammation, or irreversible and more likely due to chronic musculoskeletal damage. Irreversible functional limitations increase with the duration of RA.[16,17]

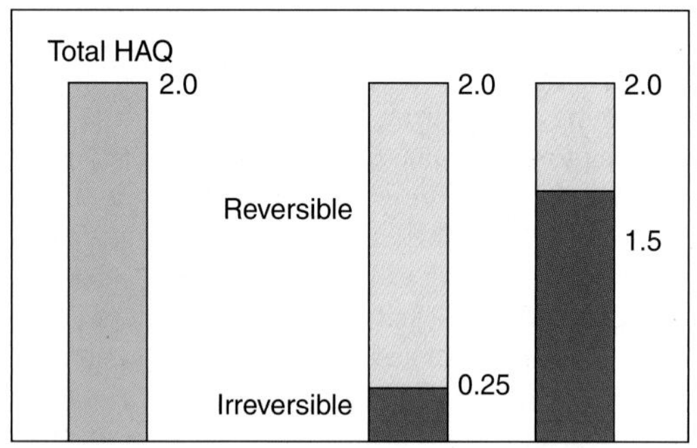

Figure 9B-2. Interpretation of measures of functional limitation. Measures characterize the degree of limitation but do not provide information about the cause of the limitation. The same degree of functional limitation may be due largely to reversible problems in one patient and irreversible problems in another patient. For example, an HAQ of 2.0 may represent someone with a small irreversible component (0.25 out of 2.0) or someone with a large irreversible component (1.5 out of 2.0).

Methods of Assessment

Three methods are used to assess physical function: performance-based measures, observation, and self-report measures (Table 9B-1). Performance-based measures test a person's ability to do prescribed tasks, most often in a timed exercise. Examples include the 50-foot walk time, button test (a timed test of unbuttoning and rebuttoning 5 buttons on a standard board), the Jebsen test of hand function (seven tests of finger dexterity, pinching, grip, and lifting), and the Moburg pick-up test (test of picking up 12 small objects).[18] Measurement of grip strength using a dynamometer is also a performance-based measure. These measures assess capacity to perform a task, but may focus on only one type of task while ignoring many others. The results are effort dependent. The need for special equipment and standardized administration tends to limit their use. These tests can predict long-term outcomes in RA, including mortality, likely because of the degree of chronic joint damage they capture—more so than the degree of active synovitis.[19] Because they are less sensitive than other measures of physical function in capturing changes in physical function and less specifically related to RA activity, performance-based measures have not been recommended as core measures of RA activity.[20,21]

Observation methods are based on assessment by a knowledgeable observer. This may be a clinician who makes an informal assessment based on the physical function of the patient in the clinic (largely based on mobility) or a more formal assessment of difficulty in performing daily tasks, in the clinic or in the home setting. The most commonly used observation measures are the Steinbrocker and the revised American College of Rheumatology functional classes.[22,23] These provide a global assessment of physical function, but the four categories of functional ability defined in these measures are too crude to be useful guides for interventions or endpoints in trials. Another observation method occurs when physical function questionnaires are completed for a patient (a child or a cognitively impaired patient) by a proxy respondent.[24]

The approach most frequently used to measure physical function is self-report questionnaires. These can range from single items ("How many days during the past month did you need to reduce your activity?") to multi-item questionnaires that assess performance in a wide range of tasks. These questionnaires can exist as standalone instruments or as components of questionnaires that assess other aspects of health status.[25] Numerous physical function measures have been developed, and several compendia of these measures are available (Table 9B-1).[25–27] Many measures, such as the Katz Index of ADL and the Physical Function scale of the Short-Form 36 (SF-36), are generic measures of physical function rather than arthritis-specific measures.[28,29] The generality of the tasks assessed and the wide range of functions impacted by RA suggest that generic measures may perform as well as arthritis-specific measures of physical function in RA. Many multi-item questionnaires have excellent measurement properties. They have also been found to be sensitive to change in clinical trials, meaning that measurements obtained before and shortly after the start of effective treatment will register an improvement in function. Physical function as assessed by self-report questionnaire has been recommended as a core measure of RA activity.[9,10,21]

The Health Assessment Questionnaire Disability Index (HAQ), the most commonly used measure of physical function

Table 9B-1. Common Measures of Physical Function		
Performance-Based	**Observation**	**Self-Reported**
50-foot walk time	Steinbrocker functional classes	Days of limited activity
Grip strength	American College of Rheumatology functional classes	Katz Index of Activities of Daily Living
Button test	Self-report questionnaire completed by proxy	Nagi scale
Jebsen test of hand function		Barthel Index
Moburg pick-up test		Short-Form 36 (physical function scale)
		Health Assessment Questionnaire Disability Index
		Arthritis Impact Measurement Scales (physical function scales)
		MACTAR Patient Preference Disability Questionnaire

in RA, is discussed in detail in the next section.[30] Three other measures—the Arthritis Impact Measurement Scales (AIMS) physical function scale, the Physical Function subscale of the SF-36, and the McMaster Toronto Arthritis Patient Preference Disability Questionnaire (MACTAR)—have also been used in RA.[29,31,32] The AIMS2 is a 28-item questionnaire that asks respondents to report how often in the past month they experienced difficulty performing tasks in six functional areas (mobility, walking and bending, hand and finger function, arm function, self-care, and household tasks). The reliability and construct validity of the AIMS2 physical function scale has been established, but it may be less sensitive to change than the HAQ.[21,33] The SF-36 physical function scale is a 10-item scale that asks about limitations in mobility and IADLs to a greater extent than limitations in ADLs. It is one of eight scales of the SF-36, the others being role limitations due to physical problems, pain, general health, mental health, vitality, social functioning, and role limitations due to emotional problems. Population-based norms are available for each scale, and for the physical component subscale (a summary of the physical function, role physical, pain, and general health scales). The SF-36 is useful in comparing health status across diseases, and because it assesses several different components of health status it has frequently been used as a secondary endpoint in RA clinical trials.[34,35]

The MACTAR differs from many other measures by eliciting and measuring changes in five functional tasks nominated by the patient as the ones he or she would most like to improve. This approach makes the assessment more relevant for each patient, and because only problematic tasks are included the MACTAR may be more sensitive to change than questionnaires (such as the HAQ and AIMS) that include a standard set of tasks. The MACTAR is administered as a semistructured interview, which reduces its ease of use.

Health Assessment Questionnaire Disability Index

The HAQ Disability Index is a 20-question index that asks respondents to report the degree of difficulty (0 = no difficulty, 1 = some difficulty, 2 = much difficulty, 3 = unable to do) they have had performing tasks in eight areas (dressing, arising, eating, walking, hygiene, reaching, gripping, and errands and chores) in the past week[30] (available at *http://aramis.stanford.edu*). The highest scores in each functional area are averaged to compute the HAQ Disability Index, which is an ordinal scale with increments of 0.125 and a possible range of 0 to 3. Use of aids or need of help from another person to perform a task can also be incorporated in the scoring. Scores for each functional area can be used as a profile to identify those areas most affected. HAQ scores of less than 1.0 are conventionally considered to represent mild limitations, scores of 1.0 to 2.0 to represent moderate limitations, and scores greater than 2.0 to represent severe limitations.

The reliability, construct, and predictive validity of the HAQ Disability Index have been extensively documented.[36] HAQ scores correlate well with other measures of physical function, with measures of RA activity such as swollen and tender joint counts, and with the degree of radiographic damage. HAQ scores predict future functional limitations, health care utilization and costs, and mortality.[5–8] In clinical trials and observational studies, the sensitivity to change of the HAQ has been found to be moderately high—although it may be lower than that of other patient-reported measures, such as pain scores and global assessments.[21,33,36,37] This lower sensitivity to change may be because the HAQ, as a measure of functional disability, includes limitations due to irreversible joint damage as well as active synovitis.

Researchers have also sought to define the degree of change in the HAQ that represents a clinically important improvement to patients, to provide a standard against which to judge the efficacy of a given treatment. A difference in HAQ scores of 0.22 has been proposed as the clinically important difference, based on a comparison of HAQ scores among patients who talked to each other and rated themselves as having either the same functional ability or somewhat different functional ability from another person.[38] This inter-patient comparison differs from the way in which clinically important change is usually conceived, which is as a within-person change, and therefore further testing of the clinically important difference is needed. It is also not clear if the size of the change in the HAQ considered clinically important differs between patients who have little functional difficulty and those who have significant functional difficulty.[39]

Several modified versions of the HAQ have been developed. The modified HAQ (MHAQ) uses only one question from each of the eight functional areas of the HAQ and is scored as an average of these items (possible range, 0–3).[40] It was designed to be brief and easily scored, and includes supplemental questions on satisfaction with function and change over the past

6 months. The RA-HAQ also uses only one question from each of the eight functional areas of the original HAQ (some different from the MHAQ), chosen to produce a measure with an interval scale.[41] These instruments discriminate levels of functional disability less well than the full index, and may be less sensitive to change.[27,42] The multidimensional HAQ (MDHAQ) adds six questions on more rigorous functions to the MHAQ to better capture differences in functional ability at the more functional end of the spectrum, but in doing so alters the standard by which functional ability is measured (as noted previously).[14] In contrast, the CLINHAQ uses the standard 20-item HAQ to assess physical function but includes measures of other domains.[43]

Future of Physical Function Measurement

The HAQ and most other measures of physical function currently used are based on classical test theory. Such measures include a range of tasks that vary in difficulty from very easy to challenging. Comparisons among patients are possible because each patient answers the same questions, and comparisons of changes over time are also possible because the questions are invariant. However, measures based on classical test theory have several important limitations.[44] First, despite their appearance the scales of these measures are not linear. That is, a HAQ of 2.0 does not represent twice the degree of functional limitation as a HAQ of 1.0, and a change from 0.75 to 0.25 likely does not represent the same degree of improvement in function as a change from 2.5 to 2.0. The relationship between scores cannot be interpreted in this strictly mathematical way, even though they are analyzed statistically as though they can be interpreted in this way. Rather, these measures provide an ordinal ranking of patients by degree of functional ability. Second, because different questionnaires have different scales, results on one questionnaire cannot be directly compared to results on another questionnaire—and studies using different questionnaires cannot be compared.[42] For example, a HAQ of 1.25 has no direct equivalent on the AIMS2 physical function scale. Third, applying the same questionnaire in different groups of patients may yield different estimates of reliability, validity, and sensitivity to change. Fourth, because long questionnaires are burdensome the list of tasks is often fairly limited. They may omit important aspects of function (e.g., writing, driving, or more vigorous activities), overemphasize tasks that are "too easy," or include tasks that are not relevant for a given patient.

The nonlinearity problem of classical tests is a consequence of not precisely knowing the relationships between different tasks and the levels of functional ability they represent. Modern measurement theory (also known as item response theory) solves this problem by considering each trait, such as physical function, to range over a single underlying scale.[45,46] Questions are designed so that each response is related to this underlying scale. In this way, responses to different questions have an intrinsic relationship to each other. Knowing the response to one question can indicate how other questions will likely be answered. For example, knowing that someone has much difficulty going up one flight of stairs would predict with a higher probability that the same person would have moderate difficulty doing errands, moderate difficulty preparing meals, and no difficulty washing their hair (Figure 9B-3). These relationships are developed from responses of a large number of patients and from examination of the probabilities and patterns of responses among different functional tasks, which can then be mapped on a single scale.

Measures developed using item response theory have several advantages. The relatedness among different questions allows for comparison across questions and provides an internal check for inconsistent responses. It can compensate efficiently for missing answers because knowing the pattern of responses informs one of what the response to the missing item would likely have been. It also allows adaptive (dynamic) testing by computer, which is increasingly used in educational testing to be used to measure health status. Computer adaptive testing (CAT) functions in conjunction with a large databank of questions about functional tasks, each pretested and with a known relationship to the single underlying trait of functional ability.[44,46] Respondents are asked a question drawn by computer from the databank, and depending on their response to the first question the computer program draws a second question most likely to narrow the range of functional ability. This process is repeated iteratively until a sufficiently precise measure of functional ability is achieved. For example, if the patient responds to the first question that she cannot dress herself, the computer will not choose subsequent questions about more difficult tasks such as doing errands or walking up stairs because the answers

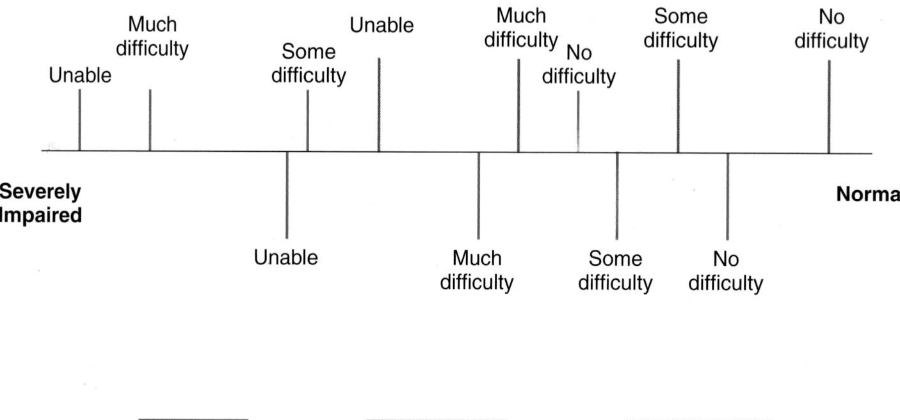

Figure 9B-3. Hypothetical example of the relationship between selected functional limitations on a single linear scale, as would be developed for measures using item response theory. The levels of difficulty in running errands, going up one flight of stairs, and washing hair are related to one another because they are related to the same underlying linear measure of physical function.

to these questions would be predictable. Rather, subsequent questions are focused on more fundamental tasks such as eating and transferring. Because questions are tailored to the individual, fewer questions need to be asked, and there are fewer problems with all questions being too hard or too easy for a given patient. In this way, CAT permits more precise discrimination of functional ability among patients, which translates into smaller sample sizes needed to demonstrate differences between groups in clinical trials. This provides greater efficiency than classical testing.

The Patient-Reported Outcomes Measurement Information System (PROMIS) initiative is currently developing a system for measuring physical function based on item-response theory.[47,48] Identification of the domains of physical function, generation of the individual test items, testing of formats and response options, and testing how responses differ among groups with different characteristics are currently in progress. Although much work remains, the goal is that this initiative will result in psychometrically sound tools and a CAT system that will be publicly available for clinical use. Given its advantages, this or other similar systems will likely replace the measures of physical function currently used.

Acknowledgments

This work was supported by the Intramural Research Program, National Institute of Arthritis and Musculoskeletal and Skin Diseases, National Institutes of Health.

References

1. Escalante A, del Rincón I. How much disability in rheumatoid arthritis is explained by rheumatoid arthritis? *Arthritis Rheum* 1999; 42:1712–1721.
2. Welsing PM, van Gestel AM, Swinkels HL, et al. The relationship between disease activity, joint destruction, and functional capacity over the course of rheumatoid arthritis. *Arthritis Rheum* 2001;44: 2009–2017.
3. Scott DL, Pugner K, Kaarela K, et al. The links between joint damage and disability in rheumatoid arthritis. *Rheumatology* 2000;39: 122–132.
4. Wolfe F. A reappraisal of HAQ disability in rheumatoid arthritis. *Arthritis Rheum* 2000;43:2751–2761.
5. Wolfe F, Michaud K, Gefeller O, et al. Predicting mortality in patients with rheumatoid arthritis. *Arthritis Rheum* 2003;48:1530–1542.
6. Yelin E, Trupin L, Wong B, et al. The impact of functional status and change in functional status on mortality over 18 years among persons with rheumatoid arthritis. *J Rheumatol* 2002;29:1851–1857.
7. Burton W, Morrison A, Maclean R, et al. Systematic review of studies of productivity loss due to rheumatoid arthritis. *Occup Med* (London) 2006;56:18–27.
8. Yelin E, Wanke LA. An assessment of the annual and long-term direct costs of rheumatoid artritis: The impact of poor function and functional decline. *Arthritis Rheum* 1999;42:1209–1218.
9. Felson DT, Anderson JJ, Boers M, et al. The American College of Rheumatology preliminary core set of disease activity measures for rheumatoid arthritis clinical trials. The Committee on Outcome Measures in Rheumatoid Arthritis Clinical Trials. *Arthritis Rheum* 1993;36:729–740.
10. Boers M, Tugwell P, Felson DT, et al. World Health Organization and International League of Associations for Rheumatology core endpoints for symptom modifying antrheumatic drugs in rheumatoid arthritis clinical trials. *J Rheumatol* 1994;41(Suppl): 86–89.
11. Felson DT, Anderson JJ, Boers M, et al. American College of Rheumatology preliminary definition of improvement in rheumatoid arthritis. *Arthritis Rheum* 1995;38:727–735.
12. World Health Organization. ICF: International Classification of Functioning, Disability, and Health. Introduction. 2001. *http://www3.who.int/icf/icftemplate.cfm*, accessed on December 9, 2007.
13. Stucki G, Cieza A, Geyh S, et al. ICF core sets for rheumatoid arthritis. *J Rehabil Med* 2004;Suppl 44:87–93.
14. Pincus T, Swearingen C, Wolfe F. Toward a multidimensional Health Assessment Questionnaire (MDHAQ): Assessment of advanced activities of daily living and psychological status in a patient-friendly health assessment questionnaire format. *Arthritis Rheum* 1999;42: 2220–2230.
15. Davidson M, de Morton N. A systematic review of the Human Activity Profile. *Clin Rehabil* 2007;21:151–162.
16. Aletaha D, Smolen J, Ward MM. Measuring function in rheumatoid arthritis: Identifying reversible and irreversible components. *Arthritis Rheum* 2006;54:2784–2792.
17. Aletaha D, Ward MM. Duration of rheumatoid arthritis influences the degree of functional improvement in clinical trials. *Ann Rheum Dis* 2006;65:227–233.
18. Stamm TA, Cieza A, Machold KP, et al. Content comparison of occupation-based instruments in adult rheumatology and musculoskeletal rehabilitation based on the International Classification of Functioning, Disability and Health. *Arthritis Rheum* 2004;51: 917–924.
19. Pincus T, Callahan LF. Rheumatology function tests: Grip strength, walking time, button tests and questionnaires document and predict longterm morbidity and mortality in rheumatoid arthritis. *J Rheumatol* 1992;19:1051–1057.
20. Gøtzsche PC. Sensitivity of effect variables in rheumatoid arthritis: A meta-analysis of 130 placebo controlled NSAID trials. *J Clin Epidemiol* 1990;43:1313–1318.
21. Verhoeven AC, Boers M, van der Linden S. Responsiveness of the core set, response critieria, and utilities in early rheumatoid arthritis. *Ann Rheum Dis* 2000;59:966–974.
22. Steinbrocker O, Traeger CH, Batterman RC. Therapeutic criteria in rheumatoid arthritis. *JAMA* 1949;140:659–662.
23. Hochberg MC, Change RW, Dwosh I, et al. The American College of Rheumatology 1991 revised criteria for the classification of global functional status in rheumatoid arthritis. *Arthritis Rheum* 1992;35: 498–502.
24. van den Ende CH, Hazes JM, Le Cessie S, et al. Discordance between objective and subjective assessment of functional ability of patients with rheumatoid arthritis. *Br J Rheumatol* 1995;34:951–955.
25. Spilker B (ed.). *Quality of Life and Pharmacoeconomics in Clinical Trials, Second Edition.* Philadelphia: Lippincott-Raven 1996.
26. Spilker B, Molinek FR Jr., Johnston KA, et al. Quality of life bibliography and indexes. *Med Care* 1990;28(Suppl):DS1–DS77.
27. Katz PP. Measures of adult general functional status. *Arthritis Rheum* 2003;49(Suppl):S15–S27.
28. Katz S, Ford AB, Moskowtiz RW, et al. The Index of ADL: A standardized measure of biological and psychosocial function. *JAMA* 1963;185:914–919.
29. Ware JE, Sherbourne CD. The MOS 36-item short-form health survey (SF–36): I. Conceptual framework and item selection. *Med Care* 1992;30:473–483.
30. Fries JF, Spitz P, Kraines RG, et al. Measurement of patient outcomes in arthritis. *Arthritis Rheum* 1980;23:137–145.

31. Meenan RF, Mason JH, Anderson JJ, et al. AIMS2: The content and properties of a revised and expanded Arthritis Impact Measurement Scales health status questionnaire. *Arthritis Rheum* 1992;35:1–10.
32. Tugwell P, Bombardier C, Buchanan WW, et al. The MACTAR patient preference disability questionnaire: An individualized functional priority approach for assessing improvements in physical disability in clinical trials in rheumatoid arthritis. *J Rheumatol* 1987;14:446–451.
33. Buchbinder R, Bombardier C, Yeung M, et al. Which outcome measures should be used in rheumatoid arthritis clinical trials? Clinical and quality-of-life measures' responsiveness to treatment in a randomized controlled trial. *Arthritis Rheum* 1995;38:1568–1580.
34. Maini RN, Breedveld FC, Kalden JR, et al. Sustained improvement over two years in physical function, structural damage, and signs and symptoms among patients with rheumatoid arthritis treated with infliximab and methotrexate. *Arthritis Rheum* 2004;50:1051–1065.
35. Strand V, Scott DL, Emery P, et al. Physical function and health related quality of life: Analysis of 2-year data from randomized controlled studies of leflunomide, sulfasalazine, or methotrexate in patients with active rheumatoid arthritis. *J Rheumatol* 2005;32:590–601.
36. Bruce B, Fries JF. The Stanford Health Assessment Questionnaire: A review of its history, issues, progress, and documentation. *J Rheumatol* 2003;30:167–178.
37. Wells GA, Li T, Maxwell L, et al. Responsiveness of patient reported outcomes including fatigue, sleep quality and activity limitations and quality of life following treatment with abatacept in patients with rheumatoid arthritis. *Ann Rheum Dis* 2008;64:260–265.
38. Redelmeier DA, Lorig K. Assessing the clinical importance of symptomatic improvements: An illustration in rheumatology. *Arch Intern Med* 1993;153:1337–1342.
39. Ward MM. Interpreting measurements of physical function in clinical trials. *Ann Rheum Dis* 2007;66(Suppl 3):iii32–iii34.
40. Pincus T, Summey JA, Soraci SA Jr., et al. Assessment of patient satisfaction in activities of daily living using a modified Stanford Health Assessment Questionnaire. *Arthritis Rheum* 1983;26:1346–1353.
41. Tennant A, Ryser L, Stucki G, et al. An 8-item international version of the HAQ: The Inter-HAQ. *Arthritis Rheum* 1999;42(Suppl):S74.
42. Wolfe F. Which HAQ is best? A comparison of the HAQ, MHAQ and RA-HAQ, a difficult 8 item HAQ (DHAQ), and a rescored 20 item HAQ (HAQ20): Analyses in 2491 rheumatoid arthritis patients following leflunomide administration. *J Rheumatol* 2001;28:982–989.
43. Wolfe F. A brief clinical health assessment instrument: The CLINHAQ. *Arthritis Rheum* 1989;32(Suppl):S9.
44. McHorney CA. Ten recommendations for advancing patient-centered outcomes measurement for older persons. *Ann Intern Med* 2003;139:403–409.
45. Chang CH, Reeve BB. Item response theory and its application to patient-reported outcomes measurement. *Eval Health Prof* 2005;28:264–282.
46. Jette AM, Haley SM. Contemporary measurement techniques for rehabilitation outcomes assessment. *J Rehabil Med* 2005;37:339–345.
47. Cella D, Yount S, Rothrock N, et al. The Patient-Reported Outcomes Measurement Information System (PROMIS): Progress of an NIH Roadmap cooperative group during its first two years. *Med Care* 2007;45(Suppl 1):S3–S11.
48. Chakravarty E, Bjorner JB, Fries JF. Improving patient reported outcomes using item response theory and computerized adaptive testing. *J Rheumatol* 2007;34:1426–1431.

Health-Related Quality of Life in Rheumatoid Arthritis

Vibeke Strand and Jasvinder A. Singh

Assessment of health-related quality of life (HRQOL) is increasingly recognized to be critical when evaluating new therapies in rheumatoid arthritis (RA). It refers to "all the ways your disease affects you today"—both physical function and "participation" (the capacity to engage in activities of life, work, home, family, and social functions). Hence, HRQOL refers to the impact of health/disease on an individual's well-being in the context of their larger financial, social, and political environment—not all of which may be ameliorated when manifestations of the underlying disease are improved.[1] Thus, we make a distinction between *HRQOL* and the broader term *quality of life* (QOL).

OMERACT, the international consensus effort regarding outcome measures in rheumatology trials, has recommended that disease-specific as well as generic measures of HRQOL be utilized.[2] In RA, the Health Assessment Questionnaire (HAQ) and its modifications, MHAQ and MDHAQ,[3] have functioned as "disease-specific" measures of physical function, reflecting the large impact of disease on performance of instrumental as well as required activities of daily living.[4] Generic measures of HRQOL—including the Medical Outcomes Study Short Form-36 (SF-36),[5–7] Euro QOL (EQ-5D), and Health Utilities Index-3 (HUI3)—are well validated (satisfying the OMERACT filter of "truth, discrimination and feasibility"[8]) and have been utilized to assess HRQOL in RA.[9] These instruments may also be used to ascertain "utilities" for pharmacoeconomic analyses, including SF-6D derived from SF-36.[10–12] Alternatively, utilities may be collected by asking patients to weight preferences for health states using "standard gamble," "time trade-off," and VAS (visual analog score) or "feeling thermometer" scores.[13] Few utility measures have been collected alongside regulatory clinical trials, with the exception of those with auranofin, leflunomide, and adalimumab.[14–17]

Seven new disease-modifying antirheumatic therapies (DMARDs) have been approved for treatment of RA since 1998. In addition, these trials have demonstrated "inhibition of radiographic disease progression" and, importantly, "improvement in physical function and HRQOL"—now established labeling claims. Data were collected in response to U.S. Food and Drug Administration (FDA) requirements for "durability of response," which requires evaluation of physical function and HRQOL over 24 months of treatment.[18] Based on this information, we now know that improvements in HAQ are closely correlated with improvements in physical as well as mental domains of HRQOL.

Short Form-36

Short Form-36 (SF-36) was developed in the 1980s to measure self-reported HRQOL, sponsored by the Rand Corporation.[19–21] A generic health survey with 36 questions, it is used in clinical research, health policy evaluations, and general population surveys to assess HRQOL. Answers to the questions yield the following eight domains [scored from 0 (low) to 100 (high)] and two summary physical and mental component scores (PCS and MCS).

- Limitations in physical activities because of health problems (physical function, PF)
- Limitations in usual role activities because of physical health problems (role physical, RP)
- Bodily pain (BP)
- General health perceptions (GHP)
- Vitality (VIT; i.e., energy and fatigue)
- Limitations in social activities because of physic or emotional problems (social functioning, SF)
- Limitations in usual role activities because of emotional problems (role emotional, RE)
- General mental health (MH; i.e., psychologic distress and well-being)

These are calculated based on positively weighting four physical domains and negatively weighting four mental domains (or vice versa) on a scale of 0 to 50—with normative values equal to 50 (as illustrated in Figure 9C-1A). SF-36 has been translated and cross culturally validated in more than 50 languages and in most rheumatic disease populations.

EQ-5D

The EuroQol Group designed EQ-5D to be a simple self-administered questionnaire for measuring HRQOL.[22–24] It provides a descriptive profile and health status index value. The descriptive profile consists of the following five dimensions:

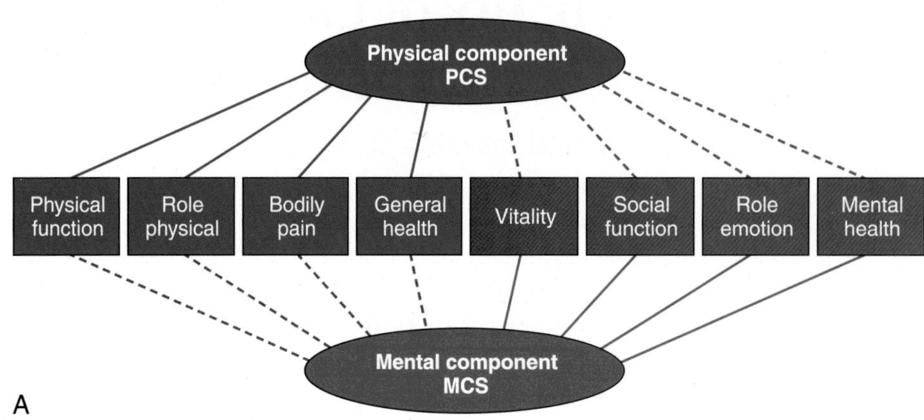

Figure 9C-1. (*A*) Illustration of how the four "physical" domains (PF, RP, BP, and GHP) of SF-36 are positively weighted and the four "mental" domains (VIT, SF, RE, and MH) negatively weighted to score PCS. The opposite is true for computing MCS scores. *Continued*

- Mobility
- Self-care
- Usual activities
- Pain/discomfort
- Anxiety/depression

Each dimension has three levels, reflecting "no," "moderate," and "extreme" health problems. EQ-5D also includes a 20-cm visual analog scale (EQ-VAS) for assessment of current general health. It is valid, reproducible, and sensitive to change in RA, and has been translated into most major languages and cross culturally validated across a variety of clinical indications.[12] EQ-5D scores differ by RA duration, DMARD use history, and presence of probable depression or anxiety.[25]

Health Utilities Index Mark 3

The Health Utilities Index Mark 3 (HUI3) is a generic health status and HRQOL measure originally developed at McMaster University for the 1990 Statistics Canada Ontario Health Survey.[26–28] It includes a health-status classification system and preference-based scoring formula based on eight attributes (vision, hearing, speech, ambulation, dexterity, emotion, cognition, and pain) with five to six levels per attribute. Categorical data are translated into single-attribute and overall utility scores, reflecting global HRQOL.

Clinically Meaningful Change

Although HRQOL questionnaires are not designed for use in daily clinical practice, information gained from their inclusion in randomized controlled trials (RCTs) has illustrated the important impact on HRQOL of pain, fatigue, and physical function due to active RA. This chapter reviews patient-reported HRQOL from RCTs with the traditional DMARDs methotrexate and leflunomide; with the biologic agents etanercept, infliximab, adalimumab, abatacept, and rituximab; and with two promising new therapies: certolizumab pegol (another TNF-α inhibitor) and tocilizumab (a monoclonal antibody to the IL-6 receptor). The relevance of these data to daily clinical practice is discussed in the material following in terms of "clinically meaningful" improvements, presented in tables and figures that follow.

Prior to introduction of the new DMARDs, longitudinal series reported progressive deterioration (at best, stabilization) in physical function in RA with standard of care (including methotrexate).[29,30] West et al. compared SF-36 in RA patients at disease onset and after 2 years in patients with long-term disease duration of 21 to 25 years.[31] Two years following diagnosis, patients reported significant improvements in role physical and bodily pain domains of SF-36 compared with disease onset. As with physical function, HRQOL is negatively impacted in early RA and improves dramatically with initiation of DMARD therapy. Patients with longer disease duration, having failed multiple DMARDs, report correspondingly greater decrements in physical function, role physical, bodily pain, general health, and vitality. In a longitudinal cohort study from the Norfolk Arthritis register, patients with mean age of 55 years, short disease duration of 6 months, and mean HAQ scores of 0.75 reported impairments in physical HRQOL—most significantly indicating that loss of HRQOL in RA occurs as early as the first few months of disease symptoms. In a systematic review of disability and joint damage, Scott et al. found that in the first years of RA there was an initial fall in HAQ scores followed by an increase over the next 4 years (a J-shaped curve) and that x-ray damage and disability became more strongly correlated with increasing disease duration (correlation coefficients 0.31–0.75 in nine studies).[32] This review concluded that "joint damage accounts for a substantial proportion of disability in RA." In an RCT comparing aggressive versus symptomatic treatment in 433 RA patients, social deprivation was significantly associated with lower HAQ scores and worse physical and emotional HRQOL scores—after adjustment for age, sex, disease duration, smoking, and treatment.[33] Therefore, comparisons of reported improvements in HRQOL across treatment groups must account for disease duration as well as baseline characteristics in protocol populations. This is similar to analyses of changes in physical function, assessed by HAQ,[34] that have considered a disease-specific measure of functional ability/limitation in patients with RA.

Clinically meaningful improvements in patient-reported outcomes have been interpreted in a variety of ways. One includes minimum clinically important differences (MCID): the amount of improvement (or deterioration) perceptible to patients as change by linking improvements in other patient-reported measures such as global disease activity (by VAS or Likert scale) or Guyatt feeling thermometer scores.[13] When mean or median changes within a treatment group well exceed MCID, it can be expected that the majority of patients have achieved clinically important improvement. The percentage of patients with improvements ≥MCID provides a means of understanding the magnitude of benefit within a treatment group, and translates group data to the level of individual impact. Values for MCID in SF-36 domain and physical (PCS) and mental component (MCS) summary scores have been derived in RA, osteoarthritis (OA), psoriatic arthritis (PsA), ankylosing spondylitis (AS), systemic lupus erythematosus (SLE), and fibromyalgia based on correlations with patient-reported improvements in global disease activity (on an individual patient basis) and are remarkably consistent. Changes of 5 to 10 points in domain scores and 2.5 to 5.0 points in PCS and MCS are considered to represent MCID.[35–39] Of importance, MCID values for deterioration are lower: –2.5 to –5.0 points in domain and –0.8 in PCS and MCS scores. These scores indicate that patients perceive small changes in worsening more readily than small changes in improvement.[40] These changes may also be used to calculate values for "number needed to treat" (NNT) to achieve clinical benefit. Although improvements ≥MCID represent levels of perceptible change, others have argued that values for "really important differences" (RID) should be defined—representing as much as three to four times MCID values.[41] For example, changes of 10 and 20 points on VASs of patient-reported pain and global assessments of disease activity have been defined to represent MCID and "important improvement," respectively—both of which add interpretations of "clinically meaningful" to statistically significant changes.

Alternatively, statistical definitions not specifically anchored to patient-reported outcomes include changes ≥0.5 standard deviations of the mean change, considered to reflect "minimally important differences" (MIDs).[27,42–44] For example, MID values for ED-5D and HUI3 were found to be 0.05 and 0.06, respectively, in a cohort of 222 RA patients with mean age 62 years, disease duration 14 years, and baseline HAQ scores of 1.1.[28]

Another interpretation of the "clinical meaningfulness" of improvements in HRQOL compares domain and summary scores of SF-36 to age- and gender-matched norms in relevant cultural populations. Baseline scores reported by RA patients in RCTs reflect large decrements in physical function, role physical, bodily pain, vitality, social function, and role emotional domains (Figure 9C-1B). In earlier RCTs, patients reported smaller decrements from normative values of 50 in MCS scores at baseline. Hence, treatment-associated improvements were not as impressive. In recent RCTs, MCS scores have also differed from baseline norms by 1 to 2 standard deviations (SD), reflecting a significant impact of active RA on mental as well as physical domains of SF-36. For example, changes at endpoint in SF-36 domain and summary scores can be evaluated by how closely they approach a "goal" of normative scores in age- and gender-matched U.S. populations. (See Figure 9C-1B as an example.)

Reported changes in specific questions in SF-36 offer another method of interpreting clinically meaningful changes attributed to treatment. These changes include decreases in walking limitations; less time lost at work due to health reasons; less inability to work because of pain; decreased, fair, or poor general health; less time felt tired or worn out; less interference of health in social activities; and fewer patients reporting feeling downhearted or blue most of the time (Table 9C-1). Answers to the "transition question" of SF-36 (i.e., "compared to a year ago ...") also offer a way of interpreting clinically meaningful treatment-associated changes. Importantly, changes from baseline in RCTs may exceed those reported in longitudinal studies, largely attributed to knowledge that a specific therapeutic intervention has occurred (e.g., "expectation bias" on the part of patients, as well as treating physicians).

HRQOL measures and HAQ provide important information in addition to traditional outcomes, such as swollen and tender joint count, and best differentiate active from placebo treatment.[45,46] In a study of randomized controlled trials, Tugwell et al. compared the standardized response mean and relative efficiency of SF-36 PCS and MCS and HAQ against tender joint count.[47,48] SF-36 PCS and HAQ had moderate effect sizes of respectively 0.42 and 0.46 and relative efficiencies of respectively 0.80 and 0.96 compared with tender joint count (set = 1.0). SF-36 MCS had a low effect size of 0.21 and a low relative efficiency of 0.20, owing to difference in domains of measurement. This review demonstrates that patient-reported HRQOL adds another dimension to outcomes assessed in RA trials. It is

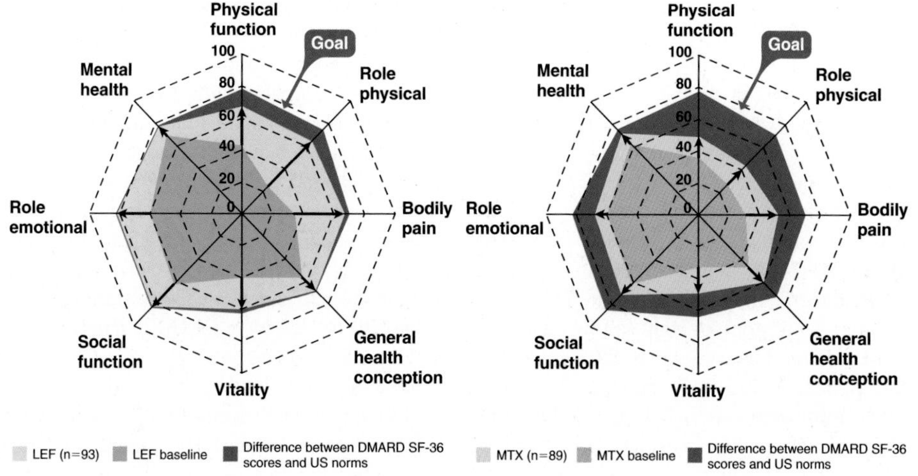

Figure 9C-1. cont'd (*B*) Baseline and final values for SF-36 domain scores in protocol U.S. 301 at 2 years in patients treated with leflunomide or methotrexate compared with U.S. normative values, representing a "goal" for treatment.

Table 9C-1. Percentage of Rheumatoid Arthritis Patients Reporting Clinically Meaningful Changes in Limitations in Physical Function by SF-36

	ERA[51,56]		**US301[49,50]**				**Phase 2B[67]**		**PREMIER[84]**			
	Rx with MTX or ETN		*Rx with MTX*		*Rx with LEF*		*Rx with ABA+MTX*		*Rx with ADA+MTX*		*Rx with MTX Only*	
	BL (%)	12 mo. (%)	BL (%)	24 mo. (%)	BL (%)	24 mo. (%)	BL (%)	12 mo. (%)	BL (%)	24 mo. (%)	BL (%)	24 mo. (%)
Limitations walking 1 block	65	36	45	38	45	17			46	8	44	13
Limitations climbing one flight of stairs	75	43	67	43	67	28			68	12	66	21
Difficulty performing at work	90	53	89	68	89	47			89	15	88	34
Less time lost at work due to health reasons							70	32	66	9	65	18
Less interference with work due to pain							51	11				
Less reported fair or poor general health							64	26				
Less time feeling tired or worn out							38	14				
Less interference of health on social activities							32	9				
Reporting feeling downhearted or blue most of the time							18	4				

important to understand the value of anchor-based approaches defining MCID and RID when assessing change in patient-reported outcomes, as well as statistical approaches—recognizing that these measures, including HAQ and HRQOL, appear more sensitive to change than traditional clinical outcome measures such as tender or swollen joint counts.

Methotrexate and Leflunomide

A 24-month placebo-controlled RCT (U.S. 301) was the first to show that SF-36 was a valid and sensitive instrument for measuring HRQOL in clinical trials in patients with active RA.[49,50] After 2 years' treatment, mean change in SF-36 PCS scores reported by patients receiving leflunomide or methotrexate were not statistically different and met or exceeded MCID in 80% of leflunomide- and 77% of methotrexate-treated patients (Table 9C-2). As baseline scores approached U.S. normative levels, improvements in SF-36 MCS did not demonstrate statistically or clinically meaningful improvements. Reported improvements in SF-36 domains were equivalent with leflunomide and methotrexate except for bodily pain, vitality, and role emotional measures—which statistically exceeded methotrexate ($p < 0.05$). With the exception of physical function, role physical, and bodily pain domain scores—with the largest decrements at baseline (Figures 9C-2A through 9C-2D)—endpoint mean scores approached age- and gender-matched U.S. norms in five of eight domains with leflunomide but none of eight following methotrexate treatment. Based on improvements in SF-36, the NNT to achieve another patient reporting normative PCS levels were 3 to 5 for leflunomide versus 6 to 17 with methotrexate versus placebo. Analysis of specific questions in the SF-36 questionnaire revealed a clinically significantly higher proportion of patients with active treatment versus placebo reporting improvement (Table 9C-1).

TNF Inhibitors: Infliximab, Etanercept, Adalimumab, and Certolizumab Pegol

Phase 3 RCTs with infliximab, etanercept, and adalimumab have demonstrated significant and clinically meaningful impact on physical function and HRQOL in patients with active RA—many of whom have failed methotrexate.[51,52] SF-36 was included in all Phase 3 RCTs with adalimumab and certolizumab pegol.

In the Anti-Tumour Necrosis Factor Trial in Rheumatoid Arthritis with Concomitant Therapy (ATTRACT), 428 patients with mean disease duration of 9 to 12 years and active RA despite treatment with methotrexate received infliximab or placebo over 2 years of treatment.[53] Baseline SF-36 PCS scores were >2 SD below U.S. norms, whereas MCS scores were within 1 SD. All active treatment groups reported statistically significant and clinically meaningful improvements in HRQOL that were evident at 6 to 10 weeks, with the greatest changes in role physical and bodily pain domains. Mean changes from baseline in all active treatment groups met or exceeded MCID in five of eight domains compared with none receiving methotrexate plus placebo (Table 9C-2). The impact of RA on MCS was not as marked at baseline, yet median changes in all active treatment groups reflected statistically and clinically meaningful improvements over 2 years of treatment versus placebo (Figures 9C-3A through 9C-3D). The Active Controlled Study of Patients Receiving Infliximab for RA of Early Onset (ASPIRE) trial enrolled 1,051 patients with a mean disease duration of 7 months. Sixty-six percent to 72% were DMARD naive, and baseline HAQ scores were 1.5. Changes in PCS and MCS are summarized in Table 9C-2. In a combined analysis of the ATTRACT and Safety Trial of Rheumatoid Arthritis with Remicade Therapy (START) trials, Han et al. analyzed 1,511 patients and reported that changes from baseline to 1 year in PCS scores were greater in infliximab versus placebo groups: 10.1 versus 4.4, and similar for MCS scores (3.2 versus 3.4, respectively).[54] Significantly more patients

Table 9C-2. Clinically Meaningful Changes from Baseline in HRQOL in Rheumatoid Arthritis Patients Receiving Various DMARDs

	n Patients	Mean Disease Duration	Mean DMARDs Failed	BL PCS Score	Mean Δ PCS at Follow-up (Time Assessment)[a]	% with Δ PCS ≥MCID	% Achieving PCS Norm	BL MCS Score	Mean Δ MCS at Follow-up (Time Assessment)	% with Δ MCS ≥MCID[a]	% Achieving MCS Norm
Leflunomide and Methotrexate: US301 Trial[49,50]											
LEF	98	7	0.8	30.9	11.9 ± 11.3[c] 10.8 ± 9.7[d]	35%[c]	NA	48.5	3.6 ± 2.9[b] 4.7 ± 4.2[d]	10%[b]	NA
MTX	101	7	0.9	30.2	8.0 ± 4.6[c] 8.4 ± 5.4[d]	28%	NA	49.8	2.5 ± 0.6[b] 2.7 ± 0.4[d]	5%	NA
TNF-Is: Infliximab: ATTRACT Trial[53]											
MTX + placebo	88	11 ± 8	NA	25.7	2.8[d]	NA	NA	48.5	1.9[d]	NA	NA
3 mg/kg INF Q8 + MTX	86	10 ± 8	NA	25.2	4.6[d]	NA	NA	46.8	3.8[d]	NA	NA
3 mg/kg INF Q4 + MTX	86	9 ± 8	NA	23.9	6.8[d]	NA	NA	49.9	2.2[d]	NA	NA
10 mg/kg INF Q8 + MTX	87	11 ± 9	NA	25.7	6.9[d]	NA	NA	47.6	2.9[d]	NA	NA
10 mg/kg INF Q4 + MTX	81	12 ± 8	NA	25.8	6.7[d]	NA	NA	47.9	3.7[d]	NA	NA
TNF-Is: Infliximab: ASPIRE Trial[83]											
3 mg/kg INF + MTX	359	1 ± 1	71% naive	28.8 ± 7.7	11.7 ± 11.6[c]	NA	NA	45.4 ± 11.5	NA	NA	NA
6 mg/kg INF + MTX	363	1 ± 1	68% naive	29.3 ± 8.2	13.2 ± 12.0[†]	NA	NA	44.2 ± 11.9	NA	NA	NA
MTX + placebo	282	1 ± 1	65% naive	29.5 ± 7.7	10.1 ± 11.4[c]	NA	NA	44.7 ± 11.9	NA	NA	NA

	n Patients	Mean Disease Duration	Mean DMARDs Failed	BL PCS Score	Mean Δ PCS at Follow-up (Time Assessment)	% with Δ PCS ≥MCID	% Achieving PCS Norm	BL MCS Score	Mean Δ MCS at Follow-up (Time Assessment)	% with Δ MCS ≥MCID[a]	% Achieving MCS Norm
TNF-Is: Etanercept: ERA[51,56]											
ETN 25 mg	198	11.9 mo.	0.5	28.2	11.2[b] 12.2[c]	NA	NA	46.4	4.9[b] 4.7[b]	NA	NA
ETN 10 mg	194	10.9 mo.	0.5	28.2	9.2[b] 8.3[c]	NA	NA	46.9	5.1[b] 4.6[b]	NA	NA
MTX	204	11.9 mo.	0.6	28.8	11.0[b] 11.2[c]	NA	NA	47.3	6.1[b] 6.0[b]	NA	NA

Continued

Table 9C-2. Clinically Meaningful Changes from Baseline in HRQOL in Rheumatoid Arthritis Patients Receiving Various DMARDs—cont'd

	n Patients	Mean Disease Duration	Mean DMARDs Failed	BL PCS Score	Mean Δ PCS at Follow-up (Time Assessment)[a]	% with Δ PCS ≥MCID	% Achieving PCS Norm	BL MCS Score	Mean Δ MCS at Follow-up (Time Assessment)	% with Δ MCS ≥MCID[a]	% Achieving MCS Norm
TNF-Is: Adalimumab: DE009 Trial[59]											
Placebo + MTX	62	11 ± 8	3.0	28.3	2.6[b]	NA	NA	NA	NA	NA	NA
20 mg ADA EOW + MTX	69	13 ± 8	3.0	27.9	7.1[b]	NA	NA	NA	NA	NA	NA
20 mg ADA EOW + MTX	69	12 ± 11	2.9	28.4	9.3[b]	NA	NA	NA	NA	NA	NA
TNF-Is: Adalimumab: DE019 Trial[60]											
Placebo + MTX	207	11 ± 9	2.4	NA	NA	NA	NA	NA	NA	NA	NA
40 mg ADA EOW + MTX	200	11 ± 9	2.4	NA	NA	NA	NA	NA	NA	NA	NA
20 mg ADA weekly + MTX	212	11 ± 9	2.4	NA	NA	NA	NA	NA	NA	NA	NA
TNF-Is: Adalimumab: PREMIER Trial[62,63]											
ADA	274	1 ± 1	67% naive	NA	NA	NA	NA	NA	NA	NA	NA
ADA + MTX	268	0.7 ± 0.8	67% naive	31.7 (7.8)	15.9[c], 16.1[d]	NA	NA	44.1 (12.5)	NA[b], 8.5[d]	NA	NA
MTX	257	0.8 ± 0.9	68% naive	32.2 (7.9)	12.0[c], 12.2[d]	NA	NA	43.5 (12.4)	NA[b], 8.5[d]	NA	NA

	n Patients	Mean Disease Duration	Mean DMARDs Failed	BL PCS Score	Mean Δ PCS at Follow-up (Time Assessment)	% with Δ PCS ≥MCID[a]	% Achieving PCS Norm	BL MCS Score	Mean Δ MCS at Follow-up (Time Assessment)	% with Δ MCS ≥MCID[a]	% Achieving MCS Norm
Abatacept: AIM[67]											
ABA + MTX	433	8.5 ± 7.3	NA	30.6 ± 7.4	8.8 ± 0.4[b]	67%[b]	47%[c]	40.9 ± 11.4	6.2 ± 0.5[b]	NA	60%
PL + MTX	219	8.9 ± 7.1	NA	30.5 ± 7.2	4.8 ± 0.6[b]	51%	31%	41.6 ± 11.2	2.8 ± 0.7[b]	NA	50%
Abatacept: ATTAIN[68]											
ABA + MTX	258	12.2 ± 8.5	NA	27.6 ± 7.0	6.5 ± 9.6[b]	NA	23%[c]	40.9 ± 11.2	5.4 ± 11.7[b]	NA	NA
PL + MTX	133	11.4 ± 8.9	NA	27.7 ± 6.4	1.0 ± 7.7[b]	NA	10%	42.9 ± 11.9	1.7 ± 10.2[b]	NA	NA
Abatacept: Phase 2B[66]											
MTX + placebo	119	7.9–10.5	NA	32.2 ± 7.5	2.6 ± 0.7[c]	NA	NA	42.2 ± 12.6	2.8 ± 0.9[b]	NA	NA
ABA 2 mg/kg + MTX	105	8.8–11.6	NA	30.7 ± 8.5	5.2 ± 0.8[c]	NA	NA	43.6 ± 12.8	3.5 ± 1.0[b]	NA	NA
ABA 10 mg/kg + MTX	115	8.6–10.1	NA	30.7 ± 8.4	8 ± 0.8[c]	NA	NA	45.6 ± 12.6	5.7 ± 0.9[b]	NA	NA

[a]6 months.
[b]12 months.
[c] 24 months.
DMARD, disease-modifying antirheumatic drug; *INF*, infliximab; *MTX*, methotrexate; *PCS*, physical component score; *MCS*, mental component score.

reported improvements ≥MCID (≥5 points) in PCS (54 versus 35%) and MCS scores (42 versus 35%), respectively, at 1 year with infliximab versus placebo treatment.

In an analysis of a subset of 48 patients completing a Phase 3 trial of etanercept 10 and 25 mg versus placebo in active RA, statistically significant improvements in SF-36 PCS scores were reported at 1, 3, and 6 months with etanercept 25 mg and 10 mg versus placebo; and in MCS at 3 and 6 months with etanercept 25 mg versus placebo.[55] In the Early Rheumatoid Arthritis (ERA) trial, 632 patients with mean disease duration of 11 months (50% to 60% of whom were DMARD naive) were randomized to receive etanercept 10 and 25 mg or methotrexate.[56] Reported improvements in SF-36 scores in domain and summary scores were significant in all treatment groups. Those in physical domain scores with etanercept treatment occurred earlier and statistically exceeded methotrexate. Despite low PCS scores at baseline, improvements at 1 and 2 years approached U.S. norms of 50—resulting in fewer patients reporting limitations in physical activities (Figures 9C-4A through 9C-4D and Tables 9C-1 and 9C-2). In the Trial of Etanercept and Methotrexate with Radiographic and Patient Outcomes (TEMPO), 682 RA patients with mean

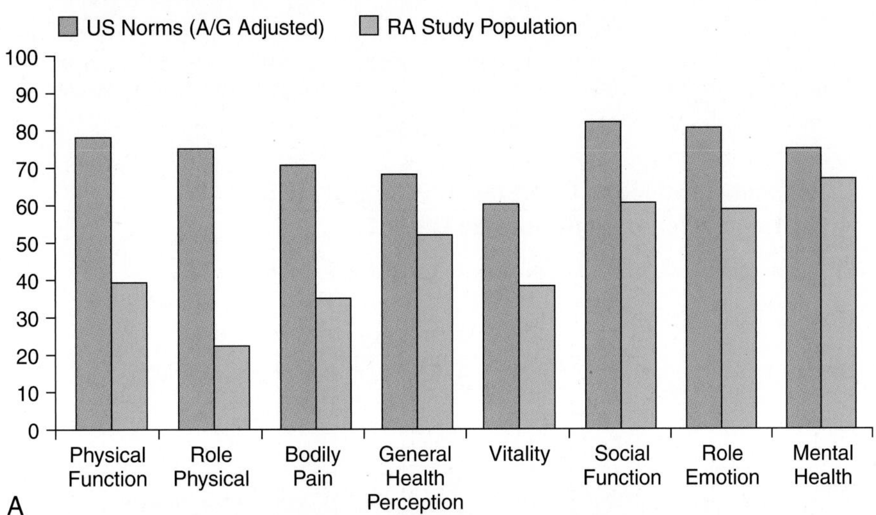

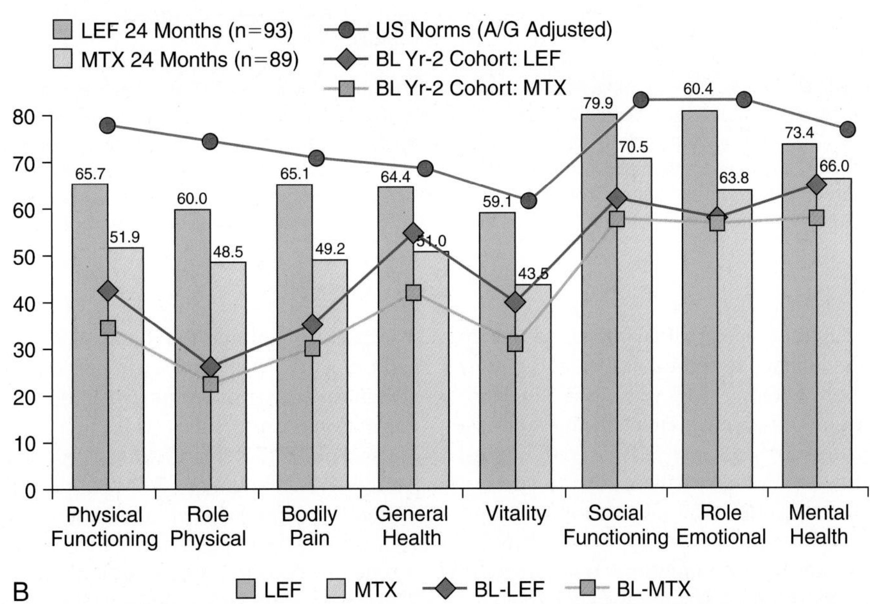

Figure 9C-2. *(A)* Baseline domain values for SF-36 for all patients enrolled in protocol U.S. 301 compared with U.S. norms, demonstrating a pattern typical across RCTs in RA. Scores are lowest in the RP, PF, BP, and VIT domains. *(B)* Baseline and final values for SF-36 domain scores in protocol U.S. 301 at 2 years in patients treated with leflunomide or methotrexate compared with U.S. norms in age- and gender-matched population. *Continued*

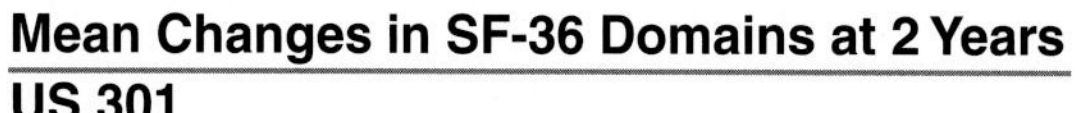

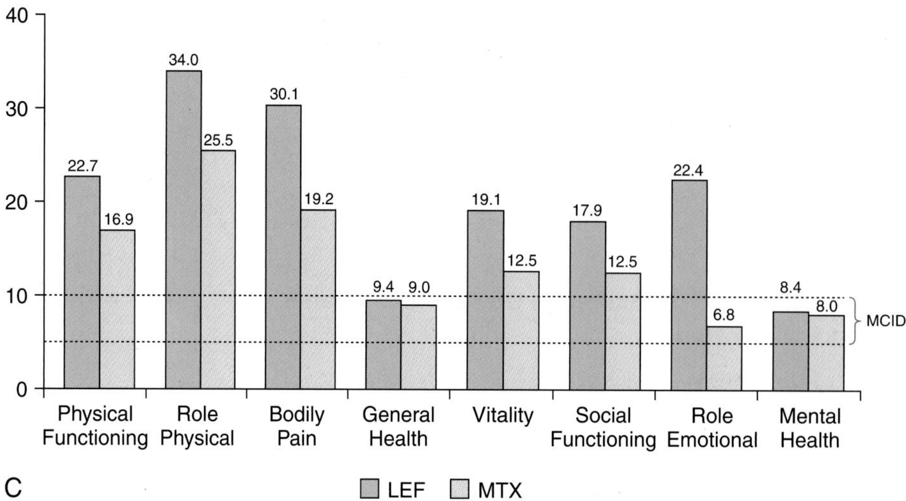

Baseline and Mean Changes in PCS and MCS at 1 and 2 Years: Leflunomide US 301

Baseline (n=93) Month 12 (n=93) Month 24 (n=93)

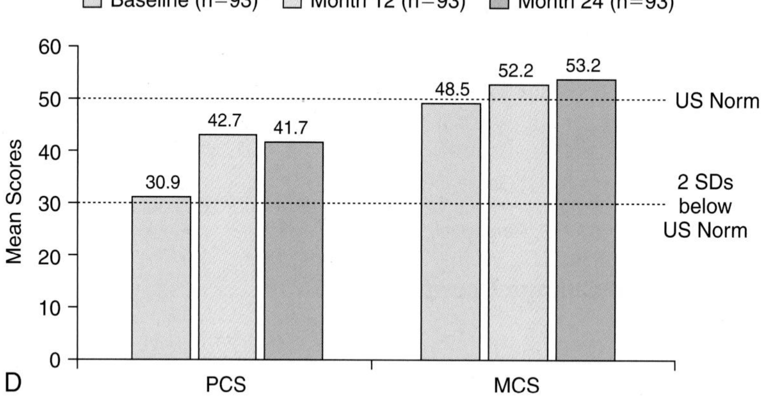

Figure 9C-2. cont'd (*C*) Mean changes from baseline in SF-36 domain scores in protocol U.S. 301 at 2 years in patients treated with leflunomide or methotrexate. All improvements with active treatment ≥MCID of 5 to 10 points. (*D*) Mean changes from baseline in SF-36 PCS scores in protocol U.S. 301 at 2 years in patients treated with leflunomide or methotrexate. Baseline values represent 2 SD below U.S. normative values (= 50). All improvements with active treatment ≥MCID of 2.5 to 5.0 points. (From Strand V, Scott DL, Emery P, et al. for the Leflunomide Rheumatoid Arthritis Investigators Groups. Physical function and health-related quality of life: Analysis of 2-year data from randomized, controlled studies of leflunomide, sulfasalazine, or methotrexate in patients with active rheumatoid arthritis. *J Rheumatol* 2005;32:590–601.)

disease duration of 6.3 to 6.8 years (having failed mean 2.3 DMARDs) were randomized to receive etanercept, methotrexate, or combination therapy.[57] At 1 year, 24%, 31%, and 41% of those receiving resepectively etanercept, methotrexate, and combination therapy reported EQ-5D VAS scores above population norms—with improvements due to combination therapy significantly better than either monotherapy. In the ADORE trial, a 16-week prospective randomized study, 315 patients with active RA despite 3 months of methotrexate therapy were randomized to add etanercept or switch to etanercept monotherapy. The mean baseline HAQ score was 1.6, the mean age was 53 years, and the disease duration was 10 years—and patients had failed a mean of 2.2 DMARDs. A similar proportion of patients in etanercept and methotrexate + etanercept groups (63% and 67%, respectively) achieved MID in EQ-5D, defined as improvements of ≥0.05. Thirty percent in each group reported EQ-5D VAS scores >82 (the population norm).[58]

The Anti-TNF Research Study Program of the Monoclonal Antibody Adalimumab (ARMADA or DE009) RCT was a 6-month comparison of adalimumab monotherapy 20 or 40 mg biweekly versus placebo in 271 patients failing methotrexate.[17,59] At 6 months, significant improvements in SF-36 PCS scores were observed—as well as improvements in seven of eight and eight of eight domains of SF-36 by patients receiving respectively 20 and 40 mg of adalimumab plus methotrexate, versus four of eight domains with placebo plus methotrexate ($p < 0.05$) (Table 9C-2). Mean increases in all domain scores exceeded MCID (5–10 points) in all active treatment groups compared with two of eight domains with placebo plus methotrexate. In DE019, a phase 3 RCT, 619 patients with active RA and inadequate responses to methotrexate were randomized to receive adalimumab (40 mg biweekly or 20 mg weekly) or placebo plus methotrexate. Secondary endpoints included changes in SF-36.[60] At 1 year, patients receiving adalimumab + methotrexate reported significant improvements in seven of eight domains at 40 mg biweekly (exceeding MCID in five domains) and in eight of eight domains at 20 mg weekly (exceeding MCID in 7 domains). These improvements contrast with only one of eight domains with placebo + methotrexate treatment (Figures 9C-5A and 9C5-B and Table 9C-2). Among those completing DE033, 505 RA patients continued long-term adalimumab treatment over a mean of 19.2 months. Mean disease duration in this population was 12.4 years, having failed a mean of four prior DMARDs. Baseline SF-36 scores in those enrolled in this study overall were ≥10 points lower than in DE033. Nonetheless, treatment-associated improvements in SF-36 scores confirmed rapid and sustained improvements in HRQOL over 6.5 months—which met or exceed MCID.[61] Mean changes in PCS scores in the entire population were similar to changes in MCS, indicating that after long-term treatment

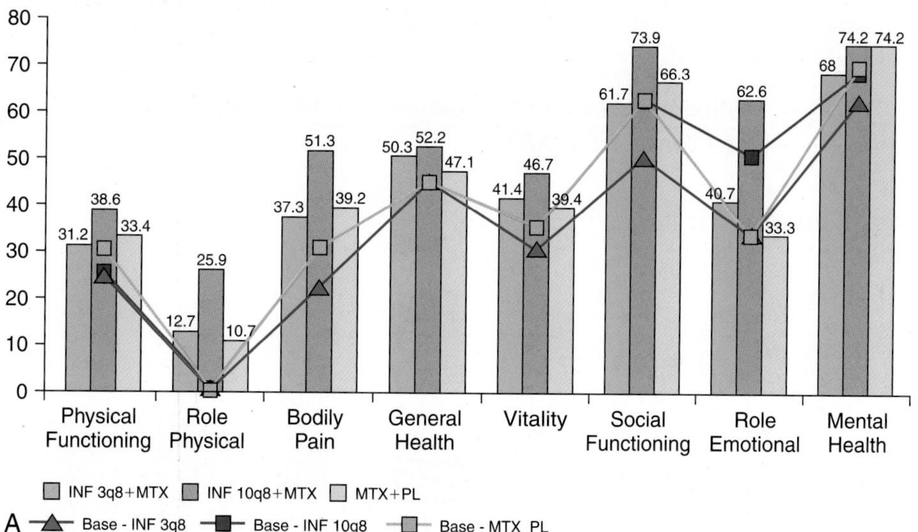

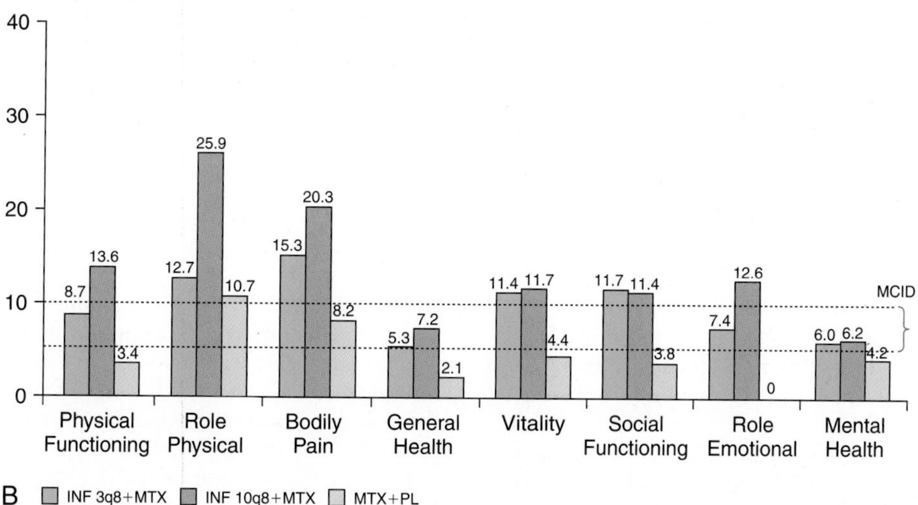

Figure 9C-3. (*A*) Baseline and median changes in SF-36 domain scores at 2 years (treatment with 3 or 10 mg/kg infliximab + methotrexate versus placebo + methotrexate in ATTRACT). Note low PF, RP, and RE baseline scores in this population with long disease duration having failed multiple DMARDs. (*B*) Median changes from baseline in SF-36 domain scores at 2 years (treatment with 3 or 10 mg/kg infliximab + methotrexate versus placebo + methotrexate in ATTRACT). All improvements with active treatment ≥MCID of 5 to 10 points.

Continued

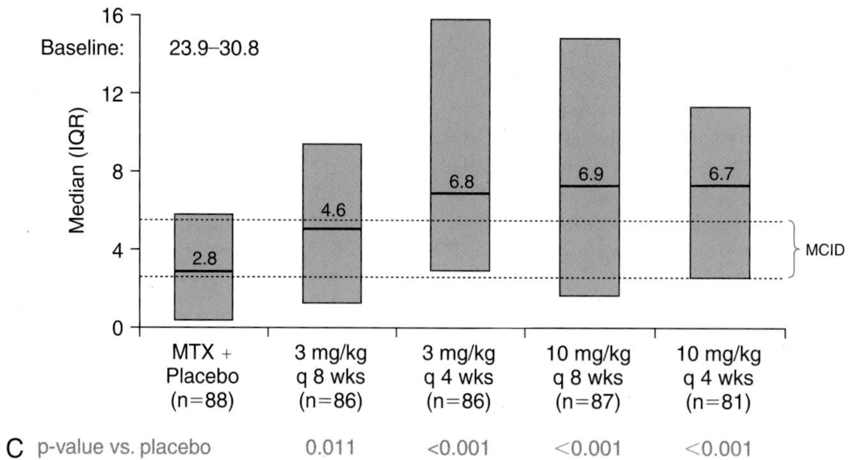

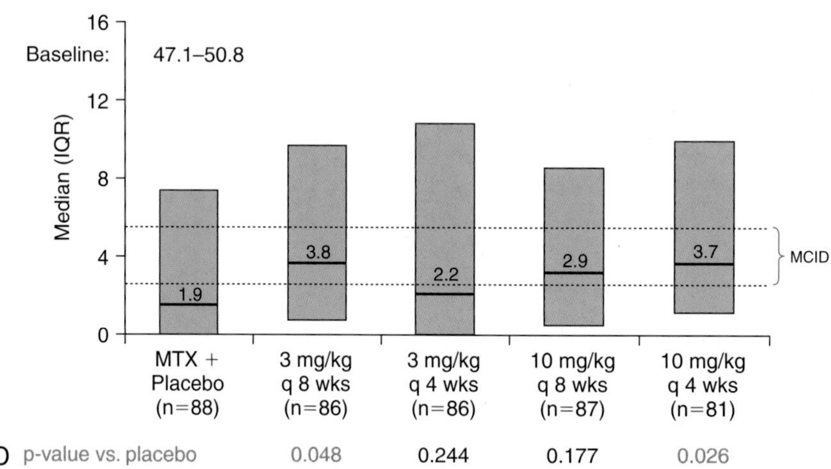

Figure 9C-3. cont'd (*C*) Median changes from baseline in SF-36 PCS scores at 2 years (treatment with 3 or 10 mg/kg infliximab + methotrexate versus placebo + methotrexate in ATTRACT). Baseline values represent ≥2 SD below U.S. normative values (= 50). All improvements with active treatment ≥MCID of 2.5 to 5.0 points. (*D*) Median changes from baseline in SF-36 MCS scores at 2 years (teatment with 3 or 10 mg/kg infliximab + methotrexate versus placebo + methotrexate in ATTRACT). Baseline values approach U.S. normative values (= 50). All improvements with active treatment ≥MCID of 2.5 to 5.0 points, but are statistically significant only in 3 mg/kg q8 weeks and 10 mg/kg q 4 weeks treatment groups. (From Maini RN, Breedveld FC, Kalden JR, et al. For the Anti-Tumor Necrosis Factor Trial in Rheumatoid Arthritis With Concomitant Therapy Study Group. Sustained improvement over two years in physical function, structural damage, and signs and symptoms among patients with rheumatoid arthritis treated with infliximab and methotrexate. *Arthritis Rheum* 2004;50:1051–1065.)

mean area-under-the-curve of SF-36 scores demonstrated sustained and clinically meaningful improvements in HRQOL. HUI scores improved by 0.18 in adalimumab versus 0.06 in the placebo group at 6 months, representing a difference of 2 times MID.

The PREMIER trial was a 2-year RCT comparing the efficacy and safety of initiating adalimumab or methotrexate monotherapy versus combination adalimumab + methotrexate treatment in patients with early RA (8 to 10 months in duration), 68% to 69% of whom were DMARD naive[62] (Figures 9C-6A through 9C-6D and Table 9C-2.). Secondary endpoints included changes from baseline in SF-36 and FACIT. Only HRQOL data comparing combination therapy with methotrexate monotherapy have been published.[63] At 3 months, improvements in five of eight domains were statistically significantly higher with combination therapy than with methotrexate alone. At 1 year, VT scores in both groups exceeded those in the general U.S. population (53.9, 52.4, and 50.4, respectively; $p < 0.001$ for combination therapy and $p = 0.03$ for MTX monotherapy) and similar in SF and MH scales; similar in combination therapy in the GH scale and significantly greater in BP (50.9 versus 49.2; $p = 0.04$). At 1 and 2 years, improvements with combination therapy as well as methotrexate monotherapy met or exceeded MCID in all domains and summary scores. PCS scores approached U.S. normative values in the combination group. A summary of changes in

SF-36 PCS and MCS scores across adalimumab trials is represented in Figures 9C-7A and 9C-7B.

Patients enrolled in a 6-month Phase 3 RCT of monotherapy with certolizumab pegol (two doses) versus placebo reported statistically significant and clinically meaningful improvements in all domain and summary scores of SF-36 (p <0.001) with active treatment.[64] A significantly greater number of certolizumab pegol–treated patients reported improvements ≥MCID in all domains and in both summary scores (p ≤0.05) as early as week 4. These results are similar to those reported in the Phase 3 RA Prevention of Structural Damage (RAPID) 1 and 2 RCTs comparing certolizumab pegol with placebo in patients with active RA despite treatment with MTX for ≥6 months.[65]

Costimulatory Molecule Inhibitor: Abatacept

Phase 3 RCTs assessing the efficacy of abatacept in RA included HAQ, SF-36, and VAS scales for pain, sleep, and fatigue.[66] In the Abatacept in Inadequate responders to Methotrexate (AIM) trial, SF-36 scores were compared in 652 patients (failing methotrexate) with mean disease duration of 9 years—randomized to receive abatacept + methotrexate or placebo + methotrexate over

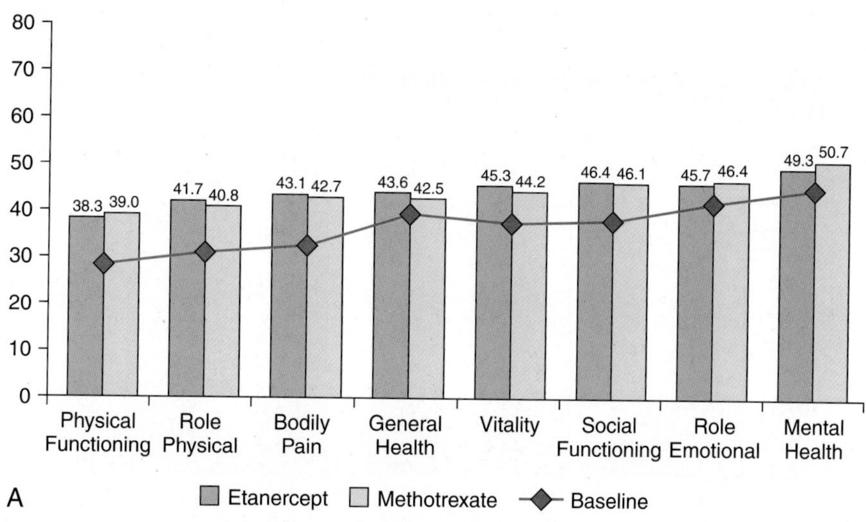

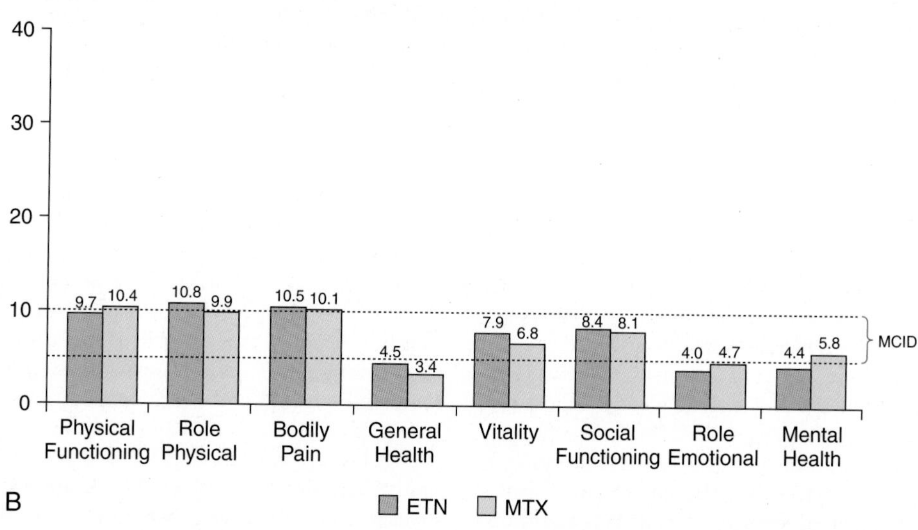

Figure 9C-4. (*A*) Baseline and mean changes in SF-36 domain scores at 1 year (treatment with etanercept 25 mg versus methotrexate in ERA). Domain scores are normalized to a scale of 0 to 50, where 50 represents U.S. normative values. (*B*) Mean changes in SF-36 domain scores at 1 year (treatment with etanercept 25 mg versus methotrexate in ERA). Domain scores are normalized to a scale of 0 to 50, where 50 represents U.S. normative values. *Continued*

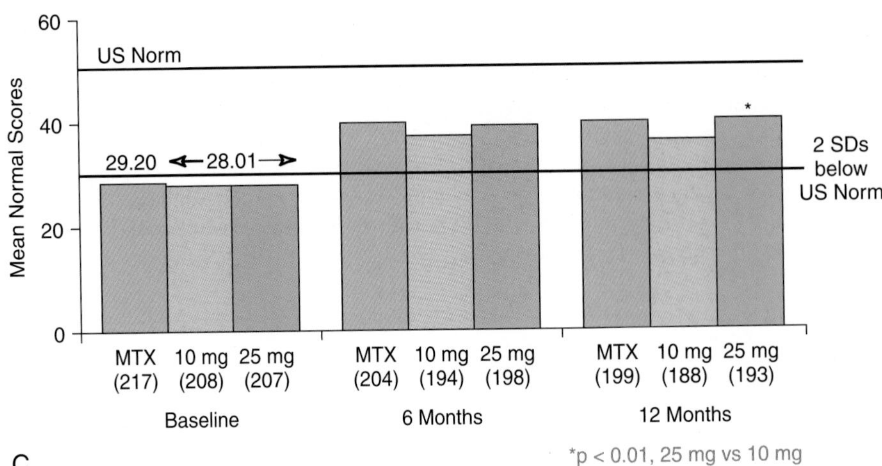

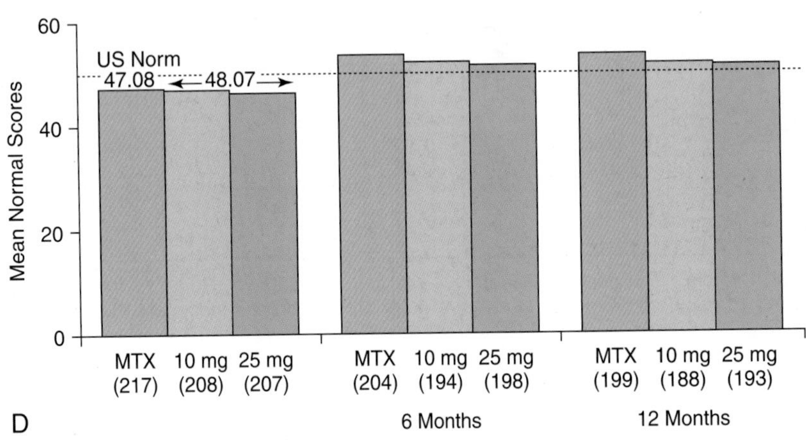

Figure 9C-4. cont'd (*C*) Mean SF-36 PCS scores at baseline, 6 months, and 1 year (treatment with etanercept 25 mg or 10 mg versus methotrexate in ERA). Baseline values represent 2 SD below U.S. normative values (= 50). All improvements with active treatment ≥MCID of 2.5 to 5.0 points. (*D*) Mean SF-36 MCS scores at baseline, 6 months, and 1 year (treatment with etanercept 25 mg or 10 mg versus methotrexate in ERA). Baseline values approach U.S. normative values (= 50), and mean changes are neither statistically significant nor clinically meaningful. (From Kosinski M, Kujawski SC, Martin R, et al. Health-related quality of life in early rheumatoid arthritis: Impact of disease and treatment response. *Am J Managed Care* 2002;8:231–240.)

1 year.[67] Mean baseline SF-36 domain scores were ≥1 SD below U.S. norms. PCS and MCS scores (PCS, 30.6; MCS, 41.8) were respectively 2 and 1 SD less than U.S. norms of 50 (Table 9C-2). Statistically significant differences between abatacept and placebo groups in reported improvements in five of eight SF-36 domains were evident as early as 1to 3 months and were sustained in eight of eight domains over 1 and 2 years of treatment (p <0.01) (Figures 9C-8A and 9C-8B). Responder analyses identified those patients who reported improvements ≥0.5 SD (MID). significantly higher with abatacept treatment (p <0.001) in PCS scores at 1 year. A significantly greater percentage of patients receiving abatacept + methotrexate reported improvements in PCS and MCS scores, which approximated U.S. age- and gender-matched norms at 6 months (p <0.01) (Table 9C-2) Based on these improvements, the NNT to achieve another patient reporting normative levels in PCS was 6, and in MCS, 10.

In the Abatacept Trial in Treatment of Anti-TNF Inadequate (ATTAIN) responders RCT, 391 patients with mean disease duration of 11.4 to 12.2 years (having failed etanercept and/or infliximab) were randomized to receive abatacept (n = 258) or placebo (n = 133) plus DMARDs over 6 months.[68] Significantly more abatacept- versus placebo-treated patients reported "clinically meaningful" improvements from baseline (defined as ≥3 points) in PCS and MCS scores (p <0.01)—with baseline scores of respectively 27.6 and 41.2, representing respectively >2 and approximately 1 SD less than norms (Table 9C-2). Statistically significant (p ≤0.013 for all) mean improvements in all SF-36 domains with abatacept treatment were reported—with ≥MCID achieved in six of eight domains. Consistently, the percentage of patients with improvements ≥MID at 6 months was significantly higher with abatacept treatment (p <0.0001). Mean changes from baseline in SF-36 PCS and

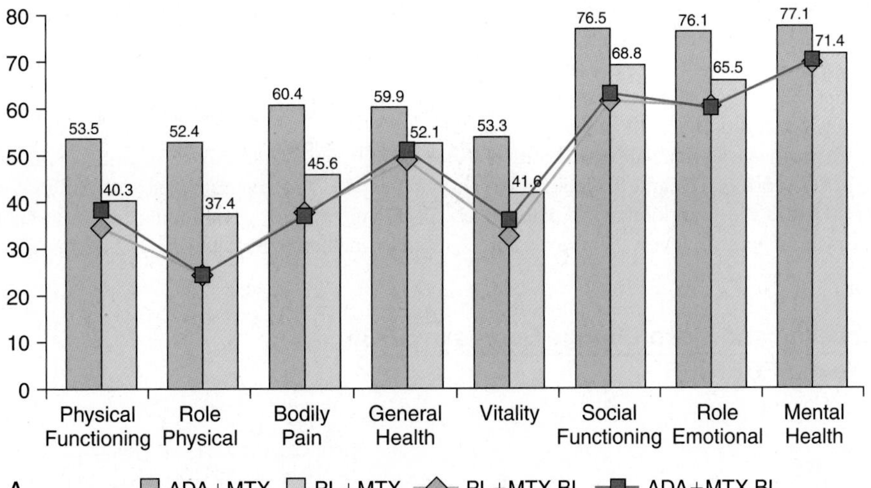

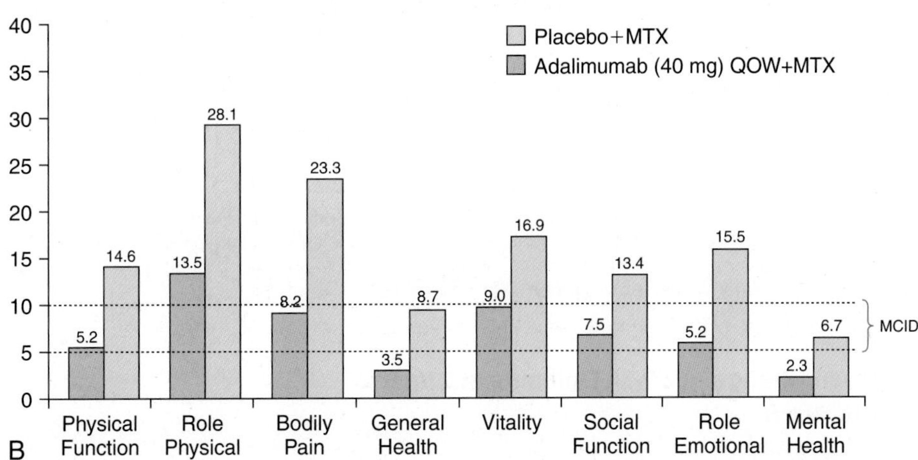

Figure 9C-5. *(A)* Baseline and mean changes in SF-36 domain scores at 1 year (teatment with adalimumab + methotrexate versus placebo + methotrexate in protocol DE019). *(B)* Mean changes in SF-36 domain scores at 1 year (treatment with adalimumab + methotrexate versus placebo + methotrexate in protocol DE019). All improvements with active treatment ≥MCID of 5 to 10 points. (From Keystone EC, Kavanaugh AF, Sharp JT, et al. Radiographic, clinical, and functional outcomes of treatment with adalimumab (a human anti-tumor necrosis factor monoclonal antibody) in patients with active rheumatoid arthritis receiving concomitant methotrexate therapy: A randomized, placebo-controlled, 52-week trial. *Arthritis Rheum* 2004;50:1400–1411.)

MCS from 6 months to 2 years in AIM and ATTAIN are presented in Figures 9C-8C and 9C-8D and Figure 9C-9A. A recent review by Michaud et al. summarizes HRQOL data at 1 and 2 years in AIM and 6 and 18 months in ATTAIN trials, shown in Figure 9C-9A.[69]

B-Cell Depletion Agent: Rituximab

In the Randomized Evaluation of Long-term Efficacy of Rituximab in RA (REFLEX) trial, 520 patients with active RA on methotrexate following inadequate responses to TNF inhibitors received rituximab or placebo for 6 months.[70] Mean disease duration was 11.7 to 12.1 years. Improvements in SF-36 PCS and MCS scores of respectively 4.7 and 5.8 were reported with rituximab versus 1.3 and 0.9, respectively, with placebo. Between-group differences were statistically significant and clinically meaningful, as they differed by >3 points (Figure 9C-9B).

Monoclonal Antibody to IL-6 Receptor: Tocilizumab

In a 6-month RCT, patients with moderate to severe RA and inadequate response to MTX were randomized to receive placebo or tocilizumab 4 or 8 mg/kg intravenously every 4 weeks in combination with methotrexate. Mean changes in both tocilizumab groups met or exceeded MCID in all SF-36 domains for PCS and MCS with active treatment. However, only bodily pain, PCS, and MCS met or exceeded MCIB with placebo.[71] Mean changes in PCS and MCS reported by patients receiving tocilizumab 4 or 8 mg/kg showed approximately twice the amount of improvement than placebo: 9.5 to 9.7 versus 5.0 and 5.7 to 7.3 versus 2.7, respectively. In addition, 1,220 patients with moderate to severe RA with mean age 53 years, disease duration 10 years, mean baseline HAQ score of 1.5, and inadequate response to conventional DMARDs were randomized to placebo or tocilizumab 8 mg/kg intravenously every 4 weeks for 6 months. Statistically significant mean changes from baseline to 6 months met or exceeded MCID in all SF-36 domains for PCS and MCS in the tocilizumab group, compared with only the bodily pain domain and MCS in the placebo group.[72]

Concordance and Discordance Among SF-36, EQ-5D, and HAQ

Intuitively, one would expect measures of physical function in RA such as HAQ to correlate well with HRQOL measures such as SF-36 and EQ-5D. This finding has been supported by several studies, including the following. EQ-5D had moderate correlations

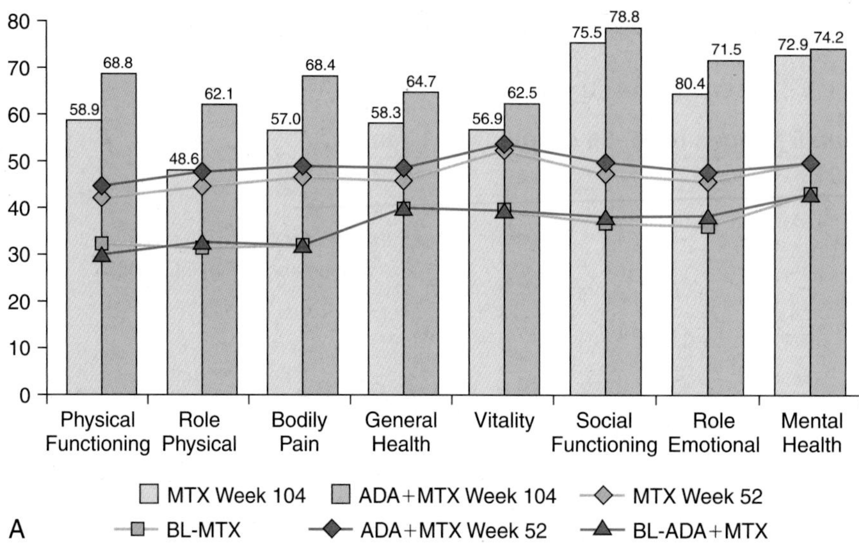

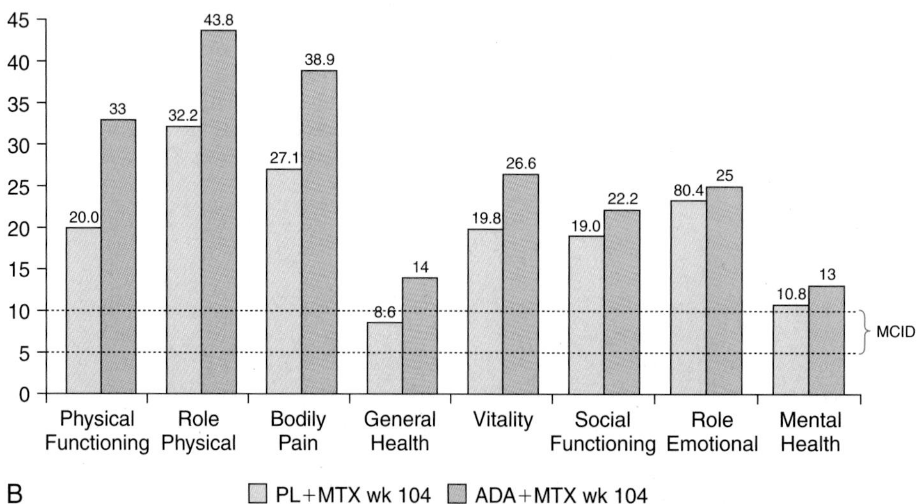

Figure 9C-6. (*A*) Baseline and mean changes in SF-36 domain scores at 1 and 2 years (teatment with adalimumab + methotrexate versus methotrexate or adalimumab monotherapy in PREMIER). (*B*) Mean changes in SF-36 domain scores at 2 years (teatment with adalimumab + methotrexate versus methotrexate or adalimumab monotherapy in PREMIER). All improvements with active treatment ≥MCID of 5 to 10 points.

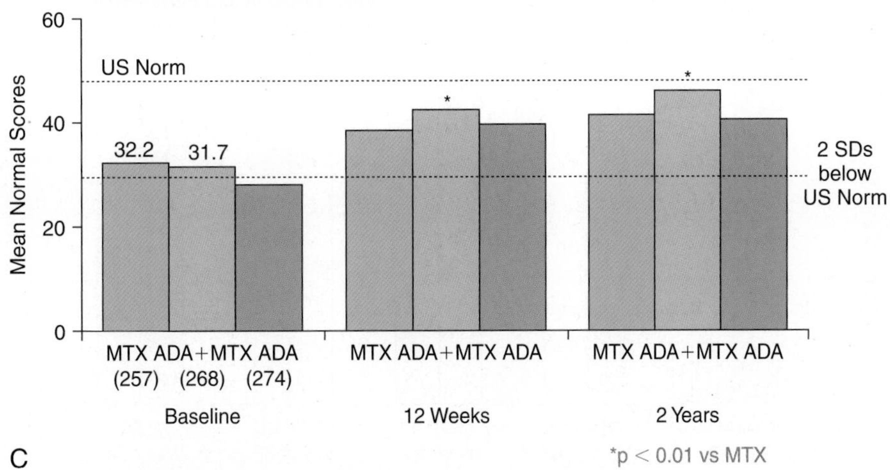

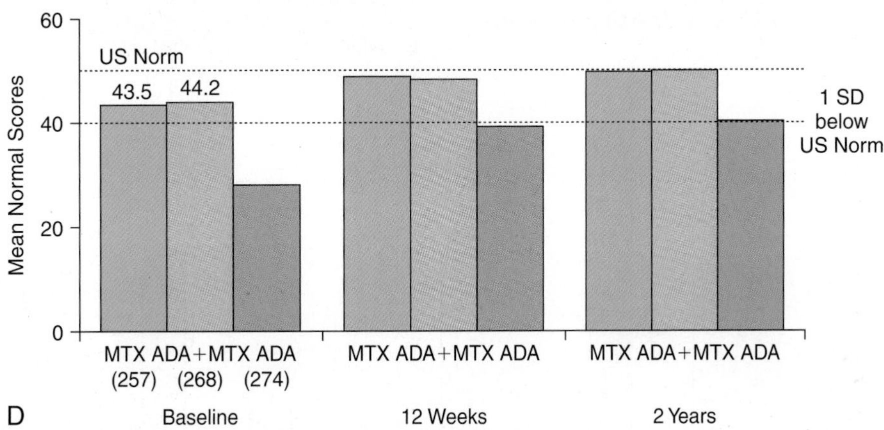

Figure 9C-6. cont'd (*C*) Baseline and mean changes in SF-36 PCS scores at 12 weeks and 2 years (teatment with adalimumab + methotrexate versus methotrexate or adalimumab monotherapy in PREMIER). Baseline values approach 2 SD below U.S. normative values (= 50). Improvements with adalimumab + methotrexate statistically exceed either monotherapy. Improvements in all groups ≥MCID of 2.5 to 5.0 points. (*D*) Baseline and mean changes in SF-36 MCS scores at 12 weeks and 2 years (teatment with adalimumab + methotrexate versus methotrexate or adalimumab monotherapy in PREMIER). Baseline values <1 SD below U.S. normative values (= 50). Improvements with adalimumab + methotrexate are not statistically different from either monotherapy. Improvements in all groups ≥MCID of 2.5 to 5.0 points. (From Weisman MH, Strand V, Cifaldi MA, et al. Adalimumab (HUMIRA) plus methotrexate is superior to MTX alone in improving physical function, as measured by the SF–36, in patients with early rheumatoid arthritis. *Arthritis Rheum* 2005;52:S395 and Kimel M, Cifaldi M, Chmiel J, et al. Relationship between health-related quality of life and employment outcomes during adalimumab (ADA) plus methotrexate (MTX) combination therapy versus MTX monotherapy in patients with early rheumatoid arthritis. *Arthritis Rheum* 2007;56:S89.)

with pain, function, and satisfaction components of HAQ and with tender and swollen joint counts in a validation study.[24] In the ATTRACT trial, patients who reported improvements in HAQ ≥MCID also had statistically greater improvements in PCS (53% versus 14%) and MCS scores (14% versus 5%) of SF-36 compared to those without.[73] In analyses of Phase 3 protocols comparing leflunomide and methotrexate, mean and median improvements in HAQ ≥MCID after 1 and 2 years closely reflected positive changes in SF-36 that met or exceeded MCID in all domains with leflunomide and methotrexate treatment.[49,50]

A recent study, however, found discordance between several measures. A nonrandomized study compared EQ-5D, SF-36, and HAQ scores in 321 consecutive patients with RA cross sectionally (mean age 60 years, disease duration 9 years) and 56 patients followed longitudinally who were receiving DMARD treatment for at least 6 months. Although baseline scores were moderately correlated, changes in HAQ and EQ-5D scores were entirely unrelated at an individual patient level—thought partially to be due to a normal distribution of HAQ but bimodal distribution of EQ-5D scores.[74] This points out that measures of HRQOL and physical function are not interchangeable on an individual level in RA, reflecting that patients perceive HRQOL and report the impact of their disease on function and HRQOL differently.

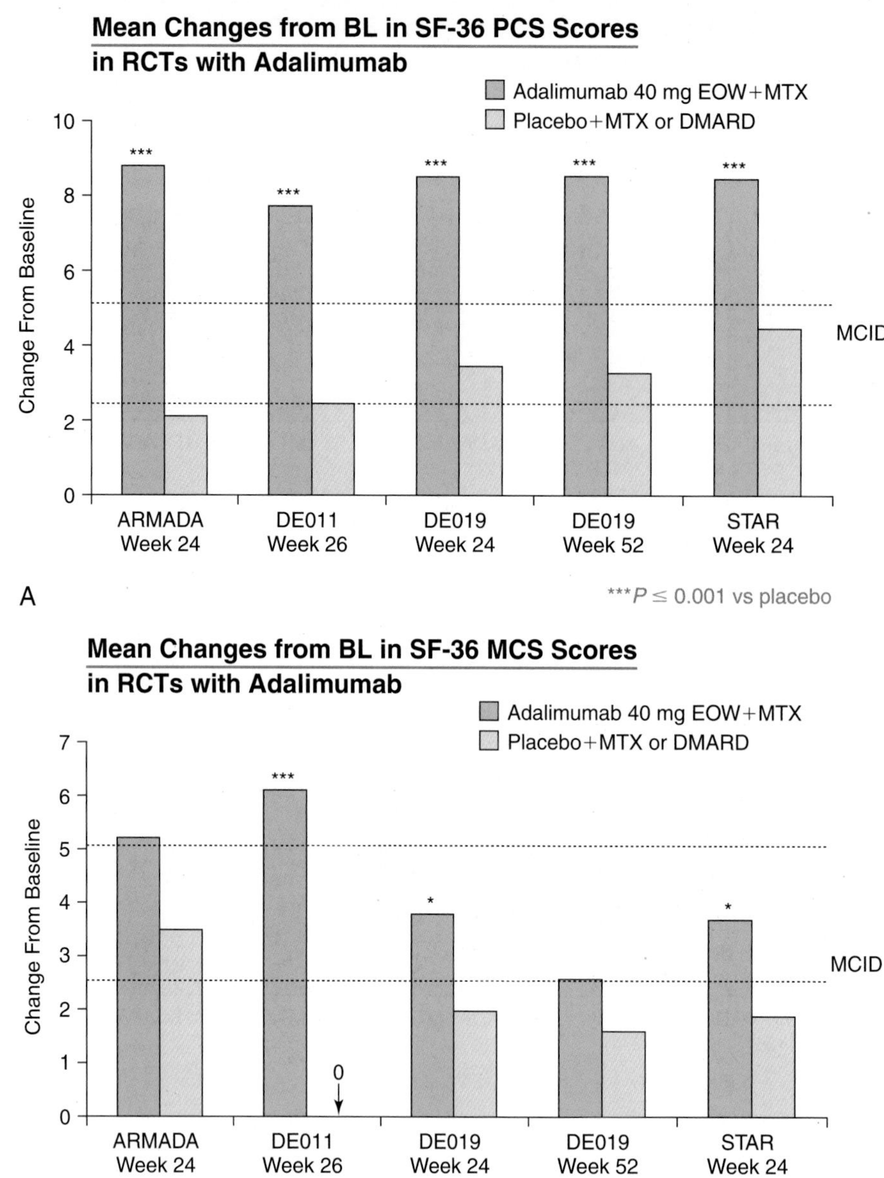

Figure 9C-7. (*A*) Mean changes from baseline in SF-36 PCS scores across Phase 3 protocols with adalimumab + methotrexate versus placebo + methotrexate (or DMARDs in STAR) at 6 months, and at 1 year in DE019. Baseline values represent SD below U.S. normative values (= 50). All improvements with active treatment are statistically significant, and ≥MCID of 2.5 to 5.0 points in three of four protocols at 6 months. (*B*) Mean changes from baseline in SF-36 MCS scores across Phase 3 protocols with adalimumab + methotrexate at 24 weeks versus placebo + methotrexate (or DMARDs in STAR) at 6 months, and at 1 year in DE019. Baseline values SD below U.S. normative values (= 50). Improvements with active treatment are statistically significant in three of four protocols at 6 months, and ≥MCID of 2.5 to 5.0 points in all four protocols. (From Strand V, Weinblatt M, Keystone E, et al. Treatment with adalimumab (D2E7), a fully human anti-TNF monoclonal antibody, improves physical function and health related quality of life (HRQOL) in patients with active rheumatoid arthritis (RA). *Ann Rheum Dis* 2002;61:S175.)

Work Productivity

Because most patients develop RA in the third to fifth decade of life, decrements in physical function experienced by many patients translate into work disability and reduced productivity in work activities outside and within the home—the latter particularly important in the 75% of RA patients who are women. Work limitations are an important component of the outcomes assessment of RA, and their associations with HRQOL were described in two recent reviews.[75,76] Disability rates were found to be twice as high in patients with RA compared with an age- and sex-matched general Dutch population.[77] In an analysis of 338 RA patients in an RCT, disease activity, disease severity, and impaired physical function were global predictors for sick leave, work disability, and confinement to bed for unemployed patients.[78] In addition, productivity costs of unemployed patients were predicted by impaired physical function and impaired mental health.

In a U.S. study of 6,649 RA patients, 28% of patients considered themselves disabled after 15 years of disease (9% of which received disability benefits).[79] A 0.25-unit difference in HAQ, considered to represent MCID, was associated with $1,095 difference in annual earnings—a value similar to earlier findings in the ARAMIS database published by Singh et al.[80] The Finnish Rheumatoid Arthritis Combination Therapy (Fin-RACo) Trial randomized 195 patients to combination or single DMARD therapy for 2 years. Patients achieving clinical remission, ACR50, ACR20 responses, and nonresponders had median (interquartile range) annual work disability days of respectively 0 (0–3), 4 (0–131), 16 (0–170), and 352 (16–365).[81] During the 5-year follow-up period, a similarly impressive trend in those reporting permanent disability was observed: 0% compared with 23% and 21% versus 56%. Data from an open-label extension study of 505 patients treated with adalimumab monotherapy who had previously failed DMARDs (DE033) were compared with a control group of RA patients receiving DMARD therapy in a Norway registry.[82] A significantly higher proportion receiving adalimumab at baseline (33%) were still working, compared with 24% in the DMARD group. Over 24 weeks of follow-up, all patients (including the subset still working at baseline) in the adalimumab group worked 2 (and 7.3) months longer than the DMARD group after controlling

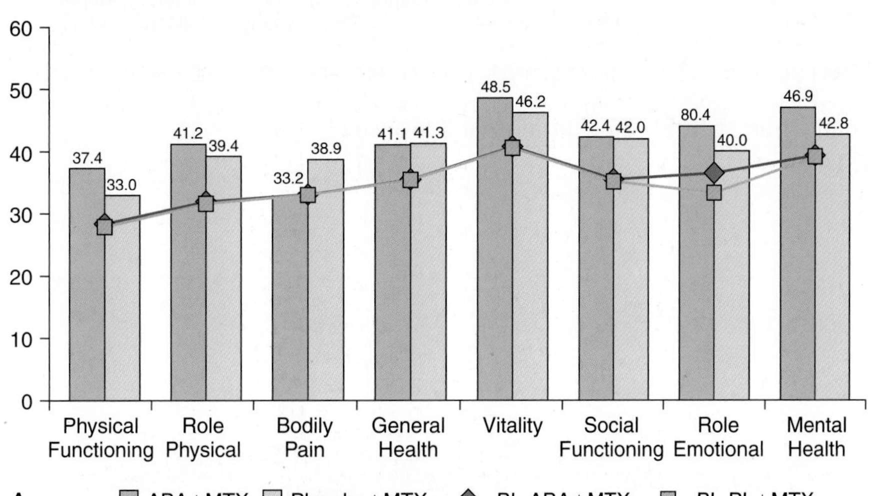

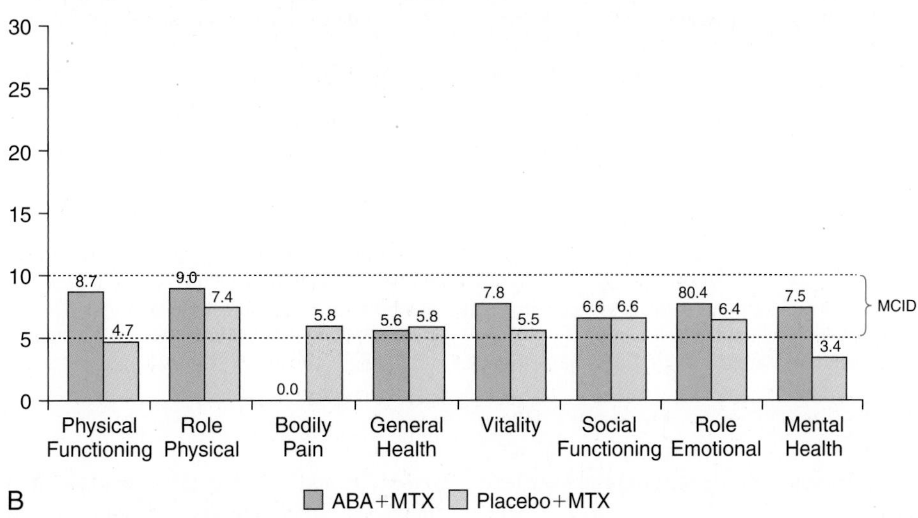

Figure 9C-8. (*A*) Baseline and mean changes in SF-36 domain scores at 1 year (treatment with abatacept + methotrexate versus placebo + methotrexate in AIM). Domain scores are normalized to a scale of 0 to 50, where 50 represents U.S. normative values. (*B*) Mean changes in SF-36 domain scores at 1 year (treatment with abatacept + methotrexate versus placebo + methotrexate in AIM). Domain scores are normalized to a scale of 0 to 50, where 50 represents U.S. normative values. All improvements with active treatment ≥MCID of 5 to 10 points.

Continued

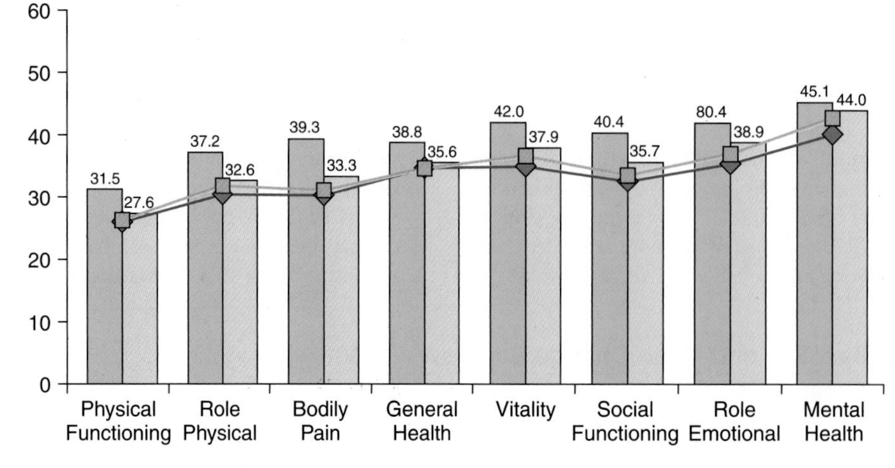

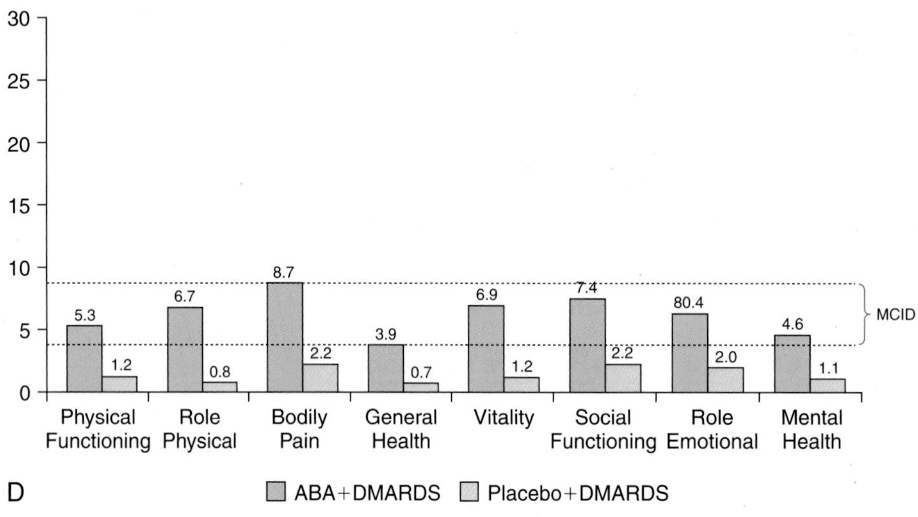

Figure 9C-8. cont'd (*C*) Baseline and mean changes in SF-36 domain scores at 6 months (treatment with abatacept + methotrexate versus placebo + methotrexate in ATTAIN). Domain scores are normalized to a scale of 0 to 50, where 50 represents U.S. normative values. (*D*) Mean changes in SF-36 domain scores at 6 months (treatment with abatacept + methotrexate versus placebo + methotrexate in ATTAIN). Domain scores are normalized to a scale of 0 to 50, where 50 represents U.S. normative values. (*A* and *B* from Russell AS, Wallenstein GV, Li T, et al. Abatacept improves both the physical and mental health of patients with rheumatoid arthritis who have inadequate response to methotrexate treatment. *Ann Rheum Dis* 2007;66:189–194 and Michaud K, Bombardier C, Emery P. Quality of life in patients with rheumatoid arthritis: Does abatacept make a difference? *Clin Exp Rheum* 2007;25:S35–S45. C and D from Westhovens R, Cole JC, Li T, et al. Improved health-related quality of life for rheumatoid arthritis patients treated with abatacept who have inadequate response to anti-TNF therapy in a double-blind, placebo-controlled, multicentre randomized clinical trial. *Rheumatology* 2006;45:1238–1246 and Michaud K, Bombardier C, Emery P. Quality of life in patients with rheumatoid arthritis: Does abatacept make a difference? *Clin Exp Rheum* 2007;25:S35–S45.)

for differences in other characteristics ($p < 0.001$) and were less likely to stop working.

In a 1-year RCT comparing leflunomide to methotrexate to placebo in >400 patients, more patients in the leflunomide and methotrexate group (≥20% and ≥50%, respectively) than in the placebo group had improvement in work productivity at 52 weeks (leflunomide versus methotrexate versus plcebo): 39 versus 38 versus 20% and 22 versus 23 versus 10%).[50] In ASPIRE, comparing infliximab + methotrexate to placebo + methotrexate in early RA patients, employability was defined by current employment or feeling well enough to work if a job were available.[83] Compared with 14% receiving methotrexate monotherapy, only 8% in the infliximab groups became unemployed at 1 year ($p = 0.05$). Patients receiving combination therapy had significantly higher

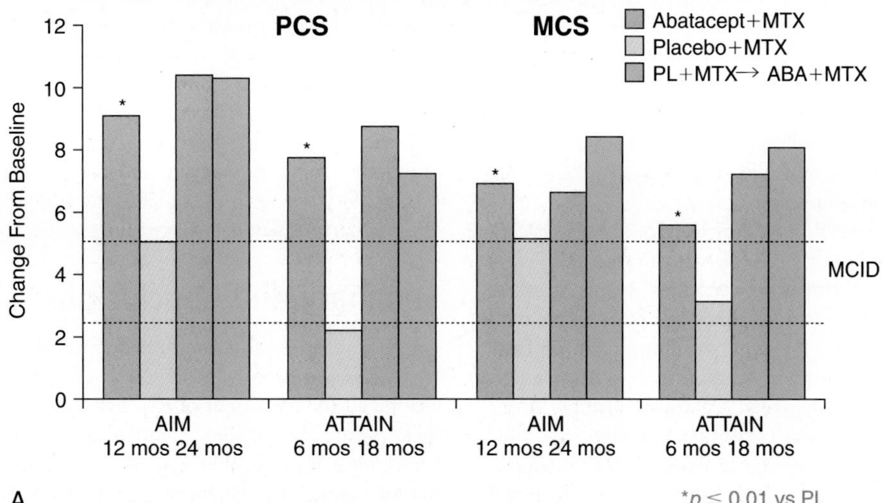

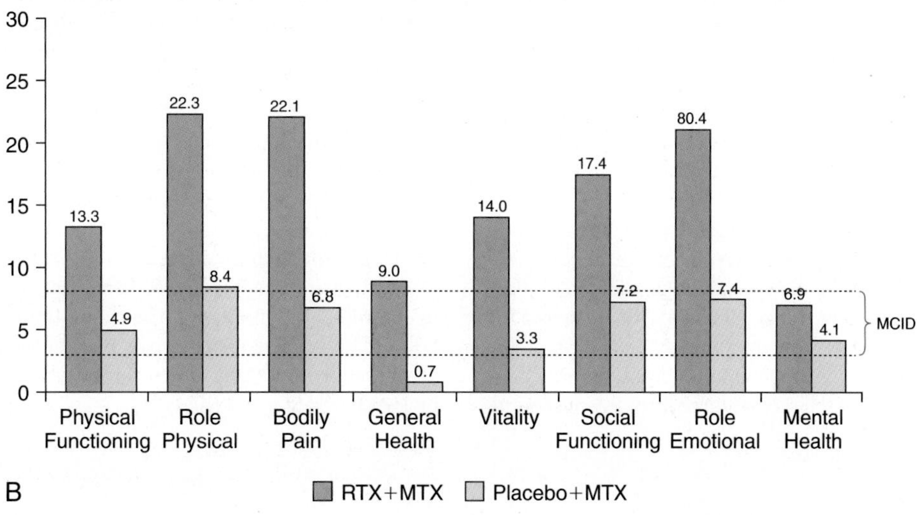

Figure 9C-9. (*A*) Baseline and mean changes in SF-36 PCS and MCS scores at 6, 12, 18, and 24 months (treatment with abatacept + methotrexate versus placebo + methotrexate in AIM and ATTAIN protocols). Patients randomized to placebo + methotrexate received abatacept after 6 months. After rescue, mean changes meet or exceed those originally assigned active therapy. In AIM, mean changes in PCS and MCS statistically significant at 12 months and ≥MCID of 2.5 to 5.0 points at 12 and 24 months. In ATTAIN, mean changes in PCS and MCS statistically significant at 6 months and ≥MCID of 2.5 to 5.0 points at 6 and 18 months. (*B*) Mean changes from baseline in SF-36 domain scores at 6 months (treatment with rituximab + methotrexate versus placebo + methotrexate in REFLEX). All improvements with active treatment ⩾MCID of 5 to 10 points. (*A* from Emery Emery P, Kosinski M, Li T, et al. Treatment of rheumatoid arthritis patients with abatacept and methotrexate significantly improved health-related quality of life. *J Rheumatol* 2006;33:681–689, Westhovens R, Cole JC, Li T, et al. Improved health-related quality of life for rheumatoid arthritis patients treated with abatacept who have inadequate response to anti-TNF therapy in a double-blind, placebo-controlled, multicentre randomized clinical trial. *Rheumatology* 2006;45:1238–1246, Russell AS, Wallenstein GV, Li T, et al. Abatacept improves both the physical and mental health of patients with rheumatoid arthritis who have inadequate response to methotrexate treatment. *Ann Rheum Dis* 2007;66:189–194; and Michaud K, Bombardier C, Emery P. Quality of life in patients with rheumatoid arthritis: Does abatacept make a difference? *Clin Exp Rheum* 2007;25:S35–S45. *B* from Cohen SB, Emery P, Greenwald MW, et al. for the REFLEX Trial Group. Rituximab for rheumatoid arthritis refractory to anti-tumor necrosis factor therapy: Results of a multicenter, randomized, double-blind, placebo-controlled, phase III trial evaluating primary efficacy and safety at twenty-four weeks. *Arthritis Rheum* 2006;54:2793–2806.)

likelihood of improved employability: odds ratio = 2.4 (95% confidence interval, 2.2–2.6; $p < 0.001$) versus nonsignificant odds ratio = 1.2 (0.7, 2.1, $p = 0.58$) with methotrexate. In PREMIER, an RCT that compared combination treatment to either monotherapy alone in patients with early RA found that a 1-unit change in PCS score was associated with an increased likelihood of employment (odds ratio = 1.08; $p < 0.0001$). Patients in the lowest PCS category ($0 \leq PCS < 30$) reported the fewest "currently employed" (21%) compared with those in the highest category ($PCS \geq 50$), where 73% were currently employed.

Another RCT, Prevention of Work Disability (PROWD), enrolled 148 patients with early RA (disease duration <2 years) and compared work impairment between those receiving adalimumab + methotrexate versus placebo + methotrexate over 1 year.[84] Although "all-cause job loss" and "imminent job loss" over weeks 16 to 56 (the primary endpoint) were not statistically significantly different between treatment groups, fewer patients receiving combination treatment reported loss and/or imminent job loss from baseline to week 56 (14 versus 29, $p = 0.005$).[85] A Phase 3 RCT of 400 mg certolizumab pegol monotherapy administered monthly reported statistically ($p \leq 0.05$) less mean productivity loss, measured by the Work Productivity Survey (WPS), as early as 4 weeks.[86] Importantly, this questionnaire asked about work within the home and family and social activities as well as productivity outside the home. Despite similar values at baseline, at 6 months those receiving anti-TNF therapy reported statistically fewer days of household work lost, fewer days of household work productivity reduced by 50%, and fewer days lost of family/social/leisure activities—true also in the minority of patients still employed outside the home.

In a systematic review of studies of work productivity loss in RA patients, increasing severity of RA, older age, and a physically more demanding type of work were predictors of work disability.[87] A median of 66% (range, 36%–84%) of employed RA patients reported work loss of 39 days (range, 7–84 days) in the past year, and 54% (range, 22%–76%) in the last 6 months. Survival analyses showed that the median time from RA onset until a 50% probability of being work disabled was 13 years (range, 4.5–22.0), and that the largest increase in work disability occurred in the first year after diagnosis.

Although work productivity is increasingly being included in RCTs, there is a need to standardize measures and to query productivity within the home as well as participation in family/social/leisure activities (as discussed in recent reviews).[77,88] This is particularly important in that a recent study in the Dutch RA population reported a seven-times higher loss of within-home productivity versus work outside the home.[89] An OMERACT effort is currently underway to address this issue.

Summary and Conclusions

Over the past decade, the introduction of seven new biologic DMARDs and two promising non-biologic DMARDs has revolutionized the treatment of RA. Importantly, administration of these agents has resulted in statistically significant and clinically meaningful improvements in physical function and HRQOL. Recent clinical studies confirm that patient-reported improvements in HRQOL are reflected by improved physical function, less fatigue, and better emotional and mental health. Work productivity surveys confirm that fewer patients stop working and that more report less impact of their disease on work within and outside of the home, as well as on family and social activities.

Although use of current instruments assessing HRQOL may not be practical in day-to-day clinical practice, their incorporation in RCTs and longitudinal observational studies has clarified the significant impact of disease on performance of necessary and instrumental activities of daily living and *all* domains of HRQOL. They have been predictive of functional, behavioral, and economic implications of disease progression—and have illustrated the important benefits now gained with effective DMARD therapies. It would be beneficial if a simple, short, easily scored, and intuitively clear questionnaire for assessing HRQOL at routine patient visits became available. This would add another important dimension to what is currently offered by HAQ, MHAQ, and MDHAQ.

References

1. Strand V, Russell AS. Workshop Report: WHO/ILAR Taskforce on Quality of Life. *J Rheumatol* 1997;24:1630–1633.
2. Bellamy N, Boers M, Felson D, et al. Health status instruments/utilities. *J Rheumatol* 1995;22:1203–1207.
3. Uhlig T, Haavardsholm EA, Kvien TK. Comparison of the Health Assessment Questionnaire (HAQ) and the modified HAQ (MHAQ) in patients with rheumatoid arthritis. *Rheumatology* 2006;45:454–458.
4. Bruce B, Fries JF. The Stanford health assessment questionnaire: A review of its history, issues, progress and documentation. *J Rheumatol* 2003;30:167–178.
5. Ware JE. SF–36 Health Survey update, Lincoln RI. QualityMetric Incorporated, 2007.
6. Talamo J, Frater A, Gallivan S, et al. Use of Short Form 36 for health status measurement in rheumatoid arthritis. *Brit J Rheumatol* 1997;36:463–469.
7. Ruta DA, Hurst NP, Kind P, et al. Measuring health status in British patients with rheumatoid arthritis: Reliability, validity and responsiveness of the short form 36-item health survey (SF–36). *Brit J Rheumatol* 1998;37:425–436.
8. Boers M, Brooks P, Strand V, et al. The OMERACT Filter for Outcome Measures in Rheumatology. *J Rheum* 1998;25:198–199.
9. Marra CA, Woolcott JC, Kopec JA, et al. A comparison of generic, indirect utility measures (the HUI2, HUI3, SF–6D, and the EQ–5D) and disease-specific instruments (the RAQoL and the HAQ) in rheumatoid arthritis. *Soc Sci Med* 2005;60:1571–1582.
10. Brazier JE, Roberts J, Deverill M. The estimation of a preference-based measure of health from the SF–36. *J Health Econ* 2002;21:271–292.
11. Crawford B, Brazier J. Evaluating direct and indirect measures of utility: Stability, validity and responsiveness of the SF–6D in a rheumatoid arthritis population. *Value in Health* 2001;4:71.
12. Brazier J, Roberts J, Tsuchiya A, et al. A comparison of the EQ–5D and SF–6D across seven patient groups. *Health Econ* 2004;13:873–884.
13. Guyatt G, Juniper E, Walter S, et al. Interpreting treatment effects in randomized trials. *BMJ* 1998;316:690–693.
14. Bombardier C, Ware J, Russell IJ, et al. Auranofin therapy and quality of life in patients with rheumatoid arthritis: Results of a multicenter trial. *Am J Med* 1986;81:565–578.

15. Ferraz MB, Maetzel A, Bombardier C. A summary of economic evaluations published in the field of rheumatology and related disciplines. *Arthritis Rheum* 1997;40:1587–1593.
16. Maetzel A, Strand V, Tugwell P, Wells G, et al. Economic comparison of leflunomide and methotrexate in patients with rheumatoid arthritis. *Pharmacoeconomics* 2002;20:61–70.
17. Torrance GW, Tugwell P, Amorosi S, et al. Improvement in health utility among patients with rheumatoid arthritis treated with adalimumab (a human anti-TNF monoclonal antibody) plus methotrexate. *Rheumatology* 2004;43:712–718.
18. FDA (U.S. Food and Drug Administration). RA Guidance document: Guidance for Industry Clinical Development Programs for Drugs, Devices, and Biological Products for the Treatment of Rheumatoid Arthritis (RA). *http://www.fda.gov/cber/gdlns/rheumcln.pdf.*
19. Ware JE, Sherbourne CD. The MOS 36-item short-form health survey (SF–36), I. Conceptual framework and item selection. *Med Care* 1992;30:473–483.
20. Ware J, Kosinski M. *SF–36 Physical and Mental Health Summary Scales: A Manual for Users of Version 1.* The Health Institute: Boston, MA, 2001.
21. Ware J, Kosinski M, Dewey JE. *How to Score Version 2 of the SF–36 Health Survey.* Lincoln RI: QualityMetric Incorporated 2000.
22. Coons SJ, Rao S, Keininger DL, et al. A comparative review of generic quality-of-life instruments. *Pharmacoeconomics* 2000;17:13–35.
23. Hurst NP, Jobanputra P, Hunter M, et al. for the Economic and Health Outcomes Research Group. Validity of Euroqol—a generic health status instrument—in patients with rheumatoid arthritis. *Br J Rheumatol* 1994;33:655–662.
24. Hurst NP, Kind P, Ruta D, et al. Measuring health-related quality of life in rheumatoid arthritis: Validity, responsiveness and reliability of EuroQol (EQ–5D). *Br J Rheumatol* 1997;36:551–559.
25. Witney AG, Treharne GJ, Tavakoli M, et al. The relationship of medical, demographic and psychosocial factors to direct and indirect health utility instruments in rheumatoid arthritis. *Rheumatology* 2006;45:975–981.
26. Boyle MH, Furlong W, Feeny D, et al. Reliability of the Health Utilities Index: Mark III used in the 1991 cycle 6 Canadian General Social Survey Health Questionnaire. *Qual Life Res* 1995;4:249–257.
27. Samsa G, Edelman D, Rothman ML, et al. Determining clinically important differences in health status measures: A general approach with illustration to the Health Utilities Index Mark II. *Pharmacoeconomics* 1999;15:141–155.
28. Marra CA, Woolcott JC, Kopec JA, et al. A comparison of generic, indirect utility measures (the HUI2, HUI3, SF–6D, and the EQ–5D) and disease-specific instruments (the RAQoL and the HAQ) in rheumatoid arthritis. *Soc Sci Med* 2005;60:1571–1582.
29. Uhlig T, Smedstad LM, Vaglum P, et al. The course of rheumatoid arthritis and predictors of psychological, physical and radiographic outcome after 5 years of follow-up. *Rheumatol* 2000;39: 732–741.
30. Young A, Dixey J, Cox N, et al. How does functional disability in early rheumatoid arthritis (RA) affect patients and their lives? Results of 5 years of follow-up in 732 patients from the Early RA Study (ERAS) *Rheumatol* 2000;39:603–611.
31. West E, Jonsson SW. Health-related quality of life in rheumatoid arthritis in Northern Sweden: A comparison between patients with early RA, patients with medium-term disease and controls, using SF–36. *Clin Rheumatol* 2005;24:117–122.
32. Scott DL, Smith C, Kingsley G. Joint damage and disability in rheumatoid arthritis: An updated systematic review. *Clin Exp Rheumatol* 2003;21:S20–S27.
33. Harrison MJ, Tricker KJ, Davies L, et al. The relationship between social deprivation, disease outcome measures, and response to treatment in patients with stable, long-standing rheumatoid arthritis. *J Rheumatol* 2005;32:2330–2336.
34. Aletaha D, Strand V, Smolen JS, et al. Treatment-related improvement in physical function varies with duration of rheumatoid arthritis: A pooled analysis of clinical trial results. *Ann Rheum Dis* 2008;67:2338–2343.
35. Tugwell P, Wells G, Strand V, et al. for the Leflunomide Rheumatoid Arthritis Investigator Group. Clinical improvement as reflected in measures of function and health-related quality of life following treatment with leflunomide compared with methotrexate in patients with rheumatoid arthritis: Sensitivity and relative efficiency to detect a treatment effect in a twelve-month placebo-controlled trial. *Arthritis Rheum* 2000;43:506–514.
36. Kosinski M, Zhao SZ, Dedhiya S, et al. Determining minimally important changes in generic and disease-specific health-related quality of life questionnaires in clinical trials of rheumatoid arthritis. *Arthritis Rheum* 2000;43:1478–1487.
37. Strand V, Bombardier C, Maetzel A, et al. Use of minimum clinically important differences (MCID) in evaluating patient responses to treatment of RA. *Arthritis Rheum* 2001;44:S187.
38. Strand V, Cannon G, Cohen S, et al. Correlation of HAQ with SF–36: Comparison of leflunomide to methotrexate in patients with active RA. *Arthritis Rheum* 2001;44:S187.
39. Zhao SZ, Fiechtner JI, Tindall EA, et al. Evaluation of health-related quality of life of rheumatoid arthritis patients treated with celecoxib. *Arthritis Care Res* 2000;13:112–121.
40. Strand V, Crawford B. Improvement in health-related quality of life in patients with systemic lupus erythematosus following sustained reductions in anti-dsDNA antibodies. *Expert Review of Pharmacoeconomics & Outcomes Research* 2006;5:317–326.
41. Wolfe F, Michaud K, Strand V. Expanding the definition of clinical differences from minimally clinically important differences (MCID) to really important differences (RID): Analyses in 8,931 patients with rheumatoid arthritis. *J Rheumatol* 2005;32:583–589.
42. Wyrwich KW, Nienaber NA, Tierney WM, et al. Linking clinical relevance and statistal significance in evaluating intra-individual changes in HRQOL. *Medical Care* 1999;37:469–478.
43. Wyrwich KW, Tierney WM, Wolinsky FD. Further evidence supporting an SEM based criterion for identifying meaningful intra-individual changes in HRQOL. *J Clin Epidemiol* 1999;52:861–873.
44. Norman GR, Sloan JA, Wyrwich KW. Interpretation of changes in health-related quality of life: The remarkable university of half a standard deviation. *Medical Care* 2003;41:582–592.
45. Strand V, Cohen S, Crawford B, et al. for the Leflunomide Investigators Groups. Patient reported outcomes better discriminate active treatment from placebo in RA clinical trials. *Rheumatology* 2004; 43:640–647.
46. Cohen S, Strand V, Aguilar D, et al. Patient versus physician-reported outcomes in rheumatoid arthritis patients treated with recombinant interleukin–1 receptor antagonist (anakinra) therapy. *Rheumatology* 2004;43:704–711.
47. Tugwell P, Wells G, Strand V, et al. Clinical improvement as reflected in measures of function and health related quality of life: Sensitivity and relative efficiency to detect a treatment effect in a 12 month placebo controlled trial comparing leflunomide with methotrexate. *Arthritis Rheum* 2000;43:506–514.
48. Tugwell P, Idzerda L, Wells G. Generic Quality of life assessment in rheumatoid arthritis. *Am J Managed Care* 2007;13:S224–S236.
49. Strand V, Tugwell P, Bombardier C, et al. for the Leflunomide Rheumatoid Arthritis Investigators Group. Function and health-related quality of life: Results from a randomized controlled trial of leflunomide versus methotrexate or placebo in patients with active rheumatoid arthritis. *Arthritis Rheum* 1999;42:1870–1878.
50. Strand V, Scott DL, Emery P, et al. for the Leflunomide Rheumatoid Arthritis Investigators Groups. Physical function and health-related quality of life: Analysis of 2-year data from randomized, controlled studies of leflunomide, sulfasalazine, or methotrexate in patients with active rheumatoid arthritis. *J Rheumatol* 2005;32:590–601.
51. Strand V. Longer term benefits of treating rheumatoid arthritis: Assessment of radiographic damage and physical function in clinical trials. *Clin Exp Rheumatol* 2004;22:S57–S64.

52. Strand V, Singh JA. Improved health-related quality of life with effective disease-modifying antirheumatic drugs: Evidence from randomized controlled trials. *Am J Managed Care* 2007;13:S237–S251.
53. Maini RN, Breedveld FC, Kalden JR, et al. for the Anti-Tumor Necrosis Factor Trial in Rheumatoid Arthritis With Concomitant Therapy Study Group. Sustained improvement over two years in physical function, structural damage, and signs and symptoms among patients with rheumatoid arthritis treated with infliximab and methotrexate. *Arthritis Rheum* 2004;50:1051–1065.
54. Han C, Smolen J, Kavanaugh A, et al. The impact of infliximab treatment on quality of life in patients with inflammatory rheumatic diseases. *Arthritis Res Ther* 2007;9:R103.
55. Mathias SD, Colwell HH, Miller DP, et al. Health-related quality of life and functional status of patients with rheumatoid arthritis randomly assigned to receive etanercept or placebo. *Clin Ther* 2000; 22:128–139.
56. Kosinski M, Kujawski SC, Martin R, et al. Health-related quality of life in early rheumatoid arthritis: Impact of disease and treatment response. *Am J Managed Care* 2002;8:231–240.
57. van der Heijde D, Klareskog L, Singh A, et al. Patient reported outcomes in a trial of combination therapy with etanercept and methotrexate for rheumatoid arthritis: The TEMPO trial. *Ann Rheum Dis* 2006;65:328–334.
58. van Riel P, Freundlich B, MacPeek D, et al. Patient-reported health outcomes in a trial of etanercept monotherapy versus combination therapy with etanercept and methotrexate for rheumatoid arthritis: The ADORE trial. *Ann Rheum Dis* 2007 doi:10.1136/ard.2006.068585.
59. Strand V, Weinblatt M, Keystone E, et al. Treatment with adalimumab (D2E7), a fully human anti-TNF monoclonal antibody, improves physical function and health related quality of life (HRQOL) in patients with active rheumatoid arthritis (RA). *Ann Rheum Dis* 2002;61:S175.
60. Keystone EC, Kavanaugh AF, Sharp JT, et al. Radiographic, clinical, and functional outcomes of treatment with adalimumab (a human anti-tumor necrosis factor monoclonal antibody) in patients with active rheumatoid arthritis receiving concomitant methotrexate therapy: A randomized, placebo-controlled, 52-week trial. *Arthritis Rheum* 2004;50:1400–1411.
61. Mittendorf T, Dietz B, Sterz R, et al. Improvement and longterm maintenance of quality of life during treatment with adalimumab in severe rheumatoid arthritis. *J Rheumatol* 2007;34:2343–2350.
62. Weisman MH, Strand V, Cifaldi MA, et al. Adalimumab (HUMIRA) plus methotrexate is superior to MTX alone in improving physical function, as measured by the SF–36, in patients with early rheumatoid arthritis. *Arthritis Rheum* 2005;52:S395.
63. Kimel M, Cifaldi M, Chmiel J, et al. Adalimumab plus methotrexate improved SF–36 scores and reduced the effect of rheumatoid arthritis on work activity for patients with early RA. *J Rheumatol* 2007;35:206–215.
64. Strand V, Keininger DL, Tahiri-Fitzgerald E, et al. Certolizumab pegol monotherapy 400 mg every 4 weeks improves health-related quality of life and relieves fatigue in patients with rheumatoid arthritis who have previously failed DMARD therapy. *Ann Rheum Dis* 2007;66:188.
65. Strand V, Keininger DL, Tahiri-Fitzgerald E. Certolizumab pegol results in clinically meaningful improvements in physical function and health related quality of life in patients with active rheumatoid arthritis despite treatment with methotrexate. *Arthritis Rheum* 2007;56:S393.
66. Emery P, Kosinski M, Li T, et al. Treatment of rheumatoid arthritis patients with abatacept and methotrexate significantly improved health-related quality of life. *J Rheumatol* 2006;33:681–689.
67. Russell AS, Wallenstein GV, Li T, et al. Abatacept improves both the physical and mental health of patients with rheumatoid arthritis who have inadequate response to methotrexate treatment. *Ann Rheum Dis* 2007;66:189–194.
68. Westhovens R, Cole JC, Li T, et al. Improved health-related quality of life for rheumatoid arthritis patients treated with abatacept who have inadequate response to anti-TNF therapy in a double-blind, placebo-controlled, multicentre randomized clinical trial. *Rheumatology* 2006;45:1238–1246.
69. Michaud K, Bombardier C, Emery P. Quality of life in patients with rheumatoid arthritis: Does abatacept make a difference? *Clin Exp Rheum* 2007;25:S35–S45.
70. Cohen SB, Emery P, Greenwald MW, et al. for the REFLEX Trial Group. Rituximab for rheumatoid arthritis refractory to anti-tumor necrosis factor therapy: Results of a multicenter, randomized, double-blind, placebo-controlled, phase III trial evaluating primary efficacy and safety at twenty-four weeks. *Arthritis Rheum* 2006; 54:2793–2806.
71. Smolen J, Rovensky J, Ramos-Remus C, et al. Inhibiting the IL–6 receptor with the monoclonal antibody tocilizumab significantly improves quality of life in patients with rheumatoid arthritis. *Arthritis Rheum* 2007;56:S162.
72. Gomez-Reino JJ, Fairfax MJ, Pavelka K, et al. Targeted inhibition of IL–6 signaling with tocilizumab improves quality of life and function in patients with rheumatoid arthritis with inadequate response to a range of DMARDs. *Arthritis Rheum* 2007;56:S522.
73. Kavanaugh A, Han C, Bala M. Functional status and radiographic joint damage are associated with health economic outcomes in patients with rheumatoid arthritis. *J Rheumatol* 2004;31:849–855.
74. Scott DL, Khoshaba B, Choy EH, et al. Limited correlation between the Health Assessment Questionnaire (HAQ) and EuroQol in rheumatoid arthritis: questionable validity of deriving quality adjusted life years from HAQ. *Ann Rheum Dis* 2007;66:1534–1537.
75. Hazes JM, Geuskens GA, Burdorf A. Work limitations in the outcome assessment of rheumatoid arthritis. *J Rheumatol* 2005;32: 980–982.
76. Brouwer WB, Meerding WJ, Lamers LM, et al. The relationship between productivity and health-related QOL: An exploration. *Pharmacoeconomics* 2005;23:209–218.
77. Verstappen SM, Boonen A, Bijlsma JW, et al. for the Utrecht Rheumatoid Arthritis Cohort Study Group. Working status among Dutch patients with rheumatoid arthritis: Work disability and working conditions. *Rheumatology* 2005;44:202–206.
78. Merkesdal S, Huelsemann JL, Mittendorf T, et al. Productivity costs of rheumatoid arthritis in Germany. Cost composition and prediction of main cost components. *J Rheumatol* 2006;65:527–534.
79. Wolfe F, Michaud K, Choi HK, et al. Household income and earnings losses among 6,396 persons with rheumatoid arthritis. *J Rheumatol* 2005;32:1875–1883.
80. Singh G, Terry R, Ramey D, et al. Long-term medical costs and outcomes are significantly associated with early changes in disability in rheumatoid arthritis. *Arthritis Rheum* 1996;39:S318.
81. Puolakka K, Kautiainen H, Möttönen T, et al. for the FIN-RACo Trial Group. Early suppression of disease activity is essential for maintenance of work capacity in patients with recent-onset rheumatoid arthritis: Five-year experience from the FIN-RACo trial. *Arthritis Rheum* 2005;52:36–41.
82. Halpern MT, Cifaldi M, Kvien T, et al. Adalimumab (HUMIRA) improves rheumatoid arthritis outcomes in an open-label extension study compared with a registry-based DMARD control group. *Arthritis Rheum* 2007;56:S349.
83. Smolen JS, Han C, van der Heijde D, et al. Infliximab treatment maintains employability in patients with early rheumatoid arthritis. *Arthritis Rheum* 2006;54:716–722.
84. Kimel M, Cifaldi M, Chmiel J, et al. Relationship between health-related quality of life and employment outcomes during adalimumab (ADA) plus methotrexate (MTX) combination therapy versus MTX monotherapy in patients with early rheumatoid arthritis. *Arthritis Rheum* 2007;56:S89.
85. Bejarano V, Quinn MA, Conaghan PG, et al. Improved work stability and reduced job loss with adalimumab plus methotrexate in early rheumatoid arthritis: Results of the prevention of work disability (PROWD) study. *Ann Rheum Dis* 2007;66:176.

86. Strand V, Brown M, Purcaru O, et al. Certolizumab pegol monotherapy improves productivity in patients with active rheumatoid arthritis: Results from a phase III randomized controlled trial. *Ann Rheum Dis* 2007;66:274.
87. Burton W, Morrison A, Maclean R, et al. Systematic review of studies of productivity loss due to rheumatoid arthritis. *Occup Med* 2006;56:18–27.
88. Escorpizo R, Bombardier C, Boonen A, et al. Worker productivity outcome measures in arthritis. *J Rheumatol* 2007;34:1372–1380.
89. Verstappen SM, Boonen A, Verkleij H, et al. for the Utrecht Rheumatoid Arthritis Cohort Study Group. Productivity costs among patients with rheumatoid arthritis: The influence of methods and sources to value loss of productivity. *Ann Rheum Dis* 2005;64:1754–1760.

Radiography

Désirée van der Heijde

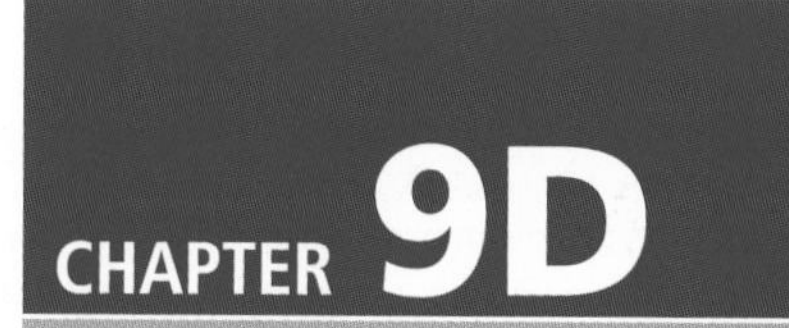

Radiography is the most widely used imaging method in making the diagnosis of rheumatoid arthritis (RA) and to follow the course of the disease and assess effectiveness of treatment. A series of radiographs constitutes the simplest and least expensive permanent record of the cumulative joint damage caused by the disease. Damage assessed on radiographs is a direct consequence of disease activity, as well as other destructive pathophysiologic processes. There is also a close relationship between radiologic damage and other outcome measures, such as functional capacity and work disability. As damage is largely irreversible, structural damage on radiographs is a reflection of cumulative disease activity. However, more and more reports become available that indicate that repair of damage is possible to some extent. More information is needed on how frequent this repair does occur, what the meaning is of this repair (e.g., is a joint with repair functioning better than a joint without signs of repair?), how long it takes to see repair, and how repair can be best assessed.

Advantages and Disadvantages of Conventional Radiographs

Conventional radiography is a widely available standardized technique for assessing structural damage of the joints. Moreover, it is inexpensive and fast and no contrast agent is necessary. Films of hands and feet provide information on many joints. An interpretation can be made by most rheumatologists themselves. Several features of structural damage can be appreciated on conventional radiographs. In addition, it has a large record as a validated and useful outcome tool. A clear disadvantage is the two-dimensional imaging of a three-dimensional joint, which may make interpretation sometimes difficult (e.g., in the wrist, caused by overprojection). Although very limited, ionizing radiation is involved. Although techniques such as magnetic resonance imaging (MRI) and ultrasound (US) (but not conventional radiographs) are able to give information on inflammation and soft-tissue involvement, conventional radiographs are able to provide an indirect assessment of cartilage involvement by joint space narrowing. This is not yet possible via MRI and US.

Abnormalities Visible on Conventional Radiographs

Many abnormalities in joints can be detected on conventional films in RA. These include soft-tissue swelling and proliferation, juxta-articular and diffuse osteoporosis, marginal bony erosions, subchondral cysts, joint space narrowing as a consequence of cartilage loss, subluxation and malalignment, ankylosis, sclerosis, and osteophytes in severely damaged joints. Erosions and joint space narrowing are the most specific features in RA, and they can be assessed in a reliable way. Moreover, they give additive information. Erosions are present in about 80% of patients in most longitudinal cohorts. The majority of patients develop the first erosions within the first year after onset.

Radiographic Technique and Views

Until recently, most centers used conventional films. However, more and more centers have converted to digital imaging. For conventional films, high-efficiency single-screen single-emulsion film-screen combinations with a focal film distance of approximately 100 cm are recommended for radiographs of hands and feet. The big advantage of digital images is that these can be easily stored and shared, and the quality can be adjusted if necessary. However, for follow-up images it is important to use the same exposure parameters and spatial resolution (matrix and image size). Especially for follow-up films, it is essential that the position of the hands and feet be as much as possible the same. Therefore, templates are recommended for a correct and consistent positioning. For the hands, a posteroanterior view is recommended, and for the feet an anteroposterior view is recommended as the only view. Although other views (e.g., the Brewerton or Nørgaard) are able to show more erosions in individual joints, the reproducibility of follow-up films is so poor that these introduce more noise than information for the use of radiographs as an outcome measure.

Films of Hands and Feet

Structural damage, especially erosions, is frequently present in the joints of hands and feet. Moreover, these are the sites in which structural damage can easily be detected because of the size of the joints. Very importantly, these are the sites that show the first erosions—and this is even more frequent in the feet than in the hands. The wrist is the predilection joint for early joint space narrowing. Therefore, it is recommended that one always take films of hands and feet. By doing so, a large number of joints are available for evaluation. It is not necessary to take films of the large joints routinely for the assessment of the course of disease because it has been proven that damage in the joints of the small joints is representative of the damage in the large joints.[1,2] Important in this respect is that Drossaers et al. showed that patients with normal radiographs of hands and feet do not have structural damage in any of the large joints.[2]

Scoring Methods: General Introduction

The information from radiographs is especially useful if this is quantified. Several scoring methods, discussed later in the chapter, are available for this purpose. The selection of the most appropriate scoring method is largely dependent on the setting in which it will be applied. For example, in clinical practice and large cohort studies feasibility is of major importance—whereas in clinical trials sensitivity to change drives the selection of method. The choice is also dependent on whether data are needed on progression (over a short or a long follow-up period) and whether a single point in time is important in the selection of the scoring method.

The methods used most frequently in recent research and clinical practice are described in the sections that follow. For a historical overview of all published scoring methods, we refer the reader to the literature.[3] The material that follows first describes the methods for applying a global score mainly based on the Larsen method. This is followed by the presentation of the more detailed scoring methods, mainly based on the Sharp method. An overview of the various characteristics of the scoring methods (such as the joints and the features included, the range per joint, and the total score) is found in Table 9D-1.[4]

Global Assessment per Joint

Larsen Score

The Larsen score applies a grade from 0 to 5 to individual joints.[5] This is the only method that can be applied to both large and small joints (a reference atlas with the grades for the various joints is available). The scoring is a combination of erosions and joint space narrowing resulting in a global grade, but this is mainly determined by erosions. The original Larsen scoring method includes soft-tissue swelling and juxta-articular osteoporosis in grade 1.[5] Only from grade 2 onward are definite abnormalities (such as erosions) present. Grade 5 represents a mutilating abnormality. Several modifications of the scoring system by the authors have been published. The most important modification is the one for use in longitudinal studies. Most studies include only the joints of the hands, wrists, and feet. The information in Table 9D-1 is based on the original method applied to hands, wrists, and feet. Originally, the wrist is evaluated as a single joint. In total, 32 joints are scored. This leads to a scoring range for hands and feet from 0 to 160. The modification published by Larsen et al in 1995 includes a change in the sites to be evaluated and a change in the grading.[6] Most striking is the deletion of soft-tissue swelling and osteoporosis for grade 1. Now erosions less than 1 mm and slight joint space narrowing are graded as 1. The number of areas in both hands and feet has been changed. The IP and MCP joint of the thumb and the IP and MTP joint of the big toe are no longer included. In this modification, the wrist is scored in quadrants. Therefore, the number of joints assessed remains 32.

Scott Modification of Larsen's Method

The modification by Scott et al. is frequently used when the Larsen method is applied.[7] They redefined the grading and applied it to the same 32 joints as in the original Larsen method. Moreover, the wrist is scored as a single joint. However, it is weighted by a factor of 5 to obtain the total score. This brings the range for hands and feet from 0 to 200.

Ratingen Score

In this modification of the Larsen score, the grading is entirely based on the surface area of the joints destructed by erosions.[8] This is graded from 0 to 5: grade 1 represents <20%, grade 2 21% to 40%, up to grade 5 >80%. In total, 38 joints of the hands are scored—resulting in a range of 0 to 190.

Detailed Scoring Methods

Sharp's Method

The sharp method was the first published method describing a detailed scoring system for erosions and joint space narrowing separately for joints in the hands and wrists.[9] The Sharp method used at present is in fact the modification described in 1985.[10] This reduced the number of joints scored from originally 27 for both erosions and joint space narrowing to 17 areas for erosions and 18 for joint space narrowing per hand. Moreover, the method was developed and validated for scoring the joints of the hands. However, these days the same methodology is also applied to the joints of the feet. Erosions are scored from 0 to 5 per joint and are counted when discrete, and surface erosions are scored according to the surface area involved. Joint space narrowing is scored on a 0 to 4 scale, representing focal narrowing (score of 1), joint space loss of <50% (score of 2), joint space loss of >50% (score of 3), and complete joint space loss or ankylosis (score of 4). Subluxation or luxation is not included in the score. The erosion score and the joint space narrowing score can be used separately, but are usually summed to obtain the total score.

Genant's Modification of Sharp's Method

The first modification of the Sharp method (by Genant) was described in 1983 and revised in 1998.[11–12] In this revision the scale for progression was extended from a 6-point scale to an 8-point scale, with 0.5-point increments from 0 to 3+ for erosions. For joint space narrowing, the system was revised from a 5-point scale to a 9-point scale (with 0.5-point increments from 0 to 4). This score is applied in 14 joints of each hand and wrist

Table 9D-1. Comparison of Radiographic Scoring Methods for Rheumatoid Arthritis

	Larsen Method	Scott Modification of Larsen Method	Ratingen Method	Sharp Method	Genant Modification of Sharp Method	van der Heijde Modification of Sharp Method	Simple Erosion Narrowing Score (SENS)
Films							
Hands	X	X	X	X	X	X	X
Feet	X	X	—	—	X	X	X
Large joints	X[a]	—	—	—	—	—	
Joints Included							
PIP/IP	X	X	X	X	X	X	X
MCP	X	X	X	X	X	X	X
Wrist	X	X	X	X	X	X	X
MTP	X	X	—	—	X	X	X
IP1	X	X	—	—	X	X	X
Features Scored							
Erosions	—	—	X	X	X	X	X
Joint space narrowing	—	—	—	X	X	X	X
Malalignment	—	—	—	—	—	X	X
Global	X	X	—	—	—	—	—
Number of Joints per Hand/Foot Scored for							
Erosions	—	—	19	17	14	22	22
Joint space narrowing	—	—	—	18	13	21	21
Malalignment	—	—	—	—	—	[c]	[c]
Global	16	16	—	—	—	—	—
Range							
Per joint for erosions	—	—	0–5	0–5	0–3+[b]	0–5/0–10[d]	0–1
Per joint for joint space narrowing	—	—	—	0–4	0–4	0–4	0–1
Per joint malalignment	—	—	—	—	—	[c]	[c]
Per joint global	0–5	0–5	—	—	—	—	—
Total	0–160	0–200	0–190	0–314	0–202	0–448	0–86

[a] Large joints are assessed separately; remaining information in this table is based on hands and feet.
[b] Scored per 0.5.
[c] Combined with the joint space narrowing score.
[d] Erosions for hands (0–5) and feet (0–10).
Reproduced with permission from van der Heijde D. Measurement of radiological outcomes. In St. Clair EW, Pisetsky D, Haynes BF (eds.), *Rheumatoid Arthritis.* Philadelphia: Lippincott Williams & Wilkins 2004:90–97.

for erosions and in 13 joints for joint space narrowing. This results in a total score range of 0 to 202.

van der Heijde's Modification of Sharp's Method

The main modification by van der Heijde was the addition of six joints per foot to the scoring system.[13,14] Moreover, two sites for erosions and two sites for joint space narrowing were deleted from the scoring areas of the 1985 Sharp method—leaving 16 sites for erosions and 15 for joint space narrowing per hand. The scoring of erosions in the hands remained the same, with a range of 0 to 5 per joint. However, for the scoring of erosions in the feet the scoring range was expanded to 10 per joint—with a maximum of 5 for the metatarsal and phalangeal site of the joint. Another major difference is that subluxation and luxation (malalignment) are integrated in the grading of joint space narrowing. Joint space narrowing is scored on a 0-to-4 scale, with the same grading as described for the Sharp method. However, in this modification a score of 3 can also be applied in the case of subluxation of a joint—and a score of 4 in the case of complete luxation. These features are for the most part scored in MCPs and MTPs. The scoring range for the total score is 0 to 448.

Simple Erosion Narrowing Score

The scoring methods previously described are used in clinical trials. In recent trials, most widely used are the (modified) Sharp methods. However, they are not very feasible for use in clinical practice. Therefore, the Simple Erosion Narrowing Score (SENS) method was developed and tested in both early and longstanding disease.[15,16] This method is based on the joints included in the van der Heijde modification of the Sharp's method for hands and feet. Instead of scoring the joints for erosions and joint space narrowing, this is a simple counting of the number of eroded joints and the number of narrowed joints. A score of 1 is applied if a site is eroded (or per narrowed site). In total, 15 joints per hand are scored for erosions and 16 for joint space narrowing. Six joints per foot for both erosions and joint space narrowing are scored. This leads to a scoring range from 0 to 86. The method is easy to learn and easy to apply in clinical practice, and takes only a few minutes. An increase of 1 in the score (equivalent to one newly eroded or narrowed joint) can be considered indicative of a progressive disease.

New Developments in the Assessment of Radiographs

Semiautomatic computerized methods of quantifying damage shown on radiographs have been tried by several investigators. Emphasis is placed on the measurement of joint space. A group of researchers has made an effort to compare the performance of various measurement methods for aspects of reliability, sensitivity to change, and discrimination between groups—mainly in patients with early disease. The results are still preliminary but sufficiently encouraging to further develop and test the methods.[17,18]

A completely different way to use the radiographs is to quantify early hand bone loss by the application of digital x-ray radiogrammetry (DXR). The value of this bone loss measure in the assessment of structural damage, or as a surrogate for structural damage as assessed by the scoring methods, is still under evaluation—but initial data are promising.[19]

Scoring for Clinical Trials

It is recommended that one always obtain films of hands and feet to analyze the efficacy on structural damage in a clinical trial. All information on the identity of the patient, clinical results, and treatment allocation are blinded to the person scoring the films. The films of the various time points are usually grouped per patient because scoring single films introduces measurement error and the focus of the evaluation is in assessing progression.[20] Absolute scores are applied to the various time points, and the scores are subtracted to obtain progression scores. For most trials, the time order of the films is also blinded to the observer. Although it is known that scoring with known time order increases the sensitivity to change, usually scoring with blinded time order is applied to minimize possible bias and to be able to judge repair in an unbiased manner. Moreover, this is required by drug registration authorities.

It is advised that two scores be obtained for all films.[21] Ideally, the same two observers score all films of all patients. However, if this is not feasible, films can be scored by three or four readers—with all films scored by at least two readers and all reader pairs preferably scoring an equal number of patients. The average score of the two readers is used as the final score for the data analysis. Recently, a process of adjudication has been applied in case of the progression score of the two readers for a particular patient exceeding a predefined limit. The films are then scored by a third reader. There are again several possibilities how to integrate this score in the final result (e.g., only the score of the adjudicator, the average of all three readers, the average of the reader closest to the adjudicator plus the adjudicator, and so on). In any event, all scores from the original readers (and the respective adjudicator) should be obtained completely independently. There is no use of consensus scoring.

If the Sharp scores are being used, the total score is suggested as the primary outcome. The erosion and joint space narrowing scores should be presented separately.[21] Only in the case of a special mode of action of a drug should one of the subscores be used as the primary outcome. The total score and the other subscore should also be presented. This methodology (together with other recommendations) is the result of a roundtable discussion published in 2002.[21] The main recommendations are outlined in Table 9D-2. Some updates that became apparent after the publication of the guidelines are added to or changed in this table.

Table 9D-2. Guidelines for Presentation of Radiographic Results in Clinical Trials
Radiographs of hands and feet
Smallest detectable change (SDC[a]) as quality control
Preferably two (2) or more observers
Kappa and/or ICC, and SDC for inter-observer agreement
Average score of observers
If one observer
Kappa and/or ICC for intra- and inter-observer agreement
SDC for intraobserver agreement
Presentation of absolute numbers
Primary endpoint: total score (erosions and joint space narrowing combined)
Secondary endpoints for Sharp methods: erosions, joint space narrowing
Primary analysis: group level
Reporting of mean, SE/SD
Box-whisker plot (median, percentiles, outliers)
Cumulative probability plot*
Secondary analysis: patient level
% of patients with progression >0.5 for two observers, >0 for one observer
% of patients with progression >SDC

[a] In the original guidelines, the SDD was proposed, but after the guidelines were published it became clear that the SDC is a more appropriate measure. The cumulative probability plot was also recommended after the publication of the guidelines and presents even more information than is already included in the box-whisker plot.

Modified from van der Heijde D, Simon L, Smolen J, et al. How to report radiographic data in randomized clinical trials in rheumatoid arthritis: Guidelines from a roundtable discussion. *Arthritis Rheum* 2002;47:215–218.

Reliability and Sensitivity to Change of Scoring Methods

For clinical trials, the reliability and sensitivity to pick-up progression in scoring methods over a relatively short period of time are of key significance. In general, the reliability for all scoring methods is acceptable to good. There is also evidence that all methods show sufficient sensitivity to change, in that all are able to discriminate between treatment arms in clinical trials. Most recent trials have employed the Sharp method, with the modifications proposed by van der Heijde and Genant. However, small differences in sensitivity to change between the methods might be of importance because these have an immediate consequence for the power of a study and thus the number of patients needed. Few direct comparisons on these aspects of the various methods have been performed. One comparison of the Larsen, Ratingen, Sharp, and van der Heijde modifications of the Sharp method showed that the repeatability was lowest for the Larsen method and best for the van der Heijde modification of the Sharp method, with the Ratingen method and Sharp method repeatability measures falling between these.[22] Precision was better for the two Sharp methods in comparison with the two Larsen methods. In another study in patients with early RA, the Scott modification of the Larsen method was compared to the van der Heijde modification of the Sharp method.[23] The discriminative capacity (0.85–0.95) and responsiveness (0.92–0.97) expressed as intraclass correlation coefficients (ICCs) were good for both methods when comparing group mean scores. However, when comparing individual patients status scores of the van der Heijde modification of the Sharp method were measured with greater precision and the method was more sensitive in detecting change over 1 year compared to the Scott modification of the Larsen method. An indirect proof of a high sensitivity to change of the van der Heijde modification of the Sharp method is the recent observation that even an interval as short as 3 months between two films is sufficient to detect changes in a considerable number of patients.[24] This might be especially helpful in Phase 2 studies to obtain an impression on the effectiveness on inhibiting radiographic progression early in the development phase.

It is well known that not all erosions visible on MRI and computerized tomography (CT) scan can be visible on conventional radiographs if compared on a joint-by-joint basis. Especially for the assessment of the wrist, multiplanar imaging methods have an advantage. However, to evaluate the usefulness of various imaging methods the comparison should be made between data typically obtained with the specific method to assess structural damage. For conventional radiographs, this applies to data of erosions and joint space narrowing of hands and feet, and for MRI information on erosions and bone edema in unilateral MCPs and wrist (although MRI is also frequently limited to one unilateral site, MCPs or wrist, but sometimes also applied to bilateral sites). Moreover, the real answer is given if the performance of both methods is compared in a clinical trial. To date, there is only one sufficiently powered dose-finding trial that included MRI (bilateral MCPs and wrists scored according a modification of the RAMRIS at baseline and 6 months) and conventional films of hands and feet (scored by the van der Heijde modified Sharp score at baseline and at 6 and 12 months).[25] MRI and conventional radiographs at 6 months showed discrimination between the high dose and placebo but not the low dose, and the conventional radiographs showed discrimination with the low dose after 12 months. Thus, in this trial no increased sensitivity by MRI could be demonstrated.

Missing Data

Because radiographs show cumulative structural joint damage, missing radiographs are an important issue in the analysis of clinical trial data. Because of the higher probability to show progression compared to improvement, and because of the risk of missing especially the films of patients who are not doing well, special attention needs to be paid to the handling of missing data. The usual method for clinical data, last observation carried forward, will by definition be an underestimation of the real progression. Most frequently used is linear extrapolation of data. However, it is important to perform several sensitivity analyses to judge the influence of missing data on results. An example of this based on a large clinical trial has been published.[26] It should be stressed that it is crucial to obtain follow-up radiographs in all patients regardless of premature discontinuation and to limit data imputation as much as possible.

Representation of Data

As outlined in Table 9D-2, the mean and median (with assessments of variation) of each trial should be represented in data. The main reason is that both give additive information. However, a graphic representation of the data in a so-called cumulative probability (or cumulative frequency) plot shows you all data in a comprehensible way.[27,28] In a probability plot, the scores per group (usually the change in scores over a defined period) are ordered from the lowest to the highest scores (Figure 9D-1). This provides an opportunity to appreciate the full range, the median, and the corresponding value for every percentile you might be interested in. This can also be used to determine the percentage of patients showing progression above a certain limit. Preferred cutoffs can be applied. This methodology is much more powerful than simply representing patients above 0.5 if the average of two observers is being used (or 0 for one observer) or above the smallest detectable change (SDC).[29] Moreover, the coherence of the data can be appreciated. In older literature, the smallest detectable difference (SDD) is considered a means of expressing measurement error in the unit of the scale. However, the SDD is the minimum number that can be used to determine if a change in patient A is different from a change in patient B. However, in trial analysis we are interested in whether patient A has progressed during the trial (progression above the measurement error). For this purpose, the SDC is the most appropriate tool. The SDC can be derived from the SDD by division of a square root of 2. The SDD is based on the 95% limits of agreement according to Bland and Altman.[30]

Repair

Although most emphasis is on detection of progression of structural damage, over the last decades it became clear that repair of damage is also possible. This could be observed in individual

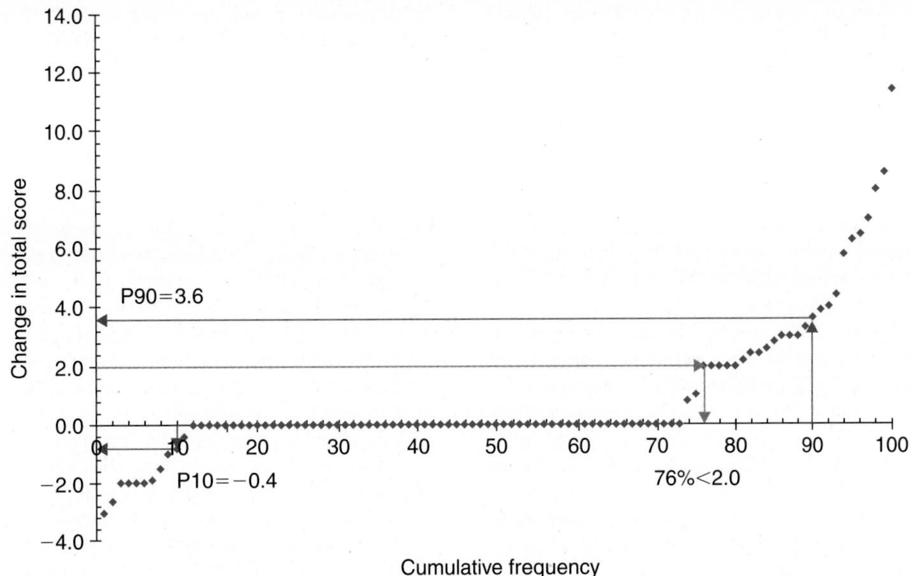

Figure 9D-1. Cumulative frequency plot showing the change in total score of the Sharp method on the Y axis and the scores of all individual patients depicted as diamonds. These are ordered from the lowest to the highest score and are presented on the X axis as cumulative frequency. If you want to read the 10th percentile, you draw a line starting at 10% cumulative frequency and connect at the crossing with the figure with the Y axis. The corresponding score on the Y axis (–0.4) can be read. Similarly, the 90th percentile corresponds to a change in score of 3.6, and the median is a change of 0. You can also start with a certain change in score (e.g., +2.0) and read the corresponding percentage on the X axis: 76% of the patients show a change in score of 2.0 or less. The magenta lines indicate scores belonging to percentiles; the orange line indicates the percentage of patients belonging to a certain score.

joints and patients, but also in studies specifically designed to test the concept of repair—as well as on the group level in clinical trials.[31–33] By definition, there is proof of repair on a group level if the mean change over time (with the entire 95% confidence interval) is below zero—indicating that there is a statistically significant improvement for the group. Determining definite repair in an individual joint or patient is more difficult. Based on data obtained in a trial, circumstantial evidence that a negative change score is indicating repair and that this is real could be deducted from the fact that negative change scores did occur almost exclusively in those joints without swelling and that this could be confirmed in independent reading sessions by different observers (unpublished data).

Summary

Conventional radiography is a well-established imaging method that remains valuable as an outcome assessment of structural damage in RA. Several widely used scoring methods applied to structural damage measurement exist. These methods have been validated and are sensitive to change over even very short periods of follow-up. Moreover, the relationship of structural damage to causal factors (such as inflammation) and to important outcome measures (such as physical function) is well known. This is an additional argument supporting the fact that conventional radiographs are useful measures of structural damage caused by RA for short-term as well as long-term outcomes.

References

1. Scott DL, Coulton BL, Popert AJ. Long term progression of joint damage in rheumatoid arthritis. *Ann Rheum Dis* 1986;45:373–378.
2. Drossaers-Bakker K, Kroon H, Zwinderman A, et al. Radiographic damage of large joints in long-term rheumatoid arthritis and its relation to function. *Rheumatology* 2000;39:998–1003.
3. van der Heijde DM. Plain X-rays in rheumatoid arthritis: Overview of scoring methods, their reliability and applicability. *Baillieres Clin Rheumatol* 1996;10:435–453.
4. van der Heijde D. Measurement of radiological outcomes. In St. Clair EW, Pisetsky D, Haynes BF (eds.), *Rheumatoid Arthritis.* Philadelphia: Lippincott Williams & Wilkins 2004:90–97.
5. Larsen A, Dale K, Eek M. Radiographic evaluation of rheumatoid arthritis and related conditions by standard reference films. *Acta Radiol Diagn Stockh* 1977;18:481–491.
6. Larsen A. How to apply Larsen score in evaluating radiographs of rheumatoid arthritis in long-term studies. *J Rheumatol* 1995;22:1974–1975.
7. Scott D, Houssien D, Laasonen L. Proposed modification to Larsen's scoring method for hand and wrist radiographs. *Br J Rheumatol* 1995; 34:56.
8. Rau R, Wassenberg S, Herborn G, et al. A new method of scoring radiographic change in rheumatoid arthritis. *J Rheumatol* 1998;25: 2094–2107.
9. Sharp JT, Lidsky MD, Collins LC, et al. Methods of scoring the progression of radiologic changes in rheumatoid arthritis: Correlation of radiologic, clinical and laboratory abnormalities. *Arthritis Rheum* 1971;14:706–720.
10. Sharp JT, Bluhm GB, Brook A, et al. Reproducibility of multiple-observer scoring of radiologic abnormalities in the hands and wrists

of patients with rheumatoid arthritis. *Arthritis Rheum* 1985;28: 16–24.

11. Genant HK. Methods of assessing radiographic change in rheumatoid arthritis. *Am J Med* 1983;75:35–47.
12. Genant HK, Jiang YB, Peterfy C, et al. Assessment of rheumatoid arthritis using a modified scoring method on digitized and original radiographs. *Arthritis and Rheumatism* 1998;41:1583–1590.
13. van der Heijde DM, van Riel PL, Nuver Zwart IH, et al. Effects of hydroxychloroquine and sulphasalazine on progression of joint damage in rheumatoid arthritis. *Lancet* 1989;8646:1036–1038.
14. van der Heijde D. How to read radiographs according to the Sharp/van der Heijde method. *J Rheumatol* 2000;27:261–263.
15. van der Heijde D, Dankert T, Nieman F, et al. Reliability and sensitivity to change of a simplification of the Sharp/van der Heijde radiological assessment in rheumatoid arthritis. *Rheumatology* 1999;38:941–947.
16. Dias, EM, Lukas C, Landewé RB, et al. Reliability and sensitivity to change of the Simple Erosion Narrowing Score compared to the Sharp/van der Heijde method for radiographs in rheumatoid arthritis. *Ann Rheum Dis* 2008;67:375–379.
17. Sharp JT, Angwin J, Boers M, et al. Computer based methods for measurement of joint space width: Update of an ongoing OMERACT project. *J Rheumatol* 2007;34:874–883.
18. Lukas C, Sharp JT, Angwin J, et al. Automated measurement of joint space width in small joints of patients with rheumatoid arthritis. *J Rheumatol* 2008 (in press).
19. Hoff M, Haugeberg G, Kvien T. Hand bone loss as an outcome measure in established rheumatoid arthritis: 2-year observational study comparing cortical and total bone loss. *Arthritis Res Ther* 2007;9:R81.
20. van der Heijde D, Boonen A, Boers M, et al. Reading radiographs in chronological order, in pairs or as single films has important implications for the discriminative power of rheumatoid arthritis clinical trials. *Rheumatology* 1999;38:1213–1220.
21. van der Heijde D, Simon L, Smolen J, et al. How to report radiographic data in randomized clinical trials in rheumatoid arthritis: Guidelines from a roundtable discussion. *Arthritis Rheum* 2002;47:215–218.
22. Wassenberg S, Herborn G, Larsen A, et al. Reliability, precision and time expense of four different radiographic scoring methods. *Arthritis and Rheum* 1998;41:S50.
23. Bruynesteyn K, van der Heijde D, Boers M, et al. The Sharp/van der Heijde method out-performed the Larsen/Scott method on the individual patient level in assessing radiographs in early rheumatoid arthritis. *J Clin Epidemiol* 2004;57:502–512.
24. Bruynesteyn K, Landewé R, van der Linden S, et al. Radiography as primary outcome in rheumatoid arthritis: Acceptable sample sizes for trials with 3 months' follow up. *Ann Rheum Dis* 2004; 63:1413–1418.
25. Cohen SB, Dore RK, Lane NA, et al. Denosumab treatment effects on structural damage, BMD, and bone turnover in rheumatoid arthritis: A randomized, placebo-controlled clinical trial. *Arthritis Rheum* 2008 10.1002/art.23417.
26. van der Heijde D, Landewé R, Klareskog L, et al. Presentation and analysis of data on radiographic outcome in clinical trials: Experience from the TEMPO study. *Arthritis Rheum* 2005;52:49–60.
27. Landewé R, van der Heijde D. Radiographic progression depicted by probability plots: Presenting data with optimal use of individual values. *Arthritis Rheum* 2004;50:699–706.
28. Landewé R, van der Heijde D. Presentation and analysis of radiographic data in clinical trials and observational studies. *Ann Rheum Dis* 2005;64(Suppl 4):iv48–iv51.
29. Bruynesteyn K, Boers M, Kostense P, et al. Deciding on progression of joint damage in paired films of individual patients: Smallest detectable difference or change. *Ann Rheum Dis* 2005;64:179–182.
30. Bland JM, Altman DG. Statistical methods for assessing agreement between two methods of clinical measurement. *Lancet* 1986;8476: 307–310.
31. van der Heijde D, Landewé R. Imaging: Do erosions heal? *Ann Rheum Dis* 2003;62(Suppl 2):ii10–ii12.
32. van der Heijde D, Sharp JT, Rau R, et al. OMERACT Workshop: Repair of structural damage in rheumatoid arthritis. *J Rheumatol* 2003;30:1108–1109.
33. van der Heijde D, Landewé R, Sharp JT for the OMERACT Subcommittee on Repair. Repair in rheumatoid arthritis, current status: Report of a workshop at OMERACT 8. *J Rheumatol* 2007;34:884–888.

Sonography

Marina Backhaus

CHAPTER 9E

Accurate assessment of disease activity and joint damage in rheumatoid arthritis (RA) is important for monitoring of treatment efficiency and predicting outcome of the disease. This requires sensitive imaging tools for detecting and monitoring of the disease course. Conventional radiography (CR) is the most well-established imaging technique in identifying progressive joint damage in RA. However, CR is insensitive in detecting soft-tissue lesions (e.g., synovitis) and early erosive bone lesions. Musculoskeletal ultrasonography (US) has become an important diagnostic technique in RA. US is able to detect both early inflammatory soft-tissue lesions (e.g., synovitis, tenosynovitis, and bursitis) and early erosive bone lesions (e.g., erosions) in arthritic joint diseases.[1–4] Studies show good correlation between US and MRI (magnetic resonance imaging) in the detection of inflammatory soft-tissue lesions and erosive bone lesions. Synovitis plays an important role in the joint-destroying process. It could be shown that no bone destruction occurs without the presence of synovitis. US allows a differentiation between exudative and proliferative synovial changes because of good soft-tissue contrast. The early detection of synovial proliferation is important in the diagnosis of early arthritis, and US is sensitive in the detection of these findings. US is able to detect superficial erosive cartilage and bone lesions earlier than CR (e.g., in the shoulder, hand, and foot joints).[1–3,5–8] US results influence further diagnostic and therapeutic procedures.[9] The application of color and power Doppler US is helpful in the detection of early inflammation. This allows the differentiation between an active and inactive joint process. Current studies with ultrasound contrast media demonstrate its benefit in the differentiation of inflammatory disorders. The use of contrast agents increases the sensitivity of the examination, enhancing the thickened, hypervascular, and inflamed joint capsule. It allows a better quantification of inflammatory disease by estimating US signal intensity changes. At present, contrast-enhanced ultrasonography (CE-US) is of particular interest for clinical studies in monitoring new anti-inflammatory drugs in RA.

Technical Requirements

Modern US devices employ multifrequency transducers. The frequency of the sound wave determines how deeply it will penetrate the tissue. The frequency also determines the resolution. For the best resolution, the highest ultrasound frequency should be used. In the next step, the penetration depth and frequency should be adapted. Musculoskeletal US is generally performed with linear transducers. The choice of transducer depends on the examined joint region. For the examination of wrist, hand, and toe joints, frequencies of 10 to 16 MHz are recommended. Middle-size joints are examined with 10- to 12-MHz transducers, and deep joints (such as hip joints) are examined with 5- to 7.5-MHz linear transducers (or for deeper penetration with curved array transducers of 3.5 MHz). Several joint regions are examined in a standardized fashion according to the guidelines of the German Society for Ultrasound in Medicine (DEGUM) and the EULAR (European League Against Rheumatism) guidelines.[10,11] US of joints is performed in multiplanar scans (e.g., the transducer navigates dynamically from proximal to distal in transverse scans and from medial to lateral in longitudinal scans). This procedure allows a complete joint scan. Dynamic imaging is necessary for the detection of smallest fluid collections in joints. In this case, the transducer should be held in a fixed position above (on top of) the examined joint while the joint is moved actively by the examiner.

Technical developments such as tissue harmonic imaging and sono-CT/cross-beam sonography have improved image quality. US results depend on the techniques employed and on the experience of the examiner. Special knowledge in musculoskeletal sonography is necessary. US courses on different levels are performed under the auspices of EULAR. Inter-observer reliabilities, sensitivities, and specificities of musculoskeletal US in comparison with MRI are moderate to good.[4,12]

The ultrasound images can be recorded and stored in the machine's data storage system and copied to media such as CD and DVD. Prints can be made using a connected black-and-white thermal printer.

Differentiation between Soft Tissue and Bone Lesions by Musculoskeletal Ultrasonography

The inflammatory soft-tissue lesions include synovitis with effusion, synovial proliferation, and tenosynovitis with effusion and/or synovial proliferation of the tendon sheath—as well as bursitis with effusion and/or synovial proliferation. Synovial proliferation of joint capsule often occurs in combination with inflammatory effusion. The combination is also called synovitis. The inflammatory bone lesion/erosion is defined as an interruption of cortical bone surface in two perpendicular scans. During the Seventh OMERACT Conference (Outcome Measurement Rheumatoid Arthritis Clinical Trial) in Monterrey, California, May 2004, the international ultrasound study group described the sonographic definitions as follows.[13]

- *Effusion:* Effusion is a hypoechoic or anechoic intra-articular material that is displaceable and compressible and without signs of Doppler signal. Echo texture is relative to subdermal fat pad (Figure 9E-1).
- *Synovial hypertrophy and synovial proliferation:* Synovial hypertrophy and synovial proliferation is an abnormal hypoechoic intra-articular tissue that is not displaceable and hardly compressible and with signs of Doppler signal. Echo texture is relative to subdermal fat pad and could also be echoic or hyperechoic (Figure 9E-2).
- *Tenosynovitis:* Tenosynovitis is an abnormal hypoechoic or anechoic material with or without fluid inside the tendon sheath with possible signs of Doppler signal in two perpendicular planes (Figure 9E-3).
- *Erosion:* Erosion is an intra-articular interruption of cortical bone surface in two perpendicular scans (Figure 9E-4).
- *Bursitis:* Bursitis is defined by OMERACT as a cyst formation with abnormal hypoechoic or anechoic material with or without fluid inside of bursa with possible signs of Doppler signals in two perpendicular planes (Figure 9E-5).

Clinical studies have shown that musculoskeletal US is more sensitive in the detection of inflammatory signs than the clinical examination.[1–3] Signs of synovitis can be detected more frequently in the palmar proximal area of the finger joints (PIP and MCP) than from the dorsal aspect.[14] Synovitis scores have been developed for the finger joints in arthritic processes.[14,15] The Synovitis score according to Szkudlarek[15] grades the inflammatory soft-tissue lesions separately for effusion and synovial proliferation. The Synovitis score according to Scheel and Backhaus combines the effusion and the synovial proliferation in one scoring system.[14,16] We could show that the best results for joint combinations were achieved using the "sum of four fingers" (second through fifth MCP and PIP joints) and "sum of three fingers" (second through fourth MCP and PIP joints) methods. Comparison to MRI results with semiquantitative US scores (grade 0 = normal; grade 1 = minimal effusion/synovial hypertrophy; grade 2 = moderate effusion/synovial hypertrophy; grade 3 = severe effusion/synovial hypertrophy) revealed high concordance to quantitative synovitis scores (measurements of joint capsule distance to bone margin in mm) (Figure 9E-6).

A tenosynovitis of the extensor carpi ulnaris tendon is an early inflammatory sign in RA that can easily be detected by US[17] (Figure 9E-3). Erosive bone lesions are also sooner detected in wrist and finger joints by US than by CR. The exact anatomic classification of bone lesions in the wrist is sometimes difficult by US. On the other hand, erosions can readily be detected by US in the finger joints—especially from the radial aspect of the second MCP and ulnar aspect of the fifth MCP joints[9,18] (Figure 9E-4).

High-resolution transducers are able to detect more erosive bone lesions on PIP joints than 0.2T MRI.[3,8] Synovitis is also evident on toes, especially in MTP joints (which can also be detected by US).[7] Of course, many other joints can be examined for the presence of synovitis by means of US.[17,19–24] Popliteal cysts are often seen in patients with RA and knee involvement. US allows a good differentiation to other causes of compression syndrome of the lower leg.

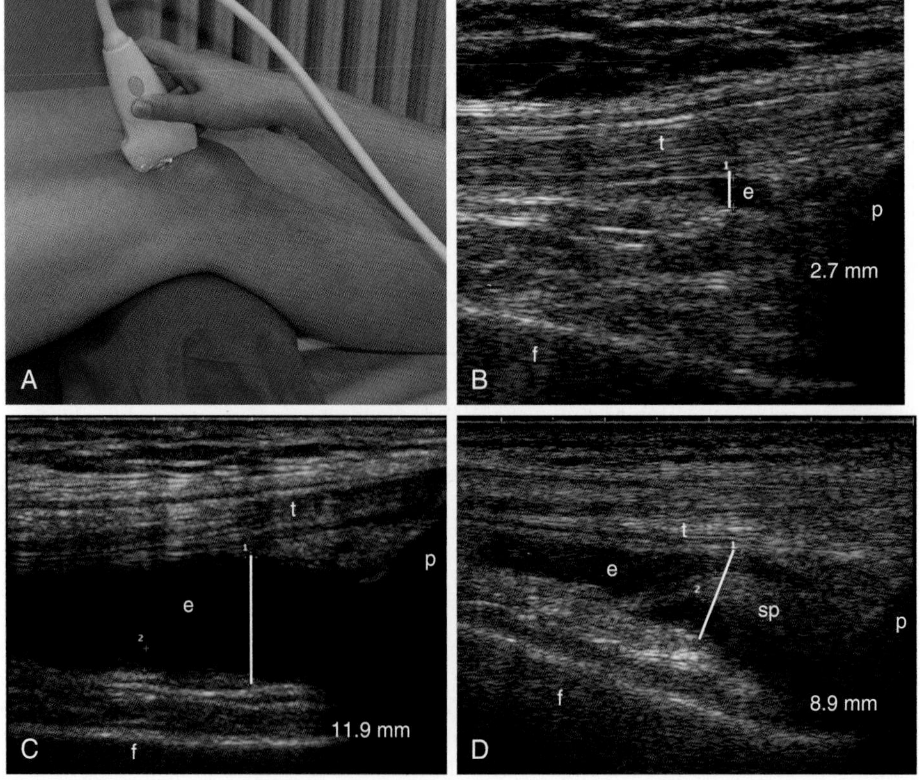

Figure 9E-1. Effusion and synovial hypertrophy of suprapatellar pouch: US probe position (*A*); longitudinal scan at suprapatellar pouch of normal knee (*B*), of knee with effusion (*C*), and with synovial hypertrophy (*D*). f, femur; p, patellar; t, tendon; e, effusion; sp, synovial hypertrophy.

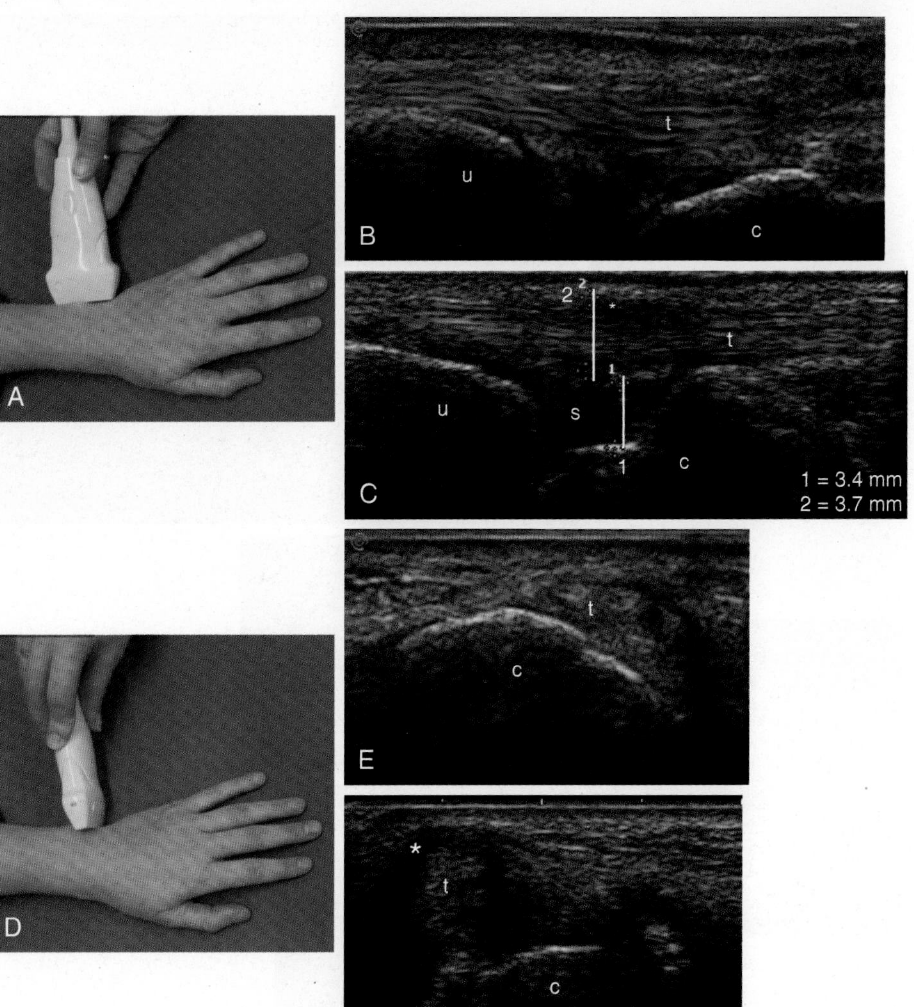

Figure 9E-2. Tenosynovitis of extensor carpi ulnaris tendon: US probe position in longitudinal (*A*) and transverse (*D*) orientation; longitudinal and transverse scan at ulnar aspect of normal wrist (*B*, *E*), and of wrist with tenosynovitis of extensor carpi ulnaris tendon in longitudinal scan (*C*) and transverse scan (*F*). u, ulna bone; c, carpal bone; t, tendon extensor carpi ulnaris; s, synovitis; *, tenosynovitis.

Color and Power Doppler Sonography in Diagnosis of Early Arthritis

The echo texture in grayscale US (B-mode) allows a first statement about the activity of the joint's process. The echo texture of synovial tissue of an active joint process is more hypoechoic, and in the case of an inactive joint process more echoic to hyperechoic. The use of color and power Doppler US facilitates a differentiation between active and inactive synovitis. Power Doppler US demonstrates the hypervascularization of inflammatory synovial tissue. The vessels of inflammatory tissue are expanded and new vessels are constituted, which is detectable by the Doppler technique. With regard to the vessel density of an inflammatory joint, it is possible to illustrate color pixels in different accumulations.

The demonstration of physiologic vascularization of healthy joints without signs of inflammation is only possible with very sensitive US devices and high-resolution scan technique (with few exceptions). The principles of diagnostic US are based on different reflexions of high-frequency ultrasound waves at the borders of tissue within the body. When ultrasound waves hit borderline areas moved to or back from their source, the frequency of reflected ultrasound waves is high (in the case of moving the reflected ultrasound waves in the direction of their source) or low (in the case of moving the reflected ultrasound waves back from their source). The change of frequency of US waves on moved borderline areas is called the "Doppler effect," a known physical phenomenon used to assess blood flow.

The reflection of US waves on the surface of corpuscular parts of blood leads to a shift of frequency (Doppler frequency shift), which is measurable and detectable. The Doppler frequency is presented in different color codes. Normally, red means a movement of US waves in the direction of the transducer and blue a movement of US waves away from the transducer. A description of blood flow in the location and direction to the anatomic structures is also possible. Modern devices use pulsed-wave Doppler (PW Doppler), which sends ultrasound waves not continuously [as with continuous-wave (CW) Doppler] but rhythmically at a certain frequency (pulse repetition frequency/PRF) in form of several "ultrasound wave packages." Doppler frequency analysis allows the measurement of respective fluid speed of blood flow. A correction of the angle of the determinate Doppler fluid curve should be considered. A combination of B-mode and Doppler sonography is called Duplex sonography.[25,26] Normally, power Doppler sonography has no direction code of blood flow—which allows a higher sensitivity

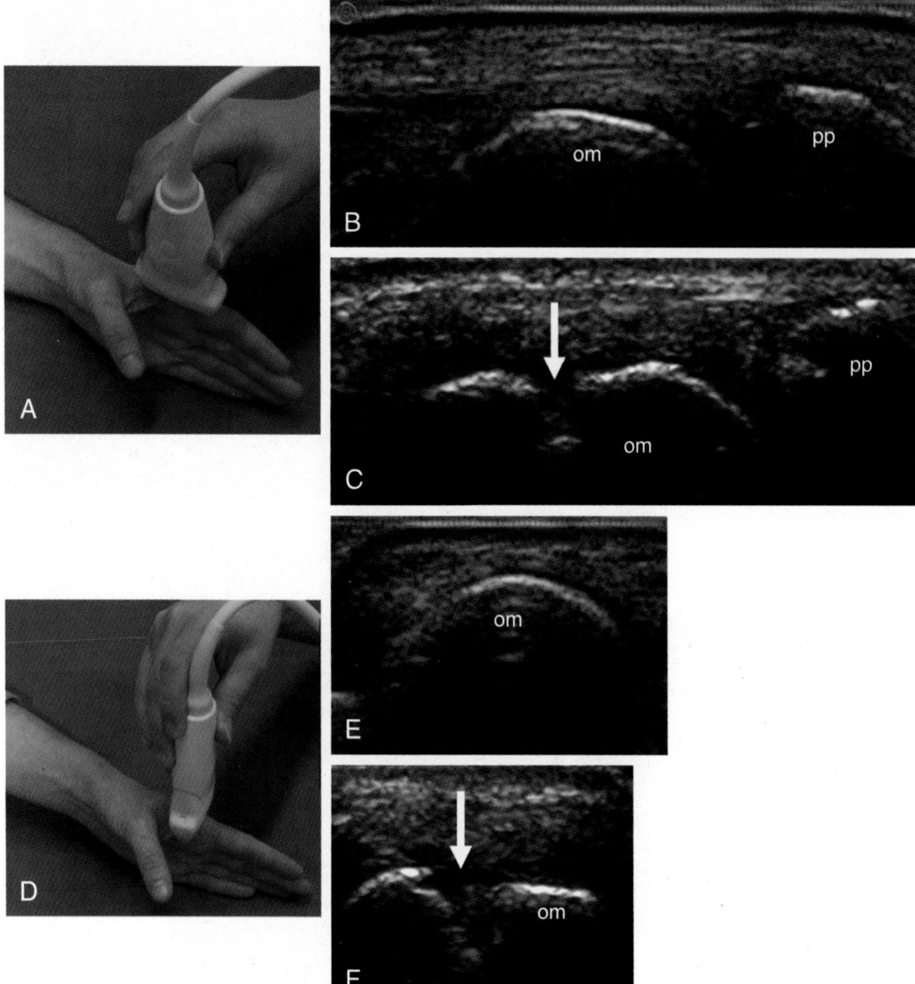

Figure 9E-3. Erosion of MCP joint 2 at the radial aspect: US probe position in longitudinal (*A*) and transverse (*D*); longitudinal and transverse scans at radial aspect of normal metacarpophalangeal joint (MCP) 2 (*B*, *E*) and with erosion (*C*, *F*). om, os metacarpale; pp, phalanx proximalis; ↓, erosion.

in the detection of blood flow with lower speed (especially in small blood vessels, such as in the case of inflammatory joints). Newer high-quality US devices use a bidirectional power doppler (PD) mode, which is able to show a direction code of blood flow according to color Doppler US but with a higher resolution (e.g., US machines from ESAOTE). Power Doppler sonography is able to represent the vascularization of pannus tissue of inflammatory joint diseases. In addition, a semiquantitative color-pixel grading system is used to represent the activity of the joint process as the following four grades[26] (Figure 9E-7).

- Grade 0 = no Doppler signal (color pixel) and no flow
- Grade 1 = single Doppler signal and little flow (three single spots or two single spots plus one confluent spot)
- Grade 2 = several Doppler signal, coherent Doppler signal, and definite flow (≤50% of color pixel of intra-articular area).
- Grade 3 = nearly complete taking up of joint area with coherent Doppler signal and strong flow (≥50% of color pixel of intra-articular area)

The intra-articular and intrasynovial color pixels are important in the description of inflamed activity of joint processes. Periarticular (outside of joint capsule) color pixels are seen as a result of hyperemia in arthritic processes. There are many studies about the use of color and power Doppler sonography in RA on hand, wrist, and knee joints. A good correlation to clinical examination and MRI with contrast enhancement as well as histopathology could be demonstrated.[22,26–28] Power Doppler sonography is also useful for therapy monitoring with new antirheumatic drugs (biologicals).[29,30]

Use of Echo Contrast Agent in Diagnosis of Early Arthritis

The differentiation between effusion and synovial proliferation with grayscale US can sometimes be difficult because both phenomena can be similar in their echo texture, ranging from hypoechoic to echoic texture. Color and power Doppler US are not able to detect slow blood flow or the blood flow in very small vessels in all cases.[31] The use of echo-contrast-enhanced US allows a functional imaging of synovial vascularization and therefore an assessment of disease activity. Blood flow with low volume in very small vessels can be detected as a result of improved signal rush ratio.[32–36] A multicenter study recently demonstrated an improvement of measurement of synovial thickness and activity of synovial processes in patients with RA by using echo-contrast-enhanced US.[34] The contrast agents are stable gas bubbles with very good reflex behavior. They are intravenously administered. The micro bubbles bind to red blood cells. There

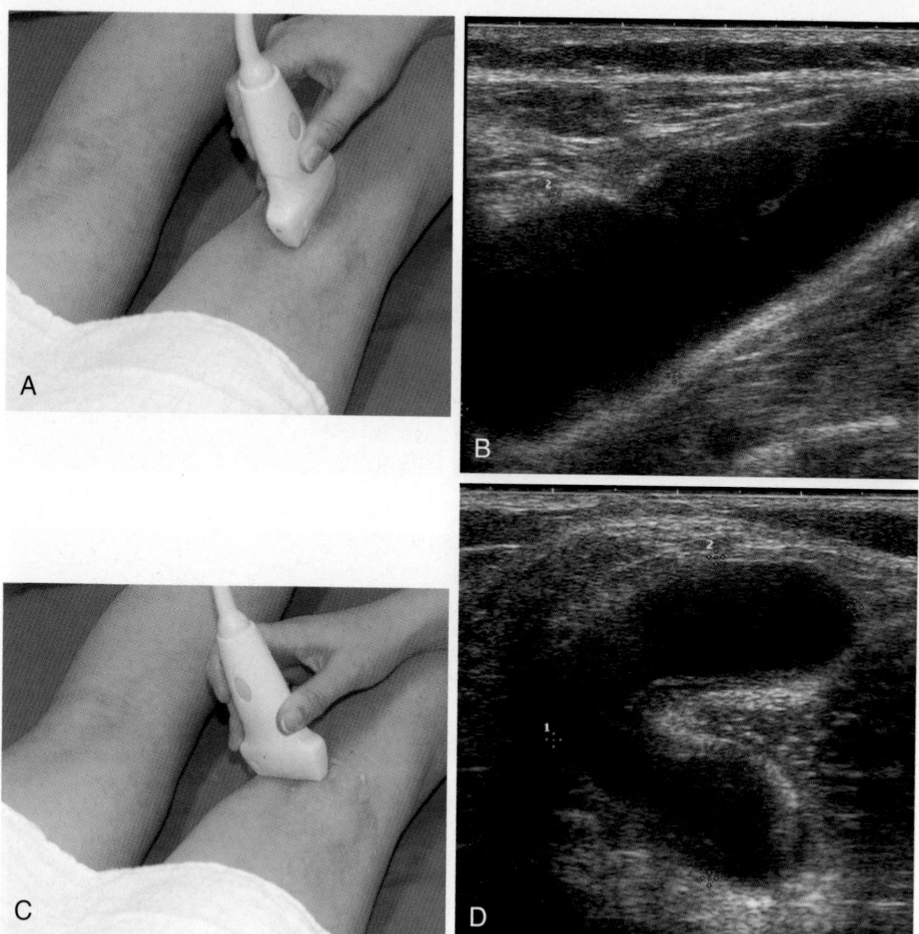

Figure 9E-4. Bursitis (popliteal cyst): US probe position in longitudinal (*A*) and transverse (*C*) orientation; popliteal cyst in longitudinal (*B*) and tansverse (*D*) plane.

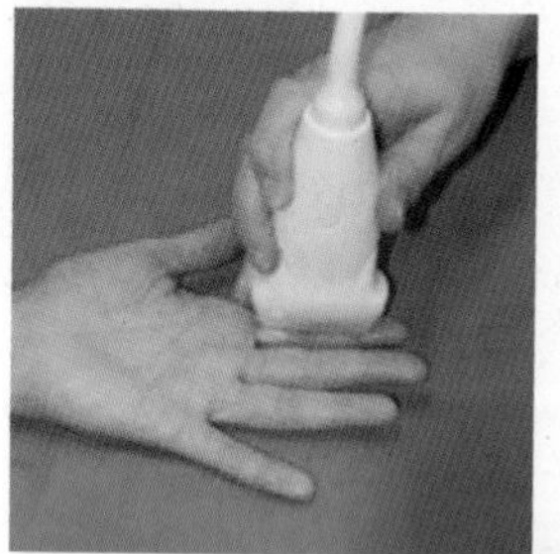

Figure 9E-5. Semiquantitative scoring in B-mode of PIP joints at palmar aspect in RA (grades 0–3). pp. phalanx proximalis.

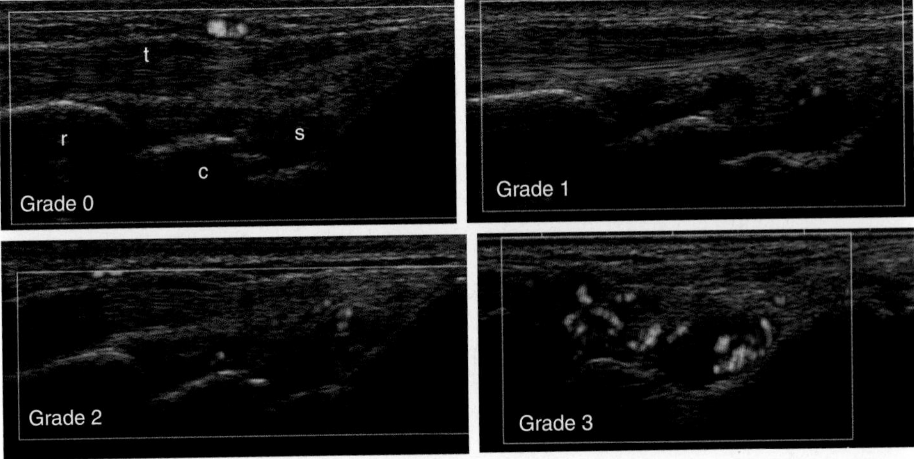

Figure 9E-6. Semiquantitative scoring in PD-US of the wrist at dorsal aspect in RA (grades 0–3). r, radius; c, carpal bone; t, tendon; s, synovitis.

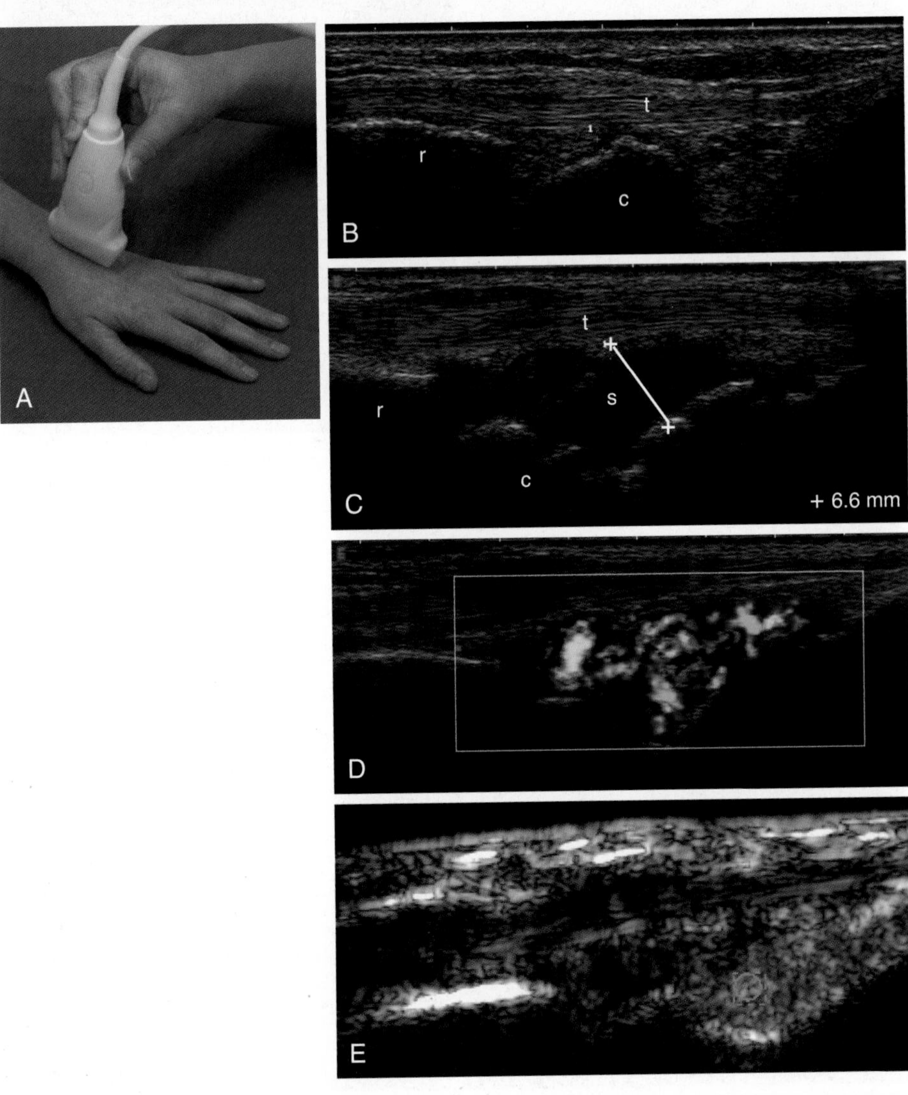

Figure 9E-7. Echo-contrast-enhanced US of the wrist in comparison to B-mode and PD-US: US probe position in longitudinal (*A*) orientation; longitudinal scan at dorsal aspect of normal wrist in B-mode (*B*), with servere synovitis of the wrist (grade 3) in B-mode (*C*), in PD-US (grade 3) (*D*), and in CE-US (grade 3) (*E*). r, radius; c, carpal bone; t, tendon; s, synovitis.

are different sizes of bubbles, which are nonrespirable or respirable. Depending on their behavior of oscillation, there are echo contrast agents of the first and second generation. Echo contrast agent of the second generation (e.g., SonoVue, Bracco, Italy) is used in studies of arthritis diagnosis. The sizes of the contrast micro bubbles are less than the size of erythrocytes (3 μm). The micro bubbles do not leave the course vessels; they are exhaled through the lung approximately 6 minutes after intravenous application. For this reason, severe diseases of heart and/or lung (e.g., lung fibrosis, coronary heart diseases NYHA state III and IV) are contraindications for using contrast-enhanced sonography. A semiquantitative grading system[34] or quantitative analysis with time intensity curves can be applied for assessment of activity of contrast-enhanced sonography. Some ultrasound devices include special software that allows a fast analysis of different parameters of US signal changes after application of the contrast agent. Parameters of interest in analysis are time intensity curves, which include the values as maximum intensity enhancement, time to peak, and "area under the curve." These parameters are suitable for follow-up examinations and could be used for accurate (control) assessment of therapy response.

The comparison of contrast agent behavior of intra- and extra-articular structures also allows a qualitative analysis of inflammatory joint activity. However, for therapy response studies an objective quantification of contrast-enhanced sonography is preferred.

Contrast-enhanced US allows a better differentiation between effusion and synovial proliferation and leads to a better assessment of disease activity of synovial processes. This differentiation is helpful in follow-up studies of therapy, especially in cases of new treatment procedures acting on the micro vascular level. For instance, fibrosis in inactive pannus tissue shows no vascularization and no accumulation of contrast agent. Current studies use contrast-enhanced sonography to evaluate inflamed synovial process in RA. A study with Levovist, a contrast agent of the first generation, on knee and MCP joints in RA shows a good correlation to clinical findings, laboratory findings, and in comparison to contrast-enhanced MRI.[28,33,37,38] No correlation was found between Levovist used in shoulder joints in comparison to MRI in patients with RA.[39] A study with SonoVue, a contrast agent of the second generation, shows a good correlation to contrast-enhanced MRI in the detection of synovitis processes of the suprapatellar recess in knee osteoarthritis (OA).[40] Contrast-enhanced sonography is inexpensive compared to contrast-enhanced MRI, with the same high resolution in the evaluation of activity in synovial processes. The time needed for examination is about 20 minutes, including preparation time. Another advantage of echo contrast agent for US compared to standard contrast agent for MRI is the fact that echo contrast agent for US does not leave the vessels and does not go into the synovial fluid or tissue. Echo contrast agents are able to precisely reflect the changes within the intravascular compartment.

Echo-contrast-enhanced ultrasonography is helpful in the differentiation and evaluation inflammatory joint processes. It is especially of interest in testing the efficacy of new antirheumatic drugs. Further studies are necessary to evaluate the new technique in assessment of joint diseases. For screening of arthritic joint processes, examination of following joints is advisable.

- Longitudinal and transverse scan of the wrist (dorsal, ulnar, palmar aspect) for signs of synovitis, tenosynovitis, and erosions
- Longitudinal and transverse scan of MCP joints and PIP joints II through IV (dorsal, palmar aspect) for signs of synovitis, tenosynovitis/tentinitis, and erosions
- Longitudinal and transverse scan of MCP joint II (radial) and MCP joint V (ulnar) for signs of erosions
- Longitudinal and transverse scan of metatarsophalangeal (MTP) joints II and V (dorsal, plantar aspect) for signs of synovitis and erosions
- Longitudinal and transverse scan of MTP joint V (lateral) for signs of erosions
- Scans of other symptomatic joints

Musculoskeletal ultrasonography is helpful in the diagnosis of early arthritis, especially in cases of normal CR but suspected clinical findings. US allows an early detection of inflamed synovial processes such as effusion and/or synovial hypertrophy, tenosynovitis, bursitis, and erosions. US is a suitable imaging technique for follow-up and for monitoring the results of therapy. US is helpful in diagnostic and therapeutic joint injection procedures. The use of color and power Doppler US as well as contrast-enhanced US achieves additional information about the activity of inflamed joint processes. US is a patient-friendly technique with high assertion and is an established method in the diagnosis and monitoring of arthritic diseases, especially in RA.

References

1. Backhaus M, Kamradt Th, Sandrock D, et al. Arthritis of the finger joints: A comprehensive approach comparing conventional radiography, scintigraphy, ultrasound, and contrast-enhanced magnetic resonance imaging. *Arthritis Rheum* 1999;42:1232–1245.
2. Backhaus M, Burmester GR, Sandrock D, et al. Prospective two-year follow-up study comparing novel and conventional imaging procedures in patients with arthritic finger joints. *Ann Rheum Dis* 2002;61:895–904.
3. Scheel AK, Hermann KG, Ohrndorf S, et al. Prospective long term follow-up imaging study comparing radiography, ultrasonography and magnetic resonance imaging in rheumatoid arthritis finger joints. *Ann Rheum Dis* 2006;65:595–600.
4. Scheel AK, Schmidt WA, Hermann KG, et al. Interobserver reliability of rheumatologists performing musculoskeletal ultrasonography: results from a EULAR "Train the trainers" course. Ann *Rheum Dis* 2005;64:1043–1049.
5. Alasaarela E, Suramo I, Lahde S, et al. Evaluation of humeral head erosions in rheumatoid arthritis: A comparison of sonography, magnetic resonance imaging, computerised tomography and plain radiography. *Br J Rheumatol* 1998;37:1152–1156.
6. Szkudlarek M, Narvestad E, Klarlund M, et al. Ultrasonography of the metatarsophalangeal joints in rheumatoid arthritis: Comparison with magnetic resonance imaging, conventional radiography, and clinical examination. *Arthritis Rheum* 2004;50:2103–2112.
7. Szkudlarek M, Narvestad E, Court-Payen M, et al. Ultrasonography of the RA finger joints is more sensitive than conventional radiography for detection of erosions without loss of specificity, with MRI as a reference method. *Ann Rheum Dis* 2004;63:82–83.
8. Wakefield RJ, Gibbon WW, Conaghan PG, et al. The value of sonography in the detection of bone erosions in patients with rheumatoid arthritis. *Arthritis Rheum* 2000;43:2762–2770.
9. Karim Z, Wakefield RJ, Conaghan PG, et al. The impact of ultrasonography on diagnosis and management of patients with musculoskeletal conditions. *Arthritis Rheum* 2001;44:2932–2933.
10. Konermann W, Gruber G. *Musculoskeletal Sonography: Guidelines of the German Society for Ultrasound in Medicine (DEGUM)*. Stuttgart: Thieme 2000.
11. Backhaus M, Burmester GR, Gerber Th, et al. Guidelines for musculoskeletal ultrasound in rheumatology. *Ann Rheum Dis* 2001;60: 641–649.

12. Naredo E, Moller I, Moragues C, et al. for the EULAR Working Group for Musculoskeletal Ultrasound. Interobserver reliability in musculoskeletal ultrasonography: Results from a "Teach the Teachers" rheumatologist course. *Ann Rheum Dis* 2006;65:14–19.
13. Wakefield RJ, Balint P, Szkudlarek M, et al. for the OMERACT 7 Special Interest Group. Musculoskeletal ultrasound including definitions for ultrasonographic pathology. *J Rheumatol* 2005;32: 2485–2487.
14. Scheel AK, Hermann KG, Kahler E, et al. A novel ultrasonographic synovitis scoring system suitable for analyzing finger joint inflammation in rheumatoid arthritis. *Arthritis Rheum* 2005;52:681–686.
15. Szkudlarek M, Court-Payen M, Jacobsen S, et al. Interobserver agreement in ultrasonography of the finger and toe joints in rheumatoid arthritis. *Arthritis Rheum* 2003;48:955–962.
16. Schell AK, Backhaus M. Ultrasonographic assessment of the finger and toe joint inflammation in rheumatoid arthritis: Comment on the article by Szkudlarek et al. *Arthritis Rheum* 2004;50:1008.
17. Backhaus M, Schmidt WA, Mellerowicz H, et al. Technique and diagnostic value of musculoskeletal ultrasonography in rheumatology. Part 6: Ultrasonography of the wrist/hand. *Z Rheumatol* 2002; 61:674–687.
18. Backhaus M, Schmidt WA, Mellerowicz H, et al. Technical aspects and value of arthrosonography in rheumatologic diagnosis. 4: Ultrasound of the elbow. *Z Rheumatol* 2002;61:415–425.
19. Joshua F, Lassere M, Bruyn GA, et al. Summary findings of a systematic review of the ultrasound assessment of synovitis. *J Rheumatol* 2007;34:839–847.
20. Hauer RW, Schmidt WA, Bohl-Bühler M, et al. Technique and value of arthrosonography in rheumatologic diagnosis. Part 1: Ultrasound diagnosis of the knee joint. *Z Rheumatol* 2001;60:139–147.
21. Mellerowicz H, Schmidt WA, Hauer RW, et al. Technique and diagnostic value of musculoskelatal ultrasonography in rheumatology. Part 5: Ultrasonography of the shoulder. *Z Rheumatol* 2002;61: 577–589.
22. Schmidt WA, Hauer RW, Banzer D, et al. Technique and value of arthrosonography in rheumatologic diagnosis. Part 2: Ultrasound diagnosis of the hip area. *Z Rheumatol* 2002;61:180–188.
23. Schmidt WA, Hauer RW, Banzer D, et al. Technique and value of arthrosonography in rheumatologic diagnosis. Part 3: Ultrasound diagnosis of the ankle joint, foot and toes. *Z Rheumatol* 2002;61: 279–290.
24. Sattler H. Sonography in rheumatology: Standard scans and dynamic examination of musculoskeletal system. *Akt Rheumatol* 2006; 31:123–127.
25. Strunk J. Color Doppler: Musculoskeletal sonography. *Akt Rheumatol* 2006;31:148–156.
26. Szkudlarek M, Court-Payen M, Strandberg C, et al. Contrast-enhanced power Doppler ultrasonography of the metacarpophalangeal joints in rheumatoid arthritis. *Eur Radiol* 2003;13:163–168.
27. Terslev L, Torp-Pedersen S, Savnik A, et al. Doppler ultrasound and magnetic resonance imaging of synovial inflammation of the hand in rheumatoid arthritis: A comparative study. *Arthritis Rheum* 2003;48:2434–2441.
28. Walther M, Harms H, Krenn V, et al. Correlation of power Doppler sonography with vascularity of the synovial tissue of the knee joint in patients with osteoarthritis and rheumatoid arthritis. *Arthritis Rheum* 2001;44:331–829.
29. Filippucci E, Iagnocco A, Salaffi F, et al. Power Doppler sonography monitoring of synovial perfusion at wrist joint in rheumatoid patients treated with adalimumab. *Ann Rheum Dis* 200665:1433–1437.
30. Ribbens C, Andre B, Marcelis S, et al. Rheumatoid hand joint synovitis: gray-scale and power Doppler US quantifications following anti-tumor necrosis factor-alpha treatment: Pilot study. *Radiology* 2003;229:562–569.
31. Goldberg BB, Liu JB, Forsberg F. Ultrasound contrast agents: A review. *Ultrasound Med Biol* 1994;20:319–333.
32. Blomley MJ, Cooke JC, Unger EC, et al. Microbubble contrast agents: A new era in ultrasound. *BMJ* 2001;322:1222–1225.
33. Klauser A, Frauscher F, Schirmer M, et al. The value of contrast-enhanced color Doppler ultrasound in the detection of vascularization of finger joints in patients with rheumatoid arthritis. *Arthritis Rheum* 2002;46:647–653.
34. Klauser A, Demharter J, De Marchi A, et al. for the IACUS study group. Contrast enhanced gray-scale sonography in assessment of joint vascularity in rheumatoid arthritis: Results from the IACUS study group. *Eur Radiol* 2005;15:2404–2410.
35. Kleffel T, Demharter J, Wohlgemuth W, et al. Comparison of contrast-enhanced low mechanical index (Low MI) sonography and unenhanced B-mode sonography for the differentiation between synovitis and joint effusion in patients with rheumatoid arthritis. *Rofo* 2005;177: 835–841.
36. Magarelli N, Guglielmi G, Di Matteo L, et al. Diagnostic utility of an echo-contrast agent in patients with synovitis using power Doppler ultrasound: A preliminary study with comparison to contrast-enhanced MRI. *Eur Radiol* 2001;11:1039–1046.
37. Carotti M, Salaffi F, Manganelli P, et al. Power Doppler sonography in the assessment of synovial tissue of the knee joint in rheumatoid arthritis: A preliminary experience. *Ann Rheum Dis* 2002;61: 877–882.
38. Zunterer H, Schirmer M, Klauser A. Contrast enhance sonography in rheumatic joint diseases. *Akt Rheumatol* 2006:31:157–161.
39. Wamser G, Bohndorf K, Vollert K, et al. Power Doppler sonography with and without echo-enhancing contrast agent and contrast-enhanced MRI for the evaluation of rheumatoid arthritis of the shoulder joint: Differentiation between synovitis and joint effusion. *Skeletal Radiol* 2003;32:351–359.
40. Song IH, Althoff CE, Hermann KG, et al. Knee OA efficacy of a new method of contrast-enhanced musculoskeletal ultrasonography in detection of synovitis in patients with knee osteoarthritis in comparison with magnetic resonance imaging. *Ann Rheum Dis* 2008; 76:19–25.

Outcome Measurement in Rheumatoid Arthritis: Magnetic Resonance Imaging

CHAPTER 9F

Jane E. Freeston and Philip G. Conaghan

To assess patient outcome in rheumatoid arthritis (RA) clinical trials, imaging techniques have been used in conjunction with markers of clinical and functional change. For many years, radiography has been the imaging modality of choice—primarily because of its ability to detect structural damage in the form of erosions and joint space narrowing as well as its reproducibility across multiple study sites. More recently, however, imaging has evolved such that simultaneous detection of both synovitis and structural damage is now possible using modalities such as magnetic resonance imaging (MRI) and ultrasound (US). Using such imaging modalities, which have an increased sensitivity for detecting pathology, has allowed dissection of the interrelationship between synovitis and bone damage[1] as well as increasing the statistical power of studies to show differences between treatment groups. As a result, MRI and US are increasingly utilized in studies both in terms of identifying features for entry into clinical trials and monitoring disease progression over time. In this chapter, we focus primarily on MRI because US has been addressed in a previous section.

MRI is arguably the most sensitive imaging modality,[2–4] and its tomographic nature allows visualization of the area of interest in three orthogonal planes. The main advantage of MRI is that it is able to provide superior detail of both the bone and surrounding soft tissue of the joint while avoiding ionizing radiation exposure for the patient.

Overview of Technical Aspects of Magnetic Resonance Imaging

The human body is primarily fat and water containing hydrogen atoms. These hydrogen atoms contain protons, each proton possessing a property known as "spin" (which acts as a small magnetic field and can produce an MR signal). When the proton is placed in an external magnetic field, the spin vector of the particle aligns itself with the external field. A magnetic field gradient allows each of the regions of spin to experience a unique magnetic field, making it possible to image their positions. MRI produces images based on spatial variations in the phase and frequency of the radio frequency energy being absorbed and emitted by the imaged object.

MRI is available in a range of field strengths. Conventional high-field machines have 1.5 or 3 Tesla (T) magnet strength, but low-field 0.2-T dedicated extremity MRI (eMRI) machines are increasingly available. High-field machines generally provide better image resolution, although this may not always be required depending on clinical need.

Pulse sequences used in musculoskeletal MR imaging include T1 weighted images that provide good anatomic detail of, for example, erosive bony change and synovial thickening but poor detection of soft-tissue edema and other T2-sensitive pathology. T2 fat suppressed and short tau inversion recovery (STIR) sequences allow detection of fluid and bone marrow edema.[5] The identification of synovitis on a T1 sequence can be enhanced by the use of intravenous gadolinium (Gd-DTPA) contrast injection. The heavy metal gadolinium exerts a paramagnetic effect on nearby water protons, causing them to relax more rapidly on T1 weighted sequences. The signal intensity increases in proportion to the concentration of Gd-DTPA, which distributes rapidly to vascular tissues. As a result, very vascular inflamed synovium (synovitis) enhances considerably.

Low-field MRI has a reduced number of image acquisition techniques and is not able to achieve frequency-selective fat saturation sequences. The low-field systems therefore use a STIR that provides a type of fat suppression image but the images are affected by poor SNR, limiting spatial resolution. To use MRI as an outcome measure, key pathologic hallmarks of RA such as erosions and synovitis are identified and followed over time. These are discussed in the material following.

Erosions and Their Measurement

A key advantage of high-field MRI over radiography is its increased sensitivity for erosion detection. The ability of MRI to identify "true" erosions has been shown by comparison with the gold standard of computed tomography (CT).[6,7] Erosion volume has also shown good correlation between these two modalities.[8] Figure 9F-1 shows an example of erosions in a rheumatoid wrist.

There are three methods currently used to measure erosions. One method is the semiquantitative method (known as the RA

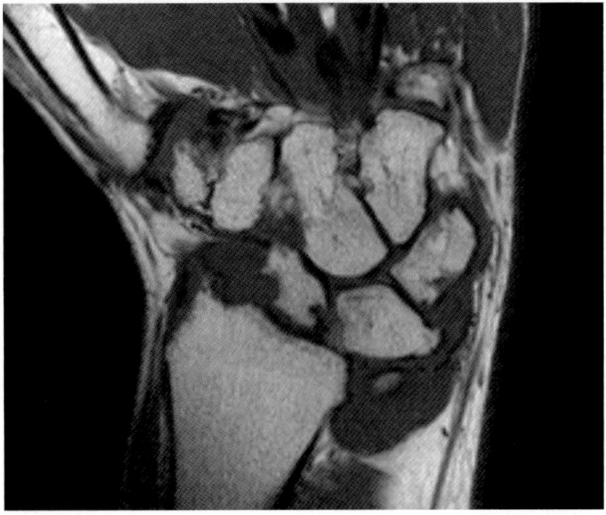

Figure 9F-1. MRI T1 SE coronal sequence of a rheumatoid wrist.

MRI score or RAMRIS) developed by the Outcome Measures in Rheumatoid Arthritis Clinical Trials (OMERACT) MRI collaborative subgroup.[9–11] Inter-reader reliability and sensitivity to change of the RAMRIS has been examined in a longitudinal setting with good results,[12] especially after training and calibration.[13] A modification of RAMRIS for use with eMRI with a reduced field of view has also been developed.[14] Other methods of erosion measurement include the numeric[1] and computer-assisted volumetric[15,16] methods.

Synovitis and Its Measurement

High-field MRI is also able to detect soft-tissue changes such as synovitis, which radiography cannot. An example of carpal synovitis in RA is shown in Figure 9F-2. The ability of MRI to detect synovitis is enhanced by the use of Gd-DTPA contrast, which allows further delineation between fluid collection and synovitis.

Measurement of synovitis can be semiquantitative (as in the RAMRIS scoring system) or quantitative. Quantitative assessment uses dynamic gadolinium-enhanced MRI (DEMRI), combining gadolinium contrast with rapid image acquisition by MRI. Analysis can be manual or semiautomated volume measures of single or multiple sections,[17] or it can be done as a dynamic estimation where the rate of Gd-DTPA enhancement and/or the maximum Gd-DTPA enhancement is measured[18,19] Both methods have been found to correlate with histologic evidence of synovitis.[20] There is still some debate as to whether the rate of enhancement as an absolute value (the E rate) should be used or whether it should be divided by the baseline signal intensity, thus incorporating an internal standard (the E ratio). Inaccuracy may occur with the latter when baseline signal intensity is low. This technique allows measurement of the rate of synovial enhancement, which can be used as a method of quantifying synovitis.[21] For example, studies such as that by Reece et al.[22] used the rate of synovial enhancement as an outcome measure to compare treatment groups in RA.

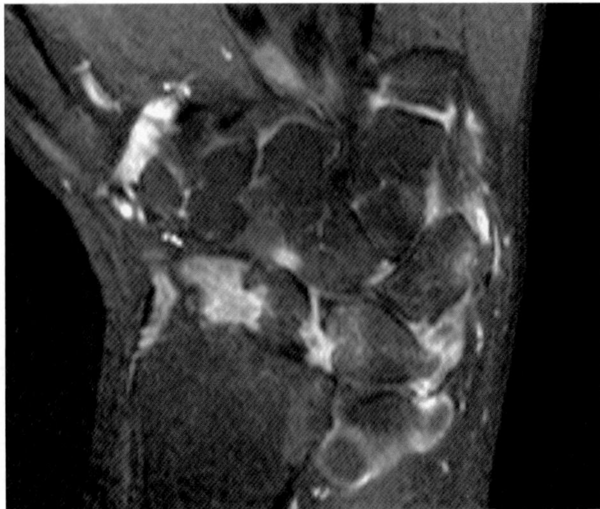

Figure 9F-2. MRI T1 SPIR postgadolinium coronal sequence of a rheumatoid wrist.

Bone Edema and Its Measurement

The term *bone edema* refers to increased signal intensity of bone on T2 weighted images after fat suppression and is due to an increased amount of water in the marrow. Bone edema was not a recognized finding in the rheumatoid joint before the advent of MRI[23] and is not associated with radiologic periarticular osteopenia.[24] Multiple studies have shown that bone edema, like synovitis, is a pre-erosive feature.[1,25] Recent validation work using bone samples obtained prior to joint replacement surgery has shown that bone edema represents osteitis (a cellular inflammatory infiltrate in subchondral bone), which represents the bone response to attack by inflamed synovium.[26,27]

Currently, bone edema is typically measured semiquantitatively, as in the RAMRIS scoring system. McQueen et al.[27] (in their recent histologic validation study of bone edema), however, used a different score combining (by multiplication) spatial extent and intensity semiquantitative scores.

Tenosynovitis and Its Measurement

MRI has been shown to be more sensitive than US[28] in detecting finger tendon inflammation in RA. Typically in studies, tendon involvement (tenosynovitis) has been reported as a dichotomous score (present or absent).[28] Recently, however, a semiquantitative tendon scoring system has been developed as an addition to RAMRIS. The system is joint/bone based, allowing more detailed assessment of tendons as part of clinical trials.[29]

Validation of Imaging Findings

As with all imaging techniques, it is important that changes seen on MRI represent true pathology—and this requires validation of imaging findings with histology. Validation in MRI has been extensively addressed using arthroscopy and synovial biopsy and comparing these with MRI synovial volume estimates.[18,19,30,31] This has been performed mainly in knees as well as mini-arthroscopy, macroscopic evaluation, and histology in the MCP joints. Ostendorf et al.[31] found that synovial enhancement post–Gd-DTPA on MRI correlated with macroscopic signs of synovitis, and joint space narrowing on MRI was significantly correlated with bony changes on arthroscopy. The validation of bone edema as osteitis was discussed previously.

Low-Field Extremity Magnetic Resonance Imaging

Dedicated eMRI using a significantly smaller 0.2 T magnet has both advantages and disadvantages compared to its high-field counterpart.[32] Cost is significantly reduced, and the machine can be situated conveniently in a suitable clinic room rather than requiring a purpose-built home setting (as for conventional MRI). The machine consists essentially of an opening in which the limb periphery containing the joints of interest is inserted, such as the metacarpophalangeal joints. There are no issues, therefore, of claustrophobia and positioning arthritic limbs that present so many problems with conventional MRI. Because of the reduction in the magnet strength, however, there is clearly some reduction in image quality—and studies have looked at whether this impacts significantly on the ability to detect synovitis and erosions.[33,34]

Use of Magnetic Resonance Imaging in Clinical Trials

Monitoring response to therapy in RA patients has been accomplished in the clinical setting and in the majority of studies by using serial plain film radiography of the hands and feet. More recently, with the advent of musculoskeletal MRI and greater accessibility to it some studies have incorporated MRI into their trial design. Ethically, trials must now compare active treatment arms resulting in slower progression and smaller differences between treatment groups. As a result, trials need to be substantially longer, with larger patient numbers, to achieve statistical significance. The advantage of using MRI compared to radiography stems from its greater sensitivity, which increases the power of a study (i.e., the ability to differentiate between two treatment arms). As a result, fewer patients are required and study duration is reduced.

The first randomized trial using MRI as an outcome measure was that by Conaghan et al. in early RA.[1] Using MRI allowed the authors to follow synovitis as well as bone erosions and to quantify synovial thickness to produce "area under the curve" results. Other examples in the literature include the study by Lee et al.,[35] who used MRI to monitor disease in 10 patients newly commenced on methotrexate and hydroxychloroquine—showing that the four patients who achieved clinical remission showed a decrease in synovial proliferation and bone marrow edema on MRI, with no new erosions over 12 months. Kalden-Nemeth[36] used MRI of wrist/knee/ankle to monitor patients treated with anti-TNF therapy, showing that changes in synovium signal intensity correlated well with clinical markers of inflammation. Ostergaard[37] used MRI of the knee to monitor changes following intra-articular corticosteroid, showing a decrease in synovial volume. Quinn et al.[38] assessed efficacy of very early treatment with infliximab in addition to methotrexate in poor-prognosis RA patients. Synovitis and structural damage in the form of erosions on MRI were significantly reduced by this therapeutic combination at 1 year when compared to the group receiving methotrexate alone.

The only published study to date using eMRI as an outcome measure for the assessment of therapeutic response was an open-label pilot protocol of RA patients who switched to infliximab after an incomplete response to etanercept.[39] In addition to standard radiography, eMRI of the metacarpophalangeal joints 2 and 3 and wrist of the most severely affected hand was performed. At week 14, there were no marked differences in the median number of erosions seen on MRI between the patients who received infliximab and those who continued on etanercept. However, the numbers in the study were small because it was a pilot design.

Summary

MRI is superior to the current gold standard of radiography as an outcome measure for clinical trials because it allows sensitive assessment of both bony and soft-tissue changes. Current disadvantages of MRI chiefly center on cost and availability, although the advent of eMRI will largely offset these problems. In the future, MRI synovitis measures could become the main outcome measure in clinical trials because better treatments are likely to reduce progressive structural joint damage to a minimum.[40]

References

1. Conaghan PG, O'Connor P, McGonagle D, et al. Elucidation of the relationship between synovitis and bone damage: A randomized magnetic resonance imaging study of individual joints in patients with early rheumatoid arthritis. *Arthritis Rheum* 2003;48(1):64–71.
2. Sugimoto H, Takeda A, Masuyama J, et al. Early-stage rheumatoid arthritis: Diagnostic accuracy of MR imaging. *Radiology* 1996;198(1): 185–192.
3. Ostergaard M, Hansen M, Stoltenberg M, et al. New radiographic bone erosions in the wrists of patients with rheumatoid arthritis are detectable with magnetic resonance imaging a median of two years earlier. *Arthritis Rheum* 2003;48(8):2128–2131.
4. Klarlund M, Ostergaard M, Jensen KE, et al. for the TIRA Group. Magnetic resonance imaging, radiography, and scintigraphy of the finger joints: One year follow up of patients with early arthritis. *Ann Rheum Dis* 2000;59(7):521–528.
5. Kaplan P, Helms C, Dussault R, et al. Basic principles of musculoskeletal MRI. *Musculoskeletal MRI.* Philadelphia: W.B. Saunders 2001:1–21.
6. Dohn UM, Ejbjerg BJ, Court-Payen M, et al. Are bone erosions detected by magnetic resonance imaging and ultrasonography true erosions? A comparison with computed tomography in rheumatoid arthritis metacarpophalangeal joints. *Arthritis Res Ther* 2006;8(4):R110.
7. Perry D, Stewart N, Benton N, et al. Detection of erosions in the rheumatoid hand: A comparative study of multidetector computerized tomography versus magnetic resonance scanning. *J Rheumatol* 2005;32(2):256–267.
8. Dohn UM, Ejbjerg BJ, Hasselquist M, et al. Rheumatoid arthritis bone erosion volumes on CT and MRI: Reliability and correlations with erosion scores on CT, MRI and radiography. *Ann Rheum Dis* 2007;66(10):1388–1392.

9. Ostergaard M, Klarlund M, Lassere M, et al. Interreader agreement in the assessment of magnetic resonance images of rheumatoid arthritis wrist and finger joints: An international multicenter study. *J Rheumatol* 2001;28(5):1143–1150.
10. Ostergaard M, Peterfy C, Conaghan P, et al. OMERACT Rheumatoid Arthritis Magnetic Resonance Imaging Studies: Core set of MRI acquisitions, joint pathology definitions, and the OMERACT RA-MRI scoring system. *J Rheumatol* 2003;30(6):1385–1386.
11. Lassere M, McQueen F, Ostergaard M, et al. OMERACT Rheumatoid Arthritis Magnetic Resonance Imaging Studies. Exercise 3: An international multicenter reliability study using the RA-MRI Score. *J Rheumatol* 2003;30(6):1366–1375.
12. Haavardsholm EA, Ostergaard M, Ejbjerg BJ, et al. Reliability and sensitivity to change of the OMERACT rheumatoid arthritis magnetic resonance imaging score in a multireader, longitudinal setting. *Arthritis Rheum* 2005;52(12):3860–3867.
13. Bird P, Joshua F, Lassere M, et al. Training and calibration improve inter-reader reliability of joint damage assessment using magnetic resonance image scoring and computerized erosion volume measurement. *J Rheumatol* 2005;32(8):1452–1458.
14. Freeston J, Olech E, Yocum D, et al. A modification of the OMERACT RA MRI score for use with an extremity MRI system with reduced field of view. *Ann Rheum Dis* 2007;66:1669–1671.
15. Bird P, Ejbjerg B, McQueen F, et al. OMERACT Rheumatoid Arthritis Magnetic Resonance Imaging Studies. Exercise 5: An international multicenter reliability study using computerized MRI erosion volume measurements. *J Rheumatol* 2003;30(6):1380–1384.
16. Bird P, Lassere M, Shnier R, et al. Computerized measurement of magnetic resonance imaging erosion volumes in patients with rheumatoid arthritis: A comparison with existing magnetic resonance imaging scoring systems and standard clinical outcome measures. *Arthritis Rheum* 2003;48(3):614–624.
17. Ostergaard M, Hansen M, Stoltenberg M, et al. Quantitative assessment of the synovial membrane in the rheumatoid wrist: An easily obtained MRI score reflects the synovial volume. *J RheumatolBr J Rheumatol* 1996;35(10):965–971.
18. Tamai K, Yamato M, Yamaguchi T, et al. Dynamic magnetic resonance imaging for the evaluation of synovitis in patients with rheumatoid arthritis. *Arthritis Rheum* 1994;37(8):1151–1157.
19. Gaffney K, Cookson J, Blake D, et al. Quantification of rheumatoid synovitis by magnetic resonance imaging. *Arthritis Rheum* 1995;38(11):1610–1617.
20. Ostergaard M, Hansen M, Stoltenberg M, et al. Magnetic resonance imaging-determined synovial membrane volume as a marker of disease activity and a predictor of progressive joint destruction in the wrists of patients with rheumatoid arthritis. *Arthritis Rheum* 1999;42(5):918–929.
21. Cimmino M, Innocenti S, Livrone F, et al. Dynamic gadolinium-enhanced magnetic resonance imaging of the wrist in patients with rheumatoid arthritis can discriminate active from inactive disease. *Arthritis Rheum* 2003;48(5):1207–1213.
22. Reece RJ, Kraan MC, Radjenovic A, et al. Comparative assessment of leflunomide and methotrexate for the treatment of rheumatoid arthritis, by dynamic enhanced magnetic resonance imaging. *Arthritis Rheum* 2002;46(2):366–372.
23. McQueen FM. Magnetic resonance imaging in early inflammatory arthritis: What is its role? *Rheumatology* (Oxford) 2000;39(7): 700–706.
24. Peterfy C. MR imaging. *Baillieres Clin Rheumatol* 1996;10:635–678.
25. McQueen FM, Stewart N, Crabbe J, et al. Magnetic resonance imaging of the wrist in early rheumatoid arthritis reveals progression of erosions despite clinical improvement. *Annals of the Rheumatic Diseases* 1999;58(3):156–163.
26. Jimenez-Boj E, Nobauer-Huhmann I, Hanslik-Schnabel B, et al. Bone erosions and bone marrow edema as defined by magnetic resonance imaging reflect true bone marrow inflammation in rheumatoid arthritis. *Arthritis Rheum* 2007;56(4):1118–1124.
27. McQueen FM, Gao A, Ostergaard M, et al. High-grade MRI bone edema is common within the surgical field in rheumatoid arthritis patients undergoing joint replacement and is associated with osteitis in subchondral bone. *Ann Rheum Dis* 2007;66(12):1581–1587.
28. Wakefield RJ, O'Connor PJ, Conaghan PG, et al. Finger tendon disease in untreated early rheumatoid arthritis: A comparison of ultrasound and magnetic resonance imaging. *Arthritis Rheum* 2007;57(7):1158–1164.
29. Haavardsholm EA, Ostergaard M, Ejbjerg BJ, et al. Introduction of a novel magnetic resonance imaging tenosynovitis score for rheumatoid arthritis: Reliability in a multireader longitudinal study. *Ann Rheum Dis* 2007;66(9):1216–1220.
30. Ostergaard M, Stoltenberg M, Lovgreen-Nielsen P, et al. Magnetic resonance imaging-determined synovial membrane and joint effusion volumes in rheumatoid arthritis and osteoarthritis: Comparison with the macroscopic and microscopic appearance of the synovium. *Arthritis Rheum* 1997;40(10):1856–1867.
31. Ostendorf B, Peters R, Dann P, et al. Magnetic resonance imaging and miniarthroscopy of metacarpophalangeal joints: Sensitive detection of morphologic changes in rheumatoid arthritis. *Arthritis Rheum* 2001;44(11):2492–2502.
32. Peterfy C, Roberts T, Genant H. Dedicated extremity MR imaging: an emerging technology. *Magn Reson Imaging Clin North Am* 1998;6(4):849–870.
33. Freeston JE, Conaghan PG, Dass S, et al. Does extremity-MRI improve erosion detection in severely damaged joints? A study of long-standing rheumatoid arthritis using three imaging modalities. *Ann Rheum Dis* 2007;66(11):1538–1540.
34. Ejbjerg B, Narvestad E, Jacobsen S, et al. Optimised, low cost, low field dedicated extremity MRI is highly specific and sensitive for synovitis and bone erosions in rheumatoid arthritis wrist and finger joints: A comparison with conventional high-field MRI and radiography. *Ann Rheum Dis* 2005;64(9):1280–1287.
35. Lee J, Lee S, Suh J, et al. Magnetic resonance imaging of the wrist in defining remission of rheumatoid arthritis. *J Rheumatol* 1997;24: 1303–1308.
36. Kalden-Nemeth D, Grebmeier J, Antoni C, et al. NMR monitoring of rheumatoid arthritis patients receiving anti-TNFα monoclonal antibody therapy. *Rheumatol Int* 1997;16:249–255.
37. Ostergaard M, Stoltenberg M, Henriksen O, et al. Quantitative assessment of synovial inflammation by dynamic gadolinium-enhanced magnetic resonance imaging: A study of the effect of intra-articular methylprednisolone on the rate of early synovial enhancement. *Br J RheumatolJ Rheumatol* 1996;35(1):50–59.
38. Quinn MA, Conaghan PG, O'Connor PJ, et al. Very early treatment with infliximab in addition to methotrexate in early, poor-prognosis rheumatoid arthritis reduces magnetic resonance imaging evidence of synovitis and damage, with sustained benefit after infliximab withdrawal: Results from a twelve-month randomized, double-blind, placebo-controlled trial. *Arthritis Rheum* 2005;52(1):27–35.
39. Furst DE, Gaylis N, Bray V, et al. Open-label, pilot protocol of patients with rheumatoid arthritis who switch to infliximab after an incomplete response to etanercept: The opposite study. *Ann Rheum Dis* 2007;66(7):893–899.
40. Ostergaard M, Duer A, Moller U, et al. Magnetic resonance imaging of peripheral joints in rheumatic diseases. *Best Pract Res Clin Rheumatol* 2004;18(6):861–879.

Physical Examination

Edward Keystone and Deborah Weber

CHAPTER 9G

Joint examination is a key element in the assessment of the clinical status of rheumatoid arthritis (RA). It is regarded by rheumatologists as the most important measure of the assessment both in clinical trials and daily practice.[1–4] The joint examination measures disease activity by the number of tender and swollen joints, functional status by the limitation of joint motion, and joint damage by deformity and bone-on-bone crepitation.

The physician's emphasis on joint counts as a measure of disease activity is supported by the inclusion of the tender and swollen joint count as prominent components of all composite indices of disease activity, such as the ACR and DAS. Any discrepancies between patient and physician global assessments within the composite indices derive mainly from the joint examination. Subjective patient disease activity measures such as pain, fatigue, and functional status are associated with patients' reporting higher disease activity than physicians—whereas swollen joints, tender joints, and ESR are associated with the physicians' reporting higher disease activity than their patients.[5]

Given the prominent role the joint examination plays in the physician global assessment it is surprising that joint counts no longer appear to be systemically conducted in clinical practice as part of the assessment of disease activity.[6] This is particularly concerning given the predictive value of the swollen joint count for radiographic damage both in early and established disease.[7,8] The modest level of correlation between the swollen joint count and radiographic progression as determined by the Sharp score likely reflects the difference between joints evaluated clinically and those evaluated radiographically. Difficulty in accurately determining joint effusions in the feet also contributes to the problem. A similar discrepancy between the joint count and physical function as determined by the health assessment questionnaire (HAQ) relates to the fact that the joint count is a reflection of disease activity and the HAQ score reflects both disease activity and joint damage. It is of significance that patients' perception of their disease activity correlates best with the tender (but not the swollen) joint count, emphasizing the concept that not all swollen joints are tender/painful (and visa versa).[9]

Although increased use of patient self-reported outcomes in routine clinical practice reflects the importance of these outcomes to patients, their use as the sole outcome in therapeutic decision making may be misleading because patient-reported outcomes do not accurately reflect the status of disease activity as determined by joint inflammation.[10] The discrepancy between patient perception and joint examination has significant implications for how patients are evaluated in therapeutic decision making. The data suggest that a formal joint count should form an essential part of a patient assessment regardless of how a patient perceives their disease activity.

Another concept not widely appreciated is the poor relationship between the joint count and ESR/CRP. Thus, several studies have documented a very low correlation (r=0.2–0.4) between the swollen joint count and ESR or CRP—suggesting that inflammation as assessed by the joint examination is not synonymous with that measured by acute-phase reactants.[11,12] It is for this reason that composite indices include physician- and patient-reported outcomes in concert with acute-phase reactants (each of the indices reflects a different element of disease activity).[13,14]

The joint count has been shown to be a valid and generally reproducible measure. Tender joint counts are reproducible, particularly, after standardization of observances. The swollen joint count is not as reproducible, and variability is only modestly reduced with training.[15] Despite its utility as a measure of disease activity, a complete 66/68 joint count is labor intensive and cumbersome in clinical practice. To simplify the count without losing validity, studies of the Fuches 28 joint count were carried out.[16,17] The studies involved reanalysis of various patient cohorts for validity and reliability to detect high and low disease activity as well as sensitivity to change in various full and reduced joint counts. The results demonstrated only small differences with respect to validity, and similar effect sizes with similar sensitivity to change for the 28 joint count compared to the full count. No advantage was demonstrated for weighting by joint size or grading of severity. On the basis of these findings by the European League Against Rheumatism (EULAR), a subcommittee of the ACR recommended the Fuches unweighted 28 joint count for use in clinical trials. Smolen et al. also investigated the validity of the 28 joint count in comparison to the 66/68 count.[18] They noted that findings from the 28 joint count correlated highly with those from the 66/68 count in all analyses. They considered the 28 joint count to be a reliable and valid measure and easier to perform than the 66/68 count in all analyses. The 28 joint count includes shoulders, elbows, wrists, MCP and PIP joints in the hands, and knees. The joints of the ankles and feet were particularly excluded because of perceived problems in reliably distinguishing joint swelling from soft-tissue swelling or edema and joint tenderness secondary to inflammation from that of secondary mechanical problems related to periarticular structures. Although the hips and feet are not part of the 28 joint count, they are important for evaluation in routine care.

More recently, Pham et al. provided recommendations regarding physical and laboratory tests in the management of RA patients for clinical practice based on published evidence and expert opinion.[1] They recommended that minimal physical data be collected for monitoring patients in order to compute the DAS28 or Simple Disease Activities Index (SDAI). They suggested that other symptomatic joints and extra-articular features be noted as well as morning stiffness. Physical variables should be collected at 3-month intervals.

Principles of Joint Examination

Clinical evaluation of joints in RA involve measures of inflammatory activity, destruction, and extra-articular features. Measures of joint inflammation include tenderness, stress pain, and synovial effusion. Measures of joint damage include collateral ligament laxity, subluxation, malalignment, bone-on-bone crepitations, and reduced range of motion. Measures of extra-articular features include assessment of skin nodules.

Inflammatory Activity

Evaluation of a joint always involves initial inspection, followed by palpation and range of motion. Inspection consists of evaluation for skin lesions and color over the joint, swelling, deformity, and periarticular muscle wasting. In RA, a severely inflamed joint has a dusky cyanotic color, erythema, and heat. Erythema is not usually a feature of RA. Erythema over the joint is more consistent with sepsis, crystal arthropathy, and spondyloarthropathies such as psoriatic arthritis or a reactive arthritis. Warmth of the joint to the touch may reflect idiopathic inflammatory arthropathy or osteoarthritis. Normally, the skin over the joint (e.g., the knee) is cooler than the regions of the leg proximal and distal to the knee. Tenderness elicited by palpation over the joint line is generally an indicator of an inflamed joint. The level of pressure to elicit tenderness can be determined by the pressure required to blanche the examiner's fingernail. In contrast, pain on joint movement may reflect inflammation or severe loss of cartilage with articulation of bone rubbing on bone. A sign specific for inflammation is stress pain. Stress pain is elicited by moving a joint to the limit of its range of motion and then pushing a little further. If performed properly, damaged joints without inflammation will not elicit stress pain. A synovial effusion is elicited by ballottement or fluctuation, where pressure is applied over one part of the joint to elicit an outward bulge in another part of the joint (Figure 9G-1). This technique is exemplified by pushing on a balloon with one hand and feeling the pressure with the other. Most joints apart from the PIP or DIP joints of the fingers are assessed using a two-finger technique (i.e., two thumbs), with the application of pressure on the joint line by one digit and sensation of an outward bulge by the other. Of importance, ballottement of larger joints (e.g., shoulders, wrists, and ankles) should be performed such that the palpating fingers (thumbs) follow the direction of muscle or tendon (Figure 9G-1). If ballottement is carried out with the palpating fingers at right angles to the direction of the muscle fibers or tendons, false positive ballottement will be elicited by pushing one muscle or tendon against the other. Ballottement with the thumbs aligned parallel to the direction of the muscle or tendon will elicit fluctuation only if fluid (and/or synovium) is present. Movement of muscles or tendons will not confound the findings. The joint that is swollen with fluid/synovium usually feels "spongy" or "boggy" in contrast to the nonfluctuant, firm, capsular thickening or boney-hard joint margins observed in patients with osteoarthritis or psoriatic arthritis. In the experience of the authors, fluid cannot be differentiated from synovial thickening.

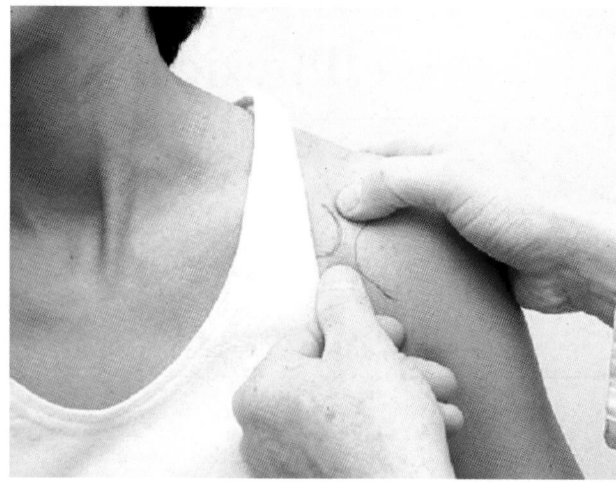

Figure 9G-1. Ballottement of shoulder joint for swelling of humeral head and coracoid.

The purpose of this chapter is to emphasize more sensitive techniques to evaluate joint tenderness and swelling. Utilization of the techniques will help in making appropriate therapeutic decisions based on sound physician-derived outcomes in concert with patient-reported outcomes and laboratory measures.

Individual Joint Evaluation: a Few Tips

The shoulder is first inspected for swelling over the joint line anteriorly. Rotator cuff involvement may exhibit swelling laterally just inferior to the lateral acromion. Fluctuency over the shoulder joint may be evaluated by two techniques: pressure over the joint line with both hands pressing back and forth anteriorly and posteriorly or a two-thumb technique with the thumbs balloting parallel to the deltoid muscle belly (Figure 9G-1). The frequency of detecting synovial fluid within the shoulders varies, with estimates varying between 10% and 30%. The low yield may reflect the technical difficulty in eliciting small amounts of fluid in this joint.[19] Tenderness is elicited by pressure over the anterior joint line. Stress pain in the shoulder is best elicited with the shoulder laterally abducted to a horizontal plane and then internally rotated to its maximum range. Stress pain elicited on internal rotation usually suggests true shoulder synovitis. Limitation of glenohumeral movement is compatible with true shoulder involvement, whereas limited scapulothoracic movement in the context of normal glenohumeral motion is in keeping with a rotator cuff disorder. Confirmation of a rotator cuff problem may be assessed by eliciting a painful arc, impingement sign, or "empty can" and "drop arm sign." Detailed descriptions of these signs are beyond the scope of this chapter and are published elsewhere.[20]

Elbow

Inspection of the elbow for an effusion is performed by evaluating the horizontal crease between the lateral epicondyle and olecranon. This is best demonstrated by extending the elbow from a flexed position to full extension and watching for the crease to fill in and then bulge outward (Figure 9G-2 and 9G-3). Palpation for an effusion is carried out in the same manner by placing the thumb in the crease of the flexed elbow and extending it to feel the fluid bulge outward (Figure 9G-3). Joint line tenderness is achieved by pressing laterally over the joint line between the lateral epicondyle of the humerus and radial head. Stress pain is best elicited with the joint in full extension.

Wrist

Careful inspection of the wrist is important to discern the nature of the swelling (i.e., a joint effusion or common extensor tenosynovitis). Wasting of the small muscles of the hand should be noted as a measure of severity of hand dysfunction.

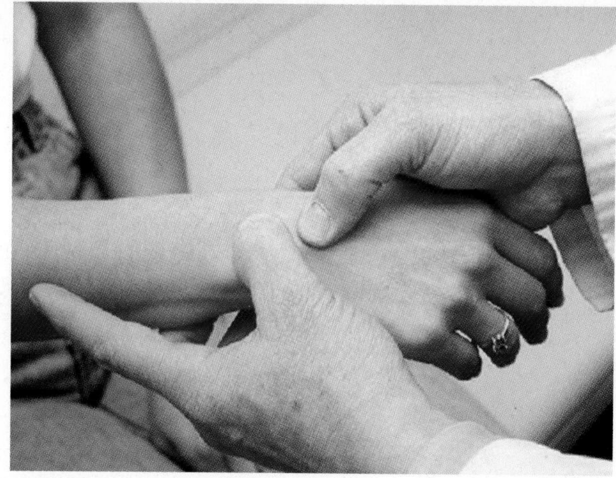

Figure 9G-4. Ballottement of wrist joint for swelling.

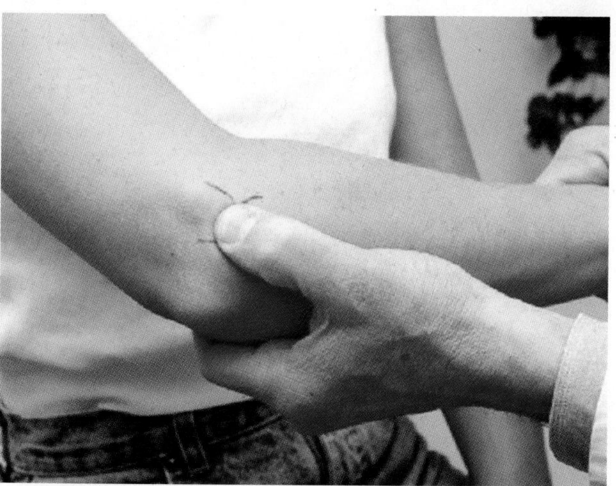

Figure 9G-2. Palpation of elbow joint for tenderness and swelling with elbow in flexion.

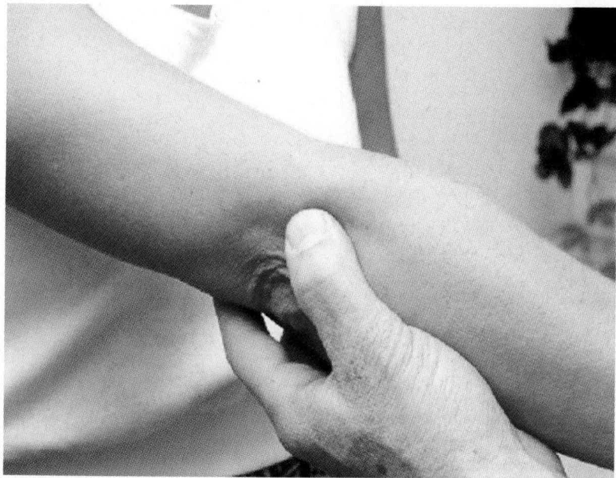

Figure 9G-3. Palpation of elbow joint for swelling with elbow in extension.

A radiocarpal joint effusion is usually seen on the radial aspect of the dorsum of the wrist extending distally. Ballottement of the wrist for swelling is performed using a two-thumb technique with the thumbs aligned parallel to the tendons (Figure 9G-4). Tenderness is elicited by pressure over the dorsal aspect of the joint line. Stress pain is best elicited with full flexion of the wrist. In contrast to the radiocarpal joint effusion, dorsal swelling of the common extensor tenosynovial sheath is detected centrally over the joint line extending distally to ⅓ the distance between the radiocarpal joint and metacarpal heads. To determine the presence of common extensor tenosynovitis, the patient is asked to perform a "tuck sign" maneuver by which they extend all their fingers with the wrist held in a neutral position. The presence of tenosynovitis will be demonstrated by increased swelling in the area and the presence of a folding or tucking of the skin under at the distal edge of the common extensor sheath swelling. No such tuck sign is observed with radiocarpal joint swelling. Ventral swelling of the wrist is particularly important in the context of carpal tunnel symptoms.

Metacarpalphalangeal Joints

Inspection of the dorsum of metacarpalphalangeal (MCP) joints for swelling has been shown to be a good predictor of a joint effusion, assuming that there is fluctuance over the joint. The most common technique for eliciting a joint effusion in the MCP is the two-thumb technique balloting on either side of the joint line for fluctuancy with the MCP slightly flexed (Figure 9G-5). Stress pain of the MCP elicited by extension may generate a false positive signal for synovitis if flexor tenosynovitis is present. Joint line tenderness or stress pain on flexion might be more reliable to distinguish between the two sites of inflammation.

Proximal Interphalangeal Joints

Inspection of the proximal interphalangeal (PIP) joints often demonstrates a fusiform swelling when a substantial joint effusion is present. Loss of the horizontal creases over the dorsum of

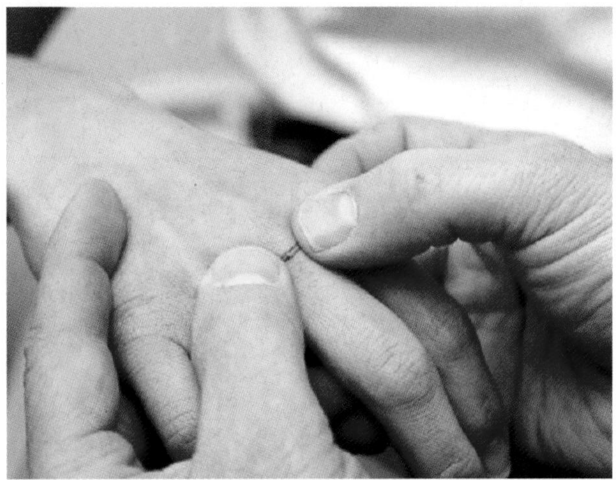

Figure 9G-5. Palpation of MCP joint for tenderness and swelling (by ballottement). Joint line is depicted between thumbs.

the joint may be the earliest sign of joint swelling. Two techniques have been utilized for detection of a PIP effusion. One technique is that of ballottement over the dorsum of an extended PIP joint with the thumbs placed dorso-medially and dorso-laterally—one being the "pressor" and the other the "sensor." A second approach is the use of four fingers (i.e., with one thumb and index finger of one hand placed dorsally and ventrally, respectively, to the joint with the other thumb and index finger on the sides of the joint). The pressors may be dorsal and ventral, with the sensors at 90 degrees to the other two fingers. A more sensitive way to detect an effusion over the PIP is to place the dorsal and ventral fingers slightly proximal over the joint so that the distal portion of the fingers are aligned over the center of the joint. The medially and laterally placed fingers should be placed slightly dorsal to the midpoint of the joint (Figure 9G-6). In this way, the fluid is captured more over the dorsal aspect of the finger away from the collateral ligaments (which may prevent detection of the joint fluid). Tenderness is elicited by squeezing the sides of the joint, whereas stress pain is elicited by extending the joint.

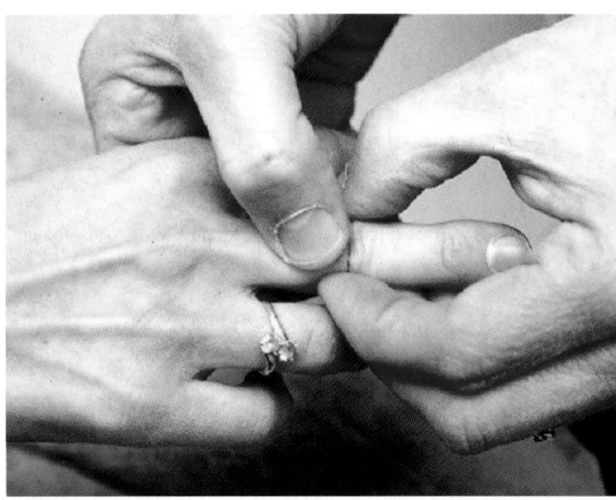

Figure 9G-6. Ballottement of PIP of the hand joint for swelling. Joint line is depicted distal to the thumb.

Knee Joint

Inspection of the knee joint involves evaluation of quadriceps wasting. A small joint effusion is detected by observing the loss of the hollow over the medial joint line with the knee extended. Palpation for a joint effusion can be assessed by one of three techniques. By the first method, a small effusion (<15 cc) is detected by the "fluid bulge" sign where fluid is pushed proximally over the medial aspect of the knee to the superpatellar pouch with one hand (Figure 9G-7) and then "milked" distally with the other hand inferiorly down the lateral aspect of the knee (Figure 9G-8). A fluid bulge is observed as a fluid wave migrates distally from the suprapatellar pouch down the medial aspect of the knee joint. Of critical importance to detecting a fluid wave is the position of the knee with the patella directly superior without external rotation of the leg. The tendency for patients to lie with the leg externally rotated for comfort makes

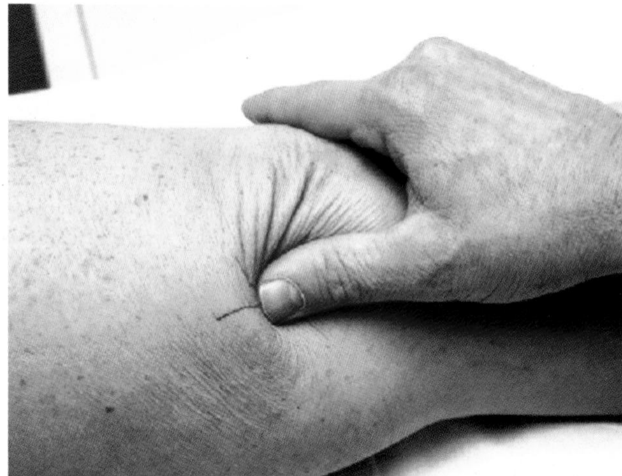

Figure 9G-7. Pushing over medial joint line to milk synovial fluid proximally into suprapatellar pouch for the "fluid bulge sign."

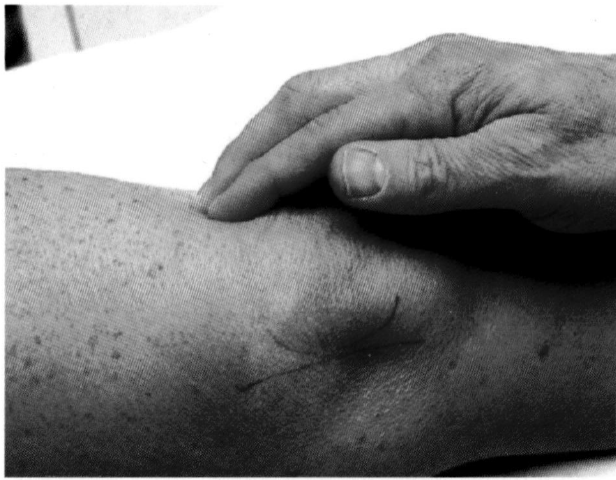

Figure 9G-8. Pushing over lateral joint line to milk synovial fluid distally into the medial aspect of joint for the "fluid bulge sign." The lines depict the patello-femoral articulation on the medial aspect of the joint.

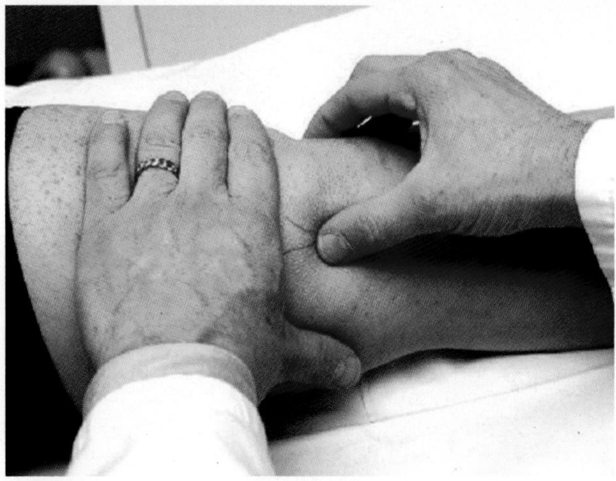

Figure 9G-9. Ballottement of the knee joint by compressing the suprapatellar space and sensing bulge with thumb and index fingers over the joint line.

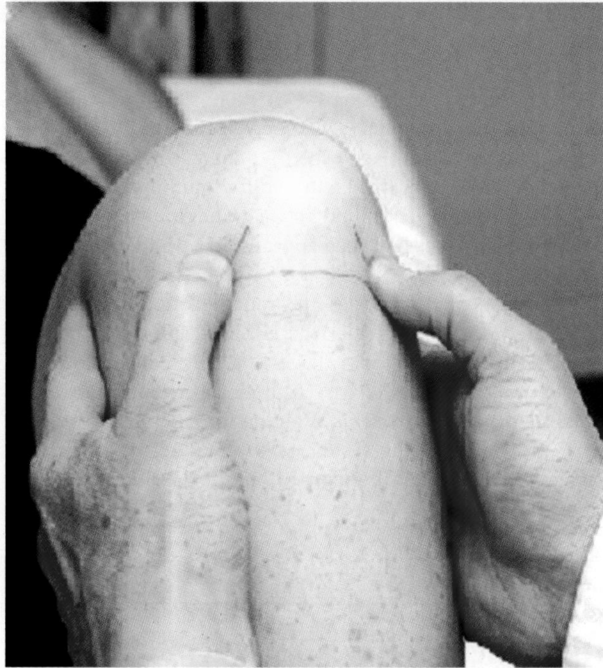

Figure 9G-10. Palpation of the knee joint in flexion for tenderness. Lines depict the femoral condyles and tibial plateau of the knee.

it difficult to illicit a fluid bulge. The second method (the most sensitive technique to elicit an effusion in the knee in which there is a substantial amount of swelling) is to ballot the joint using the thumb and index finger of one hand straddling each side of the joint (Figure 9G-9). The suprapatellar pouch is then compressed to push the fluid distally, where it is detected between the thumb and index finger (Figure 9G-9). An alternative approach for those skilled in the art is to straddle the joint with the thumb and index finger of both hands (as previously described) and ballot the joint side to side to feel the fluid fluctuate between the four fingers. The third method, the patellar tap, is the least specific technique for detection of an effusion because obesity may elicit a false positive sign. In this technique, fluid is "milked" inferiorly from the suprapatellar pouch while the patella is pushed dorsally against the joint line. If there is enough fluid to float the patella away from the joint line, a tapping sensation will be elicited on compressing the patella.

For tenderness to be elicited, the knee should be flexed approximately 90 degrees and palpated with the thumbs placed anterolaterally along the joint line (Figure 9G-10). Stress pain in the knee is carried out with the knee fully extended. Stress pain with the knee fully extended detects tibiofemoral inflammation. Stress pain with the knee fully flexed elicits more patellofemoral disease (i.e., chondromalcia patellae). Detection of knee deformity and a Bakers cyst is performed with the patient weight bearing.

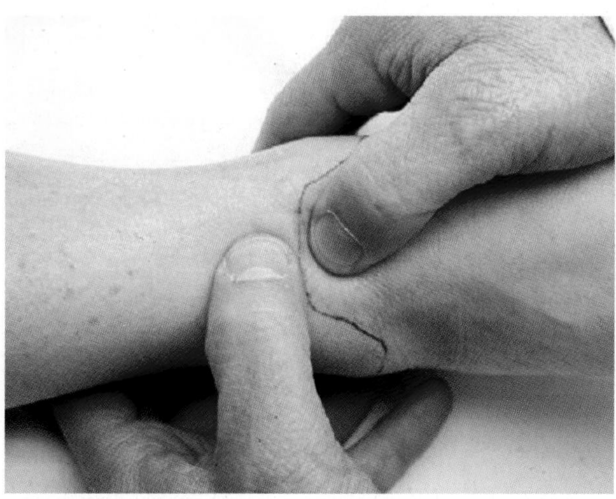

Figure 9G-11. Ballottement of the ankle joint for swelling. Joint line is depicted between the thumbs.

Ankle Joint

Swelling of the ankle joint is best detected centrally over the dorsum of the joint. Lateral or medial swelling about the ankle may denote peroneal or posterior tibial tenosynovitis, respectively. A joint effusion is best detected by evaluation of flucuancy with two thumbs aligned proximally and distally over the joint line in line with the extensor tendons (Figure 9G-11). The ankle comprises three joints that can elicit overlapping symptoms. The joints of particular interest are the true ankle joint (tibiotalar joint), subtalar joint (talocalcaneal joint), and mid-tarsal joint (talonavicular joint). Joint swelling is only readily detectable in the tibiotalar joint. In contrast, each joint can be evaluated for inflammation by stress pain. The tibiotalar joint is best evaluated for stress pain by the extremes of plantar flexion. Tenderness over the joint line anteriorily may also be elicited. Subtalar joint inflammation is detected by rocking the joint to the extremes of inversion or eversion while stabilizing the distal end of the tibia with the other hand. Tenderness just inferior to the fibula with the joint inverted may also be used. Stress pain in the mid-tarsal joint is evaluated by stabilizing the heel joint and twisting the mid-foot or pressing over the joint (Figure 9G-11).

Metatarsalphalangeal Joints

Metatarsalphalangeal (MTP) joints are the most difficult to evaluate with respect to joint swelling. Some advocate palpating the plantar aspect of the MTP for soft-tissue swelling or feeling the "thickness" of the distal foot over the MTP joint region. Another technique that may detect MTP effusions is ballottement over the dorsum of the MTP joint line using two thumbs placed parallel to the tendons (Figure 9G-12). A three-finger technique may be used with the thumb and index finger of one hand placed in a pinching configuration just proximal to the joint line and the other thumb placed distally to capture a "pocket" of fluid between the three fingers. None of these techniques has been appropriately validated by ultrasound or MRI.

Evaluation of deformities and range of motion have been adequately documented elsewhere.[21] It is critical that patients with inflammatory arthritis have a careful joint examination at each visit to assess disease activity and to monitor the effects of drug therapy. This examination should be well described, and a scoring system of the number of tender and swollen joints should be used to record the outcome in the office note.

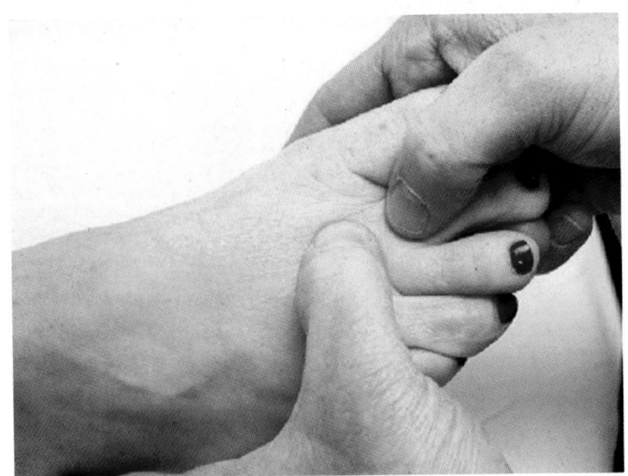

Figure 9G-12. Ballottement of the MTP joint.

References

1. Pham T, Grossec L, Fautrel B, et al. Physical examination and laboratory tests in the management of patients with rheumatoid arthritis: Development of recommendations for clinical practice based on published evidence and expert opinion. *Joint Bone Spine* 2005;72: 222–228.
2. Wolfe F, O'Dell J R, Kavanaugh A, et al. Evaluating severity and status in rheumatoid arthritis. *J Rheum* 2001;28(6):1453–1462.
3. Wolfe F, Pincus T, Thompson AK, et al. The assessment of rheumatoid arthritis and the acceptability of self-report questionnaires in clinical practice. *Arthritis Care Res* 2003;49(1):59–63.
4. van der Heide A, Johannes WG, Jacobs HJ, et al. The impact of endpoint measures in rheumatoid arthritis clinical trials. *Seminars in Arthritis and Rheumatism* 1992;21(5):287–294.
5. Leeb B, Sautner J, Leeb BA, et al. Lack of agreement between patients' and physician perspectives of rheumatoid arthritis disease activity changes. *Scand J Rheum* 2006;35:441–446.
6. Pincus T, Segurado OG. Most visits of most patients with rheumatoid arthritis to most rheumatologists do not include a formal quantitative joint count. *Ann Rheum Dis* 2006;65:820–822.
7. Thompson PW, Kirwan JR. Joint counts: A review of old and new articular indices of joint inflammation. *British Journal of Rheumatology* 1995;34:1003–1008.
8. Sokka T, Kautiainen H, Mottonen T, et al. Erosions develop rarely in joints without clinically detectable inflammation in patients with early rheumatoid arthritis. *J Rheumatol* 2003;30:2580–2584.
9. Hanley JG, Mosher D, Sutton E, et al. Self-assessment of disease activity by patients with rheumatoid arthritis. *J Rheum* 1996;23: 1531–1538.
10. Jamal S, Donka T, Kitamura C, et al. Patient derived outcomes alone are not sufficient for assessment of disease activity: The need for physical examination. *Arthritis Rheum* 2007;34(7):1391.
11. Thompson PW, Silman AJ, Kirwan JR, et al. Articular indices of joint inflammation with rheumatoid arthritis: Correlation with the acute-phase response. *Arthritis Rheum* 1987;30:618–623.
12. Wolfe F. Comparative usefulness of C-reactive protein and erythrocyte sedimentation rate in patients with rheumatoid arthritis. *J Rheumatol* 1997;24:1477–1485.
13. Felson DT, Anderson JJ, Boers M, et al. The American College of Rheumatology preliminary core set of disease activity measures for rheumatoid arthritis clinical trials. *Arthritis Rheum* 1993;36:729–740.
14. Aletaha D, Smolen J. The simplified disease activity index (SDAI) and the clinical disease activity index (CDAI): A review of their usefulness and validity in rheumatoid arthritis. *Clin Exp Rheumatol* 2005;23:S100–S108.
15. Klinkhoff AV, Bellamy N, Bombardier, et al. An experiment in reducing interobserver variability of the examination for joint tenderness. *J Rheumatol* 1988;15:492–494.
16. Fuchs HA, Pincus T. Reduced joint counts in controlled clinical trials in rheumatoid arthritis. *Arthritis and Rheumatism* 1994;37:470–475.
17. Fuchs HA, Brooks RH, Callahan LF, et al. A simplified twenty-eight quantitative articular index in rheumatoid arthritis. *Arthritis and Rheumatism* 1989;32;531–665.
18. Smolen JS, Breedveld FC, Eberl G, et al. Validity and reliability of the twenty-eight-joint count for the assessment of rheumatoid arthritis activity. *Arthritis Rheum* 1995;38:38–43.
19. Luukkainen R, Samla MT, Luukkainen P. Poor relationship between joint swelling detected by physical examination and effusions diagnosed by ultrasonography in glenohumeral joints in patients with rheumatoid arthritis. *Clin Rheumatol* 2007;26:865–867.
20. Park HB, Yokota A, Gill HS, et al. Diagnostic accuracy of clinical tests for the different degrees of subacromial impingement syndrome. *J Bone Joint Surg Am* 2005;87:1446–1455.
21. Fam A, Lawry GV, Kreder HJ. *Musculoskeletal Examination and Joint Injection Techniques*. Philadelphia: Mosby/Elsevier 2006.

Pharmacoeconomic Aspects of Rheumatoid Arthritis Management

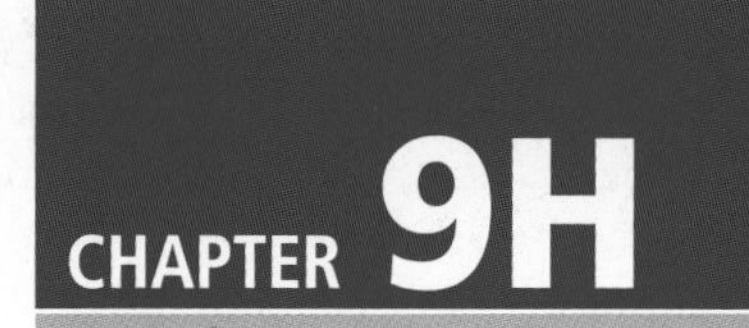

Daniel H. Solomon and Arthur Kavanaugh

Rheumatoid arthritis (RA) causes substantial morbidity and mortality as well as significant economic burden. The direct and indirect medical costs associated with RA comprise only a portion of its costs. Because it often strikes people in their fourth through sixth decades, work disability is extremely common and represents a significant part of its overall expense.[1] Lost wages from RA-related disability form an extremely important backdrop when considering the increasing cost of pharmacotherapy for RA. Biologic disease-modifying antirheumatic drugs (DMARDs) typically cost $10,000 to 20,000 per year. However, if they reduce morbidity and disability to a great enough extent they might be considered a worthwhile investment over an adequate time horizon. The growing cost of many treatments and the maturing of methods for conducting cost-effectiveness analyses have prompted many countries and health care payers to require pharmacoeconomic analyses justifying investments in healthcare innovations. Increasingly, pharmaceutical manufacturers must demonstrate the value of a given health care investment with respect to improved health and productivity.

Cost-Effectiveness Methods

Although calculating the cost effectiveness of RA management is complex and necessarily includes many assumptions, there are well-developed methods and standards for conducting such analyses.[2] Such analyses typically construct a decision analytic model to evaluate outcomes associated with treatment decisions and thus compare relevant clinical strategies, such as nonbiologic versus biologic DMARDs at different time points in the course of RA. An appropriate decision analysis can be considered an explicit representation of typical clinical decision making that addresses the uncertainty in outcomes through probabilistic simulations and the uncertainty in evidence through adequate sensitivity analyses. Cost-effectiveness ratios are calculated by multiplying the value attached to each individual outcome with the probability of an outcome. Then, the resulting expected weighted values for the branches are added to obtain the expected value of a given clinical strategy. These values are compared in a cost-effectiveness analysis to evaluate the incremental cost effectiveness of one strategy versus another.

One of the most controversial aspects of cost-effectiveness analyses is the choice of an appropriate effectiveness measure. The quality-adjusted life year (QALY) is recommended because it allows comparison of cost effectiveness across diverse conditions.[2] The QALY is based on the assumption that a year of life may have a different value based on the health state experienced. A QALY is calculated by multiplying the utility, a subjective measure of the value of a given health state ranging from 0 (no quality of life) to 1 (perfect quality of life), by the number of years lived. A perfect health state contributes a full year for every year lived. For example, RA patients report that spending 10 years with RA is equivalent to spending 7 to 8 years in full health (i.e., 10 years with RA are worth approximately 8 QALYs).[3] Incremental gains in QALYs can then be used to summarize the effects of new interventions. Although a QALY is a recommended generic effectiveness measure, other more specific metrics can be used—including clinical remission, an ACR70, working years gained, or deaths avoided.

Many different types of costs are considered when developing economic models of pharmacotherapy (Table 9H-1). Direct medical costs include the cost of care related directly to RA, such as DMARDs, visits for RA, and surgeries for RA. Direct nonmedical costs include the cost of nonmedical items that directly relate to the care of RA (e.g., the cost of modifying a home to make it more accessible to a person with disabilities). Indirect (productivity) costs are highly dependent on the estimation methods and on average are similar to direct costs.[4] Estimation of indirect costs is controversial, and current methods give insufficient weight to the potential economic gains that could be achieved by controlling a disease that more frequently affects women.[5] However, dollar valuations of these potential improvements in productivity are "potential" rather than "actual" costs to society. Counting "actual" costs is methodologically challenging—a difficulty that is partially responsible for the widespread recommendation that indirect costs be excluded from economic evaluations and included only as part of the "dys"utility of RA.[2] An alternative method for estimating "actual" indirect costs, the friction cost approach, only includes productivity costs during the period needed to restore the initial production level (generally at a fraction of 20% or less of fully valuated costs). Thus, decision makers need to be aware of the potential variation in total direct and indirect RA costs—and the fraction of the costs that may be offset by the high acquisition costs of new interventions.

Cost of Rheumatoid Arthritis

Pharmacoeconomic evaluations attempt to evaluate to what degree new agents are able to offset the cost of caring for the disease. An understanding of the cost of illness (COI) is

Table 9H-1. Components of the Cost of Rheumatoid Arthritis

Type of Cost	Definition	Examples
Direct medical costs	Resources directly related to the care of RA	Costs for drug treatments, laboratory tests, visits to physicians or nurses, hospitalizations, surgical procedures, durable medical equipment, rehabilitation services
Direct non-medical costs	Resources related to nonmedical issues arising because of RA	Costs of child care during a physician visit or hospitalization
Indirect (productivity) costs[a]	Resources related to lost wages because of RA	Costs of disability (temporary, partial, or permanent), costs of missed work because of treatments

[a]These costs are sometimes termed *indirect costs.* It is recommended that they be subtracted from quality of life, but they can also be included as costs.

therefore important to bring perspective to the pharmacoeconomic value of new agents. Several COI studies were conducted over the past 20 years to estimate the annual cost of RA.[4] The results of such studies are needed to inform policymakers about the size of the potential economic impact a disease may have at a national level. Obtaining accurate estimates, however, may be hampered by methodologic difficulties pertaining to disease definition and sampling of patients for studies, comprehensiveness of data capture,attribution of costs to target disease and other comorbid conditions, and valuation of productivity losses.

Many COI studies of arthritis conditions have relied on national surveys to estimate the costs of disease. Several recent COI studies in RA have used consecutive samples recruited from health care providers. Yelin and Wanke used the University of California at San Francisco RA Panel Study, which followed more than 1,100 patients with RA recruited from random samples of Northern California rheumatologists.[6] These patients were followed for 14 years, and 511 patients provided information for the economic evaluation in 1996. Patients underwent a comprehensive interview process to recall the use of health resources during a year prior to the interview. Annual 1996 medical costs totaled $8,500 dollars, of which $5,900 was incurred for RA. Newhall-Perry and colleagues recruited 150 consecutive patients with new-onset RA (<1 year) through the Western Consortium of Practicing Rheumatologists.[7] Patients' health assessment questionnaire (HAQ) scores were identical to the average HAQ score reported for the RA Panel Study patients at baseline. In this study, direct annual costs (1994 dollars) were estimated to be $4,400, of which $2,400 was incurred for RA. In a recent systematic review, the mean annual direct costs of patients with RA were found to be $5,800 (1996 U.S. dollars)[4]—a figure between the estimates of the studies cited previously. Estimates for the proportion of total medical costs attributable to RA vary from 55 to 70%. Thus, national forecasts of the total economic burden of RA need to account for the role of comorbidities among the total costs.

The most recent COI study for RA comes from the National Data Bank of Rheumatic Diseases in the United States[8] (Figure 9H-1). More than 7,000 patients with RA answered semiannual questionnaires, and their direct medical costs were calculated from these. Each resource was assigned a cost, and a total direct medical cost was calculated and expressed as 2001 U.S. dollars. The average cost was more than $9,000, with about two-thirds of the cost from drug treatments. For patients using biologic DMARDs, the average cost was $19,016—whereas those not receiving biologic DMARDs had average costs of $6,164.

Cost Effectiveness of Drug Treatment in Rheumatoid Arthritis

Driven in large part by the introduction of costly biologic DMARDs, there is both increasing interest as well as a growing body of data addressing the potential cost effectiveness of treatments for RA.[9–22] A number of considerations are critical to the assessment and understanding of such analyses.

In most economic studies of persons with RA, the major drivers of cost include the loss of work capacity, hospitalizations

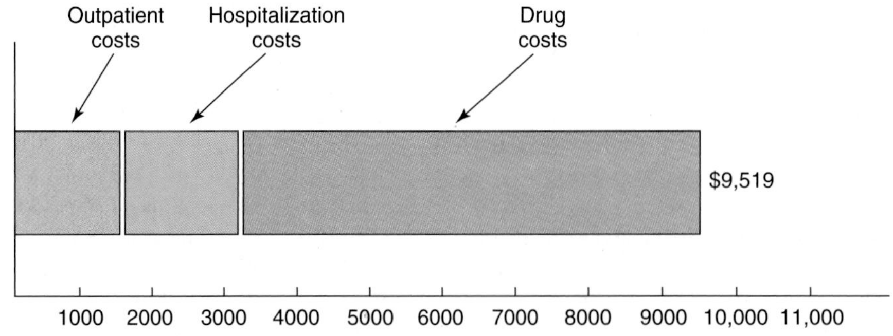

Figure 9H-1. Cost of RA. More than 7000 patients with RA answered semiannual questionnaires, and their direct medical costs were calculated from these. Each resource was assigned a cost, and a total direct medical cost was calculated and expressed as 2001 U.S. dollars. The average cost was more than $9,000, with about two-thirds of the cost from drug treatments. For patients using biologic DMARDs, the average cost was $19,016—whereas those not receiving biologic DMARDs had average costs of $6,164. (Data from Michaud K, Messer J, Choi HK, et al. Direct medical costs and their predictors in patients with rheumatoid arthritis: A three-year study of 7,527 patients. *Arthritis Rheum* 2003;48(10):2750–2762.)

related to the disease, and the acquisition costs of treatments. Work capacity is measured most readily by counting days worked, with inability to work being assessed as absenteeism. Among those employed, RA may have an important effect on their ability to perform work duties when they are at work—an effect sometimes referred to as "presenteeism." Therefore, the overall economic impact of RA may be incompletely reflected by employment as the sole metric. Nevertheless, it is used in most studies of RA because costs related to impaired function of homemakers or retired persons are more difficult to quantify. The effect of RA on individuals' ability to work is typically estimated in economic analyses based on functional ability, which is in turn measured by instruments such as the HAQ. Actual data relating HAQ score to work ability in a chronic progressive disease such as RA can be derived from longitudinal observations of RA patients over many years. However, in actual therapeutic trials it would be impractical to gain such data over a sufficient time frame. Therefore, in order to gain the long-term perspective necessary economic studies in RA must involve modeling.

Although economic models try to incorporate relevant data from epidemiologic studies and assess results from actual clinical trials, the methods utilized can vary in important ways—making comparisons among assessments potentially tenuous. A key variable with important effects on economic analyses is the specific population of RA patients under study. Patients with early RA and those who have tried fewer treatments tend to respond to therapies to a greater extent than those with more well-established ("refractory") disease. Thus, attempts at comparing across studies must take into account the populations involved. Another important factor in economic assessments is that much of the data populating the models comes from clinical trials. Differences between patients enrolled in trials and typical RA patients will likely affect the results of economic models. In addition, although modeling attempts to provide a long-term perspective for assessment it may not account for infrequent yet important events that could affect cost effectiveness. For example, hospitalizations related to joint replacement surgery are important and expensive sequelae of poorly controlled RA. Although they are not common, they must be included in economic analyses. Moreover, uncommon toxicities (i.e., opportunistic infections and cancer) that may relate to treatment could be expensive and must be part of any credible economic model.

In RA, because the biologic DMARDs have shown substantial clinical efficacy it appears that they may have an incremental cost within the range of generally accepted medical interventions. Much of these data come from follow-up of patients participating in clinical trials of infliximab, etanercept, and adalimumab in RA—and extending the time horizon through modeling. Notably, studies using distinct populations and agents have come to similar estimates; namely, treatment of patients with established RA costs roughly $30,000 per discounted QALY gained.[9,13,14,16,17] Of note, an analysis performed that did not use clinical trial data but used information from patients in a national registry of RA patients treated with tumor necrosis factor (TNF) inhibitors as well as traditional DMARDs found comparable results—with a cost per QALY of 23,882 British pounds.[18]

When considering biologic DMARDs in patients with early RA, distinct pharmacoeconomic issues might arise.[22] On the one hand, if early RA patients achieve significant incremental or sustained efficacy with biologic DMARDs these treatments may have favorable cost-effectiveness ratios compared with standard strategies. On the other hand, the need for longer-term treatment or longer-term implications of toxicity could make them less cost effective. If treatment paradigms analogous to the "induction-consolidation" approach to cancer chemotherapy were effective in RA, this might be translated into a shorter period of treatment with highly effective and sustained benefits. This could very favorably impact the costeffectiveness of biologic DMARDs or future therapies.

Additional factors may impact the health economic implications for TNF inhibitors. For example, as more agents are brought to the clinic will market forces cause their price to decline? As of 2008, there are two additional TNF inhibitors in late-phase clinical development. Competition has certainly resulted in drastically lowered prices for other classes of therapy. Similarly, will there ever be cheaper generic versions of biologic agents? Among current biologic agents, patent expiration dates are: etanercept (2012), adalimumab (2016), abatacept (2016), and infliximab (2018). The situation regarding generic versions is more complex for biologics than it is for smaller, more easily synthesized, chemicals. Factors such as variable glycosylation have been shown to affect both the efficacy and toxicity of biologic agents. These considerations will certainly impact regulatory approval and, ultimately, cost.

Conclusion

As drug treatments for RA evolve, so does the field of pharmacoeconomics. The methods are constantly being refined, and gaps in the evidence base filled in. Of particular importance for economic models in RA is the fact that therapy is continuous and that patients often require changes of DMARD regimens. Biologic DMARDs are generally not approved as first-line agents but clearly have a role in patients who fail other DMARDs. Thus, the incremental costeffectiveness of new DMARDs can be evaluated as the only DMARD[10,11] or as part of a sequence of DMARDs (a strategy) for RA management.[2,12] When evaluated within a sequence, the cost-effectiveness ratio is a property of the sequence (e.g., the one including a biologic DMARD versus one excluding them). It may thus be influenced by the combination and place of the other DMARDs, and clearly influenced by the way the evaluated DMARD is modeled to change the disease course.

Many of the clinical trials examining new biologic DMARDs use "partial responders" with an inadequate response to their current DMARD as the eligible study population. The disadvantages of using partial responders have been outlined by others.[21] Because partial responders have a very low likelihood of improvement, the relevant clinical decision in patients with inadequate response to one DMARD is not whether to continue the ineffective DMARD but whether to start new treatment A or new treatment B. A study design that would more closely mimic clinical practice would compare two new treatments (e.g., abatacept to infliximab) in methotrexate partial responders. Not only would this comparison be valuable for clinical decision making but it would provide valuable data for comparing the cost effectiveness of relevant treatment strategies.

Finally, long-term follow-up of patients taking biologic DMARDs will provide for more precise estimates of the relative rates of their potential beneficial and adverse effects. For example, it is possible that such newer agents may result in greater longevity through reducing important comorbidities (such as acute myocardial infarctions and osteoporotic fractures). On the other hand, these newer drugs may result in significant increases in rare side effects (such as atypical infections and uncommon cancers). The clinical and economic implications of such beneficial and adverse outcomes will help clarify the role of these agents.

With the advent of these newer and more expensive agents, most clinicians have learned pharmacoeconomics the hard way—through filling in "prior authorization" forms and petitioning pharmaceutical benefits programs to add these agents to the formulary. Although the published data suggest that biologic therapies have favorable incremental cost-effectiveness ratios, not all new agents look like a "good buy" for the health care system. As the portion of health care budgets devoted to drugs continues to grow, prescribing physicians will be increasingly asked to make hard decisions about which medications to prescribe to which patients. The science of pharmacoeconomics helps payers, clinicians, patients, and society at large understand the value of a given medication.

References

1. Barrett EM, Scott DG, Wiles NJ, et al. The impact of rheumatoid arthritis on employment status in the early years of disease: A UK community-based study. *Rheumatology* 2000;39(12):1403–1409.
2. Gold MR, Siegel JE, Russel LB, et al. *Cost-effectiveness in Health and Medicine.* New York: Oxford University Press 1996.
3. Marra CA, Marion SA, Guh DP, et al. Not all "quality-adjusted life years" are equal. *J Clin Epidemiol* 2007;60(6):616–624.
4. Cooper NJ. Economic burden of rheumatoid arthritis: A systematic review. *Rheumatology* 2000;39(1):28–33.
5. Clarke AE, Penrod J, St Pierre Y, et al. for the Tri-Nation Study Group. Underestimating the value of women: Assessing the indirect costs of women with systemic lupus erythematosus. *J Rheumatol* 2000;27(11):2597–2604.
6. Yelin E, Wanke LA. An assessment of the annual and long-term direct costs of rheumatoid arthritis: The impact of poor function and functional decline. *Arthritis Rheum* 1999;42(6):1209–1218.
7. Newhall-Perry K, Law NJ, Ramos B, et al. for the Western Consortium of Practicing Rheumatologists. Direct and indirect costs associated with the onset of seropositive rheumatoid arthritis. *J Rheumatol* 2000;27(5):1156–1163.
8. Michaud K, Messer J, Choi HK, et al. Direct medical costs and their predictors in patients with rheumatoid arthritis: A three-year study of 7,527 patients. *Arthritis Rheum* 2003;48(10):2750–2762.
9. Wong JB. Cost-effectiveness of anti-tumor necrosis factor agents. *Clin Exp Rheumatol* 2004;22(5/Suppl 35):S65–S70.
10. Wong JB, Singh G, Kavanaugh A. Estimating the cost-effectiveness of 54 weeks of infliximab for rheumatoid arthritis. *Am J Med* 2002; 113(5):400–408.
11. Choi HK, Seeger JD, Kuntz KM. A cost-effectiveness analysis of treatment options for patients with methotrexate-resistant rheumatoid arthritis. *Arthritis Rheum* 2000;43(10):2316–2327.
12. Choi HK, Seeger JD, Kuntz KM. A cost effectiveness analysis of treatment options for methotrexate-naive rheumatoid arthritis. *J Rheumatol* 2002;29(6):1156–1165.
13. Kobelt G, Jonsson L, Young A, et al. The cost-effectiveness of infliximab (Remicade) in the treatment of rheumatoid arthritis in Sweden and the United Kingdom based on the ATTRACT study. *Rheumatology* 2003;42(2):326–335.
14. Kobelt G, Eberhardt K, Geborek P. TNF inhibitors in the treatment of rheumatoid arthritis in clinical practice: Costs and outcomes in a follow up study of patients with RA treated with etanercept or infliximab in southern Sweden. *Ann Rheum Dis* 2004;63(1):4–10.
15. Welsing PM, Severens JL, Hartman M, et al. Modeling the 5-year cost effectiveness of treatment strategies including tumor necrosis factor-blocking agents and leflunomide for treating rheumatoid arthritis in the Netherlands. *Arthritis Rheum* 2004;51(6):964–673.
16. Brennan A, Bansback N, Reynolds A, et al. Modelling the cost-effectiveness of etanercept in adults with rheumatoid arthritis in the UK. *Rheumatology* 2004;43(1):62–72.
17. Bansback NJ, Brennan A, Ghatnekar O. Cost effectiveness of adalimumab in the treatment of patients with moderate to severe rheumatoid arthritis in Sweden. *Ann Rheum Dis* 2005;64(7):995–1002.
18. Brennan A, Bansback N, Nixon R, et al. Modelling the cost effectiveness of TNF-alpha antagonists in the management of rheumatoid arthritis: Results from the British Society for Rheumatology Biologics Registry. *Rheumatology* 2007;46(8):1345–1354.
19. Kavanaugh A, Han C, Bala M. Functional status and radiographic joint damage are associated with health economic outcomes in patients with rheumatoid arthritis. *J Rheumatol* 2004;31(5):849–855.
20. Yelin E, Trupin L, Katz P, et al. Association between etanercept use and employment outcomes among patients with rheumatoid arthritis. *Arthritis Rheum* 2003;48(11):3046–3054.
21. Fleurence R, Spackman E. Cost-effectiveness of biologic agents for treatment of autoimmune disorders: Structured review of the literature. *J Rheumatol* 2006;33(11):2124–2131.
22. Hallert E, Husberg M, Jonsson D, et al. Rheumatoid arthritis is already expensive during the first year of the disease (the Swedish TIRA project). *Rheumatology* 2004;43(11):1374–1382.

Synovial Biomarkers

Daniëlle M. Gerlag and Paul Peter Tak

Rheumatoid arthritis (RA) is a chronic inflammatory disorder affecting synovial tissue in multiple joints. Because the synovium represents the major target of the disease process,[1,2] recent studies have focused on the identification of synovial biomarkers that could be used for differential diagnosis, prediction of radiologic outcome, evaluation of novel therapies, and prediction of clinical response to treatment. A clear advantage of this approach is that tissue specificity is not a problem.

Different synovial biomarkers may be needed for diverse goals. For instance, mechanism of action studies evaluating the effects of anti–B-cell therapy would require studies on B cells, plasma cells, and immunoglobulins—whereas completely different biomarkers could be required in the diagnostic workup. Moreover, synovial biomarkers might be used as surrogate markers to predict outcome in individual patients—whereas analysis of synovial biomarkers for screening purposes during early drug development will mainly be on the group level. Thus, there may be different validation requirements depending on the specific use of the synovial biomarkers.

Feasibility of Synovial Biopsy

Many investigators have used blind needle biopsy to obtain synovial tissue samples in the past. It is a well-tolerated, safe, inexpensive, and technically easy method that yields adequate tissue samples in most cases. Measures of inflammation in tissue samples taken from clinically inflamed joints using the blind needle technique are generally similar to samples obtained by arthroscopy under vision.[3] In our experience with more than 800 Parker–Pearson biopsy procedures, we have obtained sufficient synovial tissue for histologic examination in about 85% of the patients with various forms of arthritis.[4] The procedure failed especially in joints that were not swollen. In this series, the procedure was never complicated by hemarthros or infection.

There are also limitations and disadvantages to the use of blind needle biopsy: it is usually restricted to larger joints, the operator is not able to visually select the tissue, and it is not always possible to obtain adequate tissue samples. This is especially true when clinically uninvolved joints are investigated (e.g., after successful therapy).

Therefore, most investigators have recently abandoned blind needle biopsy and used arthroscopic synovial biopsy. There are several advantages to this approach. It allows macroscopic evaluation of the synovium. Using narrow-diameter arthroscopes, small joints (such as ankles, wrists, and even metacarpophalangeal and proximal interphalangeal joints) can be evaluated.[5,6] Moreover, it is basically always possible to obtain tissue in adequate amounts—even when the synovial tissue volume has decreased as a result of effective treatment. The arthroscopic procedure is well tolerated and has a low complication rate, with 35% to 36% of patients reporting minimal pain or discomfort during the procedure.[7] In another survey, in which information from 15,682 arthroscopies performed by rheumatologists was collected, the complication rate of hemarthrosis was 0.9%, deep vein thrombosis 0.2%, and wound and joint infection 0.1%.[8] In a series of the AMC/University of Amsterdam of more than 2,000 arthroscopic synovial biopsy procedures, the complication rate was <0.3% (hemarthrosis, portal infection, and septic arthritis).[4] The procedure was generally well tolerated, and many patients preferred rheumatologic arthroscopy over closed MRI (unpublished observations). Taken together, arthroscopic synovial biopsy is feasible because it is generally safe and well tolerated. It is likely that synovial biopsy will be increasingly used in the future, especially by means of office-based mini-invasive ultrasound-guided techniques.[9]

Differential Diagnosis

A variety of biomarkers is differentially expressed in RA compared to other forms of arthritis. Multivariate models can, for instance, predict a diagnosis of RA on the basis of synovial tissue analysis with an accuracy of 85% when there is massive infiltration by plasma cells and macrophages. A diagnosis other than RA can be predicted in 97% in the case of minimal infiltration by these cells.[10] Although of pathogenetic interest, these markers cannot be used to establish the diagnosis of RA solely on the basis of the characteristics of the synovium. Therefore, the diagnosis of RA is made primarily on the basis of clinical examination, routine laboratory tests, radiographic examination, and perhaps synovial fluid analysis. The value of examination of synovial tissue as part of the diagnostic workup is mainly limited to exclusion of rare infectious, infiltrative, and deposition diseases of joints in selected cases.[11,12] It has previously been suggested that the presence of lymphoid neogenesis would support a diagnosis of RA, but their presence is not specific for this disease[13,14] nor for a clinically distinct subset of RA.[15] Similarly, citrulinated proteins have been detected in RA synovial tissue—but also in other forms of arthritis.[16–18] It has been suggested that the presence of HLA-DR shared epitope-human cartilage glycoprotein 39 (263–275) complexes may be specific for RA synovium, but the sensitivity is too low (40%–50%) to be used for differential diagnosis in the clinic.[19] Future research will focus on the identification of synovial gene signatures and protein profiles associated with the diagnosis of RA.

Prediction of Radiologic Outcome

Because demographic and clinical parameters, serologic markers, and genetic background can only partially predict disease outcome, there is still a need for better predictive biomarkers. Data on the relationship between the features of synovial tissue and radiologic outcome after follow-up are still very scarce. Studies from one center have suggested a relationship between synovial tissue macrophages and an unfavorable outcome of RA. In the first study on 12 patients, a significant correlation between the number of synovial tissue macrophages and the degree of joint erosion after 1 year was found.[20] Subsequently, a correlation between intimal lining layer depth ($r = 0.63$) and numbers of sublining macrophages ($r = 0.59$) on the one hand and progression of radiologic damage on the other was shown in 28 RA patients with a mean disease duration of 2.5 years at inclusion who were followed up for a mean of 70 months.[21] In another study on 36 patients with early RA (disease duration <1 year) who were followed up for a mean of 58 months regression analysis identified the numbers of fibroblast-like synoviocytes [relative risk (RR) = 1.7], T cells (RR = 2.7), and granzyme B positive cytotoxic cells (RR = 7.2) as discriminators for unfavorable radiologic outcome.[22] Consistent with these studies, a third study observed a correlation between intimal macrophages and CD4 positive T cells and radiologic progression.[23] Focusing on cytokine profiles, multivariate analysis demonstrated the predictive value of synovial mRNA expression of IL-1α, tumor necrosis factor (TNF), IL-17, and IL-10 for progression of joint destruction after 2 years of follow-up in 60 patients.[24] The cytokine profile explained 57% of the joint damage shown on MRI over 2 years. Another study demonstrated a correlation between the synovial expression of MMP-2 in early RA patients and erosive disease after 1 year of follow-up.[25] Thus, although no reliable single prognostic biomarkers have been identified so far several studies have provided proof of principle that the characteristics of the synovium may have predictive value. It can be anticipated that future studies will focus on the use of more extensive markers of joint degradation as well as the use of panels of biomarkers in synovial tissue samples.

Evaluation of Novel Therapies

Our usual thinking about the use of biomarkers in clinical trials has recently changed dramatically. Increasingly, clinical investigations consist of small trials with a high density of data. This approach may be instrumental in the identification of an early therapeutic effect using small numbers of patients, accelerating decisions in phase I/II studies, and enhancing dose selection before large conventional clinical trials (necessary to determine whether the biologic effects translate into clinically meaningful improvement) are conducted. The need for such innovative trial design in relatively small proof-of-concept studies is clear from the large number of compounds in the pipeline of the pharmaceutical industry, from increasing difficulty in including RA patients with active disease in clinical trials due to the success of available treatment, and from the influence of financial and ethical considerations.

The importance of collecting data on the primary site of inflammation, the synovium, to understand the effects of antirheumatic treatment is illustrated by the observation that clinical arthritis activity is accompanied by persistent histologic signs of synovitis after treatment with humanized anti-CD52 antibodies or chimeric anti-CD4 antibodies despite profound depletion of peripheral blood lymphocytes.[26,27] Similarly, recent work has shown that B cells may persist in the synovium in some RA patients after treatment with rituximab—in spite of marked depletion of peripheral blood B cells in nearly all patients.[28,29]

Using this approach, successful treatment with disease-modifying antirheumatic drugs (such as gold,[30] methotrexate,[31–33] leflunomide,[33] and corticosteroids[34–36]) was shown to be associated with decreased mononuclear cell infiltration. Similarly, successful treatment of RA patients with infliximab,[37–41] etanercept,[42] anakinra,[43] and rituximab[28,29,44] results in reduced synovial inflammation. Evaluation of serial synovial biopsies has also been used to evaluate the effects of experimental compounds for the treatment of RA, including a synthetic retinoid,[45] IL-10,[46] anti-CD4 antibodies administered intra-articularly,[47] IFNβ,[48] a CCR1 antagonist,[49] a CCR2 antagonist,[50] a C5a receptor blocker,[51] and anti-CCL2 antibody treatment.[52]

These studies highlight that it is feasible to use examination of serial biopsy samples to monitor the response to treatment and to screen for interesting biologic effects at the site of inflammation. These investigations provide two types of data: data on the specific effects related to the mechanism of action of the drug and data on biomarkers associated with active treatment independent of the primary mechanism of action. A discussion of the use of synovial tissue analysis to provide insight into the specific mechanism of action of treatment is beyond the scope of this chapter and we refer the reader to a recent review.[53]

To formally address the question of which feature in RA synovial tissue samples could be used as a biomarker for clinical efficacy in relatively small studies of short duration, we have designed a randomized clinical trial.[36] In this study, patients were treated with prednisolone according to the combination therapy in early RA (COBRA) regimen or with placebo for 2 weeks. This study identified sublining macrophages as the best biomarker associated with the clinical response to corticosteroids. Next, the utility of macrophages in the synovial sublining as a candidate biomarker was tested across discrete interventions and kinetics.[54] A strong correlation between the mean change in disease activity score (delta DAS28) and the mean change in the number of sublining macrophages was observed (Figure 9I-1). When patients from all actively treated studies were grouped ($n = 70$), the standardized response mean (SRM)—a measure of sensitivity to change—was high for the change in sublining macrophages (indicating good sensitivity to change). For a biomarker to pass the "discrimination criterion" of the OMERACT (Outcome Measures in Rheumatology Clinical Trials) filter, not only should it exhibit high sensitivity to change but it should distinguish between effective and ineffective treatment. Therefore, the data from two recently performed randomized controlled clinical trials of treatment strategies shown to be ineffective in RA were added to the data set described previously.[55] The weighted mean of the SRM for CD68-positive

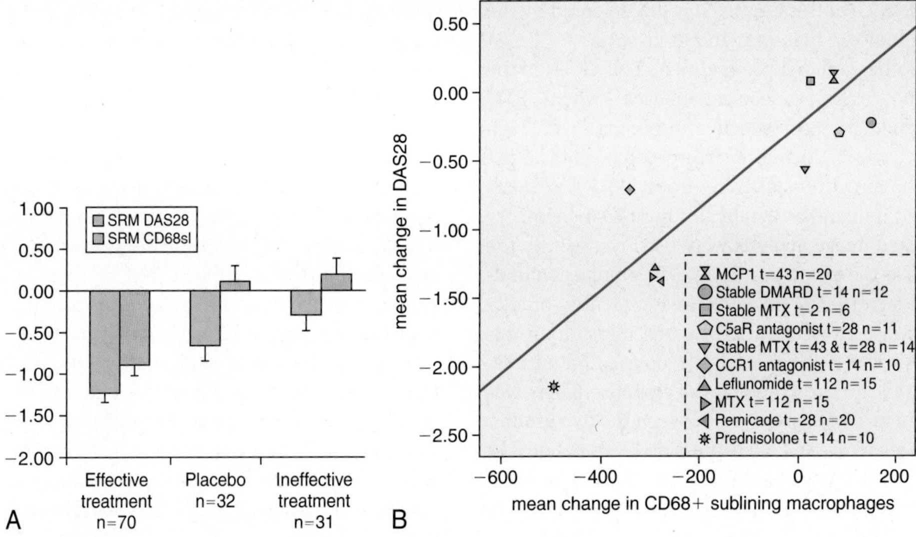

Figure 9I-1. (*A*) Weighted average and standard error of the standardized response mean (SRM) for the change in 28-joint Disease Activity Score (DAS28) and in number of CD68-positive sublining macrophages (CD68sl) among RA patients treated with effective experimental drugs, RA patients treated with placebo, and RA patients treated with ineffective experimental drugs. The biomarker CD68-positive sublining macrophages showed good sensitivity to change and were not susceptible to placebo effects in small proof-of-concept studies of relatively short duration. (*B*) Correlation between the mean change in number of CD68-positive sublining macrophages and mean change in DAS28 for each substudy (Pearson correlation = 0.895, $p < 0.001$; weighted linear regression $R^2 = 0.801$, 95% confidence interval 0.002–0.004, $p < 0.001$). There was a consistent relationship between the change in macrophage numbers and clinical improvement after treatment. The group that received DMARD therapy was treated with methotrexate (MTX), sulfasalazine, hydroxychloroquine, leflunomide, or a combination of these drugs. MCP-1 = monocyte chemotactic protein 1; t = time (days) between first biopsy and second biopsy; C5aR antagonist = C5a receptor antagonist. (From Wijbrandts CA, Vergunst CE, Haringman JJ, et al. Absence of changes in the number of synovial sublining macrophages after ineffective treatment for rheumatoid arthritis: Implications for use of synovial sublining macrophages as a biomarker. *Arthritis Rheum* 2007;56(11):3869–3871. Reproduced with permission from Wiley InterScience.)

sublining macrophages was −0.89 (±SE 0.12) in the patients receiving effective experimental treatment, 0.20 (SE 0.18) in the patients receiving ineffective experimental treatment, and 0.11 (SE 0.18) in the patients receiving placebo (Figure 9I-1). The difference in the weighted mean of the SRM between the effective treatment group and the ineffective treatment group was significant for CD68-positive sublining macrophages. Hence, a clear distinction between effective and ineffective treatment could be made. Linear regression analysis showed that the mean change in the number of sublining macrophages could predict 80% of the variance in the mean change in DAS28 in each study group. As expected, in contrast to the results obtained using the synovial biomarker the DAS28 was susceptible to placebo effects—as shown by the weighted mean of the SRM of −0.30 (SE 0.18) in the group receiving ineffective treatment.[55]

In conclusion, serial synovial biopsy can be used for selection purposes during early drug development. In proof-of-concept studies based on this approach, three types of data are obtained: clinical data, synovial biomarkers specifically related to the mechanism of action of the therapy, and quantification of the number of CD68-positive macrophages. We would recommend rethinking of the therapeutic strategy moving to large clinical trials if there is no change in DAS28, no specific effects related to the mechanism of action, and no change in macrophage numbers after treatment. The drug might not hit the target effectively or the concept behind the role of the target in the pathogenesis might be wrong.

Prediction of Clinical Response to Treatment

Although a variety of studies has shown a clear simultaneous relation between changes in synovial tissue and response to treatment, there are still only a few studies addressing the question whether the features of the synovium at baseline or changes in the synovium early after initiation of treatment can be used to predict the clinical response to treatment over time. One pioneering study on 18 RA patients found a correlation between synovial TNF expression and vascularity at baseline and the clinical response to an array of conventional disease-modifying antirheumatic drug (DMARD) treatments.[56] In another study, synovial biopsy samples were obtained from 66 patients with persistent inflammatory arthritis (rheumatoid arthritis, psoriatic arthritis, undifferentiated arthritis, and other causes of inflammatory arthritis) before treatment with combination therapy consisting of 90Y radiation synovectomy and intra-articular glucocorticoids or with intra-articular glucocorticoids.[57] Clinical response was assessed after 6 months. The number of macrophages in the synovial sublining at baseline was significantly higher in responders than in nonresponders, independent of treatment group and diagnosis. The clinical effect was positively correlated with pretreatment total macrophage numbers and expression of vascular cell adhesion molecule-1 (VCAM-1).

Prediction of clinical response to biologic treatment would obviously be very important in the context of individualized treatment. The relevance of this approach is underscored by the expanding array of biologic therapies and their costs.

Recently, we hypothesized that pretreatment TNF levels in the synovium might be related to clinical efficacy—where TNF blocking therapy could be most effective in patients with high pretreatment TNF levels.[58] Therefore, arthroscopic synovial tissue samples were obtained prospectively from 143 RA patients prior to initiation of infliximab therapy. Immunohistochemistry and computer-assisted image analysis were used to quantify the cell infiltrate as well as the expression of cytokines, adhesion molecules, and growth factors. The objective was to identify predictors of clinical response 16 weeks after the first infusion. In this study, the hypothesis was that the level of synovial TNF expression would be a significant early predictor of response. There was considerable overlap in TNF expression between the two groups. There was on average increased TNF expression levels in both the intimal lining layer and synovial sublining of responding compared to nonresponding patients (Figure 9I-2).[58] In line with these findings, there was increased infiltration by macrophages, including both CD163-positive resident tissue macrophages and MRP8-positive and MRP14-positive infiltrating macrophages—as well as T cells in responders versus nonresponders. These macrophage populations and T cells are the main source of TNF in the synovium of RA patients. Consistent with these results, large-scale gene expression profiling using microarrays has shown that patients with a high level of tissue inflammation are more likely to benefit from TNF blockade.[59] Multivariate logistic regression analysis of synovial markers showed that TNF expression could explain about 10% of the variance in response to therapy.[58] After adjusting for disease activity at baseline, this increased to 17%.

Another study was performed to investigate the kinetics of the synovial tissue response to rituximab treatment in relation to the clinical response at 6 months in 24 RA patients.[60] There were no baseline characteristics of the synovium that could reliably predict clinical response to treatment. Furthermore, the decrease in synovial B cells between baseline and 4 weeks or

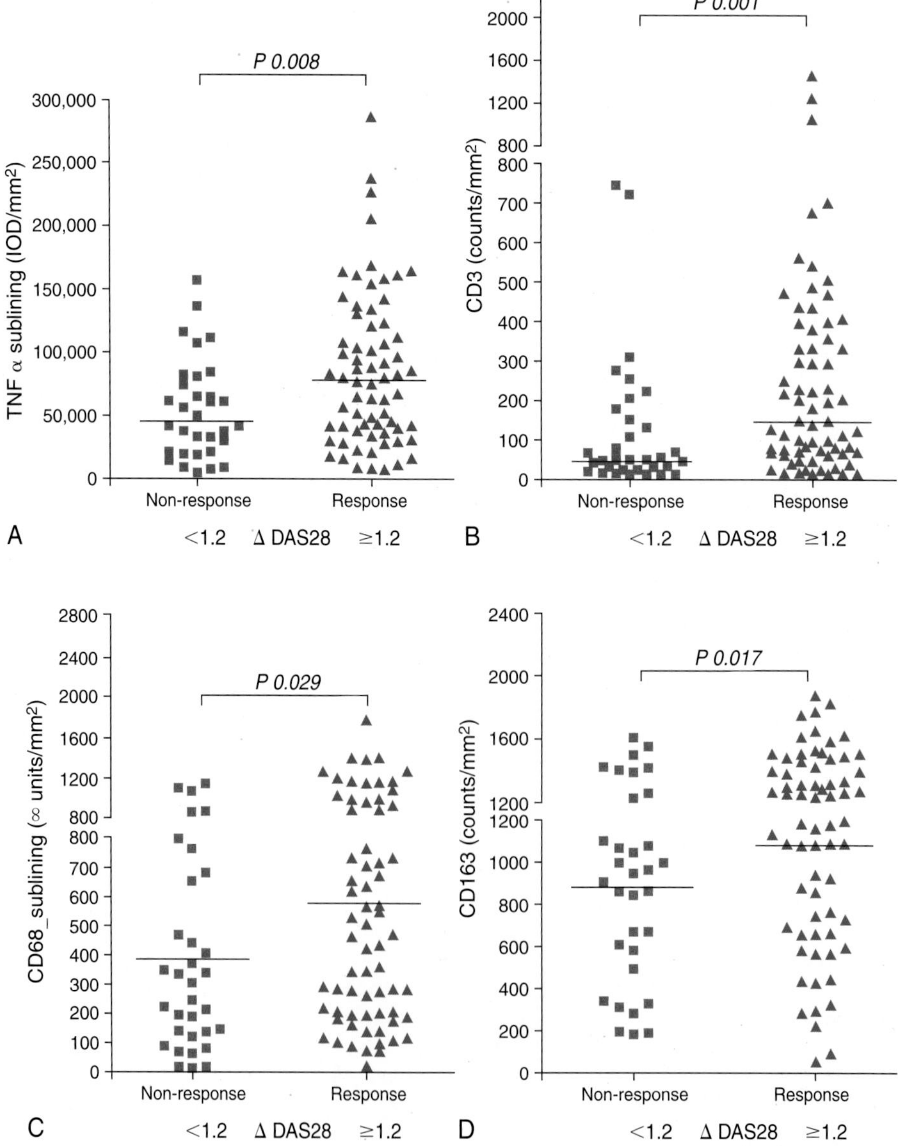

Figure 9I-2. (*A*) The median synovial sublining TNF expression was higher in responders compared to nonresponders ($p = 0.008$). (*B*) The median number of CD3-positive T cells in responders versus nonresponders ($p = 0.001$). (*C*) The mean number of CD68-positive sublining macrophages was also higher in responders (576 ± 428) than in nonresponders (387 ± 338 [$p = 0.029$]). (*D*) CD163-positive macrophages in responders versus nonresponders ($p = 0.017$). (From Wijbrandts CA, Dijkgraaf MGW, Kraan MC, et al. The clinical response to infliximab in rheumatoid arthritis is in part dependent on pre-treatment TNF-alpha expression in the synovium. *Ann Rheum Dis* 2007;. Reproduced with permission from the BMJ Group.)

between 4 weeks and 16 weeks was not significantly different between responders versus nonresponders to treatment.[60]

However, there was a highly significant difference in the change in plasma cells (derived from B cells) between responders and nonresponders. In line with these results, linear regression analysis demonstrated a positive correlation between the change in plasma cells (derived from B cells) between 4 and 16 weeks and clinical improvement after 24 weeks. This analysis also revealed that the decrease in plasma cells between 4 and 16 weeks could predict the decrease in DAS28 at 24 weeks after treatment (R2 = 0.26, P = 0.002).

The predictive value of synovial biomarkers could be of great interest in helping us understand why there is a lack of response in a subset of patients. This approach, however, cannot yet be used because there is no surrogate marker yet to reliably predict clinical response in individual patients and to guide treatment decisions. However, the results do provide proof of principle that this might be achieved by further optimization of the biomarkers or perhaps combinations with other clinical and biologic variables that need to be identified.

Conclusion

The predictive value of synovial biomarkers is of great interest to understand the lack of response in a subset of the patients, but this approach can as yet not be used as a surrogate marker to reliably predict clinical response in individual patients and guide treatment decisions." The point I want to make is that these synovial markers can already be used on the group levels as biomarkers to understands lack of response, but they cannot be used as surrogate markers (which has regulatory implications) to predict response in individual patients.

References

1. Tak PP, Bresnihan B. The pathogenesis and prevention of joint damage in rheumatoid arthritis: Advances from synovial biopsy and tissue analysis. *Arthritis Rheum* 2000;43(12):2619–2633.
2. Firestein GS. Evolving concepts of rheumatoid arthritis. *Nature* 2003;423(6937):356–361.
3. Youssef PP, Kraan M, Breedveld F, et al. Quantitative microscopic analysis of inflammation in rheumatoid arthritis synovial membrane samples selected at arthroscopy compared with samples obtained blindly by needle biopsy. *Arthritis Rheum* 1998;41(4): 663–669.
4. Gerlag D, Tak PP. Synovial biopsy. *Best Pract Res Clin Rheumatol* 2005;19(3):387–400.
5. Kraan MC, Reece RJ, Smeets TJM, et al. Comparison of synovial tissues from the knee joints and the small joints of rheumatoid arthritis patients: Implications for pathogenesis and treatment. *Arthritis Rheum* 2002;46:2034–2038.
6. Reece R, Emery P. Needle arthroscopy. *Br J Rheumatol* 1995;34: 1102–1104.
7. Baeten D, Van den Bosch F, Elewaut D, et al. Needle arthroscopy of the knee with synovial biopsy sampling: Technical experience in 150 patients. *Clin Rheumatol* 1999;18(6):434–441.
8. Kane D, Veale DJ, FitzGerald O, et al. Survey of arthroscopy performed by rheumatologists. *Rheumatology* (Oxford) 2002;41(2): 210–215.
9. Scire CA, Epis O, Codullo V, et al. Immunohistological assessment of the synovial tissue in small joints in rheumatoid arthritis: Validation of a minimally invasive ultrasound-guided synovial biopsy procedure. *Arthritis Res Ther* 2007;9(5):R101.
10. Kraan MC, Haringman JJ, Post WJ, et al. Immunohistological analysis of synovial tissue for differential diagnosis in early arthritis. *Rheumatology* 1999;38:1074–1080.
11. Gerlag DM, Tak PP. How useful are synovial biopsies for the diagnosis of rheumatic diseases? *Nat Clin Pract Rheumatol* 2007; 3(5):248–249.
12. Bresnihan B. Are synovial biopsies of diagnostic value? *Arthritis Res Ther* 2003;5(6):271–278.
13. Da RR, Qin Y, Baeten D, et al. B cell clonal expansion and somatic hypermutation of Ig variable heavy chain genes in the synovial membrane of patients with osteoarthritis. *J Immunol* 2007;178(1): 557–565.
14. Canete JD, Santiago B, Cantaert T, et al. Ectopic lymphoid neogenesis in psoriatic arthritis. *Ann Rheum Dis* 2007;66(6):720–726.
15. Thurlings RM, Wijbrandts CA, Mebius R, et al. Synovial lymphoid neogenesis does not define a specific clinical rheumatoid arthritis phenotype. *Arthritis Rheum* 2008 (in press).
16. Vossenaar ER, Smeets TJ, Kraan MC, et al. The presence of citrullinated proteins is not specific for rheumatoid synovial tissue. *Arthritis Rheum* 2004;50(11):3485–3494.
17. Chapuy-Regaud S, Sebbag M, Baeten D, et al. Fibrin deimination in synovial tissue is not specific for rheumatoid arthritis but commonly occurs during synovitides. *J Immunol* 2005;174(8): 5057–5064.
18. Makrygiannakis D, af Klint E, Lundberg IE, et al. Citrullination is an inflammation-dependent process. *Ann Rheum Dis* 2006;65(9): 1219–1222.
19. Steenbakkers PG, Baeten D, Rovers E, et al. Localization of MHC class II/human cartilage glycoprotein–39 complexes in synovia of rheumatoid arthritis patients using complex-specific monoclonal antibodies. *J Immunol* 2003;170(11):5719–5727.
20. Yanni G, Whelan A, Feighery C, et al. Synovial tissue macrophages and joint erosion in rheumatoid arthritis. *Ann Rheum Dis* 1994; 53:39–44.
21. Mulherin D, FitzGerald O, Bresnihan B. Synovial tissue macrophage populations and articular damage in rheumatoid arthritis. *Arthritis Rheum* 1996;39:115–124.
22. Kraan MC, Haringman JJ, Weedon H, et al. T cells, fibroblast-like synoviocytes, and granzyme B+ cytotoxic cells are associated with joint damage in patients with recent onset rheumatoid arthritis. *Ann Rheum Dis* 2004;63(5):483–488.
23. Fonseca JE, Cortez-Dias N, Francisco A, et al. Inflammatory cell infiltrate and RANKL/OPG expression in rheumatoid synovium: Comparison with other inflammatory arthropathies and correlation with outcome. *Clin Exp Rheumatol* 2005;23(2):185–192.
24. Kirkham BW, Lassere MN, Edmonds JP, et al. Synovial membrane cytokine expression is predictive of joint damage progression in rheumatoid arthritis: A two-year prospective study (the DAMAGE study cohort). *Arthritis Rheum* 2006;54(4):1122–1131.
25. Goldbach-Mansky R, Lee JM, Hoxworth JM, et al. Active synovial matrix metalloproteinase–2 is associated with radiographic erosions in patients with early synovitis. *Arthritis Res* 2000;2(2): 145–153.
26. Ruderman EM, Weinblatt ME, Thurmond LM, et al. Synovial tissue response to treatment with Campath–1H. *Arthritis Rheum* 1995; 38:254–258.
27. Tak PP, Van der Lubbe PA, Cauli A, et al. Reduction of synovial inflammation after anti-CD4 monoclonal antibody treatment in early rheumatoid arthritis. *Arthritis Rheum* 1995;38:1457–1465.
28. Vos K, Thurlings RM, Wijbrandts CA, et al. Early effects of rituximab on the synovial cell infiltrate in patients with rheumatoid arthritis. *Arthritis Rheum* 2007;56(3):772–778.

29. Kavanaugh A, Rosengren S, Lee SJ, et al. Assessment of rituximab's immunomodulatory synovial effects (ARISE trial). 1: Clinical and synovial biomarker results. *Ann Rheum Dis* 2008;67(3):402–408.
30. Rooney M, Whelan A, Feighery C, et al. Changes in lymphocyte infiltration of the synovial membrane and the clinical course of rheumatoid arthritis. *Arthritis Rheum* 1989;32(4):361–369.
31. Firestein GS, Paine MM, Boyle DL. Mechanisms of methotrexate action in rheumatoid arthritis: Selective decrease in synovial collagenase gene expression. *Arthritis Rheum* 1994;37:193–200.
32. Dolhain RJ, Tak PP, Dijkmans BA, et al. Methotrexate reduces inflammatory cell numbers, expression of monokines and of adhesion molecules in synovial tissue of patients with rheumatoid arthritis. *Br J Rheumatol* 1998;37(5):502–508.
33. Kraan MC, Reece RJ, Barg EC, et al. Modulation of inflammation and metalloproteinase expression in synovial tissue by leflunomide and methotrexate in patients with active rheumatoid arthritis: Findings in a prospective, randomized, double-blind, parallel-design clinical trial in thirty-nine patients at two centers. *Arthritis Rheum* 2000;43(8):1820–1830.
34. De Bois MHW, Arndt JW, Tak PP, et al. 99Tcm-labelled polyclonal human immunoglobulin G scintigraphy before and after intra-articular knee injection of triamcinolone hexacetonide in patients with rheumatoid arthritis. *Nucl Med Commun* 1993;14:883–887.
35. Youssef PP, Triantafillou S, Parker A, et al. Variability in cytokine and cell adhesion molecule staining in arthroscopic synovial biopsies: Quantification using color video image analysis. *J Rheumatol* 1997; 24(12):2291–2298.
36. Gerlag DM, Haringman JJ, Smeets TJ, et al. Effects of oral prednisolone on biomarkers in synovial tissue and clinical improvement in rheumatoid arthritis. *Arthritis Rheum* 2004;50(12):3783–3791.
37. Tak PP, Taylor PC, Breedveld FC, et al. Decrease in cellularity and expression of adhesion molecules by anti-tumor necrosis factor alpha treatment in patients with rheumatoid arthritis. *Arthritis Rheum* 1996;39:1077–1081.
38. Taylor PC, Peters AM, Paleolog E, et al. Reduction of chemokine levels and leukocyte traffic to joints by tumor necrosis factor alpha blockade in patients with rheumatoid arthritis. *Arthritis Rheum* 2000;43(1):38–47.
39. Ulfgren AK, Andersson U, Engstrom M, et al. Systemic anti-tumor necrosis factor alpha therapy in rheumatoid arthritis down-regulates synovial tumor necrosis factor alpha synthesis. *Arthritis Rheum* 2000;43(11):2391–2396.
40. Smeets TJ, Kraan MC, van Loon ME, et al. Tumor necrosis factor alpha blockade reduces the synovial cell infiltrate early after initiation of treatment, but apparently not by induction of apoptosis in synovial tissue. *Arthritis Rheum* 2003;48(8):2155–2162.
41. Lindberg J, af Klint E, Catrina AI, et al. Effect of infliximab on mRNA expression profiles in synovial tissue of rheumatoid arthritis patients. *Arthritis Res Ther* 2006;8(6):R179.
42. Verschueren PC, Markusse HM, Smeets TJ, et al. Reduced cellularity and expression of adhesion molecules and cytokines after treatment with soluble human recombinant TNF receptor (P75) in rheumatoid arthritis patients. *Arthritis Rheum* 1999;42:S197.
43. Cunnane G, Madigan A, Murphy E, et al. The effects of treatment with interleukin-1 receptor antagonist on the inflamed synovial membrane in rheumatoid arthritis. *Rheumatology* (Oxford) 2001; 40(1):62–69.
44. Teng YK, Levarht EW, Hashemi M, et al. Immunohistochemical analysis as a means to predict responsiveness to rituximab treatment. *Arthritis Rheum* 2007;56(12):3909–3918.
45. Gravallese EM, Handel ML, Coblyn J, et al. N-[4-hydroxyphenyl] retinamide in rheumatoid arthritis: A pilot study. *Arthritis Rheum* 1996;39(6):1021–1026.
46. Smeets TJ, Kraan MC, Versendaal J, et al. Analysis of serial synovial biopsies in patients with rheumatoid arthritis: Description of a control group without clinical improvement after treatment with interleukin 10 or placebo. *J Rheumatol* 1999;26(10):2089–2093.
47. Veale DJ, Reece RJ, Parsons W, et al. Intra-articular primatised anti-CD4: Efficacy in resistant rheumatoid knees. A study of combined arthroscopy, magnetic resonance imaging, and histology. *Ann Rheum Dis* 1999;58(6):342–349.
48. Tak PP, 't Hart BA, Kraan MC, et al. The effects of interferon-beta treatment on arthritis. *Rheumatology* 1999;38:362–369.
49. Haringman JJ, Kraan MC, Smeets TJ, et al. Chemokine blockade and chronic inflammatory disease: Proof of concept in patients with rheumatoid arthritis. *Ann Rheum Dis* 2003;62(8):715–721.
50. Vergunst CE, Gerlag DM, Lopatinskaya L, et al. Modulation of CCR2 in rheumatoid arthritis. *Arthritis Rheum* 2008 (in press).
51. Vergunst CE, Gerlag DM, Dinant H, et al. Blocking the receptor for C5a in patients with rheumatoid arthritis does not reduce synovial inflammation. *Rheumatology* (Oxford) 2007;46(12):1773–1778.
52. Haringman JJ, Gerlag DM, Smeets TJ, et al. A randomized controlled trial with an anti-CCL2 (anti-monocyte chemotactic protein 1) monoclonal antibody in patients with rheumatoid arthritis. *Arthritis Rheum* 2006;54(8):2387–2392.
53. Gerlag DM, Tak PP. Novel approaches for the treatment of rheumatoid arthritis: Lessons from the evaluation of synovial biomarkers in clinical trials. *Best Prac Res Clin Rheumatol* 2008;22(2):311–323.
54. Haringman JJ, Gerlag DM, Zwinderman AH, et al. Synovial tissue macrophages: A sensitive biomarker for response to treatment in patients with rheumatoid arthritis. *Ann Rheum Dis* 2005;64(6): 834–838.
55. Wijbrandts CA, Vergunst CE, Haringman JJ, et al. Absence of changes in the number of synovial sublining macrophages after ineffective treatment for rheumatoid arthritis: Implications for use of synovial sublining macrophages as a biomarker. *Arthritis Rheum* 2007;56(11):3869–3871.
56. Pettit AR, Weedon H, Ahern M, et al. Association of clinical, radiological and synovial immunopathological responses to anti-rheumatic treatment in rheumatoid arthritis. *Rheumatology* (Oxford) 2001;40(11): 1243–1255.
57. Jahangier ZN, Jacobs JW, Kraan MC, et al. Pre-treatment macrophage infiltration of the synovium predicts the clinical effect of both radiation synovectomy and intra-articular glucocorticoids. *Ann Rheum Dis* 2006;65:1286–1292.
58. Wijbrandts CA, Dijkgraaf MGW, Kraan MC, et al. The clinical response to infliximab in rheumatoid arthritis is in part dependent on pre-treatment TNF-alpha expression in the synovium. *Ann Rheum Dis* 2007 Nov 29. [Epub ahead of print].
59. van der Pouw Kraan TC, Wijbrandts CA, van Baarsen LG, et al. Responsiveness to anti-TNF alpha therapy is related to pre-treatment tissue inflammation levels in rheumatoid arthritis patients. *Ann Rheum Dis* 2008;67(4):563–566.
60. Thurlings RM, Vos K, Wijbrandts CA, et al. Synovial tissue response to rituximab: Mechanism of action and identification of biomarkers of response. *Ann Rheum Dis* 2007 Oct 26. [Epub ahead of print].

Treatment of Rheumatoid Arthritis

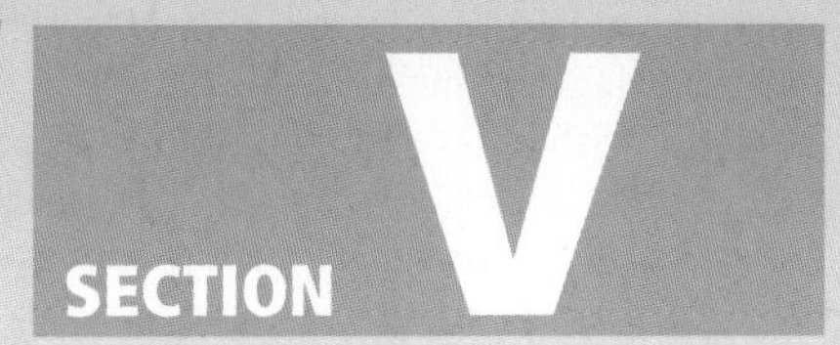

Nonsteroidal Anti-Inflammatory Drugs and Coxibs

CHAPTER 10A

Tore K. Kvien

Nonsteroidal anti-inflammatory drugs (NSAIDs) are widely used in all inflammatory and noninflammatory rheumatic diseases, including rheumatoid arthritis (RA). The treatment goal is to reduce pain and stiffness and to improve function. Patients with RA have variable levels of pain, but pain is always an area of health in which patients want to see improvement.[1] Thus, pain management is important from the patient perspective and NSAIDs and COX-2 selective NSAIDs (often called coxibs) are important parts of the pharmacologic treatment of patients with RA. However, a considerable proportion of patients with RA do not use NSAIDs—even if they report pain as a prioritized area for improvement.[1]

NSAIDs do not belong to the same or a distinctive chemical class. For example, naproxen, ibuprofen, and ketoprofen are propionic acids—whereas diclofenac is a phenylacetic acid. Nabumetone is the only nonacidic traditional NSAID. Plasma half-life varies, but some NSAIDs can be administered less frequently than expected because the tissue and synovial fluid conscentrations are sustained longer than the plasma concentrations.[2] Currently, only one coxib is on the market in United States as well as the rest of the world (celecoxib)—whereas etoricoxib is available in most countries outside the United States.

Mechanism of Action

The most important mechanism of action is to inhibit prostaglandin production by competing with arachidonic acid for binding in the cyclooxyganase (COX) catalytic site.[3] The reduced formation of prostaglandins is responsible for the anti-inflammatory, analgesic, and antipyretic effects—but also for many of the potential adverse effects. In particular, prostaglandin E2 is involved in the inflammatory process and in pain signaling.

Two isoforms of COX were discovered in the early 1990s.[4] The hypothesis was that the symptom-modifying efficacy of all NSAIDs and coxibs was mediated through inhibition of cyclooxygenase-2 (COX-2) and the reduced formation of prostaglandins, in particular prostaglandin E2.[5–7] Other COX-independent mechanisms of action have been suggested to be relevant,[8,9] and some studies also support that COX inhibition in the central nervous system contributes to pain relief.[10]

No compelling evidence supports the concept that NSAIDs and coxibs retard radiographic progression in RA, whereas one study in ankylosing spondylitis has suggested that NSAIDs may influence the development of radiographic abnormalities in this condition.[11]

A major concern with NSAIDs is the risk of severe adverse reactions, and on rare occasions death. The discovery of the two COX isoforms in the early 1990s led to the hope that selective inhibition of COX-2 would spare COX-1 without reduced formation of the prostaglandins with important "housekeeping" functions.[5–7] For example, prostaglandin E2 protects the gastric mucosa from damage. Thus, development of selective drugs targeting COX-2 without inhibition of COX-1 became an important research area. The first two COX-2 selective NSAIDs, often called coxibs, appeared on the market around 1999. However, studies from recent years have demonstrated that the pharmacologic effects are more complex than first assumed. Further, the entire area is more complicated due to dose-dependent pharmacologic effects—and the traditional NSAIDs also differ in their degree of COX-2 selectivity.[12,13] Thus, naproxen in high doses is a strong inhibitor of COX-1, whereas diclofenac is a weak inhibitor.[14]

Clinical Efficacy

Meta-analyses have demonstrated the efficacy of conventional NSAIDs in RA, but clear differences among NSAIDs have not been demonstrated.[15] Trials performed in the 1980s were often small and had an insufficient design to answer this question,[16,17] and results in comparative trials seemed often to be biased in favor of the new drug.[18]

Better studies were performed in the 1990s after the agreement of using core measures of disease activity in clinical trials. Pain and disability were included in this core set.[19] The coxibs were usually tested in phase 3, with a design that required 12 weeks of treatment. The new coxibs were compared with placebo and with an active comparator in high doses. These studies demonstrated that celecoxib,[20] rofecoxib,[21,22] valdecoxib,[23,24] etoricoxib,[25,26] and lumiracoxib[27] were superior to placebo in RA and had similar efficacy as the active comparator. Importantly, these studies have also contributed to the understanding of efficacy of conventional NSAIDs—which overall indicated that conventional NSAIDs and coxibs had similar efficacy on a group level in RA.

However, even large studies sometimes only demonstrated borderline differentiation between placebo and active drug. This observation has also been made in a systematic review of NSAID treatment of patients with knee osteoarthritis (OA)[28] and is consistent with the clinical experience that some patients perceive an important effect of NSAIDs (whereas NSAIDs are less important for many other patients). In the Oslo RA register, about half of the patients are regular users of NSAIDs/coxibs.[29] It has been suggested that patients have individual efficacy and as a result express individual preferences for different NSAIDs.[30] However, systematic reviews have not been able to confirm this observation.[15]

Another concern for interpretation of efficacy data is the daily variation in patient-reported outcomes. Many patients in stable disease will report great variations in the pain perception, even when recorded daily. A recent study of RA patients with stable disease and treatment demonstrated that daily pain on a 100-mm visual analogue scale varied within a band of 20 mm.[31]

Many patients with RA will use conventional disease-modifying antirheumatic drugs (DMARDs), corticosteroids, and/or biologic agents. Treatment with corticosteroids and DMARDs has usually not been an exclusion criterion in randomized controlled clinical trials (RCTs) examining the efficacy of NSAIDs and coxibs, but subgroup analyses based on concurrent treatment have not been adequately carried out. Thus, the magnitude of benefit from coxibs and NSAIDs is largely unknown in patients being treated with DMARDs and corticosteroids. Two studies comparing etoricoxib versus naproxen versus placebo demonstrated different treatment differences (deltas) between active drugs and placebo.[25,26] The patients in the study with the small treatment effect were more actively treated with corticosteroids and DMARDs,[25] which may indirectly support that the relative benefit of NSAID is of smaller magnitude in patients with concurrent disease-modifying therapy—at least if the patients have minor residual inflammatory activity.

It is not known how and to what extent NSAIDs and coxibs relieve symptoms in patients on anti–tumor necrosis factor (TNF) drugs and other biologic agents. These drugs have usually been listed among exclusion criteria in trials with NSAIDs and coxibs.

A practical question is whether NSAIDs should be given in a stable dosing or a variable dosing according to natural fluctuations in symptom intensity. This research question has been formally addressed in osteoarthritis, and the results suggested that flexible dosing is as effective as stable dosing with a reduced amount of drug. The flexible dosing regimen was associated with a lower number of reported adverse events.[32]

Gastrointestinal Safety

It is well recognized that NSAIDs increase the risk for gastrointestinal adverse reactions. The increased risk has been estimated to be three- to fourfold in a variety of different study designs.[33] Risk factors for ulcer disease during NSAID therapy include concomitant use of corticosteroids, use of anticoagulants, age, and previous ulcer.[34] Other risk factors (e.g., cardiovascular disease) have been suggested.[35]

Epidemiologic studies from the pre-coxib period indicated differences between NSAIDs with regard to risks for gastric ulcers.[36–39] These studies also demonstrated a clear relationship between risk and dose, and gastrointestinal toxicity was at this time considered a major risk and limitation in the treatment of RA.[34]

The main idea behind the development of COX-2–selective NSAIDs was to have NSAIDs that maintained the formation of prostaglandins with their protective effects on the gastric mucosa. Early endoscopy studies[40,41] and some pooled analyses[42] suggested that coxibs could reduce the ulcer rate by 70% to 75%, which would correspond to a level close to placebo based on the known increased risk with NSAIDs from epidemiologic studies.[33] Another endoscopy study showed a 75% reduction of endoscopic gastroduodenal ulcers after 24 weeks of therapy with celecoxib compared to diclofenac.[43] This study also suggested a lower incidence of patient-reported gastrointestinal side effects with celecoxib.[43]

The first large gastrointestinal outcome studies were published in 2000 (CLASS[44] and VIGOR[45]) and demonstrated a 50% to 60% reduction in clinical ulcers and ulcer complications compared to traditional NSAIDs. However, these studies had different primary endpoints, and the CLASS study actually failed to demonstrate statistically significant difference between celecoxib and diclofenac/ibuprofen for the primary endpoint (complicated gastrointestinal ulcers). Approximately ⅔ of the study population had osteoarthritis, and a large proportion of patients not unexpectedly stopped using the trial medication. Further, more than 20% of the patients were using concomitant low-dose aspirin—which was an exclusion criterion in the VIGOR study.[45] The failure of achieving a statistically significant reduction in complicated ulcers in the CLASS study led to a great degree of criticism.[46] However, several pooled analyses have clearly demonstrated that celecoxib is superior to conventional NSAIDs with regard to gastrointestinal safety.[47,48]

Lumiracoxib was also associated with a reduction in gastrointestinal ulcers and ulcer complications in comparison with naproxen and ibuprofen.[49] Valdecoxib was never tested in a similarly designed large outcome study, but endoscopy studies and pooled analyses of individual studies suggested an improved gastrointestinal safety profile compared to traditional NSAIDs.[50]

Etoricoxib has also never been tested in outcome studies focusing on gastrointestinal ulcers as the primary endpoint. However, gastroduodenal ulcers were adjudicated in the Multinational Etoricoxib and Diclofenac Arthritis Long-Term Study Program (MEDAL) and a reduction in the rate of clinical ulcers was observed compared to diclofenac.[51] However, the rate of complicated ulcers was not different between etoricoxib and diclofenac. Etoricoxib has been associated in endoscopy studies with a lower rate of endoscopic ulcers compared to naproxen, but the rate of ulcers was even lower in the placebo-treated compared to the etoricoxib-treated patients.[52]

Another potential benefit from coxibs is a reduced rate of gastrointestinal bleeding, which has been demonstrated for etoricoxib.[52] Less anemia was also observed with celecoxib compared to ibuprofen and diclofenac in the CLASS study,[44] and fewer lower gastrointestinal tract events were seen with rofecoxib compared to naproxen in the VIGOR study.[53]

In summary, coxibs reduce the risk for gastrointestinal events. However, the reduction compared to traditional NSAIDs does not seem to be more than 50% to 60%. Thus, patients taking coxibs also have a slightly increased risk of gastrointestinal events—which was recently also demonstrated in an explorative analysis of the Adenomatous Polyp Prevention on Vioxx (APPROVe) study.[54]

Cardiovascular Safety

Concerns about the cardiovascular safety of coxibs were raised early because coxibs inhibit the formation of vascular prostacyclin without inhibiting thromboxane.[55] It was assumed that this imbalance in formation of vasodilating and vasocostrive substances could have thrombogenic impact.[7]

The VIGOR study demonstrated that rofecoxib was associated with a fivefold increase in myocardial infarctions compared to naproxen.[45] It was first assumed that naproxen may have displayed an aspirin-like cardioprotective effect in high doses because of continuous inhibition of COX-1 and platelet aggregation,[14] with some database studies supporting a cardioprotective effect.[56–58] Several subsequent analyses from administrative databases and case control studies have demonstrated that rofecoxib was associated with an increased risk of thrombotic cardiovascular adverse events, especially in higher doses.[59] Rofecoxib was withdrawn from the market 30 September 2004 when an interim analysis of the APPROVe study showed a twofold increase in cardiovascular events compared to placebo.[60] A subsequent analysis of another colorectal adenomas study (the Adenoma Prevention with Celecoxib [APC] trial) also demonstrated an increased incidence of thrombotic cardiovascular events with celecoxib compared to placebo, and the rate was related to the dose of celecoxib.[61] Valdecoxib was also associated with increases in cardiovascular events in a placebo-controlled postoperative pain study after coronary surgery.[62]

These studies together with observational studies overall indicated that coxibs are associated with an increased risk of thrombotic cardiovascular events despite the fact that another prevention of colorectal adenomas study with 200 mg of celecoxib did not demonstrate any increased risk compared to placebo[61] and the fact that rofecoxib and placebo were associated with similar rates in a study of patients with Alzheimer's disease.[63]

A recent study with more than 30,000 patients with RA or osteoarthritis was performed to explore cardiovascular events as the primary endpoint (the MEDAL program). The rate of events was similar between etoricoxib and diclofenac in this study, which also allowed concomitant use of low-dose aspirin as well as gastroprotective medication whenever clinically indicated.[64]

A meta-analysis of placebo-controlled studies has supported the notion that coxibs are associated with an increased risk of thrombotic cardiovascular events, but conventional nonnaproxen NSAIDs had similar increased risk.[65] Other database and case-control studies have presented data in the same direction.[66] These data and the MEDAL program suggest that both coxibs and nonnaproxen NSAIDs are associated with an increased risk for thrombotic cardiovascular events.

Other Safety Issues

Other safety concerns of NSAIDs include reduced kidney function, fluid retention, edema, and hypertension—as well as cutaneous reactions. Use of NSAIDs is associated with an increase in blood pressure.[67] The rate of hypertension may differ across different NSAIDs, and in particular etoricoxib has been associated with increased risk of hypertension[64] (which has also led to a warning on the label for this particular drug).

Edema, fluid retention, and reduced renal function are also mechanistically determined through inhibition of renal COX-2. It has been suggested that celecoxib has less renal problems than other coxibs and NSAIDs,[68] and sulindac was assumed to cause less reduction in glomerular filtration than other NSAIDs.[69] However, for clinical purposes all NSAIDs should be used with caution in patients with reduced renal function and in patients with edema due to cardiac failure.

Cutaneous side effects are rare but can be severe (Steven Johnson syndrome, Lyells syndrome).[70] Severe skin reactions contributed to the withdrawal of valdecoxib from the market. All NSAIDs may also lead to liver toxicity, which is usually mild. Diclofenac is more often associated with liver enzyme elevations, sometimes quite dramatic, compared to other NSAIDs and coxibs.[51] Increased occurrence of liver enzyme elevations has also been observed in trials of lumiracoxib and has contributed to the removal of this drug from many markets.[71]

Risk/Benefit Ratio

NSAIDs and coxibs relieve pain and stiffness and improve physical function in patients with RA. Some patients simply do not experience enough relief from their standard baseline regimen and need NSAIDs to improve their quality of life and function. However, the level of perceived improvement differs across individual patients. Because NSAIDs and coxibs improve symptoms, the patient will usually be in a situation to assist the physician-patient interaction in deciding whether the treatment causes a health benefit determined important.

For clinical decision making, the next consideration must be whether this benefit exceeds the risk for gastrointestinal-tract complications, cardiovascular events, and other adverse events. The risk for cardiovascular events and gastrointestinal-tract involvement may differ across individuals based on individual risk factors such as previous ulcer disease or the presence of arteriosclerosis and vascular complications such as coronary artery disease.

Follow-up of patients in RCTs suggests that the efficacy of NSAIDs usually appear after 1 to 2 weeks. RCTs are usually performed with a flare design, which means that pain will recur when NSAIDs are stopped. These observations can be translated into clinical practice in the following way. Patients who receive a NSAID or coxib prescription may use the drug for a couple of weeks and then perceive whether important symptomatic improvement occurs. If in doubt, the drug can be stopped to observe whether symptoms recur. This process may be repeated for several different NSAIDS in a rotation so that subjective comparisons can be made. One agent may appear best or may be better tolerated than all others. If the health benefit is marginal, it will usually not be justified to be exposed for long-term treatment with NSAIDs or coxibs. If, on the other hand, the health benefit is considered important the patient will usually be recommended to use NSAIDs and coxibs in the lowest dose that provides sufficient symptom relief and/or to use the drugs in a flexible dosing regimen according to fluctuations in symptom intensity.

References

1. Heiberg T, Kvien TK. Preferences for improved health examined in 1,024 patients with rheumatoid arthritis: Pain has highest priority. *Arthritis Rheum* 2002;47(4):391–397.
2. Benson MD, do-Benson M, Brandt KD. Synovial fluid concentrations of diclofenac in patients with rheumatoid arthritis or osteoarthritis. *Semin Arthritis Rheum* 1985;15(2/Suppl 1):65–67.
3. Smith WL, DeWitt DL, Garavito RM. Cyclooxygenases: Structural, cellular, and molecular biology. *Annu Rev Biochem* 2000;69:145–182.
4. Masferrer JL, Zweifel BS, Seibert K, et al. Selective regulation of cellular cyclooxygenase by dexamethasone and endotoxin in mice. *J Clin Invest* 1990;86(4):1375–1379.
5. Hawkey CJ. COX-2 inhibitors. *Lancet* 1999;353(9149):307–314.
6. Brooks P, Emery P, Evans JF, et al. Interpreting the clinical significance of the differential inhibition of cyclooxygenase–1 and cyclooxygenase–2. *Rheumatology* (Oxford) 1999;38(8): 779–788.
7. FitzGerald GA, Patrono C. The coxibs, selective inhibitors of cyclooxygenase–2. *N Engl J Med* 2001;345(6):433–442.
8. Abramson SB, Weissmann G. The mechanisms of action of nonsteroidal antiinflammatory drugs. *Arthritis Rheum* 1989;32(1):1–9.
9. Cronstein BN, Montesinos MC, Weissmann G. Salicylates and sulfasalazine, but not glucocorticoids, inhibit leukocyte accumulation by an adenosine-dependent mechanism that is independent of inhibition of prostaglandin synthesis and p105 of NFκB. *Proc Natl Acad Sci USA* 1999;96(11):6377–6381.
10. Ek M, Engblom D, Saha S, et al. Inflammatory response: Pathway across the blood-brain barrier. *Nature* 2001;410(6827):430–431.
11. Wanders A, Heijde D, Landewe R, et al. Nonsteroidal antiinflammatory drugs reduce radiographic progression in patients with ankylosing spondylitis: A randomized clinical trial. *Arthritis Rheum* 2005; 52(6):1756–1765.
12. Solomon DH. Selective cyclooxygenase 2 inhibitors and cardiovascular events. *Arthritis Rheum* 2005;52(7):1968–1978.
13. Warner TD, Mitchell JA. COX-2 selectivity alone does not define the cardiovascular risks associated with non-steroidal anti-inflammatory drugs. *Lancet* 2008;371(9608):270–273.
14. Van HA, Schwartz JI, Depre M, et al. Comparative inhibitory activity of rofecoxib, meloxicam, diclofenac, ibuprofen, and naproxen on COX-2 versus COX-1 in healthy volunteers. *J Clin Pharmacol* 2000;40(10):1109–1120.
15. Gotzsche PC. Non-steroidal anti-inflammatory drugs. *BMJ* 2000; 320(7241):1058–1061.
16. Gotzsche PC. Meta-analysis of NSAIDs: Contribution of drugs, doses, trial designs, and meta-analytic techniques. *Scand J Rheumatol* 1993;22(6):255–260.
17. Gotzsche PC. Review of dose-response studies of NSAIDs in rheumatoid arthritis. *Dan Med Bull* 1989;36(4):395–399.
18. Gotzsche PC. Methodology and overt and hidden bias in reports of 196 double-blind trials of nonsteroidal antiinflammatory drugs in rheumatoid arthritis. *Control Clin Trials* 1989;10(1):31–56.
19. Boers M, Tugwell P, Felson DT, et al. World Health Organization and International League of Associations for Rheumatology core endpoints for symptom modifying antirheumatic drugs in rheumatoid arthritis clinical trials. *J Rheumatol Suppl* 1994;41:86–89.
20. Garner S, Fidan D, Frankish R, et al. Celecoxib for rheumatoid arthritis. *Cochrane Database Syst Rev* 2002;4:CD003831.
21. Garner SE, Fidan DD, Frankish RR, et al. Rofecoxib for rheumatoid arthritis. *Cochrane Database Syst Rev* 2005;1:CD003685.
22. Geusens PP, Truitt K, Sfikakis P, et al. A placebo and active comparator-controlled trial of rofecoxib for the treatment of rheumatoid arthritis. *Scand J Rheumatol* 2002;31(4):230–238.
23. Bensen W, Weaver A, Espinoza L, et al. Efficacy and safety of valdecoxib in treating the signs and symptoms of rheumatoid arthritis: A randomized, controlled comparison with placebo and naproxen. *Rheumatology* (Oxford) 2002;41(9):1008–1016.
24. Gibofsky A, Rodrigues J, Fiechtner J, et al. Efficacy and tolerability of valdecoxib in treating the signs and symptoms of severe rheumatoid arthritis: A 12-week, multicenter, randomized, double-blind, placebo-controlled study. *Clin Ther* 2007;29(6):1071–1085.
25. Collantes E, Curtis SP, Lee KW, et al. A multinational randomized, controlled, clinical trial of etoricoxib in the treatment of rheumatoid arthritis [ISRCTN25142273]. *BMC Fam Pract* 2002;3:10.
26. Matsumoto AK, Melian A, Mandel DR, et al. A randomized, controlled, clinical trial of etoricoxib in the treatment of rheumatoid arthritis. *J Rheumatol* 2002;29(8):1623–1630.
27. Geusens P, Alten R, Rovensky J, et al. Efficacy, safety and tolerability of lumiracoxib in patients with rheumatoid arthritis. *Int J Clin Pract* 2004;58(11):1033–1041.
28. Bjordal JM, Ljunggren AE, Klovning A, et al. Non-steroidal anti-inflammatory drugs, including cyclo-oxygenase–2 inhibitors, in osteoarthritic knee pain: meta-analysis of randomised placebo controlled trials. *BMJ* 2004;329(7478):1317.
29. Heiberg T, Finset A, Uhlig T, et al. Seven year changes in health status and priorities for improvement of health in patients with rheumatoid arthritis. *Ann Rheum Dis* 2005;64(2):191–195.
30. Huskisson EC. Four commonly prescribed non-steroidal anti-inflammatory drugs for rheumatoid arthritis. *Eur J Rheumatol Inflamm* 1991;11(2):8–12.
31. Heiberg T, Kvien TK, Dale O, et al. Daily health status registration (patient diary) in patients with rheumatoid arthritis: A comparison between personal digital assistant and paper-pencil format. *Arthritis Rheum* 2007;57(3):454–460.
32. Kvien TK, Brors O, Staff PH, et al. Improved cost-effectiveness ratio with a patient self-adjusted naproxen dosing regimen in osteoarthritis treatment. *Scand J Rheumatol* 1991;20(4):280–287.
33. Ofman JJ, MacLean CH, Straus WL, et al. A metaanalysis of severe upper gastrointestinal complications of nonsteroidal antiinflammatory drugs. *J Rheumatol* 2002;29(4):804–812.
34. Wolfe MM, Lichtenstein DR, Singh G. Gastrointestinal toxicity of nonsteroidal antiinflammatory drugs. *N Engl J Med* 1999;340(24): 1888–1899.
35. Silverstein FE, Graham DY, Senior JR, et al. Misoprostol reduces serious gastrointestinal complications in patients with rheumatoid arthritis receiving nonsteroidal anti-inflammatory drugs: A randomized, double-blind, placebo-controlled trial. *Ann Intern Med* 1995;123(4):241–249.
36. Langman MJ, Weil J, Wainwright P, et al. Risks of bleeding peptic ulcer associated with individual non-steroidal anti-inflammatory drugs. *Lancet* 1994;343(8905):1075–1078.
37. Henry D, Dobson A, Turner C. Variability in the risk of major gastrointestinal complications from nonaspirin nonsteroidal anti-inflammatory drugs. *Gastroenterology* 1993;105(4):1078–1088.

38. Henry DA, Johnston A, Dobson A, et al. Fatal peptic ulcer complications and the use of non-steroidal anti-inflammatory drugs, aspirin, and corticosteroids. *Br Med J (Clin Res Ed)* 1987;295(6608): 1227–1229.
39. Garcia Rodriguez LA, Jick H. Risk of upper gastrointestinal bleeding and perforation associated with individual non-steroidal anti-inflammatory drugs. *Lancet* 1994;343(8900):769–772.
40. Simon LS, Weaver AL, Graham DY, et al. Anti-inflammatory and upper gastrointestinal effects of celecoxib in rheumatoid arthritis: A randomized controlled trial. *JAMA* 1999;282(20):1921–1928.
41. Kivitz AJ, Nayiager S, Schimansky T, et al. Reduced incidence of gastroduodenal ulcers associated with lumiracoxib compared with ibuprofen in patients with rheumatoid arthritis. *Aliment Pharmacol Ther* 2004;19(11):1189–1198.
42. Goldstein JL, Silverstein FE, Agrawal NM, et al. Reduced risk of upper gastrointestinal ulcer complications with celecoxib, a novel COX-2 inhibitor. *Am J Gastroenterol* 2000;95(7):1681–1690.
43. Emery P, Zeidler H, Kvien TK, et al. Celecoxib versus diclofenac in long-term management of rheumatoid arthritis: Randomised double-blind comparison. *Lancet* 1999;354(9196):2106–2111.
44. Silverstein FE, Faich G, Goldstein JL, et al. Gastrointestinal toxicity with celecoxib vs nonsteroidal anti-inflammatory drugs for osteoarthritis and rheumatoid arthritis: the CLASS study: A randomized controlled trial. Celecoxib Long-term Arthritis Safety Study. *JAMA* 2000;284(10):1247–1255.
45. Bombardier C, Laine L, Reicin A, et al. for the VIGOR Study Group. Comparison of upper gastrointestinal toxicity of rofecoxib and naproxen in patients with rheumatoid arthritis. *N Engl J Med* 2000; 343(21):1520–1528.
46. Mukherjee D, Nissen SE, Topol EJ. Risk of cardiovascular events associated with selective COX-2 inhibitors. *JAMA* 2001;286(8): 954–959.
47. Deeks JJ, Smith LA, Bradley MD. Efficacy, tolerability, and upper gastrointestinal safety of celecoxib for treatment of osteoarthritis and rheumatoid arthritis: Systematic review of randomised controlled trials. *BMJ* 2002;325(7365):619.
48. Moore RA, Derry S, Makinson GT, et al. Tolerability and adverse events in clinical trials of celecoxib in osteoarthritis and rheumatoid arthritis: Systematic review and meta-analysis of information from company clinical trial reports. *Arthritis Res Ther* 2005;7(3): R644–R665.
49. Schnitzer TJ, Burmester GR, Mysler E, et al. Comparison of lumiracoxib with naproxen and ibuprofen in the Therapeutic Arthritis Research and Gastrointestinal Event Trial (TARGET), reduction in ulcer complications: randomised controlled trial. *Lancet* 2004; 364(9435):665–674.
50. Goldstein JL, Eisen GM, Agrawal N, et al. Reduced incidence of upper gastrointestinal ulcer complications with the COX-2 selective inhibitor, valdecoxib. *Aliment Pharmacol Ther* 2004;20(5):527–538.
51. Laine L, Curtis SP, Cryer B, et al. Assessment of upper gastrointestinal safety of etoricoxib and diclofenac in patients with osteoarthritis and rheumatoid arthritis in the Multinational Etoricoxib and Diclofenac Arthritis Long-term (MEDAL) programme: A randomised comparison. *Lancet* 2007;369(9560):465–473.
52. Hunt RH, Harper S, Callegari P, et al. Complementary studies of the gastrointestinal safety of the cyclo-oxygenase–2-selective inhibitor etoricoxib. *Aliment Pharmacol Ther* 2003;17(2):201–210.
53. Laine L, Connors LG, Reicin A, et al. Serious lower gastrointestinal clinical events with nonselective NSAID or coxib use. *Gastroenterology* 2003;124(2):288–292.
54. Lanas A, Baron JA, Sandler RS, et al. Peptic ulcer and bleeding events associated with rofecoxib in a 3-year colorectal adenoma chemoprevention trial. *Gastroenterology* 2007;132(2):490–497.
55. McAdam BF, Catella-Lawson F, Mardini IA, et al. Systemic biosynthesis of prostacyclin by cyclooxygenase (COX)–2: the human pharmacology of a selective inhibitor of COX-2. *Proc Natl Acad Sci USA* 1999;96(1):272–277.
56. Watson DJ, Rhodes T, Cai B, et al. Lower risk of thromboembolic cardiovascular events with naproxen among patients with rheumatoid arthritis. *Arch Intern Med* 2002;162(10):1105–1110.
57. Solomon DH, Glynn RJ, Levin R, et al. Nonsteroidal anti-inflammatory drug use and acute myocardial infarction. *Arch Intern Med* 2002; 162(10):1099–1104.
58. Rahme E, Pilote L, LeLorier J. Association between naproxen use and protection against acute myocardial infarction. *Arch Intern Med* 2002;162(10):1111–1115.
59. Juni P, Nartey L, Reichenbach S, et al. Risk of cardiovascular events and rofecoxib: Cumulative meta-analysis. *Lancet* 2004;364(9450): 2021–2029.
60. Bresalier RS, Sandler RS, Quan H, et al. Cardiovascular events associated with rofecoxib in a colorectal adenoma chemoprevention trial. *N Engl J Med* 2005;352(11):1092–1102.
61. Solomon SD, McMurray JJ, Pfeffer MA, et al. Cardiovascular risk associated with celecoxib in a clinical trial for colorectal adenoma prevention. *N Engl J Med* 2005;352(11):1071–1080.
62. Nussmeier NA, Whelton AA, Brown MT, et al. Complications of the COX-2 inhibitors parecoxib and valdecoxib after cardiac surgery. *N Engl J Med* 2005;352(11):1081–1091.
63. Salpeter SR, Gregor P, Ormiston TM, et al. Meta-analysis: Cardiovascular events associated with nonsteroidal anti-inflammatory drugs. *Am J Med* 2006;119(7):552–559.
64. Cannon CP, Curtis SP, FitzGerald GA, et al. Cardiovascular outcomes with etoricoxib and diclofenac in patients with osteoarthritis and rheumatoid arthritis in the Multinational Etoricoxib and Diclofenac Arthritis Long-term (MEDAL) programme: A randomised comparison. *Lancet* 2006;368(9549):1771–1781.
65. Kearney PM, Baigent C, Godwin J, et al. Do selective cyclo-oxygenase–2 inhibitors and traditional non-steroidal anti-inflammatory drugs increase the risk of atherothrombosis? Meta-analysis of randomised trials. *BMJ* 2006;332(7553):1302–1308.
66. McGettigan P, Henry D. Cardiovascular risk and inhibition of cyclooxygenase: A systematic review of the observational studies of selective and nonselective inhibitors of cyclooxygenase 2. *JAMA* 2006;296(13):1633–1644.
67. de Leeuw PW. Nonsteroidal anti-inflammatory drugs and hypertension: The risks in perspective. *Drugs* 1996;51(2):179–187.
68. Whelton A, Lefkowith JL, West CR, et al. Cardiorenal effects of celecoxib as compared with the nonsteroidal anti-inflammatory drugs diclofenac and ibuprofen. *Kidney Int* 2006;70(8):1495–1502.
69. Ciabattoni G, Cinotti GA, Pierucci A, et al. Effects of sulindac and ibuprofen in patients with chronic glomerular disease: Evidence for the dependence of renal function on prostacyclin. *N Engl J Med* 1984;310(5):279–283.
70. Layton D, Marshall V, Boshier A, et al.. Serious skin reactions and selective COX-2 inhibitors: A case series from prescription-event monitoring in England. *Drug Saf* 2006;29(8):687–696.
71. Shi S, Klotz U. Clinical use and pharmacological properties of selective COX-2 inhibitors. *Eur J Clin Pharmacol* 2008;64(3):233–252.

Glucocorticoids

Johannes W.J. Bijlsma and Frank Buttgereit

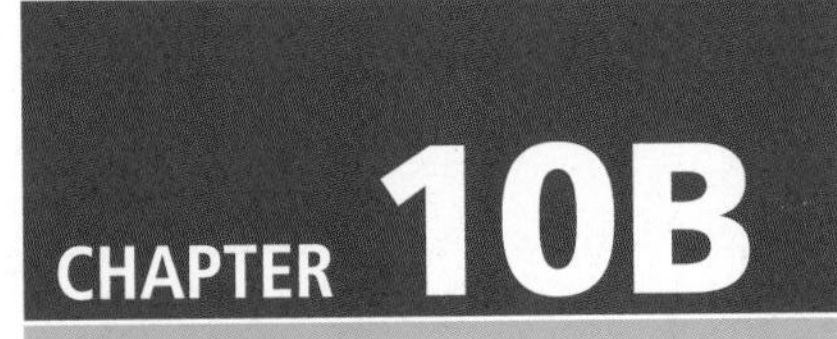

Glucocorticoids (GCs) play a pivotal role in the management of rheumatoid arthritis (RA), as well as in many other rheumatic diseases. The proportion of patients treated with GCs by practicing rheumatologists on a daily basis is clearly in excess of the usually conservative recommendations in textbooks and review papers. Nearly 60 years after their introduction into clinical practice, GCs still represent the most important and most frequently employed class of anti-inflammatory drugs. Between 25% and 75% of patients with RA are treated more or less continuously with GCs.[1] Recent studies have reestablished the disease-modifying potential of low-dose GCs in RA and have renewed the debate on the risk/benefit ratios of this treatment. There is no doubt that especially when applied incorrectly GCs have a rather high potential for frequent and serious side effects, but when used prudently many of these side effects can be dealt with. For daily practice, some suggestions are given in the European League Against Rheumatism (EULAR) recommendations on the management of systemic GC therapy in rheumatic diseases.[2]

Mechanisms of Action

The dosage of GCs used often increases based on clinical activity and severity of the RA.[3,4] The rationale for this (mostly successful) clinical decision is: higher dosages increase GC receptor saturation in a dose-dependent manner, which intensifies the therapeutically relevant genomic GC actions; and it is assumed that with increasing dosages additional and qualitatively different nonspecific nongenomic actions of GCs increasingly come into play.

Genomic Actions of Glucocorticoids

The important anti-inflammatory and immunomodulatory effects of GCs are mediated predominantly by genomic mechanisms (Figure 10B-1). Binding to cytosolic GC receptors (cGCR) ultimately induces ("transactivation") or inhibits ("transrepression") the synthesis of regulator proteins.[4] GCs influence the transcription of approximately 1% of the entire genome.[5] The lipophilic structure and low molecular mass allow GCs to pass easily through the cell membrane and to form an activated GC/cGCR complex. This receptor complex is then translocated into the nucleus, where it binds as a homodimer to consensus palindromic DNA sites, which are called GC-responsive elements (GREs)].[6] Depending on the target gene, transcription is either activated (transactivation via positive GRE) or inhibited (negative GRE). In addition to these mechanisms, the interaction of activated cGCR monomers with transcription factors such as AP-1 (activator protein-1), NF-kB (nuclear factor-kappaB), and NF-AT (nuclear factor for activated T cells) is recognized as a further important genomic mechanism of GC action.[7,8] Accordingly, although the GC/cGCR complex does not inhibit their synthesis it modulates the activity of these factors—which leads to inhibition of nuclear translocation and/or function of these transcription factors and hence to inhibition of the expression of many immunoregulatory and inflammatory factors (transrepression). There are indications that many adverse clinical effects are caused by the transactivation mechanism (i.e., induced synthesis of regulator proteins), whereas many important anti-inflammatory effects are mediated by transrepression (i.e., inhibited synthesis of regulator proteins). This differential molecular regulation provides the basis for current drug-discovery programs that aim at the development of dissociating cGCR ligands. These novel substances, also called selective GC receptor agonists (SEGRAs), are being developed in order to obtain drugs with high repression activities against inflammatory mediator production but lower transactivation activities than traditional GCs. At the moment, it cannot be reliably predicted whether SEGRAs will as "improved GCs" enter clinical medicine in the near future.[4,9,10]

Nongenomic Actions of Glucocorticoids

Some regulatory effects of GCs arise within a few seconds or minutes. Such observations cannot be explained by the previously mentioned genomic actions because of the time these require. Nongenomic mechanisms of action are thought to be responsible for these rapid effects. Three different nongenomic mechanisms have been proposed to explain rapid anti-inflammatory and immunosuppressive GC effects: nonspecific interactions of glucocorticoids with cellular membranes,[3,4] nongenomic effects that are mediated by the cGCR,[11,12] and specific interactions with membrane-bound GCR.[10,13–15]

Glucocorticoid Effects on Immune Cells

Based on the mechanisms mentioned previoulsy, GCs mediate fascinating anti-inflammatory and immunomodulatory effects when used therapeutically. There are many specific effects of the commonly used GC drugs: virtually all primary and secondary immune cells are more or less affected. A selection of the most important effects on the different cell types is outlined in Figure 10B-2.[16]

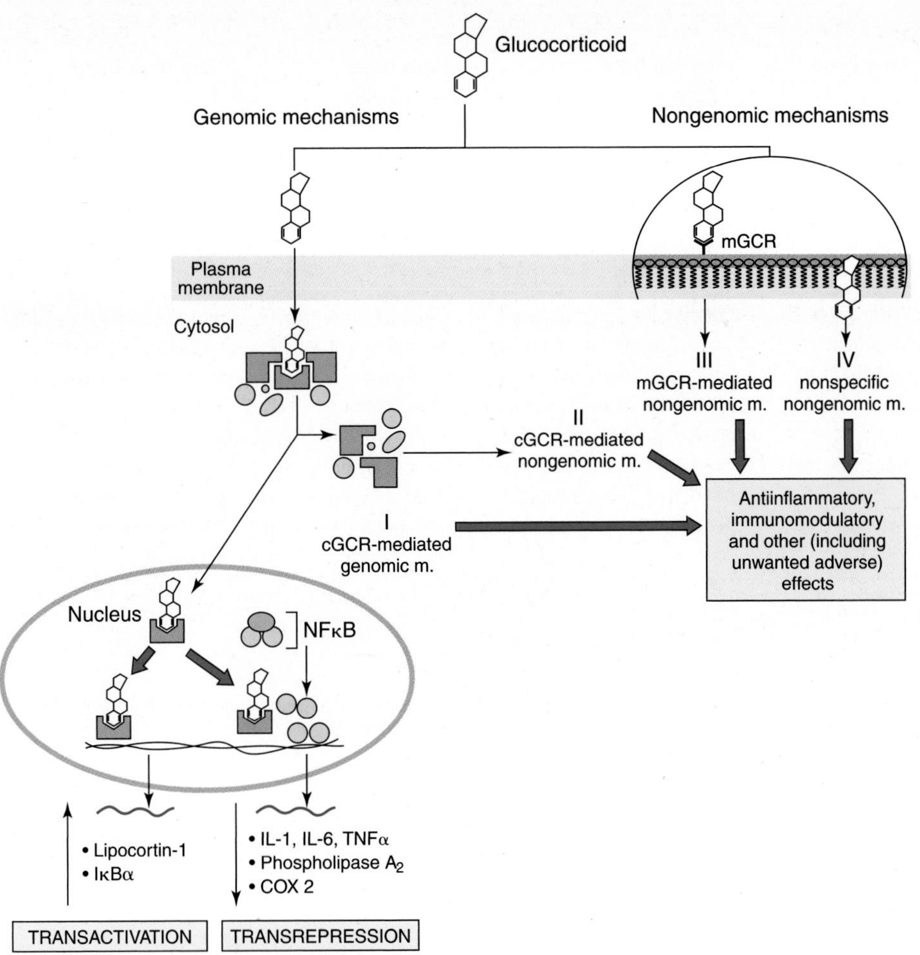

Figure 10B-1. Mechanisms of the cellular actions of glucocorticoids. As lipophilic substances, glucocorticoids pass very easily through the cell membrane into the cell, where they bind to ubiquitously expressed cytosolic glucocorticoid receptors (cGCR). This is followed by either the classical cGCR-mediated genomic effects (I) or by cGCR-mediated nongenomic effects (II). Moreover, the glucocorticoid is very likely to interact with cell membranes either specifically via membrane-bound glucocorticoid receptors (mGCR) (III) or via nonspecific interactions with cell membranes (IV). (Adapted from Buttgereit, F, Straub, RH, Wehling M, et al. Glucocorticoids in the treatment of rheumatic diseases: An update on mechanisms of action. *Arthritis Rheum* 2004;50:3408–3417.)

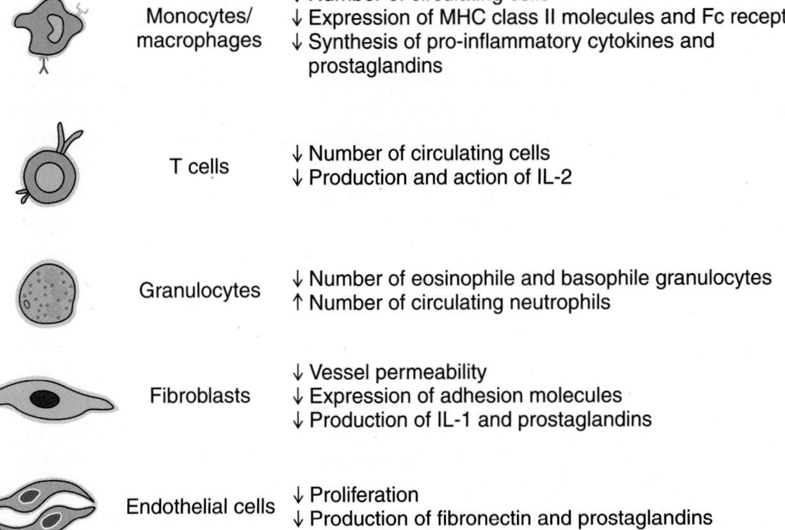

Figure 10B-2. Immunosuppressive actions of glucocorticoids. Influence of GCs on different cells of the immune cells. (Adapted from Buttgereit F, Saag K, Cutolo M, et al. The molecular basis for the effectiveness, toxicity, and resistance to glucocorticoids: focus on the treatment of rheumatoid arthritis. *Scand J Rheumatol* 2005;34:14–21.)

Therapeutic Use

There is a widespread use of different GC treatment regimens in RA and other rheumatic diseases. In addition, different GC drugs have different potencies and pharmacodynamics.[17] A recent consensus statement recommended specific definitions of GC dosages, partly based on the action of GCs via genomic and nongenomic pathways (Table 10B-1).[3] For the genomic effects, the degree of cytosolic receptor saturation is considered a direct modulator of the intensity of (therapeutic) GC actions. Higher doses (e.g., 100 mg or more) are required to result in nearly complete receptor saturation. These considerations coincide

Table 10B-1. Definitions of GC Dosages According to a Recent Consensus Statement

	Low Dose	Medium Dose	High Dose	Very High Dose[a]
Dose range (mg prednisone equivalent per day)	≤7.5	7.5–30	>30–≤100	>100
Action of GC via genomic pathways (saturation of cytosolic glucocorticoid receptors)	+ (<50%)	++ (>50–<100%)	++(+) (almost 100%)	+++ (100%)
Actions of GC via nongenomic pathways	–/?	(+)	+	++/+++
Clinical usage in RA	Often used as maintenance therapy in active disease	Effective if given initially in various conditions of the disease; used for extra-articular complications such as pericarditis and pleuritis	Initial treatment for serious exacerbations or vasculitic complications	Initial dosages for acute or life-threatening exacerbations such as vasculitis
Adverse effects	Relatively few (such as osteoporosis)	Considerably and dose dependent if given for longer periods	Cannot be administered for long-term therapy due to severe side effects	Cannot be administered for long-term therapy due to severe side effects

[a]The term *pulse therapy* describes a specific therapeutic entity using very high GC doses. It refers to the administration of ≥250 mg prednisone equivalent per day (usually IV) for a short period of time (1 to a maximum of 5 days) to quickly reduce them or stop GC treatment altogether. These doses are sometimes given to bridge the gap in RA disease activity when underlying DMARD therapy is changed. Since the introduction of biologicals, these pulses are given less frequently. The nongenomic potencies of GCs in the table come increasingly into play at such high doses, which are assumed to be the reason for the clinical observation that generally pulse therapy is successful in acute exacerbations of RA. Pulse therapy results in termination of the exacerbation or regression of severe forms of RA in a high proportion of cases with a relatively low incidence of side effects.[24] Note that intra-articular GC injections are a type of (local) pulse therapy.
GC, glucocorticoid.
Adapted from Buttgereit F, da Silva JA, Boers M, et al. Standardised nomenclature for glucocorticoid dosages and glucocorticoid treatment regimens: Current questions and tentative answers in rheumatology. *Ann Rheum Dis* 2002;61:718–722; and Buttgereit F, Scheffold A. Rapid glucocorticoid effects on immune cells. *Steroids* 2002;67:529–534.

with the fact that clinicians in their daily practice have created landmark GC doses that are still cloudy in their definition but clearly group around 7.5, 30, and 100 mg prednisolone equivalent per day.

Efficacy of Glucocorticoids in Rheumatoid Arthritis

Low-Dose Maintenance Therapy

In RA, GC therapy is often started and maintained with low dosage, most often as additional therapy. GC in doses ≤10 mg are highly effective for relieving symptoms in patients with active RA. Many patients are functionally dependent on this therapy and continue it long-term. A Cochrane review evaluated the symptomatic effect of GC in RA and concluded that when administered for a period of approximately 6 months, GCs are "very effective for the treatment of RA."[18] Improvement has been documented in all clinical parameters, including pain scales, joint scores, morning stiffness and fatigue, and in parameters of the acute-phase reaction (such as ESR and CRP). After 6 months of therapy, the beneficial effects of GC in general start to diminish. However, if this therapy is then tapered off and stopped patients often experience clear aggravation of symptoms.

Evaluating the disease-modifying properties of GC is of course particularly relevant in RA. In 1995, joint-preserving effects of 7.5-mg prednisolone for 2 years in patients with RA of short and intermediate disease duration who were also treated with nonsteroidal anti-inflammatory drugs (NSAIDs; 95%) and disease-modifying antirheumatic drugs (DMARDs, 71%) were described.[19] Since then, other trials have corroborated the potency of GCs to retard joint damage. In 2002, the Utrecht study was published: a randomized placebo controlled trial on the effects of GCs in DMARD-naive patients with early RA during 2 years.[20] Ten mg of prednisolone daily in these patients, who only received sulfasalazine therapy as a rescue, clearly inhibited the progression of radiologic joint damage. This beneficial effect was already significant after 12 months, and continued to be significant after 5 years (Figure 10B-3).[21] In this study, 40% decrease in the need for intra-articular GC injections, 49% decreased the need for acetaminophen use, and (importantly) 55% decreased the need for NSAID use in the GC group compared to the placebo group. Recently, a Cochrane meta-analysis on the effects of GCs on radiologic progression in RA was published.[22] Fifteen studies were identified that had at least one treatment arm with GCs and one without GCs, and where there was evaluation of radiographs of hands and/or feet. In total, 1,414 patients were included (the majority with early RA). The mean cumulative dose of GC was 2,300 mg prednisone equivalent over the first year. The standardized mean difference in progression was 0.40 in favor of GCs (95% CI, 0.27–0.54). In studies lasting 2 years (806 patients included), the standardized mean difference in favor of GCs at 1 year was 0.45 (0.24–0.66)—and at 2 years was 0.42 (0.30–0.55). The beneficial effects of GCs were generally achieved when used in conjunction with other DMARD treatment. It was concluded that even in the most conservative estimate the evidence that GCs given in addition to standard therapy can substantially reduce the rate of erosion

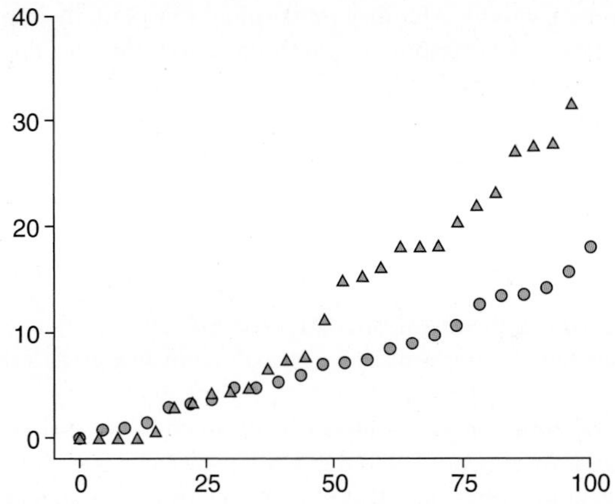

Figure 10B-3. Five years of radiologic data from the Utrecht study. Follow-up during 5 years of radiologic damage (Sharp vander Heijde score) of patients with early RA who participated in a 2-year randomized placebo-controlled study comparing 10 mg of prednisone with placebo. The erosion-retarding effects of GCs persisted even 3 years after stopping the GC treatment. (Adapted from Jacobs JW, VanEverdingen AA, Verstappen SM, et al. Follow-up radiographic data on patients with RA who participated in a two-year trial of prednisone therapy or placebo. *Arthritis Rheum* 2006;54:1422–1428.)

progression in RA is convincing. Today, GCs can be considered to have disease-modifying properties in early RA and may thus be called DMARDs.[23]

Glucocorticoid Pulse Therapy

In RA, GC pulse therapy is applied to treat some of the serious complications of the disease and to induce remission in active disease—often in the initiation phase of second-line antirheumatic treatment. In the latter patients, pulse therapy with regimens of 1,000 mg methylprednisolone intravenously, 200 mg dexamethasone, or other equivalent doses for one or several days has been proven to be effective in most studies. The beneficial effect generally lasts for about 6 weeks, with large variations in the duration of the effect.[24] It thus does not seem sensible to apply pulse therapy in active RA, unless a change in therapeutic strategy is made (e.g., with DMARD treatment aimed at stabilizing on the long-term remission induced by the pulse therapy). A mitigated form of pulse therapy is the parental use of 120 mg depot methylprednisolone acetate, which is quite popular in, among others, the United Kingdom.

Intra-Articular Glucocorticoid Injections

Intra-articular injections with GC are often used in RA. The effect depends on several factors, such as the treated joint (size, weight bearing, or non–weight bearing), the activity of arthritis and volume of synovial fluid of the treated joint, application of arthrocentesis (synovial fluid aspiration) before injection, the choice and dose of the GC preparation, the injection technique, and application of rest to the injected joint.[25] It is recommended that intra-articular GC injections be repeated no more often than once every 3 to 4 weeks and be given no more frequently than 3 to 4 times a year in a weight-bearing joint to prevent GC-induced joint damage.[26,27]

Adverse Effects

Studies of GC toxicity tend to be retrospective and observational.[9] The ability to differentiate unfavorable outcomes attributable to GCs from those occurring due to the underlying disease or other comorbidities, therefore, confounds the picture. Selection bias for GC use in patients with more severe disease, differences in dosages GCs used, and toxicity reports covering a heterogeneous group of GC-treated diseases further confound the interpretation of toxicity data. Frequent, but less serious, adverse effects (e.g., skin thinning, Cushingoid appearance) may be of great concern to patients—whereas more debilitating toxicities such as osteoporosis, cataracts, and GC-induced hypertension may initially go unrecognized or be asymptomatic.

Compared with other anti-rheumatic agents, GCs have a low incidence of short-term symptomatic toxicity and patients uncommonly discontinue therapy for these reasons. Despite nearly 60 years of use, robust data on the longer-term toxicities of GCs (such as from large randomized controlled trials with long-term follow-up) are sorely lacking.[28–30] Table 10B-2 outlines the most common GC toxicities recently published in greater detail.[2]

Cardiovascular Adverse Effects

Despite evidence that GCs rarely induce fluid retention, hypertension is a well-established adverse effect of GCs—observed in up to 20% of patients exposed to exogenous GCs.[31] Patients with essential hypertension require closer surveillance of blood pressure and may need modification of their antihypertensive regimens while on moderate to high doses of GC therapy. In patients receiving ≤10 mg/day, age and elevated pretreatment blood pressure may better explain significant hypertension than the use of GCs.[28]

Table 10B-2. Reported Adverse Events in Glucocorticoid-Treated Patients with Rheumatic Diseases, Expressed as Adverse Events per 100 Patient Years

Type of Adverse Event	Median (25th to –75th Percentile)
Cardiovascular (dyslipidemia, water and electrolyte imbalance, edema, renal and heart dysfunction, hypertension)	15 (3–28)
Infectious (viral, bacterial, skin)	15 (3–15)
Gastrointestinal (peptic ulcer disease, pancreatitis)	10 (4–20)
Psychological and behavioral (minor mood disturbances, psychosis)	9 (2–36)
Endocrine and metabolic (glucose intolerance and diabetes, fat redistribution, interference with hormone secretion)	7 (3–34)
Dermatologic (cutaneous atrophy, acne, hirsutism, alopecia)	5 (2–80)
Musculoskeletal (osteoporosis, ostenonecrosis, myopathy)	4 (3–9)
Ophtalmologic (glaucoma, cataract)	4 (0–5)

From Hoes JN, Jacobs JW, Boers M, et al. EULAR evidence-based recommendations on the management of systemic glucocorticoid therapy in rheumatic diseases. *Ann Rheum Dis* 2007;66:1560–1567.

Another potential toxicity of GCs is the development of premature atherosclerotic vascular disease. Active inflammation may modify the vascular endothelium, leading to an increased risk of cardiovascular disease. Therefore, low doses of GC used to dampen this inflammation may result in reduction in cardiovascular risk in these patients. Observational studies of patients on long-term treatment with moderate to high doses of GCs demonstrate elevations in total plasma cholesterol, low-density lipoprotein cholesterol (LDL-C), high-density lipoprotein cholesterol (HDL-C), and triglycerides. The effects of GCs on lipids seem to be dose dependent, and some studies have even suggested that GCs may reverse unfavorable lipid changes.[32] A cohort study, following 600 RA patients over 13 years, compared GC users with never users. In rheumatoid factor negative patients there was no relation between GC use and cardiovascular disease, but in rheumatoid factor positive patients there was an increased risk.[33] Another database study including 1,115 RA patients concluded that the incidence of all cardiovascular diseases (including myocardial infarction, heart failure, and cerebrovascular diseases) was not increased in patients using <7.5 mg prednisolone long term.[34] At this time, controlling inflammation (even with low dose GCs) should be the priority in reducing cardiovascular risk in RA patients.

Infectious Diseases

Medium- to high-dose GC therapy, particularly when administered for prolonged periods, may lead to an increased risk of serious infections requiring hospitalization, surgery, or both. However, no prospective studies have explored the risk of infection in patients treated with lower-dose GCs. A meta-analysis in elderly patients with RA showed that the rate of infection was not significantly increased in patients given a mean dose of <10 mg/d of prednisone but was increased in higher dosages: dosage 10 to 19 mg/day RR 2.7 and for ≥20 mg/day RR 5.5.[35]

In patients treated with GCs, physicians should anticipate the risk of infections with both typical and atypical organisms, realizing that GCs may blunt the classic clinical features and delay the diagnosis. *Pneumocystis carinii* infections and Herpes Zoster have been reported to have a higher incidence among RA patients treated with GC and (other) immunosuppressive agents.

Gastrointestinal Adverse Effects

GCs are considerably less toxic to the upper gastrointestinal (GI) tract than NSAIDs. If GCs independently increase GI events (such as gastritis, ulceration, and gastrointestinal bleeding), the effect is slight—with estimated relative risks varying from 1.1 to 1.5. GCs are frequently used concurrently with NSAIDs in RA, and meta-analyses confirm that the combination of GCs and NSAIDs synergistically results in a higher risk of GI adverse events.[36] Therefore, patients treated with GCs and concomitant NSAIDs should be given appropriate gastro-protective medication such as proton pump inhibitors (PPIs) or misoprostol—or alternatively could switch to a cyclo-oxygenase-2 selective inhibitor (coxib).[2]

Psychological and Behavioral Adverse Effects

Many patients suffering from RA report a slight increase in their overall sense of well-being when starting on low-dose GC therapy. This appears to be independent of improvement in disease activity. Memory impairment (particularly in older patients) and symptoms of akathisia, insomnia, and depression are occasionally observed in patients taking low-dose GC therapy. Daily split-dose therapy tends to be troublesome because the evening dose disrupts normal diurnal variation in endogenous GC levels and promotes sleep disturbances. True GC psychosis is distinctly uncommon at doses <20 mg/d of prednisone.[28]

Endocrine and Metabolic Adverse Effects

It is uncommon for frank diabetes to develop *de novo* as a result of low-dose GC therapy. However, patients with diabetes mellitus will commonly have higher blood glucose levels while taking GCs. At doses of 1 to 8 mg prednisone daily, the odds ratio for hyperglycemia is 1.8. This rises progressively to an odds ratio of 7 when the dose of prednisone is 25 mg daily or more. The odds ratio of requiring therapy for hyperglycemia is 1.7 during the first 45 days of GC use, falls to 1.3 between 46 and 90 days, and is merely 1.1 beyond that point.[37]

The prevalence of hypothalamic-pituitary-adrenal (HPA) insufficiency appears to depend on both the dose and duration of GC treatment. Spontaneous recovery of the HPA axis is the rule in patients on ≤5 mg of prednisone. However, low doses (≤7.5 mg/day) given for more than 4 weeks may blunt HPA responsiveness. Patients on GC therapy for longer than 1 month, who will undergo surgery, need perioperative management with adequate GC replacement to overcome potential adrenal insufficiency.[2]

Dermatologic Adverse Effects

Even at low doses, skin thinning and ecchymoses represent one of the most common GC adverse events. Catabolic skin effects during systemic GC therapy include cutaneous atrophy, and decreased vascular structural integrity determines purpura and easy bruisability. These effects were reported to affect more than 5% of those exposed to 5 mg or more of prednisone equivalent for 1 year or longer.[38] A Cushingoid appearance, with facial fullness ("moon facies"), is very troubling to patients but is uncommon at low doses. GC acne and, to a lesser extent, hirsutism and striae are other undesirable dermatologic effects that may occur at even lower doses used for RA.

Osteoporosis

Chronic GC treatment results in rapid and profound reductions in bone mineral density (BMD), with most of the bone loss occurring during the first 6 to 12 months of treatment.[9] Although BMD is considered a good overall predictor of fracture risk, GC-induced changes in bone turnover, microarchitecture, collagen content and cross-linking, and other factors are important determinants of fracture risk. The latter is greatly increased among long-term GC-using patients: 34% to 70% suffer from low-trauma fractures within the first 5 years of therapy.[39] GC-induced osteoporosis (GIOP) initially affects trabecular bone. However, with more chronic use cortical bone at sites such as the femoral neck is also affected. The mechanisms of how GCs affect bone include decreased calcium absorption, increased renal calcium loss, diminished sex and growth hormone production, muscle wasting and modulation of RANKL/OPG, NFκB, and AP-1 signaling in bone.[40] All of these factors lead to increased bone resorption.

Table 10B-3. Some of the EULAR Evidence-Based Recommendations on the Management of Systemic Glucocorticoid Therapy in Rheumatic Diseases

- The adverse effects of glucocorticoid therapy should be considered and discussed with the patient before glucocorticoid therapy is started. This advice should be reinforced by giving information regarding glucocorticoid management. If glucocorticoids are to be used for a more prolonged period of time, a "glucocorticoid card" is to be issued to every patient.
- Initial dose, dose reduction, and long-term dosing depends on the underlying disease, disease activity, risk factors, and individual responsiveness of the patient. Timing may be important with respect to the circadian rhythm of both the disease and the natural secretion of glucocorticoids.
- When it is decided to start glucocorticoid treament, comorbidities and risk factors for adverse effects should be evaluated and treated where indicated. These include hypertension, diabetes, peptic ulcer, recent fractures, presence of cataract or glaucoma, presence of (chronic) infections, dyslipidemia, and comedication with nonsteroidal anti-inflammatory drugs.
- For prolonged treatment, the glucocorticoid dosage should be kept to a minimum and a glucocorticoid taper should be attempted in case of remission or low disease activity. The reasons to continue glucocorticoid therapy should be regularly checked.
- If a patient is started on prednisone ≥7.5 mg daily and continues on prednisone for more than 3 months, calcium and vitamin D supplementation should be prescribed. Antiresorptive therapy with bisphosphonates to reduce the risk of glucocorticoid-induced osteoporosis should be based on risk factors, including bone-mineral density measurements.

From Hoes JN, Jacobs JW, Boers M, et al. EULAR evidence-based recommendations on the management of systemic glucocorticoid therapy in rheumatic diseases. *Ann Rheum Dis* 2007;66:1560–1567.

However, reduced osteoblast function (and therefore reduced bone formation) is likely to be the most important effect of GCs on skeletal health.

Osteoporosis is well established as a serious and common consequence of GC use. Fortunately, recent years have witnessed the development of effective strategies for the prevention and treatment of GC-induced osteoporosis—all of which include daily calcium, vitamin D, and specific osteotropic agents (such as bisphosphonates or parathyroid hormone).[41,42]

Ophthalmologic Adverse Effects

Posterior subcapsular cataracts are a well-described complication of prolonged GC use. Some clinicians believe there is no minimal safe dose with respect to this complication, and reports exist of cataract formation even with inhaled glucocorticoid preparations. Others note that cataracts rarely occur in patients taking <10 mg/d for <1 year.[43] Cortical cataracts have also been associated with GC use. In addition to cataracts, GC-treated patients may develop increased intraocular pressure—which can lead to minor visual disturbances. The development of frank glaucoma, particularly with low-dose therapy, is rare and tends to appear in patients who are otherwise predisposed to the condition. A higher risk for glaucoma with GCs tends to occur in families, suggesting a genetic basis.[44]

Recommendations

Recently a task force of EULAR formulated evidence-based recommendations on the management of systemic GC therapy in rheumatic diseases.[2] A multidisciplinary group from 11 European countries, Canada, and the United States consisted of 17 rheumatologists, 1 health professional, 1 patient, and 1 research fellow. A Delphi method was used to agree on 10 key propositions related to the safe use of GCs. A systematic literature search was then used to identify the best available research evidence to support each of the 10 propositions. The strength of the recommendation was given according to research evidence, clinical expertise, and perceived patient preference. The most important of these recommendations pertaining to RA are outlined in Table 10B-3. Other recommendations in the table are for specific groups such as pregnant women and children.[2]

Summary

GCs in the treatment of RA have undergone appraisal and rebuttal. Anno 2008 GCs have found their place as a DMARD, especially helpful in early RA and when used with caution (see recommendations). The balance between efficacy and adverse effects is clearly in favor of the efficacy.

References

1. Bijlsma JW, Boers M, Saag KG, et al. Glucocorticoids in the treatment of early and late RA. *Ann Rheum Dis* 2003;62:1033–1037.
2. Hoes JN, Jacobs JW, Boers M, et al. EULAR evidence based recommendations on the management of systemic glucocorticoid therapy in rheumatic diseases. *Ann Rheum Dis* 2007;66:1560–1567.
3. Buttgereit F, da Silva JA, Boers M, et al. Standardised nomenclature for glucocorticoid dosages and glucocorticoid treatment regimens: Current questions and tentative answers in rheumatology. *Ann Rheum Dis* 2002;61:718–722.
4. Buttgereit, F, Straub, R H, Wehling, M, et al. Glucocorticoids in the treatment of rheumatic diseases: An update on mechanisms of action. *Arthritis Rheum* 2004;50:3408–3417.
5. Adcock IM, Lane SJ. Mechanisms of steroid action and resistance in inflammation. Corticosteroid-insensitive asthma: molecular mechanisms. *J Endocrinol* 2003;178:347–355.
6. Almawi WY. Molecular mechanisms of glucocorticoid effects. *Mod Aspects Immunobiol* 2001;2:78–82.
7. DeBosscher K, Vanden Berghe W, Vermeulen L, et al. Glucocorticoids repress NFκB-driven genes by disturbing the interaction of p65 with the basal transcription machinery, irrespective of coactivator levels in the cell. *Proc Natl Acad Sci U S A* 2000;97: 3919–3924.
8. Vacca A, Felli MP, Farina AR, et al. Glucocorticoid receptor-mediated suppression of the interleukin 2 gene expression through impairment

of the cooperativity between nuclear factor of activated T cells and AP–1 enhancer elements. *J Exp Med* 1992;175:637–646.

9. Bijlsma, JW, Saag, KG, Buttgereit, F, et al. Developments in glucocorticoid therapy. *Rheum Dis Clin North Am* 2005;31:1–17.
10. Stahn C, Lowenberg M, Hommes DW, et al. Molecular mechanisms of glucocorticoid action and selective glucocorticoid receptor agonists. *Mol Cell Endocrinol* 2006;275:71–78.
11. Croxtall, JD, Choudhury Q, Flower RJ. Glucocorticoids act within minutes to inhibit recruitment of signalling factors to activated EGF receptors through a receptor-dependent, transcription-independent mechanism. *Br J Pharmacol* 2000;130:289–298.
12. Hafezi-Moghadam A, Simoncini T, Yang E, et al. Acute cardiovascular protective effects of corticosteroids are mediated by non-transcriptional activation of endothelial nitric oxide synthase. *Nat Med* 2002;8:473–479.
13. Lowenberg M, Verhaar AP, Bilderbeek J, et al. Glucocorticoids cause rapid dissociation of a T-cell-receptor-associated protein complex containing LCK and FYN. *EMBO Rep* 2006;7:1023–1029.
14. Bartholome B, Spies CM, Gaber T, et al. Membrane glucocorticoid receptors (mGCR) are expressed in normal peripheral blood mononuclear cells and upregulated following in vitro stimulation and in patients with rheumatoid arthritis. *FASEB J* 2004;18:70–80.
15. Spies CM, Schaumann DHS, Berki T, et al. Membrane glucocorticoid receptors (mGCR) are down-regulated by glucocorticoids in patients with systemic lupus erythematosus and use a caveolin-1-independent pathway. *Ann Rheum Dis* 2006;65:1139–1146.
16. Buttgereit F, Saag K, Cutolo M, et al. The molecular basis for the effectiveness, toxicity, and resistance to glucocorticoids: Focus on the treatment of rheumatoid arthritis. *Scand J Rheumatol* 2005; 34:14–21.
17. Lipworth BJ. Therapeutic implications of non-genomic glucocorticoid activity. *Lancet* 2000;356:87–89.
18. Criswell LA, Saag KG, Sems KM, et al. Moderate-term, low-dose corticosteroids for rheumatoid arthritis. *Cochrane Database Syst Rev* 2000;CD001158.
19. Kirwan JR for the Arthritis and Rheumatism Council Low-Dose Glucocorticoid Study Group. The effect of glucocorticoids on joint destruction in rheumatoid arthritis. *N Engl J Med* 1995;333:142–146.
20. VanEverdingen AA, Jacobs JW, Siewertsz van Reesema DR, et al. Low-dose prednisone therapy for patients with early active RA: Clinical efficacy, disease-modifying properties and side-effects. A randomized, double-blind, placebo controlled clinical trial. *Ann Intern Med* 2002;136:1–12.
21. Jacobs JW, VanEverdingen AA, Verstappen SM, et al. Follow-up radiographic data on patients with RA who participated in a two-year trial of prednisone therapy or placebo. *Arthritis Rheum* 2006; 54:1422–1428.
22. Kirwan JR, Bijlsma JWJ, Boers M, et al. Effects of glucocorticoids on radiological progression in RA. *The Cochrane Library* 2007;3.
23. Bijlsma JW, Hoes JN, VanEverdingen AA, et al. Are glucocorticoids DMARDs? *Ann NY Acad Sci* 2006;1069:268–274.
24. Weusten BL, Jacobs JW, Bijlsma JW. Corticosteroid pulse therapy in active rheumatoid arthritis. *Semin Arthritis Rheum* 1993;23:183–192.
25. Gaffney K, Ledingham J, Perry JD. Intra-articular triamcinolone hexacetonide in knee osteoarthritis: Factors influencing the clinical response. *Ann Rheum Dis* 1995;54:379–381.
26. Jahangier ZN, Jacobs JWG, Lafeber FPJG, et al. Is radiation synovectomy for arthritis of the knee more effective than intra-articular treatment with glucocorticoïds? Results of an eighteen month, randomized, doubleblind, placebo controlled crossover trial. *Arthritis Rheum* 2005;52:3391–3402.
27. Larsson E, Erlandsson HH, Larsson A, et al. Corticosteroid treatment of experimental arthritis retards cartilage destruction as determined by histology and serum COMP. *Rheumatology* 2004;43: 428–434.
28. DaSilva JAP, Jacobs JWG, Kirwan JR, et al. Long-term glucocorticoid therapy in rheumatoid arthritis: An evidence-based review of potential adverse effects. *Ann Rheum Dis* 2006;65:285–293.
29. Thiele K, Buttgereit F, Zink A. Current use of glucocorticoids in patients with rheumatoid arthritis in Germany. *Arthritis Rheum* 2005;53:740–747.
30. Curtis JR. Population-based assessment of adverse events associated with long-term glucocorticoid use. *Arthritis Care Res* 2006; 55:420–426.
31. Whitworth JA. Mechanisms of glucocorticoid-induced hypertension. *Kidney Int* 1987;31:537–549.
32. Boers M, Nurmohamed MT, Doelman CJ, et al. Influence of glucocorticoids and disease activity on total and high density lipoprotein cholesterol in patients with RA. *Ann Rheum Dis* 2003;62:842–845.
33. Davis JM, Kremers HM, Crowson CS, et al. Glucocorticoids and cardiovascular events in RA: A population-based cohort study. *Arthritis Rheum* 2007;56:820–823.
34. Wei L, MacDonald TM, Walker BR. Taking glucocorticoids by prescription is associated with subsequent cardiovascular disease. *Ann Intern Med* 2004;141:764–770.
35. Schneeweiss S, Setoguchi S, Weinblatt ME. Anti-tumor necrosis factor alpha therapy and the risk of serious bacterial infections in elderly patients with RA. *Arthritis Rheum* 2007;56:1754–1764.
36. Piper JM, Ray WA, Daugherty JR, et al. Corticosteroids use and peptic ulcer disease: Role of nonsteroidal anti-inflammatory drugs. *Ann Intern Med* 1991;114:735–740.
37. Gurwitz JH, Bohn RL, Glynn RJ, et al. Glucocorticoids and the risk for initiation of hypoglycemic therapy. *Arch Intern Med* 1994;154: 97–101.
38. Caldwell JR, Furst DE. The efficacy and safety of low-dose corticosteroids for RSA. *Semin Arthritis Rheum* 1991;21:1–11.
39. VanStaa TP, Leufkens HG, Abenhaim L, et al. Use of oral corticosteroids and risk of fractures. *J Bone Mineral Res* 2000;15: 993–1000.
40. O'Brien C, Jia D, Plotkin L, et al. Glucocorticoids act directly on osteoblasts and osteocytes to induce their apoptosis and reduce bone formation and strength. *Endocrinology* 2004;145:1835–1841.
41. DeNijs RN, Jacobs JW, Lems WF, et al. Alendronate or alfacalcidol in glucocorticoid-induced osteoporosis. *N Engl J Med* 2006;355: 675–684.
42. Geussens PP, DeNijs RN, Lems WF, et al. Prevention of glucocorticoid osteoporosis: A consensus document of the Dutch Society for Rheumatology. *Ann Rheum Dis* 2004;63:324–325.
43. Klein R, Klein BE, Lee KE, et al. Changes in visual acuity in a population over a 10 year period: The Beaver dam eye study. *Ophthalmology* 2001;108:1757–1766.
44. Tripathi RC, Parapuram SK, Tripathi BJ, et al. Corticosteroids and glaucoma risk. *Drugs Aging* 1999;15:439–450.

Methotrexate: The Foundation of Rheumatoid Arthritis Therapy

Alyssa K. Johnsen and Michael E. Weinblatt

Methotrexate (MTX), first used to treat malignant disease over 50 years ago, has since become the cornerstone of therapy of RA (RA)—being administered to at least 500,000 patients with RA worldwide.[1] Low-dose MTX has been shown to be highly efficacious, and when monitored appropriately has an excellent safety profile. For these reasons, it has become the most commonly prescribed disease-modifying antirheumatic drug (DMARD) in the treatment of RA.[1]

Mechanism of Action

MTX is an analog of folic acid and therefore can interfere with the ability of folic acid to serve as a cofactor for a variety of enzymes essential to purine and pyrimidine synthesis and cell replication. One of the first mechanisms proposed for MTX, therefore, was inhibition of proliferation of cells responsible for synovial inflammation (such as lymphocytes). Extracellular MTX is transported into the cell via folate receptors and then metabolized to polyglutamate derivatives. MTX and its polyglutamate derivatives bind to dihydrofolate reductase (DHFR) with high affinity and inhibit its action, thereby depriving the cell of tetrahydrofolate (the active coenzyme form of folate, Figure 10C-1A). However, the fact that folic acid supplementation generally does not reverse the anti-inflammatory effects of MTX has encouraged the exploration of other potential mechanisms.[2,3] One possible mechanism for the anti-inflammatory actions of MTX has recently gained favor (Figure 10C-1B). MTX-polyglutamates also bind 5-aminoimidazole-4-carboxamide ribonucleotide (AICAR) transformylase, which leads to increased levels of AICAR (a competitive inhibitor of adenosine deaminase). This is predicted to increase levels of adenosine, which will bind to cell surface receptors—leading to increased intracellular cAMP, causing downstream anti-inflammatory effects.[4,5]

Pharmacology

MTX is absorbed from the gastrointestinal tract by a saturable active transport system. At 7.5 mg/week, oral and parenteral absorption is equivalent—but at doses of 15 mg /week or more oral absorption may decrease by as much as 30% compared to parenteral dosing.[1] The majority of MTX is excreted in the urine in the first 12 hours after administration. Renal clearance is likely due to a combination of filtration and secretion in the proximal tubule, with subsequent reabsorption in the distal tubule. Renal insufficiency can therefore lead to toxicity due to impaired clearance of MTX. The drug is generally not cleared in dialysis, and dialysis is an absolute contraindication to MTX use. Excretion of MTX is inhibited by weak organic acids such as aspirin, nonsteroidal anti-inflammatory drugs, piperacillin, penicillin G, probenicid, and perhaps cephalosporins. This interaction is generally only clinically relevant with higher-dose MTX.[1] Sulfonamides may also decrease renal tubular secretion and therefore increase levels of MTX. In addition, trimethroprim/sulfamethoxazole (bactrim) interferes with folic acid metabolism and therefore may increase the risk of bone marrow suppression with concomitant MTX.

Efficacy in Rheumatoid Arthritis

The efficacy of aminopterin, the parent compound of MTX, in RA was first reported in 1951 when five of six patients treated with the drug at 1 to 2 mg per day demonstrated decreased joint pain, swelling, and stiffness.[6] Subsequent open label studies of weekly MTX with doses ranging from 7.5 to 25 mg revealed clinical improvement in a majority of treated patients.[7–15] These studies were followed by short-term randomized controlled trials demonstrating significant improvement in disease activity measures when MTX was compared to placebo.[16–19]

MTX has also been shown to be effective when compared to other DMARDs. A double-blind randomized trial comparing MTX to azathioprine in RA patients in whom parenteral gold and/or D-penicillamine treatment had been unsuccessful revealed significantly more improvement in the pain score and disease activity score in the MTX group at 24 weeks. In addition, the number of withdrawals due to side effects was significantly higher in the azathioprine group.[20] Because initial trials of MTX evaluated its efficacy in patients who had already failed gold salts or D-penicillamine, randomized controlled trials of MTX in patients not previously treated with DMARDs were initiated. Two small randomized controlled trials found weekly MTX to be equally efficacious to gold sodium thiomalate in DMARD-naïve patients.[21,22] Subsequently,

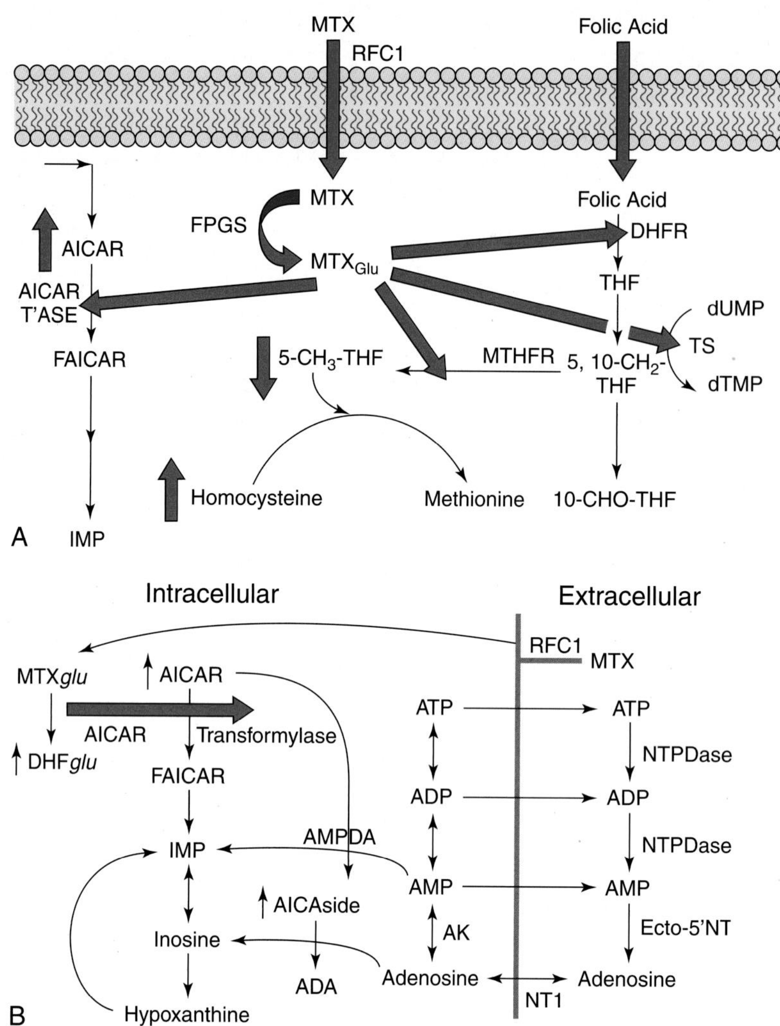

Figure 10C-1. (*A*) Methotrexate inhibits cellular synthesis of purines, pyrimidines, and methionine. *MTX,* methotrexate; *MTXGlu,* methotrexate polyglutamate; *RFC1,* reduced folate carrier 1; *DHFR,* dihydrofolate reductase; *THF,* tetrahydrofolate; *TS,* thymidylate synthase; *MTHFR,* methylene tetrahydrofolate reductase; *FPGS,* folyl polyglutamate synthase; *AICAR,* 5-aminoimidazole-4-carboxamide ribonucleotide; *AICAR T'ASE, AICAR* transformylase. (*B*) Methotrexate increases extracellular adenosine concentrations. *MTX,* methotrexate; *MTXGlu,* methotrexate polyglutamate; *DHFGlu,* dihydrofolate polyglutamate; *AICAR,* aminoimidazole carboxamidoribonucleotide; *FAICAR,* formyl AICAR; *AMPDA,* AMP deaminase; *AICAside,* aminoimidazole carboxamidoribonucleoside; *ADA,* adenosine deaminase; *AK,* adenosine kinase; *RFC1,* reduced folate carrier 1; *NTPDase,* nucleoside triphosphate dephosphorylase; *Ecto-5'NT,* ecto-5'-nucleotidase; *NT1,* nucleoside transporter 1. (Adapted from Cronstein BN. Low-dose methotrexate: A mainstay in the treatment of rheumatoid arthritis. *Pharmacol Rev* 2005;57:163–172.)

a trial of 281 RA patients randomized to MTX or auranofin showed a significantly greater response and fewer adverse events in the patients who received MTX.[23] A post hoc analysis of this study showed the ACR 20 response rate with MTX (maximum dose 15 mg/week) to be approximately 68% and the ACR 20 with auranofin to be approximately 30%.[24] More recently, MTX was shown to be superior to leflunomide with respect to disease activity measures after 1 year and radiographic progression after 2 years in a randomized double-blind trial involving 999 patients with active RA.[25] It is important to note that in most of these early comparison studies the maximum dose of MTX was 15 mg/week.

MTX slows radiographic progression of RA. In a double-blind randomized trial comparing treatment with MTX to azathioprine, patients treated with MTX showed fewer new erosions and a less pronounced change in the joint score as assessed by plain radiographs of the hands and feet at 24 and 48 weeks.[20] An open extension follow-up to 4 years showed in an intention-to-treat analysis that the beneficial effect of MTX on radiographic progression compared to azathioprine was sustained after 2 years of follow-up. Although the difference was not sustained at 4 years, this may have been due to the greater number of patients switching from azathioprine to MTX than vice versa.[26] A double-blind randomized trial comparing MTX to auranofin showed significant worsening of the erosion score on radiographs of the hands and feet in the patients treated with auranofin.[27] Similarly, a randomized clinical trial comparing MTX, auranofin, and the combination of the two showed statistically significant worsening of erosions and joint space narrowing on hand radiographs at 48 weeks in only the auranofin group.[28]

The efficacy of MTX in combination with other DMARDs has been evaluated. The combination of azathioprine[29] or auranofin[30] and MTX was not shown to be superior to treatment with either of these agents alone. However, some combination therapies have been shown to increase the effectiveness of MTX. In patients with a suboptimal response to MTX, the addition of weekly intramuscular (IM) gold[31] or cyclosporine[32] resulted in increased efficacy. In addition, DMARD-naive patients treated with the combination of MTX, intra-articular betamethasone, and cyclosporine were more likely to achieve an ACR 20 than those treated with MTX and intra-articular betamethasone alone.[33] Although no significant difference was found comparing patients treated with a combination of MTX and sulfasalazine to patients on monotherapy with these agents,[34] a study of triple therapy with MTX, hydroxychloroquine, and sulfasalazine showed that patients treated with the combination of all three were more likely to sustain clinical improvement than those treated with either MTX alone or dual therapy with hydroxychloroquine and sulfasalazine.[35] Therapy with doxycycline and MTX was also found to be superior at achieving an ACR 50 response than treatment with MTX alone.[36] The efficacy of combination therapy with leflunomide was also demonstrated in an open label study which showed improvement in patients on MTX when leflunomide was added.[37] A subsequent randomized placebo-controlled trial of MTX versus MTX plus leflunomide showed increased efficacy for the combination, with 46.2% versus 19.5% of patients achieving an ACR 20.[38]

The efficacy/safety profile of MTX in RA has made it the DMARD to which all new treatments are compared. Inhibitors of tumor necrosis factor (TNF)-α have been evaluated against and in combination with MTX. In a 12-month randomized double-blinded placebo-controlled trial comparing MTX (7.5 mg escalating to 20 mg weekly) to etanercept (10 mg or 25 mg sc twice weekly) in 652 patients with early RA, MTX was less effective than etanercept 25 mg twice weekly at achieving ACR 20, 50, and 70 during the first 4 months—but was equivalent clinically to etanercept thereafter. For example, at 12 months 72% of the patients in the group assigned to receive 25 mg of etanercept twice weekly had an ACR 20 response (compared to 65% of those in the MTX group). However, this difference was not statistically significant ($P = 0.16$). The higher dose of etanercept, however, demonstrated decreased radiographic progression compared to MTX at both 6 and 12 months.[39] The 2-year follow-up to this study using a last-observation-carried-forward analysis documented more patients achieving ACR 20 at 24 months in the higher-dose etanercept group than in the MTX group. The higher-dose etanercept group also showed less radiographic progression.[40] To evaluate the combination of MTX with anti-TNF therapy, two 24-week double-blind placebo-controlled trials comparing MTX to MTX plus etanercept or MTX plus adalimumab, respectively, showed significant improvement in disease activity measures when anti-TNF therapy was added.[41,42] Similarly, the addition of infliximab to MTX in randomized placebo-controlled trials demonstrated significant improvement in disease activity measures[43] as well as radiographic progression.[44] Subsequent studies were undertaken to directly compare MTX, anti-TNF-α therapy, and the combination of the two in the treatment of RA. In a randomized double-blind placebo-controlled trial comparing etanercept, MTX, and the combination, the combination was more efficacious with respect to measures of disease activity than either therapy alone. In addition, the combination was better at retardation of joint damage as assessed by Sharp score than MTX or etanercept alone (TEMPO).[45] These results were sustained after 2 years.[46] Similar results were found for the combination of adalimumab and MTX when compared to either drug alone (PREMIER).[47] The combination of infliximab and MTX was also found to be more efficacious than treatment with MTX plus placebo (ASPIRE).[48] These studies have been useful not only in demonstrating the efficacy of anti-TNF-α therapy and MTX in combination but in providing excellent data on the efficacy of MTX therapy as a single agent, with ACR 20 percentages ranging from 54 to 73 (Table 10C-1).

Table 10C-1. Methotrexate Efficacy as Monotherapy in Studies of Anti-TNF Efficacy

	TEMPO[a]	PREMIER[b]	ASPIRE[c]
ACR 20 (%)	75	63	54
ACR 50 (%)	43	46	32
ACR 70 (%)	19	28	21
DAS (%)	13	21	15

[a] TEMPO: Study comparing methotrexate, etanercept, and the combination of both drugs.[45]
[b] PREMIER: Study comparing methotrexate, adalimumab, and the combination of both drugs.[47]
[c] ASPIRE: Study comparing methotrexate to methotrexate plus infliximab.[48]

Although many of the studies documenting the efficacy of MTX were of relatively short duration, long-term prospective studies have demonstrated sustained effects on disease activity and radiographic progression. Weinblatt et al. prospectively followed a cohort of 26 RA patients and reported on their status after 36, 84, and 132 months of MTX therapy. For the 10 patients who completed the study to 132 months, significant improvement compared to baseline ($p < 0.001$) was noted in the number of painful joints, swollen joints, and physician and patient global assessments. There was 50% improvement in the joint pain index and joint swelling index in >65% of the patients. There was no significant difference, however, in the improvement in clinical variables between 12 and 132 months. From the original cohort, withdrawal due to MTX toxicity occurred in three patients, including two for pneumonitis and one for alopecia. There was only one withdrawal due to lack of efficacy.[49] In a study by Kremer et al., an original cohort of 29 patients was reported on after 29, 53, and 90 months of MTX therapy. For the 18 patients who were still being followed at 90 months, a significant improvement from baseline was maintained in all clinical parameters except the number of tender joints. In addition, a significant improvement compared to 53 months of treatment was found for the number of tender joints, grip strength, and functional class. In spite of continued MTX therapy, 9 of the 17 patients in whom sequential radiographs were obtained showed radiographic progression. From the original cohort, 4 patients withdrew due to MTX toxicity, including 2 for MTX pneumonitis and 2 for nausea. Two patients withdrew due to decreased efficacy.[50] An additional report after 13.3 years on 5 patients from this cohort still on MTX continued to show clinical benefit compared to baseline.[51] A larger multicenter prospective trial including 123 patients who were followed for 5 years showed significant improvement compared with baseline in all clinical disease variables, functional status, and erythrocyte sedimentation rate. Sixty-four percent of patients completed this study and were still taking MTX. Seven percent of patients withdrew due to lack of efficacy, and 7% due to adverse events.[52] It must be remembered, however, that demonstration of efficacy in long-term follow-up trials is subject to patient retention bias and can be a function of whatever alternate treatments are available for these patients.

In addition to demonstrating clinical efficacy, many clinical trials have shown that MTX decreases markers of inflammation, including the erythrocyte sedimentation rate and c-reactive protein (CRP). The decrement in CRP is rapid, with the minimum value being noted on day 3 after once-weekly dosing.[53,54]

Treatment with MTX was associated with reduced mortality in a retrospective study of 1,240 patients with RA, but only after adjustment for confounding by indication.[55] MTX was prescribed to 588 patients, and these patients were more likely to have higher disease activity. The unadjusted mortality hazard ratio of MTX compared to no MTX use was 0.8, with 95% confidence intervals of 0.6 to 1.0. However, when a weighted Cox proportional hazards model was used to adjust for potential confounders (including measures of disease activity) the adjusted mortality hazard ratio was 0.4 (0.2–0.8). Forty-four percent of the 191 deaths were due to cardiovascular causes. The hazard ratio for cardiovascular mortality was 0.3 (0.2–0.7) versus 0.6 (0.2–1.2) for noncardiovascular death.

Adverse Effects

Although MTX has clearly shown substantial benefit in the treatment of RA, an understanding of the potential adverse effects is critical for safe long-term maintenance of therapy. The most common reactions associated with low-dose weekly MTX are anorexia, nausea, vomiting, and diarrhea (reported in 10% of patients studied in early short-term controlled trials and small long-term open label studies). Most of these reactions occurred shortly after the drug was administered and were mild, although in 2.5% of patients led to discontinuation. In this same group of patients, stomatitis occurred in 6% and alopecia in 1%.[56]

Hematologic abnormalities were found in 3% of the patients in this study, which included leukopenia (most common), anemia, and thrombocytopenia.[56] A review of the literature was conducted to identify published cases of pancytopenia in response to low-dose MTX for RA. Seventy patients with pancytopenia were identified from 1980 to 1995, and 12 of these patients died. Toxicity data from long-term prospective studies showed an incidence of pancytopenia of 1.4%.[57] In a study of 481 patients followed for an average of 58 months of MTX therapy, 2 patients had thrombocytopenia and 13 patients had leukopenia—with 2/2 of the thrombocytopenic patients and 3/13 of the leukopenic patients discontinuing the drug. Hypoalbuminemia correlated independently with an increased percentage of abnormal platelet counts.[58] Other risk factors for MTX hematologic toxicity include drug overdoses, incorrect dosing (such as daily dosing), renal insufficiency, dialysis, and concomitant drugs such as trimethoprim/sulfa.

In this same population, 74 patients were noted to have an elevated aspartate aminotransferase (AST)—and this resulted in permanent discontinuation of MTX in 17. Independent predictors of a significantly higher percentage of abnormal AST values were lack of folate supplementation and untreated hyperlipidemia.[58] To determine the risk of serious liver disease in patients with RA taking MTX, members of the American College of Rheumatology were surveyed to identify cases of cirrhosis and liver failure. A case-control study was then conducted by reviewing medical records to determine prognostic factors. Twenty-four cases of cirrhosis and liver failure were identified, giving a 5-year cumulative incidence of approximately 1/1,000 treated patients. Six of the 24 patients died, including 4 who died from the initial liver disease. Late age at first use of MTX and duration of therapy with MTX were independent predictors of serious liver disease.[59] The frequency of liver disease is less in RA than in psoriasis. Some reasons for the higher rates in psoriasis could include higher alcohol consumption, higher mean body index with fatty liver disease, and higher doses of MTX.

Although the possible hepatic toxicity of MTX is well known, a potentially serious complication of MTX treatment in patients infected with hepatitis B and C virus is less appreciated. The usual picture is the development of fulminant hepatitis with MTX withdrawal. Reactivation of immune system by discontinuation of the MTX is postulated as the cause.[60]

MTX can also cause lung injury, which is generally acute interstitial pneumonitis. A retrospective combined cohort review and abstraction from the literature identified 29 cases from 1981 to 1993 who had probable or definite MTX lung injury. Predominant clinical features included shortness of breath in 93.1%, cough in 82.8%, and fever in 69.0%. Five of these patients died, and 4 of 6 patients retreated with MTX developed recurrent lung toxicity.[61] A case-control study of patients treated with MTX with and without lung injury was undertaken to identify risk factors for lung toxicity. The strongest predictors of lung injury were older age, diabetes, rheumatoid pleuropulmonary involvement, previous use of DMARDs, and hypoalbuminemia.[62] However, MTX lung toxicity is not limited to RA patients and appears to be idiosyncratic and not mechanism based.

Other potential adverse effects of MTX include an increased risk of Epstein-Barr virus (EBV)–associated lymphomas[63] that may regress upon discontinuation of MTX,[64] accelerated nodulosis,[65] and nonspecific central nervous system effects such as dizziness, headache, mood alteration, or memory impairment.[66]

The clear risk of MTX therapy during pregnancy deserves special mention. MTX is a known teratogen and can be used to induce abortion. An unfortunate case in which a fetus was exposed during the first trimester to low-dose weekly MTX resulted in multiple congenital abnormalities consistent with the "aminopterin syndrome."[67]

Folic Acid Supplementation

To prevent adverse effects of MTX, folic acid or folinic acid (leucovorin) is given concomitantly. Folinic acid is the reduced active form of folic acid. Support for this practice comes from a prospective trial in which 92 RA patients were given folinic acid or placebo 24 hours after the MTX dose (up to 30 mg each week). The patients treated with folinic acid reported fewer adverse effects but had no difference in disease activity compared to placebo,[2] in contrast to an earlier placebo-controlled trial on 27 patients in which clinical and laboratory indices of disease worsened only in the patients treated with leucovorin.[68] Folic acid has also been shown in a randomized placebo-controlled trial to decrease the toxicity without influencing efficacy of MTX, given as 5 mg or 27.5 mg each week.[3] In a larger study of 434 patients randomly assigned to receive placebo, folic acid 1 mg/day or folinic acid 2.5 mg/week in addition to MTX (dose escalation to 25 mg/week), both regimens reduced the incidence of elevated liver enzyme levels and decreased toxicity-related discontinuation. However, they had no effect on other adverse effects—including gastrointestinal and mucosal side effects. The mean dosages of MTX at the end of the 48-week study were higher in the folic acid and folinic acid groups, suggesting that a higher dose of MTX might be necessary for the same clinical effect.[69]

Pharmacogenomics

Although MTX is generally well tolerated, some patients experience adverse effects—and occasionally these are serious. In addition, although MTX is efficacious for many patients some patients do not respond. Therefore, ideally we would like to treat only those patients who will safely tolerate MTX and for whom it will have some benefit. Because the critical factors in the action and metabolism of MTX are known, it has been possible to study polymorphisms in some of these proteins to determine if they influence the drug's effects. The best studied protein polymorphisms are in methylene tetrahydrofolate reductase (MTHFR). MTHFR is a critical enzyme associated with the regeneration of 5-methyl-tetrahydrofolate from 5,10-methylene-tetrahydrofolate. 5-methyl-tetrahydrofolate contributes a methyl group to homocysteine for regeneration of methionine, and deficiency can lead to hyperhomocysteinemia and methionine deficiency. A mutation exists in the population (C677T), such that the CC genotype provides normal function—whereas the CT and TT provide 40% and 70% decrement in enzyme function, respectively.[70] In RA patients, the CT and TT genotypes have been associated with increased toxicity and MTX discontinuation.[71,72] In addition, the C allele at A1298C was shown to be associated with receiving a lower dose of MTX[72] as well as with toxicity.[73,74] MTHFR 677TT as well as serine hydroxymethyltransferase (SHMT1) 1420CC, AICAR transformylase 347GG, and thymidylate synthase (TSER) VNTR *2/*2 has been associated with adverse effects.[75]

Polymorphism in enzymes involved in folate metabolism has also been analyzed for influence on MTX efficacy. Dervieux et al. found that homozygous variant genotypes in the reduced folate carrier (RFC-1), AICAR transformylase (ATIC), and thymidylate synthase were associated with decreased disease activity on MTX.[76] In addition, MTHFR 1298AA and 677CC, AMPD1 34C, ITPA 94C, and ATIC 347C have been associated with clinical improvement.[77,78] These studies suggest that in the near future we may be able to screen patients to determine risk and benefit of MTX prior to initiating therapy. However, the small number of patients examined thus far and the lack of large prospectively controlled studies limits our current use of genetic screening for MTX efficacy and safety.

Methotrexate Use in Rheumatoid Arthritis: Recommendations

The American College of Rheumatology issued a consensus statement in 1994 providing guidelines for monitoring liver toxicity (Table 10C-2). Prior to starting MTX, the guidelines recommend obtaining liver blood tests, hepatitis B and C serologies, and other standard tests—including the complete blood count and serum creatinine. At intervals of every 4 to 8 weeks, the AST, alanine aminotransferase (ALT), and albumin levels should be monitored. Routine surveillance liver biopsies are not recommended for RA patients receiving traditional doses of MTX. However, we recommend that a biopsy should be performed if a patient develops persistent abnormalities on liver blood tests [defined as elevations in the AST of 5 of 9 determinations within a 12-month interval (6 of 12 if tests are performed monthly) or a decrease in serum albumin below the normal range].[79]

Table 10C-2. Recommendations for Monitoring for Hepatic Safety in Rheumatoid Arthritis Patients Receiving Methotrexate (MTX)

A. Baseline
   1. Tests for all patients
      a. Liver blood tests [aspartate aminotransferase (AST), alanine aminotransferase (ALT), alkaline phosphatase, albumin, bilirubin], hepatitis B and C serology studies
      b. Other standard tests, including complete blood cell count and serum creatinine
   2. Pretreatment liver biopsy (Menghini suction-type needle) only for patients with:
      a. Prior excessive alcohol consumption
      b. Persistently abnormal baseline AST values
      c. Chronic hepatitis B or C infection
B. Monitor AST, ALT, albumin at 4- to 8-week intervals
C. Perform liver biopsy if:
   1. Five of 9 determinations of AST within a given 12-month interval (6 of 12 if tests are performed monthly) are abnormal (defined as an elevation above the upper limit of normal)
   2. There is a decrease in serum albumin below the normal range (in the setting of well-controlled RA)
D. If results of liver biopsy are:
   1. Roenigk grade I, II, IIIA, resume MTX and monitor as in B, C1, and C2 above
   2. Roenigk grade IIIB or IV, discontinue MTX
E. Discontinue MTX in patients with persistent liver test abnormalities, as defined in C1 and C2 above, who refuses liver biopsy.

From Kremer JM, Alarcon GS, Lightfoot RW Jr. et al. for the American College of Rheumatology. Methotrexate for rheumatoid arthritis: Suggested guidelines for monitoring liver toxicity. *Arthritis and Rheum* 1994;37(3):316–328.

MTX is usually started at a dose of 7.5 to 10 mg weekly, and the dose is escalated every 4 to 8 weeks until disease activity is under control. The therapeutic dose is generally between 15 and 25 mg per week. Generally it takes 4 to 6 weeks after the therapeutic dose is reached for a substantial clinical effect to be noted. We generally start at 7.5 per week, and then 4 weeks later (if there has been no adverse event) the dose is increased to 15 mg (and then 4 weeks later to 20 mg per week). After another 4 weeks, if there is no clinical effect we would add another DMARD or a biologic agent. It is important to maximize the MTX dose in order to achieve the maximum efficacy with this drug. If there is an impressive clinical response, the MTX dose may be decreased. However, most patients require persistent therapy to control the arthritis. Discontinuation of MTX is generally associated with a flare of arthritis 4 to 6 weeks after stopping the drug. The maximum dose of oral MTX is generally considered to be 20 to 25 mg/week. MTX can be delivered subcutaneously in patients with gastrointestinal intolerance or in nonresponders with a predicted higher bioavailability than the oral dose. Folic acid 1 mg each day is recommended in all patients who are on MTX. If adverse effects occur, the folic acid should be increased to 2 mg per day. Outside the United States, the folic acid dose is usually 5 mg 5 to 6 days per week. If side effects continue despite folic acid, leucovorin starting at 5 mg/week should be used. The dose of leucovorin can be escalated to block side effects and should be given 8 to 24 hours after the MTX. If administered within 8 hours of the MTX, it might block the efficacy of MTX.

Patients should be aware of the adverse event profile of this drug. Generally, the drug should be held during infectious episodes. We also hold it the week of surgery and the first postoperative week. Laboratory monitoring should be done on a regular basis. Liver function tests should be measured every 4 to 8 weeks, and we monitor the creatinine and blood count at the same interval. Patients should receive routine vaccinations, including influenza vaccine, but should not receive live vaccines while on MTX. We also recommend restricting alcohol use. Women of child-bearing potential must use birth control while on the drug. The drug may lead to a reversible reduction of sperm count, which resolves with drug discontinuation. There is no data that there is a higher risk of birth defects associated with men remaining on MTX while attempting conception.

Conclusion

MTX is currently considered a first-line agent in the treatment of RA, and the "anchor drug" for combination therapy with other DMARDs and biologic agents. It has become the standard of care and the most widely used drug in the treatment of RA. When used appropriately, it has excellent efficacy and tolerability in the treatment of the signs and symptoms of RA and is the DMARD to which all new therapies should be compared.

References

1. Kremer J. Toward a better understanding of methotrexate. *Arthritis Rheum* 2004;50(5):1370–1382.
2. Shiroky JB, Neville C, Esdaile JM, et al. Low-dose methotrexate with leucovorin (folinic acid) in the management of rheumatoid arthritis: Results of a multicenter randomized, double-blind, placebo-controlled trial. *Arthritis Rheum* 1993;36:795–803.
3. Morgan SL, Baggott JE, Vaughn WH, et al. Supplementation with folic acid during methotrexate therapy for rheumatoid arthritis: A double-blind, placebo-controlled trial. *Ann Intern Med* 1994;121: 833–841.
4. Cutolo M, Sulli A, Pizzorni C, et al. Anti-inflammatory mechanisms of methotrexate in rheumatoid arthritis. *Ann Rheum Dis* 1901;60: 729–735.
5. Cronstein BN. Low-dose methotrexate: A mainstay in the treatment of rheumatoid arthritis. *Pharmacological Reviews* 2005;57: 163–172.
6. Gubner R, August S, Ginsberg V. Therapeutic suppression of tissue reactivity. II. Effect of aminopterin in rheumatoid arthritis and psoriasis. *Am J Med Sci* 1951;22:176–182.
7. Hoffmeister RT. Methotrexate in rheumatoid arthritis. *Arthritis and Rheumatism* 1972;15:114.
8. Wilke WS, Calabrese LH, Scherbel AL. Methotrexate in the treatment of rheumatoid arthritis: Pilot study. *Cleve Clin Q* 1980;47: 305–309.
9. Willkens RF, Watson MA, Paxson CS. Low dose pulse methotrexate therapy in rheumatoid arthritis. *J Rheumatol* 1980;7:501–505.
10. Willkens RF, Watson MA. Methotrexate: A perspective of its use in the treatment of rheumatic diseases. *J Lab Clin Med* 1982;100: 314–321.
11. Steinsson K, Weinstein A, Korn J, Abeles M. Low dose methotrexate in rheumatoid arthritis. *J Rheumatol* 1982;9:860–866.
12. Hoffmeister RT. Methotrexate therapy in rheumatoid arthritis: 15 years experience. *Am J Med* 1983;75:69–73.
13. Weinstein A, Marlowe S, Korn J, et al. Low-dose methotrexate treatment of rheumatoid arthritis: Long-term observations. *Am J Med* 1985;79:331–337.
14. Michaels RM, Nashel DJ, Leonard A, et al. Weekly intravenous methotrexate in the treatment of rheumatoid arthritis. *Arthritis Rheum* 1982;25:339–341.
15. Groff GD, Shenberger KN, Wilke WS, et al. Low dose oral methotrexate in rheumatoid arthritis: An uncontrolled trial and review of the literature. *Semin Arthritis Rheum* 1983;12:333–347.
16. Thompson RN, Watts C, Edelman J, et al. A controlled two-centre trial of parenteral methotrexate therapy for refractory rheumatoid arthritis. *J Rheumatol* 1984;11:760–763.
17. Weinblatt ME, Coblyn JS, Fox DA, et al. Efficacy of low-dose methotrexate in rheumatoid arthritis. *N Engl J Med* 1985;312:818–822.
18. Williams HJ, Willkens RF, Samuelson CO Jr., et al. Comparison of low-dose oral pulse methotrexate and placebo in the treatment of rheumatoid arthritis: A controlled clinical trial. *Arthritis Rheum* 1985;28:721–730.
19. Andersen PA, West SG, O'Dell JR, et al. Weekly pulse methotrexate in rheumatoid arthritis: Clinical and immunologic effects in a randomized, double-blind study. *Ann Intern Med* 1985;103:489–496.
20. Jeurissen ME, Boerbooms AM, van de Putte LB, et al. Methotrexate versus azathioprine in the treatment of rheumatoid arthritis: A forty-eight-week randomized, double-blind trial. *Arthritis & Rheumatism* 1991;34:961–972.
21. Morassut P, Goldstein R, Cyr M, et al. Gold sodium thiomalate compared to low dose methotrexate in the treatment of rheumatoid arthritis: A randomized, double blind 26-week trial. *J Rheumatol* 1989;16:302–306.
22. Suarez-Almazor ME, Fitzgerald A, Grace M, et al. A randomized controlled trial of parenteral methotrexate compared with sodium aurothiomalate (Myochrysine) in the treatment of rheumatoid arthritis. *J Rheumatol* 1988;15:753–756.
23. Weinblatt ME, Kaplan H, Germain BF, et al. Low-dose methotrexate compared with auranofin in adult rheumatoid arthritis: A thirty-six-week, double-blind trial. *Arthritis Rheum* 1990;33:330–338.
24. Felson DT, Anderson JJ, Boers M, Bombardier C, et al. American College of Rheumatology preliminary definition of improvement in rheumatoid arthritis. *Arthritis Rheum* 1995;38:727–735.
25. Emery P, Breedveld FC, Lemmel EM, et al. A comparison of the efficacy and safety of leflunomide and methotrexate for the treatment of rheumatoid arthritis. *Rheumatology* 2000;39:655–665.
26. Kerstens PJ, Boerbooms AM, Jeurissen ME, et al. Radiological and clinical results of longterm treatment of rheumatoid arthritis with methotrexate and azathioprine. *J Rheumatol* 2000;27:1148–1155.
27. Weinblatt ME, Polisson R, Blotner SD, et al. The effects of drug therapy on radiographic progression of rheumatoid arthritis: Results of a 36-week randomized trial comparing methotrexate and auranofin. *Arthritis Rheum* 1993;36:613–619.
28. López-Méndez A, Daniel WW, Reading JC, et al. Radiographic assessment of disease progression in rheumatoid arthritis patients enrolled in the cooperative systematic studies of the rheumatic diseases program randomized clinical trial of methotrexate, auranofin, or a combination of the two. *Arthritis Rheum* 1993;36:1364–1369.
29. Willkens RF, Sharp JT, Stablein D, et al. Comparison of azathioprine, methotrexate, and the combination of the two in the treatment of rheumatoid arthritis: A forty-eight-week controlled clinical

trial with radiologic outcome assessment. *Arthritis Rheum* 1995; 38:1799–1806.

30. Williams HJ, Ward JR, Reading JC, et al. Comparison of auranofin, methotrexate, and the combination of both in the treatment of rheumatoid arthritis: A controlled clinical trial. *Arthritis Rheum* 1992;35:259–269.
31. Lehman AJ, Esdaile JM, Klinkhoff AV, et al. A 48-week, randomized, double-blind, double-observer, placebo-controlled multicenter trial of combination methotrexate and intramuscular gold therapy in rheumatoid arthritis: Results of The METGO Study. *Arthritis Rheum* 2005;52(5):1360–1370.
32. Tugwell P, Pincus T, Yocum D, et al. Combination therapy with cyclosporine and methotrexate in severe rheumatoid arthritis. *N Engl J Med* 1995;333:137–141.
33. Hetland M, Stengaard-Pedersen K, Junker P, et al. Combination treatment with methotrexate, cyclosporine, and intraarticular betamethasone compared with methotrexate and intraarticular betamethasone in early active rheumatoid arthritis: An investigator-initiated, multicenter, randomized, double-blind, parallel-group, placebo-controlled study. *Arthritis Rheum* 2006;54(5):1401–1409.
34. Haagsma CJ, Van Riel PL, De Jong AJ, et al. Combination of sulphasalazine and methotrexate versus the single components in early rheumatoid arthritis: A randomized, controlled, double-blind, 52 week clinical trial. *Br J Rheumatol* 1997;36:1082–1088.
35. O'Dell JR, Haire C, Erikson N, et al. Efficacy of triple DMARD therapy in patients with RA with suboptimal response to methotrexate. *J Rheumatol* 1996;23(44):72–74.
36. O'Dell JR, Elliott JR, Mallek JA, et al. Treatment of early seropositive rheumatoid arthritis: Doxycycline plus methotrexate versus methotrexate alone. *Arthritis Rheum* 2006;54(2):621–627.
37. Weinblatt ME, Kremer JM, Coblyn JS, et al. Pharmacokinetics, safety, and efficacy of combination treatment with methotrexate and leflunomide in patients with active rheumatoid arthritis. *Arthritis Rheum* 1999;42:1322–1328.
38. Kremer JM, Genovese MC, Cannon GW, et al. Concomitant leflunomide therapy in patients with active rheumatoid arthritis despite stable doses of methotrexate: A randomized, double-blind, placebo-controlled trial. *Ann Intern Med* 2002;137(9):726–733.
39. Bathon JM, Martin RW, Fleischmann RM, et al. A comparison of etanercept and methotrexate in patients with early rheumatoid arthritis. *N Engl J Med* 2000;343:1586–1593.
40. Genovese MC, Bathon JM, Martin RW, et al. Etanercept versus methotrexate in patients with early rheumatoid arthritis: Two-year radiographic and clinical outcomes. *Arthritis Rheum* 2002;46(6): 1443–1450.
41. Weinblatt ME, Kremer JM, Bankhurst AD, et al. A trial of etanercept, a recombinant tumor necrosis factor receptor:Fc fusion protein, in patients with rheumatoid arthritis receiving methotrexate. *N Engl J Med* 1999;340:253–259.
42. Weinblatt ME, Keystone EC, Furst DE, et al. Adalimumab, a fully human anti-tumor necrosis factor a monoclonal antibody, for the treatment of rheumatoid arthritis in patients taking concomitant methotrexate: The ARMADA trial. *Arthritis Rheum* 2003;48(1):35–45.
43. Lipsky PE, van der Heijde DM, St Clair EW, et al. Infliximab and methotrexate in the treatment of rheumatoid arthritis. *N Engl J Med* 2000;343:1594–1602.
44. Smolen JS, van der Heijde DMFM, St Clair EW, et al. Predictors of joint damage in patients with early rheumatoid arthritis treated with high-dose methotrexate with or without concomitant infliximab: Results from the ASPIRE trial. *Arthritis Rheum* 2006;54(3):702–710.
45. Klareskog L, van der Heijde D, De Jager JP, et al. Therapeutic effect of the combination of etanercept and methotrexate compared with each treatment alone in patients with rheumatoid arthritis: Double-blind randomised controlled trial. *Lancet* 2004;363(9410):675–681.
46. van der Heijde D, Klareskog L, Rodriguez-Valverde V, et al. Comparison of etanercept and methotrexate, alone and combined, in the treatment of rheumatoid arthritis: Two-year clinical and radiographic results from the TEMPO study, a double-blind, randomized trial. *Arthritis Rheum* 2006;54(4):1063–1074.
47. Breedveld FC, Weisman MH, Kavanaugh AF, et al. The PREMIER study: A multicenter, randomized, double-blind clinical trial of combination therapy with adalimumab plus methotrexate versus methotrexate alone or adalimumab alone in patients with early, aggressive rheumatoid arthritis who had not had previous methotrexate treatment. *Arthritis Rheum* 2006;54(1):26–37.
48. St Clair EW, van der Heijde DM, Smolen JS, et al. Combination of infliximab and methotrexate therapy for early rheumatoid arthritis: A randomized, controlled trial. *Arthritis Rheum* 2004;50(11): 3432–3443.
49. Weinblatt ME, Trentham DE, Fraser PA, et al. Long-term prospective trial of low-dose methotrexate in rheumatoid arthritis. *Arthritis Rheum* 1988;31:167–175.
50. Kremer JM, Phelps CT. Long-term prospective study of the use of methotrexate in rheumatoid arthritis: Update after a mean of 90 months. *Arthritis Rheum* 1992;35:138–145.
51. Kremer JM. Safety, efficacy, and mortality in a long-term cohort of patients with rheumatoid arthritis taking methotrexate: Follow-up after a mean of 13.3 years. *Arthritis Rheum* 1997;40:984–985.
52. Weinblatt ME, Kaplan H, Germain BF, et al. Methotrexate in rheumatoid arthritis: A five year prospective multicenter trial. *Arthritis Rheum* 1994;37:1492–1498.
53. Segal R, Caspi D, Tishler M, et al. Short term effects of low dose methotrexate on the acute phase reaction in patients with rheumatoid arthritis. *J Rheumatol* 1989;16(7):914–917.
54. Seideman P. Better effect of methotrexate on C-reactive protein during daily compared to weekly treatment in rheumatoid arthritis. *Clin Rheumatol* 1993;12(2):210–213.
55. Choi HK, Hernán MA, Seeger JD, et al. Methotrexate and mortality in patients with rheumatoid arthritis: A prospective study. *Lancet* 2002;359(9313):1173–1177.
56. Weinblatt ME. Toxicity of low dose methotrexate in rheumatoid arthritis. *J Rheumatol* 1985;12(Suppl 12):35–39.
57. Gutierrez-Ureña S, Molina JF, García CO, et al. Pancytopenia secondary to methotrexate therapy in rheumatoid arthritis. *Arthritis Rheum* 1996;39:272–276.
58. Kent PD, Luthra HS, Michet CJ Jr. Risk factors for methotrexate-induced abnormal laboratory monitoring results in patients with rheumatoid arthritis. *J Rheumatol* 2004;31(9):1727–1731.
59. Walker AM, Funch D, Dreyer NA, et al. Determinants of serious liver disease among patients receiving low-dose methotrexate for rheumatoid arthritis. *Arthritis Rheum* 1993;36:329–335.
60. Ito S, Nakazono K, Murasawa A, et al. Development of fulminant hepatitis B (precore variant mutant type) after the discontinuation of low-dose methotrexate therapy in a rheumatoid arthritis patient. *Arthritis Rheum* 1901;44:339–342.
61. Kremer JM, Alarcón GS, Weinblatt ME, et al. Clinical, laboratory, radiographic, and histopathologic features of methotrexate-associated lung injury in patients with rheumatoid arthritis: A multicenter study with literature review. *Arthritis Rheum* 1997;40:1829–1837.
62. Alarcón GS, Kremer JM, Macaluso M, et al. Risk factors for methotrexate-induced lung injury in patients with rheumatoid arthritis: A multicenter, case-control study. *Ann Intern Med* 1997; 127:356–364.
63. Dawson TM, Starkebaum G, Wood BL, et al. Epstein-Barr virus, methotrexate, and lymphoma in patients with rheumatoid arthritis and primary Sjögren's syndrome: Case series. *J Rheumatol* 2001; 28(1):47–53.
64. Kamel OW, Van de Rijn M, Weiss LM, et al. Reversible lymphomas associated with Epstein-Barr virus occurring during methotrexate therapy for rheumatoid arthritis and dermatomyositis. *N Engl J Med* 1993;328:1317–1321.
65. Kerstens PJ, Boerbooms AM, Jeurissen ME, et al. Accelerated nodulosis during low dose methotrexate therapy for rheumatoid arthritis: An analysis of ten cases. *J Rheumatol* 1992;19(6):867–871.

66. Wernick R, Smith DL. Central nervous system toxicity associated with weekly low-dose methotrexate treatment. *Arthritis Rheum* 1989; 32:770–775.
67. Buckley LM, Bullaboy CA, Leichtman L, et al. Multiple congenital anomalies associated with weekly low-dose methotrexate treatment of the mother. *Arthritis Rheum* 1997;40:971–973.
68. Joyce DA, Will RK, Hoffman DM, et al. Exacerbation of rheumatoid arthritis in patients treated with methotrexate after administration of folinic acid. *Ann Rheum Dis* 1991;50:913–914.
69. Van Ede AE, Laan RF, Rood MJ, et al. Effect of folic or folinic acid supplementation on the toxicity and efficacy of methotrexate in rheumatoid arthritis: A forty-eight week, multicenter, randomized, double-blind, placebo-controlled study. *Arthritis Rheum* 2001;44(7): 1515–1524.
70. Kremer JM. Methotrexate pharmacogenomics. *Ann Rheum Dis* 2006;65(9):1121–1123.
71. Van Ede AE, Laan RF, Bloom HJ, et al. The C677T mutation in the methylenetetrahydrofolate reductase gene: A genetic risk factor for methotrexate-related elevation of liver enzymes in rheumatoid arthritis patients. *Arthritis Rheum* 2001;44(11):2525–2530.
72. Urano W, Taniguchi A, Yamanaka H, et al. Polymorphisms in the methylenetetrahydrofolate reductase gene were associated with both the efficacy and the toxicity of methotrexate used for the treatment of rheumatoid arthritis, as evidenced by single locus and haplotype analyses. *Pharmacogenetics* 2002;12(3):183–190.
73. Berkun Y, Levartovsky D, Rubinow A, et al. Methotrexate related adverse effects in patients with rheumatoid arthritis are associated with the A1298C polymorphism of the MTHFR gene. *Ann Rheum Dis* 2004;63(10):1227–1231.
74. Wessels JAM, Vries-Bouwstra JK, Heijmans BT, et al. Efficacy and toxicity of methotrexate in early rheumatoid arthritis are associated with single-nucleotide polymorphisms in genes coding for folate pathway enzymes. *Arthritis Rheum* 2006;54(4):1087–1095.
75. Weisman MH, Furst DE, Park GS, et al. Risk genotypes in folate-dependent enzymes and their association with methotrexate-related side effects in rheumatoid arthritis. *Arthritis Rheum* 2006; 54(2):607–612.
76. Dervieux T, Furst D, Lein DO, et al. Polyglutamation of methotrexate with common polymorphisms in reduced folate carrier, aminoimidazole carboxamide ribonucleotide transformylase, and thymidylate synthase are associated with methotrexate effects in rheumatoid arthritis. *Arthritis Rheum* 2004;50(9):2766–2774.
77. Wessels JA, de Vries-Bouwstra JK, Heijmans BT, et al. Efficacy and toxicity of methotrexate in early rheumatoid arthritis are associated with single-nucleotide polymorphisms in genes coding for folate pathway enzymes. *Arthritis Rheum* 2006;54(4):1087–1095.
78. Wessels JA, Kooloos WM, De Jonge R, et al. Relationship between genetic variants in the adenosine pathway and outcome of methotrexate treatment in patients with recent-onset rheumatoid arthritis. *Arthritis Rheum* 2006;54(9):2830–2839.
79. Kremer JM, Alarcon GS, Lightfoot RW Jr., et al. for the American College of Rheumatology. Methotrexate for rheumatoid arthritis: Suggested guidelines for monitoring liver toxicity. *Arthritis and Rheum* 1994;37(3):316–328.

Leflunomide

David L. Scott

Leflunomide is the only new disease-modifying antirheumatic drug (DMARD) to be introduced in the last two decades and the only drug to be designed and tested with this goal in mind. Overall, it is effective and safe. The balance of evidence, outlined in detail in this chapter, suggests that its place is as a second-choice DMARD to be used after methotrexate.

Pharmacology

Leflunomide is an isoxazole immunomodulatory agent. Its chemical name is N-(4'-trifluoromethylphenyl)-5-methylisoxazole-4-carboxamide (Figure 10D-1). Leflunomide is a prodrug that is rapidly converted in the gastrointestinal tact and liver into its active metabolite, an open-ring malononitrilamide.

Peak levels of its active metabolite occur between 6 and 12 hours after oral dosing. The metabolite has a long half-life, which is in the region of 2 weeks. It is mainly eliminated by further metabolism and renal excretion. Direct biliary excretion also leads to the removal of some of the active metabolite.

The long half-life of leflunomide resulted in early trials using a loading dose. In the first trial, this was 50 to 100 mg followed by daily dosing at lower levels. In the pivotal trials, it was 100 mg for 3 days. More recently, the loading dose has been avoided because its benefit of increased speed of action is outweighed by an increase in the number and severity of adverse events. As a consequence of the first large trial, the dose of leflunomide was considered to be between 10 and 25 mg daily—and most studies have used 20 mg daily.

Mechanisms of Action

The active metabolite of leflunomide at therapeutic doses reversibly inhibits dihydroorotate dehydrogenase, the rate-limiting step in the *de novo* synthesis of pyrimidines. Unlike other cells, activated lymphocytes expand their pyrimidine pool approximately eightfold during proliferation. Purine pools are increased only twofold. To meet this demand, lymphocytes must use both salvage and *de novo* synthesis pathways. Thus, the inhibition of dihydroorotate dehydrogenase prevents lymphocytes from accumulating sufficient pyrimidines to support DNA synthesis and has a consequent immunomodulatory effect.[1] Several other mechanisms of action have been proposed.[2–5] These are summarized in Table 10D-1.

Key Clinical Trials

Leflunomide is an effective DMARD that over 6 to 12 months decreases the number of active joints, improves pain, and leads to better overall assessments of disease activity. Its efficacy has been shown in an extensive clinical trials program. The first large clinical trial of leflunomide, undertaken in Europe,[6] enrolled 402 patients with active rheumatoid arthritis (RA). Patients were randomly assigned to receive leflunomide (5 mg, 10 mg, and 25 mg daily) or placebo, and treatment was given for 6 months. There were significant improvements in most clinical assessments of disease activity as well as in the American College of Rheumatology (ACR) 20% responder analysis in the 10-mg and 25-mg dosage groups for leflunomide compared to placebo. All key clinical outcomes improved over 6 months. The mean improvements in joint counts and global assessments are shown in Figure 10D-2.

Subsequently, three pivotal trials were set up in the mid 1990s. These reported their results over the next few years. Two of the trials were primarily based in Europe,[7,8] and the third was in North America.[9] The first European trial involved 358 RA patients, who were randomly assigned to receive leflunomide (20 mg daily), sulfsalazine (2 g daily), or placebo. It lasted 6 months. The second European trial compared leflunomide (20 mg daily) to methotrexate (10–15 mg weekly) and lasted 24 months. Most patients given methotrexate did not

Figure 10D-1. Structure of leflunomide.

Table 10D-1. Potential Mechanisms of Action of Leflunomide
• Pyrimidine synthesis: inhibits dihydroorotate dehydrogenase
• T-cell activation: inhibits nuclear factor kappa-B activation
• Reducing cell-cell contact: downregulates glycosylation of adhesion molecules
• Mast cell apoptosis: inhibits phosphorylation of Akt (survival signal of mast cells)
• Reduced bone marrow cell proliferation: inhibits anti CD3- and CD28-induced cytokine production
• Chondroprotective effects: increases IL-1Ra production by synovial fibroblasts and chondrocytes
• Synovial nitric oxide production: inhibited by leflunomide

receive folic acid. The North American trial involved 482 patients randomized to receive leflunomide (20 mg daily), methotrexate (7.5–15 mg weekly), or placebo. The trial lasted 12 months. In this North American trial, all patients given methotrexate also received folate supplements.

The first European study concluded that leflunomide was more effective than placebo in the treatment of RA and showed similar efficacy to sulfasalazine. The second European study concluded that both leflunomide and methotrexate were effective, but over 12 months methotrexate had some advantages over leflunomide. The North American study concluded that both leflunomide and methotrexate were better than placebo and showed equivalent efficacy. These differences among trials relates to the dosages of methotrexate used and to the co-prescription of folic acid. The prevailing opinion among rheumatologists is that the doses of methotrexate were relatively low and that in the North American trial the effect of methotrexate was possibly decreased by co-prescription of folic acid.

These trials involved two extension studies, which did not include placebo therapy and compared one active treatment against another.[10,11] Together, these four trials and two extensions were evaluated in a systematic review of the efficacy of leflunomide by Osiri and colleagues.[12] Their review included data from 2,044 RA patients. It concluded that leflunomide improves all clinical outcomes at 6 and 12 months of treatment compared to placebo. Leflunomide improved the ACR 20 response rate roughly two times over placebo both at 6 months (relative benefit 1.93; 95% CI 1.51, 2.47) and at 12 months (relative benefit 1.99; 95% CI 1.42, 2.77). All assessments of disease activity were significantly better with leflunomide than with placebo. An analysis of standardized mean differences compared to placebo at 6 months is shown in Figure 10D-3. The review also concluded that the efficacy of leflunomide after 2 years of treatment was comparable to sulfasalazine and methotrexate.

Effect on Radiologic Progression

In common with other DMARDs, leflunomide reduces radiologic progression. A systematic review of the three pivotal clinical trials by Sharp and colleagues[13] showed the leflunomide, sulfasalazine, and methotrexate reduced radiologic progression

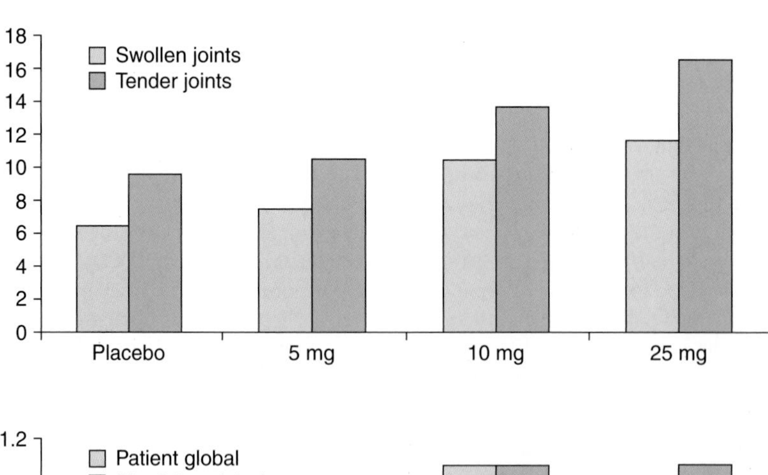

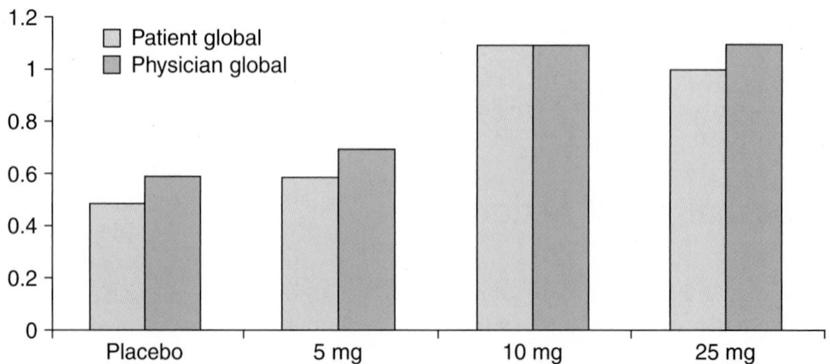

Figure 10D-2. Improvements in clinical assessments in the first large clinical trial of leflunomide. (From Palmer G, Burger D, Mezin F, et al. The active metabolite of leflunomide, A77 1726, increases the production of IL-1 receptor antagonist in human synovial fibroblasts and articular chondrocytes. *Arthritis Res Ther* 2004;6:R181–189.)

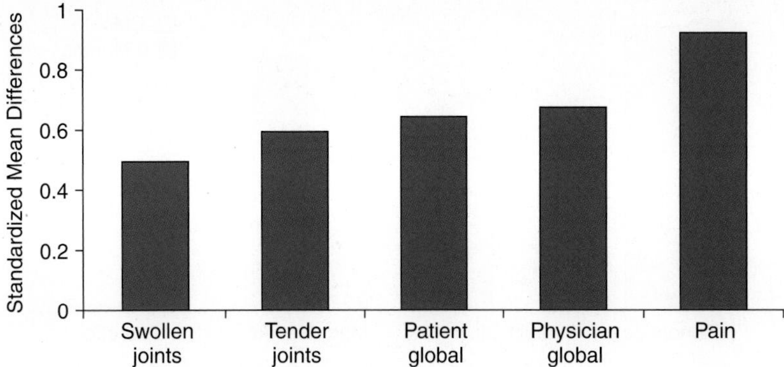

Figure 10D-3. Meta-analysis of 6-month responses to leflunomide in comparison to placebo. (From Emery P, Breedveld FC, Lemmel EM, et al. A comparison of the efficacy and safety of leflunomide and methotrexate for the treatment of rheumatoid arthritis. *Rheumatology* 2000;39:655–665.)

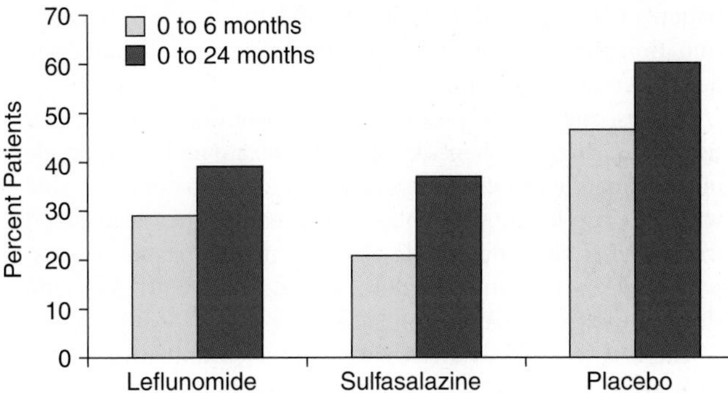

Figure 10D-4. Percentages of patients showing x-ray progression over 6 and 24 months. (From Cohen S, Cannon GW, Schiff M, et al. Two-year, blinded, randomized, controlled trial of treatment of rheumatoid arthritis with leflunomide compared with methotrexate. *Arthritis Rheum* 2001;44:1984–1992.)

compared to placebo. A subsequent systematic review by Jones et al.[14] evaluated all studies of DMARDs. They evaluated 25 trials that had enrolled 3,907 patients. This review showed that cyclosporine, sulfasalazine, leflunomide, methotrexate, parenteral gold, and auranofin were statistically better than placebo in terms of changes in erosion scores and that they were indistinguishable from one another.

The impact of leflunomide over 2 years was shown in a detailed analysis of 429 patients (evaluated using Larsen's scoring system) by Larsen and colleagues.[15] Both leflunomide and sulfasalazine reduced the numbers of patients showing any erosive progression to under 30% compared to nearly 50% in placebo-treated patients—and this magnitude of difference persisted over 2 years, as shown in Figure 10D-4.

Beyond 2 years, there is evidence from extension studies involving 128 patients taking leflunomide in the original pivotal trials that its benefits on x-ray progression persist.[16] These patients showed that using Sharp x-ray scores during treatment with leflunomide progressed by an annual average of 1.9. This contrasted with an estimated initial progression rate of 7.9 each year and an overall assessment of 7.5 per year seen in a number of longitudinal studies.[17]

Effects on Function

As with all DMARDs, leflunomide improved function as well as decreasing disease activity. In the short term, the improvements in function assessed using the Health Assessment Questionnaire (HAQ) closely mirror improvements in disease activity. These short-term changes were studied in 1,817 RA patients, including 807 patients treated with leflunomide, by Scott and Strand.[18] Over 6 months, mean HAQ scores fell by 0.38 with leflunomide and showed virtually no change with placebo (as shown in Figure 10D-5). Sulfsalazine and methotrexate showed similar changes. Over 2 years, they remained relative static on leflunomide—with a possible very small increase in the region of 1%, which is below the average annual increase in HAQ scores. Subsequent review of all 2-year results by Strand and colleagues[19] showed improvements in HAQ scores between 0.48 and 0.73 in different patient groups.

In routine clinical practice, where a broader range of patients is treated (who often have milder disease), changes in HAQ are less marked. Wolfe[20] reported changes in HAQ in 2,491 clinic RA patients with active disease at the time leflunomide was started and at subsequent follow-up, when there had been sufficient time for a response. He reported that before treatment mean HAQ scores were 1.30 and that over 6 months this fell by 0.05 as a function of treatment.

Optimal Dosing

Three questions about dosing with leflunomide have been examined separately since the key clinical trials in RA were reported. These are whether the best daily maintenance dose is 10 mg or 20 mg, whether it can be given as a single weekly dose, and whether or not the loading dose is needed.

One large 6-month trial enrolled 402 RA patients[21] and compared 10-mg and 20-mg maintenance doses. Across all clinical measures, 20 mg gave slightly better mean improvements than 10 mg—and the balance of evidence favored the use of the higher maintenance dose in most patients.

There is limited evidence about using 100 mg weekly. Two open reports suggest that it is reasonably effective.[22,23] Both involved only small groups of patients (16 and 30, respectively) and both were conducted at the same center. Nevertheless, it seems reasonable to assume that 100 mg weekly is an effective dosing regimen in some RA patients.

The loading dose issue is more complex. The balance of expert opinion is that it provides a more rapid clinical response but may increase the risk of adverse effects.[24] One small observational study of 84 RA patients from Japan suggests that the risks of adverse reactions are increased with a loading dose.[25] A similar small Spanish study of 35 patients drew the same conclusion.[26] A U.K. clinical practice survey showed that many

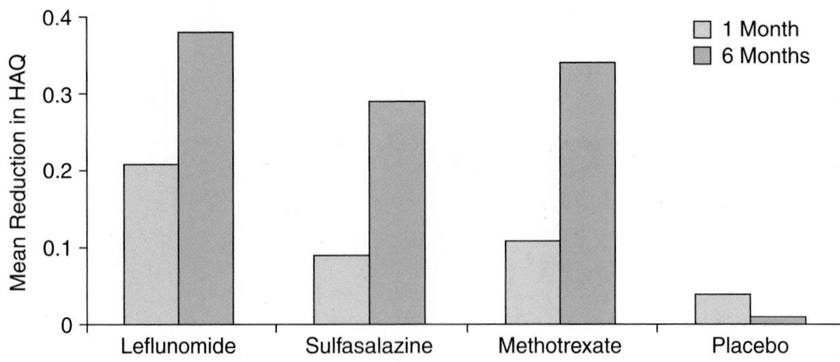

Figure 10D-5. Improvements in Health Assessment Questionnaire scores with leflunomide. (From Jones G, Halbert J, Crotty M, et al. The effect of treatment on radiological progression in rheumatoid arthritis: A systematic review of randomized placebo-controlled trials. *Rheumatology* 2003;42:6–13.)

rheumatologists do not use a loading dose[27] (and, on a personal note, this is my own approach).

Combination Therapy with Other DMARDs

There is increasing emphasis on using DMARDs in combination in active RA, and research into the optimal use of leflunomide has followed this direction.[28] A small observational study by Weinblatt and colleagues[29] evaluated the potential for combining leflunomide with methotrexate in 30 RA patients followed for 12 months. They were all patients with an inadequate response to methotrexate monotherapy. They found no significant pharmacokinetic interactions between leflunomide and methotrexate, and the combination was generally well tolerated clinically—although there were some elevations of liver enzyme levels. This study set the scene for using leflunomide in combinations.

The definitive combination trial by Kremer et al.[30] studied 263 patients who received 10 mg leflunomide or placebo in addition to methotrexate (10–20 mg weekly). The patients all had continuing active RA despite at least 6 months of treatment. ACR 20 response rates with combination therapy were 46.2% and 19.5% with methotrexate-placebo. Individual clinical assessments all favored combination therapy, as shown in Figure 10D-6. Discontinuation rates were 23% in the leflunomide group and 25% in the placebo group, and there was no evidence of an excess of adverse events with combination therapy. A subsequent open-label extension study for 12 months confirmed that the treatment effect persisted.[31] Interestingly, patients who switched from placebo to leflunomide in the continuation phase and did not have a loading dose of leflunomide had fewer adverse effects.

A subsequent observational study in routine clinical practice[32] confirmed the benefits of methotrexate and leflunomide in combination. After 30 months, 65% of 40 patients treated with this combination remained on therapy. They also found that whereas the leflunomide dosage remained stable in most patients the methotrexate dose was decreased in 35% and stopped in 28% of patients.

There is less information about other combinations. One large study has evaluated the combination of leflunomide and sulfasalazine. This was a European trial led by Dougados.[33] The design was complex. The trial enrolled 968 patients with active RA, and these all received leflunomide at standard doses. A total of 106 of these patients who showed an inadequate response were then randomized to receive sulfasalazine (2 gm daily) with continuation of the leflunomide or a matching placebo. After 6 months, 45% of patients receiving combination therapy were classified as good responders (compared with 30% on monotherapy). There was no excess of adverse events. Although too few patients were randomized to draw solid conclusions, the balance of evidence favored combination therapy.

There have been occasional reports of other combinations with leflunomide. For example, leflunomide and cyclosporine have been used together with apparent success in four patients with RA.[34] However, there are generally insufficient data to make an informed decision about the value of these other combinations.

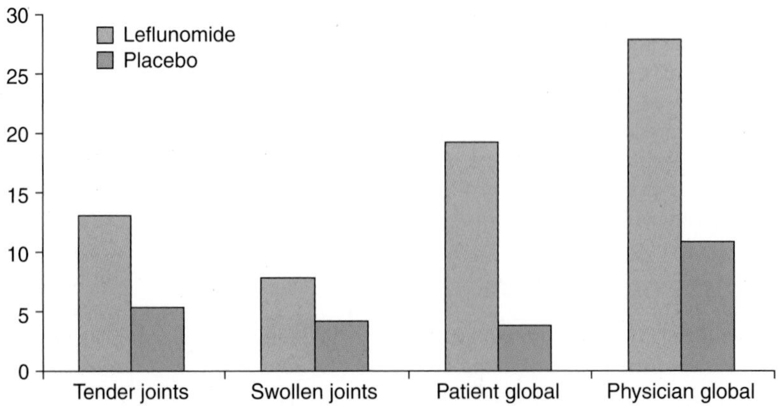

Figure 10D-6. Changes in clinical assessments with combination therapy. (From Erra A, Tomas C, Barcelo P, et al. Is the recommended dose of leflunomide the best regimen to treat rheumatoid arthritis patients? *Rheumatology* 2003;42: 1123–1124.)

Combination with Biologics

Tumor necrosis factor (TNF) inhibitors are usually given with methotrexate, and all main clinical trials have focused on this combination. There are limited data about the value of TNF inhibitor combinations with leflunomide, and the available information is mainly from observational studies. Eight separate reports have described experience with this combination.[35–42] They invariably agree on the efficacy of the combination, but there were some concerns in earlier small reports that leflunomide increased adverse events. The balance of evidence now suggests that the risk of adverse events was overemphasized in the initial reports. One of the largest observational studies reported experience with 162 RA patients started on infliximab therapy, of whom 57 were taking leflunomide (with most of the remainder taking methotrexate). There were no differences in drug survival, disease activity, or adverse events between groups. There is little information about combinations with other TNF inhibitors or other biologics. It appears rational to use leflunomide in place of methotrexate in combinations with biologics should there be a clinical need, such as intolerance to methotrexate.

Efficacy and Treatment Discontinuation in Routine Practice

Weaver and colleagues[43] studied 204 RA patients among 5,397 patients assessed prospectively in a routine practice setting. There was no difference in ACR 20 rates between leflunomide and methotrexate, confirming the results in clinical trials.

Withdrawal from treatment is generally considered a key assessment of overall efficacy and toxicity, and has been used to evaluate comparable benefits in systematic reviews.[44] There is substantial observational data comparing different DMARDs that shows that leflunomide performs similarly to methotrexate and better than sulfasalazine. Grijalva and colleagues[45] used the Tennessee Medicaid databases (1995–2004) to establish a retrospective cohort of RA patients treated with DMARDs. They found 14,932 patients and 10,547 episodes of new DMARD use. Adherence was comparable with methotrexate and leflunomide, and lower with sulfasalzine as well as combined therapies. The differences between the main DMARDs in 558 to 3,859 episodes of treatment are shown in Figure 10D-7. Methotrexate and leflunomide appear indistinguishable.

Similar data were reported by Wolfe and colleagues[46] in an evaluation of 1,431 RA patients who began taking leflunomide or methotrexate as part of their routine medical care between 1998 and 2001. The 756 patients taking leflunomide had a failure rate of 55.5 per 100 patient-years. For 675 patients taking methotrexate, the failure rate was 57.3 per 100 patient-years.

Not all studies draw similar conclusions. An observational study from Austria[47] evaluated 5,141 patient-years of DMARD treatment. Matched survival analysis showed better retention rates for methotrexate (mean survival 28 months) than either leflunomide or sulfasalazine (respective mean survivals of 20 and 23 months). Another study from France reported experience in 285 RA patients starting 515 courses of DMARDs.[48] Leflunomide was stopped in 57% of patients compared to 32% stopping methotrexate and 59% stopping sulfasalazine.

An observational study from Holland[49] studied patients starting leflunomide in 2000 to 2003 at two centers to determine predictive factors for discontinuation. During this time, 279 patients started leflunomide and 173 (62%) discontinued treatment during follow-up. Remaining on treatment was influenced by taking steroids, having an initial low erythrocyte sedimentation rate (ESR) (>35 mm/hour), and the supervising rheumatologist. The data about the impact of different clinicians are interesting but difficult to assess in detail. However, individual rheumatologists had an influence of more than fourfold on patients remaining on leflunomide. The impact of rheumatologists is so strong that it is likely to make much of this observational data difficult to interpret.

Leflunomide in Psoriatic Arthritis

The effects of leflunomide are not specific for RA, and there is strong evidence that it is also effective in psoriatic arthritis in the 6-month placebo-controlled trial by Kaltwasser and colleagues.[50] It involved 190 patients with active psoriatic arthritis and psoriasis. They received leflunomide (100 mg/day loading dose, then 20 mg/day) or placebo. The primary endpoint was the number of patients classified as responders using the Psoriatic Arthritis Response Criteria (PsARC). At 6 months, 56 (59%) of 95 leflunomide-treated patients and 27 (30%) of 91 placebo-treated patients were PsARC responders (a significant difference). Leflunomide also showed better ACR 20 responders, less psoriasis, and better quality of life. Some key outcomes in improvement are shown in Figure 10D-8.

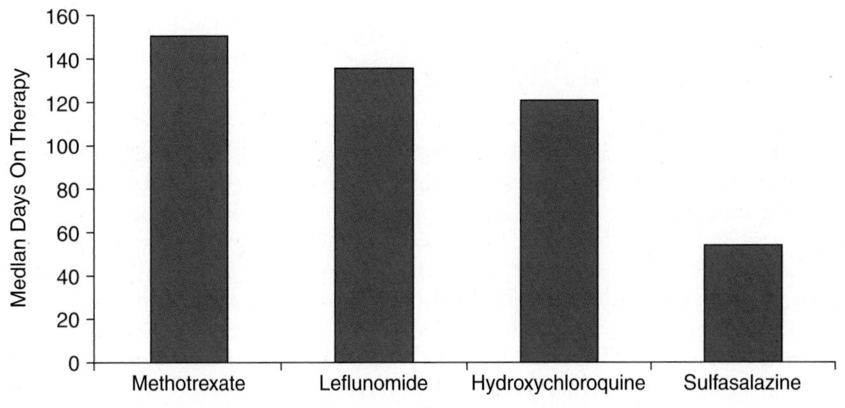

Figure 10D-7. Persistence on therapy with different DMARDs.

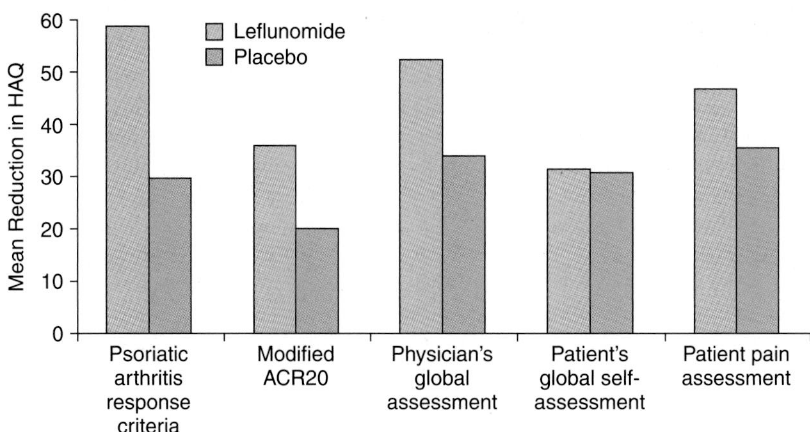

Figure 10D-8. Effects of leflunomide in trial of psoriatic arthritis.

Juvenile Arthritis

Leflunomide is also effective in juvenile RA. An open 6-month study in 27 patients with refractory polyarticular juvenile arthritis showed that 17 (63%) were able to complete 6 months of treatment.[51] Fourteen patients (52%) met the ACR Pediatric 30 response criteria. Extended treatment in 17 patients for up to 30 months showed that good responses were maintained.

A subsequent randomized controlled trial compared leflunomide and methotrexate in patients aged 3 to 17 years with polyarticular juvenile RA (94 patients were randomized and 86 completed 16 weeks of treatment).[52] By 16 weeks, more patients receiving methotrexate than leflunomide had an ACR Pediatric 30 response (89% vs. 68%). This was a significant difference. Although both methotrexate and leflunomide gave high rates of clinical improvement, methotrexate was more effective than leflunomide.

Health Economics

The data from the pivotal trial of leflunomide, methotrexate, and placebo were used to assess the comparative cost effectiveness of these DMARDs.[53] When drug monitoring and acquisition costs were excluded, leflunomide had a similar economic profile to methotrexate. At the time of the study, its acquisition and monitoring costs were higher and thus it was marginally less cost effective than methotrexate. Subsequent research in Canada modeled the 5-year cost effectiveness of adding leflunomide to a sequence of DMARDs representative of a typical RA management approach. It showed that this treatment option extended the time patients benefit from DMARD therapy with reasonable cost effectiveness and cost utility.[54] Comparable research from Germany evaluated the 3-year cost effectiveness and cost utility of introducing leflunomide into sequential therapy of frequently used DMARDs.[55] After 3 years, adding leflunomide was less costly and more effective than the strategy excluding leflunomide when both direct and indirect costs were considered. Focusing on direct costs alone showed that adding leflunomide was more costly and more effective compared with not using it. The incremental cost utility was 8,301 Euros per quality-adjusted life-year gained after 3 years.

Overall Adverse Effects in Clinical Trials

As with all DMARDs, leflunomide is associated with a range of adverse events. Most are mild, but some are serious. A U.K. consensus meeting reviewed them in detail.[56] It concluded that in clinical trials, leflunomide showed a tolerability profile intermediate between that of methotrexate and sulfasalazine in terms of all-cause withdrawal rates and infections. A summary of withdrawals due to adverse events and other serious problems is outlined in Table 10D-2. In these trials, nausea, hepatotoxicity, dermatologic problems, and hypertension were key concerns.

- Significant nausea that required withdrawal of treatment occurred in 1% of patients receiving leflunomide, which was less than methotrexate (3%) and sulfasalazine (5%).
- Diarrhea was more of a problem with leflunomide and led to withdrawal from treatment in 2% of patients compared to 1% of patients receiving methotrexate or sulfasalazine.
- Hepatic enzyme concentration elevation three times above the upper limit of normal occurred in 5% of patients taking leflunomide compared with 17% given methotrexate and 4% given sulfasalazine.
- Dermatologic adverse events occurred in 28% of patients given leflunomide compared with 32% given methotrexate and 35% given sulfasalazine. However, there were more serious dermatologic events with leflunomide.
- Withdrawals due to hypertension were uncommon. They occurred in 0.8% of patients given leflunomide compared with 0.8% receiving sulfasalazine and 0.3% receiving methotrexate.

Epidemiologic Assessment of Adverse Effects

An analysis of the Aetna-U.S. Healthcare database evaluated adverse events in 40,594 patients with RA in this large U.S. health care insurance database, which contains data on 6.5 million individuals.[57] The RA patients accumulated 83,143 person-years of follow-up. The incidence rate of all adverse events combined was lower for leflunomide monotherapy (94 events per 1000 person-years) than methotrexate (145 events per 1000 person-years) and other DMARDs (143 events per 1000 person-years. Leflunomide monotherapy also had the lowest rate of hepatic events in the DMARD monotherapy group.

Table 10D-2. Meta-Analysis of Significant Adverse Events in Pivotal Lefunomide Trials

Treatment Group	Leflunomide (*n* = 1693)	Placebo (*n* = 322)	Methotrexate (*n* = 709)	Sulfasalazine (*n* = 133)
Withdrawn due to AE	351 (21%)	26 (8%)	141 (20%)	34 (26%)
Deaths	27 (2%)	2 (0.6%)	19 (3%)	3 (2.2%)
Infection (serious)	97 (6%)	4 (1%)	58 (8%)	6 (5%)
Nausea (withdrawn)	23 (1%)	1 (0.6%)	17 (2%)	7 (5.3%)
Diarrhoea (withdrawn)	32 (2%)	5 (2%)	11 (2%)	1 (0.8%)
Liver function (withdrawn)	45 (3%)	5 (2%)	33 (5%)	2 (2%)
Dermatologic events (serious)	27 (2%)	1 (0.3%)	7 (0.9%)	1 (0.8%)
Hypertension (withdrawn)	13 (0.8%)	3 (0.9%)	2 (0.3%)	1 (0.8%)
Anaemia (withdrawn)	11 (1%)	0	4 (1%)	1 (1%)
Leucopaenia (withdrawn)	13 (1%)	2 (1%)	0	2 (2%)
Thrombocytopaenia (withdrawn)	0	0	1 (0.1%)	0
Subjects developing malignancy	17 (1%)	3 (1%)	20 (3%)	4 (3%)
Subjects developing lymphoma	3 (<1%)	0	2 (<1%)	2 (2%)

From Silverman E, Spiegel L, Hawkins D, et al. Long-term open-label preliminary study of the safety and efficacy of leflunomide in patients with polyarticular-course juvenile rheumatoid arthritis. *Arthritis Rheum* 2005;52:554–562.

Serious Liver Toxicity

Individual patients have been described in whom serious liver toxicity developed with either monotherapy[58] or combined with methotrexate.[59] It is not possible to ascertain the severity of the problem from these individual reports. However, there is less concern after large patient cohorts have suggested that hepatotoxicity is relatively uncommon.

van Roon and colleagues[60] reported the development of liver toxicity in 101 RA patients followed for a median period of 10 months on leflunomide. Minor elevations in liver function test were noted in nine patients. No serious elevations were found. None of the patients showed clinical signs of hepatotoxicity. Another study evaluated the risk of hepatic events in two cohorts of 41,885 RA patients who had been dispensed a DMARD between 1998 and 2001.[61] There were 25 cases of serious hepatic events (five per 10,000/year) and 411 nonserious hepatic events (80 per 10,000/year). Compared to methotrexate there was no increase in the rate of serious hepatic events with leflunomide (rate ratio 0.9) or traditional DMARDs (rate ratio 2.3), nor with nonserious hepatic events. Although serious liver toxicity occurs with leflunomide and other DMARDs, the evidence suggests no specific increased risk with leflunomide.

Lung Disease

There have been many occasional reports of interstitial lung disease linked to leflunomide. For example, a Japanese group described a 54-year-old woman with RA who developed acute respiratory failure 2 weeks after cessation of a 6-week treatment with leflunomide.[62] Interestingly, most of the concern about lung disease came from Japan.[63]

A subsequent detailed assessment of the risk of lung disease was performed, based on 62,734 RA patients in the PharMetrics claims database.[64] An analysis of this database found 74 patients with interstitial lung disease, corresponding to a rate of 8 of 10,000 patients per year. The risk of lung disease with leflunomide was marginally increased, with an adjusted risk ratio of 1.9. However, in patients with no previous methotrexate use and no history of interstitial lung disease there was no increased risk with leflunomide. As patients with a history of interstitial lung disease were twice as likely to have been prescribed leflunomide as any other DMARD, this indicated channeling of high-risk patients to leflunomide treatment.

The risks of leflunomide-induced lung disease and the effect of channeling remain controversial. However, a subsequent Korean report that evaluated data on 1,010 RA patients treated with leflunomide at seven university hospitals for at least 1 month found that 10 patients developed interstitial lung disease.[65] Six of these had preexisting lung disease, suggesting that it was an important risk factor. Most patients made a good recovery, and none died. The evidence favors a link between preexisting lung disease and leflunomide-induced lung damage, although channeling may be too sophisticated a concept in this clinical context.

Infections

Patients with RA are more likely to develop infections than the general population. DMARDs in general may be an additional risk factor, and one study from New Zealand has looked at leflunomide in particular.[66] This was a retrospective audit together with a review of reports to the national Pharmacovigilance Centre. They found that in one center 11 of 171 RA patients who commenced leflunomide developed infection requiring hospitalization, including for lower respiratory tract infections, cellulitis, and disseminated herpes zoster. The Pharmacovigilance Centre had received seven additional reports of severe infections in patients with RA taking leflunomide. Patients with severe disease and taking combination methotrexate and systemic steroids were at most risk. Although this rate of serious infection was considered acceptable in the context of optimally treating active RA, once established infections rapidly progress in patients taking leflunomide and early intervention is needed.

Weight Loss

Occasional studies have reported that weight loss is seen in some patients receiving leflunomide. One study from a single North American specialist center dealt with this problem in detail. It identified 5 of 70 patients who had begun leflunomide therapy and then had significant weight loss not linked to other identifiable causes.[67] They lost between 19 and 53 pounds. Thyroid-stimulating hormone levels were normal, and they had no gastrointestinal complaints. Despite this weight loss, four of the patients continued to take leflunomide due to its efficacy. It seems unlikely that this is a major concern with leflunomide therapy, although it is well documented. The mechanism is unknown.

Monitoring

Patients starting leflunomide are required to have regular monitoring of blood tests and blood pressure. Monitoring regimens vary. One example comprises:

- Full blood count and liver function tests every 2 weeks for 2 months, and then every 4 weeks
- Blood pressure check: monthly for 6 months, and then every 8 weeks

There are national monitoring guidelines from the U.K. and elsewhere,[68] although these guidelines are not always followed in clinical practice. My personal view is that they are non evidence based and largely unnecessary, but nevertheless it is usually impractical not to follow them.

Pregnancy

Leflunomide is a teratogenic drug and should not be used in pregnancy or in women who may become pregnant. Consequently, women of childbearing potential should use effective contraception during and up to 2 years after treatment. If women do become pregnant while taking leflunomide, the washout procedure may be used (see material following). In that animal studies show that leflunomide or its metabolites pass into breast milk, breast-feeding women should also not receive leflunomide. Paternal exposure is similarly advised against. The actual risk of malformations after leflunomide exposure is difficult to assess and the evidence is as follows.

- One survey[69] recorded experience from 175 North American rheumatologists who reported 10 pregnancies in women receiving leflunomide, none of which resulted in congenital malformations.
- An Italian group[70] reported experience in five women, four exposed in the first trimester and one conceived 6 months after stopping leflunomide (with one case of paternal exposure). Three women had voluntary abortions, and three had live births with healthy babies.
- A single U.K. patient has been reported in which the mother had an apparently healthy male baby born 9 weeks prematurely who was subsequently found to be blind in the right eye and to have cerebral palsy with left-sided spasticity.[71]

Other antirheumatic drugs should be used in patients who are likely to become pregnant, and there are well-known options.[72] However, when patients do conceive while taking leflunomide they need to have access to the available information to make an informed choice.

Washout Procedures

Should the need arise, due to possible pregnancy or toxicity after stopping treatment with leflunomide its removal can be enhanced by a washout procedure. This involves:

- Cholestyramine (8 g) administered three times daily for 11 days
- Activated powdered charcoal (50 g) administered four times daily for 11 days

This approach is based on the pharmacokinetics of leflunomide.[73]

Place In Clinical Practice

A U.K. consensus meeting recommended that on the basis of efficacy, safety, and cost, leflunomide should be considered in patients with RA who have failed first-line DMARD drug therapy. Whether or not it should be used before or instead of a trial of biologics in such patients is currently a matter of opinion. There are no controlled trials to guide this decision. In refractory cases, it could be used in combination with methotrexate before biologic agents—although it is realized that this is controversial in many countries. Therapy should be initiated by a specialist. Clear mechanisms are required to monitor toxicity, with good communication between the patient and rheumatologist to manage nuisance side effects and to avoid unnecessary discontinuation of leflunomide. This consensus view represents as good a definition of current opinion that can be obtained.

References

1. Breedveld FC, Dayer J-M. Leflunomide: Mode of action in the treatment of rheumatoid arthritis. *Ann Rheum Dis* 2000;59:841–849.
2. Palmer G, Burger D, Mezin F, et al. The active metabolite of leflunomide, A77 1726, increases the production of IL-1 receptor antagonist in human synovial fibroblasts and articular chondrocytes. *Arthritis Res Ther* 2004;6:R181–R189.
3. Magari K, Miyata S, Nishigaki F, et al. Comparison of anti-arthritic properties of leflunomide with methotrexate and FK506: Effect on T cell activation-induced inflammatory cytokine production in vitro and rat adjuvant-induced arthritis. *Inflamm Res* 2004;53:544–550.
4. Reddy SV, Wanchu A, Khullar M, et al. Leflunomide reduces nitric oxide production in patients with active rheumatoid arthritis. *Int Immunopharmacol* 2005;5:1085–1090.
5. Sawamukai N, Saito K, Yamaoka K, et al. Leflunomide inhibits PDK1/Akt pathway and induces apoptosis of human mast cells. *J Immunol* 2007;179:6479–6484.
6. Mladenovic V, Domljan Z, Rozman B, et al. Safety and effectiveness of leflunomide in the treatment of patients with active rheumatoid arthritis. Results of a randomized, placebo-controlled, phase II study. *Arthritis Rheum* 1995;38:1595–1603.
7. Smolen JS, Kalden JR, Scott DL, et al. For the European Leflunomide Study Group. Efficacy and safety of leflunomide compared with placebo and sulphasalazine in active rheumatoid arthritis: A double-blind, randomised, multicentre trial. *Lancet* 1999;353:259–266.
8. Emery P, Breedveld FC, Lemmel EM, et al. A comparison of the efficacy and safety of leflunomide and methotrexate for the treatment of rheumatoid arthritis. *Rheumatology* 2000;39:655–665.

9. Strand V, Cohen S, Schiff M, et al. for the Leflunomide Rheumatoid Arthritis Investigators Group. Treatment of active rheumatoid arthritis with leflunomide compared with placebo and methotrexate. *Arch Intern Med* 1999;159:2542–2550.
10. Scott DL, Smolen JS, Kalden JR, et al. Treatment of active rheumatoid arthritis with leflunomide: Two year follow-up of a double blind, placebo controlled trial versus sulfasalazine. *Ann Rheum Dis* 2001;60:913–923.
11. Cohen S, Cannon GW, Schiff M, et al. Two-year, blinded, randomized, controlled trial of treatment of rheumatoid arthritis with leflunomide compared with methotrexate. *Arthritis Rheum* 2001; 44:1984–1992.
12. Osiri M, Shea B, Robinson V, et al. Leflunomide for the treatment of rheumatoid arthritis: A systematic review and metaanalysis. *J Rheumatol* 2003;30:1182–1190.
13. Sharp JT, Strand V, Leung H, et al. for the Leflunomide Rheumatoid Arthritis Investigators Group. Treatment with leflunomide slows radiographic progression of rheumatoid arthritis: Results from three randomized controlled trials of leflunomide in patients with active rheumatoid arthritis. *Arthritis Rheum* 2000;43:495–505.
14. Jones G, Halbert J, Crotty M, et al. The effect of treatment on radiological progression in rheumatoid arthritis: A systematic review of randomized placebo-controlled trials. *Rheumatology* 2003;42:6–13.
15. Larsen A, Kvien TK, Schattenkirchner M, et al. for the European Leflunomide Study Group. Slowing of disease progression in rheumatoid arthritis patients during long-term treatment with leflunomide or sulfasalazine. *Scand J Rheumatol* 2001;30:135–142.
16. van der Heijde D, Kalden J, Scott D, et al. Long term evaluation of radiographic disease progression in a subset of patients with rheumatoid arthritis treated with leflunomide beyond 2 years. *Ann Rheum Dis* 2004;63:737–739.
17. Scott DL, Pugner K, Kaarela K, et al. The links between joint damage and disability in rheumatoid arthritis. *Rheumatology* 2000;39: 122–132.
18. Scott DL, Strand V. The effects of disease-modifying anti-rheumatic drugs on the Health Assessment Questionnaire score: Lessons from the leflunomide clinical trials database. *Rheumatology* 2002;41: 899–909.
19. Strand V, Scott DL, Emery P, et al. for the Leflunomide Rheumatoid Arthritis Investigators Groups. Physical function and health related quality of life: analysis of 2-year data from randomized, controlled studies of leflunomide, sulfasalazine, or methotrexate in patients with active rheumatoid arthritis. *J Rheumatol* 2005;32:590–601.
20. Wolfe F. Which HAQ is best? A comparison of the HAQ, MHAQ and RA-HAQ, a difficult 8 item HAQ (DHAQ), and a rescored 20 item HAQ (HAQ20): Analyses in 2,491 rheumatoid arthritis patients following leflunomide initiation. *J Rheumatol* 2001;28: 982–999.
21. Poór G, Strand V. for the Leflunomide Multinational Study Group. Efficacy and safety of leflunomide 10 mg versus 20 mg once daily in patients with active rheumatoid arthritis: Multinational double-blind, randomized trial. *Rheumatology* 2004;43:744–749.
22. Jakez-Ocampo J, Richaud-Patin Y, Simón JA, et al. Weekly dose of leflunomide for the treatment of refractory rheumatoid arthritis: An open pilot comparative study. *Joint Bone Spine* 2002;69: 307–311.
23. Jakez-Ocampo J, Richaud-Patin Y, Granados J, et al. Weekly leflunomide as monotherapy for recent-onset rheumatoid arthritis. *Arthritis Rheum* 2004;51:147–148.
24. Maddison P, Kiely P, Kirkham B, et al. Leflunomide in rheumatoid arthritis: Recommendations through a process of consensus. *Rheumatology* 2005;44:280–286.
25. Kanbe K, Inoue K, Chiba J, et al.. The side-effects and efficacy of leflunomide in Japanese patients with rheumatoid arthritis APLAR. *J Rheumatol* 2005;8:114–118.
26. Erra A, Tomas C, Barcelo P, et al. Is the recommended dose of leflunomide the best regimen to treat rheumatoid arthritis patients? *Rheumatology* 2003;42:1123–1124.
27. Rajakulendran S, Deighton C. Do guidelines for the prescribing and monitoring of leflunomide need to be modified? *Rheumatology* 2004;43:1447–1448.
28. Pincus T, O'Dell JR, Kremer JM. Combination therapy with multiple disease-modifying antirheumatic drugs in rheumatoid arthritis: A preventive strategy. *Ann Intern Med* 1999;131:768–774.
29. Weinblatt ME, Kremer JM, Coblyn JS, et al. Pharmacokinetics, safety, and efficacy of combination treatment with methotrexate and leflunomide in patients with active rheumatoid arthritis. *Arthritis Rheum* 1999;42:1322–1328.
30. Kremer JM, Genovese MC, Cannon GW, et al. Concomitant leflunomide therapy in patients with active rheumatoid arthritis despite stable doses of methotrexate. A randomized, double-blind, placebo-controlled trial. *Ann Intern Med* 2002;137:726–733.
31. Kremer J, Genovese M, Cannon GW, et al. Combination leflunomide and methotrexate (MTX) therapy for patients with active rheumatoid arthritis failing MTX monotherapy: Open-label extension of a randomized, double-blind, placebo controlled trial. *J Rheumatol* 2004; 31:1521–1531.
32. Dendooven A, De Rycke L, Verhelst X, et al. Leflunomide and methotrexate combination therapy in daily clinical practice. *Ann Rheum Dis* 2006;65:833–834.
33. Dougados M, Emery P, Lemmel EM, et al. When a DMARD fails, should patients switch to sulfasalazine or add sulfasalazine to continuing leflunomide? *Ann Rheum Dis* 2005;64:44–51.
34. Haberhauer G, Feyertag J, Dunky A. Clinical aspects of combined cyclosporin a and leflunomide therapy in rheumatoid arthritis. *J Clin Rheumatol* 2002;8:362–363.
35. Kiely PD, Johnson DM. Infliximab and leflunomide combination therapy in rheumatoid arthritis: An open-label study. *Rheumatology* 2002;41:631–637.
36. Hansen KE, Cush J, Singhal A, et al. The safety and efficacy of leflunomide in combination with infliximab in rheumatoid arthritis. *Arthritis Rheum* 2004;51:228–232.
37. Godinho F, Godfrin B, El Mahou S, et al. Safety of leflunomide plus infliximab combination therapy in rheumatoid arthritis. *Clin Exp Rheumatol* 2004;22:328–330.
38. Ortiz García AM, González-Alvaro I, Roselló Pardo R, et al. for the Infliximab and Leflunomide Study Group. Effectiveness and safety of infliximab combined with leflunomide in chronic polyarthritis. *Clin Exp Rheumatol* 2004;22:790.
39. Flendrie M, Creemers MC, Welsing PM, et al. The influence of previous and concomitant leflunomide on the efficacy and safety of infliximab therapy in patients with rheumatoid arthritis; a longitudinal observational study. *Rheumatology* 2005;44:472–478.
40. Cobo Ibáñez T, Yehia Tayel M, Balsa Criado A, et al. Safety and efficacy of leflunomide and infliximab versus methotrexate and infliximab combination therapy in rheumatoid arthritis. *Rheumatology* 2005;44:1467–1468.
41. Nordström DC, Konttinen L, Korpela M, et al. Classic disease modifying anti-rheumatic drugs (DMARDs) in combination with infliximab: The Finnish experience. *Rheumatol Int* 2006;26:741–748.
42. Perdriger A, Mariette X, Kuntz JL, et al. Safety of infliximab used in combination with leflunomide or azathioprine in daily clinical practice. *J Rheumatol* 2006;33:865–869.
43. Weaver AL, Lautzenheiser RL, Schiff MH, et al. for the RADIUS Investigators. Real-world effectiveness of select biologic and DMARD monotherapy and combination therapy in the treatment of rheumatoid arthritis: Results from the RADIUS observational registry. *Curr Med Res Opin* 2006;22:185–198.
44. Choy EH, Smith C, Doré CJ, et al. A meta-analysis of the efficacy and toxicity of combining disease-modifying anti-rheumatic drugs in rheumatoid arthritis based on patient withdrawal. *Rheumatology* 2005;44:1414–1421.
45. Grijalva CG, Chung CP, Arbogast PG, et al. Assessment of adherence to and persistence on disease-modifying antirheumatic drugs (DMARDs) in patients with rheumatoid arthritis. *Med Care* 2007;45(10/2):S66–S76.

46. Wolfe F, Michaud K, Stephenson B, et al. Toward a definition and method of assessment of treatment failure and treatment effectiveness: The case of leflunomide versus methotrexate. *J Rheumatol* 2003;30:1725–1732.
47. Aletaha D, Stamm T, Kapral T, et al. Survival and effectiveness of leflunomide compared with methotrexate and sulfasalazine in rheumatoid arthritis: A matched observational study. *Ann Rheum Dis* 2003;62:944–951.
48. Bettembourg-Brault I, Gossec L, Pham T, et al. Leflunomide in rheumatoid arthritis in daily practice: Treatment discontinuation rates in comparison with other DMARDs. *Clin Exp Rheumatol* 2006;24:168–171.
49. van Roon EN, Hoekstra M, Tobi H, et al. Leflunomide in the treatment of rheumatoid arthritis: An analysis of predictors for treatment continuation. *Br J Clin Pharmacol* 2005;60:319–325.
50. Kaltwasser JP, Nash P, Gladman D, et al. for the Treatment of Psoriatic Arthritis Study Group. Efficacy and safety of leflunomide in the treatment of psoriatic arthritis and psoriasis: A multinational, double-blind, randomized, placebo-controlled clinical trial. *Arthritis Rheum* 2004;50:1939–1950.
51. Silverman E, Spiegel L, Hawkins D, et al. Long-term open-label preliminary study of the safety and efficacy of leflunomide in patients with polyarticular-course juvenile rheumatoid arthritis. *Arthritis Rheum* 2005;52:554–562.
52. Silverman E, Mouy R, Spiegel L, et al. for the Leflunomide in Juvenile Rheumatoid Arthritis (JRA) Investigator Group. Leflunomide or methotrexate for juvenile rheumatoid arthritis. *N Engl J Med* 2005;352:1655–1666.
53. Maetzel A, Strand V, Tugwell P, et al. Economic comparison of leflunomide and methotrexate in patients with rheumatoid arthritis: An evaluation based on a 1-year randomised controlled trial. *Pharmacoeconomics* 2002;20:61–70.
54. Maetzel A, Strand V, Tugwell P, et al. Cost effectiveness of adding leflunomide to a 5-year strategy of conventional disease-modifying antirheumatic drugs in patients with rheumatoid arthritis. *Arthritis Rheum* 2002;47:655–661.
55. Schädlich PK, Zeidler H, Zink A, et al. Modelling cost effectiveness and cost utility of sequential DMARD therapy including leflunomide for rheumatoid arthritis in Germany: II. The contribution of leflunomide to efficiency. *Pharmacoeconomics* 2005;23:395–420.
56. Maddison P, Kiely P, Kirkham B, et al. Leflunomide in rheumatoid arthritis: Recommendations through a process of consensus. *Rheumatology* 2005;44:280–286.
57. Cannon GW, Holden WL, Juhaeri J, et al. Adverse events with disease modifying antirheumatic drugs (DMARD): A cohort study of leflunomide compared with other DMARD. *J Rheumatol* 2004;31:1906–1911.
58. Sevilla-Mantilla C, Ortega L, Agúndez JA, et al. Leflunomide-induced acute hepatitis. *Dig Liver Dis* 2004;36:82–84.
59. Weinblatt ME, Dixon JA, Falchuk KR. Serious liver disease in a patient receiving methotrexate and leflunomide. *Arthritis Rheum* 2000;43:2609–2611.
60. van Roon EN, Jansen TL, Houtman NM, et al. Leflunomide for the treatment of rheumatoid arthritis in clinical practice: incidence and severity of hepatotoxicity. *Drug Saf* 2004;27:345–352.
61. Suissa S, Ernst P, Hudson M, et al. Newer disease-modifying antirheumatic drugs and the risk of serious hepatic adverse events in patients with rheumatoid arthritis. *Am J Med* 2004;117:87–92.
62. Takeishi M, Akiyama Y, Akiba H, et al. Leflunomide induced acute interstitial pneumonia. *J Rheumatol* 2005;32:1160–1163.
63. Scott DL. Interstitial lung disease and disease modifying antirheumatic drugs. *Lancet* 2004;363:1239–1240.
64. Suissa S, Hudson M, Ernst P. Leflunomide use and the risk of interstitial lung disease in rheumatoid arthritis. *Arthritis Rheum* 2006;54:1435–1439.
65. Ju JH, Kim SI, Lee JH, et al. Risk of interstitial lung disease associated with leflunomide treatment in Korean patients with rheumatoid arthritis. *Arthritis Rheum* 2007;56:2094–2096.
66. Jenks KA, Stamp LK, O'Donnell JL, et al. Leflunomide-associated infections in rheumatoid arthritis. *J Rheumatol* 2007;34:2201–2203.
67. Coblyn JS, Shadick N, Helfgott S. Leflunomide-associated weight loss in rheumatoid arthritis. *Arthritis Rheum* 2001;44:1048–1051.
68. Chakravarty K, McDonald H, Pullar T, et al. BSR & BHPR guideline for disease-modifying anti-rheumatic drug (DMARD) therapy in consultation with the British Association of Dermatologists. *Rheumatology* 2008;47:924–925.
69. Chakravarty EF, Sanchez-Yamamoto D, Bush TM. The use of disease modifying antirheumatic drugs in women with rheumatoid arthritis of childbearing age: A survey of practice patterns and pregnancy outcomes. *J Rheumatol* 2003;30:241–246.
70. De Santis M, Straface G, Cavaliere A, et al. Paternal and maternal exposure to leflunomide: Pregnancy and neonatal outcome. *Ann Rheum Dis* 2005;64:1096–1097.
71. Neville CE, McNally J. Maternal exposure to leflunomide associated with blindness and cerebral palsy. *Rheumatology* 2007;46:1506.
72. Temprano KK, Bandlamudi R, Moore TL. Antirheumatic drugs in pregnancy and lactation. *Semin Arthritis Rheum* 2005;35:112–121.
73. Rozman B. Clinical pharmacokinetics of leflunomide. *Clin Pharmacokinet* 2002;41:421–430.

Other Traditional Disease-Modifying Antirheumatic Drugs: Monotherapy and Combination Therapy

CHAPTER 10E

Kevin D. Deane and Sterling G. West

In the past decade, the widespread use of methotrexate (MTX) and biologic therapies have revolutionized the management of rheumatoid arthritis (RA). However, not all patients can tolerate MTX or attain disease remission on it alone—and many patients are not appropriate candidates for biologic therapy. In addition, there is good evidence that other traditional disease-modifying antirheumatic drugs (DMARDs)—alone or in combination therapy—are effective in the management of RA.[1] As such, this chapter reviews the use of the DMARDs hydroxychloroquine (HCQ), chloroquine (CLQ), sulfasalazine (SSZ), tetracycline-derivatives, gold, d-penicillamine (DPA), azathioprine (AZA), and cyclosporine (CS) used alone and in combination with other nonbiologic DMARDs (including MTX) for the treatment of RA.

Antimalarials

Antimalarial DMARDs are derived from the compounds quinine and cinchonine, originally isolated from the bark of the Peruvian cinchona tree. The antimalarials most commonly used in RA today include HCQ and CLQ. An additional agent (quinacrine) is now only available through compounding pharmacies, and it will not be discussed here further.

The antimalarials are manufactured with the active drug (called the base) bound to sulfate for HCQ or phosphate for CLQ. The doses for these agents are based on the amount of active drug taken and ideal body weight. For HCQ, the recommended daily dose is less than 6.5 mg of base/kg/day, and for CLQ is less than 3 mg of base/kg/day based on ideal body weight. To avoid toxicity (see material following), prolonged use of these agents for RA in higher doses is not recommended. HCQ sulfate is manufactured as 200-mg tablets, with 155 mg of active drug (HCQ base) in each tablet. For RA, in most published studies and in clinical practice HCQ sulfate is dosed between 200 and 400 mg daily (equaling 155 to 310 mg of active drug per day)—which for many individuals may be under the recommended daily dose. CLQ phosphate is manufactured in 250- and 500-mg tablets. The 250-mg tablet contains 150 mg of CLQ base, and the 500-mg tablet contains 300 mg of CLQ base. For example, a 100-kg person with normal renal function could receive 3 mg/kg/day of CLQ base (or 300 mg), which would be supplied in the 500-mg CLQ phosphate tablet. HCQ and CLQ tablets can be cut in half if necessary for dosing. HCQ and CLQ have long half-lives and can take up to 3 to 4 months to reach steady-state concentrations in the blood. They can be dosed once daily, although they are often dosed twice daily to minimize gastrointestinal (GI) side effects. HCQ and CLQ are primarily cleared renally, with some clearance through the liver. As such, some recommend reducing the dose of HCQ and CLQ by 50% in renal or hepatic impairment. However, because of the risk for toxic accumulation the safest recommendation may be to avoid antimalarial use in patients with renal and/or hepatic impairment. Several drug interactions can occur with antimalarials: smoking increases and cimetidine decreases the clearance of HCQ and CLQ. In addition, antimalarials may interfere with the action of anticonvulsants and amiodarone—and may increase levels of cyclosporine.

Antimalarials modulate multiple aspects of the immune response, although the exact mechanism of their action in RA is unknown. They interfere with intracellular pathways and enzymes, possibly by increasing lysosymal and intracellular pH. This can lead to decreased prostaglandin production and inhibition of the NFκB pathway, resulting in altered cytokine production (including decreased TNFα, IL-1β, and IL-6).[2] Antimalarials also interfere with toll-like receptor (TLR) signaling, reducing inflammatory and cell proliferation responses to multiple exogenous antigens.[3]

Although no head-to-head trials have been performed, HCQ and CLQ are largely thought to be equivalent in treating RA. However, a meta-analysis suggests that CLQ may be slightly more effective.[4] In two randomized placebo-controlled trials involving approximately 240 patients, HCQ as a single treatment has been shown to improve physical functioning and reduce symptoms of RA—including pain, joint swelling, tenderness, and pain—in up to 80% of treated patients.[5,6] Open-label studies have shown that antimalarials can reduce attack frequency and delay progression to RA in patients with palindromic rheumatism.[7] For RA, most patients demonstrate response within 3 to 6 months of initiating antimalarial therapy—although it may take up to 1 year for maximal clinical response.[8] A loading dose of HCQ at 1,200 mg daily for 6 weeks has been shown to shorten the time to clinical response, although this approach was associated with increased GI side effects.[9]

In general, the antimalarials are well tolerated. GI side effects occur in up to 10% of patients and include nausea, abdominal pain, cramping, bloating, and diarrhea. If symptoms do not resolve with continued therapy or twice-daily dosing, for HCQ a trial of brand-name therapy is resonable if the patient is taking a generic prescription. Headaches and light-headedness are also seen in early therapy, but usually resolve. Erythematous maculopapular rashes can occur in up to 5% of patients, usually within the first weeks of therapy. However, these usually resolve with continued therapy. With long-term use, patients may develop hyperpigmented skin in sun-exposed areas—which can appear as blue-gray discoloration and is likely irreversible. There have been case reports of neuropathy, myopathy, and cardiomyopathy—including heart failure and conduction abnormalities—in patients taking CLQ and HCQ, especially in patients with reduced renal and/or hepatic function.[10] In cases of cardiac or skeletal muscle myopathy, biopsy can show a characteristic vacuolar lesion with curvilinear deposits in the myocytes. Rarely, hematologic abnormalities (including cytopenias) have been reported and can be screened for by a complete blood count (CBC) after 1 to 2 months of therapy (then one to two times yearly).[11]

Ocular effects of antimalarials can include double vision, usually within a few weeks of starting therapy (which is thought due to transient effects of the antimalarials on the neuromuscular apparatus of eye movement). Antimalarials can also be deposited in the cornea, leading to visual changes described by patients as "haloes" around lights. Retinal damage is the most serious ocular toxicity and is caused by antimalarial binding to the melanin of the retina, which leads to damage to the rods and cones and visual loss.

Ophthalmologic examinations are important in patients on antimalarial therapy because early eye toxicity can be unnoticed by patients. Early retinal damage can be detected with color vision and visual field testing, or on dilated funduscopic examination (which can identify macular edema and increased retinal pigmentation). Later changes on retinal examination include central macular depigmentation with surrounding hyperpigmentation, resulting in a "bull's-eye" appearance.

However, although feared, ocular toxicity with antimalarial use is rare (<1%–2%)—especially with the use of ideal body-weight-based guidelines for dosing of these agents and dose reduction or avoidance in individuals with renal or hepatic impariment.[12] As a result, screening recommendations are somewhat controversial. The guidelines for ocular screening of patients on antimalarials from the American Academy of Ophthalmology are presented in Table 10E-1, although these are not universally recognized. In the United Kingdom, the Royal College of Ophthalmologists recommends less-frequent screening.[13] Whatever screening process is used, patients should also be instructed to seek care if visual changes develop—especially if they have loss of red vision, which can be an early symptom of antimalarial retinal toxicity. In

Table 10E-1. American Academy of Ophthalmology's Recommendations for Screening for Retinopathy of Antimalarial Therapy

1. All patients on antimalarial therapy should undergo baseline ocular exam, including visual acuity, visual field testing (Amsler grid or Humphries visual fields), and funduscopic retinal exam.
2. If baseline exam is normal, within the first 5 years of therapy patients on hydroxychloroquine (HCQ) <6.5 mg base/kg/day and chloroquine (CLQ) <3 mg base/kg/day and no renal insufficiency should have:
(A) One repeat exam if under the age of 40 (during year 2–3 of therapy)
(B) Two repeat exams if between the ages of 40 and 65 (every 2 years)
3. If patients meet any of the following criteria, repeat eye examinations should be performed every 1 to 2 years:
(A) Age >65 years
(B) Duration of continuous antimalarial therapy >5 years
(C) Renal or hepatic insufficiency
(D) Doses of HCQ >6.5 mg base/kg/day or CLQ >3 mg base/kg/day

From Marmor MF, Carr RE, Easterbrook M, et al. Recommendations on screening for chloroquine and hydroxychloroquine retinopathy: A report by the American Academy of Ophthalmology. *Ophthalmology* 2002;109(7):1377–1382.

addition, patients can be given an Amsler grid for home use to periodically check their visual fields. If symptoms develop or changes are detected on examination, the antimalarial should be stopped immediately because cessation during early retinal changes may result in resolution of damage. However, if symptoms of vision loss develop and there are macular pigmentary changes damage may be irreversible.

In sum, antimalarials as single-agent therapy are useful for symptomatic improvement in mild RA and to reduce attack frequency and delay progression to RA in patients with palindromic rheumatism. However, in more severe disease antimalarials are best used as part of a combination of DMARDs. The antimalarials are well tolerated, and toxicity leading to cessation of antimalarials is infrequent in published studies. However, due to inefficacy less than 50% of patients remain on the drug at 5 years.[14] Further use of antimalarials in combination therapy is discussed in material following.

Sulfasalazine

SSZ is a conjugate of 5-aminosalicylic acid (5-ASA) and sulfapyridine (SP). The drug is absorbed in the small intestine as intact SSZ and then undergoes enterohepatic circulation, delivering SSZ to the large intestine (where it is cleaved by the action of gut flora into 5-ASA and SP). At this stage, SP is absorbed—whereas 5-ASA for the most part stays in the lumen of the large intestine.[15] The SP moiety is metabolized in the liver by hydroxylation and acetylation. There are genetic differences in the rates of acetylation, and individuals that are "slow acetylators" may have greater toxicity.

SSZ is manufactured in 500-mg tablets, and treatment is typically started at 500 mg daily (with increases by 500 mg every week with interval assessment of toxicity until the goal dose is reached, which is typically between 2000 and 3000 mg daily or 40 mg/kg/day).[16] Divided doses or an enteric-coated form of SSZ can be used to reduce GI side effects. SSZ may decrease digoxin and cyclosporine levels and increase the effect of warfarin. In theory, through inhibition of folate metabolism SSZ can potentiate the cytopenic effects of MTX. However, this adverse effect has not been seen to a significant degree in research trials or in clinical use. The use of SSZ should be avoided in patients with a history of allergy to sulfa-containing products.

There are three forms of SSZ that may act in RA: SSZ as the parent compound, and SP and 5-ASA as individual compounds. It is unclear which of these leads to benefit in RA, although it is assumed that as the 5-ASA moiety is largely unabsorbed it plays a small role.[17] SSZ (but not SP or 5-ASA) acts as a folate antagonist and may have antimetabolite effects similar to those of MTX. Intact SSZ also inhibits the binding of TNF to its membrane-bound receptor, and decreases the production of IgA and rheumatoid factor IgM.[18] SSZ and 5-ASA may decrease prostaglandin synthesis.

Two meta-analyses have evaluated the efficacy of SSZ as a single DMARD therapy in RA.[19,20] Doses ranged from 2 to 3 g of SSZ daily, and statistically significant improvements in tender and swollen joints, pain, and inflammatory markers were reported—usually by week 12 of therapy. These analyses have concluded that SSZ offered symptomatic and inflammatory benefit in RA when compared to placebo or HCQ, but its effect on the progression of radiographic erosions was unclear. However, two additional randomized studies have shown that SSZ can slow the progression of erosive disease when compared to placebo- or HCQ-treated patients.[21,22] How SSZ as monotherapy compares to MTX is debated. A randomized trial of 105 patients showed that SSZ appeared equivalent to MTX monotherapy, but the dose of MTX was lower (7.5 to 15 mg/week) than is often used clinically.[23] An additional study in 205 patients also found that clinical and radiographic responses were equivalent in SSZ- versus MTX-treated patients.[24] A meta-analysis has concluded that SSZ and MTX are equally efficacious in the treatment of RA. However, this conclusion is hampered by lower-than-maximal doses of MTX used in most studies.[4] Finally, in a phase II study comparing leflunomide (100 mg for 3 days, then 20 mg daily) to monotherapy with SSZ (2 g daily) or placebo, leflunomide and SSZ were equivalent to each other and both were superior to placebo in terms of improved joint counts ($p = 0.0001$) and radiographic progression of disease ($p < 0.01$).[22]

Nausea, vomiting, headache, nonautoimmune hemolytic anemia likely due to glucose-6-phosphate dehydrogenase (G6PD) deficiency, and methemoglobinemia can occur in patients taking high doses (>4 g daily) or with lower doses in patients who are slow acetylators. These side effects generally improve with brief cessation of SSZ and reintroduction at a lower dose. More severe reactions to SSZ, likely due to hypersensitivity/allergic responses, can occur and include rashes (which can progress to Stevens-Johnson syndrome), fever, hepatitis, pneumonitis, and aplastic anemia. A triad of these (including fever, rash, and hepatitis) has been reported, and patients should be made aware of these possible issues. Leucopenia occurs in 1% to 2% of patients treated with SSZ, and can be worsened by concomitant administration with etanercept. Most cases of leucopenia are mild and transient. However, severe granulocytopenia related to hypersensitivity can also occur and be life threatening. Most cases of this occur within the first 3 months of therapy, although some cases have been reported after several years of therapy. If idiosyncratic hypersensitivity/allergic reactions are suspected, SSZ should be stopped and not reintroduced. In general, SSZ should be avoided in patients with a history of allergy to sulfa-containing products. However, if a patient has a history of an isolated skin reaction to another sulfonamide there is a desensitization protocol available for the use of SSZ. If this approach is deemed necessary, it should be done cautiously—with assistance from an allergist.[25] Finally, male patients should be warned that SSZ can cause reversible azospermia.

Recommendations for monitoring SSZ vary, but most suggest that a CBC and liver-associated enzymes should be evaluated at baseline and every 1 to 2 weeks during the first 1 to 3 months of therapy—then every 2 to 4 weeks during the second 3 months of therapy, and then every 3 months once patients are on a stable dose. Testing for rates of acetylation is not currently recommended.

In sum, as a single agent SSZ is likely superior in reducing symptoms and inflammation of RA when compared to placebo and HCQ—and it may be equivalent to MTX and leflunomide. In addition, SSZ may be effective in slowing the rate of erosion development. As such, SSZ may be considered for use as monotherapy in mild to moderate RA or in cases where other agents are contraindicated. From pooled data, approximately 20% to 30% of patients are still on SSZ at 5 years—with most discontinuing SSZ due to side effects. Combination therapy with SSZ is discussed in the material that follows.

Tetracyclines

Tetracyclines are derivatives from *Streptomyces* species and include tetracycline, doxycycline, and minocycline. Minocyline and doxycycline are second-generation semisynthetic derivatives of tetracycline and are the best studied of these agents in RA.

Minocycline is manufactured by several companies and comes in 50-, 75-, and 100-mg tablets. In most RA trials, it has been dosed at 100 mg twice daily. Doxycycline is manufactured in multiple-dose and pill formats, but is commonly used in adults as 100-mg tablets/capsules (a 20-mg tablet is available for use in the treatment of gingivitis).

Tetracyclines have several potential mechanisms by which they can improve RA, including decreased synthesis of prostaglandins and decreased mononuclear cell phagocytosis and chemotaxis. In addition, tetracylclines decrease cellular production of matrix metalloproteinases (MMPs) and collagenase—purportedly leading to decreased joint destruction in RA.[26]

Minocycline has been shown to be effective in improving the symptoms of RA in several randomized controlled trials, although the greatest benefit was seen when used in early disease.[27] A meta-analysis on tetracycline use in RA evaluated 10 studies involving more than 500 patients, but found only three of these studies to be high-quality based on randomization, outcome measures, and analysis.[28] In this review, patients treated with minocycline or other tetracycline derivatives for ≥3 months in randomized controlled trials had statistically improved joint swelling and tenderness, pain, functional capacity, and inflammatory markers when compared to patients treated with placebo. Minocycline appeared to be superior to the other tetracyclines in controlling symptoms. In an additional study, when compared to HCQ minocycline was associated with a greater reduction in corticosteroid use and improved American College of Rheumatology-50 (ACR50) responses (60% versus 33% at 2 years, $p = 0.04$). Minocycline has not, however, been associated with decreased erosions—although the ability to detect this in published studies has been limited.[29]

In two clinical trials comparing minocycline to placebo in RA patients, adverse effects have included photosensitive rash (5%), headaches (2%–20%), dizziness (8%–40%), and GI side effects [including anorexia, nausea, and vomiting (24%–58%)]. However, discontinuation rates because of these effects have been relatively low (6% and 12.5%, respectively).[30,31] Additional rare adverse effects include antineutrophil cytoplasmic antibody (ANCA) positive vasculitis, serum sickness, systemic lupus erythematosus (SLE)–like disease with arthralgias and arthritis, pseudotumor cerebri, tooth deposition, skin rashes or hyperpigmentation, and hepatic injury. If dizziness or GI side effects occur, the dose of minocycline can be lowered to 50 mg once or twice daily and slowly increased as tolerated. However, in cases of severe reactions (including SLE or vasculitic reactions) the drug should be discontinued and not restarted.

In sum, tetracycline derivates used as single agents in the management of mild RA may result in symptomatic benefit and reduction in inflammatory markers. However, more data are needed to understand their role in the management/prevention of erosive RA. Combination therapy with tetracycline derivatives is discussed in material following.

Gold Salts

Prior to 1990, parenteral gold was the "gold" standard for RA therapy.[32] There are two parenteral gold preparations, each containing 50% gold in solution. Although not universally available, both come in multidose bottles (with 50 mg/ml concentration). Gold sodium thiomalate (GSTM) is water soluble and is rapidly absorbed after intramuscular administration, whereas gold sodium thioglucose (aurothioglucose, GSTG) is in a suspension of sesame seed oil and is more slowly absorbed. Auranofin is a gold compound formulated to be absorbed orally. Due to its poor efficacy, it is rarely used and will not be discussed.[4]

The once-weekly dosing schedule for parenteral gold starts with a test dose of 10 mg administered intramuscularly (IM) on week 1. If this is well tolerated, the next dose is 25 mg IM on week 2. In the absence of side effects, subsequent weekly doses are 50 mg a week. After 20 weekly injections (total cumulative dose $\approx$1000 mg), a clinical response should be observed. A patient who has failed to respond should have gold therapy discontinued. Patients who have responded ($\geq$ACR 20) may gain further improvement over the next several months of continued weekly injections. Once a patient has achieved optimal control, the frequency of injections can be decreased to every 2 weeks. If disease control is maintained on every 2-week therapy for 6 months, an attempt to decrease the injection frequency to every 3 (and eventually every 4) weeks can be considered—although there is a risk of loss of efficacy as the dosing interval is increased.

The mechanism of action responsible for the therapeutic benefit of gold is unknown but postulated to be its effect on macrophages and cytokine release in the rheumatoid synovium. There have been four randomized controlled trials of at least 6 months in duration totaling 415 patients that showed a significant benefit for injectable gold compared to placebo in the treatment of RA.[33] Injectable gold has been shown to be equipotent to MTX but not as well tolerated.[34] Several studies have shown that parenteral gold can retard radiographic progression more than placebo and at least a well as MTX.[35,36] However, another longer-term (5-year) observational study suggested that chrysotherapy may not significantly affect the natural course of RA.[37] In patients who fail to respond maximally to gold monotherapy, combinations with other DMARDs have been studied. A study adding hydroxychloroquine to patients with an insufficient response to gold showed no increased benefit.[38] Alternatively, a controlled trial demonstrated that adding weekly gold to the therapy of RA patients who were partial responders to MTX was beneficial.[39] Finally, the addition of cyclosporine to gold therapy showed benefit without increased toxicity at 6 months.[40]

A major drawback to gold therapy is the potential to cause adverse reactions in 30% to 40% of patients. Most toxicity occurs early ($<$ 1 year) in therapy and may be preceded by the development of eosinophilia (10%–20%). The most common side effects include mucocutaneous reactions [pruritus (30%–40%), stomatitis/dermatitis (10%)], membranous glomerulonephritis with proteinuria (1%–3%), and thrombocytopenia (1%)—which occurs most frequently in HLA–DR3-positive individuals. Post-injection reactions occur most commonly with GSTM and include post-injection arthralgias (10%–15%) and vasomotor nitritoid reactions (4%). Patients on angiotensin-converting enzyme inhibitors are more prone to develop vasomotor symptoms. Hypotension causing stroke and myocardial infarction has occurred in patients with underlying cardiovascular disease. Other rare but serious side effects include aplastic anemia, diffuse pulmonary infiltrates, enterocolitis, myokima, and cholestatic jaundice—among others.

Due to potential toxicity, treatment monitoring is crucial. Prior to an injection, patients should be asked about problems with rash, pruritus, or stomatitis. Gold injections should be held in any patient experiencing one of these symptoms. After symptoms have resolved, gold therapy can be restarted at 10 mg/week and slowly increased. Patients who experience a nitritoid reaction or post-injection flare on GSTM can often be switched to GSTG without recurrence. A CBC with platelets and a urinalysis should be done weekly the first month, and then every 2 weeks thereafter. If injections are decreased to every 3 to 4 weeks, monitoring can be done prior to each injection. Gold therapy should be held and not restarted in any patient who develops thrombocytopenia, aplastic anemia, proteinuria ($>$ 500 mg/day), or any severe side effect. Patients with mild mucocutaneous reactions and lesser degrees of proteinuria may benefit from a reduction in dose by 50%. Notably, lower doses of gold ($\leq\leq$ 25 mg/week) can result in clinical improvement when toxicity prevents use of higher doses.[41]

The sum of evidence indicates that parenteral gold is an effective therapy for RA. Overall, about 33% of RA patients will respond to gold, 33% will not respond, and 33% will develop side effects within the first year. Due to side effects or loss of efficacy, the median duration of gold therapy is less than 2 years.[42] Indeed, overall only 10% to 25% of treated RA patients remain on gold after 5 years—with 60% of these patients stopping due to side effects.[43–45] Consequently, MTX alone and in combination with other DMARDs and/or biologics has largely replaced chrysotherapy. Yet there are still RA patients who can benefit from gold therapy, including those with liver disease (alcoholic, hepatitis B), high infection risk, or intolerance to, inefficacy of, or poor access to other therapies.

D-Penicillamine

DPA is an analog of the sulfhydryl amino acid cysteine. It can be obtained by acid hydrolysis of the penicillin molecule. It is available as a 250-mg capsule. Due to potential toxicity, the mantra for dosing is "go low, go slow." It is recommended that treatment be initiated at 250 mg/day on an empty stomach. The dose can be increased by 125 to 250 mg/day every 1 to 3 months to a maximum of 1000 mg/day. The typical RA patient requires 500 to 750 mg/day for at least 3 months for improvement to occur.

DPA is neither anti-inflammatory nor immunosuppressive, and thus the exact mechanism of action in RA is unclear. Six short-term (< 6 months) randomized controlled trials involving 683 patients showed a significant benefit for DPA compared to placebo in the treatment of RA.[46] It is comparable in efficacy to parenteral gold and azathioprine, but with more toxicity.[46] There is little if any evidence that DPA slows radiographic progression or long-term disability.[35,47]

A major factor limiting DPA therapy is its potential toxicities.[48] Patients with a penicillin allergy are not more prone to develop adverse effects. The most common side effects include pruritus, rash, and stomatitis—which typically resolve with antihistamines or with stopping DPA (with reinstitution at a lower dose once symptoms resolve). Drug fever, loss of taste, nausea, and anorexia can also be seen early in therapy. Hematologic side effects include leukopenia, immune thrombocytopenia, and rarely aplastic anemia. DPA can also cause a variety of autoimmune syndromes, including membranous nephritis, Goodpasture's syndrome, bullous pemphigus, drug-induced lupus, myasthenia gravis, and polymyositis. Some of these may not resolve with discontinuation of the drug.

Due to its toxicity profile, DPA therapy must be closely monitored. Patients who experience rashes or oral ulcers should stop the drug. Once symptoms resolve, DPA can be reinstituted at a lower dose and the dose increased at a slower pace. A CBC (including platelets) and a urinalysis should be done every 2 weeks for the first 6 months. Once a stable dose is achieved, monitoring can be done monthly. DPA should be stopped indefinitely in patients who develop cytopenias, proteinuria (> 500 mg/day), or an autoimmune syndrome.

With more effective therapies available, DPA is rarely used. Due to toxicities or lack of efficacy, the median duration of DPA therapy is less than 2 years.[42] At least 20% to 30% of patients develop side effects during the first 6 months of therapy. Overall, less than 25% of RA patients treated with DPA are still on the drug 5 years later due to side effects or loss of efficacy.[43] However, some RA patients (particularly those with extraarticular manifestations such as vasculitis, severe nodulosis, Felty's syndrome, or rheumatoid lung disease) may benefit from DPA therapy if other therapies are ineffective or contraindicated.

Azathioprine

AZA is a purine analog that is rapidly converted into the active antimetabolite, 6-mercaptopurine. It is produced as a 75- and 100-mg tablet. RA patients are typically started at 50 mg/day, and the dose increased by 25 to 50 mg/day every 1 to 2 weeks to a maximum of 2.5 mg/kg/day.

Azathioprine's mechanism of action is through immunosuppression. It is converted to 6-mercaptopurine, which is then metabolized to thiopurine metabolites such as thioguanine nucleotides. These metabolites decrease the *de novo* synthesis of purine nucleotides and are incorporated into cellular DNA, leading to suppression of cellular proliferation and/or death. The onset of azathioprine's immunomodulatory effect is slow, and thus maximum clinical efficacy can take several months.

There have been three controlled trials involving 81 patients showing short-term efficacy for AZA compared to placebo for the treatment of RA.[49] Long-term follow-up studies have confirmed continued clinical benefits.[50,51] Radiographic studies have given inconsistent results on AZA's ability to retard progression. Comparison studies show that it is equipotent to parenteral gold, similarly or less potent than MTX, and less able to stop erosions than both of them.[52,53] Coadministration of AZA with MTX was no better than MTX alone.[54]

Up to 30% of patients discontinue AZA due to adverse side effects.[55] The most common toxicity is nausea, vomiting, and diarrhea. Patients experiencing these symptoms may gain relief by switching to 6-mercaptopurine. Myelosuppression is common and dose dependent. However, a subset of patients will experience severe neutroponia on low doses. This occurs in patients with low or absent thiopurine methyltransferase (TPMT) activity due to the inability to detoxify 6–mercaptopurine, resulting in increased formation of cytotoxic thioguanine metabolites.[56] In addition, there are several important drug interactions that can increase the risk of myelosuppression—including allopurinol, sulfasalazine, or trimethoprim-sulfamethoxazole. These medications should be avoided, or the dose of azathioprine reduced. AZA can also cause warfarin resistance in selected patients.[57] Other side effects include elevated liver enzymes (5%–10%), pancreatitis, and infections. Viral infections such as Herpes zoster can occur at any time, whereas bacterial infections occur more commonly in patients with neutropenia. Rarely an acute hypersensitivity syndrome occurs within the first 2 weeks, manifested by fever, rash, hepatitis, and renal failure.[58] Finally, the carcinogenic risk of AZA is debated. Although the risk of lymphoproliferative malignancy is clearly increased (50×) in renal transplant patients treated with AZA, some studies have found an increased risk in RA patients (2–9×) and others have not.[59,60]

Monitoring for AZA toxicity includes weekly CBC and monthly liver-associated enzyme tests until the patient is on a stable dose, at which time the CBC can be monitored less frequently (every 1–3 months). Monitoring can be less frequent in patients who have normal TPMT activity. This activity can be measured directly in red blood cell membranes (phenotype), or the known polymorphisms associated with low activity can be identified by polymerase chain reaction (genotype). Overall, 90% of individuals will have normal activity, 10% intermediate activity, and 0.3% absent activity (homozygous for low-activity polymorphism).[61] African Americans have lower TPMT function than Caucasians. In patients with normal TPMT activity, 6-mercaptopurine metabolites can be measured to ensure that the patient has an effective therapeutic level.

AZA appears to be as efficacious as other DMARDs but with increased toxicity.[49] The median duration a patient remains on AZA is about 2.3 years, with half stopping for inefficacy and half for toxicity.[42,62] AZA is most often used in refractory RA patients who do not improve or develop toxicities to other therapies. Patients with coexistent rheumatoid lung disease may be good candidates for AZA use. AZA can substitute for MTX in RA patients on antitumor necrosis factor therapy.[63]

Cyclosporine

CS, formerly known as cyclosporin(e) A, is a cyclic endecapeptide derived from a fungus. The best formulation is a microemulsion available in 25- and 100-mg capsules. It is variably absorbed by individuals. Grapefruit juice can dramatically increase its absorption and decrease its metabolism by inhibiting CYP3A and should be avoided. The starting dose is 2.5 mg/kg/day based on ideal body weight and given in divided doses (twice a day). The dose can be increased by 0.5 mg/kg/day every 4 to 8 weeks to a maximum dose of 4.0 mg/kg/day depending on response. Of note, the various brands of cyclosporine are not bioequivalent and should not be used interchangeably.

Cyclosporine primarily affects T-cell proliferation by impairing the production of interleukin-2 (IL-2). It binds to cyclophilin, and the complex in turn binds to calcineurin—a serine-threonine phosphatase. This inhibits calcineurin's phosphatase activity, preventing translocation of nuclear factor of activated T cells (NF-AT) from the cytoplasm to the nucleus. NF-AT is required for gene transcription for IL-2 and other cytokines necessary for T-cell activation.

Three controlled clinical trials of up to 1 year in duration totaling 318 patients demonstrated that CS is more effective than placebo in RA treatment.[64] A 2-year study showed that CS treatment is comparable to MTX both clinically and radiographically in early RA patients.[65] Two other studies showed that CS was able to retard radiographic progression.[66,67] However, most rheumatologists use CS in combination with MTX. Three controlled trials have shown that this combination caused greater and/or more rapid improvement in disease activity than MTX or sulfasalazine alone.[68,69] Another controlled study showed improved joint inflammation in RA patients who were randomized to MTX plus CS after an inadequate MTX response compared to MTX plus placebo.[70] An extension of this trial up to 1 year showed no unacceptable increase in toxicity.[71] A recent open-label study showed that CS was more effective when combined with leflunomide compared to either drug alone, without an increase in adverse events.[72]

CS is relatively well tolerated in the short term but can cause significant toxicities. Common minor side effects include nausea, hypertrichosis, gingival hyperplasia, tremor, and paresthesias. Some patients experience significant bone pain requiring dose reduction or discontinuation. Serious side effects, which typically occur within the first few months of therapy, include hypertension (20%) and an increase in serum creatinine. The hypertension and decrease in renal function are reversible with dose reduction. Irreversible nephrotoxicity is most common in patients whose serum creatinine is allowed to rise above 30% of baseline for a prolonged period. Patients on CS for greater than a year are more likely to experience this nephrotoxicity. Due to their short duration and limited number of patients, there is no evidence that CS causes increased malignancies in RA patients. However, in renal transplant recipients CS has been associated with an increased risk of skin cancer and lymphoma. Other possible side effects include hyperkalemia, hyperlipidemia, osteoporosis, and rarely drug-induced thrombotic thrombocytopenia purpura.

Patients who are to be started on CS should have a blood pressure check and CBC, chemistries, creatinine, liver-associated enzymes, uric acid, and magnesium level. The patient's blood pressure and creatinine should be monitored every 2 weeks for the first 3 months, and then monthly once on a stable dose. If the serum creatinine rises more than 30% over baseline, the CS dose should be reduced by 1 mg/kg/day. If the creatinine fails to decrease within 2 weeks, CS should be discontinued until the creatinine falls to within 15% of baseline before restarting CS at a lower dose. Notably, CS does not cause neutropenia or elevated liver-associated enzymes—precluding the need for monitoring these laboratory tests unless the patient is also on MTX. Magnesium, potassium, and lipid levels should be monitored periodically. CS blood levels do not need to be routinely monitored in RA patients.

There are several important drug interactions that can affect CS therapy. Several drugs will increase cyclosporine levels, including erythromycin (not azithromycin), azole antifungals, selected calcium channel blockers (diltiazem, verapamil), amiodarone, and others. CS concentrations can be decreased by inducers of hepatic enzymes such as rifampin, phenytoin, phenobarbitol, and St. John's wort. Nonsteroidal anti-inflammatory drugs, angiotensin-converting enzyme inhibitors, potassium-sparing diuretics, and nephrotoxic antibiotics can increase cyclosporine nephrotoxicity and/or the risk of hyperkalemia. Consequently, the best treatment of CS-induced hypertension is nifedipine or isradapine and/or beta blockers. Statin therapy and colchicine can cause neuromuscular toxicity when combined with cyclosporine.

Although a population-based study showed that 50% of RA patients were still on CS 5 years after initiation, other studies have shown that fewer than 25% were still on CS 3 years after the drug was started.[71,73] This may be due to patient selection. Indeed, many RA patients have comorbidities that preclude the use of cyclosporine. Patients with current malignancies, renal impairment, poorly controlled hypertension, or significant hepatic dysfunction or who are receiving drugs that adversely interact with CS are not good candidates. Patients without these comorbidities who have had an inadequate response to MTX may respond to the addition of CS.[70] However, this combination is best reserved for RA patients who do not respond to or are intolerant to other DMARD combinations or biologics. Other immunophilin-binding drugs (including tacrolimus, sirolimus, and everolimus) have also been used in combination with MTX to successfully treat RA patients, but data are limited.[68]

Combination DMARD Therapy

Double-Combination Therapy

When used in combination with other DMARDs (including MTX), HCQ has been shown in open-label studies to reduce glucocorticoid use in RA patients.[74] Dougadous et al. randomized 205 early RA patients (symptom <1 year and no prior DMARDs) to one of three arms: SSZ alone (2–3 g/day), MTX alone (7.5 mg/week to a maximum of 15 mg/week), or combination with SSZ and MTX. At 1 year, there were statistically significant differences in disease activity score (DAS) improvement for each of these groups—but there were no significant differences between groups in European League Against Rheumatism (EULAR) or ACR response criteria.

Triple Combination Therapy

In the COBRA (Combinatietherapie Bij Reumatoide Artritis) trial, 156 RA DMARD-naive RA patients were randomized to one of two arms.[75] The first arm received an initial 28-week period of step-down therapy with prednisolone (60 mg daily, with decrease every week until at 7.5 mg/day; which was continued until week 28 and then stopped), MTX (7.5 mg for 40 weeks gradually reduced to 0), and SSZ (2 g daily). The second arm received SSZ 2 g daily alone. In both arms, the SSZ was continued for the entire 56 weeks of the original study. The initial trial was published in 1997, with 5-year follow-up data published in 2002.[76] After the first 6 months of the study, all subjects were on SSZ. However, those who developed a flare could be treated with a variety of approaches—including adding DMARD therapy, adding corticosteroids, or reintroducing the original three-drug treatment if they had had it before. At 5 years, after adjusting for treatment differences during the post-treatment follow-up period the initial three-drug therapy arm (prednisolone, MTX, SSZ) had improved clinical symptoms and radiographic findings compared to SSZ-alone arm.[76] These results suggest that aggressive use of multiple agents in early RA is better than monotherapy, although given the multiple agents that were used it is difficult to assess which agent was most effective.

In 1996, O'Dell et al. published the results of a trial involving 102 RA patients with inadequate response to at least one DMARD who were randomized to receive either MTX alone, double therapy with HCQ and SSZ, or triple therapy with MTX (7.5–17.5 mg/week), HCQ (200 mg BID), and SSZ (500 mg BID).[77] After 2 years, 77% of the triple-therapy group versus 40% of double-therapy and 33% of MTX-alone group had 50% improvement in symptoms and physical findings ($p < 0.003$ for three-group comparison). The authors concluded that triple therapy was superior to double or single therapy in this patient population. This same group later published the results of a similar trial investigating the efficacy and tolerability of triple therapy (MTX 7.5–17.5 mg/week, SSZ 2 g/day, and HCQ 400 mg/day) versus double therapy with MTX and SSZ or MTX and HCQ.[78] The triple-therapy group had significantly increased ACR 20 responses at 2 years compared to the double-therapy groups with similar side-effect profiles [78% MTX + HCQ + SSZ versus 60% MTX + HCQ ($p = 0.05$) and 40% MTX + SSZ ($p = 0.05$)].

In the Finnish Rheumatoid Arthritis Combination Therapy Trial (FIN-RACo), 199 RA patients were randomized to receive either triple therapy with MTX (7.5–15 mg/week), SSZ (1–2 g/day), HCQ 300 mg/day, and prednisone (up to 10 mg/day) versus SSZ alone, with the option to switch to MTX and/or add prednisone in the single-therapy group.[79] At 1 year, 75% of the triple-therapy group versus 60% of the monotherapy group met the ACR 50 response criteria ($p = 0.028$).

Finally, the Tight Control for Rheumatoid Arthritis (TICORA) study demonstrated that aggressive use of traditional nonbiologic DMARDs can substantially improve disease activity, radiographic progression, physical function, and quality of life.[80] In this study, 110 patients with RA for less than 5 years were randomized to receive intensive management or routine care. The intensive group patients were seen monthly and DMARD therapy escalated according to a predefined protocol if they failed to reach remission (DAS <2.4) (Figure 10E-1). Swollen joints could be injected with intra-articular corticosteroids. The routine care group were seen every 3 months and therapy adjusted according to the discretion of the treating rheumatologist without the use of a composite disease activity measure. At the 18-month assessment, 65% of the intensively treated group had achieved remission compared to 16% of the routine care group ($p < 0.0001$). Radiographic progression was less in the intensively treated group, and mean HAQ score decreased more in

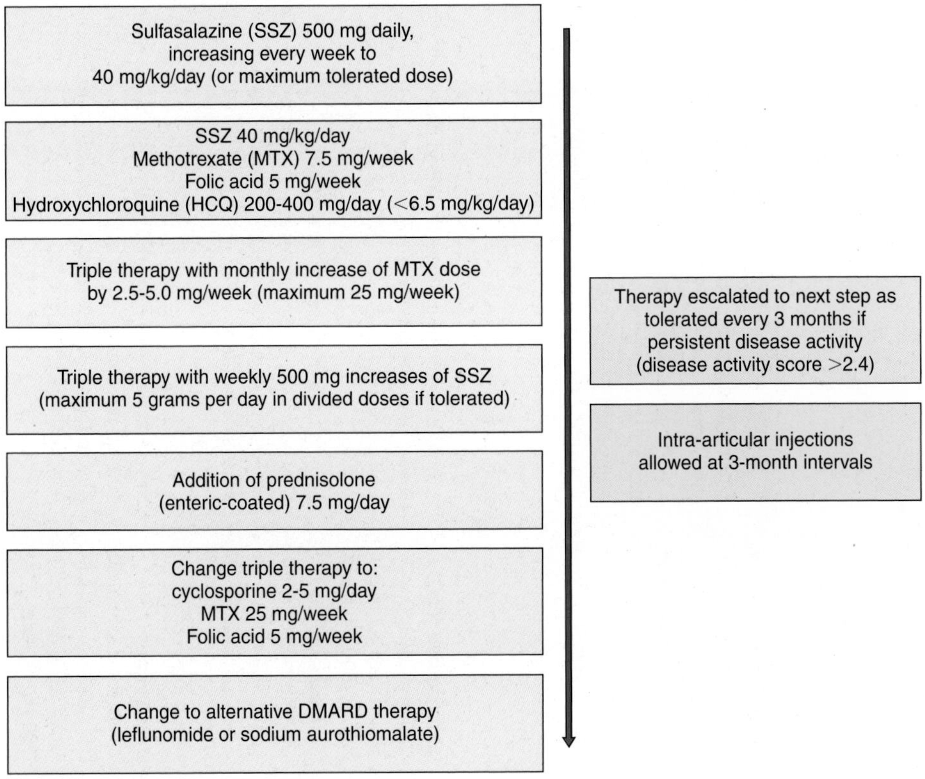

Sulfasalazine (SSZ) 500 mg daily, increasing every week to 40 mg/kg/day (or maximum tolerated dose)

SSZ 40 mg/kg/day
Methotrexate (MTX) 7.5 mg/week
Folic acid 5 mg/week
Hydroxychloroquine (HCQ) 200-400 mg/day (<6.5 mg/kg/day)

Triple therapy with monthly increase of MTX dose by 2.5-5.0 mg/week (maximum 25 mg/week)

Triple therapy with weekly 500 mg increases of SSZ (maximum 5 grams per day in divided doses if tolerated)

Addition of prednisolone (enteric-coated) 7.5 mg/day

Change triple therapy to:
cyclosporine 2-5 mg/day
MTX 25 mg/week
Folic acid 5 mg/week

Change to alternative DMARD therapy (leflunomide or sodium aurothiomalate)

Therapy escalated to next step as tolerated every 3 months if persistent disease activity (disease activity score >2.4)

Intra-articular injections allowed at 3-month intervals

Figure 10E-1. Protocol for escalation of therapy in the TICORA study. (From Grigor C, Capell H, Stirling A, et al. Effect of a treatment strategy of tight control for rheumatoid arthritis (the TICORA study): A single-blind randomised controlled trial. *Lancet* 2004; 364(9430):263–269.)

Table 10E-2. Traditional DMARDs: Dosing, Drug Interactions, Side Effects, and Monitoring

Drug	Dosing and Drug Interactions	Common Adverse Reactions	Rare Adverse Reactions	Recommendations for Monitoring Therapy
Hydroxychloroquine (HCQ) 200-mg tablets (155 mg base)	<6.5 mg of base/kg/day in single or divided doses. May interfere with action of anticonvulsants and amiodarone; decreases absorbtion of ampicillin, and may increase cyclosporine levels.	Nausea, abdominal pain/bloating, diarrhea; rash.	Ocular toxicity; neuromuscular/cardiac toxicity; cytopenias	Baseline ophthalmologic exam; then, if dose <6.5 mg/kg/day and <65 years old repeat evaluation every 2 to 4 years during first 5 years of therapy. After 5 years and if any of the following present, eye exam every 1 to 2 years: chronic kidney disease, hepatic impairment, dose >6.5 mg base/kg/day; CBC within the first month (then every 6 months). Clinical exam for neuromuscular findings and cardiomyopathy periodically.
Chloroquine (CLQ) 250-mg tablets (150 mg base), 500-mg tablets (300 mg base)	<3 mg base/kg/day in single or divided doses. Similar drug interactions as HCQ.	Similar to HCQ	Similar to HCQ	Similar to HCQ
Sulfasalazine (SSZ) 500-mg tablets, enteric-coated available	500 mg daily, increased to 40 mg/kg/day. May potentiate myelosuppression of MTX; may decrease digoxin and cyclosporine levels; may potentiate warfarin.	Nausea, vomiting, headache. Nonhypersensitivity hemolytic anemia in G6PD-deficient patients	Hypersensitivity reactions, including fever, rash, hepatitis, and granulocytopenia	Baseline CBC and liver enzymes; then, every 1 to 2 weeks for 1 to 3 months, and then every 2 to 4 weeks for 3 months, and then every 3 months once on stable dosing
Tetracycines Minocycline (Mino) 50-, 75-, 100-mg capusules Doxycycline (Doxy) 20-, 100-mg capsules	Mino 100 mg twice daily; Doxy 20 mg or 100 mg twice daily. Absorption reduced by calcium-containing products; potentiate warfarin.	Photosensitive rash, headache, anorexia, nausea, dizziness (more common with Mino)	Autoimmune syndromes/ vasculitis (including ANCA-positive); hepatic injury	Baseline liver enzymes, then 1 to 2 times yearly Monitor clinically for signs of skin disease, autoimmune syndromes

Gold 10 cc multiuse vials, 50-mg/ml concentration	IM injection: test dose 10 mg, if tolerated, next dose 25 mg/week. Increase to 50 mg IM weekly x 20 weeks (1,000 mg). If no response, discontinue therapy. May decrease dose and frequency over time. Patients on ACE-I may have increased vaso-motor side effects.	Pruritis, stomatitis/dermatitis, post-injection reactions (including vaso-motor reactions)	Membranoproliferative glomerulonephritis and proteinuria; thrombocytopenia, aplastic anemia; pulmonary injury; cholestasis	Baseline skin/membrane exam, CBC, creatinine, urinalysis (UA). Repeat weekly for first month of therapy, and then every 2 weeks. If injections are decreased in frequency to every 3 to 4 weeks, CBC, creatinine, UA can be done prior to injections.
D-penicillamine (DPA) 250-mg capsules or tablets	Starting dose 250 mg/day; increase as tolerated by 125 to 250 mg every 1 to 3 months to maximum dose 1,000 mg/day.	Pruritis, rash, stomatitis; drug fever, altered taste	Cytopenias; membranous nephritis; Goodpasture's syndrome; bullous pemphigus; drug-induced lupus; myasthenia gravis; polymyositis	Baseline CBC and UA; repeat testing every 1 to 2 weeks during the first 6 months of therapy, and then monthly once dose stable Monitor clinically for signs of skin disease, autoimmune syndromes
Azathioprine 50-, 75-, 100-mg scored tablets. Intravenous form available.	Typically start at 50 mg/day, with 50 mg/day increase every 1 to 2 weeks until maximum 2.5 mg/kg/day. Allopurinol, SSZ, trimethoprim-sulfamethoxazole may increase myelosuppression.	Nausea, vomiting, diarrhea	Cytopenias, hypersensitivity syndrome usually within 1 to 2 weeks of starting therapy (including fever, rash, hepatitis, renal failure)	Baseline CBC and liver enzymes; repeat testing every 2 to 4 weeks until dosing stable; patients with normal TPMT activity may require less-frequent testing Monitor for signs/symptoms of infection
Cyclosporine (CS) 25-, 100-mg capsules. Brand names are not bioequivalent.	Starting dose 2.5 mg/kg/day; increase as tolerated by 0.5 mg/kg/day every 1 to 2 months to a maximum dose 4.0 mg/kg/day. Multiple drug interactions; all medications need careful review. NSAIDs and ACE-I can lead to increased nephroxiticity; erythromycin, diltiazem, verapamil can increase CS levels; colchicine—neuromuscular toxicity.	Renal insufficiency, HTN, anemia; nausea, hypertrichosis, gingival hyperplasia, tremor	Bone pain; electrolyte abnormalities; thrombotic thrombocytopenic purpura	Examination for edema and HTN every 2 weeks until dose stable, then monthly; creatinine every 2 weeks for 3 months or until dose stable, then monthly; if creatinine increase >30% baseline, reduce dose; CBC, liver enzymes, potassium, magnesium, lipid levels periodically Monitor for signs/symptoms of infection

this group compared to routine care patients. Only two patients (one death, one lost to follow-up) in the intensively treated group compared to five in the routine care group did not complete the study. In sum, these studies suggest that triple therapy in early or established RA can be well tolerated and result in significant improvements in the clinical findings of RA along with delaying the progression of erosive disease.

Combination Therapy with Tetracyclines

In 2002, 66 patients with early sero-positive RA who had not been previously treated with DMARDs were randomized to receive doxycycine 100 mg twice daily plus MTX, doxycycline 20 mg twice daily plus MTX, or placebo with MTX.[81] ACR 50 responses in the high-dose versus low-dose doxycycline arms were similar. The doxycycline 20 mg twice-daily dose has been shown to not alter oral or gut flora, and thus its mechanism of action is thought to be solely matrix metalloproteinase (MMP) inhibition. Thus, the authors suggest that MTX combined with a doxycycline can result in greater improvement in disease and that it is likely due to the antimetalloproteinase effect of doxycycline.

Summary

Many rheumatologists will add biologic therapy to RA patients who do not respond maximally to MTX. However, there is significant evidence that combination therapy with traditional DMARDs is an effective and less costly alternative. In addition, the TICORA, COBRA, and other studies have demonstrated that intensive therapy with nonbiologic traditional DMARDs can improve disease activity with good tolerability and acceptable toxicity. Therefore, the use of traditional DMARDs alone or in combination continues to have a role in the treatment of RA and should be considered first-line therapy—particularly for RA patients who do not have severely aggressive disease or are not candidates for biologics (Table 10E-2).

References

1. O'Dell JR. Combinations of conventional disease-modifying antirheumatic drugs. *Rheum Dis Clin North Am* 2001;27(2):415–426.
2. Jang CH, Choi JH, Byun MS, et al. Chloroquine inhibits production of TNF-alpha, IL-1beta and IL-6 from lipopolysaccharide-stimulated human monocytes/macrophages by different modes. *Rheumatology (Oxford)* 2006;45(6):703–710.
3. Lafyatis R, York M, Marshak-Rothstein A. Antimalarial agents: Closing the gate on toll-like receptors? *Arthritis Rheum* 2006;54(10): 3068–3070.
4. Felson DT, Anderson JJ, Meenan RF. The comparative efficacy and toxicity of second-line drugs in rheumatoid arthritis: Results of two metaanalyses. *Arthritis Rheum* 1990;33(10):1449–1461.
5. A randomized trial of hydroxychloroquine in early rheumatoid arthritis: The HERA Study. *Am J Med* 1995;98(2):156–168.
6. Clark P, Casas E, Tugwell P, et al. Hydroxychloroquine compared with placebo in rheumatoid arthritis: A randomized controlled trial. *Ann Intern Med* 1993;119(11):1067–1071.
7. Sanmarti R, Canete JD, Salvador G. Palindromic rheumatism and other relapsing arthritis. *Best Pract Res Clin Rheumatol* 2004;18(5): 647–661.
8. Runge LA. Risk/benefit analysis of hydroxychloroquine sulfate treatment in rheumatoid arthritis. *Am J Med* 1983;75(1A):52–56.
9. Furst DE, Lindsley H, Baethge B, et al. Dose-loading with hydroxychloroquine improves the rate of response in early, active rheumatoid arthritis: A randomized, double-blind six-week trial with eighteen-week extension. *Arthritis Rheum* 1999;42(2):357–365.
10. Costedoat-Chalumeau N, Hulot JS, Amoura Z, et al. Cardiomyopathy related to antimalarial therapy with illustrative case report. *Cardiology* 2007;107(2):73–80.
11. Gabriel SE, Coyle D, Moreland LW. A clinical and economic review of disease-modifying antirheumatic drugs. *Pharmacoeconomics* 2001;19(7):715–728.
12. Case JP. Old and new drugs used in rheumatoid arthritis: A historical perspective. Part 1: The older drugs. *Am J Ther* 2001;8(2):123–143.
13. Marmor MF, Carr RE, Easterbrook M, et al. Recommendations on screening for chloroquine and hydroxychloroquine retinopathy: A report by the American Academy of Ophthalmology. *Ophthalmology* 2002;109(7):1377–1382.
14. Morand EF, McCloud PI, Littlejohn GO. Continuation of long term treatment with hydroxychloroquine in systemic lupus erythematosus and rheumatoid arthritis. *Ann Rheum Dis* 1992;51(12): 1318–1321.
15. Allgayer H. Sulfasalazine and 5-ASA compounds. *Gastroenterol Clin North Am* 1992;21(3):643–658.
16. Skosey JL. Comparison of responses to and adverse effects of graded doses of sulfasalazine in the treatment of rheumatoid arthritis. *J Rheumatol Suppl* 1988;16:5–8.
17. Smedegard G, Bjork J. Sulphasalazine: Mechanism of action in rheumatoid arthritis. *Br J Rheumatol* 1995;34(Suppl 2):7–15.
18. Shanahan F, Niederlehner A, Carramanzana N, et al. Sulfasalazine inhibits the binding of TNF alpha to its receptor. *Immunopharmacology* 1990;20(3):217–224.
19. Weinblatt ME, Reda D, Henderson W, et al. Sulfasalazine treatment for rheumatoid arthritis: A metaanalysis of 15 randomized trials. *JRheumatol* 1999;26(10):2123–2130.
20. Suarez-Almazor ME, Belseck E, Shea B, et al. Sulfasalazine for rheumatoid arthritis. *Cochrane Database Syst Rev* 2000(2):CD000958.
21. van der Heijde DM, van Riel PL, Nuver-Zwart IH, et al. Sulphasalazine versus hydroxychloroquine in rheumatoid arthritis: 3-year follow-up. *Lancet* 1990;335(8688):539.
22. Smolen JS, Kalden JR, Scott DL, et al. for the European Leflunomide Study Group. Efficacy and safety of leflunomide compared with placebo and sulphasalazine in active rheumatoid arthritis: A double-blind, randomised, multicentre trial. *Lancet* 1999;353(9149):259–266.
23. Haagsma CJ, van Riel PL, de Jong AJ, et al. Combination of sulphasalazine and methotrexate versus the single components in early rheumatoid arthritis: A randomized, controlled, double-blind, 52 week clinical trial. *Br J Rheumatol* 1997;36(10):1082–1088.
24. Dougados M, Combe B, Cantagrel A, et al. Combination therapy in early rheumatoid arthritis: A randomised, controlled, double blind 52 week clinical trial of sulphasalazine and methotrexate compared with the single components. *Ann Rheum Dis* 1999;58(4): 220–225.
25. Bax DE, Amos RS. Sulphasalazine in rheumatoid arthritis: Desensitising the patient with a skin rash. *Ann Rheum Dis* 1986;45(2):139–140.
26. Greenwald RA, Golub LM, Lavietes B, et al. Tetracyclines inhibit human synovial collagenase in vivo and in vitro. *J Rheumatol* 1987;14(1):28–32.
27. O'Dell JR, Haire CE, Palmer W, et al. Treatment of early rheumatoid arthritis with minocycline or placebo: Results of a randomized, double-blind, placebo-controlled trial. *Arthritis Rheum* 1997;40(5): 842–848.
28. Stone M, Fortin PR, Pacheco-Tena C, et al. Should tetracycline treatment be used more extensively for rheumatoid arthritis? Metaanalysis

demonstrates clinical benefit with reduction in disease activity. *J Rheumatol* 2003;30(10):2112–2122.
29. Bluhm GB, Sharp JT, Tilley BC, et al. Radiographic results from the Minocycline in Rheumatoid Arthritis (MIRA) Trial. *J Rheumatol* 1997;24(7):1295–1302.
30. Kloppenburg M, Terwiel JP, Mallee C, et al. Minocycline in active rheumatoid arthritis: A placebo-controlled trial. *Ann N Y Acad Sci* 19946;732:422–433.
31. Tilley BC, Alarcon GS, Heyse SP, et al. Minocycline in rheumatoid arthritis: A 48-week, double-blind, placebo-controlled trial. MIRA Trial Group. *Ann Intern Med* 1995;122(2):81–89.
32. Wolfe F. The curious case of intramuscular gold. *Rheum Dis Clin North Am* 1993;19(1):173–187.
33. Clark P, Tugwell P, Bennet K, et al. Injectable gold for rheumatoid arthritis. *Cochrane Database Syst Rev* 2000(2):CD000520.
34. Menninger H, Herborn G, Sander O, et al. A 36 month comparative trial of methotrexate and gold sodium thiomalate in the treatment of early active and erosive rheumatoid arthritis. *Br J Rheumatol* 1998;37(10):1060–1068.
35. Pincus T, Ferraccioli G, Sokka T, et al. Evidence from clinical trials and long-term observational studies that disease-modifying antirheumatic drugs slow radiographic progression in rheumatoid arthritis: Updating a 1983 review. *Rheumatology (Oxford)* 2002; 41(12):1346–1356.
36. Rau R, Herborn G, Menninger H, et al. Comparison of intramuscular methotrexate and gold sodium thiomalate in the treatment of early erosive rheumatoid arthritis: 12 month data of a double-blind parallel study of 174 patients. *Br J Rheumatol* 1997;36(3):345–352.
37. Epstein WV, Henke CJ, Yelin EH, et al. Effect of parenterally administered gold therapy on the course of adult rheumatoid arthritis. *Ann Intern Med* 1991;114(6):437–444.
38. Porter DR, Capell HA, Hunter J. Combination therapy in rheumatoid arthritis: No benefit of addition of hydroxychloroquine to patients with a suboptimal response to intramuscular gold therapy. *J Rheumatol* 1993;20(4):645–649.
39. Lehman AJ, Esdaile JM, Klinkhoff AV, et al. A 48-week, randomized, double-blind, double-observer, placebo-controlled multicenter trial of combination methotrexate and intramuscular gold therapy in rheumatoid arthritis: Results of the METGO study. *Arthritis Rheum* 2005;52(5):1360–1370.
40. Bensen W, Tugwell P, Roberts RM, et al. Combination therapy of cyclosporine with methotrexate and gold in rheumatoid arthritis (2 pilot studies). *J Rheumatol* 1994;21(11):2034–2038.
41. Klinkhoff AV, Teufel A. How low can you go? Use of very low dosage of gold in patients with mucocutaneous reactions. *J Rheumatol* 1995;22(9):1657–1659.
42. Wolfe F, Hawley DJ, Cathey MA. Termination of slow acting antirheumatic therapy in rheumatoid arthritis: A 14-year prospective evaluation of 1017 consecutive starts. *J Rheumatol* 1990;17(8):994–1002.
43. Situnayake RD, Grindulis KA, McConkey B. Long-term treatment of rheumatoid arthritis with sulphasalazine, gold, or penicillamine: A comparison using life-table methods. *Ann Rheum Dis* 1987;46(3): 177–183.
44. Bendix G, Bjelle A. A 10 year follow-up of parenteral gold therapy in patients with rheumatoid arthritis. *Ann Rheum Dis* 1996;55(3): 169–176.
45. Richter JA, Runge LA, Pinals RS, et al. Analysis of treatment terminations with gold and antimalarial compounds in rheumatoid arthritis. *J Rheumatol* 1980;7(2):153–159.
46. Suarez-Almazor ME, Spooner C, Belseck E. Penicillamine for rheumatoid arthritis. *Cochrane Database Syst Rev* 2000(2):CD001460.
47. Eberhardt K, Rydgren L, Fex E, et al. D-penicillamine in early rheumatoid arthritis: Experience from a 2-year double blind placebo controlled study. *Clin Exp Rheumatol* 1996;14(6):625–631.
48. Howard-Lock HE, Lock CJ, Mewa A, et al. D-penicillamine: Chemistry and clinical use in rheumatic disease. *Semin Arthritis Rheum* 1986;15(4):261–281.
49. Suarez-Almazor ME, Spooner C, Belseck E. Azathioprine for rheumatoid arthritis. *Cochrane Database Syst Rev* 2000(2):CD001461.
50. Hunter T, Urowitz MB, Gordon DA, et al. Azathioprine in rheumatoid arthritis: A long-term follow-up study. *Arthritis Rheum* 1975;18(1):15–20.
51. De Silva M, Hazleman BL. Long-term azathioprine in rheumatoid arthritis: A double-blind study. *Ann Rheum Dis* 1981;40(6): 560–563.
52. Alarcon GS, Lopez-Mendez A, Walter J, et al. Radiographic evidence of disease progression in methotrexate treated and nonmethotrexate disease modifying antirheumatic drug treated rheumatoid arthritis patients: A meta-analysis. *J Rheumatol* 1992;19(12):1868–1873.
53. Jeurissen ME, Boerbooms AM, van de Putte LB, et al. Influence of methotrexate and azathioprine on radiologic progression in rheumatoid arthritis: A randomized, double-blind study. *Ann Intern Med* 1991;114(12):999–1004.
54. Willkens RF, Sharp JT, Stablein D, et al. Comparison of azathioprine, methotrexate, and the combination of the two in the treatment of rheumatoid arthritis: A forty-eight-week controlled clinical trial with radiologic outcome assessment. *Arthritis Rheum* 1995;38(12): 1799–1806.
55. Singh G, Fries JF, Spitz P, et al. Toxic effects of azathioprine in rheumatoid arthritis: A national post-marketing perspective. *Arthritis Rheum* 1989;32(7):837–843.
56. Black AJ, McLeod HL, Capell HA, et al. Thiopurine methyltransferase genotype predicts therapy-limiting severe toxicity from azathioprine. *Ann Intern Med* 1998;129(9):716–718.
57. Walker J, Mendelson H, McClure A, et al. Warfarin and azathioprine: Clinically significant drug interaction. *J Rheumatol* 2002;29(2): 398–399.
58. Fields CL, Robinson JW, Roy TM, et al. Hypersensitivity reaction to azathioprine. *South Med J* 1998;91(5):471–474.
59. Silman AJ, Petrie J, Hazleman B, et al. Lymphoproliferative cancer and other malignancy in patients with rheumatoid arthritis treated with azathioprine: A 20 year follow-up study. *Ann Rheum Dis* 1988;47(12):988–992.
60. Gaffney K, Scott DG. Azathioprine and cyclophosphamide in the treatment of rheumatoid arthritis. *Br J Rheumatol* 1998;37(8): 824–836.
61. Szumlanski CL, Honchel R, Scott MC, et al. Human liver thiopurine methyltransferase pharmacogenetics: Biochemical properties, liver-erythrocyte correlation and presence of isozymes. *Pharmacogenetics* 1992;2(4):148–159.
62. Wolfe F. The epidemiology of drug treatment failure in rheumatoid arthritis. *Baillieres Clin Rheumatol* 1995;9(4):619–632.
63. Perdriger A, Mariette X, Kuntz JL, et al. Safety of infliximab used in combination with leflunomide or azathioprine in daily clinical practice. *J Rheumatol* 2006;33(5):865–869.
64. Wells G, Haguenauer D, Shea B, et al. Cyclosporine for rheumatoid arthritis. *Cochrane Database Syst Rev* 2000(2):CD001083.
65. Drosos AA, Voulgari PV, Papadopoulos IA, et al. Cyclosporine A in the treatment of early rheumatoid arthritis: A prospective, randomized 24-month study. *Clin Exp Rheumatol* 1998;16(6):695–701.
66. Forre O. for the Norwegian Arthritis Study Group. Radiologic evidence of disease modification in rheumatoid arthritis patients treated with cyclosporine: Results of a 48-week multicenter study comparing low-dose cyclosporine with placebo. *Arthritis Rheum* 1994;37(10):1506–1512.
67. Ferraccioli GF, Bambara LM, Ferraris M, et al. for the Italian Rheumatologists Study Group on Rheumatoid Arthritis. Effects of cyclosporin on joint damage in rheumatoid arthritis. *Clin Exp Rheumatol* 1997;15(Suppl 17):S83–S89.
68. Kitahara K, Kawai S. Cyclosporine and tacrolimus for the treatment of rheumatoid arthritis. *Curr Opin Rheumatol* 2007;19(3):238–245.
69. Proudman SM, Conaghan PG, Richardson C, et al. Treatment of poor-prognosis early rheumatoid arthritis: A randomized study of treatment with methotrexate, cyclosporin A, and intraarticular

corticosteroids compared with sulfasalazine alone. *Arthritis Rheum* 2000;43(8):1809–1819.
70. Tugwell P, Pincus T, Yocum D, et al. for the Methotrexate-Cyclosporine Combination Study Group. Combination therapy with cyclosporine and methotrexate in severe rheumatoid arthritis. *N Engl J Med* 1995; 333(3):137–141.
71. Stein CM, Pincus T, Yocum D, et al. for the Methotrexate-Cyclosporine Combination Study Group. Combination treatment of severe rheumatoid arthritis with cyclosporine and methotrexate for forty-eight weeks: An open-label extension study. *Arthritis Rheum* 1997;40(10): 1843–1851.
72. Karanikolas G, Charalambopoulos D, Andrianakos A, et al. Combination of cyclosporine and leflunomide versus single therapy in severe rheumatoid arthritis. *J Rheumatol* 2006;33(3):486–489.
73. Marra CA, Esdaile JM, Guh D, et al. The effectiveness and toxicity of cyclosporin A in rheumatoid arthritis: Longitudinal analysis of a population-based registry. *Arthritis Rheum* 2001;45(3):240–245.
74. Mottonen TT, Hannonen PJ, Boers M. Combination DMARD therapy including corticosteroids in early rheumatoid arthritis. *Clin Exp Rheumatol* 1999;17(Suppl 18):S59–S65.
75. Boers M, Verhoeven AC, Markusse HM, et al. Randomised comparison of combined step-down prednisolone, methotrexate and sulphasalazine with sulphasalazine alone in early rheumatoid arthritis. *Lancet* 1997;350(9074):309–318.
76. Landewe RB, Boers M, Verhoeven AC, et al. COBRA combination therapy in patients with early rheumatoid arthritis: Long-term structural benefits of a brief intervention. *Arthritis Rheum* 2002; 46(2):347–356.
77. O'Dell JR, Haire CE, Erikson N, et al. Treatment of rheumatoid arthritis with methotrexate alone, sulfasalazine and hydroxychloroquine, or a combination of all three medications. *N Engl J Med* 1996;334(20):1287–1291.
78. O'Dell JR, Leff R, Paulsen G, et al. Treatment of rheumatoid arthritis with methotrexate and hydroxychloroquine, methotrexate and sulfasalazine, or a combination of the three medications: Results of a two-year, randomized, double-blind, placebo-controlled trial. *Arthritis Rheum* 2002;46(5):1164–1170.
79. Mottonen T, Hannonen P, Leirisalo-Repo M, et al. for the FIN-RACo Trial Group. Comparison of combination therapy with single-drug therapy in early rheumatoid arthritis: A randomised trial. *Lancet* 1999;353(9164):1568–1573.
80. Grigor C, Capell H, Stirling A, et al. Effect of a treatment strategy of tight control for rheumatoid arthritis (the TICORA study): A single-blind randomised controlled trial. *Lancet* 2004;364(9430):263–269.
81. O'Dell JR, Blakely KW, Mallek JA, et al. Treatment of early seropositive rheumatoid arthritis: A two-year, double-blind comparison of minocycline and hydroxychloroquine. *Arthritis Rheum* 2001; 44(10):2235–2241.

Treatment of Rheumatoid Arthritis: Tumor Necrosis Factor Inhibitors

CHAPTER 10F

Dimitrios A. Pappas and Joan M. Bathon

The development of tumor necrosis factor-alpha (TNF-α) inhibitors has revolutionized the treatment of rheumatoid arthritis (RA). The identification of complex inflammatory cytokine pathways in the rheumatoid joint, the recognition of TNF-α hierarchic position in these pathways, and the elucidation of TNF-α central role in articular damage represent the progressive steps of bench-to-bedside investigation that led to clinical trials establishing the impressive efficacy of TNF blockade in RA. Although previously reviewed in detail elsewhere,[1] some of the most compelling preclinical studies suggesting a central role of TNF-α in RA were the TNF-α transgenic mouse model—in which overexpression of human TNF-α led to the spontaneous development of a highly inflammatory destructive arthritis-resembling RA[2] and the ability of neutralizing anti–TNF-α antibodies to downregulate collagen-induced arthritis in mice.[3] These findings were recapitulated in clinical trials in RA, thus launching the era of TNF-α antagonism in RA.

TNF-Alpha and TNF-Alpha Receptors

The ability of TNF-α to induce necrosis of tumor cells is responsible for its name.[4] It is also known as cachectin,[5] due to its unique catabolic effects on muscle.[6] The proinflammatory properties of TNF-α were also recognized rapidly after its discovery.[7] TNF-α belongs to the TNF superfamily of ligands and receptors.[8] TNF-α is primarily produced by macrophages.[9] It is initially synthesized and expressed as a transmembrane protein and is subsequently cleaved by an enzyme called TACE (TNF-α–converting enzyme). TNF-α circulates as a homotrimer and exhibits affinity for two different cysteine-rich homodimer transmembrane receptors, the 55-kd type I TNF-R (TNF-RI; p55) and 75-kd type II TNF receptor (TNF-RII; p75).[8] Data suggest that membrane-bound TNF-α, which constitutes only a minority of biologically available TNF-α, has greater binding affinity for the p75 receptor and the soluble TNF-α preferentially engages p55.[10] Most cell types express TNF receptors, thus explaining the pleotropic effects of TNF-α. TNF receptors can also be proteolytically cleaved by TACE, and as soluble TNF receptors (sTNFRs) bind circulating bioactive TNF-α and thus prevent TNF-α binding to membrane-bound receptors.[8,11] Thus, circulating sTNFRs are presumed to serve as endogenous anti-inflammatory and antiapoptotic agents. TNF and its receptors are discussed in more detail in Chapter 8.

Development of TNF-Alpha Antagonists

Two primary strategies have evolved to antagonize the actions of TNF-α: anti–TNF-α monoclonal antibodies and soluble TNF-α receptors. Both classes of agents interfere with binding of TNF-α to membrane-bound receptors, thus blocking cell signaling. The agents currently approved by the Food and Drug Administration (FDA) and in development are summarized in Table 10F-1. An alternative strategy that proved to be less successful in early clinical trials is the inhibition of TACE.[12,13]

Monoclonal Antibodies Against TNF-Alpha

Infliximab (Remicade) was the first (in 1999) monoclonal antibody (MoAb) to be approved by the FDA for use in RA. It is a chimeric molecule consisting of a human constant region of IgG1κ (75%) attached by disulfide bonds to a murine-variable region of neutralizing antihuman TNF-α antibody (25%).[14] It binds to both soluble and membrane-bound TNF-α with high affinity and has a half-life of 8 to 9.5 days. Infliximab is administered intravenously over 2 hours at an initial dose of 3mg/kg every 8 weeks, following a loading administration at 0, 2, and 6 weeks. The dose may be increased up to 10 mg/kg, and the dosing interval can be shortened to every 4 weeks if needed based on persistent disease activity. Infliximab, particularly at lower doses, has considerable immunogenicity. The development of anti-infliximab antibodies may interfere with its efficacy and induce infusion reactions but can be suppressed by concomitantly administered low-dose methotrexate (MTX). Infliximab is approved for use in moderate to severe RA in combination with MTX.[15]

Adalimimumab (Humira), approved by the FDA in 2002, contains entirely human sequences in its structure. It was produced with phage display technology and is indistinguishable from human IgG1. Its half-life approximates that of the natural human IgG

Table 10F-1. TNF Inhibitors Currently Approved or in Development

Generic Name	Description	Targets	Status
Anti-TNF-α Monoclonal Antibodies			
Infliximab	Chimeric human-murine	TNF-α	FDA approved
Adalimumab	Human	TNF-α	FDA approved
Golimumab	Human	TNF-α	In development
CDP870 (certolizumab)	PEG-linked Fab	TNF-α	In development
TNF-TeAb	Tetravalent anti-body to TNF-α	TNF-α	In development
CDP571	CDR grafted	TNF-α	Development terminated
Soluble TNF Receptors			
Etanercept	sTNF-RII: Fc	TNF-α; LTA-α	FDA approved
Lanercept	sTNF-RI: Fc	TNF-α; LTA-α	Development terminated
N/A	PEG-sTNF-RI	TNF-α; LTA-α	In development

CDR, complementarity-determining region; *FDA,* U.S. Food and Drug Administration; *PEG,* polyethylene glycol.

(15–19 days). It is administered by subcutaneous injection at a dose of 40 mg every other week but may be given weekly if disease activity persists.[16–18] Two MoAbs in clinical development currently are golimumab and certolizumab. Golimumab is a fully human MoAb in which the constant regions of heavy and light chains are identical to the corresponding regions of infliximab. However, the variable regions are also of human sequence rather than murine. In a preliminary dose-escalating study in 36 subjects, golimumab was generally well tolerated.[19] Certolizumab (CDP870) differs from the other anti-TNF MoAbs in that the Fab moiety is attached to polyethylene glycol (PEG) in an attempt to increase its half-life. Phase III trials in RA are currently in progress.[20,21] TNF-TeAb is a tetravalent antibody to TNF under investigation. It was generated by fusing the tetramerization domain of human p53 to the C terminus of anti-TNF Fab by a linking peptide derived from human albumin. Its tetramer structure increases its avidity for TNF-α. Although there have not yet been studies in man, favorable results were observed in a murine model of collagen-induced arthritis.[22] Finally, CDP571 is another humanized anti-TNF MoAb grafted to humanized complementarity-determining region (CDR).[23,24] Its development in RA was terminated, but it is under investigation for Crohn's disease.

Recombinant Soluble TNF-Alpha Receptors

Recombinant sTNFRs are molecules designed by linking the ligand-binding extracellular portion of human-derived TNF RI or TNF RII with a human immunoglobulin-Fc–like molecule. Other modifications include dimerization (which enhances affinity for secreted TNF-α) and substitution of the Fc moiety with PEG, which prolongs half-life. Although composed of human sequences, antibodies to soluble receptors may still arise—perhaps in response to non-natural sites of linkage. These engineered molecules mimic the action of the endogenous sTNFRs by binding secreted TNF-α with high affinity, thus preventing cell signaling. These molecules do not bind transmembrane TNF with the same affinity as the MoAbs.[25] However, in contrast to anti-TNF MoAbs they have the capacity to bind lymphotoxin-α (LTA-α). Etanercept (Enbrel) is currently the only FDA-approved (1998) sTNFRs for use in RA. It consists of a dimeric TNF RII bound to human Fc. Its half-life is approximately 100 hours,[26] and it is administered subcutaneously at a dose of 50 mg weekly or 25 mg twice a week. It is approved for patients with moderate to severe RA. Fusion of dimeric TNF R-I to Fc led to lenercept (sTNF R-I: Fc),[27] whereas fusion of monomeric or dimeric TNF R-I to PEG led to PEG-sTNF-RI.[28] Neither of these agents is FDA approved.

Clinical Trials of TNF Antagonists in Rheumatoid Arthritis

The pivotal double-blinded randomized placebo-controlled clinical trials in patients with RA that led to FDA approval of infliximab, adalimumab, and etanercept are summarized in Tables 10F-2 through 10F-4. All agents have been studied and proven to be effective in both early and in advanced disease, and efficacy is generally comparable for all three (although no head-to-head comparisons have ever been conducted). Although inclusion and exclusion criteria vary from study to study, clinical trials in advanced disease generally targeted patients with persistently active synovitis despite treatment with MTX. In these studies, the TNF antagonist or placebo was added to background MTX. In contrast, clinical trials of patients with early RA generally targeted individuals who were MTX naive, thus comparing the TNF antagonist head to head with MTX—except in the case of infliximab, where MTX co-therapy was required to suppress anti-infliximab antibodies.

The primary clinical response in clinical trials of TNF antagonists in RA is the American College of Rheumatology 20 (ACR 20) response. This is a composite score that requires a 20% improvement in number of tender joints and in number of swollen joints, as well as a 20% improvement in three of five other criteria[29]: patient pain assessment, patient global assessment, physician global assessment, patient self-assessed disability, and acute-phase reactant value [erythrocyte sedimentation rate (ESR) or C-reactive protein (CRP)]. ACR 50 and ACR 70 scores are derived in a similar manner, substituting a requirement for 50% and 70% improvement, respectively.

The ability of TNF antagonists to slow or halt joint damage was assessed radiographically in the majority of these clinical trials using the validated Sharp score methodology with van der Heijde modification.[30,31] Radiographic scores are calculated in specified joints in the hands, wrists, and feet at baseline and after the treatment period. The progression score reflects the increase (worsening) or decrease (improvement) in the modified Sharp score during the period of treatment.

Infliximab

The efficacy of infliximab (Table 10F-2) was studied in patients with longstanding active RA on background MTX in the ATTRACT (Anti-TNF Trial in Rheumatoid Arthritis with Concomitant Therapy) study. At both 30 and 54 weeks of treatment, the ACR 20 response rates in patients treated with infliximab (at varying doses) + MTX were two- to threefold higher

Table 10F-2. Clinical Trials with Infliximab

Study	No. of Patients	Study Arms	Study Duration	Outcomes					
				ACR Response Rates (%)	ACR Response Ratios (%)			Change in Sharp[a] Score	*p* for Change (Sharp)
Long-standing Disease				20 50 70	20 50 70			Mean ± SD	
Infliximab in combination with MTX against MTX alone									
Maini	428	MTX 15 mg (IQR:15·0–20·0) + infliximab 10 mg/kg every 4 weeks	30 weeks	58, 26, 11	2.9,	5.2,	11+	Not investigated	
ATTRACT		MTX 15 mg (IQR:12·5–17·5) + infliximab 10 mg/kg every 8 weeks		52, 31, 18	2.6,	6.2,	18+		
		MTX 15 mg (IQR:12·5–17·5) + infliximab 3 mg/kg every 4 weeks		53, 29, 11	2.7,	5.8,	11+		
		MTX 15 mg (IQR:12·5–17·5) + infliximab 3 mg/kg every 8 weeks		50, 27, 8	2.5,	5.4,	8+		
		MTX 15 mg (IQR:12·5–17·5)		20, 5, 0	1,	1,	1,		
Lipsky	428	MTX 17 ± 4 mg + infliximab 10 mg/kg every 4 weeks	54 weeks	59, 38, 19	3.5,	4.8,	9.3	−0.7 ± 3.8	<0.001
ATTRACT		MTX 16 ± 3 mg + infliximab 10 mg/kg every 8 weeks		59, 39, 25	3.5,	4.9,	12.5	0.2 ± 3.6	<0.001
		MTX 16 ± 4 mg + infliximab 3 mg/kg every 4 weeks		48, 34, 17	2.8,	4.3,	8.5	1.6 ± 8.5	<0.001
(Extension)		MTX 16 ± 4 mg + infliximab 3 mg/kg every 8 weeks		42, 21, 10	2.5,	2.6,	5	1.3 ± 6.0	<0.001
		MTX 16 ± 4 mg		17, 8, 2	1,	1,	1	7.0 ± 10.3	NS
Early Disease									
Infliximab in combination with MTX against MTX (MTX-naive patients)									
St.Clair	1049	MTX 16 ± 8 mg + infliximab 6 mg/kg every 8 weeks	54 weeks	66, 50, 37	1.2,	1.6,	1.8	0.5 ± 5.6	<0.001
ASPIRE		MTX 16 ± 8 mg + infliximab 3 mg/kg every 8 weeks		62, 46, 33	1.1,	1.4,	1.5	0.4 ± 5.8	<0.001
		MTX 16 ± 8 mg		54, 32, 21	1,	1,	1	3.7 ± 9.6	NS

Note: ACR responses are rounded.
[a]Sharp score: van Der Heijde modified. Score range: 0–440.

than those receiving placebo + MTX.[32,33] In some cases, response to infliximab was apparent as early as the second week of therapy. Improvement in quality of life, as measured by SF-36 (medical outcomes study Short Form-36 item health survey),[34] was also higher in the infliximab-treated groups compared to placebo.[33]

Infliximab in combination with MTX was also more effective than placebo + MTX in slowing radiographic progression in the ATTRACT trial. After 1 year of treatment, the mean annual progression score in the infliximab + MTX combined groups was 0.6 units/year, compared to 7.0 units/year in the placebo + MTX group ($p < 0.001$) Interestingly, 39% to 55% of patients in the combination arm had a decrease in Sharp score (compared to 14% in MTX monotherapy), suggesting the possibility of repair of joint damage. Moreover, the decrease in the rate of radiographic progression was seen in patients on infliximab + MTX even when clinical response was not present. In contrast, in the placebo + MTX arm radiographic progression occurred in some cases even in patients who had a clinical response.[33]

St.Clair et al.[35] reported the efficacy of infliximab in 1,049 patients with early RA in the ASPIRE (Active Controlled Study of Patients Receiving Infliximab for the Treatment of Rheumatoid Arthritis of Early Onset) study. This study compared the efficacy of infliximab + MTX versus MTX monotherapy in MTX-naive patients with early active disease. In terms of ACR 20%, 50%, and 70% response rates, the combination treatment exhibited a modestly better efficacy profile than MTX monotherapy (Table 10F-2). It is important to note that the differences in ACR responses of combination therapy and monotherapy in this study were not as dramatic as in the ATTRACT trial because the ASPIRE study targeted MTX-naive patients and ATTRACT targeted patients who failed MTX treatment. Radiographic progression measures also favored the combination treatment arm.[35]

Etanercept

Moreland et al.[36] compared etanercept (Table 10F-3) 25 mg subcutaneously twice a week against placebo in patients with long-standing active disease, after MTX and other DMARDs were

Table 10F-3. Clinical Trials with Etanercept

Study	No. of Patients	Study Arms	Study Duration	Outcomes			
				ACR Response Rates (%)	**ACR Response Ratios (%)**	**Change in Sharp[a] Score**	***p* for Change (Sharp)**
Longstanding Disease				20 50 70	20 50 70	Mean ± SD	
Etanercept monotherapy versus placebo after failure of at least one DMARD						median (IQR)	
Moreland	234	Etanercept 25 mg sq biw	6 months	59, 40, 15	5.4, 8, 15	Not investigated	
		Etanercept 10 mg sq biw		51, 24, 9	4.6, 4.8, 9		
		Placebo		11, 5, 1	1, 1, 1		
Etanercept alone or in combination with MTX against MTX							
Weinblatt	89	Etanercept 25 mg sq biw + MTX 15–25 mg po weekly	6 months	71, 39, 15	2.6, 13, 15+	Not investigated	
		MTX 15–25 mg po weekly		27, 3, 0	1, 1, 0		
Klareskog	682	Etanerxept 25 mg sq biw + MTX 16.9 mg po weekly	52 weeks	85, 69, 43	1.1, 1.6, 2.3	−0.54 (−1.00 – −0.07)	0.0001[b]
TEMPO		Etanerxept 25 mg sq biw		76, 48, 24	1.01, 1.1, 1.3	0.52 (−0.10 – 1.15)	0.0006[c]
		MTX 17.2 mg po weekly		75, 43, 19	1, 1, 1	2.80 (1.08 – 4.51)	0.0469[d]
Early Disease							
Etanercept monotherapy against MTX (MTX-naive patients)							
Bathon	632	Etanercept 25 mg sq biw	12 months	72, 49, 25	1.1, 1.5, 1,1	1.00 ± NS[e]	0.11
ERA		Etanercept 10 mg sq biw		61, 32, 16	0.9, 0.7, 0.7	NS	
		MTX 19 mg po weekly		65, 43, 22	1, 1, 1	1.59 ± NS[e]	

Note: ACR responses are rounded.
[a] Sharp score: van Der Heijde modified. Score range: 0–440.
[b] *p* value for combination treatment versus MTX.
[c] *p* value for combination treatment versus Etanercept.
[d] *p* value for Etanercept versus MTX.
[e] Change in Sharp score at 12 months.

washed out. Etanercept performed very well, with 5, 8, and 15 times more patients achieving ACR 20, 50, and 70 responses, respectively, at 6 months than placebo-treated patients.[36] In a second trial in patients with advanced disease, in which MTX background treatment was continued, a significantly higher proportion of patients treated with etanercept + MTX achieved the primary endpoint of ACR responses compared to patients receiving placebo + MTX.[37] The Early RA (ERA) trial targeted patients with RA of less than 3 years duration who were MTX naive, and compared etanercept monotherapy to MTX monotherapy.[38] Etanercept treatment was associated with a rapid response, with more patients achieving ACR responses during the first 6 months than in the group receiving MTX. However, this difference disappeared at later time points. Radiographically, the mean total Sharp progression scores were not different between the two treatment groups at 12 months. However, progression at 24 months was lower in the etanercept group than in the MTX group (1.3 versus 3.2, respectively; $p = 0.001$).[39]

The TEMPO (Trial of Etanercept and Methotrexate with Radiographic Patient Outcomes) study extended these findings by comparing combination treatment with etanercept + MTX to each of the individual monotherapies.[40] This study targeted RA patients with active disease who had failed at least one DMARD and who had not received MTX for at least 6 months prior to enrollment. Treatment with etanercept + MTX achieved statistically significantly higher rates of ACR 20, 50, and 70 responses, and of remission, than treatment with etanercept or MTX alone. Furthermore, mean Sharp scores for radiographic progression at 1 year were significantly lower in the combination group than in the MTX and etanercept monotherapy groups (−0.54, 2.80, and 0.52 units/year, respectively). Etanercept monotherapy was not superior to MTX in rate of ACR responses, although the response was more rapid. However, it was statistically significantly superior to MTX in slowing of radiographic progression at 1 and 2 years of follow-up.[41]

Adalimumab

Adalimumab (Table 10F-4) performed very well in longstanding active disease as monotherapy against placebo in patients in whom DMARDs were washed out.[42] Rates of ACR responses at 26 weeks in patients receiving adalimumab were at least twice as high as those on placebo. In patients with longstanding active disease despite MTX, and in whom background MTX was continued, the combination of adalimumab + MTX was associated with ACR responses two- to fourfold higher than those associated with treatment with placebo + MTX at 24 and 52 weeks in

Table 10F-4. Trials on Adalimumab

Study	No. of Patients	Study Arms	Study Duration	Outcomes					
				ACR Response Rates (%)	ACR Response Ratios (%)			Change in Sharp[a] Score	*p* for Change (Sharp)
Longstanding Disease				20 50 70	20 50 70			Mean ± SD	
Adalimumab monotherapy versus placebo after failure of at least one DMARD								median (IQR)	
Van de Putte	544	Adalimumab 40 mg sq qw	26 weeks	53, 35, 18	2.8,	4.3,	10.2	Not investigated	
		Adalimumab 40 mg sq qow		46, 22, 12	2.4,	2.7,	6.9		
		Adalimumab 20 mg sq qw		39, 21, 10	2.1,	0.3,	5.4		
		Adalimumab 20 mg sq qow		36, 19, 9	1.9,	2.3,	4.7		
		placebo		19, 8, 2	1,	1,	1		
Adalimumab in combination with MTX (12.5–25 mg weekly)									
Weinblatt	271	Adalimumab 80 mg sq qow x2 + MTX 17.2 ± 4.7 mg po qw	24 weeks	66, 43, 19	4.5,	5.2,	4	Not investigated	
ARMADA		Adalimumab 40 mg sq qow x2 + MTX 16.4 ± 4.1 mg po qw		67, 55, 27	4.6,	6.8,	5.6		
		Adalimumab 20 mg sq qow x2 + MTX 16.9 ± 4.4 mg po qw		48, 32, 10	3.3,	3.9,	2.1		
		MTX 16.5 ± 5 mg po qw		15, 8, 5	1,	1,	1		
Keystone	619	Adalimumab 40 mg sq qow + MTX 16.7 ± 4.5 mg po qw	52 weeks	59	2.5			0.1 ± 4.8	<0.001
		Adalimumab 20 mg sq qw + MTX 16.3 ± 4.6 mg po qw		55	2.3			0.8 ± 4.9	<0.001
		MTX 16.7 ± 4.1 mg po qw		24	1			2.7 ± 6.8	NS
Adalimumab in combination with standard DMARDs (most frequently, MTX)									
Furst	636	Adalimumab 40 mg sq qow + DMARD	24 weeks	53, 29, 15	1.5,	2.6,	4.2	Not investigated	
STAR		DMARD		35, 11, 4	1,	1,	1		
Early Aggressive Disease									
Adalimumab alone or in combination with MTX (20 mg weekly) in MTX-naive patients									
Breedveld	799	Adalimumab 40 mg sq qow + MTX 20 mg po qw	2 years	62	1.5			1.9 ± NS	NS
PREMIER		Adalimumab 40 mg sq qow		46	1,1			5.5 ± NS	<0.001
		MTX 20 mg po qw		41	1			10.4 ± NS	<0.001

Note: ACR responses are rounded.
[a] Sharp score: van Der Heijde modified. Score range: 0–440.

the ARMADA (Anti TNF Research Study Program of the Monoclonal Antibody Adalimumab) study.[43,44] Similarly, adalimumab in combination with other background DMARDs (STAR trial)[45] in active longstanding disease was superior to placebo +plus DMARD treatment at 24 weeks. In all of these clinical trials, the response to adalimumab was evident as early as 1 week after initiation of treatment. Importantly, in the study by Keystone et al.[44] the adalimumab plus MTX combination also had an inhibitory effect on radiographic progression of joint damage compared to MTX monotherapy in patients with longstanding active disease.[44]

In the PREMIER study of MTX-naive patients with early disease, combination treatment with adalimumab + MTX was superior to adalimumab monotherapy and MTX monotherapy in both ACR responses and in slowing of radiographic progression over 2 years of treatment. Mean total Sharp progression scores at 2 years were 1.9, 5.5, and 10.4, respectively ($p < 0.001$ for comparison of combination against either monotherapy).[46] ACR responses were comparable in the adalimumab and MTX monotherapy arms, but the adalimumab monotherapy arm had significantly less radiographic progression than the MTX arm at 6 (2.1 vs. 3.5), 12 (3.0 vs. 5.7), and 24 months (5.5 vs. 10.4) ($p < 0.001$ at all time points).

Summary of TNF Inhibitors

Overall, all three TNF inhibitors demonstrated excellent efficacy in both early and longstanding RA. They improved signs and symptoms (joint pain and swelling), laboratory parameters of inflammation (ESR and CRP), and slowed or prevented radiographic progression of joint damage. Monotherapy with TNF antagonists is modestly more efficacious than MTX, at least for slowing of radiographic progression. Combination therapy with a TNF-α antagonist and MTX is superior to monotherapy with a TNF-α inhibitor or MTX. It should be noted, however, that not all individuals with RA respond to TNF inhibitors and alternative treatments should be sought in this situation.

Safety of TNF Antagonists

Although randomized clinical trials (RCTs) are the standard mechanism to discern efficacy of a potential therapeutic agent, they are generally not sufficiently powered to detect rare adverse events related to drugs. However, meta-analyses of combined trials with a single agent or class of agents have been used recently to identify treatment-related safety signals. Other methods include the establishment of registries (longitudinal observational cohort studies) and analysis of events reported to the FDA MedWatch Adverse Events Reporting System (AERS) in patients treated with a drug or class of drugs. Each of these methods has strengths and weaknesses, which have been reviewed elsewhere.[47] All three approaches have been utilized to assess the safety of the TNF antagonists in RA. In the individual RCTs of TNF antagonists in RA, the only adverse event that was consistently and clearly increased in patients treated with TNF antagonists compared to those in the control groups was infusion or injection reactions. However, the FDA MedWatch and registry databases (and a published meta-analysis) have raised concern over additional safety issues—including infection, lymphoma, demyelinating disease, congestive heart failure, and others. These issues are discussed in material following. Because infection is covered in depth in Chapter 10L, it is only briefly dealt with here.

Infusion and Injection Reactions

In RCTs, injection reactions occurred in approximately 20% to 33% of patients treated with etanercept or adalimumab—and infusion reactions in 15% to 20% of patients treated with infliximab (versus 7%–10% in placebo). Injection site reactions generally presented as mild induration or erythema at the site of injection, and usually resolved after 1 to 3 months of treatment.[36–38,40,42–46] Antihistamines or topical corticosteroids may ameliorate symptoms. Infliximab infusions may be accompanied by nausea, headache, or less frequently by flushing or transient hypotension.[32,33,35] Most of the time, a reduction in the infusion rate and/or preadministration of antihistamines or intravenous steroids prevented recurrence of symptoms.

Immunogenicity

Infliximab treatment in some patients with RA results in anti-infliximab antibodies.[48] The presence of antibodies, especially at high titer, is associated with increased rate of infliximab clearance, reduced magnitude and duration of response, and infusion reactions.[49,50] Anti-infliximab antibodies occurred more frequently in RA patients at lower doses of infliximab.[51] Coadministration of MTX with infliximab significantly suppressed the occurrence of anti-infliximab antibodies.[51] The FDA recommends coadministration of MTX with infliximab for the treatment of RA.[50] Although not all studies on etanercept reported the incidence of antietanercept antibodies, their occurrence was reported to be rare—and, most importantly, did not alter the clinical response.[36,37,52] Antiadalimumab antibodies have also been reported, in as high as 12% of treated patients in one clinical trial,[42] but their appearance was not associated with loss of efficacy[43] or with increased levels of adverse events.[42] Loss of efficacy or the development of infusion reactions over time with treatment with a TNF-α antagonist may be due to the development of antibodies against the agent. Switching treatment to an alternative anti-TNF agent does not appear to be complicated by cross reactivity,[53] although data are limited.

Autoimmunity

The induction of systemic lupus erythematosus (SLE)–related antibodies [antinuclear (ANA) and/or anti double-stranded DNA (dsDNA) antibodies] by treatment with TNF-α antagonists is well recognized. The incidence ranges from 11% to 65% for ANA[33,54,55] and 10 to 66% for anti-dsDNA.[36,54,56] Antibodies to cardiolipin and extractable nuclear antigens have been described less frequently.[57,58] The occurrence of autoantibodies is more frequent with infliximab than with etanercept[37,52,59] or adalimumab.[55,56] Interestingly, in RCTs with adalimumab equivalent percentages of patients converted from negative to positive (and from positive to negative) status for ANA and dsDNA antibodies.[42,43,45] Fortunately, the induction of autoantibodies is only rarely associated with clinical signs and symptoms of lupus—and these are generally mild (manifested by rash) constitutional symptoms, pleurisy, and arthritis but generally not renal or other more serious organ involvement. Some investigators have argued that drug-induced lupus related to TNF antagonism may in fact represent prior unrecognized overlap of SLE with RA.[54]

Rare cases of cutaneous vasculitis have also been reported in RA patients treated with TNF-α antagonists, whereas reports of systemic vasculitis have been rare.[60] That TNF-α antagonism is causal in this process is supported by the close temporal relationship of vasculitis to anti-TNF treatment, resolution upon discontinuation of treatment, and recurrence upon re-challenge. In the case in which cutaneous vasculitis appears temporarily close to initiation of TNF inhibitors, discontinuation of the agent should be considered, histopathologic confirmation sought, and systemic involvement ruled out. Treatment may require steroids.[60]

Infection

The risk of infection associated with treatment with TNF-α antagonists is discussed extensively in another chapter. Only a brief summary of the issue is presented here. In general, in the clinical trials outlined in Tables 10F-2 through 10F-4 there was no significant increase in the rate of infections in patients treated with TNF antagonists compared to placebo or nonbiologic DMARDs. However, post-approval surveillance in RA patients treated with these agents revealed an alarmingly number of reports of opportunistic infections—most notably tuberculosis (TB), both pulmonary and disseminated.[61,62] Thus, screening for latent and active TB should be undertaken in any patient for whom anti-TNF therapy is being considered (see Chapter 10 for specific recommendations).

Patients with RA, by virtue of the disease itself, are at increased risk for serious infections with common bacterial pathogens.[63,64] Analysis of data from several national health registries[65] and a meta-analysis of clinical trials with TNF antagonists[66] have suggested that treatment with TNF-α antagonists increases this risk further, whereas other reports have not corroborated this finding.[67,68] Rates of perioperative infections in patients undergoing orthopedic surgical procedures were also reported to be increased by treatment with TNF antagonists in some[69,70] published studies.[71–73] In the absence of consistent conclusions and guidelines, a prudent approach to the use of TNF inhibitors is to avoid initiation of treatment during febrile illnesses, discontinue treatment and promptly initiate antibiotic therapy during active infections, and withhold treatment for several half-lives prior to and after major surgical procedures until wound healing is satisfactory.[74]

Preliminary data suggest that the use of TNF inhibitors may be safe in patients with hepatitis C.[75] Coadministration of etanercept with interferon and ribavirin was well tolerated in a phase II pilot study in patients with hepatitis C,[76] but close monitoring of aminotransferase levels (and arguably of viral RNA levels) is nonetheless advised.[75] Treatment of patients with hepatitis B with TNF antagonists should be avoided, however, because infliximab treatment was associated with reactivation of hepatitis B in several studies.[77–79] Patients should be screened for hepatitis B, and treated if viral infection is present, before consideration of initiation of TNF inhibitors.[75]

Malignancy

RA is associated with an increased risk of lymphoma, especially non-Hodgkin's lymphoma (NHL).[80,81] This risk is greatest in patients with longstanding severe RA.[82] There has been considerable interest in whether anti-TNF therapy modulates this risk, in that TNF is known to both promote and suppress growth of certain malignancies *in vitro* depending on the cell type.[83,84] Although it would seem reasonable to argue that by reducing chronic inflammation, anti-TNF therapy may lower the risk of lymphoma in RA, the available data on this subject are conflicting and do not provide a definitive answer. A number of lymphomas in RA patients treated with etanercept or infliximab were reported to FDA MedWatch, the majority of them non-Hodgkin's lymphomas.[85] However, the voluntary nature of this reporting system and the absence of a nonexposed comparator group do not allow for calculation of treatment-associated risk. A meta-analysis[66] of pooled data from clinical trials with the anti-TNF MoAbs infliximab and adalimumab also raised concern over an increased risk of lymphoma in patients treated with TNF inhibitors, with 10 cases of lymphomas in 3,493 anti-TNF–treated patients and none in the 1,512 patients in the control arms. However, the overall rate of malignancies was unusually low in the control arms, raising questions as to whether the increased risk in the anti-TNF–treated arms was genuine.[86,87] In data derived from a large observational study over a 3-year period, there was no evidence for an increase in the incidence of lymphoma among patients treated with any of the three approved TNF-α inhibitors compared to those treated with nonbiologic DMARDs[88] after adjusting for RA disease activity/severity and known risk factors for malignancies. These results were in agreement with previous studies,[89,90] which showed that risk of lymphoma correlated with cumulative disease-related inflammation (not with treatment). A general criticism of this methodology is that confounding by indication (in which RA patients with more severe disease who are at highest risk for lymphoma and other comorbidities are also the patients most likely to be treated with TNF antagonists) cannot be completely eradicated by statistical adjustment.

With regard to solid tumors, RA itself appears to be associated with a marginally increased risk for lung and non-melanotic skin cancers and a lower risk for breast and colorectal cancer.[91,92] In RCTs and observational studies, anti-TNF therapy appeared to independently elevate the risk for melanotic and nonmelanotic skin cancers.[66,93] Based on the existing data, the prudent approach would be avoidance of anti-TNF therapy in patients with preexisting lymphomas and melanomas—and discontinuation of anti-TNF therapy in patients who develop these cancers *de novo*. Because non-melanotic skin cancers are very common but are associated with an extremely low risk of mortality, the use of anti-TNF therapy in these patients is not contraindicated. However, long-term follow-up of these patients is warranted.

Demyelinating Disease

Preclinical and clinical data implicate TNF in the pathogenesis of multiple sclerosis (MS).[94,95] However, treatment of MS patients in a phase II study with lenercept was associated with increased frequency, duration, and severity of clinical signs and symptoms (albeit without progression in size or number of MRI plaques).[96] In RA patients treated with FDA-approved TNF antagonists, *de novo* demyelinating events have been reported along with other nonspecific neurologic complaints such as mental status changes, peripheral neuropathy, seizures, and Guillain-Barré syndrome.[97,98] TNF inhibitors should therefore not be prescribed in patients with preexisting multiple sclerosis or other demyelinating disease and should be discontinued if symptoms of demyelinating disease develop.

Congestive Heart Failure

RA patients are at higher risk for developing congestive heart failure (CHF) than age- and gender-matched controls.[99] A critical role for TNF-α in the pathogenesis of CHF has been implied by the high levels of TNF expression in the myocardia and sera of non-RA patients with CHF suggesting a therapeutic role for TNF-α inhibition in CHF. However, two large-scale studies of TNF antagonist treatment in non-RA patients with advanced CHF were terminated early due to inefficacy (etanercept)[103] or increased all-cause mortality (infliximab).[104] No clinical trials of TNF antagonists in RA patients with CHF have been performed, but some cases of *de novo* CHF and exacerbations of CHF have been reported to the FDA MedWatch database. A prospective cohort study of RA patients suggested, however, that treatment with TNF antagonists is associated with a decreased prevalence of CHF compared to patients not treated with anti-TNF agents.[105] These data are in agreement with a smaller retrospective study in which rates of incidence and exacerbation of CHF, and of CHF-associated mortality, were not different in RA patients treated with TNF antagonists compared to patients not treated with anti-TNF agents or to a non-RA control group. In fact, a trend toward lower mortality in the anti-TNF treatment group was observed.[106] Finally, a study by Curtis et al.,[107] using a health care claims utilization database, did not reveal a statistically significant difference in the risk of cumulative incident CHF in RA and Crohn's disease patients treated with TNF inhibitors compared to nonbiologic DMARDs.

Interestingly, animal studies suggest that anti-TNF therapy may be beneficial in early CHF by reducing metalloproteinase (MMP)-induced remodeling of the myocardium.[108] However, it may be harmful in fibrotic later stages.[109,110] This could explain the apparent discrepancy in results between the non-RA and RA subjects, although further investigation is clearly needed. In the meantime, TNF antagonists should not be prescribed in RA patients with CHF of New York Heart Association classes III and IV.

Morbidity and mortality due to atherosclerotic cardiovascular disease are also increased in RA populations, compared to age- and gender-matched control populations.[111] These increases are not entirely explained by traditional cardiovascular risk factors,[112] implying that the cumulative inflammatory burden of RA is a key mediator of atherosclerosis.[113] TNF-α, among other cytokines, induces an atherogenic lipid profile and insulin resistance,[114] is expressed in atherosclerogenic plaque, and likely participates in the pathology of atherosclerotic plaque rupture.[115,116] An accumulating body of evidence, based largely on RA cohort studies, suggests that treatment with TNF antagonists does not increase[117–119] and might even lower the risk for incident cardiovascular events and deaths[120,121] when compared to RA patients not treated with anti-TNF agents. These data support the notion that chronic rheumatoid inflammation plays a pivotal role in accelerated atherosclerosis in RA.

Interstitial Lung Disease

Interstitial lung disease (ILD) is a common complication of RA. Several case reports suggest that treatment of RA with infliximab is associated with stabilization or improvement of pulmonary fibrosis.[122,123] However, exacerbation and even *de novo* occurrence of ILD have also been reported in patients treated with TNF antagonists—and several of these cases were severe or fatal.[124–129] Histologic examination is sparse and the results variable, showing patterns of usual interstitial pneumonia (UIP), bronchiolitis obliterans organizing pneumonia (BOOP), and others.[124,125,128,130] Preexisting ILD was present in some affected patients and was usually mild or asymptomatic.[131] The *de novo* occurrence or worsening of pulmonary symptoms after initiation of treatment[131,132] and resolution in some cases after discontinuation of treatment lend support to a possible causal relationship between anti-TNF therapy and pulmonary toxicity, although a contributory role from concomitant MTX treatment could not be ruled out in all cases.

Interpretation of the previously cited data are difficult, and *in vitro* and *in vivo* data only add to the confusion. Increased TNF-α production has been noted by the alveolar macrophages of patients with RA, regardless of the presence or absence of ILD, compared to healthy subjects.[133] TNF-α overexpression in murine lung causes lymphocytic and fibrosing alveolitis,[134] and inhibition of TNF-α prevented silica- and bleomycin-related lung fibrosis in mice.[135] On the other hand, in other experiments overexpression of TNF-α-ameliorated bleomycin induced pulmonary fibrosis in mice.[136] It has been suggested that inhibition of TNF-α may alter the balance between fibrogenic and antifibrogenic cytokines in favor of the former.[128] Until further information is available, caution should be used in prescribing TNF inhibitors to patients with known preexisting symptomatic or asymptomatic ILD. Anti-TNF–associated pulmonary toxicity should be considered in the differential for treated patients with worsening or new pulmonary symptoms, along with infectious etiologies and MTX-associated lung toxicity.

Reproduction

RA disproportionately affects women, and onset of disease during childbearing years is common.[137] Although RA activity often decreases during pregnancy, disease flares are not uncommon during pregnancy and in the postpartum period.[138] Whether TNF antagonists are safe in pregnant women and nursing mothers with RA is a matter of debate because there are no formal clinical trials of these agents (nor of any DMARD) in pregnancy. Developmental toxicity studies in animals, however, have not revealed any embryotoxicity or teratogenicity[139,140]—even though the drugs were observed to cross the placenta. In several case reports, small series, and retrospective surveys or registries rates of miscarriages, premature births, and congenital defects were not increased in RA pregnancies exposed to TNF antagonists compared to rates in the general population or in RA patients not exposed to TNF inhibitors.[141–144] In fact, there are several case reports and small series of successful pregnancies while continuing anti-TNF therapy throughout gestation in both RA[145] and in Crohn's disease.[146] Furthermore, preliminary data on fetal outcomes from a study of 32 pregnant women with RA with first trimester exposure to etanercept or infliximab were no different from those in 77 pregnant RA patients not exposed to an anti-TNF agent.[144] Data on the safety of anti-TNF therapy during breastfeeding are scarce. Etanercept has been detected in maternal milk,[147] but the extent of oral absorption through the newborn gastrointestinal tract and subsequent bioavailability of TNF inhibitors are unknown.

In the United States, TNF inhibitors are classified by the FDA as category B (no documented human toxicity) drugs for pregnancy. British guidelines currently recommend active contraception while on TNF inhibitors, and in the case of an unexpected pregnancy consideration of cessation of anti-TNF therapy.[74] More recently, an international consensus statement on biologic agents in 2006 recommended extensive discussion with the patient about potential risks and benefits prior to decision making.[148] Avoidance of breastfeeding while receiving treatment with a TNF inhibitor has been recommended by some,[74] but this may be overly cautious.

Vaccinations

Because of the increased risk for at least some types of infections in patients with RA, prophylactic vaccination for common pathogens is generally desirable. Whether treatment with TNF antagonists impairs response to vaccinations is an important clinical question. Studies with pneumococcal vaccination have not shown a significant impact of etanercept or infliximab on the intensity of mean postvaccination antibody production in anti-TNF–treated RA patients compared to nonexposed RA controls.[149] In addition, the percentage of adalimumab-treated RA patients achieving protective levels of antibody titers compared to placebo/nonbiologic DMARD-treated RA patients did not differ.[150] It is thus appropriate to immunize RA patients against pneumococcus, preferably prior to initiation of treatment. As for influenza vaccination, the serologic response was reported to be lower in RA patients receiving anti-TNF therapy compared to nonexposed patients.[150,151] However, it was still sufficiently large as to warrant immunization on an annual basis.[152] In this case, it is more practical to immunize while continuing anti-TNF therapy. Because experience with live attenuated vaccines in RA is scarce, inactivated rather than live attenuated vaccines should be used. If live vaccination is absolutely necessary, it should be administered 4 weeks prior to commencing anti-TNF treatment.[74]

Practical Guidelines for Treatment with TNF Antagonists

In the United States, all currently available TNF inhibitors are approved for use in patients with moderate to severe RA. These are generally patients of any disease duration who have persistently active disease despite treatment with one or more nonbiologic DMARDs, administered at maximally tolerated dose (for MTX, this is up to 25 mg weekly) for several months.[148] More stringent 2005 guidelines from the British Society for Rheumatology advocate a disease activity score (DAS) higher than 5.1 for 1 month, despite treatment with two previous DMARDs at therapeutic dose for at least 2 months, before considering treatment with TNF antagonists.[74] Generally, the TNF inhibitor is added to, not substituted for, background MTX (or alternative nonbiologic DMARD) because the combination of any TNF inhibitor with MTX has proven to be superior to the TNF inhibitor alone.[40,46] If after the introduction of a TNF inhibitor there is no improvement in RA disease activity within several months, several options exist. The first is to escalate the dose: for infliximab, up to 10 mg/kg every 4 weeks; for adalimumab, up to 40 mg weekly.[153] Switching to an alternative TNF inhibitor is another option because neither inadequate response[154–156] nor hypersensitivity reaction[157] to one agent necessarily predicts a similar occurrence with a second agent. There is no evidence to suggest superiority of one TNF inhibitor versus another. Rather, the choice of a particular anti-TNF agent is frequently made on the basis of patient preference for mode or frequency of administration—and in some situations on the dictates of a third-party payer.

There are some patients for whom monotherapy with a TNF antagonist is appropriate. These include patients who cannot tolerate MTX, those with hepatitis C (because MTX and leflunomide are contraindicated), and in young women considering pregnancy (because washout of a TNF inhibitor can be performed more rapidly than for MTX or leflunomide).

Occasionally, the combination of a TNF inhibitor and MTX as initial therapy for newly diagnosed RA is justifiable.[158,159] This strategy is reserved for those patients with very aggressive disease, as indicated by one or more of the following: a large number of swollen and tender joints, very elevated ESR and/or CRP, extraarticular disease, high levels of RF and/or anti-CCP antibodies, and radiographic joint erosions. Once the disease is under adequate control or in remission, an attempt to discontinue the TNF inhibitor (or, if mild disease activity persists, substitute the TNF inhibitor with a second nonbiologic DMARD) may be undertaken. This manipulation may reduce long-term toxicity and enhance the cost effectiveness of treatment. If, however, reactivation of the disease occurs resumption of treatment with the TNF antagonist is warranted. In patients who have not responded to the combination of MTX and anti-TNF therapy, each at maximally tolerated doses, consideration should be given to alternative agents such as rituximab or abatacept.

References

1. Feldmann M, Maini RN. Discovery of TNF-alpha as a therapeutic target in rheumatoid arthritis: Preclinical and clinical studies. *Joint Bone Spine* 2002;69:12–18.
2. Keffer J, Probert L, Cazlaris H, et al. Transgenic mice expressing human tumour necrosis factor: A predictive genetic model of arthritis. *EMBO J* 1991;10:4025–4031.
3. Williams RO, Feldmann M, Maini RN. Anti-tumor necrosis factor ameliorates joint disease in murine collagen-induced arthritis. *Proc Natl Acad Sci U S A* 1992;89:9784–9788.
4. Carswell EA, Old LJ, Kassel RL, et al. An endotoxin-induced serum factor that causes necrosis of tumors. *Proc Natl Acad Sci U S A* 1975;72:3666–3670.
5. Beutler B, Greenwald D, Hulmes JD, et al. Identity of tumour necrosis factor and the macrophage-secreted factor cachectin. *Nature* 1985;316:552–554.
6. Pekala PH, Price SR, Horn CA, et al. Model for cachexia in chronic disease: Secretory products of endotoxin-stimulated macrophages induce a catabolic state in 3T3-L1 adipocytes. *Trans Assoc Am Physicians* 1984;97:251–259.
7. Dayer JM, Beutler B, Cerami A. Cachectin/tumor necrosis factor stimulates collagenase and prostaglandin E2 production by human synovial cells and dermal fibroblasts. *J Exp Med* 1985;162: 2163–2168.
8. Bazzoni F, Beutler B. The tumor necrosis factor ligand and receptor families. *N Engl J Med* 1996;334:1717–1725.
9. Heller RA, Kronke M. Tumor necrosis factor receptor-mediated signaling pathways. *J Cell Biol* 1994;126:5–9.
10. Grell M, Douni E, Wajant H, et al. The transmembrane form of tumor necrosis factor is the prime activating ligand of the 80 kDa tumor necrosis factor receptor. *Cell* 1995;83:793–802.
11. Williams LM, Gibbons DL, Gearing A, et al. Paradoxical effects of a synthetic metalloproteinase inhibitor that blocks both p55 and p75 TNF receptor shedding and TNF alpha processing in RA synovial membrane cell cultures. *J Clin Invest* 1996;97:2833–2841.
12. Newton RC, Solomon KA, Covington MB, et al. Biology of TACE inhibition. *Ann Rheum Dis* 2001;60(Suppl 3):iii25–iii32.
13. Le GT, Abbenante G. Inhibitors of TACE and caspase-1 as anti-inflammatory drugs. *Curr Med Chem* 2005;12:2963–2977.
14. Elliott MJ, Maini RN, Feldmann M, et al. Treatment of rheumatoid arthritis with chimeric monoclonal antibodies to tumor necrosis factor alpha. *Arthritis Rheum* 1993;36:1681–1690.
15. Klotz U, Teml A, Schwab M. Clinical pharmacokinetics and use of infliximab. *Clin Pharmacokinet* 2007;46:645–660.
16. den Broeder A, van de Putte L, Rau R, et al. A single dose, placebo controlled study of the fully human anti-tumor necrosis factor-alpha antibody adalimumab (D2E7) in patients with rheumatoid arthritis. *J Rheumatol* 2002;29:2288–2298.
17. Weisman MH, Moreland LW, Furst DE, et al. Efficacy, pharmacokinetic, and safety assessment of adalimumab, a fully human anti-tumor necrosis factor-alpha monoclonal antibody, in adults with rheumatoid arthritis receiving concomitant methotrexate: A pilot study. *Clin Ther* 2003;25:1700–1721.
18. Nestorov I. Clinical pharmacokinetics of tumor necrosis factor antagonists. *J Rheumatol* 2005;74(Suppl):13–18.

19. Zhou H, Jang H, Fleischmann RM, et al. Pharmacokinetics and safety of golimumab, a fully human anti-TNF-alpha monoclonal antibody, in subjects with rheumatoid arthritis. *J Clin Pharmacol* 2007;47:383–396.
20. Choy EH, Hazleman B, Smith M, et al. Efficacy of a novel PEGylated humanized anti-TNF fragment (CDP870) in patients with rheumatoid arthritis: A phase II double-blinded, randomized, dose-escalating trial. *Rheumatology (Oxford)* 2002;41:1133–1137.
21. Barnes T, Moots R. Targeting nanomedicines in the treatment of rheumatoid arthritis: Focus on certolizumab pegol. *Int J Nanomed* 2007;2:3–7.
22. Liu M, Wang X, Yin C, et al. Targeting TNF-alpha with a tetravalent mini-antibody TNF-TeAb. *Biochem J* 2007;406:237–246.
23. Rankin EC, Choy EH, Kassimos D, et al. The therapeutic effects of an engineered human anti-tumour necrosis factor alpha antibody (CDP571) in rheumatoid arthritis. *Br J Rheumatol* 1995;34:334–342.
24. ADIS International Limited. CDP 571: Anti-TNF monoclonal antibody, BAY 103356, BAY W 3356, humicade. *Drugs R D* 2003;4: 174–178.
25. Kirchner S, Holler E, Haffner S, et al. Effect of different tumor necrosis factor (TNF) reactive agents on reverse signaling of membrane integrated TNF in monocytes. *Cytokine* 2004;28:67–74.
26. Mohler KM, Torrance DS, Smith CA, et al. Soluble tumor necrosis factor (TNF) receptors are effective therapeutic agents in lethal endotoxemia and function simultaneously as both TNF carriers and TNF antagonists. *J Immunol* 1993;151:1548–1561.
27. Rau R, Sander O, van Riel P, et al. Intravenous human recombinant tumor necrosis factor receptor p55-fc IgG1 fusion protein ro 45-2081 (lenercept): A double blind, placebo controlled dose–finding study in rheumatoid arthritis. *J Rheumatol* 2003;30:680–690.
28. Edwards CK III. PEGylated recombinant human soluble tumour necrosis factor receptor type I (r-hu-sTNF-RI): Novel high affinity TNF receptor designed for chronic inflammatory diseases. *Ann Rheum Dis* 1999;58(Suppl 1):I73–I81.
29. Felson DT, Anderson JJ, Boers M, et al. American college of rheumatology. preliminary definition of improvement in rheumatoid arthritis. *Arthritis Rheum* 1995;38:727–735.
30. van der Heijde DM, van Leeuwen MA, van Riel PL, et al. Biannual radiographic assessments of hands and feet in a three-year prospective followup of patients with early rheumatoid arthritis. *Arthritis Rheum* 1992;35:26–34.
31. Sharp JT, Lidsky MD, Collins LC, et al. Methods of scoring the progression of radiologic changes in rheumatoid arthritis. correlation of radiologic, clinical and laboratory abnormalities. *Arthritis Rheum* 1971;14:706–720.
32. Maini R, St Clair EW, Breedveld F, et al. Infliximab (chimeric antitumour necrosis factor alpha monoclonal antibody) versus placebo in rheumatoid arthritis patients receiving concomitant methotrexate: A randomised phase III trial. ATTRACT Study Group. *Lancet* 1999;354:1932–1939.
33. Lipsky PE, van der Heijde DM, St Clair EW, et al. Infliximab and methotrexate in the treatment of rheumatoid arthritis: Anti-tumor necrosis factor trial in rheumatoid arthritis with concomitant therapy study group. *N Engl J Med* 2000;343:1594–1602.
34. Talamo J, Frater A, Gallivan S, et al. Use of the short form 36 (SF36) for health status measurement in rheumatoid arthritis. *Br J Rheumatol* 1997;36:463–469.
35. St Clair EW, van der Heijde DM, Smolen JS, et al. Combination of infliximab and methotrexate therapy for early rheumatoid arthritis: A randomized, controlled trial. *Arthritis Rheum* 2004;50:3432–3443.
36. Moreland LW, Schiff MH, Baumgartner SW, et al. Etanercept therapy in rheumatoid arthritis: A randomized, controlled trial. *Ann Intern Med* 1999;130:478–486.
37. Weinblatt ME, Kremer JM, Bankhurst AD, et al. A trial of etanercept, a recombinant tumor necrosis factor receptor:Fc fusion protein, in patients with rheumatoid arthritis receiving methotrexate. *N Engl J Med* 1999;340:253–259.
38. Bathon JM, Martin RW, Fleischmann RM, et al. A comparison of etanercept and methotrexate in patients with early rheumatoid arthritis. *N Engl J Med* 2000;343:1586–1593.
39. Genovese MC, Bathon JM, Fleischmann RM, et al. Long-term safety, efficacy, and radiographic outcome with etanercept treatment in patients with early rheumatoid arthritis. *J Rheumatol* 2005; 32:1232–1242.
40. Klareskog L, van der Heijde D, de Jager JP, et al. Therapeutic effect of the combination of etanercept and methotrexate compared with each treatment alone in patients with rheumatoid arthritis: Double-blind randomised controlled trial. *Lancet* 2004;363:675–681.
41. van der Heijde D, Klareskog L, Rodriguez-Valverde V, et al. Comparison of etanercept and methotrexate, alone and combined, in the treatment of rheumatoid arthritis: Two-year clinical and radiographic results from the TEMPO study, a double-blind, randomized trial. *Arthritis Rheum* 2006;54:1063–1074.
42. van de Putte LB, Atkins C, Malaise M, et al. Efficacy and safety of adalimumab as monotherapy in patients with rheumatoid arthritis for whom previous disease modifying antirheumatic drug treatment has failed. *Ann Rheum Dis* 2004;63:508–516.
43. Weinblatt ME, Keystone EC, Furst DE, et al. Adalimumab, a fully human anti-tumor necrosis factor alpha monoclonal antibody, for the treatment of rheumatoid arthritis in patients taking concomitant methotrexate: The ARMADA trial. *Arthritis Rheum* 2003;48:35–45.
44. Keystone EC, Kavanaugh AF, Sharp JT, et al. Radiographic, clinical, and functional outcomes of treatment with adalimumab (a human anti-tumor necrosis factor monoclonal antibody) in patients with active rheumatoid arthritis receiving concomitant methotrexate therapy: A randomized, placebo-controlled, 52-week trial. *Arthritis Rheum* 2004;50:1400–1411.
45. Furst DE, Schiff MH, Fleischmann RM, et al. Adalimumab, a fully human anti tumor necrosis factor-alpha monoclonal antibody, and concomitant standard antirheumatic therapy for the treatment of rheumatoid arthritis: Results of STAR (safety trial of adalimumab in rheumatoid arthritis). *J Rheumatol* 2003;30:2563–2571.
46. Breedveld FC, Weisman MH, Kavanaugh AF, et al. The PREMIER study: A multicenter, randomized, double-blind clinical trial of combination therapy with adalimumab plus methotrexate versus methotrexate alone or adalimumab alone in patients with early, aggressive rheumatoid arthritis who had not had previous methotrexate treatment. *Arthritis Rheum* 2006;54:26–37.
47. Nasir A, Greenberg JD. TNF antagonist safety in rheumatoid arthritis: Updated evidence from observational registries. *Bull Hosp Jt Dis* 2007;65:178–181.
48. LoBuglio AF, Wheeler RH, Trang J, et al. Mouse/human chimeric monoclonal antibody in man: Kinetics and immune response. *Proc Natl Acad Sci U S A* 1989;86:4220–4224.
49. Wolbink GJ, Vis M, Lems W, et al. Development of antiinfliximab antibodies and relationship to clinical response in patients with rheumatoid arthritis. *Arthritis Rheum* 2006;54:711–715.
50. Haraoui B, Cameron L, Ouellet M, et al. Anti-infliximab antibodies in patients with rheumatoid arthritis who require higher doses of infliximab to achieve or maintain a clinical response. *J Rheumatol* 2006;33:31–36.
51. Maini RN, Breedveld FC, Kalden JR, et al. Therapeutic efficacy of multiple intravenous infusions of anti-tumor necrosis factor alpha monoclonal antibody combined with low-dose weekly methotrexate in rheumatoid arthritis. *Arthritis Rheum* 1998;41:1552–1563.
52. Genovese MC, Bathon JM, Martin RW, et al. Etanercept versus methotrexate in patients with early rheumatoid arthritis: Two-year radiographic and clinical outcomes. *Arthritis Rheum* 2002;46: 1443–1450.
53. Wagner CL, Schantz A, Barnathan E, et al. Consequences of immunogenicity to the therapeutic monoclonal antibodies ReoPro and remicade. *Dev Biol (Basel)* 2003;112:37–53.
54. De Rycke L, Baeten D, Kruithof E, et al. The effect of TNFalpha blockade on the antinuclear antibody profile in patients with

chronic arthritis: Biological and clinical implications. *Lupus* 2005; 14:931–937.

55. Valesini G, Iannuccelli C, Marocchi E, et al. Biological and clinical effects of anti-TNFalpha treatment. *Autoimmun Rev* 2007;7:35–41.
56. Eriksson C, Engstrand S, Sundqvist KG, et al. Autoantibody formation in patients with rheumatoid arthritis treated with anti-TNF alpha. *Ann Rheum Dis* 2005;64:403–407.
57. Jonsdottir T, Forslid J, van Vollenhoven A, et al. Treatment with tumour necrosis factor alpha antagonists in patients with rheumatoid arthritis induces anticardiolipin antibodies. *Ann Rheum Dis* 2004;63:1075–1078.
58. De Bandt M, Sibilia J, Le Loet X, et al. Systemic lupus erythematosus induced by anti-tumour necrosis factor alpha therapy: A french national survey. *Arthritis Res Ther* 2005;7:R545–R551.
59. Shakoor N, Michalska M, Harris CA, et al. Drug-induced systemic lupus erythematosus associated with etanercept therapy. *Lancet* 2002;359:579–580.
60. Ramos-Casals M, Brito-Zeron P, Munoz S, et al. Autoimmune diseases induced by TNF-targeted therapies: Analysis of 233 cases. *Medicine (Baltimore)* 2007;86:242–251.
61. Wallis RS, Broder MS, Wong JY, et al. Granulomatous infectious diseases associated with tumor necrosis factor antagonists. *Clin Infect Dis* 2004;38:1261–1265.
62. Crum NF, Lederman ER, Wallace MR. Infections associated with tumor necrosis factor-alpha antagonists. *Medicine (Baltimore)* 2005;84:291–302.
63. Doran MF, Crowson CS, Pond GR, et al. Frequency of infection in patients with rheumatoid arthritis compared with controls: A population-based study. *Arthritis Rheum* 2002;46:2287–2293.
64. Doran MF, Crowson CS, Pond GR, et al. Predictors of infection in rheumatoid arthritis. *Arthritis Rheum* 2002;46:2294–2300.
65. Listing J, Strangfeld A, Kary S, et al. Infections in patients with rheumatoid arthritis treated with biologic agents. *Arthritis Rheum* 2005;52:3403–3412.
66. Bongartz T, Sutton AJ, Sweeting MJ, et al. Anti-TNF antibody therapy in rheumatoid arthritis and the risk of serious infections and malignancies: Systematic review and meta-analysis of rare harmful effects in randomized controlled trials. *JAMA* 2006;295: 2275–2285.
67. Wolfe F, Caplan L, Michaud K. Treatment for rheumatoid arthritis and the risk of hospitalization for pneumonia: Associations with prednisone, disease-modifying antirheumatic drugs, and anti-tumor necrosis factor therapy. *Arthritis Rheum* 2006;54:628–634.
68. Dixon WG, Watson K, Lunt M, et al. Rates of serious infection, including site-specific and bacterial intracellular infection, in rheumatoid arthritis patients receiving anti-tumor necrosis factor therapy: Results from the british society for rheumatology biologics register. *Arthritis Rheum* 2006;54:2368–2376.
69. den Broeder AA, Creemers MC, Fransen J, et al. Risk factors for surgical site infections and other complications in elective surgery in patients with rheumatoid arthritis with special attention for anti-tumor necrosis factor: A large retrospective study. *J Rheumatol* 2007;34:689–695.
70. Giles JT, Bartlett SJ, Gelber AC, et al. Tumor necrosis factor inhibitor therapy and risk of serious postoperative orthopedic infection in rheumatoid arthritis. *Arthritis Rheum* 2006;55:333–337.
71. Talwalkar SC, Grennan DM, Gray J, et al. Tumour necrosis factor alpha antagonists and early postoperative complications in patients with inflammatory joint disease undergoing elective orthopaedic surgery. *Ann Rheum Dis* 2005;64:650–651.
72. Ruyssen-Witrand A, Gossec L, Salliot C, et al. Complication rates of 127 surgical procedures performed in rheumatic patients receiving tumor necrosis factor alpha blockers. *Clin Exp Rheumatol* 2007; 25:430–436.
73. Bibbo C, Goldberg JW. Infectious and healing complications after elective orthopaedic foot and ankle surgery during tumor necrosis factor-alpha inhibition therapy. *Foot Ankle Int* 2004;25:331–335.
74. Ledingham J, Deighton C for the British Society for Rheumatology Standards, Guidelines and Audit Working Group. Update on the british society for rheumatology guidelines for prescribing TNFalpha blockers in adults with rheumatoid arthritis (update of previous guidelines of april 2001). *Rheumatology (Oxford)* 2005;44:157–163.
75. Calabrese LH, Zein N, Vassilopoulos D. Safety of antitumour necrosis factor (anti-TNF) therapy in patients with chronic viral infections: Hepatitis C, hepatitis B, and HIV infection. *Ann Rheum Dis* 2004;63(Suppl 2):ii18–ii24.
76. Zein NN for the Etanercept Study Group. Etanercept as an adjuvant to interferon and ribavirin in treatment-naive patients with chronic hepatitis C virus infection: A phase 2 randomized, double-blind, placebo-controlled study. *J Hepatol* 2005;42:315–322.
77. Wendling D, Auge B, Bettinger D, et al. Reactivation of a latent precore mutant hepatitis B virus related chronic hepatitis during infliximab treatment for severe spondyloarthropathy. *Ann Rheum Dis* 2005;64:788–789.
78. Esteve M, Saro C, Gonzalez-Huix F, et al. Chronic hepatitis B reactivation following infliximab therapy in crohn's disease patients: Need for primary prophylaxis. *Gut* 2004;53:1363–1365.
79. Michel M, Duvoux C, Hezode C, et al. Fulminant hepatitis after infliximab in a patient with hepatitis B virus treated for an adult onset Still's disease. *J Rheumatol* 2003;30:1624–1625.
80. Prior P, Symmons DP, Hawkins CF, et al. Cancer morbidity in rheumatoid arthritis. *Ann Rheum Dis* 1984;43:128–131.
81. Myllykangas-Luosujarvi R, Aho K, Isomaki H. Mortality from cancer in patients with rheumatoid arthritis. *Scand J Rheumatol* 1995;24:76–78.
82. Baecklund E, Ekbom A, Sparen P, et al. Disease activity and risk of lymphoma in patients with rheumatoid arthritis: Nested case-control study. *BMJ* 1998;317:180–181.
83. Szlosarek P, Charles KA, Balkwill FR. Tumour necrosis factor-alpha as a tumour promoter. *Eur J Cancer* 2006;42:745–750.
84. Balkwill F. Tumor necrosis factor or tumor promoting factor? *Cytokine Growth Factor Rev* 2002;13:135–141.
85. Brown SL, Greene MH, Gershon SK, et al. Tumor necrosis factor antagonist therapy and lymphoma development: Twenty-six cases reported to the food and drug administration. *Arthritis Rheum* 2002;46:3151–3158.
86. Dixon W, Silman A. Is there an association between anti-TNF monoclonal antibody therapy in rheumatoid arthritis and risk of malignancy and serious infection? Commentary on the meta-analysis by bongartz et al. *Arthritis Res Ther* 2006;8:111.
87. Matteson EL, Bongartz T, Sutton AJ, et al. Response to commentary by dixon and silman on the systematic review and meta-analysis by bongartz et al. *Arthritis Res Ther* 2006;8:404.
88. Wolfe F, Michaud K. The effect of methotrexate and anti-tumor necrosis factor therapy on the risk of lymphoma in rheumatoid arthritis in 19,562 patients during 89,710 person-years of observation. *Arthritis Rheum* 2007;56:1433–1439.
89. Askling J, Fored CM, Baecklund E, et al. Haematopoietic malignancies in rheumatoid arthritis: Lymphoma risk and characteristics after exposure to tumour necrosis factor antagonists. *Ann Rheum Dis* 2005;64:1414–1420.
90. Baecklund E, Iliadou A, Askling J, et al. Association of chronic inflammation, not its treatment, with increased lymphoma risk in rheumatoid arthritis. *Arthritis Rheum* 2006;54:692–701.
91. Mellemkjaer L, Linet MS, Gridley G, et al. Rheumatoid arthritis and cancer risk. *Eur J Cancer* 1996;32A:1753–1757.
92. Askling J, Fored CM, Brandt L, et al. Risks of solid cancers in patients with rheumatoid arthritis and after treatment with tumour necrosis factor antagonists. *Ann Rheum Dis* 2005;64:1421–1426.
93. Wolfe F, Michaud K. Biologic treatment of rheumatoid arthritis and the risk of malignancy: Analyses from a large US observational study. *Arthritis Rheum* 2007;56:2886–2895.
94. Sharief MK, Hentges R. Association between tumor necrosis factor-alpha and disease progression in patients with multiple sclerosis. *N Engl J Med* 1991;325:467–472.

95. Kuroda Y, Shimamoto Y. Human tumor necrosis factor-alpha augments experimental allergic encephalomyelitis in rats. *J Neuroimmunol* 1991;34:159–164.
96. The Lenercept Multiple Sclerosis Study Group and the University of British Columbia MS/MRI Analysis Group. TNF neutralization in MS. Results of a randomized, placebo-controlled multicenter study: The lenercept multiple sclerosis study group and the university of british columbia MS/MRI analysis group. *Neurology* 1999;53:457–465.
97. Mohan N, Edwards ET, Cupps TR, et al. Demyelination occurring during anti-tumor necrosis factor alpha therapy for inflammatory arthritides. *Arthritis Rheum* 2001;44:2862–2869.
98. Robinson WH, Genovese MC, Moreland LW. Demyelinating and neurologic events reported in association with tumor necrosis factor alpha antagonism: By what mechanisms could tumor necrosis factor alpha antagonists improve rheumatoid arthritis but exacerbate multiple sclerosis? *Arthritis Rheum* 2001;44:1977–1983.
99. Nicola PJ, Maradit-Kremers H, Roger VL, et al. The risk of congestive heart failure in rheumatoid arthritis: A population-based study over 46 years. *Arthritis Rheum* 2005;52:412–420.
100. Torre-Amione G, Kapadia S, Lee J, et al. Tumor necrosis factor-alpha and tumor necrosis factor receptors in the failing human heart. *Circulation* 1996;93:704–711.
101. Matsumori A, Yamada T, Suzuki H, et al. Increased circulating cytokines in patients with myocarditis and cardiomyopathy. *Br Heart J* 1994;72:561–566.
102. Deswal A, Bozkurt B, Seta Y, et al. Safety and efficacy of a soluble P75 tumor necrosis factor receptor (enbrel, etanercept) in patients with advanced heart failure. *Circulation* 1999;99:3224–3226.
103. Mann DL, McMurray JJ, Packer M, et al. Targeted anticytokine therapy in patients with chronic heart failure: Results of the randomized etanercept worldwide evaluation (RENEWAL). *Circulation* 2004;109:1594–1602.
104. Chung ES, Packer M, Lo KH, et al. Randomized, double-blind, placebo-controlled, pilot trial of infliximab, a chimeric monoclonal antibody to tumor necrosis factor-alpha, in patients with moderate-to-severe heart failure: Results of the anti-TNF therapy against congestive heart failure (ATTACH) trial. *Circulation* 2003;107:3133–3140.
105. Wolfe F, Michaud K. Heart failure in rheumatoid arthritis: Rates, predictors, and the effect of anti-tumor necrosis factor therapy. *Am J Med* 2004;116:305–311.
106. Cole J, Busti A, Kazi S. The incidence of new onset congestive heart failure and heart failure exacerbation in veteran's affairs patients receiving tumor necrosis factor alpha antagonists. *Rheumatol Int* 2007;27:369–373.
107. Curtis JR, Kramer JM, Martin C, et al. Heart failure among younger rheumatoid arthritis and Crohn's patients exposed to TNF-alpha antagonists. *Rheumatology (Oxford)* 2007;46:1688–1693.
108. Bradham WS, Moe G, Wendt KA, et al. TNF-alpha and myocardial matrix metalloproteinases in heart failure: Relationship to LV remodeling. *Am J Physiol Heart Circ Physiol* 2002;282:H1288–H1295.
109. Bradham WS, Moe G, Wendt KA, et al. TNF-alpha and myocardial matrix metalloproteinases in heart failure: Relationship to LV remodeling. *Am J Physiol Heart Circ Physiol* 2002;282:H1288–H1295.
110. Li YY, Kadokami T, Wang P, et al. MMP inhibition modulates TNF-alpha transgenic mouse phenotype early in the development of heart failure. *Am J Physiol Heart Circ Physiol* 2002;282:H983–H989.
111. Maradit-Kremers H, Crowson CS, Nicola PJ, et al. Increased unrecognized coronary heart disease and sudden deaths in rheumatoid arthritis: A population-based cohort study. *Arthritis Rheum* 2005;52:402–411.
112. del Rincon ID, Williams K, Stern MP, et al. High incidence of cardiovascular events in a rheumatoid arthritis cohort not explained by traditional cardiac risk factors. *Arthritis Rheum* 2001;44:2737–2745.
113. Maradit-Kremers H, Nicola PJ, Crowson CS, et al. Cardiovascular death in rheumatoid arthritis: A population-based study. *Arthritis Rheum* 2005;52:722–732.
114. Sattar N, McCarey DW, Capell H, et al. Explaining how "high-grade" systemic inflammation accelerates vascular risk in rheumatoid arthritis. *Circulation* 2003;108:2957–2963.
115. Libby P. Inflammation in atherosclerosis. *Nature* 2002;420:868–874.
116. Carter AM. Inflammation, thrombosis and acute coronary syndromes. *Diab Vasc Dis Res* 2005;2:113–121.
117. Suissa S, Bernatsky S, Hudson M. Antirheumatic drug use and the risk of acute myocardial infarction. *Arthritis Rheum* 2006;55:531–536.
118. Solomon DH, Avorn J, Katz JN, et al. Immunosuppressive medications and hospitalization for cardiovascular events in patients with rheumatoid arthritis. *Arthritis Rheum* 2006;54:3790–3798.
119. Dixon WG, Watson KD, Lunt M, et al. Reduction in the incidence of myocardial infarction in patients with rheumatoid arthritis who respond to anti-tumor necrosis factor alpha therapy: Results from the british society for rheumatology biologics register. *Arthritis Rheum* 2007;56:2905–2912.
120. Carmona L, Descalzo MA, Perez-Pampin E, et al. All-cause and cause-specific mortality in rheumatoid arthritis are not greater than expected when treated with tumour necrosis factor antagonists. *Ann Rheum Dis* 2007;66:880–885.
121. Jacobsson LT, Turesson C, Gulfe A, et al. Treatment with tumor necrosis factor blockers is associated with a lower incidence of first cardiovascular events in patients with rheumatoid arthritis. *J Rheumatol* 2005;32:1213–1218.
122. Antoniou KM, Mamoulaki M, Malagari K, et al. Infliximab therapy in pulmonary fibrosis associated with collagen vascular disease. *Clin Exp Rheumatol* 2007;25:23–28.
123. Vassallo R, Matteson E, Thomas CF Jr. Clinical response of rheumatoid arthritis-associated pulmonary fibrosis to tumor necrosis factor-alpha inhibition. *Chest* 2002;122:1093–1096.
124. Peno-Green L, Lluberas G, Kingsley T, et al. Lung injury linked to etanercept therapy. *Chest* 2002;122:1858–1860.
125. Ostor AJ, Crisp AJ, Somerville MF, et al. Fatal exacerbation of rheumatoid arthritis associated fibrosing alveolitis in patients given infliximab. *BMJ* 2004;329:1266.
126. Lindsay K, Melsom R, Jacob BK, et al. Acute progression of interstitial lung disease: A complication of etanercept particularly in the presence of rheumatoid lung and methotrexate treatment. *Rheumatology (Oxford)* 2006;45:1048–1049.
127. Schoe A, van der Laan-Baalbergen NE, Huizinga TW, et al. Pulmonary fibrosis in a patient with rheumatoid arthritis treated with adalimumab. *Arthritis Rheum* 2006;55:157–159.
128. Ostor AJ, Chilvers ER, Somerville MF, et al. Pulmonary complications of infliximab therapy in patients with rheumatoid arthritis. *J Rheumatol* 2006;33:622–628.
129. Huggett MT, Armstrong R. Adalimumab-associated pulmonary fibrosis. *Rheumatology (Oxford)* 2006;45:1312–1313.
130. Yousem SA, Dacic S. Pulmonary lymphohistiocytic reactions temporally related to etanercept therapy. *Mod Pathol* 2005;18:651–655.
131. Roos JC, Chilvers ER, Ostor AJ. Interstitial pneumonitis and anti-tumor necrosis factor-alpha therapy. *J Rheumatol* 2007;34:238–239.
132. Hagiwara K, Sato T, Takagi-Kobayashi S, et al. Acute exacerbation of preexisting interstitial lung disease after administration of etanercept for rheumatoid arthritis. *J Rheumatol* 2007;34:1151–1154.
133. Gosset P, Perez T, Lassalle P, et al. Increased TNF-alpha secretion by alveolar macrophages from patients with rheumatoid arthritis. *Am Rev Respir Dis* 1991;143:593–597.
134. Miyazaki Y, Araki K, Vesin C, et al. Expression of a tumor necrosis factor-alpha transgene in murine lung causes lymphocytic and fibrosing alveolitis: A mouse model of progressive pulmonary fibrosis. *J Clin Invest* 1995;96:250–259.

135. Piguet PF, Vesin C. Treatment by human recombinant soluble TNF receptor of pulmonary fibrosis induced by bleomycin or silica in mice. *Eur Respir J* 1994;7:515–518.
136. Fujita M, Shannon JM, Morikawa O, et al. Overexpression of tumor necrosis factor-alpha diminishes pulmonary fibrosis induced by bleomycin or transforming growth factor-beta. *Am J Respir Cell Mol Biol* 2003;29:669–676.
137. Dugowson CE, Koepsell TD, Voigt LF, et al. Rheumatoid arthritis in women: Incidence rates in group health cooperative, seattle, washington, 1987–1989. *Arthritis Rheum* 1991;34:1502–1507.
138. Nelson JL, Ostensen M. Pregnancy and rheumatoid arthritis. *Rheum Dis Clin North Am* 1997;23:195–212.
139. Treacy G. Using an analogous monoclonal antibody to evaluate the reproductive and chronic toxicity potential for a humanized anti-TNFalpha monoclonal antibody. *Hum Exp Toxicol* 2000;19: 226–228.
140. Giroir BP, Peppel K, Silva M, et al. The biosynthesis of tumor necrosis factor during pregnancy: Studies with a CAT reporter transgene and TNF inhibitors. *Eur Cytokine Netw* 1992;3:533–538.
141. Katz JA, Antoni C, Keenan GF, et al. Outcome of pregnancy in women receiving infliximab for the treatment of crohn's disease and rheumatoid arthritis. *Am J Gastroenterol* 2004;99: 2385–2392.
142. Mahadevan U, Kane S, Sandborn WJ, et al. Intentional infliximab use during pregnancy for induction or maintenance of remission in crohn's disease. *Aliment Pharmacol Ther* 2005;21:733–738.
143. Chakravarty EF, Sanchez-Yamamoto D, Bush TM. The use of disease modifying antirheumatic drugs in women with rheumatoid arthritis of childbearing age: A survey of practice patterns and pregnancy outcomes. *J Rheumatol* 2003;30:241–246.
144. Chambers CD, Tutuncu ZN, Johnson D, et al. Human pregnancy safety for agents used to treat rheumatoid arthritis: Adequacy of available information and strategies for developing post-marketing data. *Arthritis Res Ther* 2006;8:215.
145. Roux CH, Brocq O, Breuil V, et al. Pregnancy in rheumatology patients exposed to anti-tumour necrosis factor (TNF)-alpha therapy. *Rheumatology (Oxford)* 2007;46:695–698.
146. Vesga L, Terdiman JP, Mahadevan U. Adalimumab use in pregnancy. *Gut* 2005;54:890.
147. Ostensen M, Eigenmann GO. Etanercept in breast milk. *J Rheumatol* 2004;31:1017–1018.
148. Furst DE, Breedveld FC, Kalden JR, et al. Updated consensus statement on biological agents for the treatment of rheumatic diseases, 2006. *Ann Rheum Dis* 2006;65(Suppl 3):iii2–iii15.
149. Kapetanovic MC, Saxne T, Sjoholm A, et al. Influence of methotrexate, TNF blockers and prednisolone on antibody responses to pneumococcal polysaccharide vaccine in patients with rheumatoid arthritis. *Rheumatology (Oxford)* 2006;45:106–111.
150. Kaine JL, Kivitz AJ, Birbara C, et al. Immune responses following administration of influenza and pneumococcal vaccines to patients with rheumatoid arthritis receiving adalimumab. *J Rheumatol* 2007;34:272–279.
151. Gelinck LB, van der Bijl AE, Beyer WE, et al. The effect of anti-tumor necrosis factor alpha treatment on the antibody response to influenza vaccination. *Ann Rheum Dis* 2008;67:713–716.
152. Kapetanovic MC, Saxne T, Nilsson JA, et al. Influenza vaccination as model for testing immune modulation induced by anti-TNF and methotrexate therapy in rheumatoid arthritis patients. *Rheumatology (Oxford)* 2007;46:608–611.
153. Edrees AF, Misra SN, Abdou NI. Anti-tumor necrosis factor (TNF) therapy in rheumatoid arthritis: Correlation of TNF-alpha serum level with clinical response and benefit from changing dose or frequency of infliximab infusions. *Clin Exp Rheumatol* 2005;23: 469–474.
154. van Vollenhoven R, Harju A, Brannemark S, et al. Treatment with infliximab (remicade) when etanercept (enbrel) has failed or vice versa: Data from the STURE registry showing that switching tumour necrosis factor alpha blockers can make sense. *Ann Rheum Dis* 2003;62:1195–1198.
155. Wick MC, Ernestam S, Lindblad S, et al. Adalimumab (humira) restores clinical response in patients with secondary loss of efficacy from infliximab (remicade) or etanercept (enbrel): Results from the STURE registry at karolinska university hospital. *Scand J Rheumatol* 2005;34:353–358.
156. Cohen G, Courvoisier N, Cohen JD, et al. The efficiency of switching from infliximab to etanercept and vice-versa in patients with rheumatoid arthritis. *Clin Exp Rheumatol* 2005;23:795–800.
157. Ang HT, Helfgott S. Do the clinical responses and complications following etanercept or infliximab therapy predict similar outcomes with the other tumor necrosis factor-alpha antagonists in patients with rheumatoid arthritis? *J Rheumatol* 2003;30:2315–2318.
158. van der Bijl AE, Goekoop-Ruiterman YP, de Vries-Bouwstra JK, et al. Infliximab and methotrexate as induction therapy in patients with early rheumatoid arthritis. *Arthritis Rheum* 2007;56:2129–2134.
159. Allaart CF, Goekoop-Ruiterman YP, de Vries-Bouwstra JK, et al. Aiming at low disease activity in rheumatoid arthritis with initial combination therapy or initial monotherapy strategies: The BeSt study. *Clin Exp Rheumatol* 2006;24:S77–S82.

IL-1 Inhibitors in the Treatment of Rheumatoid Arthritis

CHAPTER 10G

Peter C. Taylor

Cytokines are small, short-lived proteins and important mediators of local intercellular communication. They play a key role in integrating responses to a variety of stimuli in immune and inflammatory processes. By binding their cognate receptors on target cells in their immediate vicinity or at more distant sites, a coordinated network of these molecules participates in many important biologic activities—including cell proliferation, activation, death, and differentiation.[1] IL-1 is a proinflammatory cytokine involved in the cytokine network, with an important role in the process of inflammation and tissue damage. The biologic activity of IL-1 is mediated by two cytokines produced by two different genes, IL-1α and IL-1β. They both bind to the same receptors. IL-1α is an intracellular cytokine that predominantly acts locally within cells. IL-1β has a more prominent function. It is secreted from cells and plays a subsequent role both locally and systemically as a potent inflammatory mediator. IL-1α is rapidly induced in the inflammasome of macrophages and monocytes in response to autoimmune reactions, infection, or injury.[2] Release can also be stimulated by direct cell-to-cell contact with T cells at sites of inflammation.

Once secreted, IL-1 binds to one of three different receptors expressed as either membrane-bound or soluble proteins. Binding of IL-1 to IL-1 receptor type 1 (IL-1RI) induces the recruitment of IL-1 receptor accessory protein (IL-1RAcP) and downstream cell signal transduction. Such binding to receptors on the surface of synoviocytes, chondrocytes, and bone cells in the joint leads to tissue damage and inhibition of cartilage repair. The biologic action of IL-1β is regulated by endogenous anti-inflammatory mechanisms such as binding to soluble IL-1RI or the type II "decoy" receptor (IL-1RII), which has a short cytoplasmic domain and does not transduce any intracellular signal.[3] A different type of regulation is mediated by the IL-1 receptor antagonist (IL-1ra), a naturally occurring inhibitor of IL-1 that binds competitively to IL-1 receptors.[4] It is inducible in a wide range of cell types. IL-1ra potently inhibits the various effects of IL-1, and soluble IL-1ra has been identified as a marker of disease severity.[5] Furthermore, several studies have demonstrated that the ratio of IL-1ra to IL-1β is low in RA, contributing to the perpetuation of articular inflammation and subsequent tissue destruction.[6] It is important to note that a large molar excess of IL-1ra in the order of 10- to 100-fold is required to inhibit IL-1 activity *in vitro*.[7] Similarly, blockade of the systemic responses to IL-1 in animal models requires the pre-injection of 100- to 1000-fold molar excess of IL-1ra.[8]

Implicating IL-1 in the Pathogenesis of Inflammatory Arthritis

The possibility that IL-1 and TNF-α might be implicated in the pathogenesis of inflammation and joint damage in rheumatoid arthritis (RA) arose from a number of observations on tissues and cells *in vitro* that pointed to their proinflammatory properties. IL-1 and TNF-α were shown to stimulate production of prostaglandin E and collagenase.[9,10] Both cytokines were implicated in stimulating resorption of cartilage and inhibition of synthesis of proteoglycan.[11,12] The presence of IL-1, TNF-α, and other cytokines derived principally from macrophages and fibroblasts—including granulocyte-macrophage colony-stimulating factor (GM-CSF), interleukin-6 (IL-6), and numerous chemo-attractant cytokines known as chemokines—were demonstrated in rheumatoid synovial fluid and tissues.[1] Many of these factors are important in regulating inflammatory cell migration and activation.

IL-1β directly induces arthritis when injected into murine joints and is 100 times more potent than TNF-α in inhibiting proteoglycan synthesis.[12] IL-1α and IL-1β can induce bone and cartilage destruction in murine antigen-induced arthritis.[13] In collagen-induced arthritis, the dominance of IL-1β over IL-1α has been demonstrated using IL-1β knockout mice.[14,15] IL-1β stimulates resorption of cartilage and bone through activation of osteoclasts and inhibits synthesis of proteoglycan and articular collagen.[16] It is unclear whether the dramatic effect of TNF blockade on structural damage to joints in RA is a direct one or indirect through regulation of other mediators such as IL-1. In a recent series of elegant experiments in murine models of arthritis, the effects of IL-1 were removed from a TNF-mediated inflammatory joint disease by crossing IL-1α– and IL-1β–deficient mice (IL-1-/-) with arthritic human TNF-transgenic (hTNFtg) mice.[17] Development of synovial inflammation was almost unaffected by IL-1 deficiency. However, bone erosion and osteoclast formation were significantly reduced in IL-1-/-hTNFtg mice (compared with hTNFtg mice) as a result of an intrinsic differentiation defect in IL-1-deficient monocytes. Most strikingly, cartilage damage was absent in IL-1-/-hTNFtg mice. Chimera studies revealed that cartilage preservation was the result of the absence of IL-1 on hematopoietic, but not mesenchymal, cells. These data show that in the murine hTNFtg model TNF-mediated cartilage damage is completely dependent on IL-1 and that bone damage is partially dependent.[17]

Intravenous administration of rHuIL-1ra to rabbits can prevent the synovitis and proteoglycan loss induced by intraarticular injection of recombinant IL-1α.[18] Similarly, inhibition of IL-1 by IL-1ra (administered by the intraperitoneal route) ameliorates established murine collagen-II arthritis.[19] In contrast, similar IL-1ra treatment regimens have not diminished antigen-induced arthritis in rabbits.[20] However, when administered in high dose by continuous intraperitoneal infusion IL-1ra totally prevented inhibition of proteoglycan synthesis in the murine antigen-induced arthritis model—independently of any effects on articular inflammation.[16] These observations suggested that IL-1ra may predominantly affect proteoglycan breakdown, metalloproteinase release, and cartilage damage.

Studies in animal models of arthritis have demonstrated the therapeutic potential of IL-1 blockade.[21] The dominance of IL-1β over IL-1α in the pathogenesis of collagen-induced arthritis has been demonstrated in studies of cytokine blockade[22,23] and confirmed by the finding that IL-1β gene knockout mice show markedly reduced levels of inflammation following immunization with type II collagen. The use of genetically modified mice has also helped to confirm the physiologic significance of IL-1ra (deletion of this gene in BALB/c mice results in the spontaneous development of arthritis).[24]

Clinical Studies

Proof of principle for IL-1 blockade in RA has been established using once-daily subcutaneously administered IL-1 receptor antagonist (IL-1ra: anakinra), a naturally occurring inhibitor of IL-1.[25] IL-1ra has the greatest binding affinity for IL-1R1. The off rate is slow, and binding of IL-1ra to cell surface IL-1R1 is nearly irreversible. In a phase II placebo-controlled study, 472 patients received daily subcutaneous injections of placebo or one of three different doses of human IL-1ra (30, 75, or 150 mg). Improvements were observed in all individual clinical parameters, including swollen and tender joint counts, pain score, duration of early morning stiffness, patient assessment of disease activity, and investigator assessment of disease activity—although no clear dose-response relationship was observed. At the end of the study period, significantly more patients on the higher dosage schedule achieved improvement at the ACR 20% response level than placebo-treated patients. There were also significant reductions in erythrocyte sedimentation rate (ESR) in all active treatment groups.

Of 345 patients who completed the placebo-controlled phase of the study, 309 continued in a 52-week, multicenter, double-blind, parallel-group extension phase.[26] Patients received subcutaneous injections of anakinra (30, 75, or 150 mg) once daily. A total of 218 patients completed the extension phase. Of the 91 patients who withdrew prematurely, 46 did so following adverse events and 26 withdrew because of lack of efficacy. Among patients receiving anakinra who entered the extension phase, the level of improvement was maintained for 48 weeks. The ACR 20 response was 51% at week 24 and 46% at week 48, and this effect was consistent across all dose groups. At week 48, ACR 50 and ACR 70 responses were demonstrated in 18% and 3% of patients (respectively) who continued taking anakinra (all dose groups) and in 20% and 1% of patients (respectively) who were originally receiving placebo and then were randomized to all doses of anakinra.

The efficacy and safety of anakinra in combination with methotrexate has been tested in a multicenter randomized double-blind placebo-controlled trial.[27] In this study, patients with moderate to severely active RA despite methotrexate therapy for 6 consecutive months (with stable doses for more than 3 months) were randomized to receive either single daily placebo injections or one of five different doses of anakinra. At week 12, the ACR 20 responses in the five active treatment plus methotrexate groups demonstrated a statistically significant dose-response relationship over that in the placebo plus methotrexate group—and these responses were enduring through 24 weeks. The combination of anakinra and methotrexate was safe and well tolerated. Anakinra also improved the functional status of responding RA patients[28] and led to greater improvements in patient-reported than in physician-reported outcomes.[29]

Analysis of hand radiographs obtained at baseline at 24 and 48 weeks by two different methodologies in the double-blind placebo-controlled randomized trial of anakinra versus placebo injections as a monotherapy has led to claims of retardation of the rate of development of structural damage to joints in patients receiving active drug.[30] However, the radiologic scoring methods have differing sensitivities to change. This phenomenon was noted in all rHuIL-1ra dose groups, but only reached significance in patient groups receiving the two lower doses. This benefit continues with extended therapy for 48 weeks.

Hand radiographs from the same data set were subsequently evaluated using a modified Sharp method.[31] The mean change in the total modified Sharp score of 178 patients who completed 48 weeks of treatment with anakinra, including all dosages, was significantly less than the change observed in 58 patients who received placebo for 24 weeks and anakinra for 24 weeks ($p = 0.015$). A significant reduction in the change of the total modified Sharp score was observed in the patients who received anakinra 75 and 150 mg/day. The total modified Sharp score was reduced significantly more during the second 24-week treatment period, compared to the first ($p < 0.001$). Significant reductions in the second 24-week period were observed following anakinra 75 mg/day ($p = 0.006$) and 150 mg/day ($p = 0.008$).

The heterogeneity of presentation, disease course, and response to therapeutic intervention in RA raises the possibility that a syndrome with similar phenotypic features may be driven by differing proinflammatory cytokine pathways. If so, some patients failing to respond to TNF blockade might conceivably respond to IL-1 blockade. However, in a small study of 26 patients refractory to TNF inhibition only 2 achieved ACR 20 responses after 12 weeks of anakinra given at a dose of 100 mg daily.[32] This argues against a predominantly IL-1–driven disease as the major reason for failure to respond to anti-TNF treatment.

Tolerability and Safety Aspects of IL-1 RA

No serious adverse events attributed to treatment were reported in the dose-range and frequency study,[25] but injection site reactions were noted in approximately two-thirds of participants—causing 5% to withdraw from the trial. In the long-term extension of this study, anakinra was reported to be well tolerated for up to 76 weeks. The only side effects that appeared to be treatment related were skin reactions at the injection site. There was no evidence of decreased tolerance, an increased number of withdrawals, or an increased incidence of clinical complications associated with extended anakinra therapy.[26] In the anakinra plus methotrexate study,[27] neutropenia was observed in three patients treated with anakinra—the protocol requiring that patients withdraw from the study if absolute neutrophil counts fell below $2 \times 10^3/\mu l$. None of the patients developed clinical symptoms, and the neutrophil counts normalized in each case. There is one case report of reactivation of pulmonary tuberculosis after 23 months of treatment with anakinra in a patient with severe RA who has also received treatment with 10 mg prednisolone daily along with oral methotrexate 15 mg weekly.[33]

The safety profile of daily anakinra in patients with active RA and concurrent comorbid conditions has been investigated in the context of a placebo-controlled double-blind multicenter trial in which 1,414 patients from 169 centers in nine countries with active RA were randomly assigned to receive either anakinra (100 mg) or placebo treatment by daily injection (4:1 anakinra-to-placebo allocation ratio) for 6 months.[34] Patients were considered at high risk for the occurrence of adverse events if they had a history of at least one of the following: cardiovascular event, pulmonary event, central nervous system–related event, infection, diabetes, malignancy, or renal impairment. Although the majority of patients had one or more comorbid conditions, there were no differences in the incidence of serious adverse events or infectious events between treatment groups. The incidence of serious infectious events with anakinra use was similar between high-risk patients (2.5%) and the entire study population (2.1%) and was not attributable to any single comorbidity.

Anakinra in Combination with Other Anticytokine Therapies

The widespread use of conventional disease- modifying antirheumatic drugs (DMARDs) in combination with an apparent increase in efficacy without raising significant concerns related to toxicity or tolerability has prompted the investigation of combination anticytokine therapy.[35] The potential attractions of this approach include superior immunomodulation and hence enhanced efficacy. However, in a 24-week randomized controlled trial conducted in 242 patients with RA who had not previously been treated with biologic agents and were taking background methotrexate, the combination of etanercept 25 mg twice weekly together with anakinra 100 mg once daily resulted in an incidence of serious infection of 7% and the occurrence of neutropenia in the combination group. The incidence of both infection and neutropenia was higher in the combination group than in the Enbrel-alone group, and was higher than the rate observed in studies using anakinra alone. Furthermore, there was no therapeutic benefit of the combination treatment over etanercept alone. For this reason, the concomitant use of IL-1 blockade and TNF inhibitors is not recommended.[35]

Based of Anakinra Studies: Is IL-1 A Good Therapeutic Target in RA?

The overall magnitude of clinical responses and changes in acute-phase reactants in the anakinra trials were relatively modest, at 20% to 35% from baseline, compared with those reported for TNF-α blockade. In the United Kingdom, anakinra did not receive approval from the National Institute for Clinical Excellence for use in an RA indication.

The efficacy, safety, and drug survival of anakinra has also been investigated post-licensing in the setting of routine clinical practice.[36] All RA patients who started anakinra in six hospitals between May of 2002 and February of 2004 were included in a 2-year prospective, in part retrospective, cohort study. After 3 months, 55% of the patients (n = 146) showed a European League Against Rheumatism (EULAR) response (43% moderate, 12% good). A subset of patients continuing anakinra after 18 months had a sustained clinical response compared with patients who switched to other disease-modifying antirheumatic drug treatment (DAS 28 improvement, 2.46 versus 1.79). Drug survival was 78, 54, and only 14% after 3, 6, and 24 months, respectively. The reason for discontinuation was lack of efficacy in 78% and adverse events in 22%. Adverse events were reported 206 times in 111 patients, the most common being injection site reactions (36%). Serious adverse events occurred in 12% of the patients, with one classified as related. Therefore, despite the favorable safety profile of anakinra in both clinical practice and randomized clinical studies the drug survival after 2 years is low—largely due to lack of efficacy. These observations do not necessarily imply that IL-1 is not a good target for therapy in RA. Daily administration of anakinra is reported to have the benefit of disease modification, and based on the short-term efficacy of anakinra in clinical trials, the preclinical animal model data, and current understanding of the role of IL-1β in RA pathogenesis IL-1β remains an attractive therapeutic target. However, it may be that the strategies need to be adopted to efficiently achieve this because there are a number of significant pharmacokinetic challenges for IL-1ra as a means of achieving IL-1 blockade. For example, the kidneys excrete IL-1ra rapidly, and therapeutic levels persist for a few hours only. Furthermore, IL-1 receptors are ubiquitously expressed and have a rapid turnover. As previously noted, a very large molar excess of IL-1ra is required to block the systemic effects of IL-1 *in vivo*.

Alternative Strategies for Inhibition of IL-1

Although IL-1 blockade using anakinra in combination with methotrexate has been shown to be clinically superior to methotrexate therapy alone, the disappointing magnitude and durability of clinical efficacy compared with that seen with TNF inhibitors has prompted the exploration of alternative strategies for inhibition of IL-1.

Soluble IL-1 Receptor Therapy

An alternative approach to IL-1 inhibition in RA was tested in a randomized placebo-controlled trial of recombinant human IL-1RI.[37] No significant improvement was observed at 4 weeks after treatment, whether administered by subcutaneous or intra-articular injection. This finding may reflect the fact that soluble type I receptor binds IL-1ra with greater avidity than either IL-1α or IL-1α,[38] thus potentially inhibiting binding of IL-1ra to cell-surface IL-1 receptors.

Soluble IL-1RII concentrations are elevated in RA serum and synovial fluids, and soluble IL-1RII binds IL-1α with much higher affinity than it does IL-1ra (inhibiting the interaction between IL-1α and IL-1RI).[38,39] However, although the administration of soluble IL-1RII in experimental models results in a marked inhibition of joint swelling and joint damage and demonstrates a chondroprotective effect *in vitro*[40–42] clinical trials of soluble IL-1RII for the treatment of RA have been abandoned.[4]

IL-1 Trap

IL-1 trap is a fusion protein containing some of the extracellular binding motifs of IL-1RI and IL-1RAcP coupled to the Fc fraction the human IgG (Figure 10G-1). IL-1 trap binds IL-1β and IL-1α with high affinity, and binds IL-1β with a much stronger affinity than it binds IL-1Ra—such that administration of IL-1 trap should not affect the anti-inflammatory effect of endogenous IL-1Ra. Administration of a murine form of IL-1 trap almost completely blocks the development of collagen-induced arthritis.[43]

The efficacy of IL-1 trap was assessed in a phase I randomized dose-escalating double-blind placebo-controlled trial including four groups of 15 to 20 patients with active RA. After 6 weeks, ACR 20 responses were achieved by 74% of patients receiving the highest dose of IL-1 trap compared with 36% of placebo-treated patients.[44] However, in a subsequent multicenter randomized placebo-controlled double-blind phase II trial including 200 RA patients there was no significant effect—even in patients receiving the highest (100 mg weekly) dose of IL-1 trap.[4] In contrast, IL-1 trap has been used successfully in a few patients with periodic fever syndromes.[45]

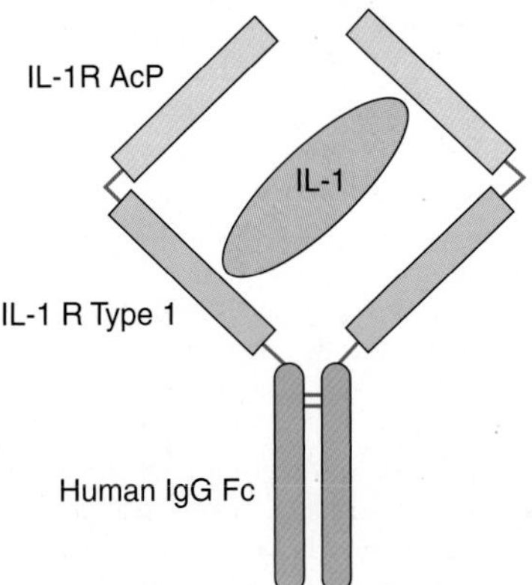

Figure 10G-1. IL-1 trap is a fusion protein containing some of the extracellular binding motifs of IL-1RI and IL-1RAcP coupled to the Fc fraction the human IgG. IL-1 trap binds IL-1β and IL-1α with high affinity.

Inhibition of IL-1β Production

A small-molecule approach to inhibition of IL-1 is to use drugs that specifically target enzymes involved in production of the cytokine such as caspase-1. Caspase-1 is responsible for cytoplasmic cleavage of an inactive precursor, 31-kDa pro-IL-1β, to generate mature bioactive 17kDa IL-1α. The same enzyme cleaves two other members (IL-18 and IL-33) of the IL-1 family of cytokines to produce the active forms.[46] Like IL-1, IL-18 plays an important role in experimental models of arthritis[47] and thus caspase-1 is viewed as a potential therapeutic target in RA. In support of this hypothesis, caspase-1 inhibitors inhibit the progression of murine collagen-induced arthritis.[48]

The efficacy of the caspase-1 inhibitor pralnacasan was investigated in a 12-week phase II placebo-controlled multicenter study in RA patients receiving concurrent disease-modifying antirheumatic drugs.[49] Disappointingly, ACR 20 responses were not significantly different in patients treated with pralnacasan from those in the placebo group. This finding may reflect the fact that other enzymes are also able to cleave pro-IL-1β and that caspase-1 does not influence the biologic effects of IL-1α.

Future Directions

Further potential approaches to the inhibition of IL-1α in RA include biologic therapies such as monoclonal antibodies targeting IL-1α. Results of future clinical trials with these monoclonal antibodies for an RA indication will be awaited with great interest. Alternative approaches to IL-1 inhibition in development include synthetic IL-1 receptor antagonists, antibodies to IL-1RI, and inhibitors of IL-1 signaling pathways (e.g., via MyD88- or IL-1R–associated kinase).

Conclusion

There is much evidence implicating Il-1 in the pathogenesis of RA, and in particular in the tissue destruction associated with joint disease. However, despite promising results in animal models anakinra displays limited efficacy in RA—even in combination therapy. This does not necessarily imply that IL-1 is an inappropriate therapeutic target in RA but might rather reflect the pharmacologic limitations of IL-1ra as an approach to IL-1 inhibition as evidenced by the immediate reversal of effects on cessation of treatment. By contrast, IL-1 blockade by anakinra is dramatically effective in systemic-onset juvenile idiopathic arthritis,[50] in adult Still's disease,[51] and in several autoinflammatory disorders—such as Muckle-Wells syndrome,[52,53] familial Mediterranean fever,[54] TNF receptor-associated periodic syndrome (TRAPS),[55] hyperimmunoglobulinemia D with periodic fever syndrome (HIDS),[56] and familial cold autoinflammatory syndrome.[57] With the exception of HIDS and TRAPS, these diseases are linked to mutations in proteins participating in the inflammasome complex. Future RA clinical trials employing new pharmacologic approaches to the inhibition of IL-1 may provide more clarity as to whether this targeted treatment approach has a clinical utility in the management of RA patients or in a defined subpopulation.

References

1. Feldmann M, Brennan FM, Maini RN. Role of cytokines in rheumatoid arthritis. *Ann Rev Immunol* 1996;14:397–440.
2. Petrilli V, Papin S, Tschopp J. The inflammasome. *Current Biology* 2005;15:R581.
3. Colotta F, Dower SK, Sims JE, et al. The type II "decoy" receptor: A novel regulatory pathway for interleukin 1. *Immunol Today* 1994; 15:562–566.
4. Burger D, Dayer JM, Palmer G, et al. Is IL-1 a good therapeutic target in the treatment of arthritis? *Best Pract Res Clin Rheumatol* 2006;2:879–896.
5. Prieur AM, Kaufmann MT, Griscelli G, et al. Specific interleukin-1 inhibitor in serum and urine of children with systemic juvenile chronic arthritis. *Lancet* 1987;2:1240–1242.
6. Deleuran BW, Chu CQ, Field M, et al. Localization of interleukin-1 alpha, type 1 interleukin-1 receptor and interleukin-1 receptor antagonist in the synovial membrane and cartilage/pannus junction in rheumatoid arthritis. *Br J Rheumatol* 1992;31:801–809.
7. Arend WP, Welgus HG, Thompson RC, et al. Biological properties of recombinant human monocyte-derived interleukin 1 receptor antagonist. *J Clin Invest* 1990;85:1694–1697.
8. Fischer E, Marano MA, Barber AE, et al. Comparison between effects of interleukin-1 alpha administration and sublethal endotoxemia in primates. *Am J Physiol* 1991;261:R442–R452.
9. Dayer JM, Beutler B, Cerami A. Cachectin/tumor necrosis factor stimulates collagenase and prostaglandin E2 production by human synovial cells and dermal fibroblasts. *J Exp Med* 1985;162: 2163–2168.
10. Dayer JM, de Rochemonteix B, Burrus B, et al. Human recombinant interleukin 1 stimulates collagenase and prostaglandin E2 production by human synovial cells and dermal fibroblasts. *J Exp Med* 1986;177:645–648.
11. Saklatvala J. Tumour necrosis factor α stimulates resorption and inhibits synthesis of proteoglycan in cartilage. *Nature* 1986;322: 547–549.
12. Pettipher ER, Higgs GA, Henderson B. Interleukin 1 induces leukocyte infiltration and cartilage proteoglycan degradation in the synovial joint. *Proc Natl Acad Sci U S A* 1986;83: 8749–8753.
13. van de Loo FAJ, Arntz OJ, Bakker AC, et al. Role of interleukin-1 in antigen-induced exacerbations of murine arthritis. *Am J Pathol* 1995;146:239–249.
14. Dinarello CA. Biologic basis for interleukin-1 in disease. *Blood* 1996;87:2095–2147.
15. Fantuzzi G, Dinarello CA. The inflammatory response in IL-1α deficient mice: Comparison with other cytokine-related knock-out mice. *J Leukocyte Biol* 1996;59:489–493.
16. van de Loo FAJ, Joosten LAB, van Lent PLEM, et al. Role of interleukin-1 tumor necrosis factor α, and interleukin-6 in cartilage proteoglycan metabolism and destruction: Effect of in situ blocking in murine antigen- and zymosan-induced arthritis. *Arthritis Rheum* 1995;38:164–172.
17. Zwerina J, Redlich K, Polzer K, et al. TNF-induced structural joint damage is mediated by IL-1. *Proc Natl Acad Sci U S A* 2007;104: 11742–11747.
18. Henderson B, Thompson RC, Hardingham T, et al. Inhibition of interleukin-1 induced synovitis and articular cartilage proteoglycan loss in the rabbit knee by recombinant human interleukin-1 receptor antagonist. *Cytokine* 1991;3:246–249.
19. van den Berg WB, Joosten LAB, Helsen M, et al. Amelioration of established murine collagen-induced arthritis with anti-IL-1 treatment. *Clin Exp Immunol* 1994;95:237–243.
20. Lewthwaite J, Blake SM, Hardingham TE, et al. The effect of recombinant human interleukin-1 receptor antagonist on the induction phase of antigen induced arthritis in the rabbit. *J Rheumatol* 1994; 21:467–472.
21. van den Berg WB. Arguments for interleukin 1 as a target in chronic arthritis. *Ann Rheum Dis* 2000;59(Suppl 1):i81–i84.
22. Joosten LA, Helsen MM, van de Loo FA, et al. Anticytokine treatment of established type II collagen-induced arthritis in DBA/1 mice: A comparative study using anti-TNF alpha, anti-IL-1 alpha/beta, and IL-1Ra. *Arthritis Rheum* 1996;39:797–809.
23. Williams RO, Marinova-Mutafchieva L, Feldmann M, et al. Evaluation of TNF-alpha and IL-1 blockade in collagen-induced arthritis and comparison with combined anti-TNF-alpha/anti-CD4 therapy. *J Immunol* 2000;165:7240–7245.
24. Horai R, Saijo S, Tanioka H, et al. Development of chronic inflammatory arthropathy resembling rheumatoid arthritis in interleukin 1 receptor antagonist-deficient mice. *J Exp Med* 2000;191:313–320.
25. Bresnihan B, Alvaro-Gracia JM, Cobby M, et al. Treatment of rheumatoid arthritis with recombinant human interleukin-1 receptor antagonist. *Arthritis Rheum* 1998;41:2196–2204.
26. Nuki G, Bresnihan B, Bear MB, et al. for the European Group of Clinical Investigators. Long-term safety and maintenance of clinical improvement following treatment with anakinra (recombinant human interleukin-1 receptor antagonist) in patients with rheumatoid arthritis: Extension phase of a randomized, double-blind, placebo-controlled trial. *Arthritis Rheum* 2002;46:2838–2846.
27. Cohen S, Hurd E, Cush J, et al. Treatment of rheumatoid arthritis with anakinra, a recombinant human interleukin-1 receptor antagonist, in combination with methotrexate: Results of a twenty-four-week, multicenter, randomized, double-blind, placebo-controlled trial. *Arthritis Rheum* 2002;46:614–624.
28. Cohen SB, Woolley JM, Chan W. Interleukin 1 receptor antagonist anakinra improves functional status in patients with rheumatoid arthritis. *J Rheumatol* 2003;30:225–231.
29. Cohen SB, Strand V, Aguilar D, et al. Patient- versus physician-reported outcomes in rheumatoid arthritis patients treated with recombinant interleukin-1 receptor antagonist (anakinra) therapy. *Rheumatology (Oxford)* 2004;43:704–711.
30. Jiang Y, Genant HK, Watt I, et al. A multicenter, double-blind, dose-ranging, randomised, placebo-controlled study of recombinant human interleukin-1 receptor antagonist in patients with rheumatoid arthritis: Radiologic progression and correlation of Genant and Larsen scores. *Arthritis Rheum* 2000;43:1001–1009.
31. Bresnihan B, Newmark R, Robbins S, et al. Effects of anakinra monotherapy on joint damage in patients with rheumatoid arthritis: Extension of a 24-week randomized, placebo-controlled trial. *J Rheumatol* 2004;31:1103–1111.
32. Buch MH, Bingham SJ, Seto Y, et al. Lack of response to anakinra in rheumatoid arthritis following failure of tumor necrosis factor alpha blockade. *Arthritis Rheum* 2004;50:725–758.
33. Settas LD, Tsimirikas G, Vosvotekas G, et al. Reactivation of pulmonary tuberculosis in a patient with rheumatoid arthritis during treatment with IL-1 receptor antagonists (anakinra). *J Clin Rheumatol* 2007;13:219–220.
34. Schiff MH, DiVittorio G, Tesser J, et al. The safety of anakinra in high-risk patients with active rheumatoid arthritis: Six-month observations of patients with comorbid conditions. *Arthritis Rheum* 2004;50:1752–1760.
35. Genovese MC, Cohen S, Moreland L, et al. Combination therapy with etanercept and anakinra in the treatment of patients with rheumatoid arthritis who have been treated unsuccessfully with methotrexate. *Arthritis Rheum* 2004;50:1412–1419.
36. den Broeder AA, de Jong E, Franssen MJ, et al. Observational study on efficacy, safety, and drug survival of anakinra in rheumatoid arthritis patients in clinical practice. *Ann Rheum Dis* 2006;65:760–762.
37. Drevlow BE, Lovis R, Haag MA, et al. Recombinant human interleukin-1 receptor type I in the treatment of patients with active rheumatoid arthritis. *Arthritis Rheum* 1996;39:257–265.

38. Arend WP, Malyak M, Smith MF Jr., et al. Binding of IL-1α, IL-1β, and IL-1 receptor antagonist by soluble IL-1 receptors and levels of soluble IL-1 receptors in synovial fluids. *J Immunol* 1994;153: 4766–4774.
39. Burger D, Chicheportiche R, Giri JG, et al. The inhibitory activity of human interleukin-1 receptor antagonist is enhanced by type II interleukin-1 soluble receptor and hindered by type I interleukin-1 soluble receptor. *J Clin Invest* 1995;96:38–41.
40. Dawson J, Engelhardt P, Kastelic T, et al. Effects of soluble interleukin-1 type II receptor on rabbit antigen-induced arthritis: Clinical, biochemical and histological assessment. *Rheumatology (Oxford)* 1999;38:401–406.
41. Bessis N, Guery L, Mantovani A, et al. The type II decoy receptor of IL-1 inhibits murine collagen-induced arthritis. *E J Immunol* 2001; 30:867–875.
42. Attur MG, Dave MN, Leung MY, et al. Functional genomic analysis of type II IL-1beta decoy receptor: Potential for gene therapy in human arthritis and inflammation. *J Immunol* 2002;168:2001–2010.
43. Economides AN, Carpenter LR, Rudge JS, et al. Cytokine traps: multi-component, high-affinity blockers of cytokine action. *Nat Med* 2003;9:47–52.
44. Guler HP, Caldwell J, Littlejohn T, et al. A phase I, single dose escalation study of IL-1 Trap in patients with rheumatoid arthritis. *Arthritis Rheum* 2001;44:S370.
45. Canna S, Gelabert A, Aksentijevich I, et al. Treatment of 4 patients with cryopyrin-associated periodic syndromes with the long-acting IL-1 inhibitor Il-1 trap. *Arthritis Rheum* 2005;52:S274.
46. Schmitz J, Owyang A, Oldham E, et al. IL-33, an interleukin-1-like cytokine that signals via the IL-1 receptor-related protein ST2 and induces T helper type 2-associated cytokines. *Immunity* 2005;23: 479–490.
47. Plater-Zyberk C, Joosten LA, Helsen MM, et al. Therapeutic effect of neutralizing endogenous IL-18 activity in the collagen-induced model of arthritis. *J Clin Invest* 2001;108:1825–1832.
48. Ku G, Faust T, Lauffer LL, et al. Interleukin-1 beta converting enzyme inhibition blocks progression of type II collagen-induced arthritis in mice. *Cytokine* 1996;8;377–386.
49. Pavelka K, Rasmussen MJ, Mikkelsen K, et al. Clinical effects of palnacasan (PRAL), an orally-active interleukin-1 beta converting enzyme (ICE) inhibitor, in a 285 patient phase II trial in rheumatoid arthritis. *Arthritis Rheum* 2002;46:LB02.
50. Pascual V, Allantaz F, Arce E, et al. Role of interleukin-1 (IL-1) in the pathogenesis of systemic onset juvenile idiopathic arthritis and clinical response to IL-1 blockade. *J Exp Med* 2005;201:1479–1486.
51. Fitzgerald AA, Leclercq SA, Yan A, et al. Rapid responses to anakinra in patients with refractory adult-onset Still's disease. *Arthritis Rheum* 2005;52:1794–1803.
52. Hawkins PN, Lachmann HJ, McDermott MF. Interleukin-1-receptor antagonist in the Muckle-Wells syndrome. *N Engl J Med* 2003;348: 2583–2584.
53. Hawkins PN, Lachmann HJ, Aganna E, et al. Spectrum of clinical features in Muckle-Wells syndrome and response to anakinra. *Arthritis Rheum* 2004;50:607–612.
54. Shoham NG, Centola M, Mansfield E, et al. Pyrin binds the PSTPIP1/ CD2BP1 protein, defining familial Mediterranean fever and PAPA syndrome as disorders in the same pathway. *Proc Natl Acad Sci U S A* 2003;100:13501–13506.
55. Simon A, Bodar EJ, van der Hilst JC, et al. Beneficial response to interleukin 1 receptor antagonist in traps. *Am J Med* 2004;117: 208–210.
56. Arkwright PD, McDermott MF, Houten SM, et al. Hyper IgD syndrome (HIDS) associated with in vitro evidence of defective monocyte TNFRSF1A shedding and partial response to TNF receptor blockade with etanercept. *Clin Exp Immunol* 2002;130:484–488.
57. Hoffman HM, Rosengren S, Boyle DL, et al. Prevention of cold-associated acute inflammation in familial cold autoinflammatory syndrome by interleukin-1 receptor antagonist. *Lancet* 2004;364: 1779–1785.

Abatacept

Sara Kaprove Penn and Larry W. Moreland

Rheumatoid arthritis (RA) is a prevalent autoimmune disease characterized primarily by inflammatory arthritis which, if left untreated, can ultimately lead to joint destruction. Adaptive immunity, including the interaction between T and B lymphocytes, is critically important in driving the process of synovitis.[1,2] By understanding the pathophysiology of the disease, one can design specific treatments to halt or diminish its progression.

The field of RA treatment has grown immensely over the past decade, with the introduction of the molecule-driven biologic treatments—including TNF-α inhibitors, an IL-1 antagonist, and most recently inhibitors of T- and B-cell function.

Abatacept (CTLA-4Ig), an inhibitor of T-cell co-stimulation, was approved by the U.S. FDA for the treatment of RA in December of 2006. This chapter reviews its role in the immunologic interaction between T cells and antigen-presenting cells (APCs), *in vitro* studies showing its down-regulation of T-cell activity, animal studies showing its effectiveness in reducing autoimmunity, and phase II and III clinical trials looking at both effectiveness and safety of abatacept in the treatment of RA.

Rheumatoid Arthritis Pathophysiology

It is well known that the synovium of patients with RA contains many types of cells, including macrophages, fibroblasts, CD4+ and CD8+ T lymphocytes, B lymphocytes, dendritic cells, and other types of APCs. The presence of activated T cells, predominantly CD4+, and proinflammatory cytokines (IL-1, IL-6, and TNF-α) perpetuates the immune response.

Lymphocytes invade the synovium and are the predominant cell type, although interaction with other cell types is critical for supporting the process of chronic inflammation. Through this interaction, activated T cells lead to structural organization of lymphoid tissue, angiogenesis, production of inflammatory cytokines, induction of synoviocyte proliferation (leading to pannus formation), and osteoclastogenesis resulting in bone loss.[3] These mechanisms, when occurring together, ultimately lead to joint destruction and loss of function.

T-Cell Costimulation and the Mechanism of Action of Abatacept

Naive T cells require at least two signals to become activated. The first is an antigen-specific signal between the T-cell receptor (TCR) and the HLA-antigen complexes on the APC. There are likely many different "second" or "costimulatory" signals, consisting of an interaction between specific receptors on the T cell and their ligands on the APC.[4] The best known of these is an interaction between CD28 on T cells and CD80 and CD86, also known as B7-1 and B7-2, which are expressed only on professional APCs[5,6] (Figure 10H-1). CD80 and CD86 have different expression on APCs (i.e., CD86 is constitutively expressed and CD80 expression is induced following more prolonged T-cell stimulation),[7] but both molecules seem to be important in the continued activation of T cells.

Costimulation of the T cell induces specific gene transcription and enhances paracrine secretion of cytokines, including IL-2—a critical T-cell growth factor.[7,8] Both signals are necessary to activate T cells to enter the cell cycle and undergo clonal expansion, rapidly producing antigen-specific T cells and generating memory T cells.[7] These antigen-specific effector T cells in turn generate proinflammatory cytokines, including TNF-α and INF-γ. Antigen recognition in the absence of CD28 costimulation results in partial activation and induces T-cell anergy, a reversible state of T-cell nonresponsiveness. CD28 is constitutively expressed on naive CD4+ T cells and is slightly upregulated after T-cell activation. CD28 signals promote T-cell differentiation into T-helper cells (Th1) and increases B-cell activity (i.e., production of antibodies) and the proliferation of activated T cells.

T cells have a mechanism to turn off uncontrolled T-cell activation. Activated T cells up-regulate cell surface expression of cytotoxic-T-lymphocyte-associated protein 4 (CTLA-4). CTLA-4 is not present on resting T cells, but surface expression of it peaks about 48 to 72 hours after T-cell stimulation. CTLA-4 is a competitive inhibitor of CD28, with which it shares approximately 30% homology, and binds CD80 and CD86 with much higher avidity than does CD28—thus allowing down-regulation of the T-cell activity (Figure 10H-2). Engagement of CTLA-4 on CD80/86 inhibits T-cell activation, resulting in reduced IL-2 and IL-2 receptor expression and leading to arrest of the cell cycle.

Based on the aforementioned information, it made sense to study this protein as a potential therapy for diseases in which T cells are central to the pathogenesis—such as transplant rejection and RA. CTLA-4Ig (abatacept) was designed to be this therapeutic molecule. Abatacept is a fusion protein developed to modulate the T-cell costimulatory signal that is mediated through the CD28-CD80/86 pathway. It consists of the extracellular binding domain of CTLA-4 fused to the heavy-chain

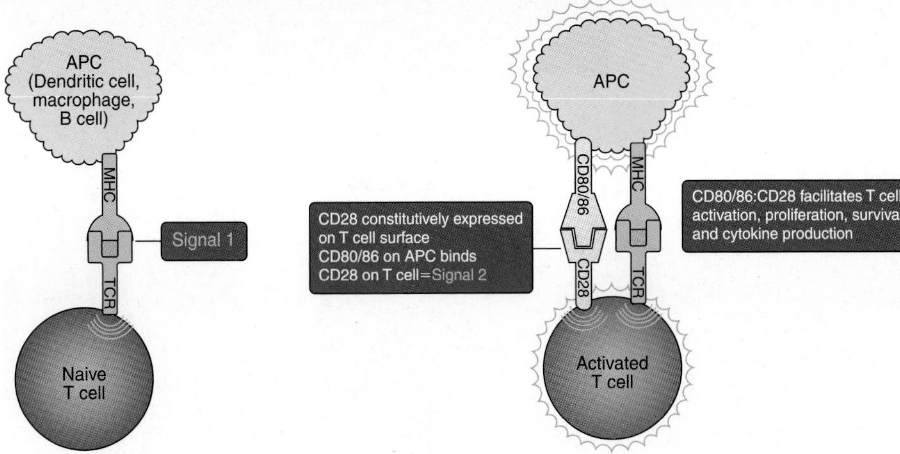

Figure 10H-1. T-cell activation requires two signals. After engagement of the T-cell receptor with the MHC-antigen complex processed by APCs (first signal), a second signal is transmitted by CD28 that interacts with either CD80 or CD86 ligands on APCs—leading to complete T-cell activation and proliferation. *APC:* antigen-presenting cell; *MHC:* major histocompatability complex; *TCR:* T-cell receptor. (Reprinted with permission from Teng GG, Turkiewicz AM, Moreland LW. Abatacept: A costimulatory inhibitor for treatment of rheumatoid arthritis. *Expert Opin Biol Ther* 2005;5(9):1247.)

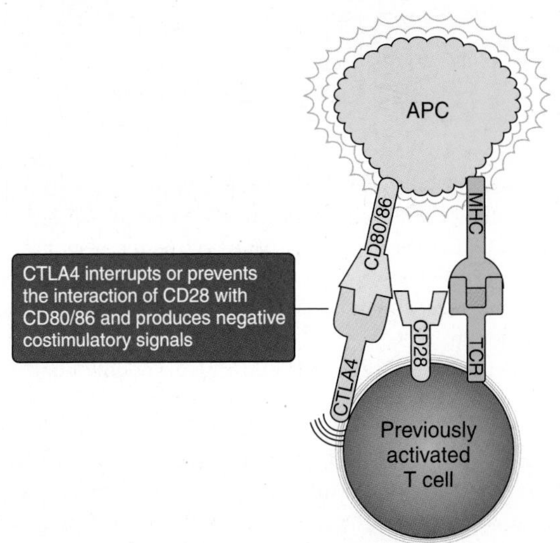

Figure 10H-2. Endogenous CTLA4 binds to CD80/86 with higher avidity than CD28 and down-regulates CD28-mediated T-cell activation. *APC:* antigen-presenting cell; *CTLA:* cytotoxic T lymphocyte antigen; *MHC:* major histocompatability complex; *TCR:* T-cell receptor. (Reprinted with permission from Teng GG, Turkiewicz AM, Moreland LW. Abatacept: A costimulatory inhibitor for treatment of rheumatoid arthritis. *Expert Opin Biol Ther* 2005;5(9):1248.)

constant region of human IgG1 (Figure 10H-3). The addition of the IgG1 domain solubilizes the CTLA-4 domain, creating a soluble receptor for CD80/C86. Abatacept binds CD80 on APCs with much higher avidity than does CD28, thus inhibiting CD28 signaling (Figure 10H-4). It does not bind CD86 as well (a second ligand for CD28), but still with much higher avidity than does CD28. The binding of abatacept to CD80/86 down-regulates T-cell proliferation and inhibits humoral immune responses.

Belatacept

Abatacept was first clinically established as a T-cell costimulation inhibitor in studies of organ transplant rejection. Although showing promise in animal models, it was not that effective in primate transplant models.[9] LEA29Y, now known as belatacept, is a second-generation CTLA-4Ig designed to bind to CD80 and CD86 more strongly than abatacept. This has been shown to be more effective in the immunosuppression necessary for transplant rejection.[10] A study was conducted comparing belatacept with cyclosporine to prevent transplant rejection in renal transplant recipients. The study confirmed non-inferiority to cyclosporine in 12-month follow-up data.

Animal Studies

There have been many animal studies investigating the role of T-cell costimulation on outcomes of immune function. Some researchers have used human CTLA-4Ig, whereas others have used antibodies against CTLA-4 or CTLA-4 knockout mice, to prove that CTLA-4 function is imperative for down-regulation of the T-cell response.

In vivo, treatment of mice with anti-CTLA-4 monoclonal antibody (mAb) boosts immunity and exacerbates autoimmunity—whereas treatment with CTLA-4Ig prevents its development. Perrin et al.[8,11] studied a murine model of experimental allergic encephalomyelitis (EAE), a demyelinating condition similar to multiple sclerosis—induced in these mice by vaccination with myelin and myelin constituents. They injected these mice with anti-CTLA-4 mAb at different times and observed the resulting T-cell activity. If given the anti-CTLA-4 mAb 2 days post-vaccination, there was mildly enhanced disease. If given the anti-CTLA-4 mAb after the onset of clinical symptoms, disease was markedly exacerbated—suggesting that CTLA-4 plays an important role in regulating T-cell activity, even after disease has been established.

Rodent models of collagen-induced arthritis (CIA) have also been used to study blockade of the CD28 costimulatory pathway. Webb et al.[12] administered CTLA-4Ig to these mice at the time of immunization and found that this prevented the development of CIA. Another observation from animal studies is that CLTA-4 knockout mice have hyperlymphoproliferative disease and do not survive beyond a few weeks.

As mentioned previously, CTLA-4 ligation to CD80 in the context of T-cell activation blocks cytokine production and cell cycle progression. This is known as the ligand competition model, and assumes that CTLA-4 inhibition occurs downstream of the initial T-cell activation. CTLA-4 also acts more proximally in the process of inhibiting T-cell activation, and does not need

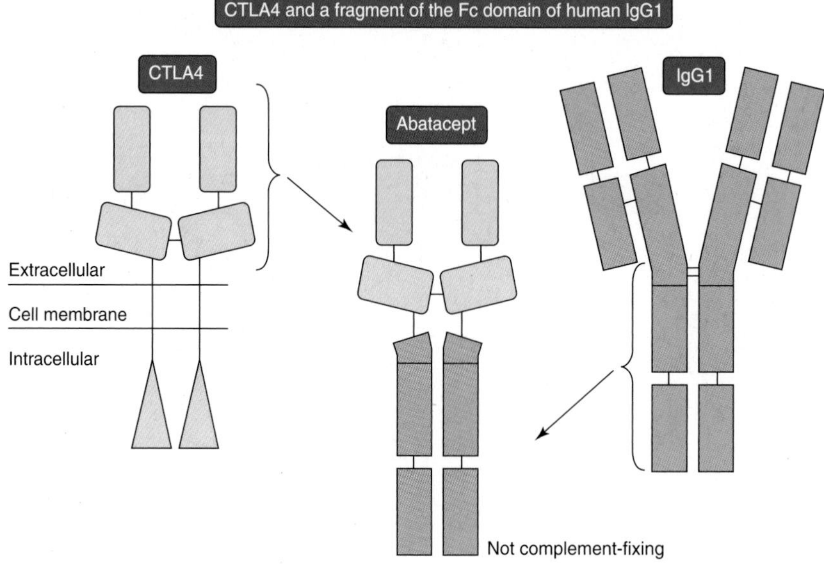

Figure 10H-3. Structure of abatacept. Abatacept consists of an extracellular domain of human CTLA4 fused to the heavy-chain constant region of human IgG1. *CTLA,* cytotoxic T lymphocyte antigen. (Reprinted with permission from Teng GG, Turkiewicz AM, Moreland LW. Abatacept: A costimulatory inhibitor for treatment of rheumatoid arthritis. *Expert Opin Biol Ther* 2005;5(9):1249.)

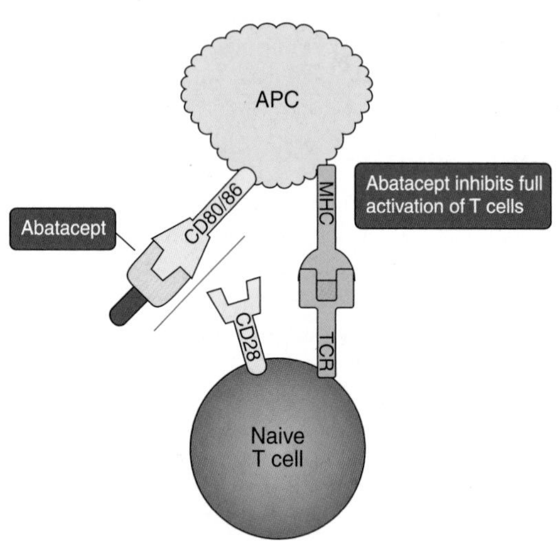

Figure 10H-4. Abatacept: mechanism of action. Abatacept binds to CD80/86 and inhibits T-cell costimulation. *APC,* antigen-presenting cell; *MHC,* major histocompatability complex; *TCR,* T-cell receptor. (Reprinted with permission from Teng GG, Turkiewicz AM, Moreland LW. Abatacept: A costimulatory inhibitor for treatment of rheumatoid arthritis. *Expert Opin Biol Ther* 2005;5(9):1249.)

to bind to B7 in order to do so. Chikuma et al. used murine models to show that expression of a B7-nonbinding CTLA-4 mutant inhibited T-cell proliferation and cytokine production in otherwise CTLA-4-deficient T cells,[13] suggesting that CLTA-4 has more than one role in the inhibition of T-cell activation.

Clinical Trials Evaluating Abatacept

Phase I

The first study evaluating abatacept in humans was conducted in patients with psoriasis. Abrams et al. investigated the role of the CD28/CTLA-4 pathway in psoriasis in a 6-month open-label dose-escalation study.[14,15] In this study, 43 patients received four infusions of abatacept at doses ranging from 0.5 to 50 mg/kg. 46% of patients achieved a 50% response rate (physician global assessment of disease activity), showing better response with higher dose. A favorable safety profile was found. These data suggest that abatacept may be effective in immunomodulation of T-cell function.

Moreland et al. subsequently performed a double-blind dose-finding placebo-controlled trial using abatacept and belatacept in RA patients who failed at least one disease-modifying antirheumatic drug (DMARD) or etanercept. A total of 214 RA patients were given four infusions of the drug at a variety of doses (0.5, 2, or 10 mg/kg). Effectiveness was evaluated at day 85. ACR 20 responses increased in a dose-dependent manner (23%, 44%, and 53% respectively for abatacept, and 34%, 45%, and 61%, respectively, for belatacept, vs. 31% in placebo).[16] The drugs were well tolerated at all dose levels, although headache was more prevalent at higher doses.

Phase II

A phase IIb 12-month randomized double-blind placebo-controlled study was conducted using CTLA-4Ig in 339 patients with RA that had remained active despite methotrexate therapy.[17,18] They were randomized to receive 2 mg/kg, 10 mg/kg, or placebo, in addition to continuation of the methotrexate. Of those who received 10 mg/kg, 62.6%, 41.7%, and 20.9% achieved ACR 20, ACR 50, and ACR 70 responses, respectively—compared with 36.1%, 20.2%, and 7.6% (respectively) of those who received placebo, which were all statistically significant. The difference in response rates between the group that received 2 mg/kg and placebo was not statistically significant. A separate analysis was performed showing that the use of abatacept led to a reduction in inflammatory biomarker response in these patients with RA.[19] Following 12 months of treatment, serum levels of IL-6, soluble IL-2 receptor, C-reactive protein, soluble E-selectin, and soluble intercellular adhesion molecule 1 were significantly lower in patients receiving abatacept 10 mg/kg versus placebo—supporting the biologic effect of this therapy.

Given the current age of biologic therapy, it was also important to study the combination of abatacept with a TNF-α inhibitor. A phase II study using abatacept in patients with active RA while receiving etanercept was performed.[20] A total of 121 patients continued etanercept and were randomized to receive abatacept at 2 mg/kg or placebo. At 6 months and 12 months, the ACR 20 response was not significantly different between groups (48.2% vs. 30.6%, $p = 0.072$). At the 1-year point, 80 patients entered a long-term extension of the trial and they all received abatacept at 10 mg/kg in combination with etanercept. Again, there was no significant difference in the ACR 20 response. More serious adverse events were experienced by the patients receiving combination treatment (16.5% vs. 2.8%).

Phase III

A 1-year international multicenter randomized double-blind placebo-controlled trial was conducted involving 652 patients with active RA despite methotrexate treatment. This Abatacept in Inadequate Responders to Methotrexate (AIM) trial compared once-monthly infusions of abatacept 10 mg/kg with placebo[21] using ACR 20 at 6 months, physical function measures (HAQ-DI), and change from baseline in joint erosion score at 1 year as co-primary outcomes. The patients had to have been on ≧15 mg/week of methotrexate for at least 3 months, and they were continued on methotrexate throughout the duration of the study. There was a 28-day washout of other DMARDs before randomization. Patients had to have met the American Rheumatology Assocation (ARA) criteria for RA and have ≧10 swollen joints, ≧12 tender joints, and c-reactive protein (CRP) levels ≧10 mg/liter. Prednisone ≤10 mg/day and NSAIDs at stable doses were allowed. At the end of 6 months, the ACR 20, ACR 50, and ACR 70 scores were higher in the abatacept group compared to placebo (e.g., ACR 20 67.9% vs. 39.7%, $p < 0.001$). Between 6 and 12 months, all ACR responses continually improved in patients receiving abatacept—whereas responses for patients receiving placebo were essentially unchanged from month 6. Physical function improvement was better in the abatacept group as well. Last, less radiographic progression from baseline was observed in the abatacept group—measured by erosion score and joint space narrowing. At 1 year, there was an approximately 50% reduction in change from baseline in Genant-modified Sharp scores compared with that of placebo. The overall incidence of adverse events was similar in both treatment groups. There were more infusion reactions in the abatacept group. The incidence of infection reported as a serious adverse event was higher with abatacept than with placebo (2.5% vs. 0.9%). The incidence of neoplasm was similar in both groups.

A 6-month randomized double-blind placebo-controlled trial was conducted in patients with active RA with an inadequate response to ≧3 months of anti–TNF-α therapy. In the Abatacept Trial in Treatment of Anti-TNF Inadequate Responders (ATTAIN) trial,[22] 391 patients were randomized to receive either abatacept 10 mg/kg or placebo at 1-month intervals. Patients had to meet ACR criteria for RA and have had RA for ≧1 year—with an inadequate response to infliximab, etanercept, or both after ≧3 months of treatment. Both current and former users of TNF-α inhibitors were included. All users were required to stop anti-TNF-α therapy during a washout period before undergoing randomization. At randomization, patients had to have ≧10 swollen joints, ≧12 tender joints, and CRP levels ≧1 mg/dL. Patients had to have been taking an oral DMARD or anakinra for ≧3 months at a stable dose. Prednisone at stable doses ≦10 mg/day was allowed. Primary outcome measures were ACR 20 response and improvement in HAQ score. Secondary outcome measures were ACR 50 and ACR 70 at 6 months. At 6 months, the rate of ACR 20, ACR 50, and ACR 70 were all significantly higher in the abatacept group versus placebo (ACR 20 50.4% vs. 19.5%, $p < 0.001$). The difference was noted as early as day 15, and the ACR responses in the abatacept group progressively increased during the duration of the trial. This result was consistent among both current and former users of anti-TNF-α therapy. Rates of remission (DAS 28 <2.6) were significantly higher in the abatacept group than in the placebo group (10.0% vs. 0.8%, $p < 0.001$). The rates of adverse events, discontinuation due to adverse events, and serious infections were similar in both groups. Infections were more frequent in the abatacept group than in the placebo group, but this was not statistically significant (37.6% vs. 32.3%, $p = 0.30$). In addition, abatacept treatment did not increase the risk of inducing ANA or anti-dsDNA. Again, acute infusion reactions were more commonly seen in the abatacept group (5% vs. 3%, $p = 0.35$)—with dizziness and headache occurring most commonly. Antibodies against abatacept developed in 1.3% of patients, all with low-level activity.

The Abatacept Study of Safety in Use with Other RA Therapies (ASSURE) trial[23] was a 1-year multinational/multicenter randomized double-blind placebo-controlled trial designed to assess the safety of abatacept at 10 mg/kg compared with placebo in 1,441 patients with active RA concurrently on one or more of the traditional nonbiologic and/or biologic DMARDs. The patients had to be on the DMARD(s) for at least 3 months prior to entry into the study, with a stable dose in the previous 28 days. To be entered into the trial, patients had to meet ACR criteria for RA and had to have active disease despite receiving background DMARDs and/or biologic therapy. Patient global assessment of disease activity measured by visual analog scale (VAS) had to be ≧20 mm at the time of screening and randomization. Patients with stable chronic medical conditions such as CHF, asthma, COPD, and diabetes mellitus (DM) were included. Primary outcome measures were the occurrence of adverse events, serious adverse events, discontinuation due to adverse events, death, clinically significant changes in vital signs, physical examination abnormalities, and clinical laboratory test abnormalities. Efficacy outcomes were secondary measures in this study. Of the 1,441 patients treated in this study, 1,231 completed 1 year of double-blind treatment. Results were presented according to background DMARD (i.e., biologic vs. nonbiologic).

Overall, the abatacept group was similar to the placebo group in terms of incidence of adverse events (90% vs. 87%), serious adverse events (SAEs) (13% vs. 12%), and severe or very severe adverse events (16% vs. 15%). Discontinuations due to adverse events were also similar in both groups (5% vs. 4%). There were five deaths (0.5%) in the abatacept group and four deaths (0.8%) in the placebo group. Seven of the nine deaths were not thought to be related to the study drug, one cause was unknown, and one in the placebo arm was due to pneumocystis pneumonia (PNP). Regardless of their treatment arm, patients who were receiving background nonbiologic DMARD therapy had similar rates of adverse events and SAEs. Those who were receiving background biologic therapy, however, did not have similar results. In this group, those receiving abatacept had more adverse events than those receiving placebo (95.1% vs. 89.1%) and had more SAEs (22.3% vs. 12.5%).

Infections were the most common adverse event in either group. The most frequent infections, including upper respiratory (URI) and nasopharyngitis, occurred at similar rates in both groups. Less than 4% of patients in each group had a severe or very severe infection, but infections that were life threatening, those resulting in hospitalization, or those resulting in death occurred more frequently in the abatacept group (2.9% vs. 1.9%). Interestingly, those patients in the abatacept group receiving background biologic therapy had more serious infections than the placebo group (5.8% vs. 1.6%)—whereas those patients in the abatacept group who received background nonbiologic DMARDs had a similar pattern, but a less substantial difference (2.6% vs. 1.7%).

The efficacy data were similar to that in the other clinical trials. That is, patients in the abatacept group did better than those in the placebo group—with those on background nonbiologic therapy having better results than those on background biologic therapy.

What Have We Learned?

Efficacy

All of the clinical trials in RA using abatacept in combination with a nonbiologic DMARD support its clinical efficacy using a 10-mg/kg 30-minute infusion on days 1, 15, and 29 (and every 28 days thereafter). The studies combining abatacept with an anti–TNF-α agent do not show any difference in efficacy.

Safety

In the three phase III trials, the rates of adverse events were similar between the treatment and placebo groups except in those patients taking both abatacept and an anti–TNF-α agent—in which there was an increase in the frequency of SAEs (particularly infections). Abatacept should therefore not be used in combination with other biologic agents. The main side effects noted with abatacept were infusion reactions, headaches, and nausea. There was a slightly higher rate of infection compared to placebo, most commonly URI and pharyngitis.

Recommendations

With the information known, first-line treatment for newly diagnosed RA remains single or combination DMARD therapy due to their long-standing use and favorable safety profile. If, however, there is lack of efficacy or partial response to treatment one could add abatacept in combination with the DMARD. At this point in time, most clinicians would first add an anti–TNF-α agent in combination with the DMARD. If that combination is not effective, they could either change to a different anti–TNF-α agent or stop the anti–TNF-α agent and add abatacept.

It is important to note that there are no published data following patients beyond 12 months of treatment, and thus long-term efficacy and safety are not clear. All of the clinical trials published thus far have studied the use of abatacept in combination with another DMARD in patients with established RA. There are currently ongoing clinical trials evaluating the safety and effectiveness of abatacept in early RA, the results of which will hopefully guide us further in making treatment decisions for these patients.

References

1. Choy E and GS Panayi. Cytokine pathoways and joint inflammation in rheumatoid arthritis. *N Engl J Med* 2001;344:907–916.
2. Vincenti F, Luggen M. T cell costimulation: A rational target in the therapeutic armamentarium for autoimmune diseases and transplantation. *Annu Rev Med* 2007;58:347–358.
3. Weyand CM, Goronzy JJ. T-cell–targeted therapies in rheumatoid arthritis. *Nat Clin Pract* 2006;2:201–210.
4. Bluestone JA, St. Clair EW, Turka LA. CTLA4Ig: Bridging the basic immunology with clinical application. *Immunity* 2006;24: 233–238.
5. Brunner-Weinzierl MC, Hoff H, Burmester G-R. Multiple functions for CD28 and cytotoxic T lymphocyte antigen-4 during different phases of T cell responses: Implications for arthritis and autoimmune diseases. *Arthritis Res Ther* 2004;6:45–54.
6. Sharpe AH, Abbas AK. T-cell costimulation: Biology, therapeutic potential, and challenges. *N Engl J Med* 2006;355:973–975.
7. Salomon B, Bluestone JA. Complexities of CD28/B7: CTLA-4 co-stimulatory pathways in autoimmunity and transplantation. *Ann Rev Immunol* 2001;19:225–252.
8. Perrin PJ, Maldanado JH, Davis TA, et al. CTLA-4 blockade enhances clinical disease and cytokine production during experimental allergic encephalomyelitis. *J Immunol* 1996;157:1333–1336.
9. Larsen CP, Pearson TC, Adams AB, et al. Rational developtment of LEA29Y (belatacept), a high-affinity variant of CTLA4-Ig with potent immunosuppressive properties. *Am J Transplant* 2005;5:443–453.
10. Vincenti F, Larsen C, Durrbach A, et al. Costimulation blockard with belatacept in renal transplantation. *N Engl J Med* 2005;353: 770–781.
11. Perrin PJ, June CH, Maldanado JH, et al. Blockade of CD28 during in vitro activation of encephalitogenic T cells or after disease onset ameliorates experimental autoimmune encephalomyelitis. *J Immunol* 1999;163:1704–1710.
12. Webb MC, Walmsley MJ, Feldmann M. Prevention and amelioration of collagen-induced arthritis by blockade of CD28 co-stimulatory pathway: Requirement for both B7-1 and By-2. *Eur J Immunol* 1996;26:2320–2328.
13. Chikuma S, Abbas AK, Bluestone JA. B7-independent inhibition of T cells by CTLA-4. *J Immunol* 2005;175:177–181.
14. Abrams JR, Kelley SL, Hayes E, et al. Blockade of T lymphocyte costimulation with cytotoxic T lymphocyte-associated antigen 4-immunoglobulin (CTLA4Ig) reverses the cellular pathology of psoriatic plaques, including the activation of keratinocytes, dendritic cells, and endothelial cells. *J Exp Med* 2000;192:681–693.
15. Abrams JR, Lebwohl MG, Guzzo CA, et al. CTLA4Ig-mediated blockade of T-cell costimulation in patients with psoriasis vulgaris. *J Clin Invest* 1999;103:1243–1252.
16. Moreland LW, Alten R, Van den Bosch F, et al. Costimulatory blockade in patients with rheumatoid arthritis: A pilot, dose-finding, double-blind, placebo-controlled clinical trial evaluating CTLA-4Ig and LEA29Y eighty-five days after the first infusion. *Arthritis Rheum* 2002;46:1470–1479.
17. Kremer JM, Dougados M, Emery P, et al. Treatment of rheumatoid arthritis with the selective costimulation modulator abatacept: Twelve-month results of a phase IIb, double-blind, randomized, placebo-controlled trial. *Arthritis Rheum* 2005;52: 2263–2271.

18. Kremer JM, Westhovens R, Leon M, et al. Treatment of rheumatoid arthritis by selective inhibition of T-cell activation with fusion protein CTLA4Ig. *N Engl J Med* 2003;349:1907–1915.
19. Weisman MH, Durez P, Hallegua D, et al. Reduction of inflammatory biomarker response by abatacept in treatment of rheumatoid arthritis. *J Rheumatol* 2006;33:2162–2166.
20. Weinblatt M, Schiff M, Goldman A, et al. Selective costimulation modulation using abatacept in patients with active rheumatoid arthritis while receiving etanercept: A randomized clinical trial. *Ann Rheum Dis* 2007;66:228–234.
21. Kremer JM, Genant HK, Moreland LW, et al. Effects of abatacept in patients with methotrexate-resistant active rheumatoid arthritis. *Ann Intern Med* 2006;144:865–876.
22. Genevese MC, Becker J-C, Schiff M, et al. Abatacept for rheumatoid arthritis refractory to tumor necrosis factor α inhibition. *N Engl J Med* 2005;353:1114–1123.
23. Weinblatt M, Combe B, Covucci A, et al. Safety of the selective costimulation modulator abatacept in rheumatoid arthritis patients receiving background biologic and nonbiologic disease-modifying antirheumatic drugs. *Arthritis Rheum* 2006;54:2807–2816.

Rituximab

Shouvik Dass, Edward M. Vital, and Paul Emery

CHAPTER 101

B Cells in Rheumatoid Arthritis

B cells are generated in bone marrow with specific antigen reactivity and are released into the circulation and become naive B cells. Upon meeting their cognate antigen, they become activated and participate in germinal center reactions. Germinal center reactions involve interaction of B and T cells by presentation of the antigen, along with other co-stimulatory molecules, by the B cell. This process leads to a number of effector mechanisms. Short-lived and long-lived plasma cells that secrete antibody are generated, as well as memory B cells.[1] Short-lived plasma cells provide an immediate antibody response, and in the case of IgM plasma cells may arise without T-cell help. Long-lived plasma cells persist for many years after migrating to the bone marrow and hence contribute to immune memory and maintenance of normal immunoglobulin levels. Memory B cells also contribute to immune memory by requiring a lower threshold for reactivation upon again encountering their cognate antigen and rapidly differentiating into plasma cells. Last, T-cell activation induced by interaction with B cells may activate effector mechanisms other than B and plasma cells—such as released inflammatory cytokines. It is not known whether the B or T cell was primarily responsible for loss of self-tolerance in rheumatoid arthritis (RA), but during germinal center reactions antibodies are modified by affinity maturation and epitope spreading—which may provide the opportunity for autoreactive antibodies to arise.

In RA, rheumatoid factor (RF) and anticyclic citrullinated peptide (anti-CCP) antibodies are produced. RF may be pathogenic by self-associating and generating immune complexes,[2] which then cause inflammation in sites where their receptor FcγRIIIa is expressed (the synovium, serosal surfaces, and sites of rheumatoid nodule formation). In addition, RF-producing B cells (which could arise by chance during germinal center reactions) have been shown to be capable of eliciting help from nonautoreactive T cells—thereby bypassing T-cell self-tolerance and proliferating. Anticitrullinated protein antibodies (anti-CCP) are highly specific to RA, and the target of ACPA is expressed in the synovium. Both of these antibodies are expressed years before clinical features of RA develop,[3] also supporting the primacy of the B cell in disease initiation.

Targeting CD20

Recent advances in understanding the central role of B cells in RA pathogenesis have been accompanied by novel therapeutic approaches. The successful use of selective B-cell depletion therapy with rituximab has led to significant insights, but many clinical and scientific questions remain unanswered.

CD20 is a 33- to 37-kDa nonglycosylated phosphoprotein expressed on the surface of mature naive B cells that have exited the bone marrow to enter blood. It is not expressed on stem cells or on plasma cells that have returned to the bone marrow. This selective expression on mature B cells but not on precursors such as stem cells or on antibody-secreting plasma cells makes it an attractive target. Thus, depletion via CD20 would be expected to permit B-cell regeneration and prevent reduction of immunoglobulin levels—at least with initial therapy. Furthermore, upon binding antibody, CD20 is neither shed nor internalized.[4–6]

CD20 has been successfully targeted using the monoclonal antibody rituximab in a variety of hematologic malignancies[7] and rheumatic autoimmune diseases.[8] However, the biology of CD20 and the mechanisms of targeting it are not completely understood. This is in part because CD20 appears to have no natural ligand and because CD20 knockout mice display an almost normal phenotype.[9,10] Various anti-CD20 monoclonal antibodies have been used in experimental settings and have induced a range of different calcium flux responses, supporting the theory that CD20 may be involved in the generation and regulation of calcium transport triggered by other receptors.[11]

Rituximab is a high-affinity chimeric monoclonal antibody specific to CD20, consisting of the fusion of light- and heavy-chain variable regions of a murine antihuman monoclonal anti-CD20 antibody with human immunoglobulin κ light-chain and γ1 heavy-chain constant regions.[12] This was originally developed for the treatment of refractory CD20+ B-cell non-Hodgkin's lymphoma, for which it has shown substantial evidence of efficacy and has now been used in more than 800,000 patients.[13] Its mechanism of B-cell depletion *in vivo* is not fully understood, but there is evidence for antibody-dependent cell-mediated cytotoxicity by effector cells, complement-dependent cytotoxicity, and apoptosis.[14]

Clinical Considerations in Rheumatoid Arthritis

Much of the clinical data regarding rituximab are drawn from three double-blind randomized placebo-controlled studies[15–17] that have subsequently entered extension phases. It should be noted that in these "placebo"-controlled studies there was never any arm that received no treatment. Rather, all investigative agents were compared to treatment with methotrexate alone—the latter representing the control arm. Rituximab was given as two infusions, 2 weeks apart. Primary outcomes were at 6 months, with clinical outcomes measured by American College of Rheumatology (ACR) improvement criteria and Disease Activity Score 28 joint assessment (DAS28) in order to determine EULAR response.

The first of these studies[15] was a phase IIa study with four arms comparing placebo, rituximab monotherapy, rituximab with cyclophosphamide, and rituximab with methotrexate. The DANCER study[16] aimed to compare two different doses of rituximab (two infusions of 500 mg vs. two infusions of 1000 mg) and to assess varying concomitant steroid regimens. The phase III REFLEX trial[17] compared the latter dose of rituximab with placebo and only included patients who had had inadequate response or toxicity following anti-TNF therapy. These studies are considered in more detail in material following.

Which Patients Receive Benefit from Rituximab?

Patients entered into these studies often had relatively severe disease, as would be expected for a novel biologic agent. Patients in the phase IIa study had active disease despite treatment with methotrexate. Patients had also failed between one and five DMARDs other than methotrexate. In the DANCER study, the mean duration of disease was 9.3 to 11.1 years—and the mean number of previous DMARDs other than methotrexate was 2.2 to 2.5. Overall, 29% of patients had received prior biologic agents. For the REFLEX study, comprising patients who had all previously received anti-TNF therapy, median disease duration was approximately 12 years, swollen joint count was 23, and DAS28 was 6.9. More than 90% of patients had previously taken either one or two anti-TNF agents, and 9% had received three anti-TNF agents. Ninety-one percent of patients had demonstrated an inadequate response to anti-TNF therapy due to lack of efficacy.

The eventual licensed dose of two infusions of rituximab of 1000 mg each (given 14 days apart), preceded by 100 mg of methylprednisolone with concomitant ongoing methotrexate therapy, demonstrated significant benefit over placebo in all of these studies (the effect of other doses and regimens is discussed in material following). In the phase IIa study, in terms of ACR 20 response all groups treated with rituximab had a significantly higher proportion of responders (65% to 76% vs. 38%, $p \leq 0.025$). With regard to EULAR response criteria, patients receiving rituximab had a significantly higher proportion of responders compared with those receiving methotrexate alone (83% to 85% vs. 50%, $p \leq 0.004$). In the DANCER study, the proportion of patients achieving ACR 20 response was significantly higher in patients receiving rituximab than placebo (54.1% rituximab vs. 27.9% placebo, $p < 0.001$). ACR 50 and ACR 70 responses were consistent with those observed for ACR 20. In the REFLEX study, at 24 weeks there was a significant difference between the two arms in the proportion of patients reaching the primary endpoint of ACR 20 response: 51% vs. 18% for the rituximab and placebo arms, respectively ($p < 0.0001$). With regard to ACR 50 and ACR 70 responses, these were also significantly increased in rituximab-treated patients (27% vs. 5% and 12% vs. 1% for ACR 50 and ACR 70, respectively). Similarly, when moderate to good EULAR responses were considered the proportion of responders was significantly higher in those who had received rituximab (65% vs. 22%, $p < 0.0001$). At week 24, 12% of patients receiving rituximab had withdrawn due to lack of efficacy in comparison to 40% of those receiving placebo. There were also significant improvements in patient-based outcomes such as pain and fatigue.

On the basis of these results, rituximab was licensed by the U.S. Food and Drug Administration (FDA) and the European Medicines Evaluation Agency (EMEA) for the treatment of severe active RA in patients with an inadequate response to anti-TNF therapy. These studies also suggest that rituximab could also be of benefit in patients who have not yet received anti-TNF therapy.

Effect of Antibody Status on Clinical Efficacy

Because autoantibody production by B cells is pivotal to their role in RA pathogenesis, the question of whether patients' autoantibody status affects clinical outcome following rituximab is potentially of key importance. The phase IIa study only included patients who were positive for rheumatoid factor. In the DANCER study, 380 patients were RF positive and 85 were RF negative. In the REFLEX study, both RF-positive (81%) and RF-negative patients were also included. The last of these found that baseline RF status had no significant effect on ACR response, although fewer RF-negative patients achieved ACR 20 (41%) than RF-positive patients (54%). When patients who were negative for both RF and anti-CCP antibody were considered, the EULAR response rate dropped to 44% (compared with 75% in seropositive patients).[18] In the DANCER study, there was a high placebo response rate (52% achieved ACR 20)—which was greater than the response rate for rituximab (48%) in seronegative patients.

What Is the Position of Rituximab in the Biologic Hierarchy?

Patients treated with an anti-TNF agent may demonstrate complete lack of response (primary nonresponse) or initial response that is subsequently lost (secondary nonresponse). It is not clear which is the most appropriate therapeutic strategy to follow subsequently in such patients. There is some evidence to suggest that switching to an alternative anti-TNF agent is beneficial in some patients.[19] In the REFLEX study, better outcomes were obtained in those patients who had only received one anti-TNF agent prior to rituximab in comparison to those who had received two or three. However, this may simply reflect less severe baseline disease activity and shorter disease duration in the former group. One observational cohort study[20] has suggested that there is greater reduction in DAS28 in patients with an inadequate response to anti-TNF therapy who then received rituximab rather than an alternative anti-TNF agent. Formal randomized controlled studies that might be stratified according to the pattern of nonresponse to anti-TNF are required before the place of rituximab in the hierarchy of biologic therapies can be more precisely identified.

What Dose of Rituximab Is Required?

The DANCER study compared two doses of rituximab (2 × 500 mg vs. 2 × 1000 mg). ACR 20 (55.3% lower-dose rituximab and 54.1% higher-dose rituximab) and ACR 50 (33% lower-dose and 34% higher-dose) responses were similar for both doses. However, ACR 70 responses were slightly higher in the higher-dose group (20% vs. 13%)—but this did not reach significance. The ACR 70 response rose during the course of the study with higher-dose rituximab, suggesting that there may be a time-related cumulative effect of this dose. With regard to EULAR responses, rituximab treatment significantly improved responses when compared to placebo ($p < 0.001$). There was no statistically significant difference between different doses of rituximab with respect to EULAR response, although a higher proportion of patients treated with the higher dose of rituximab achieved a "good" EULAR response (27.9%, 13.8%, and 4.1% for higher-dose, lower-dose, and placebo, respectively). No significant differences in safety and tolerability were identified between the two doses. The REFLEX study only used one dosing regimen of rituximab (2 × 1000 mg) and thus this became the licensed dose in this population. However, further evidence of the most appropriate dose of rituximab is warranted. The initial evidence suggests that higher doses may allow "higher-hurdle" endpoints to be reached.

What Is the Role of Concomitant Corticosteroids and DMARDs?

The DANCER study also investigated the role of concomitant steroid therapy, both intravenous (100 mg methylprednisolone prior to each infusion on days 1 and 15) and oral (prednisolone, 60 mg on days 2–7 and 30 mg on days 8–14). These were compared to placebo. Use of intravenous steroid as premedication appeared to reduce acute infusion-related reactions and is therefore recommended. However, use of oral corticosteroids appeared unnecessary in terms of improving long-term outcomes and had no effect on infusion reactions after the second infusion. Steroids did improve the initial clinical response at 4 weeks after therapy. Subsequently, the clinical improvement (ACR 20 response) continued before reaching a plateau at 12 weeks. The EULAR consensus statement regarding rituximab[21] recommends advising patients that they may experience an immediate but transient benefit after therapy followed by slower response, which may take up to 12 weeks to become apparent.

The role of concomitant DMARDs has also been investigated. Although patients who received rituximab monotherapy (i.e., without concomitant methotrexate) in the phase IIa study had significant improvement over placebo for ACR 20 at 24 weeks post-therapy, this benefit was lost by 48 weeks. In contrast, patients who received rituximab in combination with methotrexate were the only group to demonstrate significant benefits at all ACR response thresholds and at both 24 and 48 weeks. However, by week 48 responses were declining. With the refinement of retreatment strategies (discussed further in material following), it may be that with lower thresholds for retreatment than in the original studies the apparent prolongation of response with combination therapy may no longer be relevant. The duration of B-cell depletion after rituximab appears unrelated to the use of concomitant methotrexate.[22] Use of concomitant DMARDs other than methotrexate has been reported to be safe and effective in small numbers of patients.[23] Currently, rituximab is only licensed for use with methotrexate.

Repeat Treatment: Timing and Efficacy

Patients from the original large randomized studies were followed up in open-label extension studies. Patients who were deemed to be responders (by predefined criteria) were eligible for retreatment with a further cycle of two infusions of 1000 mg rituximab with preceding methylprednisolone if they subsequently had deterioration in disease activity. It is worth noting that the thresholds in studies determining both response and relapse are higher than would generally be seen in clinical practice, as reflected in the EULAR consensus statement—which defines response as a minimum improvement in DAS28 of 1.2. Due to the potentially slow onset of action of rituximab, response should not be determined earlier than 16 weeks after treatment. A subsequent increase in DAS28 of more than 0.6 is regarded as a clinically relevant deterioration, warranting retreatment. This is only recommended after 6 months have passed since the previous course.

Data are available from these open-label extension studies for up to four courses of therapy,[24] and further courses are reported in case series[25] and reports. The median treatment interval between first, second, and third courses in patients with previous anti-TNF exposure remained stable at approximately 30 weeks. Clinical responses were also sustained. ACR and DAS responses were similar after first and second courses, and the proportions of patients achieving ACR 70, DAS28 low-disease activity (DAS28 <3.2), and DAS28 remission (DAS28 <2.6) increased after the second course. The change in DAS28 after each course from baseline was consistent, implying cumulative progressive reduction in disease activity with repeated treatment.

The current paradigm of rituximab therapy is therefore one of repeated therapy if a patient deteriorates after initially improving. Inherent in this is a degree of instability, with potential clinical implications, such as more short-term steroid use and this may also be potentially detrimental to long-term outcomes. There is evidence to suggest that the less a patient's disease activity rises before retreatment the better the outcome.[26] Predictors of relapse are currently being studied. B-cell measurement by conventional sensitivity-flow cytometry has not been especially informative. The vast majority of patients have B-cell return at some point before or with relapse, but a more specific temporal relationship has not been established.[22] It has been suggested that the specific subsets of B cells at the time of repopulation may be important, with those patients who repopulate with a predominantly naive phenotype displaying longer responses.[27]

Imaging Outcomes

The REFLEX study included radiographic data as an exploratory outcome at weeks 24 and 56 after therapy. At the latter time point, significant benefit over placebo was demonstrated in preventing progression of erosions, joint space narrowing, and total Genant modified Sharp score.[28] There are also data indicating that even clinical nonresponders may derive some structural benefit, with less radiographic progression of disease than those patients receiving placebo.[29] Further imaging studies are required, with more sensitive modalities to fully define the structural effects of rituximab therapy.

Safety

No new safety signals have emerged from the use of rituximab in RA when compared with the extensive data available from hematology and oncology practice. Pertinent issues regarding rheumatologic practice are addressed in the material following.

Screening Before Therapy

It is recommended that potential patients be screened with history for chronic or concomitant comorbidity (focusing on cardiovascular and pulmonary disease as well infections) and a full physical examination. A chest x-ray may not be required in all cases. No increased risk of tuberculosis has been observed in lymphoma patients treated with rituximab,[30] and thus routine screening for this is not recommended. Screening for hepatitis B is recommended because of cases of reactivation of infection with fulminant hepatitis.[31] From the oncology literature, patients with hepatitis B have been successfully treated with antiviral prophylaxis (with lamivudine),[32] and patients with hepatitis C have been treated without prophylaxis.

Infusion Reactions

Infusion reactions are the most frequent adverse events observed with rituximab therapy. These include pruritus, urticaria, pyrexia, throat irritation, and hypo- and hypertension and are usually mild to moderate in severity. In rituximab-treated patients, it has been suggested that these reactions are due to cytokine release following B-cell lysis.[33] Such symptoms affect up to 30% of patients, but it should be noted that the incidence following the second infusion is much lower. This could be because B-cell numbers are already significantly reduced by the first infusion. The lower rate of infusion reactions in RA patients compared to non-Hodgkin's lymphoma (NHL) patients may also be related to this because the latter group often has a heavier B-cell load before therapy. A small number of patients (<1%) experienced a serious infusion reaction (anaphylaxis and bronchospasm).

Use of intravenous steroid prior to infusion of rituximab reduced infusion reactions from 37% to 29% in patients receiving a first infusion of 1000 mg rituximab.[16] Repeated courses of therapy are associated with fewer infusion reactions.[24] Infusion reactions can be managed by slowing the infusion rate, or with additional paracetamol, antihistamines, and (if required) bronchodilators and steroids.

Infections

Most infections reported in RA patients were minor and were largely upper respiratory or urinary tract infections. There was a slight increase in serious infections (5.2 vs. 3.7 per 100 patient-years) over placebo in REFLEX. There are no data to suggest an increased risk of opportunistic infections, including tuberculosis. A small number of patients with previous tuberculosis or positive Mantoux test have been treated without reactivation of disease. It has been observed that there is a cumulative reduction in immunoglobulin levels with repeated cycles of therapy. After a third course of rituximab, 23.5% of patients have a lower than normal level of IgM.[24] However, there appears to be no change in the rate of incidence of infections in these patients before and after IgM falls below the normal limit. There is an increase in infection rates after anti-TNF is administered in patients who have received rituximab, although this has not reached statistical significance.[34]

Future Issues

Rituximab has demonstrated safety and efficacy in the treatment of various RA populations, including those with severe disease that has proved refractory to all previously available therapies. However, as a relatively new agent it continues to be evaluated in wider groups of patients—and a number of issues arise that may inform future practice.

The most significant of these relates to predictors of response and relapse. These may revolve around greater understanding of B-cell depletion and repletion, as well the fundamentals of rituximab's mechanism of action. For the former, conventional sensitivity-flow cytometry suggests that all patients deplete peripheral B cells completely. Hence, this offers no correlation with response. However, more sensitive assays have revealed considerable variation in peripheral depletion, and less initial depletion has correlated with shorter duration of clinical response.[35] This may inform strategies designed to enhance B-cell depletion. With regard to repletion, it has been suggested that patients who display a predominantly naive B-cell phenotype at repletion tend to have longer responses. How far these peripheral changes at depletion and repletion reflect B cells in compartments elsewhere in the body is also unclear. B cells exist in greater numbers in compartments such as spleen, bone marrow, lymph nodes, and synovium than in peripheral blood. It is not yet known whether B cells in a certain location need to be depleted to achieve optimal clinical response or whether a pathogenic subset of B cells can be identified and targeted.

From a clinical perspective, the need to observe clinical deterioration before administering repeat courses of therapy may be an approach that can be improved. Another approach might entail fixed-interval retreatment in order to maintain stable responses. However, the safety aspects of this would need to be closely studied, particularly as this might lead to overtreatment of some patients. Ultimately, combination therapy with other targeted biologic agents might be used to enhance the effect of rituximab. The use of biomarkers to inform clinical strategies might eventually allow stable responses to be achieved using individually tailored therapy to provide patients with the smallest required dose.

References

1. Hoyer BF, Manz RA, Radbruch A, et al. Long-lived plasma cells and their contribution to autoimmunity. *Ann N Y Acad Sci* 2005;1050: 124–133.
2. Edwards JC, Cambridge G. Rheumatoid arthritis: The predictable effect of small immune complexes in which antibody is also antigen. *Br J Rheumatoly* 1998;37:126–130.
3. Rantapää-Dahlqvist S, de Jong BAW, Berglin E, et al. Antibodies against cyclic citrullinated peptide (CCP) and immunoglobulin-A rheumatoid factor predict the development of rheumatoid arthritis. *Arthritis Rheum* 2003;10:2741–2749.
4. Press OW, Howell-Clark J, Anderson S, et al. Retention of B-cell-specific monoclonal antibodies by human lymphoma cells. *Blood* 1994;83:1390–1397.
5. Press OW, Farr AG, Borroz KI, et al. Endocytosis and degradation of monoclonal antibodies targeting human B-cell malignancies. *Cancer Res* 1989;49:4906–4912.
6. Vervoordeldonk SF, Merle PA, van Leeuwen EF, et al. Preclinical studies with radiolabeled monoclonal antibodies for treatment of patients with B-cell malignancies. *Cancer* 1994;73:1006–1011.
7. Collins-Burow B, Santos ES. Rituximab and its role as maintenance therapy in non-Hodgkin lymphoma. *Expert Rev Anticancer Ther* 2007;7(3):257–273.
8. Edwards JC, Cambridge G, Leandro MJ. B cell depletion therapy in rheumatic disease. *Best Pract Res Clin Rheumatol* 2006;20(5):915–928.
9. Uchida J, Lee Y, Hasegawa M, et al. Mouse CD20 expression and function. *Int Immunol* 2004;16:119–129.

10. O'Keefe TL, Williams GT, Davies SL, et al. Mice carrying a CD20 gene disruption. *Immunogenetics* 1998;48:125–132.
11. Bubien JK, Zhou LJ, Bell PD, et al. Transfection of the CD20 cell surface molecule into ectopic cell types generates a Ca2+ conductance found constitutively in B lymphocytes. *J Cell Biol* 1993;121: 1121–1132.
12. Reff ME, Camer K, Chambers KS, et al. Depletion of B cells in vivo by a chimeric mouse human monoclonal antibody to CD20. *Blood* 1994;83(2):435–445.
13. Czuczman CS. Combination chemotherapy and rituximab. *Anti-Cancer Drugs* 2001;12(Suppl 2):S15–S19.
14. Cartron G, Watier H, Golay J, et al. From the bench to the bedside: Ways to improve rituximab efficacy. *Blood* 2004;104(9):2635–2642.
15. Edwards JC, Szczepanski L, Szechinski J, et al. Efficacy of B-cell-targeted therapy with rituximab in patients with rheumatoid arthritis. *N Engl J Med* 2004;350(25):2572–2581.
16. Emery P, Fleischmann R, Filipowicz-Sosnowska A, et al. The efficacy and safety of rituximab in patients with active rheumatoid arthritis despite methotrexate treatment: Results of a phase IIB randomized, double-blind, placebo-controlled, dose-ranging trial. *Arthritis Rheum* 2006;54(5):1390–1400.
17. Cohen SB, Emery P, Greenwald MW, et al. Rituximab for rheumatoid arthritis refractory to anti-tumor necrosis factor therapy: Results of a multicenter, randomized, double-blind, placebo-controlled, phase III trial evaluating primary efficacy and safety at twenty-four weeks. *Arthritis Rheum* 2006;54(9):2793–2806.
18. Tak PP, Cohen SB, Emery P, et al. Clinical response following the first treatment course with rituximab: Effect of baseline autoantibody status (RF, anti-CCP). *Ann Rheum Dis* 2007;66(Suppl 2):338.
19. Buch MH, Bingham SJ, Bejarano V, et al. Therapy of patients with rheumatoid arthritis: Outcome of infliximab failures switched to etanercept. *Arthritis Rheum* 2007;57(3):448–453.
20. Finckh A, Ciurea A, Brulhart L, et al. B cell depletion may be more effective than switching to an alternative anti-tumor necrosis factor agent in rheumatoid arthritis patients with inadequate response to anti-tumor necrosis factor agents. *Arthritis Rheum* 2007;56(5): 1417–1423.
21. Smolen JS, Keystone EC, Emery P, et al. Consensus statement on the use of rituximab in patients with rheumatoid arthritis. *Ann Rheum Dis* 2007;66(2):143–150.
22. Emery P, Breedveld F, Martin-Mola E, et al. Relationship between peripheral B cell levels and loss of EULAR response in rheumatoid arthritis patients treated with rituximab. *Ann Rheum Dis* 2007;66 (Suppl 2):124.
23. Dass S, Vital EM, Bingham SJ, et al. The safety and efficacy of rituximab in patients outside clinical trials. *Rheumatology* 2006;45 (Suppl 1):47.
24. Keystone E, Fleischmann R, Emery P, et al. Safety and efficacy of additional courses of rituximab in patients with active rheumatoid arthritis: An open-label extension analysis. *Arthritis Rheum* 2007; 56(12):3896–3908.
25. Popa C, Leandro MJ, Cambridge G. Repeated B lymphocyte depletion with rituximab in rheumatoid arthritis over 7 yrs. *Rheumatology* 2007;46(4):626–630.
26. Mease PJ, Keystone E, Kaell A, et al. Predicting outcome of a second course of rituximab for rheumatoid arthritis. *Ann Rheum Dis* 2007;66(Suppl 2):434.
27. Leandro MJ, Cambridge G, Ehrenstein MR, et al. Reconstitution of peripheral blood B cells after depletion with rituximab in patients with rheumatoid arthritis. *Arthritis Rheum* 2006;54(2):613–620.
28. Keystone E, Emery P, Peterfy CG, et al. Prevention of joint structural damage at 1 year with rituximab in rheumatoid arthritis patients with an inadequate response to one or more TNF inhibitors. *Ann Rheum Dis* 2006;66(Suppl 2):58.
29. Keystone E, Emery P, Peterfy CG, et al. Inhibition of radiographic progression with rituximab is not dependent on clinical efficacy: Results from a study in rheumatoid arthritis patients with an inadequate response to one or more TNF inhibitors. *Ann Rheum Dis* 2007;66 (Suppl 2):431.
30. Kimby E. Tolerability and safety of rituximab. *Cancer Treat Rev* 2005;31(6):456–473.
31. Yeo W, Johnson PJ. Diagnosis, prevention and management of hepatitis B virus reactivation during anticancer therapy. *Hepatology* 2006; 43:209–220.
32. Hamaki T, Kami M, Kusumi E, et al. Prophylaxis of hepatitis B reactivation using lamivudine in a patient receiving rituximab. *Am J Hematol* 2001;68:292–294.
33. Hainsworth JD. Safety of rituximab in the treatment of B cell malignancies: Implications for rheumatoid arthritis. *Arthritis Res Ther* 2003;5(Suppl 4):S12–S16.
34. Genovese M, Breedveld FC, Emery P, et al. TNF inhibitors in rheumatoid arthritis patients previously treated with rituximab. *Arthritis Rheum* 2007;54(9):329.
35. Dass S, Rawstron AC, Vital EM, et al. Specific peripheral blood B lineage cells predict response to rituximab in rheumatoid arthritis: A study with high sensitivity flow cytometry. *Ann Rheum Dis* 2006; 65(Suppl 2):185.

Tocilizumab

Norihiro Nishimoto and Toru Mima

CHAPTER 10J

Interleukin (IL)-6 was originally identified as B-cell stimulatory factor-2 (BSF-2), a T-cell–derived factor that induces B-cell differentiation.[1] After the cDNA for BSF-2 was found to be identical to that of interferon-β2, a hybridoma/plasmacytoma growth factor, a 26-kDa protein, and a hepatocyte stimulating factor, these entities were unified under the name IL-6.[2] IL-6 is produced not only by T cells but by B cells, monocytes, fibroblasts, keratinocytes, endothelial cells, and some tumor cells.[3] Although IL-6 plays important physiologic roles in the regulation of immune response, inflammatory reaction, and hematopoiesis, constitutive overproduction of IL-6 has been implicated in the development of immune-mediated and inflammatory diseases.[4]

In patients with rheumatoid arthritis (RA), IL-6 levels are elevated in both serum and synovial fluids.[5–8] IL-6 augments autoimmune responses through the activation of both B cells, resulting in hyper-γ-globulinemia and increased autoantibody titers, and autoreactive T cells. In animal models, it has been shown that in the presence of IL-6 transforming growth factor-β (TGF-β) induces differentiation of Th17 cells—which in turn produce IL-17, IL-6, and TNF.[9–13] In contrast, TGF-β in the absence of IL-6 induces $CD4^+CD25^+$Forkhead box P3 $(FOXP3)^+$ T regulatory cells—which inhibit autoimmune reactions. It appears that IL-6 may therefore be a key cytokine in the pathogenesis of effector Th17 cells and autoimmune responses, although further confirmatory studies will be needed in humans.

IL-6 acts synergistically with IL-1β and TNF to induce production of vascular endothelial growth factor (VEGF), which plays a role in stimulating angiogenesis in the hyperplastic synovial tissues of RA patients.[14] In the presence of soluble IL-6 receptors, IL-6 also induces osteoclast differentiation[15]—which mediates the joint destruction and osteoporosis associated with RA. As a proinflammatory mediator, IL-6 causes systemic symptoms of fever and fatigue,[16] as well as increased production of acute-phase proteins[17] such as C-reactive protein (CRP), fibrinogen, α1-antitrypsin, and serum amyloid A (SAA). Overexpression of IL-6, as a megakaryocyte-activating factor, induces thrombocytosis.[18] Finally, IL-6 induces production of the iron regulatory peptide hormone hepcidin.[19,20] By suppressing iron absorption and increasing hepatic iron storage, hepcidin promotes a hypoferremic anemia of chronic inflammation.

Recognition that IL-6 is involved in numerous inflammatory responses led to the idea that inhibition of IL-6 might be a plausible therapy for RA. Tocilizumab, a humanized antihuman IL-6 receptor (IL-6R) monoclonal antibody specifically targeting IL-6,[21] has been the subject of recent safety and efficacy trials in patients with RA.

Pharmacologic Features of Tocilizumab

Mode of Action

Tocilizumab was engineered by grafting complementarity-determining regions (CDRs) from mouse antihuman IL-6R antibody to human IgG1 to create a human IL-6R binding site on a human antibody.[21] This strategy proved effective for minimizing immunogenicity, as fewer neutralizing antibodies have been detected with repetitive tocilizumab administration than with treatments using mouse antibodies or mouse and human chimeric antibodies. This results in a prolonged half-life for tocilizumab.

IL-6 signal transduction is mediated by a ligand-binding IL-6R and a non ligand-binding but signal-transducing chain, gp130, on the surface of target cells. Soluble forms of IL-6R, found in blood and synovial fluids, are also capable of signal transduction through "trans-signaling"[22]—a signaling mechanism unique to the IL-6R system. Tocilizumab recognizes IL-6 binding sites on both the membranous and soluble forms of IL-6R, and competitively inhibits IL-6 binding to IL-6R (Figure 10J-1). Using the standard tocilizumab dosing regimen, neither antibody-dependent nor complement-dependent cellular cytotoxicity has been observed in cells that express IL-6R.

Pharmacokinetics

Serum tocilizumab concentrations showed nonlinear pharmacokinetics in the dose range of 2 to 8 mg/kg when intravenously administered by drop infusion for 2 hours.[23] The half-life of tocilizumab (t1/2) was dose dependent, and approximated the half-life of human IgG1 (241.8 ± 71.4 hours) by the third dose of 8 mg/kg. The mean area under the curve (AUC) for serum tocilizumab concentration peaked at approximately 10.66 ± 4.07 mg*hour/ml.[23]

Interestingly, CRP and SAA levels were undetectable in RA patients with serum concentrations of free tocilizumab greater than 1 μg/ml, suggesting that IL-6 is essential for CRP and SAA production *in vivo*. In fact, CRP levels have been shown to function as a surrogate marker for the level of tocilizumab activity.[23]

Clinical Studies of Tocilizumab in RA Patients

Clinical studies of tocilizumab in patients with immune-inflammatory diseases were initially performed in the Osaka University Hospital of Japan. The pilot studies, which were performed in patients with refractory disease, demonstrated the therapeutic potential of tocilizumab.[14,24,25] Tocilizumab

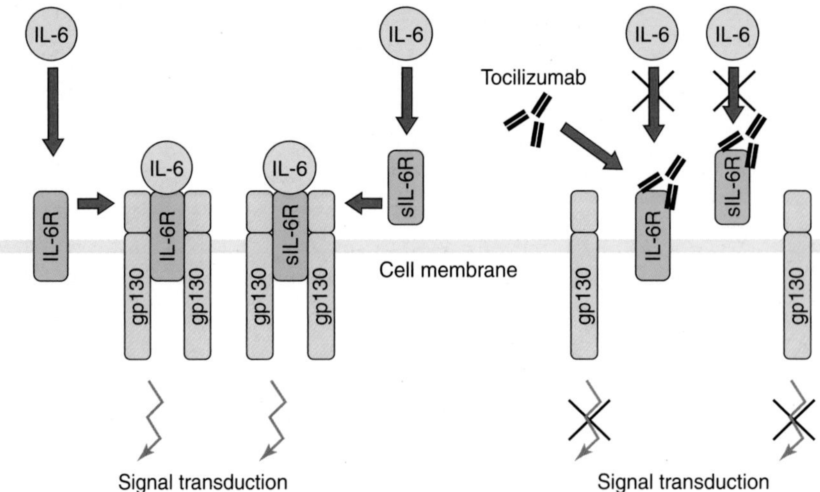

Figure 10J-1. Inhibitory action of tocilizumab in IL-6 signaling. IL-6 signal transduction is mediated by a ligand-binding IL-6R and a non–ligand-binding but signal-transducing chain, gp130, on the cell surface. Soluble IL-6R (sIL-6R) is also capable of signal transduction. Tocilizumab recognizes IL-6 binding sites on both the membranous IL-6R and sIL-6R and inhibits IL-6 signal transduction.

treatment dramatically improved both inflammatory symptoms and laboratory abnormalities, including serum levels of acute-phase proteins, albumin, hemoglobin, and VEGF. On the basis of these findings, clinical trials were designed and conducted.

Phase I/II Studies in the United Kingdom and Japan

The phase I/II study in the United Kingdom was a double-blind placebo-controlled trial testing the pharmacokinetics, safety, and efficacy of single-dose intravenous administration of tocilizumab at the following doses: 0.1, 1, 5, and 10 mg/kg.[26] The treatment was well tolerated, and normalization of CRP was achieved in the 5- and 10-mg/kg groups. In the 5-mg/kg group, 55.6% of the patients met the American College of Rheumatology (ACR) response criteria ACR 20, compared to 0% of the patients in the placebo group.

A Japanese phase I/II study then tested the pharmacokinetics, safety, and efficacy of repeated intravenous tocilizumab doses at 2, 4, and 8 mg/kg every 2 weeks in an open-label trial.[23] At 6 months, 86% and 33% of the patients had met ACR 20 and ACR 50 criteria, respectively. Treatments were again well tolerated.

Phase II Studies for RA

In 2001, the safety and efficacy of tocilizumab monotherapy for RA was evaluated in a multicenter double-blind randomized placebo-controlled phase II trial in Japan. In this study, 164 patients with refractory RA were randomized to receive intravenous treatment with placebo, tocilizumab treatment at 4 mg/kg, or tocilizumab treatment at 8 mg/kg. Treatment was administered at three sessions spaced 4 weeks apart, and the clinical responses were evaluated at 12 weeks using the ACR criteria.[27] Tocilizumab treatment significantly improved all measures of disease activity, and a dose-response relationship was observed across the 4- and 8-mg/kg groups. Patients had a mean disease duration of 8 years, and had used an average of four to five antirheumatic drugs before beginning tocilizumab treatment. Despite their advanced disease, 78% of the patients in the 8-mg/kg group met ACR 20 criteria—compared to 57% in the 4-mg/kg group ($p = 0.02$) and only 11% in the placebo group ($p < 0.001$). ACR 50 and ACR 70 responses in the 8-mg/kg group were 40% and 16%, respectively, and both were superior to those in the placebo group ($p < 0.001$, $p = 0.002$). The efficacy of tocilizumab monotherapy was also confirmed by the disease activity score in 28 joints (DAS28): 91% of patients in the 8-mg/kg group reported "good or moderate" joint scores, as opposed to 19% in the placebo group ($p < 0.001$). Complete normalization of CRP was observed in 76% of the patients in the 8-mg groups, but only 1.9% of patients in the placebo group. Significant improvement was also noted in lab values for hemoglobin, platelet count, fibrinogen, SAA, RF, albumin, bone formation markers, and bone resorption markers.

Safety data did not show a dose-dependent relationship. The overall incidence for adverse events was 56%, 59%, and 51% in the placebo, 4-, and 8-mg/kg groups, respectively. Serious adverse events were reported in three patients receiving tocilizumab (2.8%) and two patients receiving placebo (3.7%). One patient died from hemophagocytosis syndrome associated with reactivation of chronic active Epstein-Barr virus (EBV) infection after receiving a single dose of 8 mg of tocilizumab. This patient had increased serum EBV DNA levels before study enrollment, and it was later determined that she had developed Hodgkin's disease prior to tocilizumab treatment.[28] Although the mechanism of EBV reactivation is currently unclear, a careful pretreatment examination is necessary to assess whether the patient has a concurrent infectious disease. Other serious adverse events included allergic pneumonitis and super-infection of a burn, both of which were adequately treated with no long-term sequelae.

Abnormalities in laboratory values were also reported, notably including increased total cholesterol (TC) in 44% of patients receiving tocilizumab. High-density lipoprotein (HDL) cholesterol also increased, however, leaving the atherogenic index (total cholesterol − HDL cholesterol/HDL cholesterol) unchanged throughout the study period. The TC values tended to stabilize in the upper normal range, and no cardiovascular complications were reported. Similar increases in TC concentrations were also reported with TNF inhibitor treatments,[29] suggesting that the dyslipidemia may be secondary to the improvement in disease activity. Mild to moderate increases in liver function tests were observed in 14 of 109 patients (12.8%) receiving tocilizumab. They were all transient and normalized with the repeated administration of tocilizumab. There were no increases in antinuclear antibodies or anti-DNA antibodies, as is occasionally reported with TNF inhibitor treatments. These results indicate that treatment with tocilizumab was generally well tolerated.

A European phase II trial later tested the safety and efficacy of tocilizumab in combination with methotrexate (MTX) among patients with inadequate responses to MTX monotherapy.[30] This multi-arm trial randomized 359 patients into seven parallel arms. Patients received MTX (10–25 mg/week) with tocilizumab placebo; tocilizumab at 2, 4, or 8 mg/kg with MTX; or tocilizumab at 2, 4, or 8 mg/kg with MTX placebo. Tocilizumab or tocilizumab placebo was infused every 4 weeks for a total of 16 weeks.

ACR 20 criteria were met by 61% and 63% of patients, respectively, receiving 4 mg/kg and 8 mg/kg of tocilizumab as monotherapy, and by 63% and 74% of patients, respectively, receiving 4 mg/kg and 8 mg/kg of tocilizumab plus MTX. In contrast, only 41% of patients receiving placebo plus MTX satisfied the ACR 20 criteria. However, no statistical difference was observed in the ACR 20 response rate between the groups receiving monotherapy with 8 mg/kg tocilizumab and those receiving combination therapy with 8 mg/kg tocilizumab and MTX. ACR 50 and ACR 70 responses, as well as the European League Against Rheumatism (EULAR) remission rates, were significantly higher in patients receiving a combination therapy than in patients receiving MTX alone. EULAR remission was achieved in 34% of patients receiving tocilizumab 8 mg/kg plus MTX, compared to 17% in the group receiving 8 mg/kg tocilizumab monotherapy and 8% in the group receiving only MTX. The clinical benefits of tocilizumab, however, appeared to be similar with and without concomitant MTX therapy—although concomitant use of MTX increases the efficacy of TNF inhibitors.

In this study, tocilizumab was also well tolerated—with approximately 50% of patients experiencing adverse events, the majority of which were mild or moderate. No clear dose-dependent pattern was observed. Thirty-five serious adverse events were reported, with higher rates in the 2-mg/kg tocilizumab monotherapy group. Serious anaphylactic reactions were observed only in the groups receiving monotherapy with either 2 or 4 mg/kg of tocilizumab, and may be related to the development of anti-tocilizumab antibodies. Two cases of sepsis developed in patients receiving combination therapy with 8 mg/kg tocilizumab and MTX. Clinically significant laboratory abnormalities included increased transaminase levels, which seemed to be exacerbated by MTX. It is possible that tocilizumab treatment diminishes the protective effect of IL-6 on hepatocytes against MTX-induced toxicity. As in earlier trials, increased TC and decreased neutrophil counts were noted.

Phase III Studies for RA

The Japanese phase III trials consisted of two studies: The SATORI study evaluated the safety and efficacy of tocilizumab monotherapy for RA patients with inadequate responses to MTX treatment,[31] and the SAMURAI trial investigated the efficacy of tocilizumab monotherapy in slowing joint damage.[32]

In the SATORI study, 127 RA patients with inadequate responses to MTX (8 mg/week) were randomized to receive tocilizumab 8 mg/kg every 4 weeks in addition to a MTX placebo (tocilizumab group) or tocilizumab placebo in addition to MTX 8 mg/week (MTX group) for 24 weeks. ACR 20 improvement rates at 24 weeks served as the primary endpoint, with additional outcome measures including ACR 50 and ACR 70 improvement rates, DAS28, EULAR response, and ACR-N AUC.[31] At 24 weeks, ACR 20 response rates were significantly higher in the tocilizumab group than in the MTX group (80.3% vs. 25.0%, $p < 0.001$). Patients in the tocilizumab group also reported significantly higher ACR 50 and ACR 70 rates than patients treated by MTX [49.2% vs. 10.9% ($p < 0.001$) and 29.5% vs. 6.3% ($p < 0.001$), respectively]. Similarly, tocilizumab therapy was associated with improvements in both the EULAR response rates and the ACR-N AUC. Tocilizumab was very well tolerated, and withdrawals due to adverse events (tocilizumab, $n = 2$; MTX, $n = 3$) as well as the occurrence of serious adverse events (tocilizumab, $n = 4$; MTX, $n = 3$) were similar between tocilizumab and MTX groups. The frequency of liver function test abnormalities was higher in the MTX group (mean alanine transaminase [ALT] increase of 10.9%), although most cases were grade 1.

The SAMURAI study was designed to assess the change in total Sharp score (TSS), a quantitative radiographic evaluation of bone erosion and joint space narrowing in hand and foot joints of RA patients. This x-ray reader-blinded open-label randomized 1-year controlled trial enrolled RA patients who had been diagnosed less than 5 years prior to the study start date.[32] A total of 306 patients with active RA were randomly allocated to receive tocilizumab 8 mg/kg every 4 weeks or conventional disease-modifying antirheumatic drugs (DMARDs) for 52 weeks. Patients in the tocilizumab group showed significantly less radiographic progression, as measured by the change in TSS, than those receiving DMARDs (2.3 ± 5.6 versus 6.1 ± 11.4, $p = 0.001$). Tocilizumab was also superior to DMARDs in preventing both erosion and joint space narrowing ($p < 0.001$ and $p = 0.018$, respectively). The overall incidence of adverse events (including laboratory abnormalities) was 89% and 82% in the tocilizumab and DMARDs groups, respectively (serious adverse events: 18% and 13%, respectively; serious infections: 7.6% and 4.1%, respectively).

The results of two tocilizumab global phase III studies, OPTION and TOWARD, were reported in 2007.[33,34] In the OPTION study, 623 patients with moderate to severe RA received maintenance pre-study doses of MTX therapy in addition to placebo, 4 mg/kg of tocilizumab, or 8 mg/kg of tocilizumab. A significantly higher proportion of tocilizumab-treated patients achieved the primary endpoint of meeting ACR 20 criteria at 24 weeks (59% in the tocilizumab 8-mg/kg group; 48% in the tocilizumab 4-mg/kg group; 27% in the placebo group; $p < 0.0001$). ACR 50 endpoints were achieved in 44%, 32%, and 11% (respectively)—and ACR 70 endpoints were achieved in 22%, 12%, and 2% of patients in the tocilizumab 8-mg/kg group, the tocilizumab 4-mg/kg, and the placebo group, respectively.[33]

Safety profiles revealed a similar frequency of adverse events for tocilizumab and placebo groups, although serious infections were observed more frequently in the tocilizumab group (2.9% in the tocilizumab 8-mg/kg group; 1.4% in the tocilizumab 4-mg/kg group; 1% in the placebo group). Tocilizumab treatment significantly improved quality of life in patients with RA, as assessed by the health assessment questionnaire (HAQ), functional assessment of chronic illness therapy-fatigue scale (FACIT-fatigue), and short form-36 health survey (SF-36).[35]

Similarly, the TOWARD study evaluated the efficacy and safety of tocilizumab in a larger population of 1,216 RA patients with inadequate responses to a range of DMARDs.[34] Patients continued maintenance DMARD treatment while receiving intravenous tocilizumab 8 mg/kg or placebo every 4 weeks for 24 weeks. ACR 20, ACR 50, and ACR 70 responses were significantly higher in the tocilizumab group than in the placebo group (61% vs. 25%, 38% vs. 9%, and 21% vs. 3%, respectively; $p < 0.0001$). This study also confirmed that tocilizumab treatment improved physical function, fatigue, and physical and mental health scores as assessed by HAQ, the FACIT-fatigue scale, and SF-36.[36]

Tocilizumab Safety Concerns

Because IL-6 plays a crucial role in immunity regulation, IL-6 inhibition may result in increased susceptibility to infectious diseases. In addition, suppression of inflammatory symptoms and laboratory value abnormalities may delay detection of infections. Clinical trials have demonstrated that the incidence of infections is similar to that of control groups, and similar to that reported for TNF inhibitors. It is noteworthy that tuberculosis was observed in only 2 of more than 4000 patients treated with tocilizumab, without pretrial screening or prophylactic use of anti-tuberculosis drugs. In comparison, tuberculosis frequently emerges during treatment with TNF inhibitors. This may be explained by the fact that TNF plays an important role in the formation of granulomas, whereas IL-6 is largely uninvolved in this immune response.

Several reports have claimed that TNF blockade may increase the risk of malignancy in RA patients, and it is possible that suppression of IL-6 action may also be carcinogenic. To investigate the risk of malignancy in RA patients treated with tocilizumab, outcomes from patients treated with long-term tocilizumab were compared to those of a Japanese cohort of RA patients (IORRA cohort) and a Japanese population database.[37] The incidence of malignancy, adjusted for age and gender, was calculated by direct and indirect methods.

In the tocilizumab cohort (mean age 51.5, female 79.8%, mean disease duration 6.21 years), 11 malignancies (male 3, female 8) were identified among 618 patients (1,459 person-years). In the IORRA cohort (mean age 55.9, female 81.8%, mean disease duration 8.73 years), 173 malignancies (male 56, female 115) were identified among 7,656 patients (25.567 person-years). The crude incidence of malignancies was 753.7 (male 1171.3, female 664.8) per 100,000 in the tocilizumab cohort and 676.7 (male 1331.5, female 542.2) per 100,000 in the IORRA cohort. Compared to the IORRA cohort, the standardized incidence ratio (SIR) of malignancies in the tocilizumab cohort was overall 1.33 (95% CI: 0.74–2.40). The SIR for males in this study was 1.18 (95% CI: 0.38–3.66), and that for females was 1.39 (95% CI: 0.70–2.79). Compared to the Japanese population database, the SIR was overall 1.66 (95% CI: 0.92–3.00)—and for males was 1.58 (95% CI: 0.51–4.88) and for females 1.70 (95% CI: 0.85–3.39). The incidence of malignancy in the tocilizumab cohort, therefore, did not exceed those of the Japanese RA cohort nor the Japanese population database.

Conclusion

Clinical studies have demonstrated that IL-6R inhibition by tocilizumab is a promising therapeutic approach for RA. The mechanisms by which IL-6 inhibition mediates improvements in RA, however, are not yet fully understood. Because regulation of inflammatory cytokines, including IL-6, is involved in the pathogenesis of RA future research will be needed to identify compounds that may act synergistically with tocilizumab. The long-term safety of tocilizumab treatment—particularly involving infection, malignancy, and cardiovascular risk—will also require investigation.

References

1. Hirano T, Yasukawa K, Harada H, et al. Complementary DNA for a novel human interleukin (BSF-2) that induces B lymphocytes to produce immunoglobulin. *Nature* 1986;324:73–76.
2. Wolvekamp MC, Marquet RL. Interleukin-6: Historical background, genetics and biological significance. *Immunol Lett* 1990;24:1–9.
3. Kishimoto T. The biology of interleukin-6. *Blood* 1989;74:1–10.
4. Nishimoto N. Interleukin-6 in rheumatoid arthritis. *Curr Opin Rheumatol* 2006;18:277–281.
5. Hirano T, Matsuda T, Turner M, et al. Excessive production of interleukin 6/B cell stimulatory factor-2 in rheumatoid arthritis. *Eur J Immunol* 1988;18:1797–1801.
6. Houssiau FA, Devogelaer JP, Van Damme J, et al. Interleukin-6 in synovial fluid and serum of patients with rheumatoid arthritis and other inflammatory arthritis. *Arthritis Rheum* 1988;31:784–788.
7. Sack U, Kinne R, Marx T, et al. Interleukin-6 in synovial fluid is closely associated with chronic synovitis in rheumatoid arthritis. *Rheumatol Int* 1993;13:45–51.
8. Madhok R, Crilly A, Watson J, et al. Serum interleukin 6 levels in rheumatoid arthritis: Correlation with clinical and laboratory indices of disease activity. *Ann Rheum Dis* 1993;52:232–234.
9. Harrington LE, Hatton RD, Mangan PR, et al. Interleukin 17-producing CD4+ effector T cells develop via a lineage distinct from the T helper type 1 and 2 lineages. *Nat Immunol* 2005;6:1123–1132.
10. Park H, Li Z, Yang XO, et al. A distinct lineage of CD4 T cells regulates tissue inflammation by producing interleukin 17. *Nat Immunol* 2005;6:1133–1141.
11. Nakae S, Nambu A, Sudo K, et al. Suppression of immune induction of collagen-induced arthritis in IL-17-deficient mice. *J Immunol* 2003;171:6173– 6177.
12. Mangan PR, Harrington LE, O'Quinn DB, et al. Transforming growth factor-beta induces development of the T(H)17 lineage. *Nature* 2006;441:231–234.
13. Bettelli E, Carrier Y, Gao W, et al. Reciprocal developmental pathways for the generation of pathogenic effector TH17 and regulatory T cells. *Nature* 2006;441:235–238.
14. Nakahara H, Song J, Sugimoto M, et al. Anti-interleukin-6 receptor antibody therapy reduces vascular endothelial growth factor production in rheumatoid arthritis. *Arthritis Rheum* 2003;48:1521–1529.
15. Tamura T, Udagawa N, Takahashi N, et al. Soluble interleukin-6 receptor triggers osteoclast formation by interleukin 6. *Proc Natl Acad Sci U S A* 1993;90:11924–11928.
16. van Gameren MM, Willemse PH, Mulder NH, et al. Effects of recombinant human interleukin-6 in cancer patients: A phase I–II study. *Blood* 1994;84:1434–1441.
17. Castell JV, Gomez-Lechon MJ, David M, et al. Recombinant human interleukin-6(IL-6/BSF-2/HSF) regulates the synthesis of acute phase proteins in human hepatocytes. *FEBS Lett* 1988;232:347–350.
18. Ishibashi T, Kimura H, Shikama Y, et al. Interleukin-6 is a potent thrombopoietic factor in vivo in mice. *Blood* 1989;74:1241–1244.
19. Nemeth E, Rivera S, Gabayan V, et al. IL-6 mediates hypoferremia of inflammation by inducing the synthesis of the iron regulatory hormone hepcidin. *J Clin Invest* 2004;113:1271–1276.
20. Lee P, Peng H, Gelbart T, et al. Regulation of hepcidin transcription by interleukin-1 and interleukin-6. *Proc Natl Acad Sci U S A* 2005; 102:1906–1910.
21. Sato K, Tsuchiya M, Saldanha J, et al. Reshaping a human antibody to inhibit the interleukin 6-dependent tumor cell growth. *Cancer Res* 1993;53:851–856.

22. Scheller J, Ohnesorge N, Rose-John S. Interleukin-6 trans-signalling in chronic inflammation and cancer. *Scand J Immunol* 2006;63: 321–329.
23. Nishimoto N, Yoshizaki K, Maeda K, et al. Toxicity, pharmacokinetics, and dose finding study of repetitive treatment with humanized anti-interleukin 6 receptor antibody, MRA, in rheumatoid arthritis: Phase I/II clinical study. *J Rheumatol* 2003;30:1426–1435.
24. Nishimoto N, Kishimoto T, Yoshizaki K. Anti-interleukin 6 receptor antibody treatment in rheumatic disease. *Ann Rheum Dis* 2000;59 (Suppl 1):i21–i27.
25. Nishimoto N, Sasai M, Shima Y, et al. Improvement in Castleman's disease by humanized anti-IL-6 receptor antibody therapy. *Blood* 2000;95:56–61.
26. Choy EH, Isenberg DA, Garrood T, et al. Therapeutic benefit after blocking interleukin-6 activity in rheumatoid arthritis with an anti-interleukin-6 receptor monoclonal antibody. *Arthritis Rheum* 2002; 46:3143–3150.
27. Nishimoto N, Yoshizaki K, Miyasaka N, et al. Treatment of rheumatoid arthritis with humanized anti-interleukin-6 receptor antibody: A multicenter, double-blind, placebo-controlled trial. *Arthritis Rheum* 2004;50:1761–1769.
28. Ogawa J, Harigai M, Akashi T, et al. Exacerbation of chronic active Epstein-Barr virus infection in a patient with rheumatoid arthritis receiving humanised anti-interleukin-6 receptor monoclonal antibody. *Ann Rheum Dis* 2006;65:1667–1669.
29. Seriolo B, Paolino S, Sulli A, et al. Effects of anti-TNF-alpha treatment on lipid profile in patients with active rheumatoid arthritis. *Ann N Y Acad Sci* 2006;1069:414–419.
30. Maini RN, Taylor PC, Szechinski J, et al. for the CHARISMA Study Group. Double-blind randomized controlled clinical trial of the interleukin-6 receptor antagonist, tocilizumab, in European patients with rheumatoid arthritis who had an incomplete response to methotrexate. *Arthritis Rheum* 2006;54:2817–2829.
31. Nishimoto N, Miyasaka N, Yamamoto K, et al. Efficacy and safety of tocilizumab in monotherapy, an anti–IL-6 receptor monoclonal antibody, in patients with active rheumatoid arthritis: Results from a 24 week double-blind phase III study. *Ann Rheum Dis* 2006;65 (Suppl II):59.
32. Nishimoto N, Hashimoto J, Miyasaka N, et al. Study of active controlled monotherapy used for rheumatoid arthritis, an IL-6 inhibitor (SAMURAI): Evidence of clinical and radiographic benefit from an x-ray reader-blinded randomized controlled trial of tocilizumab. *Ann Rheum Dis* 2007;66:1162–1167.
33. Smolen J, Beaulieu A, Rubbert-Ruth A, et al. Tocilizumab, a novel monoclonal antibody targeting IL-6 signalling, significantly reduces disease activity in patients with rheumatoid arthritis. *Ann Rheum Dis* 2007;66(Suppl):88.
34. Genovese M, McKay J, Nasonov E, et al. IL-6 receptor inhibition with tocilizumab reduces disease activity in patients with rheumatoid arthritis with inadequate response to a range of DMARDs: The TOWARD Study. *Arthritis Rheum* 2007;52(Suppl):L15.
35. Smolen J, Rovensky J, Ramos-Remus C, et al. Targeting the IL-6 receptor with the monoclonal antibody tocilizumab significantly improves quality of life in patients with rheumatoid arthritis. *Arthritis Rheum* 2007;52(Suppl):S162.
36. Gomez-Reino JJ, Fairfax MJ, Pavelka K, et al. Targeted inhibition of IL-6 signalling with tocilizumab improves quality of life and function in patients with rheumatoid arthritis with inadequate response to a range of DMARDs. *Arthritis Rheum* 2007;52(Suppl):L6.
37. Yamanaka H, Nishimoto N, Inoue E, et al. Incidence of malignancies in Japanese rheumatoid arthritis patients treated with tocilizumab in comparison to those in an observational cohort of Japanese patients and a Japanese population database. *Ann Rheum Dis* 2007;66 (Suppl):122.

Promising Biologic Agents and Small Chemical Compounds

Christopher G. Meyer and E. William St. Clair

Biologics	Small Chemical Compounds

Substantial progress has been made in the treatment of rheumatoid arthritis (RA) over the past decade with the addition of biologic agents to the therapeutic armamentarium. The approved agents for this indication are the tumor necrosis factor α (TNF-α) inhibitors (etanercept, infliximab, and adalimumab), anakinra (IL-1 receptor antagonist), abatacept (CTLA4Ig), and rituximab (anti-CD20)—with certolizumab pegol (pegylated Fab' fragment of an anti-TNF antibody) and tocilizumab (anti–IL-6 receptor) looming on the horizon. Propelled by an unmet need for effective RA therapies and the wealth of attractive therapeutic targets, companies are aggressively exploring novel interventions to favorably impact care of this disease. Among the innovative drugs under development are the biologics targeting IL-15, -17, -18, and -12/23. Given the success of rituximab in the clinic, companies are looking beyond anti-CD20-induced B-cell depletion to strategies that fine tune B-cell function by inhibiting B-cell costimulation and survival. Protein kinases that mediate the proinflammatory signals of TNF and IL-1 are also attracting attention as potential sites of intervention, as are inhibitors of leukocyte migration. With these innovative therapies coming into view, we examine herein the biologics and small molecules under development that could dramatically impact the landscape of RA therapy over the next several years.

Biologics

Novel TNF Antagonists

Two novel TNF antagonists, certolizumab pegol and golimumab, had progressed to late-phase clinical development at the time of this writing. Certolizumab pegol is a pegylated humanized Fab' fragment of an anti-TNF monoclonal antibody, and as such excludes an Fc portion that can trigger complement activation, antibody-dependent cytotoxicity, or apoptosis. Based on results from two phase III placebo-controlled, double-blind randomized trials, subcutaneously administered certolizumab pegol in combination with weekly methotrexate (MTX) has been shown to be significantly more effective than MTX alone for reducing RA activity.[1,2] Golimumab, a human monoclonal antibody to TNF, had produced similarly favorable therapeutic responses through phase II of development.

Anti-Interleukin-15

Anti-interleukin-15 (IL-15) has emerged as a possible therapeutic target in RA because of its ability to stimulate proinflammatory cytokine production. The receptor for IL-15 has two subunits in common with the receptor for IL-2, drawing frequent comparisons between the two cytokines. The IL-15 receptor consists of the IL-15-specific subunit, IL-15α, the IL-2/IL-15β subunit, and the common γ-chain (γ_c).[3] Unlike IL-2, IL-15 is only secreted in small quantities and exists mainly in a membrane-bound form. IL-15 has been shown to stimulate the proliferation of natural killer (NK) cells, and T and B cells; maintain the survival of CD8$^+$-memory T cells; regulate the secretory activities and survival of neutrophils and eosinophils; serve as a growth factor for mast cells; stimulate monocyte/macrophges to produce TNF, IL-6, IL-8, and IL-12; promote phagocytosis and bacterial clearance; induce dendritic cells to increase expression of CD86, CD40, and MHC II; stimulate release of interferon-γ; and protect fibroblasts and endothelial cells from apoptosis.[4]

IL-15 inhibition has been shown to decrease joint inflammation and articular destruction in murine collagen-induced arthritis (CIA).[5,6] In RA, synovial biopsies show up-regulated expression of IL-15 by macrophage-like and fibroblast-like synovial cells and endothelial cells—suggesting a possible role for this cytokine in promoting synovitis. Furthermore, IL-15 has also been shown *in vitro* to promote cytokine and chemokine release directly via effects on synovial T cells and indirectly through maintenance of cytokine-activated T-cell cognate interactions with synovial macrophages.[7] IL-15 is also a potent inducer of IL-17 (see material following) and promotes osteoclastogenesis.[8,9]

The clinical efficacy and safety of a fully human IgG1 anti-IL-15 monoclonal antibody (AMG714) has been examined in a placebo-controlled, double-blind, placebo-controlled trial involving 180 patients with active RA on background MTX therapy. Although the primary efficacy endpoint was not met in this trial, American College of Rheumatology (ACR) responses trended higher than those of placebo in the highest-dose AMG714 group.[10] Because the IL-15 pathway is distinct from the pathways used by TNF, IL-1, and IL-6 to drive joint inflammation, its blockade has been deemed a potentially attractive strategy for treating anti-TNF nonresponders.

Targeting the IL-23/IL-17 Axis

For more than a decade, the differentiation of CD4$^+$-naive T cells into T helper (Th) 1 and Th2 subsets was the dominant paradigm in models of autoimmunity. IL-12 was the key player driving Th1 cell development, whereas IL-4 was the principal stimulator of Th2 cell differentiation. Th1 cells predominately secreted interferon (IFN)-γ, IL-2, and TNF. By comparison,

Th2 cells mainly produced IL-4, IL-5, and IL-13. Although RA had been generally viewed as a Th1-driven disease, the evidence for such a concept had been far from conclusive. The discovery of IL-23 and Th17 cells, a third type of differentiation pathway for T cells, has dramatically altered this perspective. IL-23 bears a structural relationship to IL-12, as they both are members of the type 1 cytokine family.[11] IL-12, a heterodimer, consists of a p35 and p40 subunit. The IL-23 complex, also a heterodimer, contains the IL-12 p40 subunit and a unique p19 subunit. The receptors for these two cytokines also have structural similarities. The receptor for IL-12 consists of IL-12Rβ1 and IL-12Rβ2 chains, whereas the IL-23 receptor (IL-23R) consists of an IL-12Rβ1 chain and a unique IL-23R chain.

The sharing of subunits between IL-12 and IL-23 and their receptors explains some of the paradoxical findings that had confused researchers in the past. Based on studies using anti-p40 antibodies and p40-deficient mice, the development of CIA was believed to be critically dependent on IL-12 and Th1 cells. However, mice deficient in IFN-γ (a product of Th1 cells) had more severe CIA than wild-type mice. The discovery that the p40 subunit was shared between IL-12 and IL-23 resolved this inconsistency. Indeed, later studies using p19-deficient mice (IL-23 deficient, but IL-12 intact) were found to be resistant to the development of CIA.[12]

In mice, IL-23 is intimately linked to the development of Th17 cells.[13] TGF-β and IL-6 are required initially to induce the differentiation of naive $CD4^+$ T cells into mature Th17 cells. IL-23 acts subsequently to expand the memory-effector Th17 population. Th1 and Th2 cells strongly suppress Th17 development and function. Although TGF-β plays a critical role in mouse Th17 differentiation, initial studies had shown that it was not required for induction of Th17 cells in humans.[14] In humans, IL-1 potently triggers naive $CD4^+$ T cells to differentiate into Th17 cells, whereas IL-6 alone is a relatively poor inducer of Th17 development—which differs from the situation in the mouse.

Mouse T cells activated by IL-23 express high levels of transcripts for IL-17, IL-6, IL-22, TNF, GM-CSF, CXCL1, CCL7, CCL20, CCL22, and α_3 integrin.[13] Evidence from animal studies suggests that IL-23 and IL-17 are intimately linked in the mechanisms of inflammatory arthritis. In one study, IL-23 mediated the surplus of IL-1 signals in an IL-1 receptor antagonist-deficient model of arthritis by promoting the differentiation of $CD4^+$ T cells into Th17 cells.[15] Moreover, experiments using IL-17 blocking antibodies, IL-17-soluble receptor, and IL-4-producing dendritic cells showed suppression of CIA[16–18]—supporting a prominent role for Th17 cells in the pathogenesis of experimental arthritis.

In RA, serum and synovial fluid levels of IL-23p19 levels correlate with serum and synovial fluid concentrations of IL-17.[19] IL-17 synthesis has been detected in the T-cell–rich areas of RA synovium.[20] The IL-17 receptor is expressed on several different cell types, including epithelial cells, endothelial cells, and fibroblasts. Upon ligand binding, it has been shown to activate the NFκB pathway and stimulate the secretion of IL-6, IL-8, G-CSF, monocyte chemotactic protein 1, prostaglandin E2, TNF, IL-1,[13] and MMP-1.[21] Th17 cells also promote osteoclastogenesis by inducing receptor activator of nuclear factor kappa B ligand (RANKL) on the mesenchymal cells that support osteoclast differentiation.[22]

A human IL-12/23 p40 antibody has been tested in a phase II randomized, placebo-controlled trial of 320 patients with moderate to severe plaque psoriasis.[23] The scientific rationale for this approach had derived from the finding of increased expression of both IL-23p19 and IL-12p40 in lesional skin, mainly from keratinocytes and Langerhans cells.[13] In this trial, subjects who received the IL-12/23 antibody achieved levels of clinical benefit on the order of responses previously described using the TNF inhibitors. Because this antibody inhibits both IL-12 and IL-23, specific inhibitors of IL-23 will be needed to determine if neutralizing IL-23 and impeding Th17 cell development were the basis for its clinical efficacy. The IL-23/Th17 axis will likely be a target of novel RA therapies in the future.

Blocking IL-1 and Related Family Members

IL-1 has long been considered an important player in the pathogenesis of joint inflammation. However, the modest clinical efficacy of anakinra (an IL-1 receptor antagonist) has cast doubt on the validity of this hypothesis. The disappointing clinical responses in RA using anakinra may derive from the unfavorable pharmacokinetics of this drug and the requirement for it to occupy 99% of the IL-1 receptors on the cell surface in order to effectively block signaling. Anti-IL-1 monoclonal antibodies have been developed to overcome these drawbacks and are currently being tested in RA trials.

IL-18, another member of the IL-1 superfamily of cytokines, is produced mainly by macrophages and dendritic cells. IL-18 induces expression of many cytokines (such as IFN-γ, TNF, IL-6, and IL-32), as well as an array of chemokines and angiogenic factors. It also activates neutrophils, stimulates cartilage destruction indirectly via IL-1, and accelerates the development of osteoclasts by inducing TNF, IL-1, and IL-6.[24,25] Studies in animal models of arthritis strongly support a pathogenic role for IL-18 in joint inflammation. IL-18 binds to a heterodimeric receptor consisting of IL-18Rα and IL-18Rβ chains, which in turn induces signaling pathways shared with the IL-1R and toll-like receptors (TLRs). IL-18 can also be regulated by IL-18 binding protein (IL-18BP), an endogenous ligand with high binding affinity for IL-18 that prevents binding to the IL-18R.

Phase I studies using a recombinant human IL-18BP have been performed in healthy volunteers and in patients with psoriasis and RA.[26] Given the lack of larger trials of IL-18BP in RA, this approach will require further study.

Lymphotoxin β Receptor Ig (LTβR-Ig) Fusion Protein

The lymphotoxins (LTs) are members of the TNF superfamily.[27] LTα homotrimers bind to the TNF receptors 1 and 2 (TNF-R1 and TNFR-2), although their role in the mechanisms of inflammatory arthritis remain unclear (e.g., etanercept binds LTα). LTα also binds to LTβ, forming membrane-bound $LT\alpha_1\beta_2$ heterotrimers. LTαβ is expressed on activated T, B, and NK cells and binds to the LTβ receptor—which is expressed on the stromal cells of lymphoid tissues, follicular dendritic cells, monocytes, and dendritic cells. In mice, LTαβ is essential for proper organization of the splenic and lymph node microarchitecture.

Human LTβR-Ig (baminercept) has been developed for clinical use as an inhibitor of the LTαβ pathway. The idea that inhibiting the LTαβ pathway may improve joint inflammation comes in part from the fact that rheumatoid synovitis displays immunohistologic features of ectopic lymphoid tissue. Fibroblast-like synoviocytes have been shown to express the LTβR, which upon ligation with LTαβ induces the expression of cell adhesion molecules and secretion of the CCL2 and CCL5 chemokines.

LTαβ may therefore be an important factor in recruitment and retention of lymphocytes in the synovial microenvironment.[28] This approach gains further support from studies of murine CIA, where administration of LTβR-Ig has been found to ameliorate the arthritis.[29]

The efficacy and safety of baminercept was recently examined in a randomized, placebo-controlled phase IIa study of patients with active RA on background MTX therapy.[30] Subjects in this study received subcutaneously administered doses of baminercept ranging from 0.01 to 3 mg/kg once weekly for 4 weeks. Baminercept-treated patients had 60% and 47% improvements in swollen and tender joint count, respectively, as opposed to 4.6% and 7.6% reductions for these measures in the placebo group. The most common side effect was a flu-like infusion reaction of mild to moderate intensity. Further trials of baminercept have been initiated based on these early promising results.

Other Cytokine Targets

Other cytokines are being evaluated as possible therapeutic targets, including GM-CSF, TWEAK (TNF-like weak inducer of apoptosis), and IL-32. As of this writing, the evaluation of a human anti-GM-CSF monoclonal antibody was in phase I studies—whereas inhibitors of TWEAK and IL-32 were still in preclinical development.

Emerging B-Cell Targets

The success of rituximab (chimeric anti-CD20 monoclonal antibody) therapy for RA has validated the B cell as a crucial player in the pathogenesis of RA. Second-generation human anti-CD20 monoclonal antibodies are under clinical development to improve upon this approach. These include ocrelizumab and ofatumumab. Another CD20-directed technology utilizes single-chain polypeptides customized with specifc targeting and effector functions. These molecules are termed *small modular immunopharmaceuticals* (SMIPs). TRU-015, the first SMIP to enter clinical development, binds CD20 and is designed with potent antibody-dependent cellular cytotoxicity but limited complement-dependent cytotoxicity. So far, TRU-015 has progressed to phase II studies in RA—with preliminary evidence of clinical efficacy and good tolerability.[31]

Belimumab is a human monoclonal antibodies to soluble B-cell–activating factor belonging to the TNF family (BAFF) (also known as BLyS). BAFF is expressed by myeloid lineage cells in both membrane-bound and soluble forms.[32] B cells express three known receptors for BAFF (BAFFR or BR3, transmembrane activator and calcium modulator and cyclophilin ligand interactor [TACI], and B-cell maturation protein [BCMA]).[33] The binding of BAFF to the BAFFR on B cells is essential for the full development of B cells. Several lines of evidence implicate excessive BAFF in the mechanisms of autoimmune diseases, including those of RA. However, belimumab has shown only modest clinical efficacy for the treatment of RA in phase II studies.[34] Atacicept, a recombinant fusion protein engineered along the lines of etanercept, consists of TACI in covalent linkage with the Fc portion of IgG1. It binds to BAFF and to APRIL, a ligand for both TACI and BCMA. Results from phase I studies have shown that single and repeated subcutaneous injections of atacicept decrease serum levels of rheumatoid factor and anti-CCP antibodies, and alter the numbers of circulating B cells—with favorable trends observed for clinical efficacy.[35]

Integrin and Chemokine Inhibitors

A key checkpoint in cellular migration is the interaction between cell surface receptors, termed *integrins*, on leukocytes and a diverse set of ligands on endothelial cells and leukocytes themselves—as well as within the extracellular matrix.[36] Integrins also serve as a means by which cellular adhesion can regulate lymphocyte responses. Integrin signaling occurs in two phases: inside-out and outside-in. Inside-out signaling through engagement of receptors on the cell surface enables leukocytes to adhere to vascular endothelium and communicate with other cells. By comparison, outside-in signaling affects leukocyte effector functions. Based on several lines of evidence, β2-integrin lymphocyte function antigen-1 (LFA-1) has been postulated to play a critical role in inflammatory disease.[37] It is expressed on the surface of T cells and interacts with intracellular adhesion molecule-1 (ICAM-1) on antigen-presenting cells, synovial fibroblasts, and endothelial cells. Many signaling pathways increase LFA-1 binding to ICAM-1, including those downstream of the T-cell receptor and chemokine receptors. Thus, LFA-1 interactions may foster an activating environment inside the rheumatoid joint. However, a phase II trial of efalizumab (anti-LFA-1 monoclonal antibody) for the treatment of RA was halted after this biologic failed to show any significant clinical benefits.

Natilizumab, a humanized anti-α4 integrin monoclonal antibody, inhibits cell binding mediated by $\alpha_4\beta_1$ and $\alpha_4\beta_7$ to vascular cell adhesion molecule 1 (VCAM-1). Because the expression of VCAM-1 is up-regulated on synovial tissue from patients with RA, interfering with α_4 integrin binding may reduce migration of leukocytes to the synovial tissue. A phase II randomized, placebo-controlled trial of natilizumab therapy for RA was prematurely stopped after two patients with multiple sclerosis and one patient with Crohn's disease developed progressive multifocal leukoencephalopathy in other clinical trials of this antibody.[38] After 6 months of treatment, a nonsignificant trend toward clinical improvement was observed in the patients receiving natalizumab compared to the placebo group (ACR 20 response: 43% vs. 33%).

Chemokines are also critical mediators of cell migration.[39] CCL2 (monocyte chemotractic protein 1, MCP-1) has been considered a relevant therapeutic target in RA because its levels are increased in the peripheral blood, synovial fluid, and synovial tissue of patients with this disease. CCL2 mediates the migration of monocytes and T cells, and for this reason may regulate joint inflammation in RA. However, a recent phase II trial found that an anti-CCL2 monoclonal antibody was ineffective for the treatment of RA.[40]

Specific Inhibitors of Structural Damage

Denosumab is a human anti-RANK ligand (RANKL) monoclonal antibody that has been developed to inhibit osteoclasts. In addition to its applications in osteoporosis and cancer, denosumab may protect against joint destruction in RA. RANKL is a key mediator of osteoclast formation, function, and survival. A recent phase II study of patients with erosive RA found that denosumab treatment every 6 months significantly slowed radiographic progression of disease in comparison to placebo, as measured by the total Sharp score.[41] Not unexpectedly, denosumab treatment had no effect on the signs and symptoms of joint inflammation.

Small Chemical Compounds

Whereas the major advances in new therapies for RA have come from biologically based interventions, efforts in drug discovery have been increasingly directed toward targets amenable to intervention with small-molecule inhibitors. In principle, small molecules may have several advantages relative to biologics—such as more straightforward manufacturing, easier dose titration, added convenience of oral deliverability, and lower cost. However, a significant hurdle for some of the small molecules in development has been the occurrence of nonspecific drug-related toxicities.

p38MAP Kinase Inhibitors

Proinflammatory signals from diverse cell surface receptors culminate in the activation of mitogen-activated protein kinases (MAPKs) (Figure 10K-1). The MAPKs consists of four subfamilies with distinct upstream signaling cascades: extracellular-signal-regulated kinases (ERKs), ERK5, JUN N-terminal kinases (JNKs), and p38 kinases.[42] The substrates of MAPKs impact a wide range of biologic processes controlling the cell cycle, cell differentiation, cell proliferation, and the inflammatory response. The p38 MAP kinase family includes four isoforms encoded by separate genes: p38α, p38β, p38γ, and p38δ. Many protein kinases are involved in the MAPK cascade upstream of the p38 family members and may also therefore be amenable to inhibition. The α and γ isoforms of p38 predominate in the inflamed synovium of patients with RA, with expression predominately localized to the synovial lining cells and endothelium.[43] In rheumatoid synovial cells, p38 MAP kinase has been shown to regulate TNF production by post-transcriptional control of mRNA stability and translation—as well as by NF-κB-mediated effects on TNF gene transcription.[44]

Single-dose studies of p38 MAP kinase inhibitors (including BIRB-796, VX-745, and RO19) have shown good oral biovailability and pharmacokinetic profiles. However, repeated dose studies of these small-molecule inhibitors have revealed significant toxicities. BIRB-796 progressed through phase II studies before its further development was stopped because of liver toxicity. VX-745 proceeded to a phase II study in RA, where it showed some evidence of clinical benefit. However, its development came to an end as a result of drug-related central nervous system (CNS) toxicity in a parallel animal study. After VX-745 failed to move forward in development, VX-702 (a structurally related compound without CNS penetration) was advanced into clinical trials. A preliminary report from a 12-week phase II study of VX-702 involving 315 patients with active RA showed that this oral p38 inhibitor had modest clinical efficacy and good tolerability.[45] SCIO-469, an oral p38 inhibitor, has also moved forward to phase II studies. Several other oral p38 inhibitors remain in clinical development despite the less than encouraging results thus far.

Janus Kinase 3 (Jak3) Inhibitors

The Janus kinase family of tyrosine kinases consists of Jak1, Jak2, Jak3, and Tyk2.[46] All of the family members are ubiquitously expressed except for Jak3, which is expressed exclusively in leukocytes. Jak3 associates with the common γ_c, which is a component of the IL-2 receptor as well as other cytokine receptors (including IL-4, IL-7, IL-9, IL-15, and IL-21). In humans, mutations in Jak3 have been associated with severe combined immunodeficiency disease.

In particular, Jak3 plays a crucial role in regulating leukocyte function—becoming activated following ligand binding to the IL-2 receptor. Once activated, Jak3 phosphorylates specific tyrosine residues on the receptor—leading to the recruitment of specific signal transducers and activators of transcription (STATs)[46,47] (Figure 10K-2). The STATs are then phosphorylated and then reorient as dimers, followed by their release from the receptor and translocation to the nucleus (where they act as powerful regulators of gene transcription). One study showed Jak3, STAT1, STAT4, and STAT6 to be expressed in the synovial tissue of patients with RA.[48]

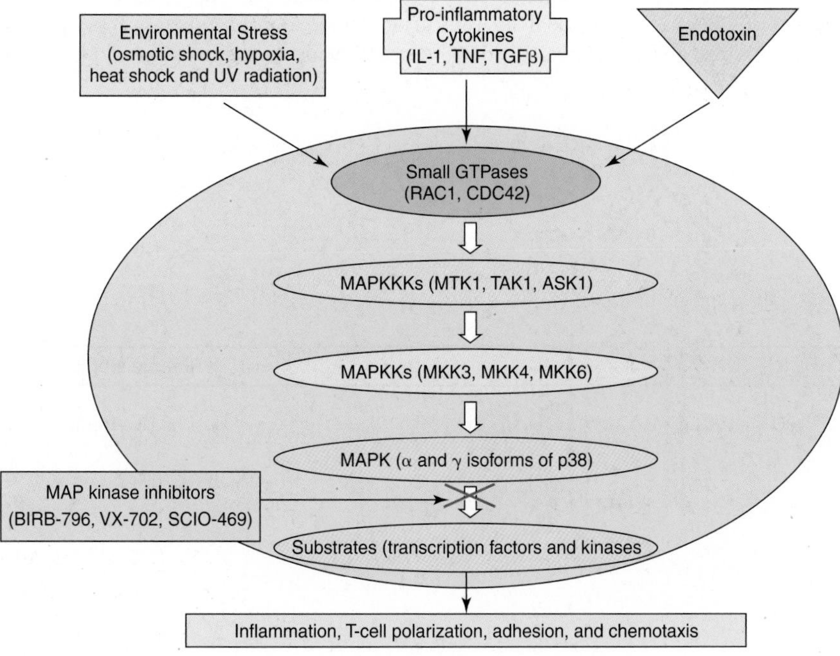

Figure 10K-1. Mitogen-activated protein kinase (MAPK) inhibitors block activation of p38 family members. Proinflammatory cytokines are among the external stimuli that initiate GTPase-dependent activation of mitogen-activated protein kinase kinase kinases (MAPKKKs), which in turn active the mitogen-activated protein kinase kinases (MAPKKs). The MAPKKs then phosphorylate and activate p38, leading to increased expression of mRNAs for cytokines and receptors involved in inflammation and immunity. Abbreviations: MAPKKK4 (also known as MTK1 in humans), apoptosis signal regulating kinase 1 (ASK1), TGFβ-activated protein kinase 1 (TAK1), kinases MAPKK3 (MKK3), MKK4, and MKK6. (Adapted from Ashwell JD. The many paths to p38 mitogen-activated protein kinase activation in the immune system. *Nat Rev Immunol* 2006;6:532–540.)

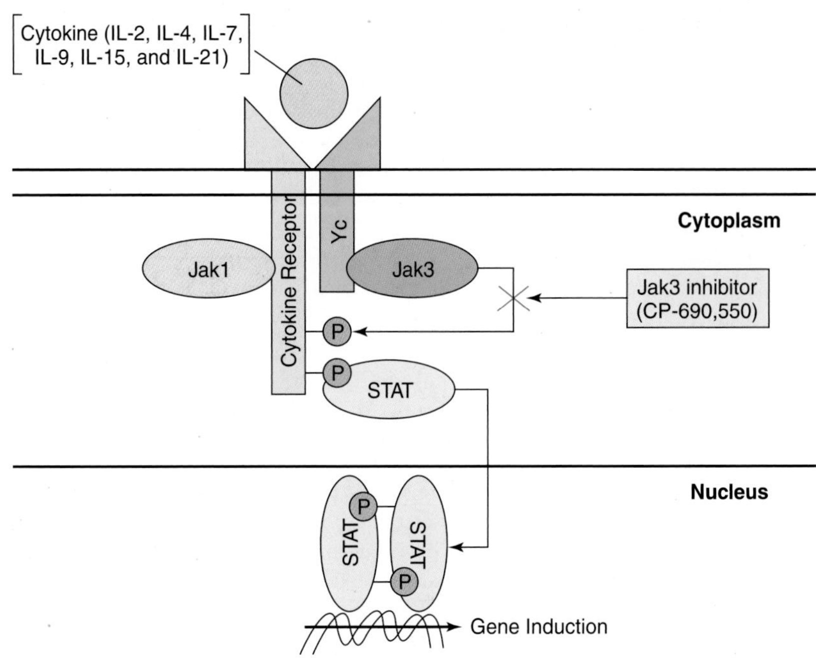

Figure 10K-2. The inhibition of Jak3 blocks the recruitment of STATs. Jak3 associates with the common γc, which is a component of cytokine receptors—including IL-2, IL-4, IL-7, IL-9, IL-15, and IL-21. Jak3 becomes activated after ligand binding to the cytokine receptor. Once activated, Jak3 phosphorylates specific tyrosine residues on the receptor—leading to the recruitment of specific signal transducers and activators of transcription (STATs). The STATs are then phosphorylated and then reorient as dimers, followed by their release from the receptor and translocation to the nucleus (where they act as powerful regulators of gene transcription). (Adapted from Fantini MC, Becker C, Kiesslich R, et al. Drug insight: Novel small molecules and drugs for immunosuppression. *Nat Clin Pract Gastroenterol Hepatol* 2006;3:633–644.)

A phase II trial of an oral Jak3 inhibitor in 264 patients with active RA has shown promising results.[49] In this study, treatment of subjects with three different doses of CP-690,550 was compared to a placebo over a 6-week period. At the 15-mg twice-daily dose, ACR 20, ACR 50, and ACR 70 responses were found to be 81%, 54%, and 22%, respectively—which compared to response rates in the placebo group of, respectively, 29%, 6%, and 3%. There was a dose-related reduction in neutrophil counts (<1000/mm^3 in one case) during the study, but no significant increase in the incidence of infections.

Spleen Tyrosine Kinase Inhibitors

Spleen tyrosine inase (Syk), an intracellular tyrosine kinase, is a key mediator of Fc receptor and B-cell receptor signaling[50] (Figure 10K-3). In CIA, treatment using an oral Syk inhibitor (R406) has been shown to decrease joint inflammation, bone erosions, and pannus formation.[51] A short-term study of R406 in healthy volunteers has provided evidence of *ex vivo* biologic activity.[52] In a preliminary report from a 12-week dose-ranging phase II study, an oral Syk inhibitor (R788) produced ACR 20 response rates for the three different dose groups ranging from 32% to 72%—which compared to a response rate of 38% in the placebo group.[53] The most common side effects in this trial were dose-related neutropenia and elevated liver enzymes.

Other kinases have been considered as possible targets for RA therapy. The remarkable success of imatinib mesylate for the treatment of Philadelphia chromosome-positive (translocation between chromosomes 9 and 22) chronic myeloid leukemia has highlighted the potential for molecular targeting of the kinases for therapeutic purposes. This particular translocation gives rise to the BCR-ABL1 gene, leading to a constitutively active protein kinase. Imatinib mesylate binds to the activation loop of the

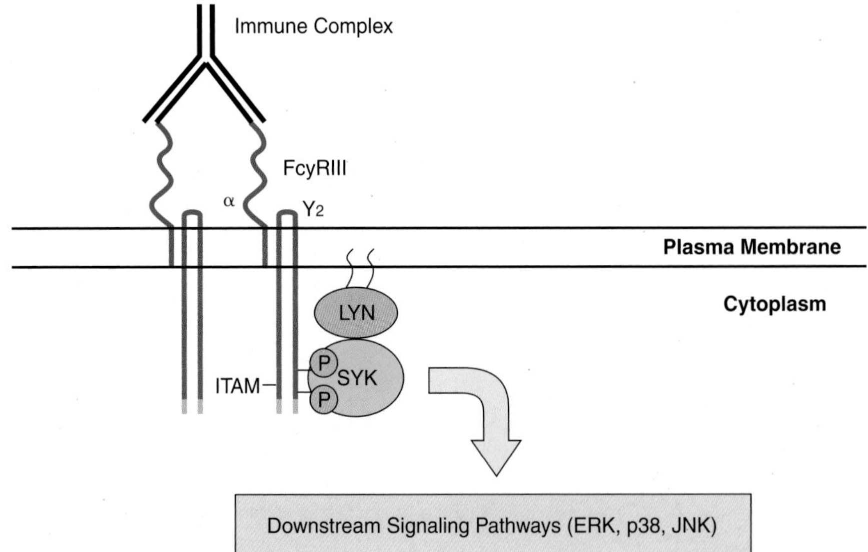

Figure 10K-3. Spleen tyrosine kinase (SYK) recruitment. Immune complexes that cross-link the Fcγ receptor III lead to tyrosine phosphorylation of the immunoreceptor tyrosine-based activation motif (ITAM) by kinases of the Src family. This creates docking sites for SYK, which in turn activates downstream signaling pathways that result in cell activation, cytokine release, and oxidative burst. (Adapted from Nimmerjahn F, Ravetch JV. Fcγ receptors as regulators of immune responses. *Nat Rev Immunol* 2008;8:34–47.)

ABL kinase, trapping the kinase in an inactive confirmation.[54] It also binds to other kinases, including c-kit and platelet-derived growth factor receptor. Because administration of imatinib mesylate has been effective in CIA,[55] it is being considered as a possible treatment for RA. Bruton's tyrosine kinase is another example in this category of an attractive therapeutic target because of its critical role in B-cell lineage development and cell signaling.

CCR1 Antagonists

As mentioned previously, the chemokine receptors and their ligands play important roles in the migration of leukocytes to sites of inflammation. CCR1 is a chemokine receptor expressed on monocytes, T cells, dendritic cells, and neutrophils that interacts with multiple ligands—including CCL3 (macrophage inflammatory protein-1α, MIP-1α), CCL5 (RANTES, regulated on activation, normal T-cell expressed and secreted), CCL7 (monocyte chemotactic protein-3, MCP-3), CCL14 (hemofiltrate C-C chemokine-1), CCL8 (monocyte chemotactic protein-2, MCP-2), CCL15 (leucotactin-1), and CCL23 (myeoloid progenitor inhibitory factor-1, MPIF).[39] CCR1 also induces up-regulation of integrins to stimulate firm adhesion of inflammatory cells to the endothelium. In RA, the CCR1 ligands CCL3 and CCL5 are believed to play an important role in attracting monocyte/macrophages to the inflamed joint—where these cells secrete proinflammatory mediators and tissue-damaging enzymes.

Several companies are developing small-molecule CCR1 antagonists that have advanced as far as phase II clinical trials. These candidates include BX471; CP-481,715; and MLN3897. In a proof-of-concept study, patients with active RA who were treated with a 14-day course of CP-481,715 had a significant decrease between baseline and post-treatment in the overall cellularity of synovial biopsies and the number of synovial macrophages.[56]

Other Oral Agents

Many other small-molecule inhibitors are under development for the treatment of RA. Among this group, oral antagonists of toll-like receptors are appealing because they may interfere with the release of inflammatory mediators. Oral CD80 inhibitors are also promising drugs for the treatment of RA because they inhibit T-cell costimulation and might be expected to mimic the favorable effects of abatacept. Oral inhibitors of the P_2X_7 purinergic receptor and the A3 adenosine receptor are also being investigated for an RA indication.

Summary

The field of RA therapy has been invigorated by a robust pipeline of new biologics and small molecules. The outlook is bright for an expanded array of therapeutic biologics that will enable the clinician to control disease progression in more patients than possible with the approved agents. Novel oral inhibitors will only further diversify the treatment options. The bar for success of any new drug will continue to rise with the tide of therapeutic advances. Further improvements in therapy will undoubtedly require a better understanding of patient variation in treatment response such that biomarkers can be used to individually tailor prescriptions that enhance the likelihood of treatment success.

References

1. Keystone E, Mason D, Combe B, et al. The anti-TNF certolizumab pegol in combination with methotrexate is significantly more effective than methotrexate alone in the treatment of patients with active RA: 1-year results from the RAPID 1 study. *Arthritis Rheum* 2007; 56(Suppl):S300.
2. van der Heijde D, Strand V, Keystone E, et al. Inhibition of radiographic progression by lyophyilized certolizumab pegol added to methotrexate in comparison with methotrexate alone in patients with rheumatoid arthritis: The RAPID 1 trial. *Arthritis Rheum* 2007;56(Suppl):S390.
3. Waldman TA. Targeting the interleukin-15 system in rheumatoid arthritis. *Arthritis Rheum* 2005;52:2585–2588.
4. Budagian V, Bulanova E, Paus R, et al. IL-15/IL-15 receptor biology: A guided tour through an expanding universe. *Cytokine Growth Factor Rev* 2006;17:259–280.
5. Ferrari-Lacraz S, Zanelli E, Neuberg M, et al. Targeting IL-15 receptor-bearing cells with an antagonist mutant IL-15/Fc protein prevents disease development and progression in murine collagen-induced arthritis. *J Immunol* 2004;173:5818–5826.
6. Ruchatz H, Leung BP, Wei X, et al. Soluble IL-15 receptor α-chain administration prevents murine collagen-induced arthritis: A role for IL-15 in development of antigen-induced immunopathology. *J Immunol* 1998;160:5654–5660.
7. Baslund B, Tvede N, Danneskiold-Samsoe B, et al. Targeting interleukin-15 in patients with rheumatoid arthritis: A proof-of-concept study. *Arthritis Rheum* 2005;52:2686–2692.
8. Miranda-Carús M, Balsa A, Benito-Miguel M, et al. IL-15 and the initiation of cell contact-dependent synovial fibroblast–T lymphocyte cross-talk in rheumatoid arthritis: Effect of methotrexate. *J Immunol* 2004;173:1463–1476.
9. Miranda-Carús M, Benito-Miguel M, Balsa A, et al. Peripheral blood T lymphocytes from patients with early rheumatoid arthritis express RANKL and interleukin-15 on the cell surface and promote osteoclastogenesis in autologous monocytes. *Arthritis Rheum* 2006;54:1151–1164.
10. McInnes I, Martin R, Zimmermann-Gorska I, et al. Safety and efficacy of a human monoclonal antibody to IL-15 (AMG 714) in patients with rheumatoid arthritis: Results of a multicenter, randomized, double-blind, placebo-controlled trial. *Ann Rheum Dis* 2006;65(Suppl II):60.
11. Kastelein RA, Hunter CA, Cua DJ. Discovery and biology of IL-23 and IL-27: Related but functionally distinct regulators of inflammation. *Annu Rev Immunol* 2007;25:221–242.
12. Murphy CA, Langrish CL, Chen Y, et al. Divergent pro- and anti-inflammatory roles for IL-23 and IL-12 in joint autoimmune inflammation. *J Exp Med* 2003;198:1951–1957.
13. Kikly K, Liu L, Na S, et al. The IL-23/Th_{17} axis: Therapeutic targets for autoimmune inflammation. *Curr Opin Immunol* 2006;18:670–675.
14. Laurence A, O'Shea JJ. T_H-17 differentiation: Of mice and men. *Nat Immunol* 2007;8:903–905.
15. Cho M, Kang J, Moon Y, et al. STAT3 and NF-κB signal pathway is required for IL-23-mediated IL-17 production in spontaneous arthritis animal model IL-1 receptor antagonist-deficient mice. *J Immunol* 2006;176:5652–5661.
16. Lubberts E, Joosten LAB, Oppers B, et al. IL-1-independent role of IL-17 in synovial inflammation and joint destruction during collagen-induced arthritis. *J Immunol* 2001;167:1004–1013.
17. Lubberts E, Koenders MI, Oppers-Walgreen B, et al. Treatment with a neutralizing anti-murine interleukin-17 antibody after the onset of collagen-induced arthritis reduces joint inflammation,

cartilage destruction, and bone erosion. *Arthritis Rheum* 2004; 50:650–659.

18. Sarkar S, Tesmer LA, Hindnavis V, et al. Interelukin-17 as a molecular target in immune-mediated arthritis: Immunoregulatory properties of genetically modified murine dendritic cells that secrete interleukin-4. *Arthritis Rheum* 2007;56:89–100.
19. Kim HR, Kim HS, Park MK, et al. The clinical role of IL-23p19 in patients with rheumatoid arthritis. *Scand J Rheumatol* 2007;36: 259–264.
20. Chabaud M, Durand JM, Buchs N, et al. Human interleukin-17: A T cell-derived proinflammatory cytokine produced by the rheumatoid synovium. *Arthritis Rheum* 1999;42:963–970.
21. Chabaud M, Garnero P, Dayer JM, et al. Contribution of interleukin 17 to synovium matrix destruction in rheumatoid arthritis. *Cytokine* 2000;12:1092–1099.
22. Sato K, Suematsu A, Okamoto K, et al. Th17 functions as an osteoclastogenic helper T cell subset that links T cell activation and bone destruction. *J Exp Med* 2006;203:2673–2682.
23. Krueger GG, Langley RG, Leonardi C, et al. A human interleukin-12/23 monoclonal antibody for the treatment of psoriasis. *N Engl J Med* 2007;356:580–592.
24. McInnes IB, Liew FY, Gracie JA. Interleukin-18: A therapeutic target in rheumatoid arthritis? *Arthritis Res Ther* 2005;7:38–41.
25. Dai S, Shan Z, Xu H, et al. Cellular targets of interleukin-18 in rheumatoid arthritis. *Ann Rheum Dis* 2007;66:1411–1418.
26. Tak PP, Bacchi M, Bertolino M. Pharmacokineteics of IL-18 binding protein in healthy volunteers and subjects with rheumatoid arthritis and plaque psoriasis. *Eur J Drug Metab Pharmacokinet* 2006;31: 109–116.
27. McCarthy DD, Summers-Deluca L, Vu F, et al. The lymphotoxin pathway: Beyond lymph node development. *Immunol Res* 2006; 35:41–53.
28. Braun A, Takemura S, Vallejo AN, et al. Lymphotoxin β-mediated stimulation of synoviocytes in rheumatoid arthritis. *Arthritis Rheum* 2004;50:2140–2150.
29. Fava RA, Notidis E, Hunt J, et al. A role for the lymphotoxin/literIGHT axis in the pathogenesis of murine collagen-induced arthritis. *J Immunol* 2003;171:115–126.
30. Baldassare A, Feichtner J, Filipowicz-Sosnowska A, et al. Preliminary safety and efficacy of LTβR-Ig (BG9924) in the treatment of rheumatoid arthritis. *Arthritis Rheum* 2007;56(Suppl):S394.
31. Burge D, Chopiak V, Dvoretskiy L, et al. TRU-015 improves rheumatoid arthritis disease activity in a randomized, double-blind, placebo-controlled, multicenter phase II dose ranging trial. Presented at the 2007 Annual Scientific Meeting of the American College of Rheumatology, Boston, MA, November 6–11, 2007.
32. Nardelli B, Belvedere O, Roschke V, et al. Synthesis and release of B-lymphocyte stimulator from myeloid cells. *Blood* 2001;97:198–204.
33. Mackay F, Silveira PA, Brink R. B cells and the BAFF/APRIL axis: Fast forward on autoimmunity and signaling. *Curr Opin Immunol* 2007;19:327–336.
34. McKay J, Chwalinska-Sadowska H, Boling E, et al. Belimumab (BmAb), a fully human monoclonal antibody to B-lymphocyte stimulator (BLyS), combined with standard of care therapy reduces the signs and symptoms of rheumatoid arthritis in a heterogenous subject population. *Arthritis Rheum* 2005;52(Suppl):S710.
35. Tak PP, Thurlings RM, Rossier C, et al. Atacicept in patients with rheumatoid arthritis. *Arthritis Rheum* 2008;68:61–72.
36. Abram CL, Lowell CA. Convergence of immunoreceptor and integrin signaling. *Immunol Rev* 2007;218:29–44.
37. Watts GM, Beurskens FJM, Martin-Padura I, et al. Manifestations of inflammatory arthritis are critically dependent on LFA-1. *J Immunol* 2005;174:3668–3675.
38. Cohen S, Birgara C, Pazdur J, et al. A phase 2 study of natalizumab in subjects with moderate to severe rheumatoid arthritis. *Arthritis Rheum* 2006;54(Suppl):S243.
39. Allen SJ, Crown SE, Handel TM. Chemokine:receptor structure, interactions, and antagonism. *Annu Rev Immunol* 2007;25:787–820.
40. Haringhan JJ, Gerlag DM, Smeets TJM, et al. A randomized controlled trial with an anti-CCL2 (anti-monocyte chemotactic protein 1) monoclonal antibody in patients with rheumatoid arthritis. *Arthritis Rheum* 2006;54:2387–2392.
41. van der Heijde D, Cohen S, Sharp JT, et al. Denosumab inhibits RANKL, reducing progression of the total Sharp score and bone erosions in patients with rheumatoid arthritis: 12-month x-ray results. *Arthritis Rheum* 2007;56(Suppl):S299.
42. Ashwell JD. The many paths to p38 mitogen-activated protein kinase activation in the immune system. *Nat Rev Immunol* 2006;6:532–540.
43. Korb A, Tohidast-Akrad M, Cetin E, et al. Differential expression and activation of p38 MAPK α, β, γ, and δ isoforms in rheumatoid arthritis. *Arthritis Rheum* 2006;54:2745–2756.
44. Campbell J, Ciesielski CJ, Hunt AE, et al. A novel mechanism for TNF-α regulation by p38 MAPK: Involvement of NF-κB with implications for therapy in rheumatoid arthritis. *J Immunol* 2004;173: 6928–6937.
45. Vertex. Vertex Reports Investigational p38 MAP Kinase Inhibitor, VX-702, Meets Primary Objectives in Phase II Clinical Study in Rheumatoid Arthritis. January 23, 2008. http://investor.shareholder.com/vrtx/releasedetail.cfm?releaseid=233051.
46. Schindler C, Levy DE, Decker T. JAK-STAT signaling: From interferons to cytokines. *J Biol Chem* 2007;282:20059–20063.
47. Fantini MC, Becker C, Kiesslich R, et al. Drug insight: Novel small molecules and drugs for immunosuppression. *Nat Clin Pract Gastroenterol Hepatol* 2006;3:633–644.
48. Walker JG, Ahern MJ, Coleman M, et al. Changes in synovial tissue Jak-STAT expression in rheumatoid arthritis in response to successful DMARD treatment. *Ann Rheum Dis* 2006;65:1558–1564.
49. Kremer JM, Bloom BJ, Breedveld FC, et al. A randomized, double-blind, placebo-controlled trial of 3 dose levels of CP-690,550 versus placebo in the treatment of rheumatoid arthritis. Presented at the 2007 Annual Scientific Meeting of the American College of Rheumatology, Boston, MA, November 6–11, 2007.
50. Nimmerjahn F, Ravetch JV. Fcγ receptors as regulators of immune responses. *Nat Rev Immunol* 2008;8:34–47.
51. Pine PR, Chang B, Schoettler N, et al. Inflammation and bone erosion are suppressed in models of rheumatoid arthritis following treatment with a novel Syk inhibitor. *Clin Immunol* 2007;124:244–257.
52. Braselmann S, Taylor V, Zhao H, et al. R406, an orally available spleen tyrosine kinase inhibitor blocks Fc receptor signaling and reduces immune complex-mediated inflammation. *J Pharmacol Exp Ther* 2006;319:998–1008.
53. *http://www.bio-medicine.org/medicine-technology-1/Rigels-R788-Demonstrates-Significant-Improvement-in-Rheumatoid-Arthritis-in-Phase-2-Clinical-Study-1057-1.* Rigel's R788 Demonstrates Significant Improvement in Rheumatoid Arthritis in Phase 2 Clinical Study. January 22, 2008.
54. Quintás-Cardama A, Kantarjian H, Cortes J. Flying uder the radar: The new wave of BCR-ABL inhibitors. *Nat Rev Drug Disc* 2007; 6:834–848.
55. Paniagua RT, Sharpe O, Ho PP. Selective tyrosine kinase inhibition by imatinib mesylate for the reatment of autoimmune arthritis. *J Clin Invest* 2006;116:2633–2642.
56. Haringman JJ, Kraan MC, Smeets TJM, et al. Chemokine blockade and chronic inflammatory disease: Proof of concept in patients with rheumatoid arthritis. *Ann Rheum Dis* 2003;62:715–721.

Infections and Rheumatoid Arthritis: Old Bugs and New Drugs

CHAPTER 10L

Kevin L. Winthrop

Infectious diseases have long challenged patients with rheumatoid arthritis. The underlying immune cell dysfunction associated with the disease, and the therapies directed against it, predispose patients to infection and early infectious mortality. New biologic therapies directed against rheumatoid arthritis (RA) bring both tremendous clinical benefit and significant challenge to patients and their physicians with regard to infection prevention. This chapter reviews the relationships among RA, its therapies, and the infections typical of this patient population, and provides the treating rheumatologist with tools to prevent infectious morbidity in RA patients.

An Evolution of Infectious Explanations

In the early 20th century, owing to the histologic appearance of rheumatoid synovitis, Forestier postulated that RA was due to tuberculosis (TB).[1] Since then, a variety of other infectious agents have been proposed as either the cause or trigger for RA,[2] and some even speculated that this infectious disease originated in the New World, and later affected the colonizers from the Old World. In modern times, with better understanding of RA's immunopathology, infectious explanations for RA have lost traction. In hindsight, however, an alternative infectious explanation is perhaps plausible. The modern epidemiology of RA bears striking similarity to the historic epidemiology of tuberculosis.[3] Populations suffering high rates of tuberculosis mortality in the last 250 years, are those who today generally have high prevalence rates of RA. This includes some Native-American populations in the United States who have the highest rates of RA in the world. With the relatively recent understanding of the importance of tumor necrosis factor-alpha (TNF-α) in the immune response against TB and in the pathogenesis of RA, this cytokine provides a hypothetical explanation for this observation.[4] In historic populations evolving under heavy selective pressure from TB, it is possible that people with relatively more robust TNF immune responses were better protected from TB and more likely to survive, and that a by-product of this evolutionary process led to populations today with higher numbers of patients suffering from RA. It is unknown whether this intriguing evolutionary hypothesis is actually true or could explain RA in populations without a history of heavy TB mortality. Nonetheless, it seems that we have come full circle from the time of Forestier, and it is still not clear what, if any infectious process triggers RA. What is clear, however, is that patients with RA are at increasingly higher risk for infectious morbidity and mortality in modern times.

Infectious Morbidity and Mortality

Case series and anecdotal reports in the latter 20th century suggested that RA patients suffered greater infectious morbidity than the general population. When reviewing these reports, a consistent theme emerges, as most report increased numbers of bone and joint, pulmonary, and skin/soft tissue infections.[5–8] In addition, numerous studies have shown that RA patients suffer early death when compared to healthy counterparts, and that at least some of this excess mortality results from infection.[9–11] In one of the first large epidemiologic studies in the United States to address this issue, Wolfe et al. showed that RA patients were five times more likely to die of pneumonia than the general population.[10]

While it is presumed that some of these serious infections could be adverse sequelae of either corticosteroid use (both oral and intra-articular) or orthopedic surgery, until recently it was unclear what proportion of these infections could be attributed to the underlying immune dysfunction of RA itself. Doran et al. are responsible for perhaps the first and most elegant population-based assessment of this question, a 2002 retrospective cohort study of RA patients within Minnesota's Mayo Clinic patient population. At the time, this population had virtually no exposure to biologic therapy. They selected over 600 RA patients and appropriately matched non-RA controls, and documented culture proven (or radiographic findings) infections and serious infection (those requiring hospitalization) to be nearly twofold higher in RA patients, even after controlling for the effects of important comorbidities also known to increase the risk of infection including smoking, diabetes, and chronic lung disease.[12] Consistent with historical reports, they found that RA patients frequently suffered from serious pulmonary and skin infections (Table 10L-1). Their RA patients were hospitalized for

Table 10L-1. Frequency of Infection among Rheumatoid Arthritis Patients and Healthy Controls from Minnesota Cohort Before Widespread Use of Biologic Therapies

	Incidence per 100 Patient-Years		
Infection Type	**Rheumatoid Arthritis**	**Non–Rheumatoid Arthritis**	**Relative Risk (95% confidence interval)**
Pneumonia	4.0	2.4	1.7 (1.5–1.9)
Skin	3.0	0.9	3.3 (2.7–4.1)
Sepsis	0.78	0.51	1.5 (1.1–2.1)
Septic joint	0.40	0.02	14.9 (6.1–73.7)
Intra-abdominal	0.22	0.08	2.8 (1.4–6.2)
Osteomyelitis	0.17	0.01	10.6 (3.4–126.8)

Source: Adapted from Doran MF, Crowson CS, Pond GR, et al. Frequency of infection in patients with rheumatoid arthritis compared with controls: A population-based study. *Arthritis Rheum* 2002;46:2287–2293.

serious infections on average at a rate of 9/100 patients per year, a rate nearly double their non-RA counterparts. While bone and joint infections occurred much less frequently than skin or lung infections, they were strongly associated with RA and occurred 10 to 15 times more frequently than in healthy controls, and approximately one-third of septic arthritis occurred in prosthetic joints. This study went further to document that worsened RA severity and older age further increased the risk of these infections. These increases were independent of diabetes, prednisone use, smoking, and other risk factors, and for the first time, documented the risks seemingly attributable to the RA disease state itself and irrespective of its therapy.[12,13]

Immune Dysfunction and Predisposition to Infection

The precise immune derangements of RA that decrease the host's ability to fight infection are not yet clearly delineated. Certainly, the immunopathology of RA is complex, as are the various aspects of innate and adaptive immunity that protect one from various pathogens. There is evidence that with time, RA patients develop an overabundance of CD28 null cells and a lack of CD28-positive T cells, a process driven by overproduction of TNF-α.[14] CD 28 null cells are T cells that have lost their CD28 marker due to repeated antigenic stimulation over time, and without, have lost their capacity to stimulate B cells and appear to downregulate the function of antigen-presenting dendritic cells. Given CD28's known costimulatory role in the activation and proliferation of T lymphocytes, it is plausible that RA patients have diminished T-lymphocyte responses in the face of antigen presentation. RA patients are known to have reduced capacity to generate new T lymphocytes, and that their T-lymphocyte repertoire becomes severely contracted over time.[15] This T-lymphocyte senescence appears similar to that seen in the normal aging host, and might explain too why the elderly are more prone to infectious diseases in general.[16]

Lastly, the physical derangements due to RA might also impair local immunity or provide a respite for circulating pathogens. Destruction of articular or bony surfaces, prosthetic surfaces, RA lung and skin defects, all likely contribute to the increased risk of infection attributable to the disease state of RA.

Serious Infections Related to the Therapy of RA

Corticosteroids and Methotrexate

Serious risks of corticosteroids are well known, but until recently, have not been well quantified in RA patients and other populations. As an example, the 2000 TB-targeted screening and treatment statement issued by the U.S. Centers for Disease Control and Prevention (CDC) stated that prednisone treatment at doses of 15 mg/day for more than 1 month increases the risk of TB.[17] However, at the time of that statement, there were no prospective or retrospective studies supporting the idea, and in fact, a variety of small studies prior to that time failed to demonstrate a link between corticosteroids and TB.[18] This idea was supported only as an extrapolation from two studies that showed suppression of tuberculin skin test reactivity at these prednisone doses.[17] Recently, however, a large, controlled epidemiologic study from the UK's population database provided the needed data. They demonstrated an increase in TB risk among corticosteroid users, even at doses lower than 15 mg/day. They reviewed all cases of TB in the UK occurring during 1990 to 2001, and after adjustment for TB risk factors and antirheumatic therapy, patients with TB were nearly five times more likely to be using corticosteroids at the time of their diagnosis.[19] The study provides the best data to date suggesting that even "low-dose" corticosteroids and TB go "hand-in-hand."

In RA populations, beginning with the Doran study, several other recent observational studies have examined the relationship of low-dose corticosteroids and serious infection. Most find that steroids elevate the risk of serious infections 1.5- to 2-fold.[12,20] In 2006, Wolfe et al. reviewed the national data bank for rheumatic diseases in the United States and found a dose–response relationship with risk at doses less than 5 mg/day (hazard ratio [HR] 1.4, 95% confidence interval [CI] 1.1–1.6) increasing with higher doses of 10 to 15 mg/day (HR 2.3 95% CI 1.6–3.2).[20] These risks were also recently documented in prospective fashion in a UK primary care cohort of inflammatory arthritis patients, where corticosteroids doubled the risk of serious infection.[21] Interestingly, despite these infectious risks and the advent of newer biologic therapies, corticosteroid use in RA remains quite prevalent. Recent point estimates of prednisone use range from 47% of RA patients in the United States before the widespread usage of biologic therapy,[8] to 49% in a recent survey of RA patients in the UK.[22]

Perhaps the most frequent agent used to treat RA is methotrexate. One recent survey found that 54% of patients were taking this drug either alone or in combination with other antirheumatic therapies.[12] Methotrexate is known to decrease neutrophil chemotaxis and superoxide generation, antigen-stimulated T-cell proliferation, and even TNF-α and INF-gamma release from T cells in RA patients. Like with many immunosuppressive agents, the scientific literature is studded with infectious case reports in methotrexate-treated RA patients, including reports of *Pneumocyctis carinii* (now *jarvecii*) pneumonia, histoplasmosis, nocardiosis, and others.[23–25] In addition, small case series have reported increases in self-reported skin infections and antibiotic use, and even herpes zoster.[26,27] However, unlike prednisone, there are no large observational or prospective studies that definitively link methotrexate to an increased risk of infection in RA patients. In fact, the two recent large observational studies that have examined this question failed to find any independent risk for serious infection associated with methotrexate.[13,20]

Biologic Therapy

The opportunity to effectively treat RA has greatly expanded in the last 10 years due to the advent of targeted biologic therapy. To date, these include those compounds that inhibit TNF-α (infliximab, adalimumab, and etanercept), IL-1 (Anakinra), and the newly approved CTLR-4 ligand (abatacept) and CD20+ B-cell antibody (rituximab). With regard to infection, the most publicized story to date has involved the association of TB with the widely used anti-TNF therapies.[28–31] While the majority of these cases have been reported in association with the monocloncal antibody infliximab, cases have also been reported in patients taking the monoclonal antibody adalimumab and the soluble p-75 receptor etanercept. For the clinician, it is very important to recognize that TB associated with any of these agents often presents atypically. Many patients have extrapulmonary (50%) or disseminated disease (15%), and accordingly, can be difficult to diagnose with TB. As variety of other intracellular and extracellular infections have also been reported in this setting, it is clear that TNF plays an important role in the defense against a number of different pathogens.[32]

TNF and Its Immune Function

This proinflammatory cytokine is expressed by activated macrophages, T lymphocytes, and other immune cells, and plays a crucial role in the host response against a variety of infections, and in particular *Mycobacterium tuberculosis* and other intracellular pathogens.[33,34] TNF is essential in the control and containment of intracellular pathogens by stimulating inflammatory cell recruitment to the area of infection, and by stimulating the formation and maintenance of granulomas that contain infection. In murine models of TB infection, mice deficient in either TNF or p55 TNF receptors fail to recruit inflammatory cells to the site of infection and fail to form functioning granulomas.[35–37] Similarly, neutralization of TNF interferes with the development of granulomas during bacille Calmette-Guerin (BCG) infection of mice,[38] and in those mice already infected with BCG or TB, causes lysis of formed granulomas leading to mycobacterial spread and death.[38,39]

In addition, TNF also directly activates macrophages to phagocytose and kill mycobacteria and other pathogens.[40] Mice deficient in this signaling pathway are highly susceptible to listeria infection,[41] histoplasmosis,[42] and numerous other pathogens including extracellular bacterial organisms like *Klebsiella pneumoniae* and *Streptococcus pneumoniae*, both frequent causes of pneumonia in humans.[43,44]

Infectious Risk in Anti-TNF Setting

While relatively few infections were reported during clinical trials with these agents, sporadic case reports of serious infections in the postmarketing period helped trigger the establishment of biologic registries, primarily in Europe. With the epidemiologic luxury of national health-care databases, investigators are able to compare outcomes between RA patients treated or untreated with anti-TNF therapy. To date, most of these registries have reported some increase in serious infections in patients using anti-TNF therapies. German investigators found that the rate of serious infection in RA patients taking anti-TNF drugs was 6/100 patient-years and more than 2.5-fold higher than the rate seen in unexposed patients.[45] The UK registry examined rates of site-specific infections and found similar rates of serious infections overall in anti-TNF treated patients, including a statistically significant fourfold increase in osteomyelitis (as compared to RA patients not receiving anti-TNF drugs). With other site-specific infections, however, they did not find elevated risk associated with anti-TNF therapy. With regard to intracellular infections specifically, however, UK researchers found a strong association with anti-TNF agents. During their study, they documented 19 cases of intracellular infection (incidence of 2/1000 patient-years), and all occurred exclusively in anti-TNF users, including 10 cases of TB (rate varied between 50 and 150 per 100,000 person-years depending on the anti-TNF compound, with higher, but not statistically significant rates seen with the monoclonal antibodies).[46] Other intracellular infections captured in this study included nontuberculous mycobacteria (n=3), salmonella (n=3), listeria (n=3) and legionella (n=3), and nontuberculous mycobacteria (n=1). Interestingly, the UK registry recently published a follow-up reanalysis of their original study. By restricting their definition of "time at risk" for patients using anti-TNF therapy to the first 90 days after initiation, they demonstrated a four-fold increase in all serious infections with no differences noted among the three agents.[47]

In the United States, less population-level data are available to compare. One recent study using claims data in the southeastern United States also found a fourfold elevated infectious risk in the 6 months after starting anti-TNF agents,[48] although these investigators did not evaluate the risk of TB or other organism-specific infections. Regarding TB and other opportunistic infections, little information exists outside of the cases reported passively to the Food and Drug Administration's Medwatch system, where the most recent review of cases through September 2002 found a variety of granulomatous infections reported, with TB the most numerous.[29] A recent nationwide survey of infectious diseases consultants in the United States suggested that nontuberculous mycobacterium (most frequently *M. avium*), histoplasmosis, and invasive *S. aureus* all occur more frequently than TB in this country[49]; perhaps not surprising given the relatively low background TB prevalence in the United States (Figure 10L-1).

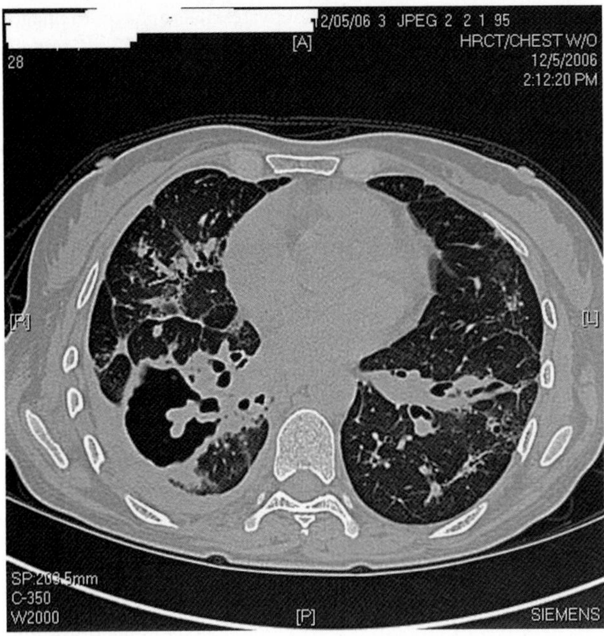

Figure 10L-1. Pulmonary *M. avium* disease in a 57-year-old woman with rheumatoid arthritis treated with anti-TNF agents. She was first diagnosed with pulmonary MAC while receiving infliximab. She subsequently initiated antimycobacterial therapy, briefly received adalimumab without good clinical response, and then continued to use etanercept for 1 year. Despite antimycobacterial therapy, her pulmonary disease continued to progress. Chest CT shows extensive infiltrate and cavitary destruction of the right lung with lesser areas of infiltrate and lung destruction noted on the left. (Courtesy of Michael Iseman, MD, National Jewish Medical Center.)

Infections of Rheumatoid Arthritis and their Prevention

Skin/Soft Tissue, Bone/Joint, and Pulmonary Infections

Unfortunately, there is a paucity of organism-level data for most of these infections, but it is presumed that most of these infections are caused by the same types of organisms seen in the general public. Most skin/soft tissue infections are likely due to *S. aureus* and *Streptococcus sp.*, and it is suggested that up to two-thirds of septic arthritis in RA patients is due to *S. aureus*.[50] RA patients are known to have higher rates of colonization with *S. aureus*, as high as 50% compared to 30% for the general public,[51,52] and colonization rates might even be higher in patients concurrently receiving anti-TNF therapy and methotrexate.[53] The risk of this colonization with regard to subsequent infection has not been clarified, but rather, is presumed based on a demonstrable risk in other medical settings (ICU, presurgical, hemodialysis).[54] Of particular concern is the rise of methicillin-resistant *S. aureus* (MRSA) within the general public. Emergency department–based surveillance from across the United States suggests that nearly 60% of presenting soft tissue infections are now caused by MRSA.[55] There are no data yet to suggest that MRSA is of greater concern to RA populations than the general public; however, given RA patients' increased risk of *S. aureus* colonization and propensity for skin/soft tissue infections, this trend deserves monitoring. MRSA should be high in the differential diagnosis for any RA patient presenting with signs of skin infection, particularly when accompanied by furuncles or abscess formation. In our clinical practice, we frequently see anti-TNF–treated patients with chronic *S. aureus* furunculosis. We frequently screen these patients by culture (nares, oropharynx, perineum) for *S. aureus* colonization and then attempt to decolonize them prior to their resumption of anti-TNF therapy. It should be noted that while it is presumed that *S. aureus* colonization precedes subsequent infection, there is not yet definitive data to support this assertion or any systematic policy of screening and decolonizing patients prior to anti-TNF therapy.

A significant number of RA patients are also hospitalized each year with community-acquired pneumonia.[12,20,45] Similar to soft tissue infections, studies of pneumonia in RA patients have not reported organism level data, although it is suspected that the same types of bacteria are implicated as in the general population: *S. pneumoniae, Haemophilus influenzae, S. aureus*, gram-negative bacilli, and influenza are some of the most common etiologies. Of these, although less frequent, *S. aureus* and notably again MRSA seem to be on the rise.[56]

With regard to *S. pneumoniae*, it is widely recommended that patients receive 23-valent pneumococcal vaccine prior to initiating anti-TNF therapies and other long-term immunosuppressive therapies, primarily because it protects against invasive pneumococcal disease.[57] It should be noted that immunogenecity to this vaccine is poor and can be diminished by methotrexate, so if possible, patients should be vaccinated while not exposed to methotrexate.[58] RA patients are known to have some reduction in their response to influenza vaccine, although this appears to be unrelated to methotrexate, prednisone, or anti-TNF therapy. Despite this, most achieve protective levels of antibodies, and therefore should be immunized annually before the onset of influenza season.[59]

TB, Dimorphic Fungi, and Other Intracellular Pathogens

These infections appear to be particularly important in RA patients treated with anti-TNF therapy[46] and include a variety of organisms: coccidioidies, listeria, salmonella, histoplasma, aspergillus, nocardia, nontuberculous mycobacterium, and others.[29] Of serious concern is the development of active tuberculosis (TB) disease in some patients receiving these drugs.[32] Similar to HIV patients who develop TB, patients using anti-TNF compounds frequently present "atypically," with extrapulmonary or disseminated disease. Accordingly, TNF antagonists should be used with caution in any person with risk factors for TB, and screening for latent TB infection (LTBI) should be undertaken before starting anti-TNF therapy. Recommendation for TB screening have been issued by various public health authorities and professional societies.[28,60,61] (See CDC recommendations in Table 10L-2 for the United States.) In general, these recommendations vary according to region based on the background prevalence of TB and the use of BCG vaccination, which can interfere with interpretation of the tuberculin skin test. Recently, interferon-gamma release assays have been developed in response to the latter concern, and offer a more specific diagnostic test for latent TB infection. In some areas, these assays have replaced the TST in initial screening,[60] although it should be noted that little data exists by which to judge the relative sensitivities of the two methodologies in immunosuppressed patients with rheumatic arthritis and other inflammatory auto-immune diseases.[32,62] Use of either test may still result in false-negative results due to immunosuppression, and negative results should

Table 10L-2. CDC Recommendations for Screening, Diagnosis, and Treatment of Latent Tuberculosis Infection and Tuberculosis in Patients Administered or Scheduled to Receive TNF Antagonists

Screen patients for risk factors for *Mycobacterium tuberculosis* and test them for infection before initiating immunosuppressive therapies, including TNF antagonists. Risk factors include birth or extended living in a country where TB is prevalent, or history of any of the following: residence in a congregate setting (e.g., jail or prison, homeless shelter, or chronic-care facility), a positive tuberculin skin test (TST) result, substance abuse (injection or noninjection), health-care employment in settings with TB patients, and chest radiographic findings consistent with previous TB.[17]
Diagnosis and treatment of LTBI and TB disease should be in accordance with published guidelines.[17,71,72]
In patients who are immunocompromised (e.g., because of therapy or other medical conditions), interpret a TST induration of >5 mm as a positive result and evidence of *M. tuberculosis* infection.
Interpret a TST induration of <5 mm as a negative result but not an exclusion for *M. tuberculosis* infection.
Anergy panel testing is not recommended. Results from control-antigen skin testing (e.g., *Candida*) should not alter the interpretation of a negative TST result.
Test to exclude TB disease before starting treatment for LTBI.[17,72]
Start treatment for LTBI before commencing TNF-blocking agents, preferably with 9 months of daily isoniazid.[17,72]
Consider treatment for LTBI in patients who have negative TST results, but whose epidemiologic and clinical circumstances suggest a probability of LTBI.
Pursue TB disease as a potential cause of febrile or respiratory illness in all patients receiving TNF-blocking agents.
Consider postponement of TNF-antagonist therapy until the conclusion of treatment for LTBI or TB disease if possible. If not clinically possible, withhold TNF-antagonist therapy until the patient has demonstrated LTBI treatment adherence and tolerance, or in the case of TB disease, until the patient has shown adherence to appropriate anti-TB drugs to which the specific organism is known to be sensitive.

CDC, Centers for Disease Control and Prevention; *LTBI,* latent tuberculosis infection; *TNF,* tumor necrosis factor.
Source: Winthrop KL, Seigel JN, Jereb J, et al. Tuberculosis associated with therapy against tumor necrosis factor-alpha. *Arthritis Rheum* 2005;52:2968–2974.

be guarded with suspicion in any patient with a history of TB exposure. For now, clinicians should refer to local TB expertise and guidelines on this issue, as recommendations will continue to evolve as further data becomes available by which to judge the sensitivity of IGRAs in immunosuppressed populations.

Histoplasma capsulatum is a dimorphic fungus endemic to Midwestern regions of North America, South America, Asia, and parts of Europe and Africa. Recent work suggests that it might be the most commonly reported granulomatous pathogen in the United States associated with TNF blockade.[49] Like TB, it can exist in a slowly progressive or latent state, and can progress to active disease during immunosuppression. While granuloma seen on chest radiograph might raise the likelihood of previous infection, granulomas are nonspecific and could represent a variety of previous infectious states like latent tuberculosis. Evidence of previous infection by serologic testing or histoplasmin skin testing could be obtained before drug start; however, it is unclear how useful these tests are, and whether positive results would indicate a need for prophylaxis or avoidance of TNF blockade. Currently, skin or serologic testing for histoplasmosis is not routinely recommended in HIV-infected persons.[63] Prophylaxis is to be considered in severely immunosuppressed HIV patients (CD4 <150) who live in highly endemic areas where histoplasmosis disease incidence exceeds 10 cases per 100 patient-years.[64] On the contrary, a study of over 500 bone marrow or organ transplant patients living in a hyperendemic area failed to show any benefit for itraconazole prophylaxis.[65] Given the large number of people likely exposed to histoplasmosis during anti-TNF therapy, and the relative paucity of reported cases, screening and prophylaxis prior to anti-TNF therapy is probably not warranted.

Coccidioides immitis is a dimorphic fungus endemic to the southwestern United States, and Central and South America. It is a common cause of community-acquired pneumonia is highly endemic areas like Arizona in the United States.[66] Like histoplasmosis, it too can exist in a latent or subclinical infectious state after exposure, and can later progress to disease during immunosuppression. In this setting, disease generally disseminates from the lung to involve other viscera including skin, bone, lymph, and central nervous system, and is associated with fairly high mortality rates, particularly in patients of Asian and African descent.[67] Patients in endemic areas could potentially be screened with serology prior to initiation of TNF blockade, although many of the coccidiodomycosis cases thus far reported in association with TNF blockade appear to be cases of acute infection and not reactivation making the utility of such an approach unknown.[66] One large transplant center in Arizona uses serologic monitoring in both pre- and post-transplant settings, coupled with fluconazole treatment, in an effort to prevent coccidiodomycosis, although little data are yet available by which to judge this strategy's success.[69] Further, HIV-infected individuals living in endemic areas are not routinely screened for coccidiocomycosis, and given the relative paucity of reported coccidiodomycosis cases in association with TNF blockade, it is unclear whether a need exists to screen before initiation of such therapy.

Intracellular Bacterial Pathogens

Fatal cases of listeriosis have occurred in people taking TNF-blocking agents.[29,70] *Listeria monocytogenes* is an intracellular pathogen acquired via the ingestion of contaminated meats and dairy products. Accordingly, we routinely advise patients under TNF blockade to avoid undercooked meat, delicatessen meat, and unpasteurized milk products. *Salmonella sp.* are also known to cause serious infection in those receiving anti-TNF therapy.[29,46] It is typically transmitted by contaminated raw or undercooked foods including fresh produce, cheese made from

Table 10L-3. Frequently Asked Questions for ID Consultant

QUESTION: My patient is about to have surgery. Should the anti-TNF therapy be stopped?
ANSWER: There are several small, retrospective case series focused on this question that reported no increase in perioperative infection risk. Recently, however, two larger retrospective studies evaluating this question documented either a small increase in postorthopedic operation infection risk or a delay in wound healing in patients who did not discontinue anti-TNF drugs before surgery. For now, it seems prudent to discontinue anti-TNF therapy several weeks before surgery (depending on the drug's half-life) if possible until the patient's surgical wounds are healed.[73]
QUESTION: My patient was screened for TB before starting anti-TNF therapy, do I need to rescreen them annually?
ANSWER: Currently, there are no guidelines or recommendations to serially test any group of immunosuppressed patients for TB, except in HIV patients who belong to populations in which there is a substantial risk for exposure to TB.[63] We recommend re-testing of anti-TNF treated patients who have negative initial evaluations only if they are potentially exposed to TB. This would include foreign travel to, or living in, areas of high TB prevalence or prolonged exposure to other settings where TB is known to be more common.
QUESTION: My patient developed active TB disease while on anti-TNF therapy and it was discontinued. When is it safe to resume anti-TNF therapy?
ANSWER: While it seems prudent to discontinue anti-TNF therapy when a patient is diagnosed with TB, it is unclear whether this is necessary presuming the patient is on a correct multidrug anti-TB therapeutic regimen. There are case reports of immune reconstitution inflammatory syndrome (IRIS) occurring in TB patients in whom anti-TNF therapy was stopped,[74] although a recent national survey of infectious disease specialists found few cases of IRIS in such individuals. There is also very limited evidence that concurrent therapy of TB with anti-TNF compounds might be safe.[75] Further, if anti-TNF therapy is stopped, there is no data to suggest when it is safe to resume such therapy. Clearly, these questions deserve further study. Until then, it seems prudent to stop anti-TNF therapy when TB is diagnosed and remain vigilant for IRIS (and the potential need to institute immunosuppressive therapy for IRIS), and resume anti-TNF therapy after the patient has demonstrated clinical improvement while adhering to an appropriate anti-TB regimen.
QUESTION: I think my patient has latent TB infection and I have started treating him with Isoniazid (INH). How long do I have to wait to institute anti-TNF therapy?
ANSWER: It is presumed that the bacillary burden in latent TB infection is quite low, so it is unlikely that one would need to wait nine months until treatment of LTBI is complete before initiating anti-TNF therapy. It seems reasonable to wait some time period, however, to ensure compliance and tolerance of INH. Observational data from Spain suggests that waiting to initiate anti-TNF therapy until one month after starting INH treatment is successful in reducing the rate of TB disease associated with anti-TNF therapy.[76] We have adopted a similar approach in our practice. There are other data that suggest waiting lesser time periods might also be appropriate.[77]

Source: Cohen J, Powderly W, Opal S. *Infectious Diseases*, 3rd ed. London: Mosby, 2008.

raw milk, and even reptiles sold as pets. Patients should be advised to wash produce, cook meat thoroughly, and practice good hand hygiene in general.

Conclusion

RA patients are at higher risk for serious infections and death from infection than the general public. Anti-TNF agents and prednisone seem to further raise this risk, particularly with regard to skin/soft tissue, bone/joint, lung, and opportunistic infections. Clinicians should remain vigilant for these infections in any RA patient undergoing long-term immunosuppressive therapy of any kind. Some of these infections are preventable with screening (i.e., TB), vaccination, and patient education. Certainly, as newer biologic targeted therapies are developed, new infectious challenges will arise with either established or emerging pathogens. Future postmarketing surveillance efforts will remain key to detecting these infectious signals early, so that physicians and patients can minimize the infectious risks of RA and its therapy (Table 10L-3).

References

1. Forestier J. Rheumatoid arthritis and its treatment with gold salts. *J Lab Clin Med* 1935;20:827–840.
2. Carty SM, Snowden N, Silman AJ. Should infection still be considered as the most likely triggering factor for rheumatoid arthritis? *Ann Rheum Dis* 2004;63(Suppl 2):ii46–ii49.
3. Mobley JL. Is rheumatoid arthritis a consequence of natural selection for enhanced tuberculosis resistance? *Med Hypotheses* 2004;62: 839–843.
4. Correa PA, Gomez LM, Cadena J, et al. Autoimmunity and tuberculosis. Opposite association with TNF polymorphism. *J Rheumatol* 2005;32:219–224.
5. Baum J. Infection in rheumatoid arthritis. *Arthritis Rheum* 1971; 14:135–137.
6. Mitchell WS, Brooks PM, Stevenson RD, et al. Septic arthritis in patients with rheumatoid disease: A still underdiagnosed complication. *J Rheumatol* 1976;3:124–133.
7. Hernandez-Cruz B, Cardiel MH, Villa AR, et al. Development, recurrence, and severity of infections in Mexican patients with rheumatoid arthritis: A nested case–control study. *J Rheumatol* 1998;25: 1900–1907.
8. Goldenberg DL. Infectious arthritis complicating rheumatoid arthritis and other chronic rheumatic disorders. *Arthritis Rheum.* 1989;32:496–502.
9. Mutru O, Laakso M, Isomaki H, et al. Ten year mortality and causes of death in patients with rheumatoid arthritis. *BMJ (Clin Res Ed)* 1985;290:1797–1799.

10. Wolfe F, Mitchell DM, Sibley JT, et al. The mortality of rheumatoid arthritis. *Arthritis Rheum* 1994;37:481–494.
11. Sihvonen, S, Korpela M, Laippala P, et al. Death rates and causes of death in patients with rheumatoid arthritis: A population-based study. *Scand J Rheumatol* 2004;33:221–227.
12. Doran MF, Crowson CS, Pond GR, et al. Frequency of infection in patients with rheumatoid arthritis compared with controls: A population-based study. *Arthritis Rheum* 2002;46:2287–2293.
13. Doran MF, Crowson CS, Pond GR, et al. Predictors of infection in rheumatoid arthritis. *Arthritis Rheum* 2002;46:2294–2300.
14. Bryl E, Vallejo, Matteson EL, et al. Modulation of C28 expression with anti-tumor necrosis factor alpha therapy in rheumatoid arthiritis. *Arthritis Rheum* 2205;52:2996–3003.
15. Wagner UG, Koetz K, Weyland CM, et al. Perturbation of the T cell repertoire in rheumatoid arthritis. *Proc Natl Acad Sci U S A* 1998; 95:1447–1452.
16. Vallejo AN, Weyand CM, Goronzy JJ. T-cell senescence: A culprit of immune abnormalities in chronic inflammation and persistent infection. *Trends Mol Med* 2004;10:119–124.
17. Centers for Disease Control and Prevention. Targeted tuberculin testing and treatment of latent tuberculosis infection. American Thoracic Society. *MMWR Morb Mort Wkly Rep* 2000;49(RR-6):1–51.
18. Bateman ED. Is tuberculosis chemoprophylaxis necessary for patients receiving corticosteroids for respiratory disease? *Respir Med* 1993;87:485–487.
19. Jick SS. Lieberman ES, Rahman MU, et al. Glucocorticoid use, other associated factors, and the risk of tuberculosis. *Arthritis Rheum* 2006;55:19–26.
20. Wolfe F, Caplan L, Michaeud K. Treatment for rheumatoid arthritis and the risk of hospitalization for pneumonia. *Arthritis Rheum* 2006;54:628–634.
21. Franklin J, Lunt M, Bunn D, et al. Risk and predictors of infection leading to hospitalization in a large primary-care–derived cohort of patients with inflammatory polyarthritis. *Ann Rheum Dis* 2007;66: 308–312.
22. Hyrich K, Symmons D, Watson K, et al. Baseline comorbidity levels in biologic and standard DMARD treated patients with rheumatoid arthritis: Results from a national patient register. *Ann Rheum Dis* 2006;65(7):895–898.
23. Arunkumar P, Crook T, Ballard J. Disseminated histoplasmosis presenting as pancytopenia in a methotrexate-treated patient. *Am J Hematol* 2004;77:86–87.
24. Keegan JM, Byrd J. Nocardiosis associated with low dose methotrexate for rheumatoid arthritis. *J Rheumatol* 1988;15: 1585–1586.
25. Lang B, Riegel W, Peters T, et al. Low dose methotrexate therapy for rhematoid arthritis complicated by pancytopenia and Pneumocystis carinii pneumonia. *J Rheumatol* 1991;18:1257–1258.
26. Antonelli MA, Moreland LW, Brick JE. Herpes zoster in patients with rheumatoid arthritis treated with weekly, low-dose methotrexate. *Am J Med* 1991;90:295–298.
27. Van der Veen MJ, van der Heide A, Kruize AA, et al. Infection rate and use of antibiotics in patients with rheumatoid arthritis treated with methotrexate. *Ann Rheum Dis* 1994;53:224–228.
28. Winthrop KL, Seigel JN, Jereb J, et al. Tuberculosis associated with therapy against tumor necrosis factor-alpha. *Arthritis Rheum* 2005;52:2968–2974.
29. Wallis RS, Broder MS, Wong JY, et al. Granulomatous infectious diseases associated with tumor necrosis factor antagonists. *Clin Infect Dis* 2004;38:1261–1265.;(Erratum in *Clin Infect Dis* 2004; 39:1254–1255.)
30. Keane J, Gershon S, Wise RP, et al. Tuberculosis associated with infliximab, a tumor necrosis factor-α neutralizing agent. *N Engl J Med* 2001;345:1098–1104.
31. Mohan AK, Cote TR, Block JA, et al. Tuberculosis following the use of etanercept, a tumor necrosis factor inhibitor. *Clin Infect Dis* 2004;39:295–299.
32. Winthrop KL. Risk and prevention of tuberculosis and other serious opportunistic infections associated with the inhibition of tumor necrosis factor. *Nat Clin Pract Rheumatol* 2006;2:602–610.
33. Ehlers S. Tumor necrosis factor and its blockade in granulomatous infections: differential modes of action of infliximab and etanercept? *Clin Infect Dis* 2005;41(Suppl 3):S199–S203.
34. Wajant H, Pfizenmaier K, Scheurich P. Tumor necrosis factor signaling. *Cell Death Differ* 2003;10:45–65.
35. Flynn JL, Goldstein MM, Chan J, et al. Tumor necrosis factor-alpha is required in the protective immune response against *Mycobacterium tuberculosis* in mice. *Immunity* 1995;2:561–572.
36. Algood HM, Lin PL, Flynn JL. Tumor necrosis factor and chemokine interactions in the formation and maintenance of granulomas in tuberculosis. *Clin Infect Dis* 2005;41(Suppl 3):S189–S193.
37. Roach RR, Bean AGD, Demangel C, et al. TNF regulates chemokine induction essential for cell recruitment, granuloma formation, and clearance of mycobacterial infection. *J Immunol* 2002;168: 4620–4627.
38. Kindler V, Sappino AP, Grau GE, et al. The inducing role of tumor necrosis factor in the development of bactericidal gramulomas during BCG infection. *Cell* 1989;56:731–740.
39. Mohan VP, Scanga CA, Yu K, et al. Effects of tumor necrosis factor alpha on host immune response in chronic persistent tuberculosis: Possible role for limiting patholology. *Infect Immun* 2001;69: 1847–1855.
40. Bekker LG, Freeman S, Murray PJ, et al. TNF-α controls intracellular mycobacterial growth by both inducible nitric oxide synthase–dependent and inducible nitric oxide synthase–independent path ways. *J Immunol* 2001;166:6728–6734.
41. Rothe J, Lesslauer W, Lotscher H, et al. Mice lacking the tumour necrosis factor receptor 1 are resistant to TNF-mediated toxicity but highly susceptible to infection by Listeria monocytogenes. *Nature* 1993;364:798–802.
42. Deepe GS Jr. Modulation of infection with Histoplasma capsulatum by inhibition of tumor necrosis factor–alpha activity. *Clin Infect Dis* 2005;41(Suppl 3):S204–S207.
43. O'Brien DP, Briles DE, Szalai AJ, et al. Tumor necrosis factor alpha receptor I is important for survival from *Streptococcus pneumoniae* infections. *Infect Immun* 1999;67:595–601.
44. Moore TA, Lau HY, Cogen AL, et al. Defective innate antibacterial host responses during murine *Klebsiella pneumoniae* bacteremia: Tumor necrosis factor (TNF) receptor 1 deficiency versus therapy with anti–TNF-alpha. *Clin Infect Dis* 2005;41(Suppl 3):S213–S217.
45. Listing J, Strangfeld A, Kary S, et al. Infections in patients with rheumatoid arthritis treated with biologic agents. *Arthritis Rheum* 2005;52:3403–3412.
46. Dixon WG, Watson K, Lunt M, et al. Rates of serious infection, including site-specific and bacterial intracellular infection, in rheumatoid arthritis patients receiving anti-tumor necrosis factor therapy: results from the British Society for Rheumatology Biologics Register. *Arthritis Rheum* 2006;54:2368–2376.
47. Dixon WG, Symmons DP, Lunt M, et al. Serious infection following anti-tumor necrosis factor alpha therapy in patients with rheumatoid arthritis: Lessons from interpreting data from observational studies. *Arthritis Rheum* 2007;56(9):2896–2904.
48. Curtis J, Patkar N, Xie A, et al. Risk of serious bacterial infections among rheumatoid arthritis patients exposed to tumor necrosis factor alpha antagonists. *Arthritis Rheum* 2007;56:1125–1133.
49. Winthrop KL, Yamashita S, Beekman SE, Polgreen PM. Infectious Diseases Society of America Emerging Infections Network. Mycobacterial and other serious infections in patients receiving anti-tumor necrosis factor and other newly approved biologic therapies: Case finding through the Emerging Infections Network. *Clin Infect Dis* 2008;46:1738–1740.
50. Dubost JJ, Soubrier M, De Champs C, et al. No changes in the distribution of organisms responsible for septic arthritis over a 20 year period. *Ann Rheum Dis* 2002;61:267–269.

51. Jackson MS, Bagg J, Gupta MN, et al. Oral carriage of staphylococci in patients with rheumatoid arthritis. *Rheumatology (Oxford)* 1999;38:572–575.
52. Tabarya D, Hoffman WL. *Staphylococcus aureus* nasal carriage in rheumatoid arthritis: Antibody response to toxic shock syndrome toxin-1. *Ann Rheum Dis* 1996;55:823–828.
53. Bassetti S, Wasmer S, Hasler P, et al. Staphylococcus aureus in patients with rheumatoid arthritis under conventional and anti–tumor necrosis factor-alpha treatment.*J Rheumatol* 2005;32:2125–2129.
54. Kluytmans J, van Belkum A, Verbugh H. Nasal carriage of *Staphylococcus aureus*: Epidemiology, unerlying mechanisms, and associated risks. *Clin Microbiol Rev* 19997;10:505–520.
55. Moran GJ, Krishnadasan A, Gorwitz RJ, et al. Methicillin-resistant *S. aureus* infections among patients in the emergency department. *N Engl J Med* 2006;355:666–674.
56. Kollef MH, Shorr A, Tabak YP, et al. Epidemiology and outcomes of health-care–associated pneumonia: Results from a large US database of culture-positive pneumonia. *Chest* 2005;128:3854–3862. (Erratum in: *Chest* 2006;129:831.)
57. Targonski PV, Poland GA. Pneumococcal vaccination in adults: Recommendations, trends, and prospects. *Cleve Clin J Med* 2007;74: 401–406, 408–410, 413–414.
58. Kapetanovic MC, Saxne T, Sjoholm A, et al. Influence of methotrexate, TNF blockers and prednisolone on antibody responses to pneumococcal polysaccharide vaccine in patients with rheumatoid arthritis. *Rheumatology (Oxford)* 2006;45:106–111.
59. Fomin I, Caspi D, Levy V, et al. Vaccination against influenza in rheumatoid arthritis: the effect of disease modifying drugs, including TNF blockers. *Ann Rheum Dis* 2006;65:191–194.
60. Beglinger C, Dudler J, Mottet C, et al. Screening for tuberculosis infection before the initiation of an anti–TNF-alpha therapy. *Swiss Med Wkly* 2007;137:620–622.
61. British Thoracic Society Standards for Care Committee. BTS recommendations for assessing risk and for managing Mycobacterium tuberculosis infection and disease in patients due to start anti–TNF-alpha treatment. *Thorax* 2005;60:800–805.
62. Mazurek GH, Jereb J, Lobue P, et al. Guidelines for using the QuantiFERON-TB Gold test for detecting Mycobacterium tuberculosis infection, United States. *MMWR Recomm Rep* 2005;54(RR-15): 49–55. (Erratum in: *MMWR Morb Mort Wkly Rep* 2005;54:1288.)
63. Kaplan JE, Masur H, Holmes KK. USPHS. Infectious Disease Society of America. Guidelines for preventing opportunisitic infections among HIV-infected persons—2002. *MMWR Recomm Rep* 2002;51 (RR-8):1–52.
64. Wheat JL, Freifeld AG, Kleiman MB, et al. Clinical practice guidelines for the managment of patients with histoplasmosis: 2007 update by the infectious diseases society of America. *Clin Infect Dis* 2007;45: 807–825.
65. Vail GM, Young RS, Wheat LJ, et al. Incidence of histoplasmosis following allogeneic bone marrow transplant or solid organ transplant in a hyperendmic area. *Transpl Infect Dis* 2002;4:148–151.
66. Valdivia L, Nix D, Wright M, et al. Coccidioidomycosis as a common cause of community-acquired pneumonia. *Emerg Infect Dis* 2006;12:958–962. (Erratum in *Emerg Infect Dis* 2006;12:1307.)
67. Saubolle MA, McKellar PP, Sussland D. Epidemiologic, clinical, and diagnostic aspects of coccidioidomycosis. *J Clin Microbiol* 2007;45: 26–30.
68. Bergstrom L, Yocum DE, Ampel NM, et al. Increased risk of coccidioidomycosis in patients treated with tumor necrosis factor alpha antagonists. *Arthritis Rheum* 2004;50:1959–1966.
69. Blair JE, Douglas DD, Mulligan DC. Early results of targeted prophylaxis for coccidioidomycosis in patients undergoing orthotopic liver transplantation within an endemic area. *Transpl Infect Dis* 2003;5:3–8.
70. Slifman NR, Gershon SK, Lee JH, et al. Listeria monocytogenes infection as a complication of treatment with tumor necrosis factor alpha–neutralizing agents. *Arthritis Rheum* 2003;48:319–324.
71. Centers for Disease Control and Prevention. Update: Adverse event data and revised American Thoracic Society/CDC recommendations against the use of rifampin and pyrazinamide for treatment of latent tuberculosis infection—United States, 2003. *MMWR Morb Mort Wkly Rep* 2003;52:735–739.
72. Centers for Disease Control and Prevention. Treatment of tuberculosis: American Thoracic Society, CDC, and Infectious Diseases Society of America. *MMWR Morb Mort Wkly Rep* 2003;52:RR-11.
73. Wendling D. Do patients with RA receiving anti-TNF agents have an increased risk of surgical site infections? *Nat Clin Pract Rheumatol* 2007:8:432–433.
74. Belknap R, Reves R, Burman W. Immune reconstitution to *Mycobacterium tuberculosis* after discontinuing infliximab. *Int J Tuberc Lung Dis* 2005;9(9):1057–1058.
75. Wallis RS, Kyambadde P, Johnson JL, et al. A study of the safety, immunology, virology, and microbiology of adjunctive etanercept in HIV-1–associated tuberculosis. *AIDS* 2004;18:257–264.
76. Carmona L, Gomez-Reino JJ, Rodriguez-Valverde V, et al. Effectiveness of recommendations to prevent reactivation of latent tuberculosis infection in patients treated with tumor necrosis factor antagonists. *Arthritis Rheum* 2005;52:1766–1772.
77. Westhovens R, Yocum D, Han J, et al. The safety of infliximab, combined with background treatments, among patients with rheumatoid arthritis and various comorbidities: A large, randomized, placebo-controlled trial. *Arthritis Rheum* 2006;54:1075–1086.

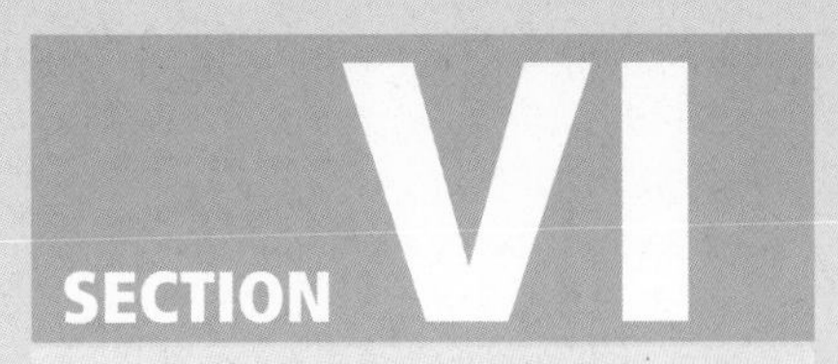

Design of Trials for New Therapies in Patients with Rheumatoid Arthritis

CHAPTER 11A

Lee S. Simon and Maarten Boers

The development of therapies for the treatment of rheumatoid arthritis (RA) is fundamentally dependent on the use of the appropriate clinical trial design to define the risk and benefit of a putative new therapy. Regulatory authorities specify the design of the studies necessary for approval of a drug. To answer the demands of the clinical **community** and patients who are interested in the extent of the benefit in the context of risk, however, other trial designs are often necessary.

Currently many trials are designed to be used in some fashion for regulatory approval. These trials will often restrict inclusion to selected patients to ensure, for example, homogeneous patient population and lack of comorbidity, among other design factors. Such designs for proving efficacy and assessing risk within the regulatory context are less suited to help clinicians and patients to make informed choices on the benefits and risks of new therapies compared to what is already available. Thus, approval trials need to be followed by "pragmatic" randomized trials that mimic standard practice in large unselected patient populations and observational studies.

It is important to consider in the design of clinical trials, what the patients or the investigators may expect as an outcome, since expectation bias may inflate the results, especially when outcome measures are subjective.[1] To minimize this potential problem, ideally separate blinded assessors of safety and efficacy are often desired, and for certain types of drugs such as biologic response modifiers premedication and slowing of infusion times to reduce treatment-associated reactions are used when the effects of these agents are to be studied.[2]

RA patients have significantly benefited from the early application of disease-modifying antirheumatic drugs (DMARDs, including both small-molecules and biologic therapies) as soon as the diagnosis becomes confirmed. This chapter reviews what we have accomplished upon outlining available clinical trial designs.

The Randomized Controlled Trial

Randomized, double-blind, controlled trials (RCTs) are the essential component of the clinical development program for new drugs including both small molecules and biologic agents. Open-label trials often yield positive results, especially in diseases such as RA where therapeutic options are limited, the natural course of disease in the specific patient is difficult to predict, and the underlying disease activity is variable. Placebo responses are regularly observed, even in patients with longstanding active disease, which may partly be due to the trial providing both more regulated therapy as well as structured physician office visits in addition to expectation bias. Because treatment effects may be small, use of an appropriate comparison group is essential, whether placebo or active comparator.[2] Random assignment to active or placebo treatment should be performed on a "by-patient" basis and must be concealed from all study personnel.[3] As noted previously, separate blinded assessors for safety and efficacy should be utilized to minimize unblinding due to rapid response, and infusion or injection site reactions observed with some biologic therapies. Other pitfalls include failure to clearly define the hypothesis to be addressed by the RCT and/or attempting to answer too many questions in a single protocol (Table 11A-1). It is important to define the hypothesized outcome a priori, design the trial to recruit adequate numbers of patients with similar disease characteristics to generate a more homogeneous patient population, accept a reasonable amount of patient dropout, and develop a plan to significantly educate potential investigators how to consistently

Table 11A-1. Issues Specific to Biologic Agents
Immunologically active molecules may downregulate other immune functions.
Mechanism of action may be altered by redundant cytokine cascades and cellular interactions.
In vitro or *ex vivo* tests may not predict *in vivo* responses.
Interference with other immune surveillance functions may lead to infections, autoimmune manifestations, and/or lymphoproliferative disorders.
Parenteral administration.
Limited preclinical and toxicology data due to species specificity.

identify the appropriate patient to be studied, how to consistently perform safety and efficacy assessments, and how to improve patient retention.

Guidance documents developed by the U.S. Food and Drug Administration (FDA) and European Medicines Agency (EMEA) have facilitated new product development, especially in RA.[4,5] These "road maps" allow companies to prepare for the hurdles of regulatory approval and what trial designs have been successful.

Trial Design

As treatment options multiply, so does the complexity of trial design. Most drug trials published in major journals are pivotal phase III registration trials and are designed considering the needs for regulatory approval. Such "efficacy trials" are quite straightforward in comparing the novel drug with an accepted alternative to answer the following questions: Does the new drug have an effect? Does it meet minimum safety standards? Is the risk of harm worth the potential benefit in an ideal population? In contrast, in "effectiveness" (or "pragmatic") trials, the research question becomes, in terms of efficacy or safety: Is the drug better than current practice? In this review, there is an attempt to create a taxonomy that categorizes the various dimensions trials may have (Table 11A-2). This taxonomy considers the number and kind of comparisons, the regimens, and whether and how changes are handled within the regimen. Table 11A-3 summarizes the essential issues required for an RCT of a new agent.

Table 11A-2. Taxonomy of Trial Designs
Comparison Dimension
Parallel/crossover
Two or multiple groups
Simple or (partial or full) factorial
Regimen Dimension
Single drug
Fixed combination
Step-up
Step-down (includes total withdrawal)
Regimen Change Dimension
No change
Fixed: changes at specified timepoints
Flexible: based on criterion (usually disease activity: tight control)

Table 11A-3. Essential Components of Randomized-Double-Blinded Controlled Trial for New Agent
Appropriate control treatment group
Adequate sample size
Selection of appropriate patient population
Sufficient duration of treatment to demonstrate effect
Prospectively defined outcome measure assessed on a by-patient basis
Prospectively defined statistical analysis plan
Central randomization on a by-patient basis, concealed from all study personnel
Separate blinded assessors for safety and efficacy
Means to reduce treatment-associated toxicities
Clearly defined hypothesis

Number and Kind of Comparisons

The comparison dimension describes the setup and the number of trial arms (Figure 11A-1). Most trials have a parallel design where two or more arms are compared. With more than two arms, the number of potential comparisons increases, and these must be prioritized in the design stage to optimize statistical analysis. For example, the standard extension of the *t*-test for more than two groups is analysis of variance (ANOVA), but this test has as the null hypothesis "there is no difference between the groups." There is more interest in all the two-by-two comparisons between the groups, but unfortunately these cannot all be answered with the same power. An example of what can be learned in such a design is observed from studies aiming to compare leflunomide with methotrexate.[6] When combinations of drugs are studied, a factorial design can be used when the individual drug effects are thought to be independent and there is the need to define the contribution to both efficacy and safety of each component. Thus, with two drugs A and B, the four trial arms are placebo, A, B, and A+B; ANOVA increases efficiency in the

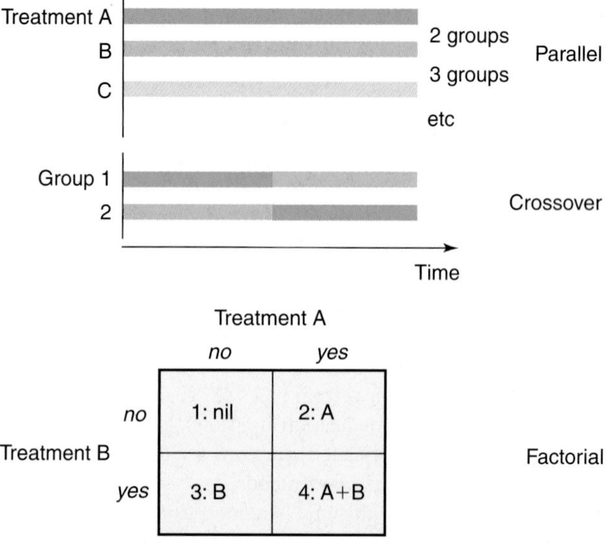

Figure 11A-1. Examples of comparison dimension designs, illustrating parallel, crossover, and factorial displays.

analysis. This design is frequently employed in dose-ranging studies where the arms could, for example, be dose 1, twice dose 1, thrice dose 1 (= dose 1 + twice dose 1), and placebo. One way to increase efficiency is the crossover design, where patients are switched to the other arm after a prespecified period. Thus, each patient is her own, perfectly matched control. One disadvantage of this design is the potential for "carryover" effects, meaning that the effects of the first drug linger after it is stopped, potentially interacting and interfering with the measurement of the effects of the second agent. To minimize this, extensive periods of washout of the former drug are necessary. Another problem arises when the outcome is primarily patient reported. After completing the first therapeutic period, the expectation regarding response has been changed. This may bias the response in the second phase. For this reason the crossover design is rarely used in RA. However, such a design demonstrated the superiority of nonsteroidal anti-inflammatory drugs (NSAIDs) over acetaminophen for the treatment of osteoarthritis.[7,8]

Nature of Interventions: Regimen

The regimen dimension considers what is applied in each of the trial arms (Figure 11A-2). The simplest design is a single drug. Next in complexity is a fixed combination of two or more drugs. Finally, drugs can be applied in a step-up or step-down schedule (also called "bridge"), where drugs are added or dosages increased, drugs stopped or dosages decreased according to prespecified rules.[9] A relatively new design twist in this dimension is the comparison of continued treatment versus stopping patients currently on the drug. This type of trial is referred to as a withdrawal trial and many pediatric rheumatology trials are examples of such.

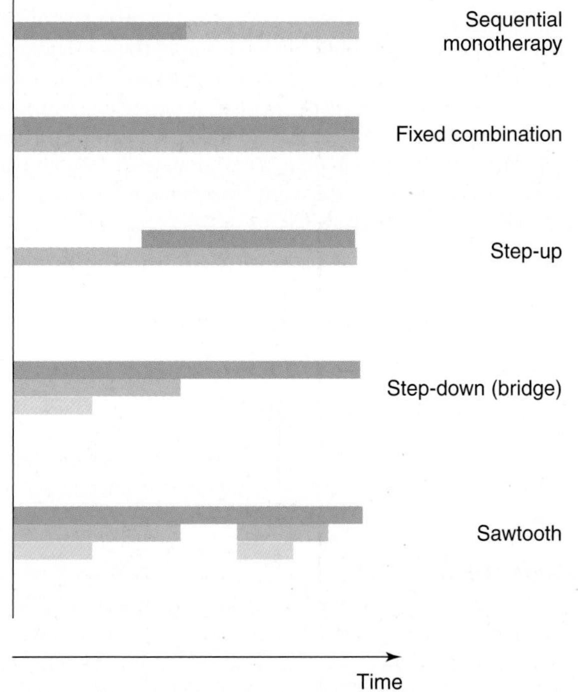

Figure 11A-2. Examples of regimen and regimen-change dimension designs, illustrating the sequential monotherapy (single drug), fixed combination, step-up, step-down ("bridge"), and "saw-tooth" displays.

The change dimension describes whether and how the regimen can change. The big disadvantage of parallel group trials with a fixed regimen is that if a patient fails to respond or experiences toxicity, there is no other option than to discontinue trial treatment. Such patients may still be followed for outcome assessment, but usually they will be treated with another drug outside the trial that will confound the interpretation of the end result. Thus a trial that compares regimens that can change according to the condition of the patient is not only much more practical but also allows much more flexibility to keep patients in the trial. The simplest setup (but inflexible) is one where the regimen is intensified or eased at specific time points. In such a design, usually an opt-out rule is included that allows the patient to stay on the same regimen if necessary (e.g., no increase if the patient is experiencing side effects).

More complicated, but also potentially more relevant, are trials that make regimen changes dependent on meeting a certain success or failure criterion. Although informative, it is difficult to use such trials for regulatory approval; they are quite effective, however, in teaching about specific therapeutic regimens for the clinician to determine the best and more appropriate approaches. Recent investigator-driven trials in RA have been of this type; as a group they can be labeled as "tight-control" trials, a term pioneered by Capell et al.[10] Patients are put on a certain regimen for a certain period, and then their disease activity is assessed. If the disease activity is not below a certain threshold, treatment is intensified or switched. Patients experiencing toxicity are also moved to the next treatment step (but of course not treated with a higher dose). The regimen lays out many treatment steps, allowing ongoing treatment often for at least 2 years. Such a tight-control regimen can then be compared to "usual practice" (TICORA[11]), but also to other more or less intensive regimens (BeSt[12]). BeSt is to date unique because each of the four regimens had both an "intensify/change" option (in case of too high disease activity) but also a "reduce" option (in case of remission). However informative, these trials have designs that are not conducive to being blinded, although they maintain a randomization strategy; thus they are randomized but unblinded. The "saw-tooth" is another strategy that uses a fixed step-down regimen as a way of induction; rather than change the regimen it is repeated if disease activity recurs.

Use of Placebo

Regulatory approval of a new therapeutic product in a given clinical indication frequently requires it to demonstrate superiority of specific effect to the placebo or is at least equivalent to the standard of care. The use of placebo for any length of time is controversial, especially in diseases where irreversible morbidity may occur if active treatment is withheld, and in general other effective therapies exist. However, placebo comparisons are essential at some time in the clinical development process to meet minimum standards of safety. A true placebo arm allows a comparison with no biologically active therapy, although often it would be unethical to design a longer term study with the expectation that a progressive inflammatory disease, such as RA, is not treated with at least standard of care as comparator.

Add-On Design

The "add-on" design has become an informal standard for phase III trials of many agents recently approved for RA.[13,14] Such trials select patients who have active disease despite stable treatment with a DMARD, usually methotrexate. These patients are then randomized to receive additionally the test drug or placebo. The patients are called "partial responders," but this is misleading in most cases because they have very active disease. The design has many practical advantages, the main one being that the FDA has accepted this design as a "placebo-controlled" trial. However, this design also carries many disadvantages that are insufficiently recognized,[15] including (1) testing of the efficacy of the new drug and the efficacy of the combination in the same trial; (2) a priori selection of suboptimal or nonresponders, thus a biased population at least to the old drug; (3) testing the new drug in a fixed combination for the benefit–risk ratio is unknown; and (4) unexpectedly high "placebo" response when the background drug is actually working, that is, when patients are truly "partial responders." For example, the patient may only be a partial responder to methotrexate due to taking the therapy at an inadequate dose or for too short a period of time. Once within the confines of a clinical trial, a response to methotrexate taken appropriately is then observed. Effect size calculations become critical in this circumstance. Finally, as a thinly disguised placebo trial, all the disadvantages of this design apply as well. Active controlled trials using a gold standard such as methotrexate or even one of the newly approved biologic agents, are considered more ethically appropriate and may yield information more relevant for day-to-day practice. Even in the context of an RCT, collection of data allowing relative cost-effectiveness comparison of the experimental agent with an existing therapy will offer additional information important to clinicians, payers, and health-care regulators.[16]

Equivalence Trials

Proving equivalence to presently available therapies presents unique problems. Equivalence trials require much larger sample sizes; a good estimate is roughly six times those required for a placebo RCT designed to demonstrate superiority. Equivalence is best defined using confidence intervals, where the null hypothesis of nonequivalence is rejected.[17] Unfortunately, demonstration of equivalence between two treatments does not necessarily indicate that they both are effective; each therapy may be equally ineffective and it is critical to understand how the comparator therapy has been anchored to measured clinical responsiveness.[18,19] It is therefore preferable to select an active comparator approved for use in the specified clinical indication that, more importantly, has previously been demonstrated to be efficacious compared with placebo. Ideally, an equivalence RCT should attempt to mimic the earlier "anchoring" placebo-controlled trial so that the active comparator can again be shown effective to a similar degree as when it was compared with placebo. This may not be easy to accomplish: Clinical practice may have evolved, utilizing different doses or dosing schedules than what is specified in the product label; concomitant use of medications, patient populations eligible for treatment with the agent, and even outcome measures may have changed.

RCTs in RA are now expected to be at least 3 months in duration; there is a clear need to demonstrate durability subsequent to those 3 months of active therapy and composite outcomes such as the American College of Rheumatology (ACR) response criteria or the Disease Activity Score (DAS) are used. It is important that if noninferiority designs are employed that rigorous margins of noninferiority are a priori defined to provide as much useful evidence of benefit as possible suggesting that the new therapy is at least as effective as the older more established therapy.

RCTs designed to demonstrate superiority of the experimental agent compared to the standard of care may be preferable as they will require smaller sample sizes. Given that a breakthrough therapy with profound-disease altering characteristics does not exist on a background of treating heterogeneous populations with variable disease courses, it is therefore difficult to demonstrate statistical superiority of an experimental treatment over an accepted therapy, and such designs are potentially a risk.

Another alternative study design is a three way comparison of monotherapy with a "gold standard of care" or the experimental agent versus combination of the two. This design may satisfy obvious questions on the part of treating physicians and care providers once the product is approved, but may prove of risk to the sponsor of the development program. By what criterion should nonequivalence be defined? Despite more rapid onset of benefit and resulting differences in area under the curve of "response," thus far it has been difficult to show statistical differences using our accepted outcome criteria.[20]

Selection of Appropriate Patient Population

Crucial to the success of a well-designed RCT is enrollment of a sufficient number of patients with likely active disease to demonstrate a true treatment difference. The patient has to have enough active disease at baseline for differences in effect of different therapies within the trial to be appreciated. Placebo responses are uniformly observed; RA as a disease is heterogeneous; and small pilot studies may not predict clinical responses once larger populations with more variable disease manifestations as required for regulatory approval are studied. Discontinuation rates can be as large as 40% to 50% in protocols of long duration. Reasons for dropout in longer-term trials are not only due to adverse events or lack of efficacy, but also include convenience, change in insurance and/or geographic relocation, change of health care provider, and interference with work activities, particularly in trials of long duration. Such dropout rates commonly require that long-term assessments of efficacy in RCTs are analyzed through the use of detailed and extensive sensitivity analyzes.

Randomized Controlled Trials in Rheumatoid Arthritis: Issues with Biologic Therapies

Randomized controlled trials with biologic agents must take into account issues that distinguish them from small molecules (Table 11A-4).

Adverse Events

Biologic agents are developed to achieve an effect by altering a relevant immune response or target. However, they may also have concomitant off-target effects on other immune functions that may be associated with possibly compromising immune function. The desired biologic effect may alter immune surveillance. Finally, this downregulation of surveillance due to either cause may lead to an increased burden of infections, the emergence of new autoimmuninty as measured by antibodies with or

Table 11A-4. Confounding Characteristics of Biologic Agents
Potential unblinding due to rapid onset of action, possible first-dose and infusion reactions
Immunogenicity
Injection site reactions
Concomitant effects of background therapy
Expectation bias

without new concomitant symptoms, and importantly, increased risk for lymphoproliferative disorders or solid tumor development. Rare adverse events such as these may not be observed during the typical clinical development program of a product, since exposure of a large number of patients will be required for such an event to be observed. Recently regulatory agencies have emphasized the importance of a large safety database prior to approval, including studies designed to assess the safety of the product in patients receiving usual care. Table 11A-4 outlines issues that may confound uniquely trials which include biologic therapies.

Biomarkers of Effect

It is possible that clinical development programs for both biologic agents and small molecules could become more efficient if biologic markers indicating successful delivery of the therapeutic and resultant effects of administration were available. Although these measurements may not correlate directly with clinical responses, biomarkers could be utilized to predict on and off effects of the experimental agent. They may be utilized with minimal pharmacokinetic (PK) data to reveal important pharmacodynamic (PD) information. They may also help in understanding other effects which persist beyond the measurable half-life of the administered agent. Unfortunately no biologic marker has been good enough at predicting clinical responses to serve as a true surrogate marker—even rapid and profound decreases in CRP levels following administration of a TNF-α inhibitor in RA do not always identify patients who achieve clinical benefit.[13]

Conduct of Randomized Controlled Trial

Just as design of an RCT requires careful consideration to detail, so must its conduct be carefully controlled. Statistical analysis plans are critical, the identification of primary and secondary outcomes all must be prospectively defined. Rules applied governing the implementation of a clinical trial include appropriate methods to ensure randomization, and equal distribution of baseline demographic and disease characteristics, as well as all efforts to avoid selection bias.

Simple Randomization or Stratification

Central randomization is recommended. Use of an analysis model that accounts for multiple potential parameters of variability is typically preferable to stratification of enrollment based on fewer predefined characteristics. It is difficult to predict clinical responses in heterogeneous rheumatic disease populations, and full stratification may interfere with convenient and efficient protocol enrollment. True patient stratification will also require far greater numbers of patients to ensure adequate powering of a trial as opposed to applying the characteristics of balanced randomization. If necessary, balanced enrollment by one or two parameters can be applied, and other potential covariates should be included in the model to analyze efficacy according to enrollment site, geographic distribution, baseline disease characteristics, and prior treatment.

Analysis and Therapy Change

In clinical indications where treatment options are limited and those treatments rarely result in cures, definitions of standard of care may change, even during conduct of an RCT with limited duration. The statistical analysis plan must therefore include appropriate rules allowing for modification based on accumulated new clinical information, which might include changes in therapeutic practice that may become available only after protocol treatment is initiated.[21] These issues must be identified prospectively, such that statistical analyzes remain robust and retain a valid reflection of day-to-day clinical practice. It is possible that applying adaptive design will allow for arms of the trial to be dropped if efficacy or safety issues become evident. If this is considered, then strict a priori–defined rules will need to be followed and may alter the powering of the trial. An interim analysis needs to be prespecified in this circumstance, and thus an adaptive design may be more appropriate for phase II trials rather than pivotal phase III trials when the latter are predicated on regulatory needs.

Sample Size Calculation

Clinical indications with limited available treatments and no definitive cures make it difficult to calculate sample sizes to identify statistically significant and/or clinically meaningful efficacy of an experimental therapy compared with a placebo and/or active control therapy. Data from phase I and II trials offer important information, but are often conducted in patient populations of insufficient size and may be limited to a small number of clinical practices that may not reflect more generally observed patients. Based on imperfect estimates of required sample size, blinded interim analyzes can assure protocol populations of sufficient size and/or treatments of sufficient duration to demonstrate statistical significance. Nonetheless these blinded analyzes alter the conduct of the protocol, even when a blinded adjudication committee is utilized—although they offer no additional clinical information to the sponsor, they include recommendations on whether the RCT should continue either enrollment and/or treatment or be stopped. Conduct of these interim analyzes will therefore require adjustment of the p-value.[22,23]

Outcome Measures

In rheumatoid arthritis, the Outcome Measures in Rheumatology Clinical Trials (OMERACT) consensus process, initiated in 1991, identified a minimum number (core set) of outcome measures to be used in RCTs[24]; other attempts to develop consensus resulted in validation and use of two "responder indices" in RCTs in patients with active RA: ACR20 response and EULAR improvement criteria based on the DAS.[25,26] Use of both criteria facilitated U.S. and EU regulatory approvals of new biologic and small-molecules therapies for the treatment of RA, and, more importantly, established precedents for subsequent development and approval strategies.

Whereas the ACR index relies on a certain combination of changes in core set measures to define response, the EULAR criteria combine a change in DAS with an achieved DAS state. Data from recent RCTs in RA have demonstrated several points:

- Utilization of DAS can "stratify" patient populations at baseline, and help to identify those who respond to treatment; unfortunately they continue to not emphasize outcomes that are often considered important to patients.
- Although the ACR ≥20/50/70 definition of response is not a continuous measure; its measured components are continuous measures. Recent RCTs of newly approved therapies in RA demonstrate that improvement, by ACR ≥20 or DAS definitions of "good and moderate" responses are closely correlated, identifying plus/minus 10% of the same population.
- Increasingly, there has been recognition of the importance of "patient reported" outcome measures.[27–29] These differ according to patient expectations, including understanding, and acceptance of the unfortunate circumstance that they suffer a presently incurable chronic disease that requires them to allow the recognition of a new reality. This affects not only performance of required daily activities but also perception of self, within the home and social situations, as well as work-related and public activities. Now that new therapies in RA have demonstrated statistically as well as clinically significant improvements in performance of physical and psychosocial activities important to patients, we better comprehend the multiple ways that diseases such as RA impact everyday living and its associated activities—health-related quality of life.

Conclusion

Randomized controlled trials are the only way to determine true response when developing new therapies. In studying treatment effects in patients with rheumatic diseases, significant placebo responses are expected. The introduction of biologic therapies has begun a new era of product development in rheumatology. These therapies provide early responses, frequently after the first or second dose, when previously at least 3 months of DMARD administration were required before confirming treatment failure. Adherence to careful trial design will be required to minimize some of the effects of these newer therapies.

Parallel-designed RCTs and randomized withdrawal RCTs are the most powerful methods to define response today whether against placebo or active comparator. However, trial designs for uses other than for regulatory approval, including step-up or step-down trials and randomized open-label pragmatic trials with prespecified and predetermined outcomes, as well as simple pragmatic open-label observations may provide useful clinical information to inform patients and clinicians about the relative risk and benefits of both new and older therapies.

References

1. Epstein WV. Expectation bias in rheumatoid arthritis clinical trials. The anti CD4 monoclonal antibody experience. *Arthritis Rheum* 1996;39:1773–1779.
2. Strand V, Scott DL, Panayi GS. Editorial: Evaluating biologic agents in rheumatoid arthritis: A framework for clinical trials. *J Rheumatol* 1994;21:1390–1392.
3. Schulz KF. Assessing allocation concealment and blinding in randomized controlled trials: why bother? *ACP J Club* 2000;132: A11–A12.
4. Food and Drug Administration. Clinical development programs for drugs, devices, and biological products for the treatment of rheumatoid arthritis (RA). http://www.fda.gov/cder/guidance/1208fnl.htm.
5. European Commission, Enterprise Directorate General, Pharmaceuticals Unit. Points to consider on clinical investigation of slow-acting anti-rheumatic medicinal products in rheumatoid arthritis. London, December 17, 1998. http://www.eudra.org/emea.html.
6. Strand V, Cohen S, Schiff M, et al. Treatment of active rheumatoid arthritis with leflunomide compared with placebo and methotrexate. Leflunomide Rheumatoid Arthritis Investigators Group. *Arch Intern Med* 1999;159:2542–2550.
7. Pincus T, Koch GG, Sokka T, et al. A randomized, double-blind, crossover clinical trial of diclofenac plus misoprostol versus acetaminophen in patients with osteoarthritis of the hip or knee. *Arthritis Rheum* 2001;44:1477–1480.
8. Pincus T, Koch G, Lei H, et al. Two randomized placebo-controlled cross-over clinical trials in patients with osteoarthritis of the knee or hip. Placebo, Acetaminophen (Paracetamol) or Celecoxib Efficacy Studies (PACES). *Ann Rheum Dis* 2004;63:897–900.
9. Boers M, Verhoeven AC, Markusse HM, et al. Randomized comparison of combined step-down prednisolone, methotrexate and sulphasalazine with sulphasalazine alone in early rheumatoid arthritis. *Lancet* 1997;350:309–318.
10. Capell HA, Madhok R, Porter DR, et al. Combination therapy with sulfasalazine and methotrexate is more effective than either drug alone in patients with rheumatoid arthritis with a suboptimal response to sulfasalazine: Results from the double-blind placebo-controlled MASCOT study. *Ann Rheum Dis* 2007;66(2): 235–241.
11. Grigor C, Capell H, Stirling A, et al. Effect of a treatment strategy of tight control for rheumatoid arthritis (the TICORA study): A single-blind randomised controlled trial. *Lancet* 2004;364:263–269.
12. Allaart CF, Goekoop-Ruiterman YP, de Vries-Bouwstra JK, et al. Aiming at low disease activity in rheumatoid arthritis with initial combination therapy or initial monotherapy strategies: The BeSt study. *Clin Exp Rheumatol* 2006;24(Suppl 43):S77–S82.
13. Lipsky PE, van der Heijde DM, St Clair EW, et al. Infliximab and methotrexate in the treatment of rheumatoid arthritis. Anti-Tumor Necrosis Factor Trial in rheumatoid arthritis with concomitant therapy study group. *N Engl J Med* 2000;343:1594–1602.
14. Weinblatt ME, Kremer JM, Bankhurst AD, et al. A trial of etanercept, a recombinant tumor necrosis factor receptor–Fc fusion protein, in patients with rheumatoid arthritis receiving methotrexate. *N Engl J Med* 1999;340:253–259.
15. Boers M. Add-on or step-up trials for new drug development in rheumatoid arthritis: A new standard? *Arthritis Rheum* 2003;48: 1481–1483.
16. Cohen S, Cannon G, Schiff M, et al. Two-year treatment of active rheumatoid arthritis with leflunomide compared with methotrexate. *Arthritis Rheum* 2001;40:1984–1992.
17. Jones B, Jarvis P, Lewis JA, et al. Trials to assess equivalence: the importance of rigorous methods. *BMJ* 1996;313:36–39.
18. Temple R, Ellenberg SS. Placebo controlled trials and active control trials in the evaluation of new treatments. Part 1: Ethical and scientific issues. *Ann Intern Med* 2000;133:455–463.

19. Temple R, Ellenberg SS. Placebo controlled trials and active control trials in the evaluation of new treatments. Part 2: Practical issues and specific cases. *Ann Intern Med* 2000;133:464–470.
20. Bathon JM, Martin RW, Fleischmann RM, et al. A comparison of etanercept and methotrexate in patients with early rheumatoid arthritis. *N Engl J Med* 2000;343(22):1586–1593.
21. Wittes J, Lachenbruch PA. Opening the adaptive toolbox. *Biom J* 2006;48:598–603.
22. O'Brien PC, Fleming TR. A multiple testing procedure for clinical trials. *Biometrics* 1979;35:549–556.
23. Lan KKG, DeMets DL, Halperin M. More flexible sequential and non-sequential designs in long-term clinical trials. *Commun Stats A Theory Methods* 1984;13:2339–2353.
24. Boers M, Tugwell P, Felson DT, et al. World Health Organization and International League of Associations for Rheumatology core endpoints for symptom modifying antirheumatic drugs in rheumatoid arthritis clinical trials. *J Rheumatol* 1994;21:86–89.
25. Weinblatt ME, Coblyn JS, Fox DA, et al. Efficacy of low-dose methotrexate in rheumatoid arthritis *N Engl J Med* 1985;312:818–822.
26. Olsen NJ, Brooks RH, Cush JJ, et al. A double blind placebo controlled study of anti-CD5 immunoconjugate in patients with rheumatoid arthritis. *Arthritis Rheum* 1996;39:1102–1108.
27. Goldsmith C, Boers M, Bombardier C, et al. Criteria for clinically important changes in outcomes: development, scoring and evaluation of rheumatoid arthritis patient and trial profiles. *J Rheumatol* 1993;20:561–565.
28. Wells GA, Tugwell P, Kraag GR, et al. Minimum important differences between patients with rheumatoid arthritis: The patient's perspective. *J Rheumatol* 1993;20:557–560.
29. Kosinski M, Zhao SZ, Didhiya S, et al. Determining minimum clinically important changes in generic and disease-specific health-related quality of life questionnaires in clinical trials of rheumatoid arthritis. *Arthritis Rheum* 2000;43:1478–1487.

What Should Be Reported in Clinical Trials?

CHAPTER **11B**

Robert Landewe

- **Make Clear That You Appreciate the Difference Between Internal Validity and External Validity**
- **Do Not Report about Efficacy Trials as if They Are Effectiveness Trials and Vice Versa**
- **Find Out Whether Your Trial Patients Resemble the "Average Patient in Clinical Practice"**
- **Realize That Low Disease-Activity State Rather Than Clinical Response Is Main Aim of Rheumatoid Arthritis Treatment**
- **The Null Hypothesis Is Not Only for Statisticians**
- **Statistical Power Considerations Are Not Only for Statisticians**
- **Appreciate Missing Data as Carefully as Present Data**
- **Design an Appropriate Trial Flow Chart**
- **Intention-to-Treat Analysis Is a Means Rather Than a Dogma**
- **An Appropriate Look Tells More Than an Appropriate Statistical Test**
- **Use Statistical Tests Modestly and Avoid *p*-Value Fetishism**
- **Longitudinal Trial Data Can Be Informative, but Analysis and Interpretation Require Caution**
- **The Most Dangerous Drugs May Have the Most Reassuring Trial Safety Data**
- **Do Not Embellish Trial Report with Subgroup Analyses**

The cornerstone of medical experimentation in human beings is the randomized clinical trial (RCT). It is commonly accepted that RCTs provide the highest level of evidence with regard to efficacy of treatments or treatment strategies. The most important feature of an RCT is the randomized treatment allocation. This probabilistic process aims at creating treatment groups (two or more) that are prognostically similar for all known and unknown—either prognostically important or irrelevant—variables except the treatment. Prognostic similarity at baseline allows the investigator to attribute an observed difference between treatment groups to a particular treatment. While fundamental theory underlying the RCT—and the primary analysis of an RCT—is relatively simple, practical trial conduct faces a lot of potential pitfalls that may eventually result in the violation of prognostic similarity and introduce bias. Well-known examples are inadvertent unblinding of study drug (e.g., if the study treatment is very effective while the placebo is not), unbalanced nonrandom discontinuation (e.g., if the study drug is responsible for adverse drug reactions that cause selective dropout), or simply poor trial conduct or overt misconduct (e.g., if patients do not show up for visits, assessors do not measure with scrutiny, or at worst nonexisting or virtual patients with faked response patterns are reported). It is the investigators' responsibility to optimize trial conduct and data collection, to perform correct analysis of the data, and to transparently describe the process and results of the trial in reports and peer-reviewed articles in the medical literature (known as "good clinical practice"). The consumers of these reports, peer-reviewers, scientists, clinicians, workers in the pharmaceutical industry, regulatory authorities, and others have their own responsibilities. They have the obligation to interpret the data carefully, weighing their integrity and importance, unprejudiced with respect to the investigators' interpretations, and to translate trial information into useful, clinically applicable information. This process has gained attention as "critical appraisal," and the literature provides superb guidance as to how to critically appraise the report of an RCT.

Ideally, good clinical practice and critical appraisal are supplementary in getting important new medical developments where they belong: the patient. An essential part of this interplay is the trial report with which information from the investigator is transferred to the consumer. Medical journals have agreed on guidelines with respect to trial-report (e.g., CONSORT guidelines). Pharmaceutical industries and regulatory authorities use their own guidelines that go far beyond the requirements of scientists and clinicians in terms of comprehensiveness, and these guidelines serve the purpose of public health responsibility in the process of drug registration.

This chapter deals with the article in medical literature that describes the results of a clinical trial. What information/data should such an article include and why? The focus of this chapter is the clinical investigator who has completed a trial and has to write a manuscript. In order to increase comprehension, the chapter provides 14 points to consider. The reader is referred to the literature to obtain detailed and structured information about methodologic details to be included in the report of clinical trials. The 14 points to consider cover the entire area of trial reporting, but are by no means a complete representation of what is important in writing a trial report. They rather reflect the author's opinion, inspired by experience in designing, describing, and reading numerous clinical trials. Sometimes the points to consider touch existing guidelines, and sometimes they do not.

In view of the title of this book, the discussion has been written against a background of rheumatoid arthritis (RA) clinical trials.

Make Clear That You Appreciate the Difference Between Internal Validity and External Validity

A trial is a rather artificial construct that usually serves a single major purpose: to investigate whether a particular treatment is efficacious or not. In general, elements of trial-design, such as the selection of patients, the sample size, the choice of the comparative intervention and the duration of the trial, are chosen in such a manner that the trial can optimally demonstrate a treatment effect, that is, a difference in efficacy between the new treatment and the control intervention. The methodologic robustness of a trial, which is dependent on these elements of trial design, is referred to as internal validity.

Understandably, trials do often not resemble clinical practice. RA trials, for example, often include patients with a high level of disease activity, who represent only a minority in clinical practice. The extent to which clinical trial results can be extrapolated to the common clinical practice is referred to as external validity. External validity is much more diffuse than internal validity. It depends on how the consumers of the data interpret the results, how these results are presented to them, how convincingly the investigators have argued their message, and how credible they are in the eyes of the beholders. It depends on whether readers think the data of the trial are applicable to an individual patient in their own practice. Undoubtedly, external validity will be judged as unsatisfactory if internal validity falls short. The opposite is not necessarily true. A trial with high internal validity can easily have insufficient external validity. An increasingly common example in RA is the RCT with 1000 patients with high disease activity that tests a new treatment against the "currently best available disease-modifying treatment for RA," and finds a subtle, not very relevant but nevertheless statistically significant difference in favor of the new treatment. Such a new treatment will probably be approved by drug registration authorities if it is considered safe, since it has proven superiority in a well-conducted trial with high internal validity. Needless to say, this effective treatment with doubtful advantage over existing treatments should not be broadly applied in common clinical practice without further consideration (external validation). A second example that has ethical implications beyond the discussion of this chapter, arises if—for reasons of inclusion rates—this 1000-patient drug trial has been conducted in countries with health care systems that cannot regularly afford the "currently best available treatment for RA" in view of costs. Undoubtedly, patients in that trial do not necessarily resemble patients in western countries with respect to previous treatment, comorbidity, cultural differences, genetic differences, and so on, and it is very difficult to judge if the results of such a trial are still applicable to patients in Western countries.

Trial reports should discuss the balance between internal and external validity, about which of both prevails, where one falls short in favor of the other, and which elements are important in translating the trial result into clinical practice.

Do Not Report about Efficacy Trials as if They Are Effectiveness Trials and Vice Versa

It is obligatory to be informed about the underlying aim of the trial, which is not necessarily the same as the primary study objective. Drug registration trials under the auspices of the pharmaceutical industry serve a different purpose than investigator-driven trials with treatment strategies. The former are often referred to as explanatory or efficacy trials, and are characterized by a high level of internal validity, while the latter—pragmatic trials or effectiveness trials—more closely resemble clinical practice, often find their basis in questions emerging from clinical practice, and as a consequence have a higher level of external validity.

The results of explanatory trials are often very robust and confirm the efficacy of the tested drug beyond statistical doubt, but may fall short in terms of clinical significance. Examples are numerous and include any trial that presents results of a "new drug" tested against placebo or an active comparator.

Effectiveness trials often have a more understandable trial result that is more easily applicable in individual patients, but results may be biased, for example, by imperfections in blinding and changes in kind and intensity of treatment during the trial. An interesting type of trial that belongs to this group is the benchmark trial in RA. The essential characteristic of the benchmark trial is that treatment (kind and/or intensity) is not kept constant during the course of the trial, but is dependent on the clinical response of the individual patient (e.g., whether the benchmark is met or not). Such a trial mimics every day clinical practice very well, but is in conflict with fundamental theory underlying RCTs that patient groups in a trial are prognostically similar during the trial. The methodologic robustness of the trial is to some extent jeopardized by increased clinical face validity.

Trial investigators should discuss these important elements since they are relevant for the interpretation of the results by the consumers of the report who have to decide about their usefulness for application in individual patients.

Find Out Whether Your Trial Patients Resemble the "Average Patient in Clinical Practice"

As argued before, the type of patients included in the trial is of pivotal importance with respect to the interpretation of the trial results. In efficacy trials, statistical power—the probability that the trial confirms the superiority of a new treatment if this superiority truly exists—is of eminent importance. Discriminatory ability and sensitivity to change of outcome measures are determinants of statistical power. The outcome measures propagated for clinical trials in RA, such as the American College of Rheumatology (ACR) and European League Against Rheumatism (EULAR) response criteria, perform best—and have been validated—in patient groups with high levels of disease activity, which is why most efficacy trials include these patients. In the spectrum of patients with RA, however, these patients do not constitute a majority, which may have implications for the interpretation of trial results. It is possible, if not likely, that many RA patients with less active disease do not necessarily need the "new treatment" that tested most effectively in the efficacy trial, but can do very well with the comparator drug.

Another prevalent discrepancy between clinical practice and RCT is the paucity of clinically relevant comorbid conditions in RCTs as compared to clinical practice, because patients with relevant comorbidities are usually excluded. Similar reasoning can be followed regarding compliance, or in general any reason that increases the probability of premature discontinuation and/or nonresponse.

It is very important when reading a report of a clinical trial to realize that the patients in the trial do not necessarily resemble the individual patient in clinical practice, and that such discrepancies may have consequences for the translation of trial results. Trial reports should include all necessary information about disease activity, severity, and prognosis (which they often do), but also information about relevant comorbidity and comedication (which they often exclude).

Realize That Low Disease-Activity State Rather Than Clinical Response Is Main Aim of Rheumatoid Arthritis Treatment

The primary outcome measure of RCT is a measure that is used for technical reasons to determine whether the null hypothesis is met or should be rejected. Therefore, the primary outcome measure is usually used in sample-size calculations. By far, most clinical trials in RA make use of the ACR response criteria for 20% improvement (ACR20), 50% improvement (ACR50), and 70% improvement (ACR70). Only the ACR20 is formally validated for this goal, and is therefore usually applied as the primary outcome measure for assessing drug efficacy on signs and symptoms of RA in most drug registration trials. The ACR20 response criteria have been very instrumental in the demonstration of drug efficacy, because they are sensitive and highly discriminatory. However, it would be negligent to limit the report of a clinical trial to only these response criteria for several reasons. First, since an ACR20 (or 50 or 70) can be met in different ways, it does not truly express what has changed in the patients. Second, ACR20 is a change measure. There is accumulating evidence that the true outcome of RA is determined by the actual level of disease activity, rather than by change. If a patient starts with a very high level of disease activity, even an ACR70 response results in significant residual disease activity that may lead to further radiographic progression and functional impairment. Third, many in the field believe that ACR20 does not reflect a clinically meaningful response (anymore). This opinion should be weighed in light of the increased number of highly effective antirheumatic treatments that have become available.

These arguments certainly do not disregard the scientific value of ACR20 as a primary outcome measure in a trial, but point to the importance of reporting additional clinical outcome measures that describe a state of disease rather than change in disease activity state. There is consensus about reporting the core-set variables, the single-item components necessary to determine an ACR20 response, such as level of pain, swollen/tender joint count, acute-phase reactant (C-reactive protein [CRP] and/or erythrocyte sedimentation rate [ESR]), and health assessment questionnaire (HAQ) score. Especially in Europe, there is a lot of appreciation for the indices describing a disease activity state: the Disease Activity Score (DAS) (the original and comprehensive form as well as the "truncated" 28-joint form), and its derivatives, the Clinical Disease Activity Index (CDAI) and Simple Disease Activity Index (SDAI). These indices of disease activity, which have validated cut-off levels for clinically important states such as remission, low-, moderate-, and high-disease activity, have face validity, show better correlation with long-term consequences of RA, and can be used as benchmarks. Indices of disease activity should therefore be reported in clinical trials of RA.

The Null Hypothesis Is Not Only for Statisticians

Textbooks in clinical trial design teach that the underlying null hypothesis should be carefully formulated during the design-phase of the trial. The formulation of the null hypothesis, which is in theory the hypothesis that is challenged by experimentation (the trial), tells immediately whether the basic design of the RCT aims at proving superior efficacy of a new treatment (the superiority design) or at proving that a new drug treatment is as effective as a comparator drug, for ethical reasons often the current standard of therapy (the noninferiority design). The RCTs we have seen during the last decade in RA most often had a superiority design, with the null hypothesis that the new treatment was as efficacious as a placebo or a comparator treatment. The design of the trial and the sample size are dependent on a minimally important difference, which is determined up front by the investigators, and serves as the basis for sample size calculations. In the context of RA, many consecutive RCTs have resulted in a number of treatments that have proven efficacy against placebo or against the standard of care therapy (usually methotrexate).

This affluence of effective treatments in RA has its other side of the coin. First, there is increasing sympathy for the ethical argument that progress in the treatment of RA should have its consequences for the standard of care in this disease. The immediate implication with regard to trial design is that conventional RCTs with placebo, or even methotrexate, as therapy in the control group will be considered unethical. The more effective the therapy in the control group is, the more difficult it is to surpass the effect in the control group with a new treatment: The classic superiority trial will be increasingly unfeasible in RA.

Second, while we have that affluence of effective drugs in RA, there is a knowledge gap with respect to drug efficacy in mutual comparison. Using previous argumentation, these pregnant clinical questions cannot be solved with classic trial designs.

Consequently, we will probably see an increasing number of noninferiority trials in RA in the near future. Such trials have as a null hypothesis that the new drug is inferior to the effective treatment in the control arm, and embark on the determination of an appropriate noninferiority margin. More than the choice of a minimally important difference in superiority trials, the choice of a noninferiority margin in a noninferiority trial is a highly subjective decision that includes elements of efficacy, safety and costs, and can make or break the interpretability of such a trial.

It is crucial that elements of the null hypothesis, such as choices and considerations relating to the design type of the trial (superiority vs. noninferiority) and relating to levels of minimally important difference and noninferiority margin, are properly described and justified in the trial report.

Statistical Power Considerations Are Not Only for Statisticians

Every RCT in patients with RA should technically be able to reject the null hypothesis if the alternative hypothesis reflects the truth: It should have sufficient statistical power. One could justifiably argue, at least in the field of RA, that trials with insufficient power should not have been executed. It is unethical to expose patients to potentially harmful drugs if the trial is not able to demonstrate superiority or noninferiority of that drug; it fills medical literature with data that are inconclusive, with the risk of misinterpretation and inappropriate application for patient care, and it is extremely cost-ineffective to execute trials that do not meet their goals. So, it seems obvious that the trial investigator ensures sufficient statistical power and that the reader of a clinical trial report ascertains that statistical power was appropriate. Many do not realize that statistical power is more than sample size alone. Although the latter is of great importance, statistical power is—among others—dependent on the outcome measure (the responsiveness and discriminatory capacity) and the expected effect size (the anticipated difference between the new treatment and the control treatment). The wording justifying the sample size of the trial gives to some extent resolution about the power considerations. In sample size calculations, patient numbers are calculated for a given primary outcome measure with an assumption for its variability, for given values of beta (statistical power) and for a predefined effect size. Sometimes, the anticipated effect size is based on realistic assumptions stemming from previous studies, but all too often an effect is chosen that has no scientific precedent ("20% between-group difference"). Some investigators want 80% statistical power, others choose 90% power as a preference, and all too often the reader is left with the impression that convenience outweighs theoretical arguments about power: "The calculation should fit."

Rather than only describing the sample size calculation per se (which is often done inappropriately), the trial report should include argumentation for the chosen assumptions such as the level of the minimal clinically important difference, the noninferiority margin, the level of beta, the historic precedents, and so on.

Appreciate Missing Data as Carefully as Present Data

Ideally, an RCT provides complete data. Practically, RCTs without missing data do not exist.

Patients miss visits for whatever reason, and do that more frequently than any investigator would consider acceptable. Patients withdraw consent, lose motivation, and drop out. Patients report adverse events to the investigator, who decides to discontinue the patient from the trial. The investigator and the patient are disappointed with regard to the drug effect, and decide to stop. The patient moves and gets lost to follow-up. All these examples create missing data. Although the examples given here will be very familiar to every reader (and will be considered inherent to clinical practice), trial methodology, statistical analysis, and interpretation of trial results do not very well comply with the problem of missing data. It is crucial to realize the issue of missing data before the trial starts, and to consider scenarios of how to handle missing data. There is no single acceptable generic solution, but by far the worst solution is to entirely withdraw the patient from the analysis. Usually, trial discontinuation is a nonrandom process, which means that the reason why patients withdraw is somehow associated with disease severity, and therefore with the probability of achieving a treatment response (confounding). Ignoring these patients means that treatment groups cannot be considered prognostically similar anymore, which is probably the most important violation of trial methodology that you can commit.

Data imputation is the only alternative. Imputation means that an imaginary value is attributed to missing assessments, so that the patient with missing data remains in the analysis, but the question obviously is what to impute. Nonresponder imputation is a popular and conservative means of data imputation in clinical trials with a response measure (e.g., ACR20) as primary outcome variable. It simply attributes nonresponse to every patient who discontinues from the trial, irrespective of the reason for discontinuation. Last-observation-carried forward (LOCF) is a popular means of imputing continuous data, in which the last value that was actually measured is imputed as a substitute for subsequent missing assessments. Worst-case scenarios impute the worst group value or the value representing the 95th percentile. Imputation of group means or group medians are also used. Linear interpolation can be useful if in-between data points are missed, and linear extrapolation is used if the expected time course follows an approximately linear trend. Finally, sophisticated computer algorithms (e.g., Bayesian Markov chain Monte Carlo multiple imputation procedure exist that use multiple imputation techniques.[1] A discussion of such techniques is beyond the scope of this chapter.

As argued, there is not a single acceptable means of imputation. Nonresponder imputation usually works well if a predefined response is the outcome of interest, and LOCF seems a reasonably conservative approach for imputation of missing continuous data in a setting in which treatment should improve a pre-existent state (e.g., disease activity, physical function). Linear extrapolation is frequently used to impute missing radiographic data, since the natural course of radiographic damage is compatible with worsening, and LOCF would result in a spurious inhibition of progression. In theory, trial results (treatment contrast) should not be dependent on what means of data imputation for missing data is used. The only transparent way of confirming the robustness of the trial result is to perform and show sensitivity analyzes for missing data. This means that you perform different means of imputation and check the consequences with regard to the treatment effect.

Recently, the handling of dropout and missing data has gained increasing attention because of the introduction of the placebo-controlled trial with early escape option in RA and ankylosing spondylitis. The characteristic feature of such a trial is that—after a prespecified time period—patients are allowed to switch to open active treatment (usually the treatment given in the active treatment arm) in order to avoid the withholding of treatment for an ethically unacceptable period of time. Usually, the trial endpoint to assess efficacy with respect to signs and symptoms is at the time-point of early escape, but patients continue the trial for other endpoints. In order to maintain the trial blinding, early escape is allowed in both trial arms, and patients following this option are considered nonresponders. Recent experience has shown that more than 70% of patients in the placebo group, and up to 30% of patients in the active drug group may take the route of early escape. This implies that for the remainder of the trial more than 50% of the patients originally randomized are analyzed with imputed data, which may have implications for the interpretation of prognostic similarity, and therefore the results of the trial.

Design an Appropriate Trial Flow Chart

Under the influence of the CONSORT guidelines, the trial flow chart in the report of the clinical trial has become ubiquitous. The flow chart describes the course of the study, starting before randomization with a box containing the number of screened patients and ending with boxes containing the numbers of patients completing the study in the treatment group they were allocated to by randomization. In between, a number of boxes deviate from the "straight course," including patients who for some reason have discontinued the trial. Usually, there is a brief motivation for the reason why patients have discontinued, e.g., lack of efficacy, adverse drug reaction, lost to follow-up, and others.

The flow chart is a useful tool for the reader to obtain a first impression about the course of the study. A number of screened patients that is many times higher than the number of eligible patients tells something about patient selection and has implications for external validity. Sometimes, patients are randomized but do not receive the study drug for any reason. It is important to find out about their fate in the analysis. Unbalanced withdrawal (e.g., 10% in the intervention group vs. 50% in the control group) can be the first sign of drug efficacy, or may tell us something about adverse events, but we should also focus particular attention on how these patients are handled in the analysis. Unbalanced withdrawal is a feature of nonrandom discontinuation and a potential source for bias. Finally, a flow chart should give resolution about the number of patients actually included in the analysis (see following Intention-to-Treat section).

Intention-to-Treat Analysis Is a Means Rather Than a Dogma

Every investigator, every trial designer, and every clinician knows about the dogmatic character of the intention-to-treat (ITT) principle underlying the main analysis of a clinical trial. Although occasionally a paper mentions a surrogate of ITT, such as "modified ITT analysis," the definition of ITT is crystal clear. It means that every patient in the trial is considered to belong to the group that he or she was originally allocated to by randomization, regardless of what has happened with this patient during the trial. The justification for this somewhat dogmatic principle is that the ITT analysis is the most conservative analysis because it preserves at least the prognostic similarity that was created at baseline by randomization. All other types of analyses, including "modified ITT," are second-rate since they allow retrograde patient selection at baseline. The typical completers analysis, for example, only includes those patients that have done well on the allocated study treatment, and ignores the patients that have discontinued, and may differ from the completing patients in terms of prognosis (prognostic dissimilarity).

ITT is not a certificate for an appropriate trial analysis. The trial report should spell out how patients that do not actually provide measured trial data are handled (see "Appreciate Missing Data" section). It should mention how data generated by patients that discontinued trial medication but showed up at visits are handled. And last but not least, there is no generic means of data manipulation in this regard. For example, considering every dropout as not having changed (improved) in a clinical trial with RA patients and ACR20 as the primary outcome measure is probably conservative, since a proportion of these patients will have had a clinical response. However, considering these dropouts as not having changed, in a clinical trial with radiographic progression as the outcome measure, is conservative, since it looks as if the dropouts do not have progression, and a trial arm with a high proportion of premature discontinuations may be spuriously benefited.

In summary, ITT together with appropriate handling of data, including appropriate imputation, works conservatively in that it tends to reduce a treatment contrast. Conservatism, however, is not necessarily a guarantee for a more truthful trial result. In the noninferiority trial, ITT may spuriously lead to a conclusion of noninferiority, while in truth unbalanced withdrawal, poor trial conduct or unintended cointerventions may be responsible for the absence of a difference between treatment groups. This is clarified by the example shown in Table 11B-1. Suppose that two analgesic drugs (A and B) are compared with respect to their ability to relieve pain in an RCT, and that drug A is in truth more effective than drug B (which, of course, you do not know in reality). The primary outcome measure is the number of patients with a 40% decrease in pain on a visual analog scale. Suppose also that patients take additional acetaminophen if they experience too much pain. Expectedly, the proportion of patients taking additional medication is lower in group A (the better treatment) as compared to group B (10 patients vs. 30 patients). Also expectedly, only 2 of these 10 patients in group A needing additional drug experienced a response (the severe cases), while 20 of the 30 patients needing additional drug (the milder cases) in group B experienced a response (attributable to comedication). Table 11B-1 shows how different types of analysis (ITT vs. per protocol) work with regard to response percentages and treatment effect. Keep in mind that in truth drug A is more efficacious than drug B. The unbalanced use of comedication resulted in a treatment effect of (only) 5% more responses in group A versus group B if analyzed by ITT. This is a small difference,

Table 11B-1. Imaginary Clinical Trial Data with Two Types of Analysis

Intention-to-Treat Analysis		
	Treatment A (n = 100)	**Treatment B (n = 100)**
Number of patients who entered the trial	100	100
Without clinical response	55	60
With clinical response	45	40
Response percentage based on intent-to-treat analysis	45% (45/100)	40% (40/100)
Per-Protocol Analysis		
	Treatment A (n = 100)	**Treatment B (n = 100)**
Number of patients who completed the trial and did not receive co-medication	90	70
Without clinical response	47	50
With clinical response	43	20
Response percentages based on per-protocol analysis	48% (43/90)	29% (20/70)

probably not compatible with a conclusion of superiority of drug A in a trial with a superiority design, but easily compatible with a conclusion of noninferiority of drug B in a trial with a noninferiority design. The picture changes, however, if you repeat the analysis on a per-protocol basis. Now, the treatment effect is almost 20% more responders in group A versus group B, probably compatible with the superiority of drug A in a trial with a superiority design and incompatible with noninferiority of drug B in a trial with a noninferiority design: ITT analysis is conservative with respect to concluding superiority of a drug in a superiority design (even if in truth superiority exists). Per-protocol analysis is conservative with respect to concluding noninferiority in a noninferiority design.

The analysis of noninferiority trials is not yet a closed book, but most are in favor of simultaneously presenting ITT and per-protocol analyses, so that readers can judge for themselves. It is always wise to be careful with interpretation if both analyses differ importantly (like in this example).

An Appropriate Look Tells More Than an Appropriate Statistical Test

Probably the most important means of communicating trial results is by graphs. A well-designed graph provides far more information than a statistical analysis, or a table with comprehensive descriptive data, such as means, standard deviations, and so on. An appropriate graphical representation of treatment results can give you a good idea, at first glance, about the relative efficacy of a new treatment in comparison with a control drug. Every reader of RA clinical trial articles will be familiar with the informative bar-graph representation of ACR20/50/70 responses per group. More cumbersome is the graphical representation of radiographic progression. The most frequently used Sharp–van der Heijde progression score usually has a skewed distribution, meaning that the data are not normally distributed. Very often, a data set of radiographic progression scores includes a high number of zero scores, and a relatively low number of positive scores with a minority of extreme progression scores at the right side of the spectrum. This feature means that the usual parametric descriptive statistics such as means and standard deviations do not appropriately reflect what has actually happened in the group. Medians and percentiles (25%, 75%) do a better job in that respect, but median progression in modern clinical trials in RA is often zero in the intervention as well as the control group, while progression is statistically significantly different. Recently, probability plots have been proposed to fill in this gap of communication. A probability plot shows every individual change score per trial arm that is ordered, from the lowest through the highest observed value, and is plotted against its cumulative probability. By superimposing the plots of the trial arms in a single graph, it is clear at first glance how the groups have performed with respect to radiographic progression.

Tabulation of data is important for several reasons: first, of course, to underscore the author's conclusions and make them transparent to critical appraisal; second, to make additional inferences for data interpretation (examples are calculations for number-needed-to-treat [NNT] and effect sizes for researchers interested in the performance of outcome measures), and third, as a source for the meta-analyst. It is critical that the authors of a trial report realize that their data may be used for several scientific purposes, and they should provide sufficient information. It is difficult to give exact guidelines, since prerequisites are different for different outcome measures, but a few examples may help. When ACR response is used as the outcome measure, it is crucial to not only report proportions, but also crude numbers (nominator as well as denominator). When continuous outcome measures (swollen joint count, DAS, etc.) are reported, data about status and change should be provided as means and appropriate standard deviations (rather than standard errors of the mean), as well as the actual number of patients who were used in the analysis. When distributions of continuous outcome measures are overtly skewed (such as radiographic progression scores), the investigators should not only present means and standard deviations but also medians and key percentiles (e.g., 25 and 50). With regard to reporting on radiographic progression there is consensus that—in the interest of the meta-analyst—also logarithmically transformed progression scores are reported in the tables.

Use Statistical Tests Modestly and Avoid *p*-Value Fetishism

The main goal of the statistical analysis in the report of the clinical trial is to challenge the null hypothesis, or in other words: to find probabilistic support for a difference observed between treatments. A second aim of statistical testing is to find out about the robustness of a demonstrated treatment effect (defined as the difference in an outcome variable between treatment groups in a trial).

In flagrant contrast to what is often done, in reality the statistical analysis should only take a modest place in the report of a clinical trial. But in the "era of *p*-values and overpowered trials," many authors cannot resist the attractiveness of "$p < 0.0001$," and build their article around the statistical test result rather than the opposite. Unfortunately, many of these authors are unable to reproduce the correct interpretation of $p < 0.0001$, and counter critical questions about the relevance of the difference with, "It is highly statistically significant, though, isn't it?," implying that the difference is important.

The *p*-value is a probability, namely the probability that, assuming that the null hypothesis is correct, this null hypothesis is nevertheless rejected. This sentence is only comprehensible if one realizes that the clinical trial one is looking at is only one (random) example of many, let's say 1000 imaginary similar trials. Who accepts this will also accept that all 1000 imaginary trials will have 1000 different results. The majority only slightly differs, but a few will have more deviant results, simply by coincidence, and a very few will even have extremely deviant results in either direction, while in truth the difference should be zero! In theory, such differences could be of such a magnitude that they lead to rejecting the null hypothesis. We talk about erroneous rejection of the null hypothesis, or type I error. The *p*-value is the probability of type I error: $p < 0.0001$ means that there is very, very small chance of a type I error. You could say that the result is very robust, and such a *p*-value adds to the credibility of the trial (internal validity). It does not say that the difference that was found is a relevant difference, or that an effect is meaningful. Current efficacy trials are often so powerful in statistically underscoring small differences that very good *p*-values can be obtained with treatment effects that are negligible when considered in the context of patient care. So, statistically significant does not imply clinically relevant. The opposite is also true: Not statistically significant does not mean not relevant. In other words, "The absence of evidence is not the same as the evidence of absence (of a meaningful effect)," a statement referring to type II error. Type II error will be discussed in more detail below.

The second aim of statistical analysis is to find out about how robust the trial results are. You could use the *p*-value for that, but that has a number of limitations. Actually you are not interested in the statistical robustness itself, but rather in the implications with respect to the size of the treatment effect. Usually, a 95% confidence interval (CI) is used to describe the bandwidth for the estimate of the treatment effect. Elaborating on the discussion about *p*-value, the 95% CI is best understandable by imagining that a particular trial is done 1000 times. In 95% of the times the trial result (the estimate of the treatment effect) will lie between the limits of the 95% CI, but in 5% of the times the treatment effect will take a more extreme value. The relation between *p*-value and 95% CI is further clarified in Figure 11B-1. Suppose a clinical trial in RA patients with two treatment arms (A vs. B) and (improvement in) disease activity score as the outcome measure. Three possible treatment effects are plotted in a diagram that a reader of meta-analysis may be familiar with. The zero treatment effect reflects the level of equivalence. All three scenarios represent a trial result in which treatment B is better than treatment A (more improvement in DAS with B as compared to A). The *p*-values are presented per scenario. The arrows represent the 95% confidence intervals around the mean improvements in DAS. Note that the 95% CIs of scenarios A and C lie entirely right from zero. Both treatment effects are statistically significant ($p < 0.05$): The null hypothesis of "no difference" is rejected. Note that the 95% CI in scenario B crosses zero. The treatment effect is not statistically significant ($p > 0.05$); the null hypothesis is not rejected. Note also that notwithstanding a smaller treatment effect in scenario C as compared to B, the treatment effect in C is statistically significant, as represented by a narrower 95% CI. We say that the trial result is more precise. It is the combination of statistical information and information about the preciseness of the treatment effect that make 95% CIs such attractive tools in clinical trials. In order to improve information exchange and interpretation of trial results, it is almost mandatory to present 95% CIs around the mean treatment effects, and not only *p*-values. As with many generic rules, occasionally, the balance dips to the other side: It is not particularly useful and often confusing to present 95% CIs of variables not related to treatment effects (or related to hypothesis testing). An example is the presentation of a 95% CIs around the mean DAS28 at baseline.

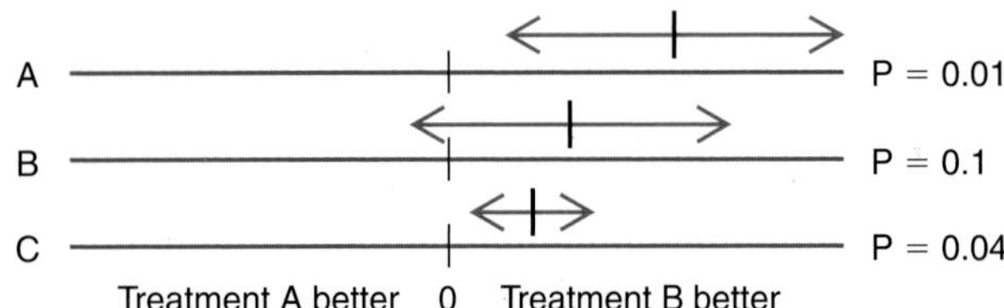

Figure 11B-1. Treatment effects and 95% confidence intervals of three potential scenarios (*A*, *B*, and *C*) for an imaginary clinical trial comparing treatment A and treatment B.

Longitudinal Trial Data Can Be Informative, but Analysis and Interpretation Require Caution

Most clinical trials have a primary endpoint that is evaluated at a certain time point. In efficacy trials for the approval of new drugs, such time points are usually defined. A trial "meets its endpoint" if the hypothesized effect is indeed demonstrated at the endpoint, but this information leaves the development of a response out of consideration. The development of a response may conceal important information, as shown in Figure 11B-2.

Both treatments arrive at the same DAS28 at week 24. But treatment A showed a gradual improvement over time, whereas there was a 16-week delay in improvement with treatment B. Such information may be important for the reader who has the task of interpreting the results of this trial in the context of clinical practice. The question is how longitudinal information from RA clinical trials can best be conveyed. Very often, investigators present proportions of ACR20/50/70 per treatment arm at different time points, as well as statistical tests per time point. Although such a policy may give insight into how a response develops, it is methodologically not entirely correct. First, an ACR response is a relative measure and the response in an individual patient is dependent on the patient's baseline values. Carrying forward ACR response over time gives too much weight to the baseline value, and the consequences of doing so are not known. Second, ACR responses over time do not guarantee that it is always the same set of patients who fulfill the response criteria. Third, statistically testing the between-group difference at every time point ignores the within-patient dependence (the phenomenon that the probability of a response at a certain time point is higher if one knows that this patient had a response at the previous time point) and bears a risk of multiple testing (i.e., inflated type I error). As such, the (statistical) results may look better than they really are.

It is very informative to present longitudinal data in the report of the clinical trial, but it is better to present continuous-state scores (e.g., DAS, swollen joint count, ESR) instead of response proportions, and to refrain from multiple time-points

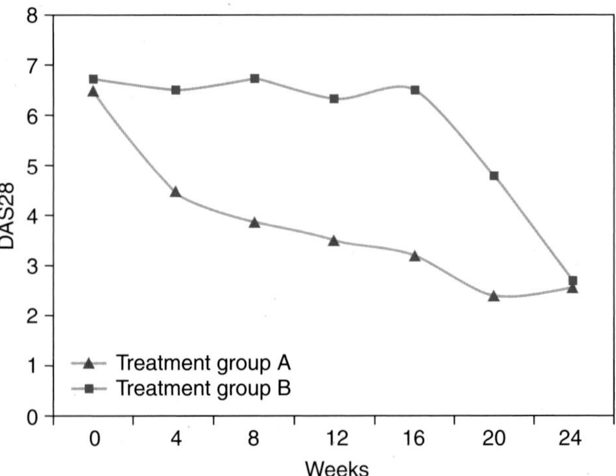

Figure 11B-2. Longitudinal trial results of an imaginary clinical trial comparing treatment *A* and treatment *B*.

statistical testing. Alternatively, and preferably if there is a focus on the longitudinal development of a response or an effect, the investigators could apply models for longitudinal data analysis that adjust for within-patient dependence.

The Most Dangerous Drugs May Have the Most Reassuring Trial Safety Data

Suppose a highly effective drug for the treatment of RA is associated with a relatively common cardiovascular complication in such a manner that one out of every 200 patients who is treated with that drug for 5 years will die of that complication. Almost certainly, clinicians and registration authorities would consider this an unacceptable safety risk. You may, however, question how likely it is that such relevant information regarding the safety of a new drug emerges from clinical trial results.

Let us take a placebo-controlled RCT with two arms and 500 RA patients per trial arm. Let us consider a background cardiovascular mortality rate of 0.5% per year. You can calculate that statistically 2.5 patients will die during the course of the trial due to "natural comorbidity." The drug we talk about has an excess mortality of 1/200 patients/5 years, or 0.1% per year, and you can calculate a mortality ratio of 1.2 (20% excess mortality). Table 11B-2 shows these figures translated into patient numbers.

The interpretation of the data coming from this simple exercise is that you need at least 4 of such trials to find a single additional case of mortality to be attributed to the new treatment. Needless to say that this subtle safety signal will be missed by trial analysts, especially if you realize that the distribution of deaths across these four consecutive trials could, for example, be 2 versus 1, 1 versus 2, 1 versus 2, and 1 versus 1 (placebo group vs. active drug group), and still arrive at 5 versus 6 deaths in total. While it is commonly accepted that RCTs are insensitive with respect to detecting small risks, almost every trial report mentions a very reassuring picture of adverse drug reactions, and if deaths or serious adverse events occur during the course of the trial, the tone of the description always reflects a strong belief that the occurrence is not related to trial medication. Important examples of such adverse events that may too easily be ascribed to coincidence rather than trial medication in RA clinical trials are cardiovascular death, lymphoma, and opportunistic infections. It should be recommended that the authors of clinical trial reports refrain from tendentious (even statistical) comparisons of rare adverse events between groups, or at least bring to the readers' notice that such comparisons in RCTs are unreliable. Once again, the absence of evidence is not the evidence of absence.

Table 11B-2. Mortality Data from Imaginary Placebo-Controlled Clinical Trial with Active Drug That Causes One Case of Cardiovascular Mortality in Every 200 Patients Treated with Drug for 5 Years

	Placebo Group (n = 500)	Active Drug Group (n = 500)
Number of patients dying of unrelated causes	1.25 patients	1.25 patients
Number of patients dying of drug-related causes	0 patients	0.25 patients

Note: Unrelated cardiovascular mortality of 0.5% per year assumed.

Do Not Embellish Trial Report with Subgroup Analyses

Subgroup analysis in clinical trials is a topic of considerable controversy. The proponents of subgroup analysis point to its hypothesis-generating potential. Opponents argue that subgroup analysis is irresponsible data mining, looking for statistically significant differences by splitting up the trial population into smaller subgroups. Both parties are right to some extent. Subgroup analysis can sometimes help to disentangle incomprehensible trial results, and can raise attention to new, previously unacknowledged phenomena. But inappropriate subgroup analysis can also provide spurious results, either by coincidence (multiple testing effects) or by unintended patient selection mechanisms. An example of the latter follows. Suppose that the investigators of an RCT compare radiographic progression in a subgroup of patients with an early clinical response and a subgroup of patients without an early response, and find that progression is significantly lower in the first subgroup. This result, however, may easily be confounded by less severe disease at baseline in the favorable subgroup.

It is relevant to some extent to divide subgroup analysis into preplanned and post-hoc subgroup analysis. The former refers to the design phase of the trial and includes analyses in subgroups that are of potential relevance, such as the treatment effect tested in men and women separately, or in rheumatoid factor–positive and –negative patients. Importantly, and in contrast with post-hoc subgroup analysis, the decision to perform and report such an analysis cannot be driven by knowing the data. In practice, however, it is often difficult to find out whether a preplanned subgroup analysis is truly preplanned or not. Methodologically, preplanned subgroup analysis is only superior to post-hoc analysis if subgroups of interest were created by stratified randomization, which means randomization within the subgroups. Stratified randomization hopefully creates prognostic similarity within the strata (a trial within a trial), and—if performed appropriately—provides sufficient statistical power to detect a meaningful difference within the subgroup.

Usually, subgroup analysis is not performed in subgroups created by stratified randomization. If subgroup analysis is performed, and the question of interest is whether a particular treatment performs differently in subgroup X as compared to subgroup Y, it is important to realize that the analytical translation of this question refers to testing statistical interaction.

Figure 11B-3 shows an example of such an interaction. In the first panel, treatment A is less effective than treatment B, both in the subgroup of patients with high disease activity and in the subgroup of patients with low disease activity. The treatment effect is similar in both subgroups: no interaction.

In the second panel, however, the treatment effect is dependent on the subgroup of disease activity. While treatment A seems effective in patients with low disease activity, though less effective than treatment B, it seems completely ineffective in patients with high disease activity, while treatment B is still effective in this subgroup: interaction. Very often, the absence of efficacy in the subgroup of patients with high disease activity is found and reported, while the other subgroup is ignored, so that

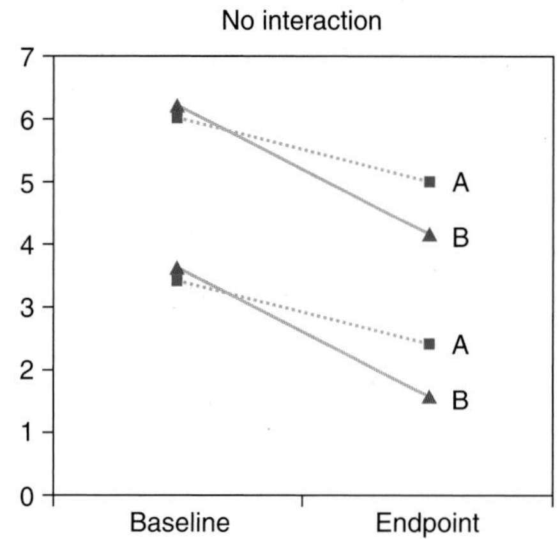

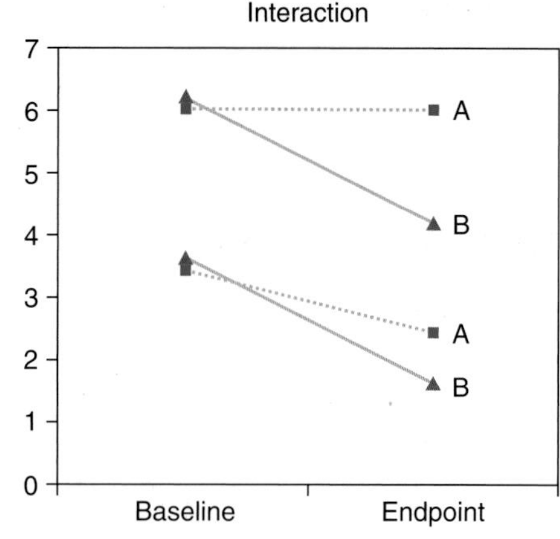

Figure 11B-3. An example of interaction. Results of a subgroup analysis of an imaginary clinical trial comparing two treatments (dashed line with squares, treatment *A*; solid line with triangles, treatment *B*) in a subgroup with high baseline disease activity and a subgroup with low baseline disease activity.

it is not clear whether a presumed effect is truly attributable to a specific subgroup. This type of subgroup analysis only makes sense if the interaction is demonstrated and confirmed statistically. The issue of how to statistically test interaction is beyond the scope of this chapter.

In summary, subgroup analysis can be informative, but there are certain rules of play, among which the most important is probably "Choose your subgroup analyses cautiously and with reservation."

Conclusion

In this chapter, a wide array of points to consider have been addressed that may be important in reporting about clinical trials in RA. Some are theoretical and others are more practical. Often a particular issue is raised with some theoretical background, and the reader is referred to the literature for further information about how to apply. Examples are missing data analysis, statistical power, and subgroup analysis. Other points to consider, such as reporting disease activity states and descriptive statistics are easily to apply in trial reports.

Emphasis is laid on issues referring to generalizability, because that is what most consumers need to know. Generalizability requires particular attention in the discussion section of the report, and authors should take it seriously.

As mentioned in the introduction of this chapter, the choice of points to consider is rather subjective and is by no means intended to cover everything that is important in reporting clinical trial data. It is hoped that the points that are raised will increase the awareness of the importance of the interplay between the clinical investigator responsible for the trial report and the consumer of the data, often the clinician, who has to decide about the application of trial results in the area of clinical medicine: the individual patient. Only an appropriate communication in this area will ultimately improve patient care. The trial report plays a pivotal role in that process.

Reference

1. Kenward MG, Carpenter J. Multiple imputation: Current perspectives. *Stat Methods Med Res* 2007;16(3):199–218.

Regulatory View: U.S. Food and Drug Administration

CHAPTER 11C

Sarah Okada and Jeffrey N. Siegel

The last decade has witnessed major advances in the treatment of a number of rheumatic diseases. Beginning with the approval of the TNF-blocking agents infliximab, etanercept, and adalimumab, effective therapies became available for patients with rheumatoid arthritis (RA) who previously had no effective treatments available (Table 11C-1). In addition, disease-modifying antirheumatic drugs (DMARDs), including other biologic agents, with novel mechanisms of action were approved for treating signs and symptoms of RA, including the antimetabolite leflunomide, the IL-1 blocker anakinra, the T-cell costimulation blocker abatacept and the B-cell–depleting agent rituximab. Many of these agents have also been shown to decrease the structural damage to joints that leads to physical impairment and disability over time if it is not adequately treated. Use of the TNF blockers has also proven effective in the treatment of other inflammatory arthritides, including psoriatic arthritis and ankylosing spondylitis. However, important challenges remain in the treatment of rheumatic diseases as not all patients with RA are adequately treated with current therapies and new modalities of treatment are sorely needed for osteoarthritis, systemic lupus erythematosus (SLE), scleroderma, and other conditions.

The major advances seen in the treatment of rheumatic disease over the last decade can be attributed to several factors. Important advances in basic science have improved our understanding of the pathogenesis of rheumatic disease and allowed for the development of therapeutics that target those pathogenic mechanisms. In addition, advances in clinical science have defined the components of disease that should be assessed in determining the effects of new therapies and have defined clinically meaningful outcome measures to assess efficacy of new treatments in clinical trials. These scientific advances were then applied in rigorously designed clinical trials to assess the safety and efficacy of these new products.

Regulatory agencies have played an important role in aiding recent advances in the treatment of rheumatic diseases. The U.S. Food and Drug Administration (FDA) is responsible for reviewing the safety and the design of clinical trials proposed by industry and academic investigators and for determining whether the data obtained for an investigational product indicate a favorable risk-benefit relationship. Before approving a new product the FDA must determine whether treatment provides a meaningful clinical benefit to patients and, if it does, what those benefits are. The FDA has aided the development of new products for rheumatic disease by communicating the types of clinical benefits that would be adequate for approval both in advice to industry sponsors and in the form of publicly available guidance documents. In this chapter, we will cover several topics relating to the role of the FDA in regulating new products for rheumatic disease. We will review considerations regarding the assessment of efficacy of new products for RA, considerations regarding the assessment of safety of new products and considerations for assessing safety and efficacy of new therapies for children. In this chapter, the term sponsor is intended to describe the group responsible for carrying out clinical trials and would include pharmaceutical company or biotechnology company sponsors as well as sponsor-investigators.

Assessment of Labeling Claims for Rheumatoid Arthritis

The central purpose of labeling claims is to inform prescribers and patients about the documented benefits of a product. Because RA is a chronic, symptomatic disease that can result in a variety of outcomes with different chronologies, severities, and overall patient effects, a number of different clinical outcomes could provide the basis for labeling claims (Table 11C-2).

Reduction in Signs and Symptoms of RA

This claim is intended to reflect the demonstration of symptomatic benefit or benefits that includes improvement in signs of disease activity as well as symptoms. Acceptable outcome measures include validated composite endpoints, such as the ACR response criteria or the DAS. Reduction in signs and symptoms may ordinarily be the initial claim granted for marketing approval.

Ordinarily, this claim is established by trials with a controlled period of at least three months duration. However, longer-term treatment data are often required for adequate assessment of the safety profile of biologics and other immunosuppressives (see following "Safety" section). Longer-term open-label treatment data demonstrating the durability of responses have been described in the clinical studies section of the product label when those data were robust.

In evaluating signs and symptoms, clinical trials of RA frequently use analyses that evaluate the response at a final time point compared to baseline. However, collection of data on the response to treatment over the course of the trial, such as at

Table 11C-1. FDA-Approved Drugs/Biologics for Rheumatoid Arthritis

Drug Name	Approved for RA[a]	Approved for Juvenile RA/Juvenile Idiopathic Arthritis	Current[b] Indicated Population and Claims
Sulfasalazine	Date unknown	Yes, >6 years	RA with inadequate response to salicylates or other NSAIDs
Methotrexate	10/31/1988	Yes, >2 years	Patients with severe, active RA who have had insufficient response to, or are intolerant of, NSAIDs
Hydroxychloroquine	Date unknown	No	RA
Azathioprine	Date unknown	No	Active RA, to reduce signs and symptoms
Penicillamine	Date unknown	No	Severe, active RA with failure to respond to conventional therapy
Cyclosporine	5/22/1997	No	Severe, active RA with inadequate response to MTX
Auranofin	Date unknown	No	Adults with active RA who have had insufficient response to, or are intolerant of, NSAIDs
Leflunomide	9/10/1998	No Some info in label	Adults with active RA, to reduce signs and symptoms, inhibit structural damage, and improve physical function
Etanercept	11/2/1998	Yes, >2 years	Reducing signs and symptoms, inducing major clinical response, inhibiting the progression of structural damage, and improving physical function in patients with moderately to severely active RA
Infliximab	11/10/1999	No Some info in label	In combination with MTX, for reducing signs and symptoms, inhibiting the progression of structural damage, and improving physical function in patients with moderately to severely active RA
Anakinra	11/14/2001	No	Reducing signs and symptoms and slowing the progression of structural damage in moderately to severely active RA, in patients >18 years who have failed one or more DMARDs
Adalimumab	12/31/2002	Yes, >4 years	Reducing signs and symptoms, inducing major clinical response, inhibiting the progression of structural damage, and improving physical function in adults with moderately to severely active RA
Abatacept	12/23/2005	Yes, >6 years	Reducing signs and symptoms, inducing major clinical response, inhibiting the progression of structural damage, and improving physical function in adults with moderately to severely active RA who have had inadequate response to one or more DMARDs
Rituximab	2/28/2006	No	In combination with MTX, for reducing signs and symptoms in patients with moderately to severely active RA who have had inadequate response to one or more TNF antagonist therapies

[a] Approval dates can only be verified from 1984 to the present.
[b] Approved label as of November 28, 2007.
DMARDs, disease-modifying antirheumatic drugs; *MTX,* methotrexate; *NSAID,* nonsteroidal anti-inflammatory drugs; *TNF,* tumor necrosis factor.
Sources: Food and Drug Administration, http://www.accessdata.fda.gov/scripts/cder/drugsatfda/index.cfm; National Library of Medicine, http://dailymed.nlm.nih.gov/dailymed/about.cfm; Center for Drug Evaluation and Research, http://cdernet.cder.fda.gov/cder/da/da/htm

monthly intervals, is important to incorporate in the trial design in order to assess the time course of the clinical response.

Major Clinical Response

When the RA guidance document was first being developed, some clinicians expressed a concern that while products were available that improved signs and symptoms, the level of response was often modest. To define a response that was larger in magnitude, the FDA used data indicating that an ACR70 response was rarely seen among patients receiving placebo in randomized clinical trials. Based on this information, the RA guidance document defined a major clinical response as an ACR70 response lasting for 6 consecutive months. A trial demonstrating a major clinical response would be one where a greater proportion of patients in the treatment arm achieved a major clinical response during the study than in the control arm. Major clinical responses have subsequently been documented in clinical trials of etanercept (10% of patients on monotherapy; 24% in combination with MTX), infliximab (8% to 18% of patients, in combination with MTX), adalimumab (25% of patients on monotherapy; 49% in combination with MTX), and abatacept (14% when added to background MTX).[1–4]

Complete Clinical Response/Remission

Although it is uncommon to achieve a response with a complete absence of signs and symptoms of RA with currently available therapies, the RA guidance document defines a claim for a product capable of reducing measurable disease activity to zero for a sustained period. A complete clinical response is defined as a response with both remission by ACR criteria and no progression in radiographic changes for a continuous 6-month period. A trial demonstrating a complete clinical response would be one where a greater proportion of patients in the treatment arm achieve a complete clinical

Table 11C-2. FDA Guidance on Design and Conduct for RA Trials

Claim	Trial Duration	Endpoints
Reduction in signs and symptoms	≧3 months	ACR response criteria or other well-accepted composite endpoints or sign/symptoms measures
Major clinical response	≧6 months	ACR70 for 6 consecutive months
Complete clinical response	≧6 months	Remission by ACR criteria and no radiographic progression for 6 consecutive months
Remission	≧6 months	Remission by ACR criteria and no radiographic progression for 6 consecutive months while off all antirheumatic therapy
Improvement in physical function	≧3 months	HAQ or AIMS and SF-36
Slowing or inhibition of progression of structural damage	≧1 year	Modifed Sharp score or other validated radiographic index

ACR, American College of Rheumatology; *AIMS,* Arthritis Impact Measure Scales; *HAQ,* Health Assessment Questionnaire.

response during the study than in the control arm. Remission is defined identically to complete clinical response, except that patients must be off all antirheumatic medications to be considered to be in remission.

Improvement in Physical Function

This claim is intended to reflect the effect of treatment in improving patients' functional capabilities as a result of control of joint inflammation in the short term and preservation of the structural integrity of the joints in the long term. Currently, the Health Assessment Questionnaire (HAQ)[5] and the Arthritis Impact Measure Scales (AIMS)[6] are adequately validated measures for use as the primary outcome measure in these trials. Studies in support of this claim are expected to have a randomized controlled period of at least 3 months in duration showing clinically meaningful improvement in one of these outcome measures, for example the proportion of subjects achieving a decrease in HAQ score of more than 0.3 units from baseline.[5–7] After the magnitude of treatment effect is demonstrated in a controlled period, durability of treatment effect could be assessed by maintenance of or continued improvement in these measures on open-label treatment for the remainder of a study, ideally out to at least 2 years. The FDA encourages use of the physical component summary score of the Medical Outcomes Survey 36-Item Short Form (SF-36 PCS) as a secondary endpoint to support this claim. Typically, this claim is only considered in cases where sponsors have demonstrated improvement in signs and symptoms, either previously or concomitantly.

Inhibition of Progression of Structural Damage

Prevention of structural damage is an important goal of RA therapy. However, inhibition or slowing of radiographic progression does not in itself define a clinical benefit; therefore, it is expected that the claim of inhibiting the progression of structural damage would be sought for an agent that has been shown (previously or concomitantly) to be effective for one of the other claims (e.g., reduction in signs and symptoms).

Studies supporting a claim of inhibition of progression of structural damage are expected:

- To be of at least 1 year in duration
- Show a decrease in the rate of progression compared to control utilizing a validated index of radiographic damage, such as the total Sharp score or the Larsen score

Experience with highly effective therapies has shown that it is possible to demonstrate a statistically significant difference in mean radiographic scores between the study therapy and a placebo control group as early as 6 months. After 6 months, patients in the placebo control group could be crossed over to active treatment with the therapy under investigation. An efficacious treatment would be expected to reduce progression of structural damage in the controlled portion of the trial. If patients are permitted to cross over from placebo to study drug after month 6, that crossover would be expected to reduce the rate of progression in the control group in the second 6 months of the study compared to the first 6 months. In addition, to ensure that the results are durable out to 1 year if a 6-month primary endpoint is chosen for the comparison of study drug to control, the study is also expected to document that the slope of radiographic progression does not increase on study drug between month 6 and month 12. Trials designed to assess superiority of an investigational treatment to an active control could also be acceptable without a crossover component.

In addition, the FDA will consider a number of key issues in regarding this area:

1. Robustness of radiographic data

It is important that studies of structural damage be conducted in a rigorous manner to avoid confounding factors that can raise questions about the robustness of the results. Studies are expected to specify how films should be taken and quality ensured. Quality control measures, such as assessing the adequacy of films before patients leave the radiology suite, may increase the proportion of high-quality films. Obtaining a relatively complete data set in radiographic studies in RA is a practical goal. Inclusion of provisions to maximize collection of x-rays, such as those described above, has led to substantial improvements in data completeness. In contrast to earlier radiographic studies where one-third or more of the data was not available at 1 year, more recent studies of biologic agents have demonstrated high levels of completeness. For the etanercept ERA study in early RA, over 90% of films were available at 1 year and 72% at 24 months. For the infliximab ATTRACT study, 80% of films were available at 1 year.[1]

2. Relationship to clinical benefit

Some agents are not intended to affect acute inflammation, but are designed to prevent or slow joint destruction by other means. An agent that inhibits structural damage without also having anti-inflammatory effects is not expected to provide a short-term clinical benefit to patients, but it may provide clinical benefits in the long-term to the extent that it prevents the destruction of joints over time that is observed in patients with RA who do not receive adequate treatment. Therefore, slowing radiographic progression of disease is considered a surrogate marker for overall patient benefit in RA. Federal regulations could allow an approval based on a demonstration of significant slowing of radiographic progression in a seriously affected population of RA patients under some circumstances.

3. Use of other imaging modalities

Since radiographic progression based on plain films is an accepted surrogate marker, could other imaging modalities be used similarly? Magnetic resonance imaging (MRI) has great potential as an outcome measure in RA due to its ability to allow direct visualization and assessment of synovitis, as well as possible early markers of structural damage such as bone marrow edema and early erosive changes. MRI outcomes, including scoring systems, definitions of important joint pathologies and core sets of basic MRI acquisition sequences, have been proposed and are being evaluated and validated.[8] Once standardization and validation of MRI assessments is achieved, the potential for earlier detection of inflammation and damage with MRI could be useful in a number of ways; for example, in proof of concept studies for new therapies, optimization of dose, selection of early arthritis patients in need of more aggressive therapy, stratification of RA patients in clinical trials, or as a means to characterize therapies that alleviate signs and symptoms but that do not reduce the risk of structural damage.

A number of questions need to be answered before MRI data can be used as a primary outcome measure to support a radiographic claim in RA. Because of the technique's potential for identifying small, albeit statistically significant changes, the magnitude of the difference that would reflect actual patient benefit is still unclear and needs to be established. Also, the relationship between MRI inflammation and the progression to structural damage has not yet been defined; therefore, an effect on synovitis alone might not support a structural damage claim. Finally, the relationship of improvement in MRI inflammation and clinical benefit is not clear—treatments that differ on improvement in MRI inflammation may have similar effects on signs and symptoms.

Issues in Rheumatoid Arthritis Clinical Trial Design

Clinical trials in RA can be designed in a variety of ways. More than one claim can be pursued in the same trial, and claims can be submitted singly or together. Trials can be designed to test a difference—demonstrating that the investigational product is superior to control (e.g., placebo, lower test dose, sham treatment, another active agent, etc.), or they can be designed to test no difference—demonstrating that the product is adequately similar in efficacy to active control. Placebo-, dose-, concentration-, sham-, or active-controlled designs can be used.

Since the persuasiveness of trials showing a difference is, in general, much greater than that of noninferiority trials, the FDA usually expects a claim to be convincingly demonstrated in at least one trial showing superiority of the test agent over placebo or active control.[9] If a claim of superiority over a specific comparator is sought, substantial evidence is required via two adequate and well-controlled trials showing superiority. Such trials can also be the basis for demonstrating the product's efficacy.

Superiority Trials

The availability of highly effective therapies for RA and evidence suggesting that early treatment with DMARDs can improve the disease course[10] has made it more difficult to justify the use of placebo or placebo/nonsteroidal anti-inflammatory drugs (NSAID)–only treatment arms. Placebo or placebo/NSAID-only treatment arms could be acceptable in certain limited situations, such as a population of patients with very mild RA without the presence of prognostic markers that suggest aggressive disease; however, sponsors are advised to discuss this with the Agency beforehand, and provisions should be included in such a trial to ensure that patients may receive early escape from the assigned treatment regimen if disease activity is significant and not adequately controlled.

The standard two-arm design, with an investigational agent versus placebo added on to background DMARD therapy has been the most common RA trial design and is the most straightforward. The details of trial design will depend on the population tested. If the population targeted has failed the background DMARD therapy, then early escape provisions are recommended so these patients do not continue to do poorly on a failed therapy for a prolonged period of time.

Alternatives to the two-arm difference design are a standard dose-response study and a superior-to-active-control design. These designs may also accommodate the need to provide active treatment to patient groups where randomization to placebo is infeasible.

Noninferiority Trials

Noninferiority trials are designed to demonstrate that the investigational agent is adequately similar to (i.e., no worse than) an active control by a prespecified amount (the noninferiority margin). The basis of the decision on an appropriate noninferiority margin in RA trials remains, fundamentally, a clinical one. It represents a consensus, in that particular circumstance and for that particular claim, on what small potential difference can be considered clinically insignificant, to allow the treatments to be considered clinically equivalent. Obviously, the allowed margin of inferiority should not be larger than the effect size that the active comparator can reliably be expected to have in the setting of the planned trial. In some cases, the allowed margin of inferiority should be considerably less than the effect size of the active comparator to be able to conclude that most of the efficacy is retained.

A major problem in noninferiority trials lacking a placebo arm is ensuring that both treatments are equally effective, rather than equally ineffective. Comparative trials intended to show noninferiority to treatments that have fairly small effects, when not anchored by a placebo control group, may lack credibility. Thus, it is desirable in noninferiority designs to select highly effective comparative agents. In addition, it is desirable to select comparator agents which are either the standard of care or well accepted as effective agents. If possible, use of a third (placebo or lower-dose) arm, so that a treatment difference can be shown, is a desirable strategy in noninferiority trials. This arm would not necessarily have as many patients or as long a duration as the active comparator. If a placebo arm is present, both the test and active arms need to statistically exceed placebo for a finding of noninferiority to have meaning.

If the noninferiority trial will not be using a concurrent placebo arm, it is crucial that the active comparator has reliably shown an effect of at least some defined size on a particular endpoint in previous appropriately designed, sized, and conducted trials. A noninferiority trial based upon this information would need to be of similar design and enroll a similar patient population, in order to be able to determine whether the estimated effect of the comparator still holds true.

Strict attention to numerous aspects of trial design and conduct are important to ensure accurate inferences from noninferiority trials. Design decisions regarding patient population, dosing, and efficacy and safety assessments should be done in a manner that is unbiased against the control to ensure a fair comparison. Furthermore, attention to certain problems in trial conduct, such as minimizing dropouts, noncompliance, and missing data is essential to the reliability of the inference. These aspects of trial conduct may obscure differences and lead to a false conclusion of noninferiority. This is the opposite of their effect in a difference design to show superiority, where they work against trial success.

Given the many potential pitfalls in the design and conduct of noninferiority trials, the FDA recommends that industry sponsors consult with relevant Agency staff before embarking on trials of this nature.

Randomized Withdrawal Trials

Although not traditionally used in the study of new RA treatments, the randomized withdrawal design can be considered in certain circumstances, and has proven to be particularly useful in populations where placebo control groups are problematic, such as in juvenile idiopathic arthritis (JIA). In this design, patients in both arms of a study are treated with the investigational agent, which is then blindly withdrawn from one arm, after which patient outcomes are compared. Showing that patients who are taken off the investigational drug become worse provides the demonstration of effectiveness. Natural endpoints for withdrawal designs are time to (predefined) worsening using standard time-to-occurrence statistical tests or a simple comparison of the proportion of outcomes in the two arms. Withdrawal studies may be performed with both arms on background therapy.

In general terms, a randomized withdrawal design has certain limitations compared to a standard randomized induction design. Since patients are initially exposed to therapy in an open-label fashion, it does not provide blinded data on the magnitude of treatment response. To optimize the interpretability of the results of the open-label period it would be important to have prespecified criteria for the definition of response. It also does not provide randomized controlled data on adverse event rates. Nonetheless, a randomized withdrawal trial can provide evidence of efficacy.

There are a number of caveats about withdrawal designs. If the product is very toxic, so that only a small (tolerant) subset of the original population remains at the end of the trial and is available for the double-blind withdrawal phase, the generalization of any inference from the withdrawal design is limited to that tolerant subset. Additionally, it should be noted that for some patients or products withdrawal or rebound phenomena may make withdrawn patients worse. The likelihood of this possibility should be taken into consideration when utilization of this trial design is entertained.

Pediatric Rheumatic Disease

In the past, pharmaceutical products that were approved for use in adults were often not studied in children. As a consequence, pediatricians often had to treat children with medications for which there was inadequate information about appropriate dosing in children or about safety and efficacy. To remedy this unfortunate situation, pharmaceutical companies were urged to study drugs in children for which there was a use. When voluntary measures proved ineffective at obtaining information on pediatric use, congress passed a series of laws to provide incentives for sponsors to conduct studies in children or to require that studies be done. These laws—the Best Pharmaceuticals for Children Act (BPCA) and the Pediatric Research Equity Act (PREA)—form the current basis for obtaining information on pediatric use of newly approved drugs and biologics and for certain drugs that were approved before these laws were passed.

In 2002, the BPCA was signed into law and was reauthorized under the FDA Amendments Act of 2007 (FDAAA). The BPCA reauthorized the incentive program established by the FDA Modernization Act of 1997 which offered additional marketing protection in return for conducting FDA-requested pediatric studies. This incentive only applies to drugs, not biologics. If a drug is under patent or has existing exclusivity (e.g., for orphan indications), the FDA may issue a Written Request for studies in children. If the sponsor conducts the study(ies) and adequately responds to the terms of the Written Request then they qualify for an additional 6 months of exclusivity. For those sponsors who decline to conduct the pediatric studies in response to a Written Request, the BPCA provides for other mechanisms by which these pediatric studies may be conducted.

The BPCA also contains provisions to promote the conduct of pediatric studies for drugs with no existing patent or marketing exclusivity ("off-patent drugs"). Under this provision, the National Institutes of Health (NIH), in consultation with FDA and experts in pediatric research, issues a priority list of off-patent drugs for which a need for pediatric studies exists. Based on this list, the FDA, in consultation with NIH, issues a Written Request to all approved holders of the drug. If the holders of the drug decline to perform the pediatric studies in the Written Request, it is referred to the NIH, which utilizes mechanisms provided for in the BPCA in order to get the studies conducted. When completed, the study results are submitted to the public docket and to the FDA for review.

In 2003, the PREA was signed into law and was also reauthorized under FDAAA. The PREA codified many of the elements of the Pediatric Rule, a final rule issued by FDA in 1998. Under the Pediatric Rule, approval actions taken or applications submitted on or after April 1, 1999, for changes in active ingredient, indication, dosage form, dosing regimen, or route of administration were required to include pediatric assessments for indications for which sponsors were receiving or seeking approval in adults, unless the requirement was waived or deferred. This requirement affects both drugs and biologic products.

In situations where the nature of the disease is similar, effectiveness in children can be extrapolated from adequate and well-controlled studies in adults, when supplemented with other information, such as pharmacokinetic and safety data. If efficacy in adults cannot be extrapolated to children, then separate studies need to be carried out to establish effectiveness in children. In that case, sponsors could apply for a deferral by describing what studies they plan to carry out in the pediatric population and submitting evidence that the studies are either being done or will be conducted at the earliest possible time. The FDA may grant a full waiver when the condition does not occur in the pediatric population, where the necessary studies would be impossible or highly impractical (e.g., there are too few children with the condition to conduct a study), if there is evidence that the product would be unsafe or ineffective in children, or if the product does not represent a meaningful advance over existing therapies and the product would not be used in substantial numbers of children. Examples of condition for which full waivers may be granted are osteoarthritis and gout.

Both BPCA and PREA are designed to work in conjunction with one another, and both have had a substantial impact for products for rheumatic disease. For example, celecoxib (Celebrex) was studied in children under a Pediatric Written Request, as were leflunomide and several nonsteroidal anti-inflammatory drugs (NSAIDs). Etanercept (Enbrel) was studied in children with juvenile idiopathic arthritis (JIA) under the Pediatric Rule, and is now approved for children with polyarticular JIA. The Enbrel label contains dosing information for children down to age 2. Studies of anakinra (Kineret) and infliximab (Remicade) in children with JIA conducted based on the Pediatric Rule did not lead to indications in children since the data were insufficient to establish efficacy. Nonetheless, these studies led to the incorporation of information on pediatric use in the Kineret and Remicade labels.

Carrying out controlled efficacy studies in children entails unique challenges. Since children represent a vulnerable population, there is particular concern about the use of placebo for the control arm, particularly if there is a known efficacious treatment available. Where feasible, a noninferiority design may be considered. A noninferiority design was used to demonstrate efficacy of celecoxib in children with JIA by comparing celecoxib to naproxen, which was already approved for use in children .[11] However, in designing a noninferiority study in children, it is critical take into account that placebo responses can be quite high in JIA. For example, in the infliximab study the proportion of patients with a response at week 14 (JIA30) in the placebo control arm was 45%. Therefore, it is critical in designing such a study to specify an active comparator that works consistently and a noninferiority margin that is small enough that a positive result can be interpreted as truly demonstrating efficacy of the new product.[12]

Alternative clinical trial designs can also be considered to establish efficacy in children for a product already demonstrated efficacious in adults. For example, a randomized withdrawal design has been used in several studies in JIA. In these randomized withdrawal studies children were initially treated with the product in an open-label fashion. Children who had a response (e.g., JIA30) were then randomized to continue on drug or to switch to placebo. If the study demonstrates a significantly greater proportion of children who flare or a shorter time to flare when the study drug is withdrawn than when the study drug is continued, this provides evidence of efficacy for the product. Other trial designs that may provide evidence of efficacy while still offering all study subjects the opportunity to receive study drug include the placebo phase design[13] and a study of dose response.

Patient-Reported Outcomes

Outcome measures in clinical trials may be objective laboratory measures (e.g., ESR, CRP), physician-assessed measures (e.g., swollen, tender joint counts) or patient-reported outcomes. Patient-reported outcomes (PROs) are particularly valuable because some treatment effects are known only to the patient and because there is a desire to know the patient's perspective on the effectiveness of the treatment. PRO instruments (e.g., standardized questionnaires) are useful in that they provide a systematic assessment of the patient's point of view that is not filtered through a clinician's evaluation of a patient's response to interview questions. Examples of PROs used in rheumatology include the health assessment questionnaire (HAQ) and child's health assessment questionnaire (CHAQ) in RA and JIA, respectively, the SF-36 health-related quality-of-life instrument and various instruments that measure fatigue.

PRO instruments measure concepts ranging from specific symptoms (e.g., pain) to the overall state of a condition, where specific symptoms and the impact of the condition are measured or feelings about the condition are assessed. PRO instruments also differ in whether they are generic (e.g., the SF-36) or specific to a condition (e.g., the HAQ, which is specific to arthritis). It is important for PRO instruments to be validated to ensure that they accurately measure the concept they are intended to measure.

The FDA has published a draft guidance document on the use of PROs in clinical development of therapeutic products to support labeling claims.[14] The PRO draft guidance document describes the different ways that PRO instruments may be developed and validated, and offers recommendations on how to incorporate PRO instruments in clinical development so that the data generated in clinical trials is optimal to support the claims that are sought by the sponsor. In general, the expectations to support labeling claims for PROs do not differ from those for other labeling claims, that is, there should be substantial evidence from adequate and well-controlled trials. As for other claims the statistical analytic plan for the PRO instrument should be prespecified and should take into account multiplicity resulting from multiple endpoints and multiple study arms. The FDA recommends that industry sponsors proposing a novel PRO for use in a clinical development program consult the appropriate FDA review division early in development.

Critical Path Initiatives

Biomarkers

A biomarker is a characteristic that is objectively measured and evaluated as an indicator of normal biological processes, pathogenic processes, or pharmacologic responses to a therapeutic intervention.[15] Biomarkers can assist in the development and evaluation of novel therapies for RA and may serve as supportive evidence of efficacy in clinical trials. In conjunction with clinical measures, biomarkers may play a role in assessing clinical outcomes and identifying potential clinical benefit from new therapies.

Surrogate endpoints are a subset of biomarkers which are expected to predict clinical benefit (or harm or lack of benefit) and are intended to substitute for a clinical endpoint.[16] For example, in RA, assessment of structural damage via radiographic outcomes (e.g., total Sharp score) has been accepted as a surrogate for the long-term clinical outcomes associated with joint structural integrity, such as physical functional ability or need for joint replacement. However, thus far, radiographic outcomes have been utilized as a basis for an adjunctive claim for products already demonstrating a clinical benefit in reducing signs and symptoms.

In certain situations, FDA may grant marketing approval for a new drug product on the basis of adequate and well-controlled clinical trials establishing that the drug product has an effect on a surrogate endpoint that is reasonably likely, based on epidemiologic, therapeutic, pathophysiologic, or other evidence, to predict clinical benefit (accelerated approval). Approval under these circumstances will be subject to the requirement that the applicant study the drug further, to verify and describe its clinical benefit, where there is uncertainty as to the relation of the surrogate endpoint to clinical benefit, or of the observed clinical benefit to ultimate outcome. The FDA recommends that sponsors proposing use of surrogate endpoints discuss these on a case-by-case basis with the appropriate review division.

The FDA recommends that sponsors consult the appropriate FDA center—either CBER (Center for Biologics Evaluation and Research) or CDRH's (Center for Devices and Radiographic Health) Office of In Vitro Diagnostic Devices Evaluation and Safety—if a biomarker used in clinical trials could be used in prescribing the product if it is approved, such as for selection of patients or for monitoring safety or effectiveness.

Adaptive Design Trials

In conventional clinical trial design, overall sample size, the size of the individual study arms, and the analysis of the primary endpoint are all kept constant to avoid potential bias. In the traditional scheme of clinical development, final data from a previous study is used to plan a separate, next study, with an inherent lag time. Therefore, great interest has been expressed in alternative methods that might allow for a "seamless" transition between trial phases. Adaptive trials are one such method.

An adaptive trial is a prospectively designed study that allows for future prespecified design modifications depending on the data accrued in the trial up to some interim time, but in a manner that appropriately controls the type I error for the multiple options and possibilities that these adaptations will allow.

Possible adaptations include change in sample sizes, choice of test statistic, choice of hypothesis (inferiority to superiority), choice of dose groups, choice of endpoints, the ability to drop or add treatment arms, or the ability to stop the study early for efficacy or harm.

Although adaptive designs have the potential for making clinical development more efficient, they also raise issues of the potential for bias, given the possibility of unblinding, and multiplicity. To minimize these risks, certain principles have been recommended, including:

- All possible adaptations should be prespecified and analysis plans developed to handle multiplicity, bias, and estimation of effects.
- Strict precautions should be undertaken to minimize bias due to unblinding, such as limited and secured access to the interim data, documentation, and other assurances on the integrity of a trial.
- The evidentiary weight given to the exploratory phase and the confirmation phase of the trial should be clarified.

Some adaptations are more flexible when done early in product development, rather than in phase III. The FDA advises sponsors considering adaptive design trials to involve FDA early in the planning of these trials.

Safety Assessment

When the FDA considers a new product for approval for marketing, information is available about the safety of the product in the population that was studied in the clinical trials. The available safety data are carefully scrutinized to determine whether the clinical benefits to the patient population outweigh the potential risks.

Unfortunately, the safety profile observed during clinical trials may not fully reflect the safety of new products after they are marketed. Among the important factors accounting for this are the limited size of the safety database at the time of approval and differences between the patients studied in clinical development and the population that receives the product after it is marketed.

Size of Safety Database

One of the main reasons that new safety concerns emerge after marketing is that rare, but serious, adverse events may occur at a frequency that is too small to detect with the limited number of patients treated during clinical development. The "Rule of Three" provides an estimate of how confidently we can rule out that a product is associated with a serious adverse event (SAE) if that event is not observed in clinical trials. If no SAE is seen in a trial of 100 subjects, using the upper bound of the 95% confidence interval allows us to state that it is unlikely the SAE occurs at an incidence of 3% or greater. Similarly, an SAE with a true incidence of 0.3% is unlikely to go unobserved in a trial of 1000 subjects. Since marketed products used in RA can be used in hundreds of thousands of people, it would take a study of over 100,000 patients to assess all the rare but serious adverse events that may occur. Clearly this is impractical since the number of patients exposed to new products prior to approval never approaches the numbers who may receive the product when it is marketed. Also of note, very rare events may have a limited impact on the desirability of using a therapy with substantial efficacy in a serious disease such as RA.

The E1 document of the International Conference on Harmonization (ICH), which is also an FDA guidance document, provides recommendations for the safety information that should be available for new drugs and biologic products intended for chronic use.[17] Overall, the ICH E1 document recommends safety data on at least 1500 patients treated for any duration. To assess longer-term safety, the E1 document recommends collecting information on 300-600 patients treated for 6 months, and 100 patients treated for 1 year (Table 11C-3). However,

Table 11C-3. Safety Database Recommended for Drugs and Biologics Intended for Chronic Use for Non–Life-Threatening Conditions[a]

Duration of Exposure	Number of Subjects
Any	1500
3–6 months	300–600
≧1 year	100

[a] Size of safety database may need to be larger if there are specific safety concerns based on preclinical data, or concerns related to the drug class or on other sources of concern.

larger and/or longer-term safety databases may be necessary to adequately characterize the safety profile if safety signals emerge or in the case of agents with known or potential safety problems, such as immunosuppressive products.

Experience from Anti-TNF Agents

The approvals of the first TNF blockers illustrate when a larger database may be necessary to fully evaluate safety. For etanercept (Enbrel) and infliximab (Remicade), the minimum ICH recommendations were not large enough to capture the safety signals related to serious infection and malignancy. These adverse events were not fully appreciated until the postmarketing period. Despite the fact that their mechanism of action is to inhibit an important arm of host defenses, the clinical trial data from etanercept and infliximab did not clearly show an increase in infections at the time of their approvals. After approval, reports of serious infections with both etanercept and infliximab led to the addition of bold warnings of rare but serious infections that were occasionally fatal. Later still, reports of reactivation of latent tuberculosis infection led to revisions to both labels. A boxed warning was added to the Remicade label (and subsequently to the Humira [adalimumab] and Enbrel labels) recommending screening of all patients for latent tuberculosis infection prior to initiating treatment and treatment with antituberculous medications for any patient testing positive. In addition, the FDA became aware of cases of multiple sclerosis (MS) and other demyelinating syndromes in patients treated with TNF blockers, leading to the addition of warnings to both the Enbrel and Remicade labels. Because these SAEs are uncommon, the risk–benefit ratio is still favorable for both these agents in selected patients with RA.

Long-Term Safety

Some adverse events are observed only after prolonged exposure to therapeutic agents. Unfortunately, even studies of 1 or 2 years in duration may not reveal adverse events that appear only with long-term use. One recent example is the issue of whether the use of azathioprine and methotrexate is associated with an increase in the risk of lymphoma. Reports of lymphoma in RA patients receiving chronic treatment with these agents suggested that the risk might be increased. However, careful epidemiologic studies revealed that the background rate of lymphoma may be increased in RA patients. Furthermore, two studies have suggested that the risk of lymphoma is particularly increased in RA patients with high levels of inflammation, suggesting that the association with azathioprine and methotrexate may be related to the severe nature of the disease rather than to the drugs themselves.[18,19] This example illustrates how difficult it may be to determine accurately the safety of long-term use of therapeutic agents. It also illustrates how critical it is to systematically collect data to address long-term safety issues. Since immune surveillance against tumors is an important role of the immune system, immunomodulatory and immunosuppressive agents could increase the risk of malignancy. The agency encourages sponsors to collect long-term safety data for immunosuppressive products intended for chronic use for rheumatic diseases over a span of at least 3 to 5 years in a sufficient number of patients to evaluate the risk of malignancies, serious infections and the induction of new autoimmune diseases.

Other Safety Concerns

Clinical trials of novel therapeutic agents are typically more restrictive compared to usual clinical practice with respect to the patients who are included in trials and the concomitant medications that are allowed. The strict rules followed in clinical trials provide a relatively homogeneous patient population that maximizes the ability to discern the treatment effect of a new agent and to assess adverse events that are associated with use of the product. Unfortunately, because of the way these strict rules define the patient population in clinical trials, the safety data may not be fully generalizable to patients in usual clinical practice. For example, there may be important interactions between the novel product and other antirheumatic medications and with concomitant medical conditions that are missed during drug development. Unexpected SAEs associated with specific concomitant medical conditions have been observed in several recent examples. Studies in preclinical models suggested that TNF-α blockade may be beneficial for MS. Based on this information, studies of lenercept (an investigational soluble TNF receptor) and infliximab were carried out in patients with MS. Surprisingly, both studies observed a worsening of disease activity.[20,21] These studies, along with postmarketing adverse event reports, led to a warning in the package insert for both etanercept and inflximab (and subsequently for adalimumab) to avoid use in patients with pre-existing MS. A second example is the use of TNF antagonists in patients with CHF. Again, preclinical models suggested that TNF-α was harmful in CHF and that TNF blockade may ameliorate disease. However, instead of seeing benefit, two clinical trials of etanercept in patients with CHF were stopped early because of futility, and one study showed a suggestion of possible worsening. A clinical trial of infliximab in patients with class III and IV CHF was also stopped early because of evidence of worsening of CHF and increased mortality in infliximab-treated patients.

How can we ensure that the safety data available at the time of approval of new agents more fully reflect the safety of the products when they are marketed? One way to address this issue is to carry out randomized safety studies prior to approval with flexible inclusion and exclusion criteria that enroll a patient population closer to typical clinical practice. For a product for RA, such a study could include any patient with active disease with liberal inclusion and exclusion criteria. Unless there are specific, known safety concerns, any medication and combination of medications could be allowed. Patients with concomitant medical conditions could be enrolled so long as there were no specific contraindications. Finally, while complete adverse event data would be collected, other data collection could be kept to a minimum to encourage enrollment of patients who might not otherwise participate in clinical trials because of the inconvenience factor.

For several products recently approved for RA, there have been relatively large randomized safety trials carried out prior to approval. Amgen carried out a randomized safety study of anakinra as part of their clinical development program prior to its approval. In addition to phase II studies that enrolled a total of 892 patients and a 506-patient phase III trial, Amgen carried out a randomized, placebo-controlled safety study with 1414 subjects. The study included patients receiving a wide range of concomitant DMARDs, including methotrexate, hydroxychloroquine, sulfasalazine, leflunomide, and others, alone and in combination. A significant proportion (5% to 10% each) had a variety of common concomitant medical conditions, including COPD, asthma, coronary artery disease, and diabetes. The study demonstrated a higher incidence of serious infection among anakinra-treated patients, a result that had not been apparent from earlier studies. The data did not indicate any association between serious infections and either concomitant DMARDs or concomitant medical conditions, with the exception of a higher incidence of serious infections in patients with underlying asthma.

Data from the usual types of clinical trials conducted during drug development may not fully reflect the safety of new products when they are marketed. The experience with the anakinra safety trial demonstrates that it is feasible to gather safety data on the use of new agents in a patient population more similar to that seen in usual clinical practice. Safety studies of this type would provide additional data on the safety of new products in a variety of clinical settings, may pinpoint subsets of patients who should avoid the new agent and may decrease the frequency of occurrence of unexpected SAEs in the postmarketing experience. The sponsors of etanercept, infliximab, adalimumab and abatacept all carried out randomized studies assessing safety of those products in a setting closer to actual use.[22–25]

Longer studies of potentially immunogenic products are important to determine whether antibodies to the product diminish the clinical activity over time and whether adverse events develop related to the antibodies. Finally, some adverse drug reactions are only observed with a longer duration of exposure.

Conclusion

Advances in biomedical research hold out the promise of improving the health of patients with rheumatic disease. Translating those research advances into safe and effective therapies requires rigorous clinical development programs to characterize the benefits and risks of therapy. In this chapter, we reviewed the approach the FDA has taken in assessing clinical benefits of products in RA and the information needed to characterize the safety of new products. Since all therapies have the potential for toxicity, approving a new therapy involves a careful weighing of potential benefits against potential risks. When the risks and benefits of new therapies are fully communicated clinicians can choose therapies for individual patients that optimize the benefits and minimize the potential for toxicity.

Despite the significant advances of the past several years, there remain important areas of unmet medical need in rheumatology, including diseases for which there are no approved therapies and new therapies for patients who are inadequately treated by currently available therapies. Hopefully, new insights into disease pathogenesis will help to identify promising candidate treatments. At the same time, advances in other areas may facilitate the clinical development of these products. Advances in clinical science have defined outcome measures to optimally measure benefits in clinical trials. Biomarkers hold promise in identifying clinically active agents early in development and in determining which patients are most likely to benefit from specific agents. Finally, advances in clinical trial design, including adaptive design, should help streamline clinical trials to shorten the time and resources required to demonstrate the clinical benefits of new products.

Acknowledgment

The views presented in this chapter do not necessarily reflect those of the Food and Drug Administration.

References

1. Amgen and Wyeth Pharmaceuticals. Prescribing Information. http://www.enbrel.com/prescribing-information.jsp. (Accessed December 5, 2007.)
2. Food and Drug Administration: Remicade product label. Center for Drug Evaluation and Research. http://www.accessdata.fda.gov/scripts/cder/drugsatfda/index.cfm. (Accessed December 5, 2007.)
3. Abbott Laboratories. Information about Humira. http://www.humira.com/. (Accessed December 5, 2007.)
4. Bristol-Meyers Squib. ORENCIA® (Abatacept). http://www.orencia.com/. (Accessed December 5, 2007.)
5. Fries JF, Spitz PW, Young DY. The dimensions of health outcomes: The Health Assessment Questionnaire, Disability, and Pain Scales. *J Rheumatol* 1982;9:789–793.
6. Meenan RF, Gertman PM, Mason JH, et al. The Arthritis Impact Measurement Scales: Further investigations of a health status measure. *Arthritis Rheumatol* 1982;25:1048–1053.
7. Wells GA, Tugwell P, Kraag GR, et al. Minimum important difference between patients with rheumatoid arthritis: The patient's perspective. *J Rheumatol* 20:3, 557–560, 1993.
8. Østergaard M, Peterfy C, Conaghan P, et al. OMERACT RA MRI studies: Core set of MRI acquisitions, joint pathology definitions, and the OMERACT RA-MRI scoring system. *J Rheumatol* 2003; 30:1385–1386.
9. International Conference on Harmonisation of Technical Requirements for Registration of Pharmaceuticals for Human Use E10. Choice of Control Group and Related Issues in Clinical Trials. FDA Guidance Document, May 2001. http://www.ich.org/cache/compo/276-254-1.html.
10. O'Dell JR. Treating rheumatoid arthritis early: A window of opportunity? *Arthritis Rheum* 2002;46(2):283–285.
11. Food and Drug Administration. November 29, 2006 meeting of the Arthritis Advisory Committee, FDA Briefing Document. http://www.fda.gov/ohrms/dockets/ac/06/briefing/2006-4252b1-00-index.htm.
12. Food and Drug Administration. *FDA Guidance for Industry: Providing Clinical Evidence of Effectiveness for Human Drug and Biological Products.* 1998. http://www.fda.gov/cder/guidance/index.htm.
13. Feldman B, Wang E, Willan A, et al. The randomized placebo-phase design for clinical trials. *J Clin Epidemiol* 2001;54(6):550–557.
14. Food and Drug Administration. *FDA Draft Guidance for Industry: Patient-Reported Outcome Measures: Use in Medical Product Development to Support Labeling Claims.* 2006. http://www.fda.gov/cder/guidance/index.htm.
15. Biomarkers Definitions Working Group. Biomarkers and surrogate endpoints: preferred definitions and conceptual framework. *Clin Pharmacol Ther* 2001;69(3):89–95.
16. Food and Drug Modernization Act of 1977. Title 21, Code of Federal Regulations, Part 314, Subpart H, Section 314.500.
17. Food and Drug Administration. *FDA Guidance for Industry. International Conference on Harmonization E1A: The Extent of Population Exposure to Assess Clinical Safety: For Drugs Intended for Long-term Treatment of Non-Life-Threatening Conditions.* 2005. http://www.fda.gov/cder/guidance/index.htm#ICH_efficacy.
18. Baecklund E, Ekbom A, Sparen P, et al. Disease activity and risk of lymphoma in patients with rheumatoid arthritis: nested case–control study. *BMJ* 1998;517:180–181.

19. Wolfe F, Michaud K. Lymphoma in rheumatoid arthritis: The effect of methotrexate and anti-tumor necrosis factor therapy in 18,572 patients. *Arthritis Rheum* 2004;50(6):1740–1751.
20. Lenercept Multiple Sclerosis Study Group, University of British Columbia MS/MRI Analysis Group. TNF neutralization in MS: Results of a randomized, placebo-controlled multicenter study. *Neurology* 1999;53(3):457–465.
21. van Oosten BW, Barkhof F, Truyen L, et al. Increased MRI activity and immune activation in two multiple sclerosis patients treated with the monoclonal anti-tumor necrosis factor antibody cA2. *Neurology* 1996;47(6):1531–1534.
22. Weisman MH, Paulus HE, Burch FX, et al. A placebo-controlled, randomized, double-blinded study evaluating the safety of etanercept in patients with rheumatoid arthritis and concomitant comorbid diseases. *Rheumatology (Oxford)* 2007;46(7):1122–1125.
23. Westhovens R, Yocum D, Han J, et al. The safety of infliximab, combined with background treatments, among patients with rheumatoid arthritis and various comorbidities: A large, randomized, placebo-controlled trial. *Arthritis Rheum* 2006;54(4):1075–1086.
24. Furst DE, Schiff MH, Fleischmann RM, et al. Adalimumab, a fully human anti tumor necrosis factor-alpha monoclonal antibody, and concomitant standard antirheumatic therapy for the treatment of rheumatoid arthritis: results of STAR (Safety Trial of Adalimumab in Rheumatoid Arthritis). *J Rheumatol* 2003;30(12):2563–2571.
25. Weinblatt M, Combe B, Covucci A, et al. Safety of the selective costimulation modulator abatacept in rheumatoid arthritis patients receiving background biologic and nonbiologic disease-modifying antirheumatic drugs: A one-year randomized, placebo-controlled study. *Arthritis Rheum* 2006;54(9):2807–2816.

Ethics in Clinical Trials

C. Ronald MacKenzie and Stephen A. Paget

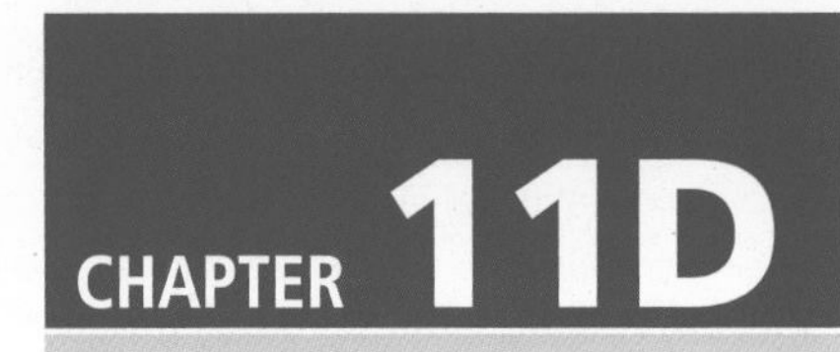

The objective of clinical research is the acquisition of generalizable knowledge in order to increase understanding of human biology or to improve health. Although the participation of human subjects is required to achieve these ends, the attainment of the goals of clinical research does not ensure benefit to those who participate. Indeed it is self-evident that the research subject may be placed at some risk for the good of others, a reality at the core of the ethical dilemmas in human subject's research. It is therefore incumbent on those who formulate, conduct, and report such research that their work adhere to the highest of ethical standards. This chapter reviews the ethical dilemmas arising in the research setting and presents principles that should guide this activity, referencing clinical trials in rheumatoid arthritis (RA) where applicable.

General Ethical Principles

Extensive literature and experience serves to inform the philosophical and practical paradigms that guide current human subject's research.[1–6] Theorists interested in this area have looked to the field of moral philosophy and ethical theory to derive principles that provide a foundation for ethical judgments concerning research involving human subjects.[7] Rooted in the Nazi experimentation revealed in Nuremberg, these efforts have been bolstered by a number of seminal documents beginning with the Nuremberg Code (1947),[8] the Declaration of Helsinki (1964),[9] the Belmont Report (1979),[10] the International Ethical Guidelines for Biomedical Research Involving Human Subjects,[11] and most recently, Guidelines for Good Clinical Practice for Trials on Pharmaceutical Products of the World Health Organization.[12] Malfeasance and ethical lapses typified by the Tuskegee study have also provided a potent stimulus for change.[1,2,13] Thus, ethically designed and conducted research now rests on principles articulated in these foundational documents. The Belmont Report, a particularly influential statement in the current era, added the notions of respect for persons, beneficence, and justice to the enduring principle of informed consent established in Nuremberg over 30 years before. Indeed these core ethical tenants provide the foundational elements guiding the current regulation of human subject's research, whether that be of the Department of Health and Human Services, the Food and Drug Administrations, or locally at the level of the Institutional Review Board.

What Is Ethical Research?

The multifaceted nature and broad scope of ethical controversy concerning the conduct of human subject's research cannot simply be articulated by an examination of these principles. For instance, the reconsideration of the ban on the use of women[14] and children,[15] the unresolved debate about the appropriate role of placebos,[16–19] and the problems arising from the globalization of clinical research,[20–22] cite just a few of the current ethical challenges that impel discourse beyond an analysis of general principles.

A systematic framework for understanding the ethics of human subject's research has been developed by Emanuel et al.[23] Derived from an examination of the relevant literature and incorporating the concepts espoused in the aforementioned declarations and codes, seven requirements are presented to ensure that research subjects are treated with respect and are not exploited in doing so. Table 11D-1 summarizes the seven requirements, their rationale, and the ethical value justifying their inclusion. The ethical considerations inherent in these requirements could be framed in the form of questions[6,23]:

1. Does the anticipated societal and scientific value of the research justify the resources required to conduct the research?
2. Does the research employ valid scientific methodology and is it practically feasible?
3. Is the selection of subjects fair and equitable?
4. What potential harms and risks are imposed on the research subjects? Are the risks minimized? Are the potential societal benefits in proportion to the risks imposed on the participants?
5. Has the study undergone independent review?
6. Is informed consent sought from the research subjects?
7. Are there safeguards to ensure the respect for research subjects during their participation in the research?

These requirements and the questions derived from them are premised on ethical values that include those of the Belmont Report but also other defining statements concerning research ethics. Introduced are such considerations as exploitation, public accountability, and conflict of interest.

In the setting of drug trials, the traditional stages (phases I to VI) of scientific development present phase-specific ethical challenges.[3,5] While all of the aforementioned ethical constructs apply at each level of drug development, there is some fluidity concerning which constructs are dominant as a drug (device)

Table 11D-1. Requirements for Ethical Research

Requirement	Ethical Values
Social or scientific value	Scarce resources, nonexploitation
Scientific validity	Scarce resources, nonexploitation
Fair subject selection	Justice
Favorable risk-benefit ratio	Nonmaleficence, beneficence, and nonexploitation
Independent review	Public accountability, minimizing influence of potential conflicts of interest
Informed consent	Respect for autonomy
Respect for potential and enrolled subjects	Respect for autonomy and welfare

works it way through the approval cycle. Phase I trials represent the phase of drug or device development in which therapeutic intervention is first being introduced for testing in human subjects. Such trials are characterized by small number of subjects who are often, but not always, healthy volunteers. As such safety and toxicity in contrast to efficacy are the primary objectives. Given these characteristics, the ethical concepts of informed consent, risk-benefit, and scientific validity are particularly relevant. As they receive no benefit and may experience significant adverse consequences, subjects participating in phase I clinical trials are dedicating themselves to the "greater good." Phase II clinical trials differ from phase I studies in that they include more subjects who suffer from the disease for which the treatment is intended and may include efficacy as an active endpoint. The ethical considerations are similar to those of the phase I investigation. Phase III trials begin to involve not only larger numbers of patients but also an ever-widening range of participants, bringing the ethical construct of fair subject selection to the forefront. Clinical trials at this stage of development focus on efficacy and safety. With both phase III and IV clinical investigations, the latter conducted after the drug has been approved, respect for enrolled subjects becomes a primary consideration raising concerns such as voluntary withdrawal from participation, privacy protection, informing subjects of new risks and benefits as well as the results of the research. Further, an ethical concern of particular relevance to the phase IV clinical trial is the postmarketing investigations conducted by the pharmaceutical industry. While a subject of some criticism, these are considered justified because they may provide important data on serious but low-prevalence adverse advents associated with the approved therapy.

The Randomized Clinical Trial

Randomized clinical trials (RCTs) remain the "gold standard" methodology for the demonstration of efficacy and safety in the development of new therapies. This format is defined by a number of design characteristics including randomization, blinding, and the comparison of two (or more) interventions, utilized in order to demonstrate therapeutic equivalence or superiority of one treatment over another. Despite the advantages, this research design presents a unique spectrum of ethical challenges to the investigator.[3,24] These include such considerations as the treatment versus research dichotomy,[25–28] equipoise (no convincing evidence that one intervention is superior to another),[6,29] choice of control (the use of placebo is one aspect of this issue),[3,5,16–19] randomization (which does not allow for autonomous preferences in treatment),[3] blinding,[3] and the sharing of preliminary information. Each ethical challenge disserves more discussion.

Trials and Clinical Practice

Levine defines "practice" as activities "designed solely to enhance the well-being of an individual patient," whereas the intent of "research" is to contribute to a base of knowledge that can be generalized to all those who suffer from the disease under investigation.[28] In the setting of clinical research, this distinction can be easily blurred, especially when existing treatments for the disease in question are unsatisfactory or when the proposed treatment under study is highly innovative. As practice and research commonly coexist—most often with new cancer therapies but also in the care and treatment of patients with RA and the biologics—in these circumstances it is virtually instinctive that physicians might wish to employ such therapy despite the lack of formal validation. In so doing, the line that demarcates research from treatment may be breached.

Of all the principles that unite codes of medical ethics, the physician's duty to the individual patient remains a central doctrine. Dating back to Hippocrates, this notion is deeply embedded in how medicine expresses its professionalism. The physician's duty is communicated primarily through the clinical transaction, a patient-centered exercise that relies on physician-based characteristics that could be considered virtuous.[30–32] Against this backdrop, there is the contrasting duty of the researcher—the promotion of human welfare through the rigorous application of the scientific methods in the conduct of research. Tension between these roles and conflicting points of view are especially evident when one considers the RCT. An important and problematic feature of this trial design arises from the randomization itself, a practice in which treatment is apportioned by chance rather than the physician recommendation of clinical practice. While there are scientific, ethical, and practical advantages to the random of assignment of treatment, it can be argued that a patient's needs and values become subverted and sacrificed for the greater good of others. An approach to resolving this dilemma is the concept of "clinical equipoise," first articulated by Freedman.[29] The construct of equipoise requires a researcher to have no justifiable reason for preferring one treatment arm of the study over another. Clinical equipoise expands this concept examining it from a broader perspective, taking the focus off the researcher and placing it on the greater community of physicians. Instead of the requirement that the treatments being compared exist in exact balance (circumstances in which the researcher would have no preference), clinical equipoise is based on an honest disagreement amongst knowledgeable professionals; as long as a genuine dispute exists concerning the superiority of one treatment over another, a RCT can be considered permissible.

Use of Placebos

Another problematic aspect of clinical trials has to do with controls, particularly the use of placebos. In the setting of new therapies, or where current treatment is ineffective or unsatisfactory for a condition, the use of placebos does not raise ethical concern. However, their use becomes increasingly more problematic when new therapies are being compared to established treatment, circumstances in which currently accepted therapy could be employed as the comparator. The authors of the Declaration of Helsinki may have recognized this issue when they state that the "benefits, risk, burdens, and effectiveness of a new method should be tested against those of the best current ... methods."[9] The FDA, however, has generally been supportive of the use of placebos as studies designed in this fashion produce more "purified" knowledge.[16] Thus, the role of placebos in clinical research continues to provoke active ethical debate.[16–19] An approach toward a reconciliation of these conflicting positions has been to suggest that the burden of proof lies with those who propose depriving patients of standard care.[16] In addition a "middle ground" has been advocated by Emanuel and Miller.[19] In their analysis these polarized views—the "placebo orthodoxy" that promotes the use of placebos based on methodologic considerations is contrasted to the "active-control orthodoxy" in which placebos are viewed as sacrificing the rights and welfare of patients in the name of scientific rigor—can be reconciled if specific ethical and methodologic criteria are met. Thus, situations in which life-saving therapy is available, placebo-controlled studies are prime facie unethical. In contrast, for conditions that are not thought to be serious, and the risk associated with the use of placebos seems minimal, a placebo comparator can be ethically employed. Placebo use becomes most problematic in those conditions in which effective treatments do exist and some potential for harm may arise as a consequence of using a placebo. In these circumstances, compelling methodologic advantages must exist in order to justify the use of a placebo control. This would include the study of conditions in which there is a high placebo response rate; a waxing and waning course or frequent spontaneous remissions; those for which existing therapies are only partly effective or have very serious side effects; or the low frequency of the condition means that an equivalency trial would have to be so large as to compromise enrollment and completion of the trial.[19] Many of these disease characteristics are germane to RA.

Randomization

Other methodologic features of the RCT raise ethical concerns. For instance, there is the defining element of the RCT, the randomization. Randomization is usually performed in a blinded manner, either single (subject does not know what treatment/intervention he/she is receiving), or double (neither subjects nor investigators know which treatment/intervention is being employed). Random assignment and blinding are employed to minimize bias and to enhance study validity. While compatible with the goals of the RCT (to enhance generalizable knowledge), such procedures are not necessarily compatible with the patient's best interests and desires, nor does it respect the subject's autonomy.[5] Two ethical concerns arise from this procedure: (1) Preferences and information concerning what intervention the subject is receiving is necessary for autonomous decision making; and (2) information pertaining to which intervention the subject is receiving may be important in the assessment of adverse events or medial emergency. Informed consent addresses the first concern, while providing the appropriate safeguards concerning adverse events requires specification in the research protocol of the conditions, thresholds, and consequences of breaking the code (unblinding the study). A related problem with ethical implications is the sharing of preliminary information. As evidence accumulates in a clinical trial, the understanding of the risks and benefits of the study therapy may change, potentially altering equipoise. Study monitors and independent data safety–monitoring boards (DSMBs) are therefore employed to make decisions regarding the early termination of a clinical investigation, thus taking the decision out of the hands of the investigator. Arising in the context of international research, a more recent problem with important ethical dimensions has to do with the investigator's (and sponsor's) obligation to study subjects to ensure ongoing access to the investigational therapy upon completion of the clinical trial.[5,33]

Role of Contract Research Organizations

Another recent phenomenon of relevance to clinical trials is the advent of the role of contract research organizations (CROs) in drug development.[34] CROs are commercial organizations that, as independent contractors, offer clients (usually drug companies) a wide range of pharmaceutical research services. These may include some or all of the following: protocol design, clinical trial (phases I through IV) management, centralized laboratory services for processing of clinical trial samples, data analysis, and assistance with the approval status of a drug through the FDA. In effect, they offer an important "outsourcing" function to the pharmaceutical industry, which provides for cost savings while bypassing the academic medical center, the traditional (and possibly safer) site for the conduct of clinical trials. CRO industry revenues have grown dramatically since their inception in the early 1990s.[34] However, along with their development, ethical questions have also arisen. Problems such as the preferential enrollment of the economically disadvantaged (through pretrial monetary inducements); "back-loading" payment approaches in which the largest payments are made to study subjects at the end of the trial (inhibiting patients who may wish to terminate their participation); disquiet pertaining to the comprehension of nonprimary English-speaking subjects (raising concerns regarding informed consent); inadequate monitoring of adverse events; and concerns about the depth, diversity, and medical knowledge of the CRO workforce. Further, whether this model, premised mainly on the desire to reduce costs, compromises oversight remains open to question. Lastly, uncertainty exists with respect to the role and scope of the regulatory mechanisms that oversee the activity of the CROs—that is, do CROs answer to the federal agencies responsible for monitoring clinical trials (a mandated requirement for academic medical centers) or to the drug company for whom they are clients? Little data exist on the degree to which clinical trials in RA may have been affected by the phenomenon of the CRO. However, reliance on this model remains strong and this practice is likely to grow.

Conflict of Interest

The term "conflict of interest" encompasses a spectrum of behaviors and actions involving personal gain, usually but not limited to financial benefit.[35,36] Arising over the last two decades from the complex relationships which have developed between industry,[37,38] investigators,[37,38] and the academic institutions where they are employed,[39] such conflicts raise a variety of ethical challenges. That financial and other inducements might influence, and at times overpower, professional judgment comes as no surprise given the pressures accompanying modern life, yet the circumstances and determinants of such behavior are not fully understood. Barnes and Florencio[39] cite a number of considerations including that conflict of interest increases with the value of the secondary interest, as professional judgment becomes more specialized and less amenable to supervision, as the decision-making process becomes less transparent, and when there is a long-standing relationship between the participants. It is well documented that financial and other incentives influence physicians in the clinical environment.[40,41] While their influence in other arenas of academic medicine may be less appreciated, nevertheless such influences are pervasive and affect virtually every corner of the academic medical enterprise: physician–industry interactions, investigator–industry relationships, and the academic center itself. Journal publication and continuing medical education are likewise not immune.[42–44]

Efforts to control or manage these conflicts have taken center stage at academic institutions. Initially, simple disclosure was considered sufficient. Whether the context was clinical research, a lecture or grand rounds, physicians were expected to disclose outside financial interests. More recently however institutions have established committees to develop policy, review reported conflicts, and on occasion require the divestment of equities, the termination of consulting relationships, and the imposition of methods of monitoring. Medical journals have also followed suit requiring disclosure and implementing other methods such as the rejection of medical reviews by those believed to have conflicts.[36] Despite these safeguards, breaches are often seen, supporting the need to be ever vigilant.

Clinical Trials in Rheumatoid Arthritis: A Case Report

Due to its systemic nature and propensity to early progression and joint damage, current RA treatment paradigms have increasingly focused on aggressive therapy employing multiple disease-modifying drugs (DMARDs) that are administered early in the onset of disease. While methotrexate (MTX) remains the "anchor" drug on which combination regimes have been superimposed, newer approaches to the suppression of the inflammatory response have focused on a variety of potential targets including cytokines, B and T cells, osteoclasts, and additional immunologic factors that may be important in the perpetuation of the disease state.[45] As many of these new therapies have potential significant toxicities, patient safety and the ethical considerations arising in context of clinical trial participation will be at the forefront of the effort to find more effective treatment for this disease. In order to discuss some of the important ethical considerations which arise in the research setting, a recent RA clinical trial, the analysis of which is as yet incomplete, is illustrative. The clinical details of this case are summarized in Table 11D-2.

As a consequence of this tragic experience, this protocol has undergone intense scrutiny both from the lay press,[46,47] and the scientific community, an assessment that has included an examination by the NIH Recombinant DNA Advisory Committee. Numerous questions have arisen: Was the science underlying the proposed therapy flawed? What factors or conditions associated with the clinical trial contributed to this outcome? Was the patient adequately informed about the risks of participation? Was the patient sufficiently protected against these risks?

An ethical analysis of this event begins with the informed consent. Under the current guidelines for research participation in the United States, all research subjects must be informed of the risks and the benefits of their participation in a research study, a requirement fulfilled by the process of informed consent.[48] It is in this process that respect for the research subject as a person and recognition of their autonomy is demonstrated. Three primary elements support this process: information, comprehension, and voluntariness. Once these elements are achieved the subject's authorization is sought.[10,48] Information provided to the research subject should be adequate to explain the rationale for and the procedures involved in the study and should meet a "reasonable volunteer" standard. In order to do so, the investigator may need to consider factors such as the subject's age and educational level, and other barriers to communication such as language. Informed consent continues throughout the subject's participation in the research.

Table 11D-2. Case Study
The patient was a 36-year-old Caucasian female enrolled in an open-label phase I/II clinical trial (safety/efficacy study) of a genetically engineered adenovirus encoded with a TNF-receptor construct under development by a biotech company as an intra-articular injection for RA. The patient had developed RA 15 years before her enrollment, had previously been treated with etanercept (2002–2004) and at the time of her recruitment to the study had been managed with adalimumab, methotrexate, and prednisone. She previously had surgery on her toe but not her knee, although she had been treated with multiple (10) knee injections of corticosteroids. Randomized to the highest-dose group, she received her first dosage of the study drug on February 26, 2007 without incident. Her second intra-articular injection was administered on July 2, 2007, and on the same evening the patient developed fever and diarrhea. Due to the persistence of the fever, Levaquin was prescribed (July 5, 2007), but the patient remained febrile (104° F), and was experiencing nausea and vomiting. By July 9, 2007 her knee had become tender, she was tachycardic, and had a WBC of 29,000/mm^3 (predominantly lymphocytes), and exhibited mild liver function abnormalities. Her fever persisted despite aggressive antibiotic therapy, and subsequently (July 16, 2007) her liver function was further deteriorating, she remained febrile, and Hgb was noted to be dropping (to a low of 4.6). Hypotension and respiratory distress ensued and she was transferred to another center.
By July 19, additional laboratory and radiologic testing revealed a coagulopathy, retroperitoneal hemorrhage, and further deterioration in the liver function. At this time, the question of liver transplantation was raised but dismissed. Serologies for HSV-1 were negative as were nasopharyngeal cultures. On July 19, a liver biopsy was performed and revealed small areas of acute necrosis and inflammatory lesions, and was positive for histoplasma. Her deterioration continued and she expired on July 24, 2007. An autopsy revealed disseminated histoplasma capsulatum involving all organs without granuloma (a feature typical for histoplasmosis in the immunocompromised), a large retroperitoneal hematoma, and minimal swelling of the knees.

Early indications have suggested that there may have been problems with respect to the informed consent process in the case under discussion. For instance, it has been reported that the subject participated in the clinical trial because of a perceived benefit, primarily the alleviation of her knee pain.[46,47] This problem, often referred to as the therapeutic misconception, is not uncommon.[24,25] It refers to a mistaken belief held by the research subject that his or her participation will directly benefit them and certainly produce no harm. Thus, it is possible that this patient believed she was receiving state-of-the-art, even novel therapy, to which others would not have access. Such beliefs are strong inducements to participation and have to be adequately tempered by the primary investigator through a thoughtful, considered process of informed consent. Statements such as "you cannot expect to benefit directly from your participation in this study," so often found in consent forms, cannot be regarded as sufficient to mitigate the problem of therapeutic misconception.

Another important consideration relates to the pretrial risk assessment of the developers of the drug and the primary investigators. Although this subject's death may not be a direct consequence of the study drug (and unrelated to the adenovirus vector employed to deliver it), the magnitude of the patient's immunosuppression, a consequence of the totality of her therapy, as well as this risk of infection with histoplasmosis in a patient living in an endemic region for this condition may not have been sufficiently appreciated by the investigators. Just as with tuberculosis, the risk of which took several years to be realized, the risk of fungal infections, and histoplasma specifically, has been reported in this setting.[50,51] As such, a greater appreciation of this potential risk might have been indicated in this subject.

Compounding the concerns pertaining to the scientific oversight of this investigation is the approval of the protocol by an independent IRB, one unaffiliated with an academic medical center. Two issues are raised in this context. First is the quality of scientific review given the complexities of therapy in this disease setting. Was there sufficient rheumatologic, immunologic, and infectious disease expertise on the IRB to adequately assess the potential for adverse outcomes with this new therapy? The second concern pertains to the for-profit nature of this IRB. Could the IRB process have been influenced by circumstances in which they are being paid directly by the company seeking approval for the drug?

A third issue has also been raised having to do with coercion. In the case presented, the research subject was approached directly by her rheumatologist concerning her willingness to participate in this investigation. In the trial presented, the study sponsor had agreed in principle to the use of a neutral party in the recruitment of patients, although this procedure was not employed.[52] This practice has the potential for placing undue influence on the patient to agree to enroll in the study. In order to reduce this form of influence, the National Institutes of Health recommends that physicians should not recruit their own patients into clinical trials they are conducting. In circumstances where this cannot be avoided, it has been suggested that an impartial third party explain the study and obtain informed consent.[49] This practice is particularly relevant to studies involving novel therapies which are deemed risky, in circumstances when the individual's condition is not life-threatening, and is especially of interest in studies in which the investigator has a financial interest (as was the case in the RA trial discussed herein).

A final concern has to do with the assumption of risk. As in the case of an earlier and now well-documented study involving gene therapy with fatal consequences,[53,54] the RA study subject had a mild, or at least well-controlled disease, with standard therapy. Thus, the degree of assumed risk may have been out of proportion to the potential benefit, provoking concern in general as to which diseases should even be considered for innovative therapies that employ emerging technologies.[52]

References

1. Beecher HK. Ethics and clinical research. *N Engl J Med* 1966;274: 1354–1360.
2. Rothman D. Ethics and human experimentation. *N Engl J Med* 1987; 317:1195–1199.
3. Emanuel EJ, Crouch RA, Arras JD, et al. *Ethical and Regulatory Aspects of Clinical Research: Readings and Commentary*. Baltimore, MD: Johns Hopkins University Press, 2003.
4. Vanderpool HY, ed. *The Ethics of Research Involving Human Subjects: Facing the 21st Century*. Frederick, MD: University Publishing Group, 1996.
5. Grady C. Ethical principles in clinical research. In: Gallin JI, Ognibene FP, eds. *Principles and Practice of Clinical Research*, 2nd ed. Amsterdam and Boston: Elsevier/Academic Press, 2007.
6. Derenzo E, Moss J. *Writing Clinical Research Protocols: Ethical Considerations*. Amsterdam and Boston: Elsevier/Academic Press, 2006.
7. Beauchamp TL, Childress JF. *Principles of Biomedical Ethics*, 5th ed. New York: Oxford University Press, 2001.
8. The Nuremberg Code, 1949. www.hhs.gov/ohrp/references/nurcode.htm.
9. World Medical Assembly. Declaration of Helsinki 2000. www.wma.net/e/ethicsunit/helsinki.htm.
10. National Commission for the Protection of Human Subjects of Biomedial and Behavioral Research. *The Belmont Report: Ethical Principles and Guidelines for the Protection of Human Subjects of Research*. Washington, DC: U.S. Government Printing Office, 1979.
11. Council for International Organizations of Medical Sciences (CIOMS). *International Ethical Guidelines for Biomedical Research Involving Human Subjects*. Geneva: CIOMS/SHO, 2002. www.cioms.ch.
12. International Conference on Harmonisation of Technical Requirements for Registration of Pharmaceuticals for Human Use. ICH Harmonised Tripartite Guideline—Guideline for Good Clinical Practice (ICH-GCP Guideline), Geneva, 1996. www.vadscorner.com/internet29.html.
13. Brandt AM. Racism and research: The case of the Tuskegee Syphilis Study. *Hastings Center Rep* 1978;6:21–29.
14. National Institutes of Health. *Recruitment and Retention of Women in Clinical Studies*. A Report of the Workshop Sponsored by the Office of Research on Women's Health. NIH Publication No. 95-3756. Bethesda, MD: U.S. Department of Health and Human Services, NIH, 1995.
15. National Institutes of Health. NIH Policy and Guidelines on the Inclusion of Children as Participants in Research Involving Human

Subjects, Notice 98-024. March 6, 1998. http://grants.nih.gov/grants/guide/notice-files/not98-024.html.
16. Rothman KJ, Michels KB. The continuing unethical use of placebo controls. *N Engl J Med* 1994;331:394–398.
17. Temple R, Ellenberg SS. Placebo-controlled trials and active-control trials in the evaluation of new treatments. Part I: Ethical and scientific issues. *Ann Intern Med* 2000;133:455–463.
18. Freedman B. Placebo-controlled trials and the logic of clinical purpose. *IRB Rev Hum Subj Res* 1990;12:1–6.
19. Emanuel EJ, Miller FG. The ethics of placebo-controlled trials: A middle ground. *N Engl J Med* 2001;345:915–919.
20. Glantz LH, Annas GJ, Grodin MA, Mariner W. Research in developing countries: Taking "benefit" seriously. *Hastings Center Report* 1998;28(6):38–42.
21. Koski G, Nightingale SL. Research involving human subjects in developing countries. *N Engl J Med* 2001;345:136–138.
22. Shapiro HT, Meslin EM. Ethical issues in the design and conduct of clinical trials in developing countries. *N Engl J Med* 2003;345:139–142.
23. Emanuel EJ, Wendler D, Grady C. What makes clinical research ethical? *JAMA* 2000;283:2701–2711.
24. Hellman S, Hellman DS. Of mice but not men: Problems of the randomized clinical trial. *N Engl J Med* 1991;324:1585–1589.
25. Appelbaum PS, Roth LH, Lidz CW, et al. False hopes and best data: Consent to research and the therapeutic misconception. *Hastings Center Rep* 1987;17:20–24.
26. Hochhauser M. Therapeutic misconception and recruiting doublespeak in the informed consent process. *IRB Ethics Hum Res* 2002;24:11–12.
27. Freedman B, Fuks A, Weijer C. Demarcating research and treatment: A systemic approach for the analysis of the ethics of clinical research. *Clin Res* 1992;40:653–660.
28. Levine RJ. *Ethics and Regulation of Clinical Research*, 2nd ed. Baltimore: Urban & Schwarzenberg, 1986.
29. Freedman B. Equipoise and the ethics of clinical research. *N Engl J Med* 1987;317:141–145.
30. Barondess JA. Medicine and professionalism. *Arch Intern Med* 2003;163:145–149.
31. Pellegrino ED. Professionalism, profession and the virtues of the good physician. *Mt Sinai J Med* 2002;69:378–384.
32. MacKenzie CR. Professionalism and medicine. *Hosp Special Surg J* 2007;3:222–227.
33. Grady C. The challenge of assuring continued post-trial access to beneficial treatment. *Yale J Health Policy Law Ethics* 2005;5(1):425–435.
34. Shuchman M. Commercializing clinical trials—risks and benefits of the CRO boom. *N Engl J Med* 2007;537:1365–1368.
35. Thompson D. Understanding financial conflicts of interest. *N Engl J Med* 1993;329:573–576.
36. MacKenzie CR, Cronstein BN. Conflict of interest. *Hosp Special Surg J* 2006;2:198–201.
37. Korn D. Conflicts of interest in biomedical research. *JAMA* 2000;284:2234–2237.
38. Bekelman JE, Li Y, Gross CP. Scope and impact of financial conflicts of interest in biomedical research. *JAMA* 2003;289:453–465.
39. Barnes M, Florencio P. Financial conflicts of interest in human subjects research: The problem of institutional conflicts. *J Law Med Ethics* 2002;30:1–13.
40. Hillman AL, Pauly MV, Kerslein B. How do financial incentives affect physician's clinical decisions and the financial performance of health maintenance organizations. *N Engl J Med* 1989;321:86–89.
41. Hillman AL, Joseph CA, Mabry MR, et al. Frequency and costs of diagnostic imaging in office practice: Comparison of sel-referring and radiologist referring physicians. *N Engl J Med* 1990;323:1604–1608.
42. Chren MM, Landefeld CS. Physicians behavior and their interactions with drug companies: A controlled study of physicians who request additions to a hospital formulary. *JAMA* 1994;271:684–689.
43. International Committee of Medical Journal Editors. Uniform Requirements for Manuscripts Submitted to Biomedical Journals. November 2001. www.icmje.org.
44. New England Journal of Medicine Editors. Financial associations of authors. *N Engl J Med* 2002;346:1901–1902.
45. Savage C, St. Clair W. New therapeutics in rheumatoid arthritis. *Rheum Dis Clin North Am* 2006;32:57–74.
46. Weiss R. Death points to risks in research. *Washington Post*, 8/6/07, p. A01.
47. Weiss R. Fungus infected woman who died after gene therapy. *Washington Post*, 8/17/07, p. A10.
48. U.S. Department of Health and Human Services, National Institutes of Health, Office for Human Research Protections. The Common Rule, Title 45 (Public Welfare), Code of Federal Regulations, Part 46 (Protection of Human Subjects). Washington, DC: Department of Health and Human Services, revised November 13, 2001, effective December 13, 2001.
49. Editorial. Uninformed consent? *Nat Med* 2007;13:999.
50. Lee JH, Slifman NR, Gersho SK, et al. Life-threatening histoplasmosis complicating immunotherapy with tumor necrosis factor alpha antagonists infliximab and etanercept. *Arthritis Rheum* 2002;46:2565–2570.
51. Wook KL, Hage CA, Know KS, et al. Histoplasmosis after treatment with anti-tumor necrosis factor-alpha therapy. *Am J Respir Crit Care Med* 2003;167:1279–1282.
52. Hughes V. Therapy on trial. *Nat Med* 2007;13(9):1008–1009.
53. Baron J. *Against Bioethics*. Cambridge, MA: MIT Press, 2006.
54. Stolberg SG. "The biotech death of Jesse Gelsinger." *NY Times Magazine*, November 28, 1999.

European Biologics Registers

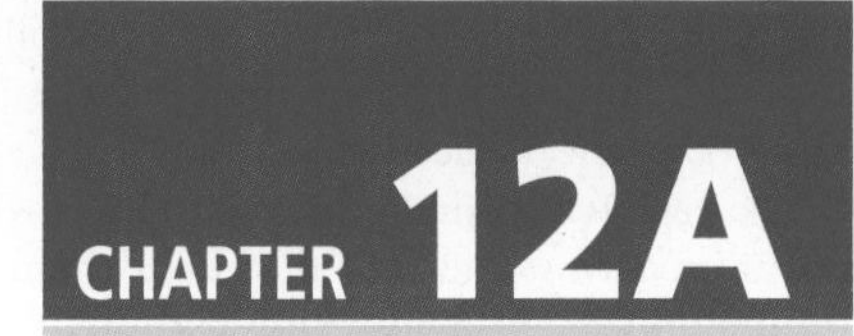

Angela Zink

During the past decade, it has become increasingly clear that randomized clinical trials and spontaneous reporting systems are inadequate instruments to detect rare, unexpected, or long-term adverse outcomes of new drugs. Additionally, important clinical questions concerning flexibility in dosage, combination of drugs, application in patients with severe comorbidities, or reasons for switching therapies will never be subject to clinical trials. These questions can only be approached in well-designed, long-term observational studies.

In 2000, the first two biologic agents, etanercept and infliximab, became available for routine treatment of patients with severe rheumatoid arthritis (RA). Due to their novel mode of action and the limited data on safety and long-term effectiveness from clinical trials, registers of patients treated with biologic agents were initiated in several European countries. They follow the methodologic approach of epidemiologic cohort studies in order to overcome the drawbacks of either spontaneous reporting systems or open-label extensions of clinical trials. While spontaneous notification of adverse events to the national pharmaco-vigilance systems leads to significant under-reporting of events and lacks any opportunity to relate the events to the number of patients treated with the substance, open label extensions have the limitation that they only observe patients previously included in randomized clinical trials which have been shown not to be equal to those treated in real practice.

Common Features of European Registers

Biologics registers have been established in several European countries such as the UK, Sweden, Germany, Spain, Norway, Denmark, and the Netherlands. Other countries are currently setting up registers. Even though these registers are heterogeneous in some aspects, they do share a number of common features, which are summarized below:

The registers were initiated by the national rheumatology societies of respective countries.

The advent of biologic agents for the treatment of severe, refractory RA conferred the opportunity to influence the course of the disease in a previously unknown manner. This had the potential to change rheumatology as a whole. However, a number of important open questions regarding the long-term safety and effectiveness of the drugs in real practice remained. Therefore, the rheumatology societies in several European countries felt that the medical profession should take the lead and initiated independent observational studies in order to assess the long-term outcomes of biologic treatment.

The registers are not drug-specific, but instead include all licensed biologics.

With the increasing number of licensed biologic agents, a considerable proportion of patients will be treated with more than one biologic agent. Drug-specific registers, maintained by the respective pharmaceutical company, are not appropriate to answer questions related to the risks conferred by exposure to multiple biologic agents. Therefore, all registers include all licensed biologic agents.

The registers are epidemiologic cohort studies.

This means that each patient ever enrolled in the register will be followed-up, irrespective of whether or not the patient remains under the initial drug. This is an indispensable prerequisite for both the comparability of exposed and unexposed patients and for the identification of long-term effects. Events that occur after treatment has ended can only be captured if the observation period is independent of the time under treatment.

Most of the registers have established comparator cohorts.

In order to put the prevalence of observed adverse events into perspective, having an adequate control group is indispensable. These control cohorts are either part of the register itself (Germany) or collected at specific rheumatologic sites (UK). Other countries use previously collected cohorts as comparators. In the UK, Sweden and Denmark national register data on cancer and death, in Sweden and Denmark also on hospitalization, can be linked to the register data. Each kind of comparator cohort has its specific strengths, and this will be discussed for the individual registers.

The registers are supported by unconditional grants from all companies whose products are under observation.

After having been approached by the rheumatology societies, the pharmaceutical companies agreed to support the registers with unconditional joint grants. This innovative approach led to both a long-term commitment of several competing companies and a collaboration on the national as well as international level. The companies support the registers with substantial amounts of grant money for many years, since long-term observational designs are expensive and are usually not covered by any research organization.

The registers are independent in design, conduct, and publication of results.

The registers have contracts with the companies that ensure that the conduct and publication of results is not influenced by any of the companies. The companies usually have the right to see and comment on publications before submission but they cannot prevent publication.

The registers provide the companies with semianual reports on adverse events that help them to fulfill the requirements of the health authorities.

The British, Swedish, and German registers, and the pharmaceutical companies have agreed on a standardized reporting system following the "Manchester Template." This system includes the biannual reporting of the incidence of serious adverse events in all treatment groups and control cohorts. The companies use the reports to fulfill the requirements of the European drug agency EMEA. In Denmark, all serious adverse events in all treatment groups are reported four times yearly to the companies.

Since their inception, the registers have worked together closely and met regularly.

The registers have met once each year since 2002 in Manchester/UK, Stockholm, and Uppsala/Sweden, or Berlin/Germany. The meetings were initiated by the British, Swedish, and German registers. These registers share a particularly close collaboration with one other. All other registers have been invited to participate in these workshops.[1]

Individual Registers

British Society of Rheumatology Biologics Register

The British Society of Rheumatology Biologics Register (BSRBR) was established in October 2001 by the British Society for Rheumatology, and is coordinated by the ARC Epidemiology Unit University of Manchester.[2] The goal is to register all patients in the United Kingdom with rheumatic diseases newly starting treatment with one of the biologic agents up to a maximum of 4000 per drug and to follow them up for an individual observation period of 5 years. This number allows detection of a doubling in the incidence of lymphoma. Following a requirement from the NICE institute in 2002 to enroll patients treated with biologics in the BSRBR, it grew rapidly and is today by far the world's largest biologic register.[3–7] More than 14,000 patients treated with biologics (among them about 12,000 with RA), and a comparator cohort of more than 3,000 patients with active RA treated with conventional DMARDs have been enrolled. The patients are followed-up at 6, 12, 18, 24, 30, 36, 48, and 60 months with clinical data and for the first three years with patient data. They are followed-up for their entire lifetime for malignancy and death via the national registers.

Website: http://www.medicine.manchester.ac.uk/arc/BSRBR

German Biologics Register: Rheumatoid Arthritis: Observation of Biologic Therapy

The German biologics register, Rheumatoid Arthritis: Observation of Biologic Therapy (RABBIT), was established in May 2001 following an initiative of the German Society of Rheumatology.[8–11] It is coordinated at the Epidemiology Unit of the German Rheumatism Research Centre in Berlin. Patients beginning new treatments with any of the currently six biologic agents licensed in Germany for the treatment of RA or a conventional DMARD after failure of at least one other (control group) are followed-up for an individual observation period of up to 10 years. The German register includes control cases in the identical manner and at the same sites as the biologics cases. About 6,000 patients have been enrolled. Since January 1, 2007, recruitment has been ongoing for only rituximab and abatacept. All other cohorts are closed and will be followed up until end of 2011. The patients are followed up at 3, 6, 12, 18, 24, 30, and 36 months, and annually thereafter with clinical data and patient data.

Website: http://www.biologika-register.de

Swedish Biologics Register

The Swedish biologics register ARTIS was initiated by the Swedish Rheumatology Association in 1999, when biologic agents were first available.[12–16] Patients are entered in the ARTIS register at the start of treatment. They are followed up at 3, 6, and 12 months, and biannually thereafter. Since 2003, it has been possible to enter the data through a Web-based format.

Two regional registers contribute to the national data set: the STURE register in the Stockholm area and the South Swedish Register (SSATG).[17–20] Although initially restricted to patients with RA, all rheumatologic indications for biologic therapy are now covered. Some 15,000 treatments (11,000 patients of whom 8,000 have RA) have been enrolled in ARTIS.

The ARTIS data are linked to national registers tracking status, causes of death, inpatient and outpatient care, and cancer via an individual subject ID issued to all Swedish residents.

Spanish BIOBADASER Register

BIOBADASER was initiated in 2000 by the Spanish Society for Rheumatology.[21–26] It receives funding from five pharmaceutical companies and the Spanish Agency for Medicines and Medical Devices. The short clinical record form contains gender, age, diagnosis, date of diagnosis, and dates of treatment start and discontinuation. Since the register aims to detect relevant and unexpected adverse events while on drug treatment and after the cessation of therapy, as well as to identify risk factors of adverse events, no clinical effectiveness data or patient-derived data are collected.

In the first phase of BIOBADASER (2000–2006), the number of participating hospitals was not limited. Roughly 50% of all patients being treated with biologic agents in Spanish rheumatology centres were included. After on-site monitoring in autumn of 2006, the number of participating sites was reduced and the intensity of monitoring has been increased. In the second phase of BIOBADASER, all patients beginning treatment with biologic agents for any rheumatic disease in 14 participating hospitals are going to be included. The centers were selected based on the number of patients enrolled in the first phase and the quality of their data. For comparison, a large cohort of RA patients (EMECAR) for whom the most relevant comorbidities were collected is used.

Website: http://www.biobadaser.ser.es

Danish Rheumatological Database

The Danish Rheumatological Database (DANBIO) was introduced in 2000 in collaboration with the Danish Society of Rheumatology and the Institute for Rational Pharmacotherapy.[27–31] It covers all 26 rheumatologic departments in the country and more than 90% of all biologics prescriptions in Denmark. More than 3500 RA patients have been enrolled so far; patient inclusion continues. Patients with AS, psoriatic arthritis, and other inflammatory diseases are routinely enrolled as well. The patients will be further followed up as long as they are seen in the documenting units. Comparison cohorts of patients with early

RA and with RA treated with conventional DMARDs have been established.

Data are entered via the Internet (80%) or on paper (20%). The items recorded include age, gender, diagnosis, the year of diagnosis, DMARD history, disease activity, patient assessments of function (HAQ), pain, global health, current treatment, date and reasons for withdrawal, adverse events, and x-rays.

DANBIO can be linked to national registers such as the cause-of-death register, the inpatient register and the cancer register via an individual subject ID.

Website: http://danbio-online.dk

Norwegian DMARD Register

The Norwegian DMARD Register (NOR-DMARD) was established in 2000 with five rheumatology centers.[32] It is not restricted to biologic agents, but comprises all DMARD prescriptions, including biologics, for patients with inflammatory arthropathies. This offers the opportunity to compare effectiveness between RA and other inflammatory arthropathies[33] and between biologics and conventional DMARDs in a real-life setting.[34]

Dutch Rheumatoid Arthritis Monitoring Register

The Dutch Rheumatoid Arthritis Monitoring Register (DREAM) was started in 2003 in 11 rheumatology centers in the Netherlands. It is managed by the Radboud University Nijmegen Medical Centre.[35] Patients can be included if they have active RA and no prior exposure to a biologic agent (anti–TNF-α therapies), or inadequate response to anti–TNF-α therapy (abatacept and ritixumab). About 1000 patients have been enrolled so far.

The Nijmegen inception cohort of early RA cases not previously treated with DMARDs is available as a comparator cohort. The adverse events are reported by the patients. There is no coding system for AEs in place. The register is supported by the Dutch National Health Insurance Board and the companies producing the agents under observation.

Swiss Clinical Quality Management Database

Not originally a biologics register but set up as quality monitoring system, the SCQM database enrolls patients treated with biologics prior to the initiation of therapy.[36,37] Rheumatologists can deduct the costs of biologic therapy from their treatment expenditure by enrolling the patients which is an incentive for registration. There are no fixed follow-up time points but rather ongoing registration at visits to the rheumatologist, at least one per year. Clinical, patient-derived, and safety data are recorded.

Differences Among Registers

Although there are similarities, the description of the various registers made a number of differences apparent. First are comparisons drawn from specific cohorts or from national registers. The British and the German registers have built up specific comparison cohorts for the biologics patients. In the German register, the control patients are enrolled using the same system as the biologics patients, in the UK the control patients are gathered at specific sites. This enables the two registers to draw direct comparisons between patients treated with biologics and controls. The British register enrolls patients on DMARD therapy, irrespective of previous failure. The German register has previous DMARD failure and start of a new DMARD therapy as an inclusion criterion for the control group. In Sweden and Denmark, due to the various population-based registers, comparison data are gained from national routine registration of deaths, hospitalization, or cancer. Additionally, various cohorts assembled for other reasons are available in Sweden. Other countries use cohorts established for other reasons as comparators.

Second is coding of adverse events. Uniform coding and reporting of adverse events is a critical prerequisite for the comparability of results across registers. The British, Spanish, and German registers work with the uniform coding system MedDRA,[38] which enables them to ensure that the same events are summarized under the same heading. The Swedish register uses ICD-10 in order to be comparable to the national registers.

Next, diseases included are different. Most of the registers focus on rheumatoid arthritis (RA). The Spanish register enrolls patients with any form of chronic arthritis who are treated with biologics. In the British register, 2313 out of 14,058 patients enrolled in July 2007 had diseases other than RA. The Danish register comprises all adult rheumatologic patients treated with biologics regardless of diagnosis. Almost all publications from the registers so far deal with RA. The following summarized results therefore refer to this disease if not indicated otherwise.

Major Results

Effectiveness of Anti–TNF-α Treatment in Daily Practice

The registers have contributed significantly to our understanding of the effectiveness of treatment with biologics under the conditions of everyday clinical practice. Six major topics have been raised.

What Is the Survival Rate for Individual Anti–TNF-α Treatments?

Several registers have analyzed treatment continuation in daily practice. In Denmark, the 12-month survival rates for a first treatment were 70% for etanercept or infliximab.[29] In Germany, the figures were 65% for infliximab (INF) and 69% for ETA.[8] In Spain, the range was from 81% to 88% for INF, adalimumab (ADA), and ETA.[26] After 2 years, 72% of ETA, 59% of INF and only 50% of ADA courses in the Swedish register were still continuing. If only first treatment courses were considered, however, there was no difference among the drugs (about 80% after 1 year[39]). The Spanish register compared drug survival rates in different rheumatic diseases and found 83%, 72%, and 65% for drug survival over 1, 2, and 3 years in RA, and 88%, 82%, and 76% for the same times in ankylosing spondylitis, respectively.[24]

Several analyses showed that combination with methotrexate (MTX) or another DMARD like leflunomide (LEF) increases treatment continuation. Drug survival over 6 months in the British register was 84% for ETA plus MTX and 78% for ETA monotherapy compared to 79% for INF plus MTX and 70% for INF monotherapy.[5] The 12-month survival rates in the German register were 82% for ETA/MTX and 77% for INF/MTX, compared to 71% and 67% for monotherapy.[8] Survival rates for the combination of anti–TNF-α therapies with LEF were comparable to MTX.[40]

What Is the Effectiveness of Anti–TNF-α Treatments in Real Life?

Two groups compared effectiveness data from the registers with the results of major clinical trials.[10,35] Both groups showed that the effectiveness in clinical practice in total was lower than that in clinical trials. If the inclusion criteria of the major trials were applied, however, the patients fulfilling the criteria for a given trial had a clinical response similar to those in the trial.

Less than one-third of the German patients treated in real practice would have been eligible for the trials.[10] Ineligible patients had lower disease activity, lower functional status, and higher comorbidity than eligible patients. However, this difference was mainly due to the fact that the ACR response measures relative improvement and, therefore, patients who begin treatment with very high disease activity have a better chance of reaching large improvement. If the EULAR (DAS28) response was applied, the absolute level of disease activity reached was equal in both groups.

The South Swedish register found ACR50 responses at 12 months in about 45% of patients treated with ETA and 40% of patients treated with INF.[17]

The Danish register found that the fraction of patients who achieved a good EULAR response after 1 year of treatment had increased from 28% in the 2000/2001 cohort to 50% in the 2005 cohort, and the fraction with no response decreased from 29% in 2000/2001 to 16% in 2005. Similarly, ACR20/50/70 response rates have increased from 53%/31%/13% to 69%/51%/30% in 2005.[41]

How Successful Is Switching of Biologic Therapies?

The British register showed that 12% of patients stopped treatment due to inefficacy and 15% due to adverse events at a mean of 15 months of follow-up. Sixty percent of the patients who had stopped due to inefficacy, and 35% of those who had stopped due to toxicity received a second anti–TNF-α treatment. Survival of the second agent was comparable to the first for those patients who had stopped for inefficacy and lower for those who had stopped for adverse events. The reasons for stopping a second treatment cycle were associated with the reasons for the first termination.[7]

In the Spanish register BIOBADASER, the survival rates for a second treatment cycle with biologics were significantly lower than those for the first. ETA and ADA showed better survival rates (76% and 67%) than INF (34%) over 1 year after switching.[26] In contrast to the British data, survival was better if the first drug had been terminated because of adverse events.

The Swedish register[42] has shown that switching due to secondary loss of efficacy is only a minor problem. About 40% of the patients reached low disease activity or remission at 6 months. Of the remaining 60%, one-third were EULAR nonresponders and two-thirds were partial responders. Switching in these patients depends on the availability of alternative drugs and on the judgment of the treating physician. This finding agrees with earlier data from the Swedish register, which showed that switching biologics can lead to a DAS28 response that is almost as good as the one reached in first treatment cycles.[43]

The Danish register found that patients who switched because of lack of efficacy had a better clinical response to the second treatment. Those who switched because of adverse events responded equally well to both treatments, with a low risk of discontinuing the second drug as a result of adverse events.[30]

How Frequent Is Remission?

The national guidelines of the various European countries require previous treatment failure with DMARDs, among them MTX, before treatment with biologics can be started. Therefore, the patients enrolled in the registers form a selection of patients with poor prognosis. It is not surprising that the rates of remission (measured with the DAS28 or the ACR criteria) are quite low (9% to 16%[6,11]). After controlling for differences in baseline status, the German register showed that (1) the chance of remission for patients receiving anti–TNF-α treatment was double that of those treated with conventional DMARDs, and (2) the chance of patients with severe functional disability to reach a good physical function was fourfold.

What Are Predictors of Response?

The British register found a EULAR good response in 18% and moderate response in 50% of the patients after 6 months of treatment with either ETA or INF.[6] Lower response rates were found for current smokers, specifically those treated with INF.

What Is the Cost-Effectiveness of Anti–TNF-α Treatment?

Data on cost-effectiveness have been published from the South Swedish and the British registers. In an economic analysis of 160 patients treated with ETA or INF for at least 1 year in Sweden, the cost per quality-adjusted life year (QALY) was estimated to be 53,600 euros.[44] A much larger analysis based on 8284 patient-years of observation was performed by the British register.[45] Using a simulation model with a time horizon over the full patient lifetime, the cost-effectiveness of TNF-α inhibitors as a group versus traditional DMARDs was quantified. The main outcome was an incremental cost per QALY gained. The estimated discounted lifetime cost of therapy with TNF-α inhibitors was nearly £58,000 ($116,000, €89,000) compared to £21,000 ($42,000, €31,000) for conventional DMARDs. The incremental cost per QALY gained from using TNF-α inhibitors was estimated at £24,000 ($47,700, €35,000). There was a probability of 84% that treatments were cost-effective at a threshold of £30,000 ($60,000, € 44,000).

Safety of Anti–TNF-α Therapies

The major reason driving the creation of the biologics registers was the need to evaluate the long-term safety of these novel agents. Due to their modes of action, specific concerns existed regarding whether the agents would trigger the development of lymphoproliferative disorders, solid tumors or autoimmune diseases or lead to an increase in infections. Today, we can provide some intermediate answers to the majority of these questions.

Infections

Three registers have thus far published data describing the risk of infections in patients treated with TNF-α inhibitors compared to that in control patients. The first data came from the German register, and it showed an incidence of serious infections of about six per 100 patient-years. This was twofold higher than the incidence in the control group of patients treated with conventional DMARDs after controlling for confounding factors.[9] The British register described very similar absolute rates concerning the active treatment (5.1 to 5.5 per 100 person=years for the three anti–TNF-α agents). However, there was no increase compared to the control group (4.1 per 100 person-years).[3] The Swedish register analyzed the risk of hospitalization for serious infections using record linkage with the Swedish Inpatient Register. They found a risk for hospitalization of 4.7 per 100 person-years. The relative risk was increased during the first year of treatment (RR=1.43), but equaled the population risk thereafter.[15]

An explanation for the time-dependent risk of infection was offered recently by the British register.[46] Dixon re-analyzed the British data and found that the decreasing risk with time was due to an increased risk at start of therapy. This can be, at least in part, explained by the selection of patients with lower risks remaining on the therapy. Since the decision to stop or continue a therapy in an observational study is made by the physician according to the clinical situation of the patient, a patient who experiences an infection is most likely to be taken off the drug and may not be restarted after the infection has passed. This explains why the lowest rates of infection were found when only patients on-drug at the time of the infection were considered; the risk increased with longer follow-up after treatment cessation. A fourfold increase in risk was found when only the first 3 months of therapy were considered. This is an important example of the pitfalls of observational designs and the importance of observing—and standardizing where possible—the assumptions made.

Cardiovascular Events

Patients with RA have a twofold greater risk of experiencing a myocardial infarction.[47] It is well established that atherosclerosis is an inflammatory condition associated with elevated acute-phase reactants. Reducing the inflammatory burden should therefore lead to a decrease in morbidity and mortality from atherosclerosis. Data from the registers support this view.

The Spanish register found (1) a decrease in mortality from cardiovascular events compared to that in a clinical cohort of conventionally treated patients, and (2) mortality similar to that of the general population of the same age and gender.[23]

The South Swedish register compared first cardiovascular events in patients treated versus not treated with TNF-α blockers using register data, data from a population cohort, and data from the national inpatient care register. The age and sex adjusted incidence was significantly lower in patients with RA treated with TNF-α blockers.[20]

The British register compared the rate of myocardial infarction in 8670 patients treated with TNF-α inhibitors to that of 2170 patients treated with traditional DMARDs. The rates were 5.9 and 4.8 events per 1000 person-years, respectively. After adjustment for baseline risk factors, there was no difference between the two groups. However, those patients who responded to the anti–TNF-α treatment within 6 months had a significantly lower rate of MI than those who did not.[48]

The German register analyzed the risk of heart failure for patients treated with anti–TNF-α and a control group. Patients treated with TNF-α inhibitors showed no increased risk of developing heart failure. More importantly, patients with prevalent heart failure at start of treatment did not have a higher risk of worsening when treated with TNF-α inhibitors.[49]

Lymphomas

An early report from the South Swedish register of an 11.5-fold increase in the occurrence of lymphoma among patients treated with TNF-α inhibitors raised concerns about the induction of lymphoproliferative disorders by anti–TNF-α treatments.[50] When the data were included in the larger Swedish register and linked to the National Cancer Register, however, the increase in risk disappeared.[51] Since it is known that the risk of lymphoma is strongly associated with disease activity,[52] and patients with higher disease activity are more likely to receive anti–TNF-α treatment, current available data do not suggest that this treatment confers an additional risk for lymphomas. However, further observation is needed.

Solid Tumors

By linkage with the Cancer and Census Registers, the Swedish biologic register found no difference in the risk for solid cancers between patients treated with anti–TNF-α agents and other RA patients.[53] No increased risk of new malignancies of recurrence of prior malignancy was found in the German biologics register.[54,55]

Pregnancies

The British register reported that 23 women were directly exposed to anti–TNF-α treatment at the time of conception.[4] All except two stopped treatment within the first trimester. There were six first-trimester miscarriages and three elective first-trimester terminations. Furthermore, nine women stopped anti–TNF-α treatment prior to conception. Of these 32 women who became pregnant, 91% decided to continue the pregnancy and 76% delivered healthy infants. However, the rate of 24% first-trimester miscarriages appears high.

The German register analyzed 42 pregnancies in 31 women. In 24 pregnancies, women were exposed to anti–TNF-α treatment during the first trimester. In nine pregnancies each, the women had stopped anti–TNF-α treatment before conception or were anti–TNF-α naive.[56] The data suggest the presence of no serious adverse birth outcomes for any of the groups. Interestingly, the birth weight for the control group was significantly lower than that for the two groups of women exposed to anti–TNF-α treatment before or at onset of pregnancy. However, the available data on pregnancies remain too limited to allow any conclusions regarding the risk conferred by anti–TNF-α treatment to be drawn.

Deaths

Two registers have reported on mortality risk under TNF-α blockade so far. The Spanish register found decreased age- and sex-adjusted cardiovascular disease and cancer mortality rates compared to the population. The mortality rate from infections was significantly elevated, but it was not higher than that of an external cohort of RA patients from several sites in Spain.[23]

The South Swedish register found a lower mortality risk for patients with RA treated with anti–TNF-α agents after controlling for age, gender, and disease severity markers. This decrease was specifically seen in women.[19]

Both studies support the assumption that successful suppression of inflammatory activity increases survival in patients with RA.

Challenges and Limitations of Drug Registers

Drug registers like those operating in several European countries are methodologically demanding and have a number of limitations. The most obvious limitation involves channeling bias or confounding by indication. Guidelines effective in all European countries limit the prescription of anti–TNF-α agents to patients with severe disease and the failure of previous DMARD therapies. Regardless of the control group chosen, therefore, there is a high likelihood that the anti–TNF-α group will still have a poorer a priori prognosis. Additionally, as seen with the infection example, selective treatment dropout by patients with poor prognosis may lead to a better average prognosis for those patients remaining on therapy.

Methods for controlling these biases and adjusting for confounding must be applied at several stages of the research process:

1. Decisions involving the control group

Since treatment history, disease severity, and comorbidity influence treatment decisions and outcomes, patients in the control group should be as similar as possible to biologics patients. These similarities should include age, gender, disease duration, clinical measures of disease activity and severity, and treatment history. Therefore, it is adequate to require previous failures on traditional DMARDs as an inclusion criterion for the control group. Early DMARD-naive patients therefore seem inadequate as a control group. However, since there is no guarantee that the patients are comparable and key outcomes may be influenced by the heterogeneity of the groups, statistical methods controlling for confounding by indication must be in place at the analysis stage.

2. Process of follow-up

It is essential to follow the control group with the same rigidity and protocol as the biologics group. Differences in ascertainment of adverse events, for example, inevitably lead to noncomparable results.

The unblinded nature of the study bears in itself the risk of differential awareness and reporting. If a physician is aware of an increased risk of certain infections in patients treated with biologics, she might be more careful in examining for this in biologics patients than in controls. Also, she might consider it more important to report it if a biologics patient is involved.

Therefore, any form of spontaneous reporting necessarily leads to biased results. Even within the framework of an intensively monitored observational study, this problem cannot be completely ruled out.

The researchers have to communicate to the participating physicians to follow their control patients in an identical manner as the patients on biologics. Additionally, data derived from external sources, e.g., register linkages, can be used. Patient reports can be used to complement the reports from physicians; however, without verification by a physician they are not adequate to assess treatment risks.

3. Data analysis

The greatest challenge lies in the adequate statistical analysis of the observational data. Several methods controlling for confounding by indication have been applied during the past decade. Propensity-score risk adjustment and propensity-based matching are the most widely used methods. The propensity score reflects the probability of receiving a specific treatment based on prognostically relevant baseline data. Patients treated with biologics and controls are stratified according to their propensity score value. Within propensity score strata, the covariates in biologics and control patients are equally distributed.[57]

Propensity-based matching means that the propensity score is used to select patients from the control group who are similar with respect to their propensity scores to the biologics patients. The problem here is that atypical patients are chosen from the biologics and the control group due to the unequal distributions among cases and controls. These patients may therefore no longer represent the patients in each respective group.

Conclusion

The European biologics registers represent a novel generation of pharmaco-epidemiologic cohort studies. They were all initiated by epidemiologists and rheumatologists, and all are conducted under the auspices of the respective national rheumatology societies. They have already tremendously increased our knowledge from randomized clinical trials. In total, the intermediate results from the registers are reassuring. No new signals that had not already been observed in clinical trials have been identified. The intermediate results regarding defined outcomes are reassuring. The registers have provided important data regarding what to expect when new treatments are used in patients who would never be included in clinical trials due to comorbidity, severe functional disability, or currently low disease activity.

The registers also contribute to the further development of research methodology. Differences in results between registers have driven analyses leading to more complex explanations of time-dependent risks. Therefore, it is extremely useful that we have different registers in Europe that produce their results independent of each other but collaborate closely. For rare events or for defined exposures there is also the option to pool the experience, such as by pooling data from register-specific, nested case–control studies.

Rheumatologists prescribing the new biologic agents now have better information on the balance of their benefits and risks, including aspects of costs to society. When new treatments arise, it is necessary to both evaluate them in the same manner as those currently on the market and compare the effectiveness and safety of the different agents. With longer exposure to multiple biologic treatments and more frequent switches, however, it will be increasingly difficult or even impossible to establish the influence of individual substances. The methodologic challenges of these approaches have only just begun.

References

1. Zink A, Silman A, Klareskog L. Summary of report of the 3rd Workshop of European Biologics Registries. *Ann Rheum Dis* 2005; 64(4):644.
2. Silman A, Symmons D, Scott DG, et al. British Society for Rheumatology Biologics Register. *Ann Rheum Dis* 2003;62(Suppl 2):ii28—ii29.
3. Dixon WG, Watson K, Lunt M, et al. Rates of serious infection, including site-specific and bacterial intracellular infection, in rheumatoid arthritis patients receiving anti-tumor necrosis factor therapy: Results from the British Society for Rheumatology Biologics Register. *Arthritis Rheum* 2006;54(8):2368–2376.
4. Hyrich KL, Symmons DP, Watson KD, et al. Pregnancy outcome in women who were exposed to anti-tumor necrosis factor agents: results from a national population register. *Arthritis Rheum* 2006;54(8):2701–2702.
5. Hyrich KL, Symmons DP, Watson KD, et al. Comparison of the response to infliximab or etanercept monotherapy with the response

to cotherapy with methotrexate or another disease-modifying antirheumatic drug in patients with rheumatoid arthritis: results from the British Society for Rheumatology Biologics Register. *Arthritis Rheum* 2006;54(6):1786–1794.

6. Hyrich KL, Watson KD, Silman AJ, et al. Predictors of response to anti-TNF-alpha therapy among patients with rheumatoid arthritis: Results from the British Society for Rheumatology Biologics Register. *Rheumatology (Oxford)* 2006;45(12):1558–1565.
7. Hyrich KL, Lunt M, Watson KD, et al. Outcomes after switching from one anti-tumor necrosis factor alpha agent to a second anti-tumor necrosis factor alpha agent in patients with rheumatoid arthritis: results from a large UK national cohort study. *Arthritis Rheum* 2007;56(1):13–20.
8. Zink A, Listing J, Kary S, et al. Treatment continuation in patients receiving biological agents or conventional DMARD therapy. *Ann Rheum Dis* 2005;64(9):1274–1279.
9. Listing J, Strangfeld A, Kary S, et al. Infections in patients with rheumatoid arthritis treated with biologic agents. *Arthritis Rheum* 2005;52(11):3403–3412.
10. Zink A, Strangfeld A, Schneider M, et al. Effectiveness of tumor necrosis factor inhibitors in rheumatoid arthritis in an observational cohort study: Comparison of patients according to their eligibility for major randomized clinical trials. *Arthritis Rheum* 2006;54(11):3399–3407.
11. Listing J, Strangfeld A, Rau R, et al. Clinical and functional remission: Even though biologics are superior to conventional DMARDs overall success rates remain low—results from RABBIT, the German biologics register. *Arthritis Res Ther* 2006;8(3):R66.
12. van Vollenhoven RF, Askling J. Rheumatoid arthritis registries in Sweden. *Clin Exp Rheumatol* 2005;23(Suppl 39):S195—S200.
13. Askling J, Fored CM, Geborek P, et al. Swedish registers to examine drug safety and clinical issues in RA. *Ann Rheum Dis* 2006;65(6): 707–712.
14. van Vollenhoven RF, Klareskog L. Clinical responses to tumor necrosis factor alpha antagonists do not show a bimodal distribution: Data from the Stockholm tumor necrosis factor alpha followup registry. *Arthritis Rheum* 2003;48(6):1500–1503.
15. Askling J, Fored CM, Brandt L, et al. Time-dependent increase in risk of hospitalisation with infection among swedish RA patients treated with TNF-antagonists. *Ann Rheum Dis* 2007;66(10):1339–1344.
16. van Vollenhoven RF, Ernestam S, Harju A, et al. Etanercept versus etanercept plus methotrexate: A registry-based study suggesting that the combination is clinically more efficacious. *Arthritis Res Ther* 2003;5(6):R347—R351.
17. Geborek P, Crnkic M, Petersson IF, et al. Etanercept, infliximab, and leflunomide in established rheumatoid arthritis: Clinical experience using a structured follow-up programme in southern Sweden. *Ann Rheum Dis* 2002;61(9):793–798.
18. Kristensen LE, Saxne T, Nilsson JA, et al. Impact of concomitant DMARD therapy on adherence to treatment with etanercept and infliximab in rheumatoid arthritis. Results from a six-year observational study in southern Sweden. *Arthritis Res Ther* 2006;8(6):R174.
19. Jacobsson LT, Turesson C, Nilsson JA, et al. Treatment with TNF blockers and mortality risk in patients with rheumatoid arthritis. *Ann Rheum Dis* 2007;66(5):670–675.
20. Jacobsson LT, Turesson C, Gulfe A, et al. Treatment with tumor necrosis factor blockers is associated with a lower incidence of first cardiovascular events in patients with rheumatoid arthritis. *J Rheumatol* 2005;32(7):1213–1218.
21. Gomez-Reino JJ, Carmona L, Valverde VR, et al. Treatment of rheumatoid arthritis with tumor necrosis factor inhibitors may predispose to significant increase in tuberculosis risk: A multicenter active-surveillance report. *Arthritis Rheum* 2003;48(8):2122–2127.
22. Carmona L, Gomez-Reino JJ, Rodriguez-Valverde V, et al. Effectiveness of recommendations to prevent reactivation of latent tuberculosis infection in patients treated with tumor necrosis factor antagonists. *Arthritis Rheum* 2005;52(6):1766–1772.
23. Carmona L, Descalzo MA, Perez-Pampin E, et al. All-cause and cause-specific mortality in rheumatoid arthritis are not greater than expected when treated with tumour necrosis factor antagonists. *Ann Rheum Dis* 2007;66(7):880–885.
24. Carmona L, Gomez-Reino JJ. Survival of TNF antagonists in spondylarthritis is better than in rheumatoid arthritis. Data from the Spanish registry BIOBADASER. *Arthritis Res Ther* 2006;8(3):R72.
25. Gomez-Reino JJ, Carmona L, Angel DM. Risk of tuberculosis in patients treated with tumor necrosis factor antagonists due to incomplete prevention of reactivation of latent infection. *Arthritis Rheum* 2007;57(5):756–761.
26. Gomez-Reino JJ, Carmona L. Switching TNF antagonists in patients with chronic arthritis: An observational study of 488 patients over a four-year period. *Arthritis Res Ther* 2006;8(1):R29.
27. Hetland ML, Unkerskov J, Ravn T, et al. Routine database registration of biological therapy increases the reporting of adverse events twentyfold in clinical practice. First results from the Danish Database (DANBIO). *Scand J Rheumatol* 2005;34(1):40–44.
28. Hetland ML. DANBIO: A nationwide registry of biological therapies in Denmark. *Clin Exp Rheumatol* 2005;23(Suppl 39):S205—S207.
29. Ostergaard M, Unkerskov J, Linde L, et al. Low remission rates but long drug survival in rheumatoid arthritis patients treated with infliximab or etanercept: results from the nationwide Danish DANBIO database. *Scand J Rheumatol* 2007;36(2):151–154.
30. Hjardem E, Ostergaard M, Podenphant J, et al. Do rheumatoid arthritis patients in clinical practice benefit from switching from infliximab to a second tumor necrosis factor alpha inhibitor? *Ann Rheum Dis* 2007;66(9):1184–1189.
31. Hjardem E, Hetland ML, Ostergaard M, et al. Prescription practice of biological drugs in rheumatoid arthritis during the first 3 years of post-marketing use in Denmark and Norway: Criteria are becoming less stringent. *Ann Rheum Dis* 2005;64(8):1220–1223.
32. Kvien TK, Heiberg, Lie E, et al. A Norwegian DMARD register: prescriptions of DMARDs and biological agents to patients with inflammatory rheumatic diseases. *Clin Exp Rheumatol* 2005;23 (Suppl 39):S188—S194.
33. Heiberg MS, Koldingsnes W, Mikkelsen K, et al. The comparative one-year performance of anti-tumor necrosis factor alpha drugs in patients with rheumatoid arthritis, psoriatic arthritis, and ankylosing spondylitis: Results from a longitudinal, observational, multicenter study. *Arthritis Rheum* 2008;59(2):234–240.
34. Heiberg MS, Kaufmann C, Rodevand E, et al. The comparative effectiveness of anti-TNF therapy and methotrexate in patients with psoriatic arthritis: 6-month results from a longitudinal, observational, multicentre study. *Ann Rheum Dis* 2007;66(8):1038–1042.
35. Kievit W, Fransen J, Oerlemans AJ, et al. The efficacy of anti-TNF in rheumatoid arthritis: A comparison between randomized controlled trials and clinical practice. *Ann Rheum Dis* 2007;66(11): 1473–1478.
36. Genevay S, Finckh A, Ciurea A, et al. Tolerance and effectiveness of anti-tumor necrosis factor alpha therapies in elderly patients with rheumatoid arthritis: A population-based cohort study. *Arthritis Rheum* 2007;57(4):679–685.
37. Finckh A, Dehler S, Gabay C. The effectiveness of leflunomide as co-therapy of TNF inhibitors in rheumatoid arthritis. A population-based study. *Ann Rheum Dis* 2008, January 29 (epub ahead of print).
38. MedDRA Maintenance and Support Services Organization. Home page. www.meddramsso.org. (Accessed on December 12, 2007.)
39. Van Vollenhoven RF, Cullinane CC, Bratt J, et al. Six-year report of the STURE registry for biologicals in rheumatology: satisfactory overall results, but plenty of room for improvement. *Arthritis Rheum* 2005;52(Suppl):S135 (Abstract).
40. Zink A, Strangfeld A, Herzer P, et al. Leflunomide is an acceptable combination partner for TNF inhibitors if methotrexate is not tolerated–results from the German biologics register. *Arthritis Rheum* 2007;56(Suppl):S181 (Abstract).

41. Hetland ML, Lindegaard HM, Hansen A, et al. Do changes in prescription practice in patients with rheumatoid arthritis treated with biologics affect treatment response and adherence to therapy? Results from the nationwide Danish DANBIO registry. *Ann Rheum Dis* 2008 (in press).
42. van Vollenhoven RF. Switching between anti-tumour necrosis factors: trying to get a handle on a complex issue. *Ann Rheum Dis* 2007;66(7):849–851.
43. van Vollenhoven RF. Switching between biological agents. *Clin Exp Rheumatol* 2004;22(Suppl 35):S115—S121.
44. Kobelt G, Eberhardt K, Geborek P. TNF inhibitors in the treatment of rheumatoid arthritis in clinical practice: costs and outcomes in a follow up study of patients with RA treated with etanercept or infliximab in southern Sweden. *Ann Rheum Dis* 2004;63(1):4–10.
45. Brennan A, Bansback N, Nixon R, et al. Modelling the cost effectiveness of TNF-{alpha} antagonists in the management of rheumatoid arthritis: results from the British Society for Rheumatology Biologics Registry. *Rheumatology (Oxford)* 2007;46(8):1345–1354.
46. Dixon WG, Symmons DP, Lunt M, et al. Serious infection following anti-tumor necrosis factor alpha therapy in patients with rheumatoid arthritis: Lessons from interpreting data from observational studies. *Arthritis Rheum* 2007;56(9):2896–2904.
47. Dixon WG, Symmons DP. What effects might anti-TNFα treatment be expected to have on cardiovascular morbidity and mortality in rheumatoid arthritis? A review of the role of TNFα in cardiovascular pathophysiology. *Ann Rheum Dis* 2007;66(9):1132–1136.
48. Dixon WG, Watson KD, Lunt M, et al. Reduction in the incidence of myocardial infarction in patients with rheumatoid arthritis who respond to anti-tumor necrosis factor alpha therapy: Results from the British Society for Rheumatology Biologics Register. *Arthritis Rheum* 2007;56(9):2905–2912.
49. Listing J, Strangfeld A, Kekow J, et al. Does tumor necrosis factor alpha inhibition promote or prevent heart failure in patients with rheumatoid arthritis? *Arthritis Rheum* 2008;58(3):637–640.
50. Geborek P, Bladstrom A, Turesson C, et al. Tumour necrosis factor blockers do not increase overall tumour risk in patients with rheumatoid arthritis, but may be associated with an increased risk of lymphomas. *Ann Rheum Dis* 2005;64(5):699–703.
51. Askling J, Fored CM, Baecklund E, et al. Haematopoietic malignancies in rheumatoid arthritis: Lymphoma risk and characteristics after exposure to tumour necrosis factor antagonists. *Ann Rheum Dis* 2005;64(10):1414–1420.
52. Ekstrom K, Hjalgrim H, Brandt L, et al. Risk of malignant lymphomas in patients with rheumatoid arthritis and in their first-degree relatives. *Arthritis Rheum* 2003;48(4):963–970.
53. Askling J, Fored CM, Brandt L, et al. Risks of solid cancers in patients with rheumatoid arthritis and after treatment with tumour necrosis factor antagonists. *Ann Rheum Dis* 2005;64(10):1421–1426.
54. Strangfeld A, Zink A, Rau R, et al. No increased risk of solid tumors in patients treated with biologics–a nested case-control study from the German biologics register RABBIT. *Ann Rheum Dis 67* 2008(2); Abstract No. FRI0143), EULAR Congress, Paris 2008.
55. Strangfeld A, Listing J, Herzer D, et al. RA patients with prior malignancy under treatment with biologics. *Ann Rheum Dis 67* 2008(2): Abstract No FRI0142), EULAR Congress, Paris 2008.
56. Strangfeld A, Listing J, Rau R, et al. Pregnancy outcome after exposure to biologics: Results from the German Biologics Register RABBIT. *Arthritis Rheum* 2007;56(Suppl):S311—S312 (Abstract).
57. D'Agostino RB. Propensity score methods for bias reduction in the comparison of a treatment to a non-randomized control group. *Stats Med* 1998;17(19):2265–2281.

Registries in Rheumatic Disease Epidemiology

CHAPTER 12B

Joel Kremer

At the time of this writing, six biologic agents had been approved for use by the Food and Drug Administration (FDA) for use in the United States, including etanercept, infliximab, anakinra, adalimumab, abatacept, and rituximab. Several additional biologic agents are in phase III, and it is likely that there will soon be several other new agents approved.

All of the new biologic drugs are quite expensive, and society has the right to expect that data on "real-world" safety and effectiveness are aggressively pursued after these agents are approved. Newly developed drugs must be tested in rigorous phase III randomized, controlled trials (RCTs) over limited treatment intervals because of the mandated need for a placebo control. As has been reviewed by others,[1–3] RCTs typically enroll selected populations of patients without significant comorbidities. Patients entered in these trials typically discontinue their prior medications, a practice generally not followed in the course of clinical practice. Another difference from clinical practice is that patients entered in RCTs must meet entry criteria for disease activity, which ensures that they have more active disease than is more commonly seen in patients who may be considered for treatment with these same drugs in the United States.[3,4] There are thus significant differences between the kinds of patients entered into RCTs and those treated with the same drugs in clinical practice.

Because less common side effects may be missed in short-term trials involving only limited numbers of patients, it is necessary to gather information on a large number of patients who receive new drugs for longer treatment intervals than are typical in RCTs. A robust experience with patient exposure to new biologic agents is to study up to approximately 2000 to 3000 patients prior to drug approval. While these numbers are usually enough to detect common toxicities, they may not be sufficient to determine if less common side effects will emerge over longer treatment intervals. Therefore, it is apparent that other methods for data collection on biologic agents are needed in order to enhance many of the data elements of RCTs.

Longitudinal Observational Studies

Longitudinal observational studies (LOS) can fill some of the gaps left by RCTs. These studies can be conducted using a variety of data sources including:

- Drug and/or disease registries that may be embedded in a national health-care system as is the case in Sweden and the United Kingdom[5,6]
- Administrative databases of patients with Medicare or Medicaid insurance that may include prescription, inpatient and outpatient data[7]
- Privately run voluntary drug and/or disease registries that are privately administered without government involvement[8,9]
- Pharmaceutical (pharma) company–sponsored drug registries

Administrative databases that contain data on state Medicare or Medicaid recipients are, of course, not designed for the purpose of later analysis, as is the case with a registry in which the cohort is planned and assembled for the purpose of collecting and analyzing data. Administrative databases also make certain assumptions such as patients who are prescribed drugs actually take them and hospitalization discharge diagnosis codes are accurate. It is possible that pharma registries may have inherent pressures to represent data on a drug which they market in a positive manner. It is therefore advantageous if outcomes from pharma registries can be overseen by neutral committees of medical professionals who have no stake in the success or failure of the particular agent which is being evaluated.

The Agency for Healthcare Research and Quality (AHRQ) has recently recognized the need for uniform definitions of data collection quality, and published a white paper primer describing how to design, implement, run, and mine registries, while ensuring quality.[10] Many nations in Europe, Japan, and Canada now have, or are developing, national databases in rheumatology.[5,6,11–18] For a summary and comparison of these systems, see Table 12B-1. It has thus become apparent that registries fulfill several fundamental needs which are shared worldwide. The differences between the kinds of information derived from RCTs and registries are compared in Table 12B-2.[1]

Table 12B-1. Comparative Characteristics of International Registries of Patients with Rheumatoid Arthritis

Country/ Registry	Sponsor	Individual from Sponsor in Charter	Number Patients	Number Patients on Biologic Data	Physician-Derived Clinical Data	Patient-Derived Data	Frequency of Data Collection	Strengths	Weaknesses
Europe									
Great Britain BSRBR	Pharma funds through British Society for Rheumatology	Yes	9018[6]	7664[6]	ACR/DAS-28 core set	Demographics/ HAQ	q6 months	Mandatory enrollment in order to access biologic agents; cross link with U.K. death registry	Only 8% of RA patients in U.K. treated with biologics; must have DAS28 >5.1 and failed 2 DMARDs to enter
Norfolk	Norwich Health Authority (primary care inception cohort)	NA	1236[11]	1236[11]	NA	Demographics/ HAQ	At death	Comparison cohort of .5 million patients in Norwich, U.K. with link to U.K. death registry	No MD-derived data
Sweden ARTIS	Swedish Medical Products Authority; Swedish Society for Rheumatology	NA	-20,000[a,1]	-12,000[a,1]	ACR/DAS-28 core set	Demographics/ HAQ	0, 3, 6, and then q6 months	Extensive linkage with other national databases including Ca and hospitalization, among others; mandatory enrollment for biologic access	Control group of partially different population (inpatients), <12%–15% of patients receive biologic agents
Germany Rabbit	Pharm through Germany Rheumatism Assoc.	Yes	5481[b]	3645[b]	ACR/DAS-28 core set	Demographics, Hanover Functional	0, 3, 6, and then q6 months	Standard definitions of AE provided to MD	
Switzerland SCQM	Swiss Clinical Quality Management Program for RA	NA	4400[c]	1700[c]	ACR/DAS-28 core set	Self-assessment of symptoms	Variable	Mandatory registration for patients on biologics; 80% of all anti-TNFs	
Spain Blobadaser	Spanish Society of Rheumatology, Spanish Medicines Agency	NA	4459[13]	4459[13]	No	Demographics, toxicities	NS	AE by World Health Organization criteria	No MD-derived data; No comparison group not on biologics
EMECAR	Spanish Society of Rheumatology	NA	789[13]	NS	Yes	Yes	Not available	Representation of Spanish population	Few patients on biologic agents
Austria	2 Vienna Rheumatism Clinics	NA	1214[14]	NS	No	No	NS		Two hospitals; no clinical measures
Denmark	Danish Nationwide	NA	1021[15]	NS	DAS28	NS	NS	Physician-derived outcomes	Small numbers

North America									
Canada									
Ontario (OBR)	Canadian Institutes of Health Research	Yes	Start-up	Start-up	ACR/DAS28 core set	Demographics/ HAQ, fatigue, work status	0, 6, and then every 6 months for MD measures	Linkage with other administrative data sources in Canada	Nascent stage
United States									
Administrative	NIH, Arthritis Foundation, AHRQ	Yes	3500[7]–15,000[7]	469[7]–494[7]	No	No	NA	Very large numbers	No physician-derived data; little data on nonhospitalization events; mean age 75-81 years
National Databank	Pharma	Yes	19,562[8]	>10,000[8]	No	HAQ, demographics	q6 months	Very large numbers, excellent publication record, work status, demographics, patient-reported toxicities	No MD-derived clinical outcomes; no x-ray, labs, quality measures; mail/ telephone contact with patients only; representativeness a challenge
CORRONA	Pharma	Yes	15,240 (RA)	7962 (RA)	ACR/DAS-28 core set, Dexa, radiographs	mHAQ, demographics, ROS	q3 months	Very large numbers; both MD and patient-derived data; labs, quality >40% of patients receive biologics reflecting U.S. experience	Representativeness a challenge

[a]Personal communication, Lars Klareskog;
[b]Personal communication, Angela Zink;
[c]Personal communication, Axel Finkh.
AHRQ, Agency for Healthcare Research and Quality; *NA,* not available; *NIH,* National Institutes of Health; *NS,* not stated; *USPHS,* U.S. Public Health Service.

Table 12B-2. Strengths and Weaknesses of Randomized Controlled Trials and Longitudinal Observational Registry Studies

Trial Type	Strengths	Weaknesses
Randomized controlled trials	Study groups very similar before treatment Conducted by well-established methodologic rules Considered gold standard for assisting efficacy Can be registered to prevent selective reporting	Costly, cumbersome Involve limited number of participants Often under-represent key patient groups Short duration Comparator (or placebo) often irrelevant May measure surrogate end points rather than clinical outcomes Protocol may not reflect typical clinical care
Registries	Can involve large numbers of typical patients in settings of routine care Can focus on specific vulnerable populations Can be performed relatively quickly and at modest cost Can identify rare adverse events Can follow patients over many years Can compare outcomes of several treatment alternatives	Susceptible to confounding caused by underlying differences among patients treated with different drugs Confounding (especially due to patient selection and differences in compliance can generate drug-outcome associations that are not truly causal) Methodologically difficult to do well Difficult to identify selective reporting findings Difficult to require registration

Registry Challenges

At the same time, longitudinal observational studies face many potential challenges. Internal validity is maximized in a double-blind RCT that effectively avoids issues of potential bias and unmeasured confounding that may threaten observational studies. However, as has been stated, external validity can be severely compromised in RCTs due to a variety of factors.[19] Recent publications have suggested that RCTs of biologic agents in RA patients are selecting a skewed subset of RA patients based on disease activity levels.[20,21] While this strategy may reduce the number of patients required by selecting a subset of patients who may be more likely to show a significant difference (delta) from baseline status, studying patients with severe disease may simultaneously compromise the external validity of the RCT.

However, issues of external validity may also be relevant to registries. The patient populations for a longitudinal observational registry study should ideally be representative of the population at large in the country or area from which the database is derived. In order to achieve "representativeness," either the majority of patients in a particular area, or an appropriately selected random sample, should be studied. This is a challenge for U.S. databases in which registration in these LOS are not mandated by the government, as is the case in certain European countries including Sweden, and the UK, where registry enrollment is required in order to prescribe biologic agents.[5,6]

Long-term follow-up is an additional challenge for all clinical studies, particularly LOS that may follow patients for multiple years. Patients may be lost to follow-up and their fate needs to be determined in a reliable manner. There is no centralized, reliable system within the United States to determine if a patient has died, moved, or is simply lost to follow-up. The health-care system in the United States is presently a hodgepodge of various payers and government-funded systems for the elderly (Medicare) and indigent (Medicaid). Because there is not a single insurance provider that can mandate uniform metrics for following patients, studies based on a single insurance plan data set in a particular geographic area can lead to attrition of follow-up with no ability to fill gaps. Moreover, linkage between outpatient and inpatient records is not possible, except within a limited set of U.S. health care systems such as the Veterans Health Administration.

In contrast, the Swedish health care system supports national registries which simultaneously records inpatient hospitalizations, cancer, deaths, and drug prescribing. All of these systems are available to researchers who are able to perform cross-linkage studies between these nationally maintained registries to determine if patients have died or experienced any number of important comorbidities or hospitalizations. Standard ICD-9 codes at the time of hospital discharge are used to establish the existence of comorbidities. Independent studies have established the accuracy of this means of assessing diagnoses. Patients lost to follow-up in a drug or disease registry can be cross-referenced with the death registry so that this important information on patients without follow-up will not be missed.

In the United States, events which occur outside of the research setting of the outpatient registry require a labor-intensive search of hospitalization and other medical records. There are therefore additional challenges in the United States that are not found elsewhere where national health-care systems and cross-talking databases exist.

As a tangible example of the value of cross linkage with other established health-care databases within the same country or region, the Swedish system has been able to ascertain the incidence of lymphomas[22] and tuberculosis[23] using cross-linkages with the national inpatient and cancer registries. Information on tumor histology or culture characteristics from sputa or other tissue can be requested directly from linkages with the in-patient hospitalization records from within the national system which can be routinely scanned for the presence of data on patients in the RA registry. In the United States, the information would be obtained first from the patient, and researchers would then have to request the data from the hospitalization records. There is a death registry for patients on Medicare (65 years old and older) within the United States, but access to information is typically delayed for 18 months.

Drug versus Disease Registries

In establishing a registry for conducting longitudinal observational studies, organizers must decide whether to design the registry around a specific disease or a particular drug or class of drugs. Successful registries have been established using both registry models. Prior to launching a registry, it is critical to establish its primary objectives. A set of study design possibilities and considerations are described in Table 12B-3. A drug registry with a carefully selected drug comparator cohort may be well-positioned to answer pharmaco-epidemiologic questions on the drug of interest, but may be less well-suited to study the natural history and epidemiology of disease. A registry which collects data on only one drug may have significant channeling bias, and thus it would be difficult to derive meaningful comparative efficacy or toxicity conclusions with other agents. For example, an epidemiologic study in RA patients based on a "biologics only" registry could have a biased representation of disease activity and severity.

Another important consideration for pharmaco-epidemiologic studies is the selection of comparator patients. Regardless of whether the registry uses a drug or a disease LOS design, it is critical to carefully consider the comorbidities and risk factors of patients in a comparator group in evaluating a drug's toxicities. There may be inherent biases of prescribing patterns and patient characteristics which would influence the validity of comparisons between these groups. Various techniques have been used to deal with these biases, including propensity modeling,[1,24] but it is also possible that patients within the database may not have sufficiently similar profiles to be compared.[1]

Principles of Longitudinal Observational Registry Study Design

The abiding principles of patient registries are covered in detail in Gliklich and Dreyer.[10] Many real-world case studies are also included in this richly documented publication. A review of these principles is beyond the scope of this publication, but the interested reader may learn more about the principles of planning a registry,[25–29] design,[30,31] data elements to be included,[32] and the importance of standardization of data elements,[33] as well as a summary of the relative merits of RCTs versus LOS.[34,35]

CORRONA: An Example of a Disease-Based Registry Established in the United States

Busy physicians may not see the need to collect data at the time of a clinical encounter if data collection is not mandated by a national system. As already noted, if completion of registry forms are necessary in order to allow access to biologic agents, there is a built-in incentive to encourage data collection. In the United States, however, although participation in LOS is becoming more common, there are presently no such incentives to encourage physician participation. It was therefore evident to the Consortium of Rheumatology Researchers of North America (CORRONA) organizers that a variety of incentives would be needed in order to encourage widespread participation. One of the incentives for participation therefore adopted by CORRONA was to provide a Web-based interactive reporting system that provides participating physicians with the ability to receive detailed reports on data entered on patients at their site. In addition, rheumatologists could provide needed documentation for billing purposes as well as elements of quality being defined by national administrative efforts. It was felt that U.S. rheumatologists would be unlikely to adopt the process of collecting data at regular intervals on a widespread basis without these incentives, even though leaders in the field of data collection had been proselytizing the use of standard data collection forms for many years.[36,37]

The "Quality" Incentive

The process of motivating physicians through incentives has worked in Europe and is becoming more successful in the United States, although the mechanisms are quite different. Long-discussed initiatives to reward quality have matured within the United States. The Center for Medicare and Medicaid Services (CMS) has stated that by mid-2008, monetary rewards will be provided to physicians who have at least 80% of their patients followed in a quality system. Quality will have a variety of definitions depending on which disease is considered. This definition is still in development for virtually all rheumatologic primary

Table 12B-3 Research Implications for Drug versus Disease Registries

	Disease Registry	Drug Registry
1. Enrollment/eligibility	All patients with disease of interest are eligible	Enrollment limited to drug(s) of interest and selected comparison drug(s)
2. Usefulness for studies of disease epidemiology	Depends on whether patients enrolled and study sites are representative of population to be studied	Similar to disease registries. However, if drug(s) of the registry are prescribed to patients with higher disease severity, estimates may be skewed
3. Usefulness for studies of drug effectiveness and safety	a. Depends on ability to recruit adequate numbers of patients on drug of interest b. May be easier to identify patients on comparison drugs with similar risk factors for outcome of interest	a. More focused approach may increase patients exposed to the drug of interest (assuming a fixed study budget) b. Achieving adequate number of patients on a comparator drug with similar risk factors may be more challenging if the study outcome was not considered in the selection criteria for comparison drug(s)
4. Data collection requirements	May be more comprehensive and therefore burdensome if a broader set of research questions are planned	May be more streamlined if the research questions are limited to a specific drug or drug class

diagnoses, including RA. However, quality measures will inevitably include regular monitoring of standardized, validated outcomes, preferably in an electronic format. It is therefore apparent that in spite of some of the impediments to the widespread use of registries found in the United States, there will also ironically be additional incentives for these systems in this country which will not be found abroad, and these additional "carrots" will be linked to quality documentation. It is apparent that registries are well-positioned to take on quality documentation needs in the United States.[38]

Funding of CORRONA

In order for CORRONA to pay physicians for participation while providing customized software reporting patient outcomes to participating physician sites, funds were required. CORRONA is funded by allowing pharmaceutical sponsors to access the aggregate data in the database by submitting queries to the CORRONA biostatisticians. This model of pharmaceutical support for database activities with complete independence of the registry exists elsewhere, including the UK (where funding is derived from the pharmaceutical industry through the British Society of Rheumatology),[6] Germany (where funding is also industry derived through the administration of the German Rheumatism Research Center), and The National Databank for the Rheumatic Diseases.[8] Like CORRONA, these registries share a charter philosophy of independence from industry influence on any of the research findings and publications derived from the registry data.

When CORRONA–pharma academic collaborations occur, a CORRONA investigator must take the lead on the effort and standards of objectivity and academic independence are critically reviewed and maintained. This stipulation is written in to each CORRONA–pharma contract and procedures for maintenance of independence are reviewed and fortified frequently. CORRONA's own researchers must take the lead on any collaboration with the pharmaceutical industry and bear complete responsibility for the final content and wording of any abstract or manuscript produced.

In European registries, pharmaceutical support is independent of actual access to any data generated by the database. This is made possible because of the frequent government mandates indicating that it was necessary for pharma to support independent mechanisms of gathering data on their products after approval. This mandate is not surprising in a system in which the government treasury pays the bills for all patients receiving these medications in the national health care systems, as is the case in Sweden and the UK.

Pharma and Registries

While pharma in the United States are also mandated to collect postapproval data, the efforts have largely taken the form of phase IV studies of up to a few thousand patients, or pharma-sponsored drug registries of patients receiving the agent manufactured by the company. Because the U.S. government only pays for a minority of patients who receive expensive biologic interventions, regulatory agencies have not yet been as aggressive in mandating enrollment in large registry studies as in many European countries, although this situation shows signs of changing.[39] There are many examples of successful, independent pharma-sponsored registries in the United States,[10] although pharma registries that collect dense data on drugs other than the ones produced by the company sponsoring the effort are understandably unusual.

Pharma sponsorship of the CORRONA database allows the sponsoring company to pose queries to the database. These queries are directed to CORRONA-supported biostatisticians who provide answers to questions without allowing access to raw data from the registry database. In addition, if pharma wishes to publish data on products that are not their own, they need to identify a CORRONA-independent investigator and allow that individual to take complete control over the content and integrity of the academic product. Thus, independence of CORRONA from industry influence or potential bias is ensured.

CORRONA collects data at the time of the clinical encounter from both physicians and patients with the diagnoses of RA and psoriatic arthritis (PsA), as well as osteoporosis and osteoporosis risk in the setting of the two primary diagnoses. ACR and DAS28 core data are collected by the physician, along with information on hospitalizations, infections, malignancies, and cardiovascular comorbidities. In addition, standard laboratory assessments are collected, along with CRP, anti-CCP and RF, with bone density scores and the results of hand radiographs.

Patients complete a modified HAQ (mHAQ) and visual analog scales for pain and global activity, as well as an updated review of systems including new comorbidities, work status, smoking and alcohol habits, and the use of over-the-counter medications not found in administrative databases, which contain only information on physician prescribed medications (Table 12B-1). Patients can also access their data on mHAQ scores, ESR, and tender and swollen joint counts on the Web using their own pass-code. It is posited that involving patients in their own care by allowing them access to a chronology of their own graphic data will enhance cooperation with the physician and improve compliance. Using these tools, the patient is encouraged to become a partner with the physician in their own care and well-being, instead of observing the system as an outsider.

Physicians may also access a Web-based system using their office computer, which provides routine tabular summaries for each patient of DAS28 and CDAI scores, swollen and tender joints, ESR, CRP, hemoglobin, and Dexa scores, as well as summaries of erosions found on radiographs. These summaries can be used to monitor progress from visit to visit and provide documentation evidence of disease status of individual patients with time. The system may also be used for documentation for billing and is likely to satisfy quality documentation requirements once they are established.

As reflected in Table 12B-1, there are presently more than 15,000 patients with RA in the database and more than 2100 patients with psoriatic arthritis. CORRONA encourages the enrollment of every RA patient at a site, so that patient data can consist of a range of clinical disease severity reflecting "real-world" conditions in patients on a variety of disease-modifying antirheumatic drugs (DMARDs), including both biologic and nonbiologic agents. No particular treatment strategy is advocated, but the aim, as in all registries, is to accurately capture the unadulterated patterns of drug prescribing and coincidental effectiveness and toxicity.

Future of Registries in United States

It is apparent that an independent registry such as CORRONA faces a variety of challenges that are uniquely endemic to the political and economic realities in the United States with its collection of many payers in a competitive, sometimes chaotic, and rapidly changing health care marketplace. As noted, however, it is likely that increasing pressure from a variety of sources with a stake in health care, including payers, patients, physicians, researchers, legislators, and regulators, will result in increased collaborative efforts. At the time of this writing, the FDA was expanding its cooperation with epidemiologic investigators and a variety of private, industry-sponsored, and medical professional organizations[38,39] in what promises to be another uniquely American response to the challenge of collecting data on large numbers of patients treated with expensive biologic agents after they are approved.

References

1. van Vollenhoven RF, Askling J. Rheumatoid arthritis registries in Sweden. *Clin Exp Rheumatol* 2005;23(Suppl 39):S195–S200.
2. Pincus T, Stein CM. Why randomized controlled clinical trials do not depict accurately long-term outcomes in rheumatoid arthritis: Some explanations and suggestions for future studies. *Clin Exp Rheumatol* 1997;15:S27–S38.
3. Pincus R. Limitations of randomized clinical trials in chronic diseases. Explanations and recommendations. *Adv Mind Body Med* 2002;18:14–21.
4. Greenberg JD, Kishimoto M, Cohen SB, et al. Low baseline joint count attenuates response to anti-TNF agents: What are the goals of biologic therapy? *Arthritis Rheum* 2005;52(9):S562.
5. Feltilius N, Fored M, Blomqvist P, et al. Results from a nationwide post marketing cohort study of patients in Sweden treated with etanercept. *Ann Rheum Dis* 2005;64:246–252.
6. Hyrich KL, Luna M, Watson KD, et al. Outcomes after switching from one anti-tumor necrosis factor alpha agent to a second anti-tumor necrosis factor alpha agent in patients with rheumatoid arthritis. Results from a large UK national cohort. *Arthritis Rheum* 2007;56:13–20.
7. Schneeweiss S, Setoguchi S, Weinblatt ME, et al. Anti-tumor necrosis factor alpha therapy and the risk of serious bacterial infections in elderly patients with rheumatoid arthritis. *Arthritis Rheum* 2007;56: 1754–1764.
8. Wolfe F, Michaud K. The effect of methotrexate and anti-tumor necrosis factor therapy on the risk of lymphoma in rheumatoid arthritis in 19,562 patients during 89,710 person-years of observation. *Arthritis Rheum* 2007;56:1433–1439.
9. Kremer JM. The CORRONA database. *Ann Rheum Dis* 2005;64: iv37–iv41.
10. Gliklich RE, Dreyer NA, eds. *Registries for Evaluating Patient Outcomes: A User's Guide.* AHRQ publication no. 07-EHC001-1. Washington, DC: Agency for Healthcare Research and Quality, April 2007.
11. Listing J, Strangfeld A, Kary S, et al. Infections in patients with rheumatoid arthritis treated with biologic agents. *Arthritis Rheum* 2005;52:3403–3412.
12. Finckh A, Ciurea A, Brulhart L, et al. On behalf of the Swiss clinical quality management program for rheumatoid arthritis. *Arthritis Rheum* 2007;56:1417–1423.
13. Carmona L, Descalzo MA, Perez-Pampin E, et al. All-cause and cause-specific mortality in rheumatoid arthritis are not greater than expected when treated with tumour necrosis factor antagonists. *Ann Rheum Dis* 2007;66:880–885.
14. Schoels M, Kapral T, Stamm T, et al. Step-up combination versus switching of non-biological disease-modifying antirheumatic drugs in rheumatoid arthritis: Results from a retrospective observational study. *Ann Rheum Dis* 2007;66:1059–1065.
15. Hjardem E, Ostergaard M, Podenphant J, et al. Do rheumatoid arthritis patients in clinical practice benefit from switching from infliximab to a second tumor necrosis factor alpha inhibitor? *Ann Rheum Dis* 2007:66:1184–1189.
16. Wessels JAM, van der Kooij S, le Cessie S, et al. A clinical pharmacogenetic model to predict the efficacy of methotrexate monotherapy in recent-onset rheumatoid arthritis. *Arthritis Rheum* 2007;56: 1765–1775.
17. Matsui T, Kuga Y, Kaneko A, et al. Disease activity store 28 (DAS28) using C-reactive protein underestimates disease activity and overestimates EULAR response criteria compared with DAS28 using erythrocyte sedimentation rate in a large observational cohort of rheumatoid arthritis patients in Japan. *Ann Rheum Dis* 2007;66: 1221–1226.
18. Goodson NJ, Wiles NJ, Luna M, et al. Mortality in early inflammatory polyarthritis. Cardiovascular mortality is increased in seropositive patients. *Arthritis Rheum* 2002;46:2010–2019.
19. Leber PD, Davis CS. Threats to the validity of clinical trials employing enrichment strategies for sample selection. *Control Clin Trials* 1998;19(2):178–187.
20. Sokka T, Pincus T. Most patients receiving routine care for rheumatoid arthritis in 2001 did not meet inclusion criteria for most recent clinical trials or American College of Rheumatology criteria for remission. *J Rheumatol* 2003;30(6):1138–1146.
21. Gogus F, Yazici Y, Yazici H. Inclusion criteria as widely used for rheumatoid arthritis clinical trials: Patient eligibility in a Turkish cohort. *Clin Exp Rheumatol* 2005;23(5):681–684.
22. Baecklund E, Sundstrom C, Ekbom A, et al. Lymphoma subtypes in patients with rheumatoid arthritis. Increased proportion of diffuse large B cell lymphoma. *Arthritis Rheum* 2003;48:1543–1550.
23. Askling J, Fored MC, Brandt L, et al. Risk and case characteristics of tuberculosis in rheumatoid arthritis associated with tumor necrosis factor antagonists in Sweden. *Arthritis Rheum* 2005;52:1986–1992.
24. Landewe RB. The benefits of early treatment in rheumatoid arthritis: confounding by indication, and the issue of timing. *Arthritis Rheum* 2003:48:1–5.
25. Epstein M. Guidelines for good pharmacoepidemiology practice. ISPE commentary. *Pharmacoepidemiol Drug Saf* 2005;14:589–595.
26. Centers for Disease Control and Prevention. Updated guidelines for evaluating public health surveillance systems. *MMWR Recomm Rep* 2001;50(RR-13):1–5.
27. Solomon DJ, Herny RC, Hogan JG, et al. Evaluation and implementation of public health registries. *Public Health Rep* 1991;106(2): 142–150.
28. Kennedy L, Craig A. Global registries for measuring pharmacoeconimic and quality-of-life outcomes: Focus on design and data collection, analysis, and interpretation. *Pharmacoeconimics* 2004;22(9): 551–568.

29. Kremer JM, Gross T, McDonough GC. Planning a registry. In: Gliklich RE, Dreyer NA, eds. *Registries for Evaluating Patient Outcomes: A User's Guide.* AHRQ publication no. 07-EHC001-1. Washington, DC: Agency for Healthcare Research and Quality, April 2007.
30. Good PI. *A Manager's Guide to the Design and Conduct of Clinical Trials.* New York: John Wiley and Sons, 2002.
31. Dreyer NA, Guggirala HJ, Samsa G, et al. Registry design. In: Gliklich RE, Dreyer NA, eds. *Registries for Evaluating Patient Outcomes: A User's Guide.* AHRQ publication no. 07-EHC001-1. Washington, DC: Agency for Healthcare Research and Quality, April 2007.
32. Institute of Medicine. *Crossing the Quality Chasm: A New Health System for the Twenty-First Century.* Washington, DC: National Academy Press, 2001.
33. Kim K. Clinical data standards in health care: Five case studies. *iHealthReports.* California HealthCare Foundation. http://www.chcf.org/topics/view.cfm?itemID5112795.
34. Benson K, Hartz AJ. A comparison of observational studies and randomized, controlled trials. *N Engl J Med* 2000;342:1878–1886.
35. Black N. Why we need observational studies to evaluate the effectiveness of health care. *BMJ* 1996;11;212:1215–1218.
36. Wolfe F, Pincus T. Standard self-report questionnaires in routine clinical and research practice-an opportunity for patients and rheumatologists. *J Rheumatol* 1991;18:643–646.
37. Pincus T. Why should rheumatologists collect patient self-report questionnaires in routine clinical care? *Rheum Dis Clin North Am* 1995;21:271–319.
38. Ault A. CMS urged to use registry data for quality reporting. *Rheumatology News,* June 2007, p. 3.
39. Pear R. Senate approves tighter policing of drug makers. *New York Times,* May 9, 2007.

Index